Fundamentals of
Aerospace
Medicine

Second Edition

Fundamentals of
Aerospace
Medicine

Second Edition

Roy L. DeHart, M.D., M.P.H.

Professor and Chairman of the Department
   of Family and Preventive Medicine
University of Oklahoma
Health Sciences Center
Oklahoma City, Oklahoma

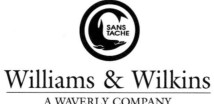

Williams & Wilkins
A WAVERLY COMPANY

BALTIMORE • PHILADELPHIA • LONDON • PARIS • BANGKOK
BUENOS AIRES • HONG KONG • MUNICH • SYDNEY • TOKYO • WROCLAW

Editor: Kathleen Courtney Millet
Managing Editor: Joyce Murphy
Production Coordinator: Barbara J. Felton
Designer: Diane Buric
Illustration Planner: Wayne Hubbel
Typesetter: Maryland Composition
Printer: Port City Press

Accurate indications, adverse reactions and dosage schedules for drugs are provided in this book, but it is possible that they may change. The reader is urged to review the package information data of the manufacturers of the medications mentioned.

Printed in the United States of America

First Edition, 1986

Library of Congress Cataloging-in-Publication Data

Fundamentals of aerospace medicine / [edited by] Roy L. DeHart. -- 2nd
  ed.
     p. cm.
  Includes bibliographical references and index.
  ISBN 0-683-02396-9
  1. Aviation medicine. 2. Space medicine.   I. DeHart, Roy L.
  [DNLM: 1. Aerospace Medicine.   WD 700 F981 1996]
  RC1062.F86 1996
  618.9'8021--dc20
  DNLM/DLC
  for Library of Congress   96-3274
                                             CIP

The publishers have made every effort to trace the copyright holders for borrowed material. If they have inadvertently overlooked any, they will be pleased to make the necessary arrangements at the first opportunity.

To purchase additional copies of this book, call our customer service department at **(800) 638-0672** or fax orders to **(800) 447-8438.** For other book services, including chapter reprints and large quantity sales, ask for the Special Sales department.

Canadian customers should call **(800) 268-4178**, or fax **(905) 470-6780.** For all other calls originating outside of the United States, please call **(410) 528-4223** or fax us at **(410) 528-8550.**

Visit Williams & Wilkins on the Internet: http://www.wwilkins.com or contact our customer service department at **custserv@wwilkins.com**. Williams & Wilkins customer service representatives are available from 8:30 am to 6:00 pm, EST, Monday through Friday, for telephone access.

97 96 97 98 99
1 2 3 4 5 6 7 8 9 10

Julia
Evelyn
John

This edition is dedicated to those aerospace medical practitioners and scientists, whose lives were lost in the practice of their profession, in the care of their patients, or in the pursuit of knowledge.

Foreword

In introducing this impressive volume, I believe it most important to begin with a definition of the subject. **Aerospace medicine is that specialty area of medicine concerned with the determination and maintenance of the health, safety, and performance of those who fly in the air or in space.** This specialty is necessary because such flight subjects humans, with their earth-bound anatomy, physiology and psychology, to the *hostile* environment of air and space. Humans must adapt to or be protected from the changes in total environment pressure, reduced partial pressures of vital gases, accelerative forces of flight, and changes in gravitational forces, to name just a few of the hazards encountered in flight.

Historically, the early balloon flights in the late 1700's produced reports of physical effects on the humans engaged in such ascents, but they were treated as interesting physiological observations. The advent of powered flight 92 years later by the Wright brothers on December 17, 1903 and then human spaceflight by Gagarin on April 12, 1961 revealed additional effects and potential obstacles to human performance in this new environment. However, these obstacles were viewed as challenges to be solved by those individuals supporting the explorers of these environments. They learned that the environments of air and space were a continuum and that basic physiologic fundamentals applied throughout this continuum. It is these environmental and vehicular stresses upon those who fly which are of ultimate concern to the aerospace medicine specialist.

The specialty area of aerospace medicine is young compared to some other medical specialties. Even though physicians had supported those who flew from the beginning, the specialty was not recognized until 1953. Though relatively young, aerospace medical research and extensive operational experience has been accumulated and well documented. These dates are in numerous scientific journals, reports, and books.

Specialized knowledge in many medical as well as non-medical areas is required of the practitioner of aerospace medicine. The medical specialties of otolaryngology, ophthalmology, cardiology, neurology, psychiatry/psychology, and pathology are of particular importance. The human can not be separated from the vehicle, therefore certain engineering principles are also important. The total support of those who fly becomes a team effort. The aerospace medicine specialist must be knowledgeable in these areas and be able to communicate with other specialists. He or she must be able to gather all of this information and evaluate it's impact on the health status of the pilot, relate this to the flying environment, and render a decision regarding fitness for flying. Therefore, the *Fundamentals of Aerospace Medicine* must cover a large amount of information. Aerospace medicine is of necessity very dynamic. It must keep pace with the ever-increasing technology of both medicine and aviation. Increases in fighter aircraft capabilities have forced a re-evaluation of a physiologic problem once thought to be solved. Current social assaults on the necessity of physical standards for those who fly have even forced a re-evaluation of medical standards. Aircraft are getting larger, and faster, and more and more people are flying. Such dynamic changes indicated the necessity for a current, comprehensive text. Dr. DeHart built upon the efforts of his predecessors, such as General Harry Armstrong, in gathering material for the first edition of *Fundamentals of Aerospace Medicine*. In the second edition, he has assembled the aid of respected authorities in their individual areas to add new chapters, update others with recent data and completely rewrite others.

We must understand our past if we are not to repeat the errors of the past. The section ''Aerospace Medicine in Perspective'' covers some of this important history very well. The sections ''Physiology of the Flight Environment,'' ''Clinical Practice of Aerospace Medicine'' and ''Operational Aerospace Medicine,'' have chapters providing fundamentals with basic references. The section ''Impact of the Aerospace Industry on Community Health'' includes a chapter concerning transmission of disease by aircraft with current concerns about an old and nearly forgotten nemesis, tuberculosis. Fundamentals revisited again. New chapters have appropriately been added: ''Thermal Stress,'' ''International Aviation Medicine'' and ''Management of Human Resources in Air Transport Operations.''

It is the rare individual today who does not have some contact with the aviation environment in some manner. All physicians should have some basic knowledge of aerospace medi-

cal problems they or their patients might experience, as well as understand the breadth of knowledge possessed by the specialist in aerospace medicine. This text can serve as the basis of this knowledge for the general physician, the aerospace medicine specialist, the student, or anyone dealing with the medical support of military, general, or airline aviation, spaceflight, or the aerospace industry.

It has been my privilege in 45 years of practice in Aerospace Medicine to participate in the Air Force, NASA, and civilian areas. I congratulate Dr. DeHart and his authors for their excellent coverage of all these areas. If we adhere to the fundamentals and provide proper aerospace medical support, the human will continue to be able to adapt to zero gravity and re-adapt to earth's gravity with ever longer sojourns in space. I believe we will see many of earth's inhabitants experiencing spaceflight and even one day living in far flung space stations and colonies. The fundamentals will be the basic knowledge and the stepping stones making such progress possible. This knowledge must be used by the planners, designers, operators, and participants in achieving safe flight. This volume makes that knowledge available.

Charles A. Berry, M.D., M.P.H.
President, Preventive & Aerospace Medicine
   Consultants, P.A.
Past President, Aerospace Medical Association
Past President, International Academy of
   Aviation and Space Medicine
Past President, University of Texas Health
   Science Center in Houston, Texas
Former Director of Life Sciences-NASA

Preface

In the ten years that have passed since the first edition of this text, much that is new has occurred in aerospace medicine and yet much remains the same. The military aviation environment continues to increase in its complexity and its demands on systems operators. Technology has increased aircraft performance, placing additional physiological demands on crew. Electronic and sensor systems have complicated, rather than simplified, environmental awareness, further adding to mental overload and psychological stress. Operational integration has heightened the requirement for human factors management.

Commercial aviation has seen the introduction of new aircraft with advanced avionic and guidance systems. More people than ever before are traveling by air, both domestically and internationally. Air travel has become a victim of international terrorism. Commerce has become dependent upon aviation with overnight delivery of letters and parcels becoming both routine and expected, even on an international scale.

The Mir Space Station sets new records for endurance with each orbit. International collaboration, including multi-national crews, has become the norm. The launch and recovery of the space shuttle has become so routine that it has lost much of its news-worthiness; no longer is there the excitement and interest of the past.

For the most part, there has been little change in human physiology or our broad understanding of the body's response to the stressors of flight.

We continue to strive for better techniques and procedures to protect the crew in both the aviation and space environments. Women are now involved in all aspects of aerospace operations.

In this second edition, much that was written remains the same. Chapters have been reviewed and updated, and where needed, new material has been included. The format of the first edition has been retained, thus similar topics are grouped together.

Section I moves us from history toward the future. Projections are made which carry us into the 21st century.

Section II defines the operational environment and addresses operational stressors, both from the perspective of the adverse effects on the crew and mechanisms of protection and coping. A new chapter addressing the thermal environment in aerospace has been included.

Section III updates our knowledge of medical issues dealing with selection and retention of air crew. Chapters have been revised to address new clinical knowledge and techniques for the diagnosis and management of medical and surgical conditions of aerospace medical interest.

Section IV brings together many of the agencies and activities engaged in aerospace operations. The material on aviation medical support to airlines has been significantly revised. New chapter topics include international aviation medicine and the management of human resources in air transport operations. New authors and a different approach is evident in the aircraft accidents, survival, and rescue chapter.

Section V is the concluding section discussing the impact of the aerospace industry on community health. All three chapters in this section have undergone significant revision and have new authors.

In preparing the second edition, I was fortunate that many of the original authors were available and interested in assisting with this revised text. I believe the reader will find that our new contributors bring their insight and unique experience to the text and thus enhance its value, both as a readable volume and an enduring reference.

Roy L. DeHart, M.D., M.P.H.

Acknowledgments

There is only one reason for publishing a second edition, and that is that the first edition has been well received and that there is a readership demand for a new, revised and updated edition. The first edition has served as a textbook in the training of aviation medical examiners, flight surgeons, and residents in aerospace medicine. It has served as a reference for physicians, physiologists, and human factors specialists. I have found the book in the outback of Australia, the deserts of Egypt, the jungles of Malaysia, a clinic in India, and on the shelf of a small flight operations office in Oklahoma. The success of the first edition represents the effort and enthusiasm of its contributors.

The birthing of the second edition went through no less a protracted labor than its predecessor. The fact that this volume is available for your reading is due to the forbearance of the scientists and physicians who put aside other things in their busy schedules to put pen to paper and give you the best that they had. I am indebted to each for their dedication to this common effort.

The section heading illustrations that were present in the first edition are retained with this effort. These line drawings created by the medical illustrator, Melvan Jordan, have been duplicated in many forms and appear throughout the aerospace medical community. I am delighted that they have become so identified with this textbook, and we wish that to continue.

During the preparation of this edition, the publishing house of Lea & Febiger was purchased by Williams & Wilkins. I am delighted that this text is back with Williams & Wilkins, which was the original publisher of the first major text in the United States, edited by Henry Armstrong—*Aviation Medicine*. My appreciation to the editorial staff who made the transition smooth and for their constant prodding to complete the manuscript before we had to write a chapter on intergalactic travel.

During the several years of the revision process, Ms. Paula Gullion was my secretary and staff assistant and played a key role in manuscript preparation, initiating correspondence with contributors, and serving as a coordinator of the numerous activities related to this second edition. When a project of this magnitude is undertaken, it is recognized that the time commitment will be enormous. Perhaps for those with good time management skills the tasks associated with being a text editor can be shoehorned into the normal day's activities. In my case, it was difficult to find a normal day, thus much of the work was done spread over the dining room table, on weekends, and evenings. Always supportive and ready to proof a manuscript, serve as the first source of feedback, and to give support and understanding during moments of frustration; it is with love and devotion that I recognize the contributions of my lifelong partner, Julia DeHart.

In recent years, my professional activities have not been primarily directed in the discipline of aerospace medicine. However, working on this book has time and again brought me back to this discipline and to the science, the scholarship, and the clinical practice that is the exciting and dynamic field of aerospace medicine—I thank each of you for that opportunity.

Recognizing the importance of continuing the educational process for those new to the field, the majority of the proceeds of this edition will be distributed in a manner similar to the first edition: to the schools and scholarship programs, nationally and internationally, that are educating and training physicians and other professionals in the discipline of aerospace medicine.

Roy L. DeHart, M.D., M.P.H.

Contributors

James W. Brinkley, SES
Director
Crew Systems Directorate
Armstrong Laboratory
Wright-Patterson AFB, Ohio

Russell R. Burton, D.V.M., Ph.D.
Chief Scientist
Armstrong Laboratory
Brooks AFB, Texas

Warren L. Carpenter, M.D., M.P.H.
Colonel, USAF (MC)
Command Surgeon
Space Command
Peterson AFB, Colorado

N. Bruce Chase, M.D., M.P.H.
Colonel, USA (Retired)
Morgantown, West Virginia

Roy L. DeHart, M.D., M.P.H.
Professor and Chairman
Department of Family and Preventive
  Medicine
University of Oklahoma Health Sciences
  Center
Oklahoma City, Oklahoma

Silvio Finkelstein, M.D., M.S.
Former Chief, Aviation Medicine Section
International Civil Aviation Organization
Past President, International Academy of
  Aviation and Space Medicine
Buenos Aires, Argentina

Karen K. Gaiser
Site Manager
Lockheed Engineering and Sciences
Ames Research Center
Moffett Fields, California

Harry L. Gibbons, M.D., M.P.H.
Chief, Aerospace Medicine
Salt Lake City, Utah

Kent K. Gillingham, M.D., Ph.D.,
  (Deceased)
Flight Motion Effects Branch
Crew Technology Division
Armstrong Laboratory
Brooks AFB, Texas

Gary W. Gray, M.D., Ph.D., F.R.C.P.C.
Consultant in Medicine
Canadian Forces Central Medical Board
Defense and Civil Institute of Environmental
  Medicine
Toronto, Canada

H. H. Hanna, M.D.
Former Chief
Otolaryngology Branch
USAF, School of Aerospace Medicine
Brooks AFB, Texas

William H. Hark, M.D., M.P.H.
Deputy Federal Air Surgeon
Federal Aviation Administration
Washington, D.C.

Kenneth R. Hart, D.O., M.P.H.
Clinical Associate Professor
Department of Family and Preventive
   Medicine
University of Oklahoma Health Sciences
   Center
Oklahoma City, Oklahoma

Richard Heimbach, M.D., Ph.D.
Medical Director
Jefferson C. Davis Wound Care and
   Hyperbaric Medicine Center
San Antonio, Texas

James Hickman, Jr., M.D., M.P.H.
Colonel USAF (MC) (Retired)
Consultant, Divisions of Preventive
   Medicine & Cardiovascular Disease
Mayo Clinic
Rochester, Minnesota

David H. Hull, M.D., F.R.C.P., Q.H.S.
Air Vice Marshall, RAF
Dean of Air Force Medicine
RAF Central Medical Establishment
London, UK

David R. Jones, M.D., M.P.H.
Aeropsych Associates
San Antonio, Texas

Jon L. Jordan, M.D., J.D.
Federal Air Surgeon
Federal Aviation Administration
Washington, D.C.

Marc S. Katchen, M.D.
Practice of Neurology
Galesburg, Illinois

Gary M. Kohn, M.D., M.H.A.
Corporate Medical Director
United Airlines
Chicago, Illinois

Robert J. Kreutzmann, M.D., M.P.H.
Colonel, USA
United States Army Reserve Surgeon
Atlanta, Georgia

Richard L. Masters, M.D., M.P.H.
Medical Director
Aviation and Preventive Medicine Associate
Englewood, Colorado

Robert R. McMeekin, M.D.
Colonel, USA
Former Federal Air Surgeon
Armed Forces Institute of Pathology
Washington, D.C.

Glenn W. Mitchell, M.D., M.P.H.
Colonel, USA
United States Army Aeromedical Center
Fort Rucker, Alabama

Stanley R. Mohler, M.D.
Professor and Vice Chair
Director, Aerospace Medicine
Department of Community Health
Wright State University, School of Medicine
Dayton, Ohio

George C. Mohr, M.D., M.P.H.
Former Commander
Air Force Aerospace Medical Research
   Laboratory
Wright-Patterson AFB, Ohio

Royce Moser, Jr., M.D., M.P.H.
Professor and Director
Rocky Mountain Center for Occupational and
   Environmental Health
Department of Family and Preventive
   Medicine
University of Utah School of Medicine
Salt Lake City, Utah

Arnauld E. Nicogossian, M.D.
Chief Medical Officer
National Aeronautics and Space
   Administration
Washington, D.C.

Charles W. Nixon, Ph.D.
Chief, Bioacoustics and Biocommunications
Biodynamics and Biocommunications Division
Crew Systems Directorate
Armstrong Laboratory
Wright-Patterson AFB, Ohio

Sarah A. Nunneley, M.D., M.S.
Crew Technology Division
Armstrong Laboratory
Brooks AFB, Texas

Ronald K. Ohslund
Captain (MC) USN (Retired)
Camarillo, California

James F. Parker, Jr., Ph.D.
President
BioTechnology, Inc.
Falls Church, Virginia

A. J. Parmet, M.D., M.P.H.
Medical Director
Trans World Airlines
Kansas City, Missouri

John C. Patterson, Ph.D.
Chief, Aerospace Clinical Psychology
USAF Consultation Service
Armstrong Laboratory
Brooks AFB, Texas

Fred H. Previc, Ph.D.
Flight Motion Effects Branch
Crew Technology Division
Armstrong Laboratory
Brooks AFB, Texas

James H. Raddin, Jr., M.D., S.M.
Director and Principal Consultant
Biodynamic Research Corporation
San Antonio, Texas

Russell B. Rayman, M.D., M.P.H.
Executive Director
Aerospace Medical Association
Alexandria, Virginia

Michael Rea, Ph.D.
Director
Biological Rhythms and Integrative
   Neuroscience Institute
Armstrong Laboratory
Brooks AFB, Texas

Mark A. Roberts, M.D., Ph.D.
Chairman
Department of Preventive Medicine
Medical College of Wisconsin
Milwaukee, Wisconsin

Guillermo J. Salazar, M.D., M.P.H.
Regional Flight Surgeon, Southwest Region
Federal Aviation Division
Fort Worth, Texas

Paul J. Sheffield, Ph.D.
Director, Research & Education
Jefferson C. Davis Wound Care and
   Hyperbaric Medicine Center
San Antonio, Texas

William T. Shepherd, Ph.D.
Manager
Biomedical and Behavioral Sciences Program
Office of Aviation Medicine
Federal Aviation Administration
Washington, D.C.

Thomas B. Sheridan, Ph.D.
Ford Professor of Engineering and Applied
   Psychology
Department of Mechanical Engineering
Massachusetts Institute of Technology
Cambridge, Massachusetts

Richard G. Snyder, Ph.D.
President
Biodynamics International
Tucson, Arizona

Roger L. Stork, Colonel, USAF, BSC
Chief, Aerospace Physiology Division
HQ Air Education & Training Command
Randolph AFB, Texas

Gil D. Tolan, M.D.
Medical Director for Quality Improvement
Princeton Medical Group
San Antonio, Texas

Thomas J. Tredici, M.D.
Senior Scientist, Ophthalmology Branch
USAF Armstrong Laboratory
USAF School of Aerospace Medicine
San Antonio, Texas

Henning E. von Gierke, Dr. Eng.
Director Emeritus
Biodynamics and Bioengineering Division,
Armstrong Laboratory
Wright-Patterson AFB, Ohio

James E. Whinnery, M.D.
Brigadier General USAF, (MC) (Retired)
Amarillo, Texas

C. T. Yarington, Jr., M.D., F.A.C.S.
Clinical Professor Otolaryngology,
University of Washington
The Virginia Mason Medical Center
Seattle, Washington

Laurence R. Young
Apollo Program Professor of Astronautics
Department of Aeronautics and Astronautics
Massachusetts Institute of Technology
Cambridge, Massachusetts

Contents

SECTION III.   Clinical Practice of Aerospace Medicine

SECTION IV.   Operational Aerospace Medicine

SECTION V. Impact of the Aerospace Industry on Community Health

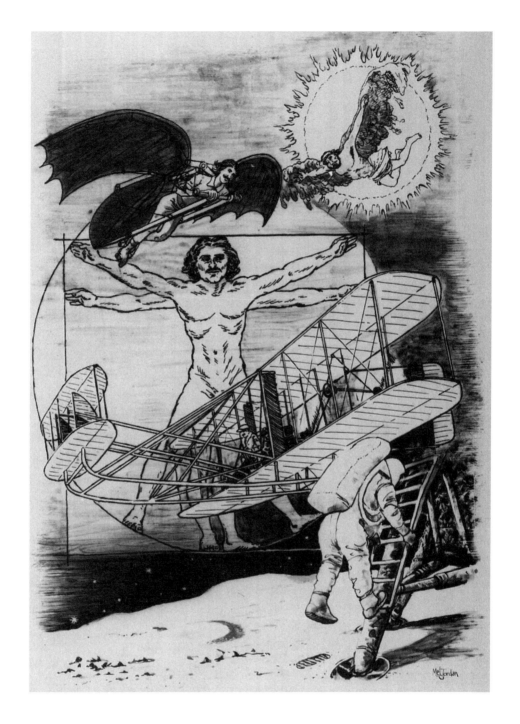

SECTION I

Aerospace Medicine in Perspective

Vision, dreams, and tall tales were humanity's first creative musings in anticipation of joining the birds in flight. Intellectual curiosity and scientific inquiry made it possible to leave earth using spheres of hot air of rarified gas. There then followed flimsy contraptions of wood, paper, and cloth that allowed many to sail and glide for short distances on the sea of air. At Kill Devil Hill an engine was added to one of these gliders, and the Wright Brothers introduced controlled-powered flight to the world. Humankind's launch into space, a man's first step on the moon, and our orbiting workshops and laboratories are part of this ongoing human aerospace activity. We have moved from dream to design to development toward our aerospace destiny.

Medicine's contribution to aviation and space flight parallels the technology and scientific achievements necessary to lift our vision above the horizon. Many of the fundamentals that form the foundation for the practice of Aerospace Medicine become evident as the perspectives of past, modern, and future activities are discussed. From the historical perspective, one can view the triumphs and tragedies as man probes the ocean of air. The modern perspective reviews man's ingenuity in meeting the environmental challenges of flight. It is during this period that this discipline of medicine became defined and requirements in training, education, and clinical skills were established through the certification process.

The future perspective offers an opportunity to consider the possibilities and the difficulties of tomorrow and beyond. As in each branch of medical science and practice, the fundamentals of Aerospace Medicine must be understood in the perspective of the dynamic dimension of time.

Recommended Readings

Anderson HG. The medical and surgical aspects of aviation. London: Oxford University Press, 1919.

Armstrong HG. Principles and practice of aviation medicine. 3rd ed. Baltimore: Williams and Wilkins, 1952.

Bilstein RE. Flight patterns—Trends of aeronautical development in the United States, 1918–1929. Athens, GA: The University of Georgia Press, 1983.

Bilstein, RE. Orders of magnitude. A history of the NACA and NASA, 1915–1990. (NAA SP-4406). Washington: US Government Printing Office, 1989.

Combs H. Kill Devil Hill. Boston: Houghton Mifflin Co, 1979.

Dhenin G, ed. Aviation medicine. London: Tri-Med Books Ltd, 1978.

Ernsting J, King P, eds. Aviation medicine. 2nd ed. London: Butterworths, 1988.

Gibson TM, Harrison MH. Into thin air. London: Robert Hale, 1984.

Gillies JA, ed. A textbook of aviation physiology. London: Pergamon Press Ltd, 1965.

Harding RM, Mills FJ, eds. Aviation medicine. 2nd ed. London: British Medical Journal, 1989.

Josephy AM. The American Heritage history of flight. New York: American Heritage, 1962.

Last JM, ed. Maxcy-Rosenau public health and preventive medicine. 13th ed. Norwalk, CN: Appleton and Lange, 1991.

McFarland RA. Human factors in air transport design. New York: McGraw-Hill Book Co, 1946.

Tierney RK. Forty years of army aviation. US Army Aviation Digest, 1982:228(8);514–524.

Chapter 1

The Historical Perspective

Roy L. DeHart

Lend me the stone strength of the past, and I will lend you the wings of the future.

Robinson Jeffers

The building blocks of an institution are laid upon a foundation of events past. Aerospace medicine's foundation was laid by those who discovered, designed, and developed the means for man to take his first steps toward the heavens.

DREAMS, LEGENDS, AND RELIGION

In prehistoric times, man turned his face skyward and followed the majesty of birds in flight, observed the beauty of billowing clouds coursing across the sky, and was in awe of the grandeur of the celestial heavens evident in the night sky. His desire to soar above the earth took form in dreams, fantasies, legends, and religion. The desire to fly, although not to be fulfilled for untold centuries, received expression in numerous ways. The Chinese provide the earliest recorded story of man in flight. The Emperor Shun escaped from the clutches of his captors when only a boy by "donning the work clothes of a bird" and flying to freedom. The legends and folklore of early civilizations all had their flying deities, heroes, and creations of the imagination.

Among those associated with aviation, perhaps the best known of the flying legends is the story of Daedalus and his son, Icarus. Held captive on the isle of Crete by King Minos, the two set to work to fashion wings of feathers attached to their bodies by hardened wax. From their site of imprisonment, Daedalus watched the soaring gulls as they flew on the updrafts rising from the steep cliffs about the island. Anticipating the dangerous heat from the sun, Daedalus warned Icarus not to soar too close to that fiery body, lest the wax become softened and the feathers detached. The moment for the escape arrived and the two captives flung themselves from their prison onto the updrafts and soared skyward. Icarus, being younger and perhaps somewhat foolhardy, surrendered to the ecstasy of the moment and soared ever higher, ignoring both advice and warning, with predictable results. As many were to learn in years to come, flying can be an unforgiving pursuit. The story goes that, with reason ruling emotion and wisdom supplanting enthusiasm, Daedalus made successful his escape.

In most cultures, similar stories are found of gods riding the winds in aerial chariots and angels with wings of eagles soaring to the music of the spheres. The ancient poets wrote wonderful descriptive odes of man flying through the air, and their contemporary artists portrayed these dreams on stone and parchment. Elijah, the Hebrew prophet, was transported alive to the heavens. For the Greeks, Apollo carried the sun in a flying chariot across the heavens on his daily obligation to the people of earth. The Romans created Mercury to serve as the rapid courier

3

of messages between the deities. In the western hemisphere, Ayar Utso, a chief of the early Peruvian Incas, grew wings and flew away to escape imprisonment, and, even today, we turn to tradition as on Christmas Eve we await the arrival of Santa Claus, drawn across the heavens in his sleigh by his eight reindeer.

THINGS THAT FLY

Occasionally, it has been found that legends are based on fact, or may, at the very least, stimulate a discovery. The concept that the propeller was understood and used in ancient Rome is best appreciated when described as a windmill. Over 2000 years ago, the Chinese invented the kite, and it is reported to have been used in military signaling. A contemporary of Confucius, Kung-suhu Tse, built a wooden and bamboo magpie that flew for 3 days. This flying contraption was most probably a kite. In southern Italy before the Christian era, there is a report of a mysterious wooden pigeon. This dove, or pigeon, developed by Archytas, is believed to have been a model of a bird suspended by wires from a revolving arm operated by a type of steam reactive device.

Another flying toy invented by the Chinese used the helicopter principle. It apparently consisted of a lightweight spindle of wood with feathers inserted at one end. When thrown or dropped, it rapidly rotated and slowly descended to earth.

The notebooks of Leonardo da Vinci, the "universal man" of the Renaissance, were filled with material related to flight. He designed a model helicopter with a helix, or spiral screw, driven by a spring mechanism. The suggestion is that he actually flew this model. Tradition also identifies da Vinci with experiments involving hot air balloons; however, these were more likely small kites, although he was certainly aware of the physical fact that hot air rises. Among his sketches is a pyramid-shaped parachute, consisting of a tent made of linen, with the measurements provided to allow construction of a device that would enable a man to "throw himself down from any great height without sustaining any injury." Da Vinci's fascination with the flight of birds took practical form in the dozens of drawings he made of ornithopters with the operator located in various positions. Within the 5000 manuscript pages left by Leonardo da Vinci were some 150 separate sketches of flying machines.

A Venetian mathematician, Giovanni Danti, constructed gliders composed of "wings in proportion to the gravity of his body," which were flown from the roofs of houses in Perugia. It would appear that these were models launched from the rooftops because there is no documentation of manned flight associated with these launches. For his efforts, Danti was exiled as a sorcerer.

Although Renaissance history is rife with tales and legends of rooftop, hill, and tower jumpers, few have been chronicled in such a way as to establish their authenticity. One such report may be accurate. It is documented that the Marquis de Bacqueville leaped from the roof of his Paris house in 1742 assisted by a glider-like device. He displayed more discretion than most potential aviators by aiming his flight path toward the Seine. Although his flight path was well established, the flight was short-lived due to some minor structural failure, causing him to fall upon the deck of a washerwoman's barge. Although described as a humiliating landing, it nevertheless was survivable, and the Marquis escaped with only a broken leg.

Wings of feathers, paper, and linen or strange mechanical devices combined with intestinal fortitude were tried and all failed in man's attempt for sustained flight. The physical principles of gas displacement and density would first allow man the privilege of soaring with the birds and introduce to him a new and potentially hazardous environment.

Balloons

The climb to free flight began with the thirteenth century scientist, Roger Bacon, who prepared an elaborate treatise on the navigation of air. He suggested that flying machines built of large, hollow, metal spheres be constructed light enough to be supported by the density of the atmosphere. His major thesis was that air was capable of supporting a craft in the same manner that water supports a ship.

The next step upward was achieved by the English chemist, Henry Cavendish, who read a paper before the Royal Society in 1766 describing the weight of hydrogen, a gas. He called this gas "inflammable air" and announced that it was considerably lighter than ordinary air. The aeronautic significance of this finding was not realized by Cavendish. Although others recognized this potential, the immediate proof of this "lighter than air" property and the realization of flight was not to be. The intellectual curiosity and the inquiring minds of two French brothers led them to combine principle and practicality and attain sustained manned flight.

The Montgolfiers

Joseph Priestly's treatise, *Experiments and Observations on Different Kinds of Air*, served as the stimulus for experimentation by Joseph Montgolfier (Fig. 1.1). The legends and stories surrounding the beginnings of Joseph's interest are both fanciful and interesting. One story has it that Madame Montgolfier's chemise took off when placed before the fire to air; a second story maintains that it was Joseph's own shirt which was raised in this way; and yet a third story tells of Madame Montgolfier placing a conical paper wrapping from a sugar loaf into the fire, where upon Joseph observed it filling with hot air and flying up the chimney without igniting (1).

Montgolfier learned the chemistry behind the production of hydrogen and used the hydrogen to fill small paper balloons or globes. He discovered, as had others before him, that the gas passes through the paper as fast as the container is filled. Silk was tried but was abandoned when it was no more successful at holding the gas. Montgolfier then turned to heated air, or what he referred to as "rarified air," as the lifting

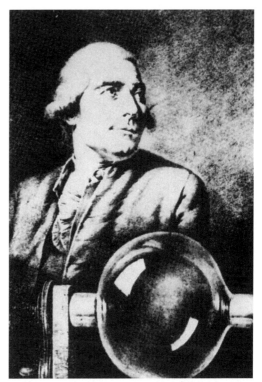

Figure 1.1. Joseph Montgolfier, the designer of the large-capacity hot air balloon (Library of Congress).

agent. Joseph was joined by his younger brother, Etienne, in the further pursuit of sustained aerial flight. The family's fortune had been made in the papermaking industry. The experience of these two brothers in paper manufacturing was essential as the size and volume of their "rarified air" balloons expanded. The Montgolfier family name was prophetic in the annals of aeronauts because it means "master of the mountain."

In November, 1782, Joseph began his first small-scale experiments with hot air balloons. A paralellepiped was made of fine silk with an open throat that, when held over an open flame, caused the envelope to inflate and to fly about the ceiling of his apartment. In the next experiment, Etienne joined his brother outdoors, where a small balloon was inflated and rose to a height of approximately 21 m.

The brothers then constructed a much larger experimental balloon with a capacity of 18 m^3.

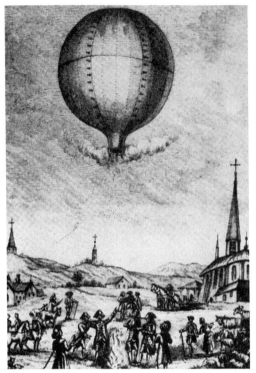

Figure 1.2. First hot air balloon ascent, June, 1783 (courtesy of The Aeronauts, L. T. C. Rolt, Walker & Co., 1966.)

This device rose successfully to a height of 183 m. In April, 1783, a balloon was constructed of a combination of paper and cloth that had a calculated lifting capacity of 204 kg. The balloon made a perfect ascent to 305 m, traveling a distance on the wind in excess of 1.2 km (Fig 1.2).

J.A.C. Charles

While the Montgolfiers experimented with larger-capacity hot air balloons, the members of the Paris Academy of Science were pursuing another alternative by supporting a young physicist by the name of J.A.C. Charles (Fig 1.3). It was Charles' intent to use the "inflammable air" as the lifting agent in his experiments. To this end, he constructed a perfect sphere that was 3.65 m in diameter and had a capacity of 26 m³. To generate sufficient hydrogen required nearly 226 kg of sulfuric acid and over 450 kg of iron fil-

ings. Repeated complications and delays in the gassing process occurred, but on August 27, 1783, Charles' hydrogen-filled balloon soared from the heart of Paris to a height of 1000 m.

Among the spectators for Charles' "inflammable air" balloon was Benjamin Franklin, who heard a skeptic in the crowd remark, "interesting, but what use is it?" The envoy from the United States growled, "What use is a newborn baby?"

Nearly an hour later and 24 km from Paris, the balloon returned to earth in a field near the village of Genesse; however, because frightened villagers attacked the balloon with pitchforks, muskets, and whatever other weapons were available, little of the balloon was left to recover.

Pilâtre de Rozier

The Montgolfier brothers' experience with large hot air balloons had reached the ear of the monarch of France. King Louis XVI and Queen Marie Antoinette requested that a command performance be conducted at Versailles. A colorfully decorated balloon was constructed that measured 17 m high and 13 m in diameter, with a capacity of 1080 m³. Although rumors were rampant that this would be a manned flight, the King had directed otherwise, considering such

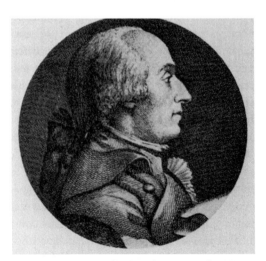

Figure 1.3. J. A. C. Charles, the young physicist who harnessed hydrogen as a lifting agent (Library of Congress).

a venture too perilous. The flight would indeed be special, however, because, as often the case in aerospace medicine today, animals were to precede man in flight. A large wicker cage was attached to the balloon and contained a sheep, a cock, and a duck. The first aeronautic instrument was attached to the cage—a barometer. The similarity to some events of today's aerospace achievements is remarkable. On this occasion, a dramatic countdown of three cannon shots took place, and with the echo of the third firing still resounding about the walls of the palace, the balloon took flight. The balloon is estimated to have achieved a height of 518 m before it began a gradual descent. One of the first to reach the downed balloon, a young scientist and physician from Metz, Pilâtre de Rozier, observed that the sheep had become free and was quietly grazing, the duck appeared no worse for the experience, and the cock had suffered a damaged wing. Much as now, an investigation was conducted into the mishap that caused the cock's injured wing. Ten witnesses testified that the sheep had kicked the cock prior to takeoff, thus explaining the injury and alleviating concern for the perils of flight.

Manned Flight

The Montgolfiers began the construction of a third giant balloon. This one was designed to carry a brazier below its throat and a two-man crew to stoke it. The young physician de Rozier volunteered persistently to crew this next historic flight (Fig. 1.4). During October, he made several tethered flights to acquaint himself with the criticality of balance and the difficulties inherent in feeding a fire attached to a paper and linen structure. De Rozier was born in Lorraine, was a member of the Academy of Sciences, and proved his scientific brilliance very early by developing a breathing apparatus that was the forerunner of the gas mask. He had a theatrical sense about him; one of his favorite lecture demonstrations was to inhale hydrogen and ignite the gas as he exhaled.

The first manned balloon was 23 m by 15 m

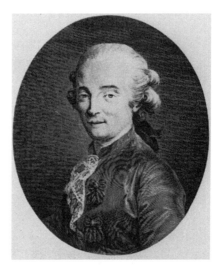

Figure 1.4. The physician, Pilâtre de Rozier, one of the first to fly in free ascent (Library of Congress).

with a neck 5 m in diameter. A one meter circular gallery was suspended beneath the balloon by cords sewn into the fabric. Beneath the gallery hung a fire basket made of wrought iron wire. When completed, the balloon weighed 725 kg with a capacity of 2250 m^3 and an estimated lift, or payload, of 770 kg.

On October 15, 1783, the balloon was ready for its first trial flight. De Rozier stepped into the gallery and, after only a few feet of rope had been released, the importance of balance became self-evident, and it was necessary to add ballasts to offset his weight. Further tethered flights were made, and de Rozier learned to regulate vertical movement and to extinguish the small fires that occurred on the balloon. Becoming confident in controlling his vertical ascent, de Rozier accepted single passengers. The Marquis d'Arlandes was such a passenger and was to join de Rozier in the first free ascent. At 13:54 on November 21, 1783, de Rozier and the Marquis ascended in free flight to a height of 85 m. Recognizing the significant danger, the two aeronauts each carried a pail of water and a sponge as major safety equipment. The fire suspended below them occasionally sent a shower of sparks onto the fragile fabric of painted cloth and paper.

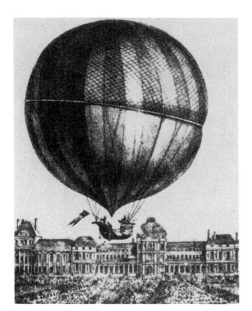

Figure 1.5. The first manned hydrogen balloon ascent, December, 1783 (courtesy of the Aeronauts, L.T.C. Rolt, Walker & Co.,1966.)

The two men had little opportunity for boredom because they were frequently involved in self-preservation by extinguishing the many little fires that were burning holes in their balloon. In all, the journey lasted some 25 minutes and took them more than 8 km across the city of Paris. The first sustained, free flight was made by a physician and a military officer.

Ten days later, on December 1, J.A.C. Charles manned the first free ascent in a hydrogen balloon with a passenger and a gondola equipped with food, extra clothing, scientific instruments, including a thermometer and barometer, and bags of sand for ballast (Fig. 1.5). The two men lifted off from the Tuileries Gardens in midafternoon. After flying on the winds for 2 hours and covering some 43 km, the balloon landed and the passenger departed. Charles decided to make a solo ascent and rapidly ascended to 2750 m, where he began to experience physiologically some of the realities of this new environment. He complained of the penetrating cold at this altitude and a sharp pressure pain in one ear as he descended. Not only did this represent the first solo flight, but Charles described clearly

some of the physiologic perils that can best be managed by those combining interests in aeronautics and medicine.

Once the trail was broken to sustained aerial flight, many an aeronaut followed on both sides of the English channel. In 1785, the next major, dynamic event occurred in balloon flight, and a major contributor to the event was an American physician.

John Jeffries

Dr. John Jeffries (Fig. 1.6), although an American, was a loyalist during the Revolutionary War and thus found it advantageous to practice medicine in England for a while. He was intrigued and fascinated by aerial flight and sought out a Frenchman, Jean-Pierre François Blanchard, who was in England demonstrating ballooning. A flight was agreed to, and Jeffries proceeded to assemble a collection of scientific paraphernalia to take aloft. This paraphernalia included vacuum flasks that were prepared by Cavendish for

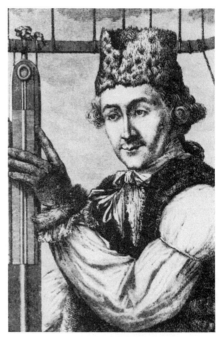

Figure 1.6. Dr. John Jeffries, an American physician, readying for his flight across the English channel (courtesy of the National Air and Space Museum).

collecting upper air samples. In addition to the quality of the air, Jeffries measured air currents and temperature changes during the flight. After the successful ascent, Jeffries learned of Blanchard's plans to attempt a crossing of the English channel. Determined to crew on the flight, Jeffries organized the adventure, provided the funds, and even agreed to get out of the gondola at any point if lightening the craft became necessary. Despite numerous personality conflicts between the two men, the flight was launched on January 7, 1785. Before successfully reaching Calais, it was necessary to strip the gondola of everything movable, including all outer garments and, according to Jeffries' own estimate, some 6 lb of urine.

The First Fatality

The first 2 years of aerial flight were miraculously free of fatal accidents, but this safety record was not to be sustained. Pilâtre de Rozier, one of the first men to achieve sustained flight, was to achieve notoriety with yet another first. Ignoring the advice of many, de Rozier created a hybrid balloon, combining Charles' "inflammable air" with a hot air Montgolfier design. The concept was pitifully simple—the pilot would be able to vary the lift simply by controlling the fire. The results were tragically predictable. In the summer of 1785, observers noticed de Rozier, while airborne at an altitude of 1000 m, doing something to the fire basket when a blue flame appeared, a muffled explosion occurred, and the gondola, trailing smoke and shreds of silk, plummeted to the earth. Both de Rozier and his passenger died.

American Ballooning

A 13-year-old boy by the name of Edward Warren made the first balloon ascent in the United States on June 24, 1784. Mr. Peter Carnes had constructed the balloon in Baltimore, Maryland. The youth was playing around, apparently in the basket, when the balloon became untethered and began an unplanned ascent. A month later, Mr. Carnes attempted an ascent in Phila-

delphia from the Walnut Street prison yard. The balloon rose 3 m, struck the prison wall severely, and knocked Carnes from the basket. The flight ended spectacularly as the lightened balloon shot skyward and caught on fire.

Benjamin Rush

The Frenchman Jean-Pierre François Blanchard, the greatest balloonist of the time, having completed 44 ascents in Europe, arrived in the United States to make his forty-fifth ascent. Being an entrepreneur and exhibitionist, Blanchard advertised his plans widely in Philadelphia, attempting to raise sufficient funds to cover the cost. The Walnut Street prison yard was again designated the launch site, and the date was set for January 9, 1793. Dr. Benjamin Rush made the acquaintance of Blanchard and was on hand for the flight. Dr. Rush reported: "I went to Mr. Blanchard and requested him to examine the state of his pulse in his aerial voyage which he was to undertake the next day. He promised to do so and accepted the use of my pulse glass for that purpose." Blanchard himself noted in his journal of the event: "I passed on the observation which Dr. Rush had requested me to make upon the pulsation of the artery when I should be arrived at my greatest height. I found it impossible to make use of the quarter minute glass which he had provided for that purpose, but supplied its place by an excellent second watch; and the result of my observations gave me 92 pulsations in the minute, the average of four observations made at the place of my highest elevation, whereas, on the ground, I had experienced no more than 84 in the same given time." This marked the first recorded contribution made in America to that branch of science that was to become known as aerospace medicine (2).

Rush continued his inquiries of Blanchard and, upon meeting him 15 days later, inquired of discomforts he may have experienced at altitude. Blanchard related that at an altitude of 9 km blood came into his mouth and that he experienced great thirst and sleepiness from the lightness of the air. This journal entry is questionable because it is extremely doubtful that Blanchard attained an altitude as high as 9 km. As balloon ascents became more frequent, both in Europe and the United States, and the scientific knowledge gained was made known to the public, Rush incorporated this new data in his medical lectures. His manuscripts recorded comments regarding suffering from severe cold, discomfort from an enlarged chest, and reports of epistaxis and rapid pulse rate.

Physiology at Altitude

In 1804, the hazards of high altitude flight became graphically demonstrated when three Italians, Andreoli, Brasette, and Zambeccari, attained an altitude well in excess of 6000 m, received frostbite of both their hands and feet, experienced vomiting, and each man lost consciousness. While still conscious, Andreoli had difficulty in reading the barometer because as they ascended in altitude, the candle in the lantern grew dimmer and finally went out. The flight ended with the balloon's descent into the Adriatic Sea, but, fortunately, the men were rescued.

Acosta

Prior to the first balloon ascent, the effects of altitude on physiology were beginning to be understood. In 1590, the Jesuit father, Acosta, may have been the first to suspect that the physical distress caused by altitude was associated with the rarefaction of air. He stated, ''There is no doubt that the cause of this distress and strange affliction is the wind or air current there . . . I am convinced that the element of the air is in this place so thin and so delicate that it is not proportioned to human breathing which requires extensive and more temperate air . . .'' For over 150 years, no similar ideas were reported, but, unfortunately, Acousta's observations went unheeded. It is evident from other reports that the natives of the South American Andes were well aware of particular illnesses they associated with mountain climbs and re-

ferred to these afflictions by terms such as Veta, Soroche, la Puna, or Moreo de la Cordillera. Typical of explanations for the unknown, the Indians frequently attributed these illnesses to evil spirits.

Glaisher and Coxwell

The first detailed attempt to describe altered physiology at altitude was accomplished by two Englishmen, Glaisher and Coxwell, on their ascent to 9450 m (Fig.1.7). The diary recording their flight in 1862 reports that at 5640 m their pulses had quickened to 100 beats/min. At 5850 m, breathing was affected, and palpitations were experienced. Their hands and lips had turned bluish, and they were having difficulty in reading the onboard instruments. At 6510 m, Glaisher experienced seasickness, although there was no rolling or pitching motion to the

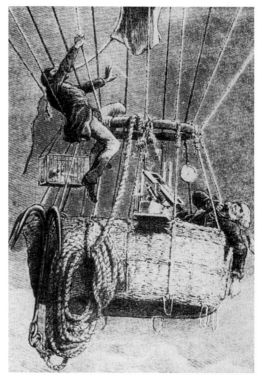

Figure 1.7. The two scientists, Glaisher and Coxwell, nearly unconscious at 8833 m as Coxwell seizes the valve cord with his teeth (courtesy of the United States Air Force School of Aerospace Medicine).

balloon. At 8700 m, the men experienced extreme muscle fatigue. Glaisher wrote, ''I seem to have no limbs.'' And then he fell back, insensible for 7 minutes. Coxwell was likewise weak and had little control of his arms or hands because of the extreme cold; however, realizing the enormity of their predicament, he was able to raise his head sufficiently to grab the valve cord with his teeth, releasing hydrogen. The ascent of the balloon ceased. Glaisher made significant contributions to the science of meteorology and was one of the founders of the Royal Aeronautical Society.

Paul Bert

The experience and reports of Glaisher and Coxwell served as a strong stimulus to the physiologist-physician, Paul Bert. He would be identified by many in the years to come as the ''Father of Aviation Medicine'' and by all as the father of altitude physiology (3). Bert, a Frenchman, received his Doctor of Medicine degree in 1864. He continued his education and was awarded a Doctor of Natural Sciences degree in 1866, followed by an appointment as professor of zoology at the University of Bordeaux. In many respects, Bert was a reincarnation of the universal man of the Renaissance. He was not only a physician but a naturalist, a zoologist, an anatomist, and, perhaps most importantly, a physiologist. His classic treatise, which was a major contribution to the field of physiology, was entitled *Barometric Pressure—Researches in Experimental Physiology*. The book consisted of both a historical review of earlier work in the field and Bert's own experiments. The contents included chapters concerning the effects of decreased and increased pressure on blood gases and the effect of changes in barometric pressure on a variety of biologic specimens. One of his important conclusions was that, regardless of the barometric pressure, air cannot support life when the partial pressure of oxygen reaches a certain low level. Based on experimentation, that level was determined to be 45 mm Hg. His significant conclusions influencing the field of

aerospace medicine included the observations that ''the diminution of barometric pressure acts upon the living being only by lowering the oxygen tension in the air, in the breath, and in the blood which supplies their tissues . . .''. ''The increase in barometric pressure acts only by increasing oxygen tension in the air and blood . . .''; and that ''Sudden decompression beginning with several atmospheres had an effect . . . only by allowing to return to a free state the nitrogen which had become dissolved in the blood and the tissues under the influence of this pressure.''

It is clear from the review of his experiments that Paul Bert was the first to elucidate the causes of altitude sickness, oxygen poisoning, and the bends.

Altitude Chamber

In his review of Paul Bert's contributions to aviation medicine, Dr. Fred Hitchock (4) identifies Bert as the first practicing flight surgeon. Two of Bert's friends who were aeronauts, Crocé-Spinelli and Sivel, were anxious to pursue and, if possible, exceed the altitude record established by Glaisher and Coxwell in 1862. Bert had constructed a chamber that would reproduce the barometric pressure of altitude (Fig 1.8). He used this chamber in a number of experiments and was to employ it for the first time as a physiologic training chamber. In this decompression or altitude chamber, he demonstrated to Crocé-Spinelli and Sivel the effects of decreased oxygen partial pressure and the beneficial effects of breathing oxygen at altitude. This instruction convinced the two aeronauts of the value and importance of oxygen, and they carried this life-giving gas with them on future flights.

In March 1874, Crocé-Spinelli and Sivel carried supplemental oxygen with them on their high-altitude flight. They discovered, however, that Bert's chamber did not reproduce all the effects of altitude; the temperature at altitude was much lower than that in the chamber, far more physical activity was required on the flight than was needed in the chamber, and the

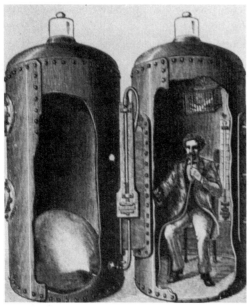

Figure 1.8. The physician Paul Bert breathing oxygen-enriched air in his altitude chamber, (1878) (courtesy of the United States Air Force School of Aerospace Medicine).

exposure to altitude was longer than the chamber training session. Nevertheless, the successful use of oxygen encouraged these two adventurers to attempt a flight to an even greater altitude.

Fatalities at Altitude

On their next flight, Crocé-Spinelli and Sivel were joined by the scientist, Gaston Tissandier. The balloon was equipped with three gas bags containing 72% oxygen, the total amount available for the three men equaling 440 L. A letter was written to Bert outlining the preparations for this high-altitude flight. Bert immediately responded, warning that the supply of oxygen was entirely inadequate for the flight as planned. Not anticipating the consequences of their decision, the aeronauts chose to make the flight in any case, waiting until the absolute last moment before using their vital and short supply of oxygen. The flight was launched on April 15, 1875, and when the balloon was recovered, only one of the three men had survived. Both Crocé-Spinelli and Sivel died of hypoxia. Tissandier, upon his re-

covery, wrote a classic description of the physiologic effects of hypoxia and is quoted in Bert's text (5). Although many aeronauts had died in descent, these two men were the first to succumb while ascending.

The frailty of man was only second to the frailty of the large, flimsy gas-filled spheres that carried him aloft. These lighter-than-air balloons were shortly to be supplemented by the frail, unstable, heavier-than-air machines that aeronautic science and engineering were about to produce.

Machines

The historic event that occurred at Kill Devil Hill 4 miles south of Kitty Hawk, North Carolina, at 10:35 A.M. on December 17, 1903 was only a spike on an endless graph of events.

Models and Gliders

Early in the nineteenth century, George Cayley was conducting research and publishing his works while laying the foundation for modern aerodynamics. In 1809, he wrote regarding the principle of powered flight: " . . . make a surface support a given weight by the application of power to the resistance of air." His designs included a wing set at a slight dihedral, a fuselage, a tail assembly, including vertical and horizontal stabilizers, and a power source that he recognized was not then technologically available. Cayley did build monoplane and triplane gliders. It is reported that in 1849, a small 10-year-old boy was lifted off the ground and flew for several yards downhill on one such glider.

Another Englishman, Samuel Henson, further developed the work of Cayley. In 1842, he patented plans for the design for an ''aerial steam carriage.'' The design described a monoplane with a wingspan of 50 m, a tail plane as a stabilizer, a vertical rudder, and tricycle landing gear. Power was to be provided by two steam-driven pusher propellers. The design was never converted to reality.

A colleague, Stringfellow, following a Henson design, constructed a small flying monoplane model that used a miniature steam engine. Throughout the mid-nineteenth century, numerous powered models were constructed, and several of these models are reported to have raised themselves unaided from the ground, thus achieving flight.

Two events are worth noting. The first event occurred around 1874 when a fullscale flying machine with a tractor propeller driven by a hot air engine, designed and built by Du Temple, may have departed the ground from an incline ramp under full power while carrying a young man onboard. The second event occurred in Russia in 1884. A steam-driven airplane, built by Mozhaiski, was launched down a long incline ramp and may have attained flight. Neither of these claims, however, are considered to represent sustained self-powered flight.

Toward the end of the nineteenth century, many names were associated with heavier-than-air machine flight and include engineers, scientists, inventors, and wealthy adventurers. Among this group were Sir Hiram Maxim, Clément Ader, Louis-Pierre Mouillard, and Otto Lilienthal.

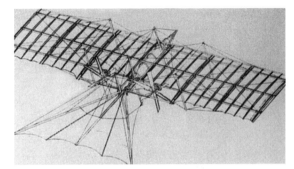

Figure 1.9. An early engineering drawing of a cambered wing flying machine conceived in 1842 (courtesy of the National Air and Space Museum).

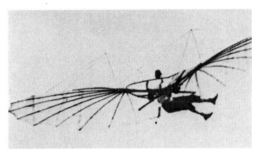

Figure 1.10. Otto Lilienthal flying his Type 2 monoplane hang glider in Germany in 1894 (courtesy of Wright State University).

Otto Lilienthal

Otto Lilienthal was the nineteenth century's major contributor to the art of gliding and directly influenced Wilbur and Orville Wright. Lilienthal's enthusiasm for gliding was motivated by two factors: first, his desire to discover, to design, and to build, and second, his need to master the art of flying so that he was prepared when adequate propulsion technology became available.

Many of Lilienthal's gliders were monoplanes in which the pilot was supported in a system that resembled the trapeze system used on today's hang gliders (Figs. 1.9 and 1.10). Flight control was thus achieved by shifting the body's weight forward or back and side to side. Beginning in 1891 and continuing for 5 years, Lilienthal made over 2000 glides, occasionally achieving flight

distances in excess of several hundred feet. While testing a glider, the craft stalled and crashed to earth, and Lilienthal received injuries from which he succumbed the following day. Lilienthal was one of many who lost their lives while pursuing flight. During this period, little consideration was given to body or head protection or to any form of restraint system. The exhilaration experienced by these adventurers risking so much can, in part, be appreciated by reading the following report from Lilienthal: ''I often reach positions in the air which are much higher than my starting point. At the climax of such a line of flight, I sometimes come to a standstill for some time, so that I am enabled whilst floating to speak with the gentlemen who wish to photograph me regarding the best position for the photographee.''

Octave Chanute

Another glider enthusiast, Octave Chanute born in Paris but raised in New York, was a self styled inventor with a keen interest in flight. Using the sand dunes near Lake Michigan as a launch site, he began testing man-carrying gliders. Starting with a monstrosity of five wings, he eventually discovered the advantage of a two wing craft—the biplane. Both the aircraft design and the concept of testing near water where there is sand and wind were to be adopted by two brothers from Ohio who had collaborated with Chanute. Unfortunately such collaboration would soon end under the pressure of litigation.

Samuel Pierpont Langley

Samuel Pierpont Langley was simply unlucky. For over a decade, extending into the twentieth century, Langley pursued aviation with a passion. He convinced the United States War Department of the military potential of a controllable, power-driven airplane. He received from Congress a grant of $50,000 to fund his pursuit of the concept. Other support was provided by the noted inventor Alexander Graham Bell. He constructed his "Aerodrome," a monoplane with two main wings in tandem, a horizontal stabilizer, and a vertical fin, which was powered by a relatively lightweight, radial, gasoline engine capable of 53 hp.

Two launches of this aircraft were conducted from a catapult mounted aboard a houseboat floating in the Potomac River. On October 7, 1903, and again on December 8, 1903, launchings were attempted, but in each case, the catapult apparently fouled and the aircraft crashed into the river. Only 9 days later, those two mechanics from Ohio, the Wright brothers, would cross the threshold of self-powered, sustained, heavier-than-air flight.

Powered Flight

The Wrights

The two Dayton, Ohio bicycle manufacturers, Wilbur and Orville Wright, had been fascinated

by Lilienthal's gliding experiences (Fig 1.11). They were also well aware of Langley's interest in powered flight using steam-driven models. Their appetites whetted, the Wrights used some of their business capital to finance their growing interest in aviation.

From the beginning, the Wrights identified three central problems for controlled power flight: the importance of the wing shape in producing lift, three-dimensional dynamic control in the air, and the application of adequate power to drive wind over the wing.

Two major contributions to aeronautics were engineered by the Wrights (6). The first, and most important, resulting in a patent, was "wing warping," as used by large birds to maintain direction and stability while soaring. The technique was first proven in the glider the Wrights developed and ultimately applied to the airplane. After reviewing the work of Maxim and Langley and other aeronautic pioneers, the Wrights abandoned the concept of "automatic equilibrium,"

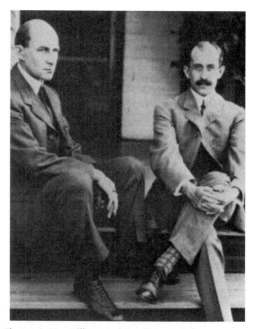

Figure 1.11. Wilbur and Orville Wright on the back porch of their home in Dayton, Ohio (courtesy of Wright State University).

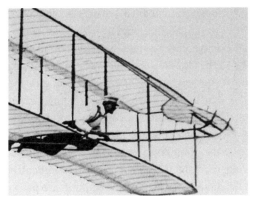

Figure 1.12. Wilbur Wright flying a sophisticated biwing glider during early trials at Kitty Hawk, North Carolina in October, 1902 (Library of Congress).

where the aircraft seeks straight and level flight, for an intentionally unstable but more flyable aircraft in which the aviator had to control direction. The Wright brothers' second major contribution was a single control system that simultaneously warped the wings and interconnected the rudder controls, thus automatically counteracting the drag produced by the downwarped wing.

Realizing the need for strong, steady, and predictable winds for their gliding test, the Wrights requested information from the National Weather Bureau. They were advised to try the beaches of North Carolina, where winds from the sea were strong and steady and the open space for gliding was plentiful. In October, 1900, they made the first of their periodic pilgrimages to Kitty Hawk, North Carolina (Fig. 1.12).

Through trial and error, ingenuity and engineering, persistence and daring, these two brothers solved the aeronautic riddle of directional stability and control in the air. One major problem remained—the power plant. A simple 12 hp water-cooled gasoline engine was developed to drive two counter-rotating propellers. After an initial unsuccessful trial, the stage was set, the photographer that was so important for documenting this historic event was in place, and at

10:35 A.M. on December 17, 1903, man lifted into the air and for 12 seconds was airborne over a distance of 40 m. Three more flights were conducted that morning, the final one lasting nearly 1 minute. The legends, fantasies, and dreams of man were realized as he attained sustained, controlled, powered flight.

By the time man had experienced powered flight, he had already been exposed to low temperatures, hypoxia, pressure changes, motion sickness, crash injuries, and death. Powered flight would further broaden the horizons and increase the hazards of the aeronautic environment.

Within a decade of that flight at Kitty Hawk, every industrial nation in the world had witnessed powered flight within its own boundaries. By 1918, thousands of flying machines would be swarming over the continent of Europe, engaged in the "great war."

AVIATION MEDICINE—THE FLEDGLING

Frequently, tragedy begets solution. During a demonstration of one of the Wright flying machines, Lieutenant Thomas Selfridge of the United States Army became the first fatal airplane accident victim. The lieutenant suffered massive and fatal head injuries. The subsequent investigation, which included input from the United States Army medical corps, recommended that head protection be developed and worn by aviators. The recommendation was not documented in the medical literature and may only represent tradition as other forms of documentation are lacking.

One year earlier, in 1907, the first series of papers to deal with the physiological factors associated with the airplane were published. The papers were written in France and addressed the subject of airsickness. Armstrong (7), in his review of the world medical literature in the early twentieth century, cites a total of 32 medical publications devoted to some aspect of aviation medicine prior to the onset of World War I.

Medical Standards

As early as 1910, countries in Europe were considering the medical ramifications of aviation. Minimum medical standards were developed for military pilots in Germany. In Great Britain, with the formation of the Naval and Military wings of the Royal Flying Corps in 1912, two service medical officers were appointed. Both learned to fly and provided the rudiments of aviation medicine support to their units. The United States War Department published its first instructions on the physical examination of candidates for aviation duty in February, 1912. Several months later, the United States Navy issued similar instructions.

The War Department's initial instructions provided that:

1. All candidates for aviation duty shall be subjected to a rigorous physical examination to determine their fitness for such duty.
2. The visual acuity without glasses should be normal. Any error of refraction requiring correction by glasses or any other cause diminishing acuity of vision below normal will be a cause for rejection. The candidates' ability to estimate distances should be tested. Color blindness for red, green, or violet is a cause for rejection.
3. The acuity of hearing should be carefully tested and the ears carefully examined with the aid of the speculum and mirror. Any diminution of the acuity of hearing below normal will be a cause for rejection. Any disease of the middle ear, either acute or chronic, or any sclerosed condition of the eardrum resulting from a former acute condition will be a cause for rejection. Any disease of the internal ear or of the auditory nerve will be a cause for rejection. The following tests for equilibrium to detect otherwise obscure diseased conditions of the internal ear should be made:
   a. Have the candidate stand with knees, heels, and toes touching.
   b. Have the candidate walk forward, backward, and in a circle.
   c. Have the candidate hop around the room. These tests should be made first with the eyes open and then closed, on both feet and then on one foot, and hopping forward and backward, the candidate trying to hop or walk in a straight line. Any deviation to the right or left from the straight line or from the arc of the circle should be noted. Any persistent deviation, either to the right or left, is evidence of a diseased condition of the internal ear, and nystagmus is also frequently associated with such condition. These symptoms, therefore, should be regarded as cause for rejection.
4. The organs of respiration and the circulatory system should be carefully examined. Any diseased condition of the circulatory system, either of the heart or the arterial system, is a cause for rejection. Any disease of the nervous system is a cause for rejection.
5. The precision of the movements of the limbs should be especially carefully tested, following the order outlined in paragraph 17, General Order, 60, War Department, 1909.
6. Any candidate whose history may show that he is afflicted with chronic digestive disturbances, chronic constipation or indigestion, or intestinal disorders tending to produce dizziness, headache, or to impair his vision should be rejected (7).

Rapidly expanding technology in the field of aeronautics was increasing the speed, altitude, performance, and complexity of the flying machine. Consequently, the demands on the aviator were likewise increasing. Although the aircraft's potential in a variety of commercial service and military roles was identified, this infant of heavier-than-air flight had yet to mature.

Aeronautics first received strong governmental support because of its potential military role. An Italian reconnaissance flight during the Trip-

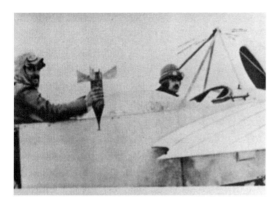

Figure 1.13. Hand-dropped bombs used in the first Balkan War in 1912 (courtesy of the United States Air Force National Archives).

olitan War in 1911 marked the first military use of the airplane. Bulgarian aviators hand-dropped small bombs over Turkish-held Adrianople during the first Balkan War of 1912 (Fig. 1.13). Prior to the outbreak of World War I, Germany possessed 1200 combat aircraft, as compared with the 1000 flown by France and Britain—no small number.

Early in World War I, the stress of high altitude flight was first experienced not by pilots of airplanes but by military crews of the lighter-than-air German zeppelins. These airships were safe from pursuit aircraft but crews experienced hypoxia and cold. Primitive oxygen equipment was installed to maintain crew performance.

The first year following the onset of hostilities, Great Britain reviewed its casualty list. Out of every 100 flyers killed, two had met their death at the hands of the enemy, eight from some defect in the airplane, and 90 deaths were ascribed to individual deficiencies, including physical defects, recklessness, and carelessness. In further refinement, it became clear that 60% of the aviation casualties were due to physical defects of the aviators. This resulted in the strongest impetus to date for the establishment of aviation medicine, and the British developed a special service for the care of the flyer. The results of this initial aviation medicine program were spectacular. Deaths due to physical defects were reduced by the end of the second year from 60% to 20%, and were down to 12% by the third year.

In 1914, the head of the aviation section of the United States Signal Corps requested advice of the United States Army Surgeon General as to how to determine fitness for flight. The Surgeon General's office responded promptly and prepared requirements for the examination and standards to be met by the candidates. Within a few months, the Surgeon General was requested to lower his standards because they were so high no applicant was able to pass the examination and, therefore, the aviation section was unable to obtain personnel. Standards were lowered, and Major Theodore Lyster, the father of American military aviation medicine, established physical examination units and developed realistic medical selection standards.

Rumors and gossip about the tough physical examinations were rampant. There was the so-called "needle test," during which the blindfolded applicant held a needle between his thumb and forefinger and a pistol was fired unexpectedly behind him. If the candidate was so startled by the sudden noise that he drew blood by puncturing his finger with the needle, he was disqualified because of excessive excitability. The rumors told of another test in which the applicant was hit over the head by a mallet when he least expected it. If he were coherent within the first 15 seconds after being struck, he was considered sufficiently resistant to concussion to make a good candidate. The French actually developed a test for nervous shock. They measured the changes in respiration, heart rate, and vasomotor response of a candidate when a revolver was fired near his ear.

Eventually, 67 examination centers were established in the larger cities of America. Approximately 100,000 applicants for the air service were examined. Of the cadet applicants examined, approximately 30% were disqualified for medical reasons. Table 1.1 lists the causes for those rejections (7). Then, as now, one of the major causes for medical rejection was related to

Table 1.1.
**The Causes For Medical Rejection For All Men
Who Applied as Cadet Flyers During World War I**

Reason for Rejection	Percent
Disqualified on three or more tests	29
Disqualified on two tests	24
Eye	20
Equilibrium	7
Other and general subnormalities	7
Vascular system	5
Ear	4
Nose and throat	3
Urinalysis	1
Total	100

vision. Defects of vision accounted for 20% of all rejections and were frequently among the multiple defects.

The physical standards established for aviators by Lyster and his co-workers were based on empirical grounds, and they felt the question needed further study. Following the lead of the British, an aviation medical research board was established by the United States Army. The responsibilities of this board were:

1. To investigate all conditions that affect the efficiency of pilots.
2. To institute and carry out such experiments and tests as will determine the ability of pilots to fly at high altitudes.
3. To carry out experiments and tests to provide suitable apparatus for the supply of oxygen to pilots at high altitudes.
4. To act as a standing medical board for the consideration of all matters relating to the physical fitness of pilots.

For every medical standard established, there was the anecdote of the successful hero who would not have been fit enough to pass the standard. Britain's greatest ace, Edward Mannock, had severe astigmatism and was essentially blind in one eye. Guynemer, a French ace, had pulmonary tuberculosis. The German ace, Oswald Boelcke, had periodic attacks of severe asthma. William Thaw, of ''Escadrille Lafayette'' fame,

had good vision in only one eye. Frank Luke, the American ace, would have failed a psychiatric examination due to his moodiness and antisocial behavior. A Canadian aviator, Leeche, was a successful combat pilot despite the inconvenience of a wooden leg. In a crash that he survived, his wooden leg was broken, and he had to bear the expenses of repair himself. Nevertheless, the accident rates did improve, in large measure due to the selection of more medically qualified aviators.

The Flight Surgeon

Parallel to the establishment of the medical research board, an American medical mission to Europe revealed that American aviators were not receiving appropriate medical support. Flying accident rates were high. Fatalities from crashes were three times the deaths due to enemy action. Accidents were occurring at the rate of one for every 241 flying hours, and a death occurred for every 721 flight hours. Medical conditions caused or complicated by flying were not recognized or understood by the assigned medical officers. This was understandable because none of the medical officers had experience or training in aviation medicine. To add insult to injury, an aviator could not see a medical officer without the permission of his commanding officer. When these reports reached Lyster, who had by now become the first Chief Surgeon of the Aviation Section of the Signal Corps of the United States Army, he immediately undertook plans for medical officers to become trained in aviation medicine. Until a school for flight surgeons could be created, manpower was dispatched from the Air Service Medical Research Laboratory (Fig. 1.14). Among those in this cadre was Major Robert Ray Hampton who, on September 17, 1918, became the first practicing flight surgeon to the American expeditionary force.

Flight Medical Training
The informal but effective training of flight surgeons commenced immediately, and these physicians were assigned to flying fields in both the

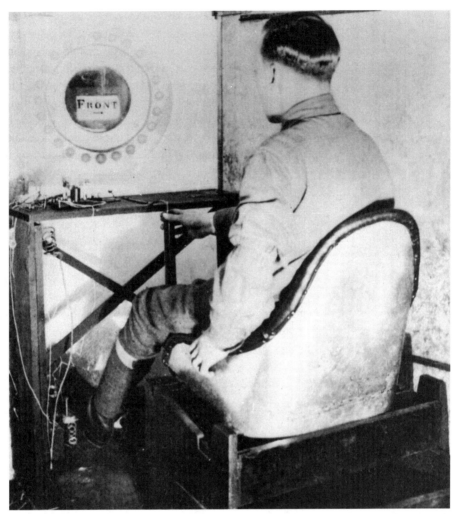

Figure 1.14. The low-pressure chamber at the School of Aviation Medicine being used for psychologic testing at altitude in 1918 (official United States Air Force photograph).

United States and Europe. By the end of the war, a complete medical service for the aviation arm of the United States Army was organized and functioning. This service provided for the medical selection of the aviator, for his classification, and, once on flight duty, for his health maintenance, all of which led to the formation of the new medical specialty in aviation medicine.

Simultaneously, in both the United States and Europe, operational flight medicine was being practiced and research, development, and testing conducted. The need for assessment procedures for balance, vision, cardiovascular efficiency, psychologic aptitude, and neurologic functioning were required. Solutions were needed for the problems of cold, hypoxia, disorientation, and fear of flying. Devices were needed to restrain the pilot in crash landings, to protect his head from crash injury, to protect his eyes from windblast, and to provide oxygen and warmth (Fig. 1.15). Such were the challenges to this new field of aviation medicine.

Interwar Period

During World War I, aviation medicine as a fledgling first tried its wings. A large historical

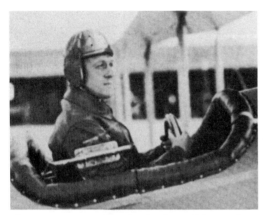

Figure 1.15. Army flyer Benjamin Foulois wearing his own football helmet for head protection (courtesy of the United States Air Force National Archives).

volume, *Air Service Medical*, was published in 1919 by the United States War Department. In that same year, H. Graeme Anderson of the British Royal Navy authored one of the first texts on aviation medicine, a fascinating treatise entitled *The Medical and Surgical Aspects of Aviation*. The War Department was again responsible, in 1920, for publishing *Aviation Medicine in the A.E.F.* The first Commandant of the School of Aviation Medicine, Louis H. Bauer, authored the text *Aviation Medicine* in 1926.

Following the conclusion of World War I, many military pilots continued to fly, both as an avocation and a vocation. Surplus aircraft were plentiful and relatively inexpensive, and soon every city, town, and hamlet became the site for Jennies performing acrobatics, an activity that was to become known as "barnstorming."

While the American public was becoming fascinated by aviation, the development and manufacturing of new aircraft were coming to a standstill. The impetus of the war years was no longer stimulating aeronautics, and all associated programs, including military aviation medicine, were undergoing belt tightening. The possibility of aircraft carrying passengers and mail did receive support, both from the returning military pilots and from the commercial sector.

Civil Aviation Medicine

President Calvin Coolidge signed the Air Commerce Act on May 20, 1926, assigning federal responsibilities in civil aviation to the United States Department of Commerce. One of the draft proposals circulated for review that same year included a requirement for physical examinations as part of the pilot licensing procedure. It is interesting to note that up to that time no physical standard existed.

In the fall of that year, the United States Department of Commerce, recognizing the need for an expert in the field of aviation medicine, requested the Army to release Dr. Lewis Bauer so that he might serve in the civil aviation arena. He immediately set about the task of developing the first physical standard for civilian pilots and establishing a medical examination system for the United States. The physical standard was promulgated one year later in air commerce regulation, and in 1927, Dr. Bauer contacted 60 physicians, later appointing 57 as aviation medical examiners (AMEs). In addition to the AMEs, Army and Navy flight surgeons were authorized to perform civil aircrew examinations, as were several United States Public Health Service hospitals. By the third decade, over 800 AMEs had been appointed, both in the United States and overseas.

Civil Physical Standards

Dr. Bauer proposed physical standards for three categories of pilots.

Private Pilots. The physical requirements were the absence of organic disease or defect that would interfere with the safe handling of an airplane under the conditions of private flying, visual acuity of at least 20/40 in each eye (less than 20/40 may be accepted if the pilot wears a corrective lens in his goggles and has normal judgment of distance without correction), good judgment of distance, no diplopia in any position, normal visual fields and color vision, and no organic disease of the eye or internal ear.

Industrial Pilots. The physical requirements were the absence of any organic disease or defect that would interfere with the safe handling of an airplane, visual acuity of not less than 20/30 in each eye, although in certain incidences, less than 20/30 may be accepted if the applicant wears corrective lens to 20/20 in his goggles and has good judgment of distance without correction, good judgment of distance, no diplopia in any field, normal visual fields and color vision, and no organic disease of the eye, ear, nose, or throat.

Transport Pilots. The physical requirements were good past history, sound pulmonary, cardiovascular, gastrointestinal, central nervous, and genitourinary systems, freedom from material structural defects or limitations, freedom from disease of the ductless glands, normal central, peripheral, and color vision, normal judgment of distance, only slight defects of ocular muscle balance, freedom from ocular disease, absence of obstructive or diseased conditions of the ear, nose, and throat, and no abnormalities of equilibrium that would interfere with flying.

Medical certification rapidly grew. In 1928, the first year, 11,688 applications were processed. By 1930, nearly 44,000 certifications had been issued.

The training of designated civil aviation medical examiners was a key part of the original plan developed by Dr. Bauer. In 1930, 12 conferences were conducted for training AMEs. In addition, Dr. Bauer requested the appointment of district or regional flight surgeons to instruct and oversee the work being performed by AMEs. This did not occur until 1931, when the first district flight surgeon was assigned to Kansas City, Missouri.

Military Aviation Medicine

Van Patten, in reviewing early physiological challenges to flight, relates how an army aviator, Rudolph Schroeder, experienced a number of life threatening events during high altitude flight in 1918 (8). Using a pipestem connected to an oxygen flask by a rubber hose, he simply titrated his hypoxic symptoms by opening a manual value to the flask. Without an indicator, he used his tongue to check the oxygen flow. At 8,230 m (27,000 ft) he was unable to see through his goggles due to frosting—ambient temp was − 60C. On another flight at 10,000 m (33,000 ft) he apparently experienced oxygen valve problems and was becoming hypoxic. He raised his goggles to better see but the moisture in his eyes immediately froze, blinding him. He pushed the nose of his aircraft over and dove for a lower altitude and survived. In 1921, another Army aviator Lieutenant Macready reached approximately 12,200 m (40,000 ft). Fortunately his aircraft reached its ceiling before he did; there was no provision for pressure breathing.

Throughout this interwar period, the military continued the development of newer, high-performance aircraft. Every year, records in altitude, speed, performance, endurance, and reliability were being established. Man was beginning to experience accelerated forces, or ''G'' forces, which were interfering dangerously with cerebral circulation. Balloon flights were reaching into the stratosphere, requiring a gondola with a sealed, pressure- and temperature-controlled environment. Aircraft were reaching altitudes where the availability of even 100% oxygen was inadequate to prevent hypoxia. Special masks were developed that were connected to a compressor system which would force oxygen into the pilot's lungs, introducing and proving the concept of positive pressure breathing. Man had reached the limit where he could safely be exposed to the elements in an open cockpit, and aircraft designers were forced to consider an enclosed cabin or cockpit for the aviator.

Aeromedical Research and Development

Throughout these years, the School of Aviation Medicine continued to train military flight surgeons and served as a focal point for research regarding the selection and maintenance of aircrews. In 1934, the Aeromedical Research Laboratory was founded at Wright Field in Dayton, Ohio. The charter for this laboratory was to study the effects of flight on man and to develop methods for eliminating or neutralizing the adverse effects that would prove detrimental to mission efficiency in military aviation. Dr. Harry G. Armstrong, the laboratory's first commander, in one of his numerous technical reports, stated: "It is concluded that sealed aircraft compartments offer the best solution for the protection of flying personnel at high altitude, and the only practical method of flight above 40,000 feet. It is recommended that projects be initiated to study, collect data, and develop aircraft incorporating the principles of pressure, oxygen, and oxygen pressure compartments." Dr. Armstrong has received credit for significant research and technology that eventually led to the pressure cabin that is so vital to both commercial and military aviation today.

On November 20, 1939, the United States Navy established its School of Aviation Medicine and Research at Pensacola, Florida. This school continues to be the premier institution conducting biomedical research in aviation medicine for the Navy.

Since World War I, the center for aviation medicine, both in education and research, for the Royal Air Force in Great Britain has been at Farnborough. This organization has supported military development, as well as satisfying British Air Ministry needs.

With the approach of the end of the fourth decade, only 35 years after the first flight at Kitty Hawk, a war was to begin in which aviation would prove decisive. Aeronautic engineering would respond with an exponential growth in technology. Larger, higher-performance aircraft, jet engines, rocket propulsion, and advances in communication and avionics would all culminate in the modern world of aerospace technology. As the handmaiden to this technology, aviation medicine would expand and change, as it made the transition to aerospace medicine in the modern era.

REFERENCES

1. Rolt LTC. The aeronauts. New York: Walker and Company, 1966.
2. Carlson ET, Heveran BT. Benjamin Rush and the birth of American aviation medicine. Aerospace Med 1974; 45:1083.
3. Engle E, Lott A. Man in flight. Annapolis, Maryland: Leeward Publications, 1970.
4. Hitchcock FA. Paul Bert and the beginnings of aviation medicine. Aerospace Med 1971;42:1101.
5. Gillies JA. A textbook of aviation physiology. London: Pergamon Press, 1965.
6. Combs H. Kill Devil Hill. Boston: Houghton Mifflin, 1979.
7. Armstrong HG. Principles and practice of aviation medicine. 3rd Ed. Baltimore: Williams & Wilkins, 1952.
8. Van Patten RE. Pioneers at high altitude. Air Force Magazine, April:88–90, 1991.

Chapter 2

The Modern Perspective

Roy L. DeHart

Invention breeds invention.

Ralph Waldo Emerson

With the advent of aviation, new professions developed, established professions evolved, and technology accelerated the demise of still others. The turn of the twentieth century saw the dawning of modern medicine and the birth of aerospace medicine.

The birth pains had occurred when man first was borne aloft under globes of hot air or flammable gas. Labor ensued with the onset of World War I and the need to reduce the carnage of thousands of young men who were enthusiastic but unfit to become military aviators. A product of that delivery was the flight surgeon, a title still given with pride to those physicians directly supporting our military flyers.

In the years following World War I, the medical requirements of the aviation industry caused an evolution in a small segment of the profession of medicine, led by those fledgling flight surgeons. In addition to the military practice of aviation medicine, other physicians entered the federal service or joined the expanding airlines. An association was formed and a journal established.

The technological developments of World War II forced new efforts in aeromedical research, and the enormous increase in the numbers of aircrew resulted in a concomitant increase in physicians involved in aviation medicine. Following that war, technological advances were applied to the civil sector, resulting

in an exponential growth of airline passenger miles flown.

Special training, a new vocabulary, and the peculiar trappings of the trade all gave legitimacy to the establishment of aviation medicine as a medical specialty. The evolutionary process, however, was not yet complete because technology and man were not to be limited to operations in an ocean of air. By the 1960s, it became clear that man was on his way into space and that medical support would be required to get him there. Within 10 years of the establishment of the specialty of aviation medicine, it was necessary for the science to further evolve into aerospace medicine—a specialty that extends literally "out of this world."

THE PRACTICE OF AEROSPACE MEDICINE

Classically, medicine has been concerned with the care and cure of the patients experiencing disease in their usual surroundings. Disease in this context can be considered the demonstration of disrupted or abnormal physiological processes. The patient is considered in the environment of the home or hospital. Thus, the patient is seen as experiencing abnormal physiological processes in a normal, terrestrial environment.

An approach to understanding the art and science of aerospace medicine is to contrast it with

23

this classic approach to medicine. Aerospace medicine most often deals with healthy individuals; in fact, the medical selection process for aviators presupposes health. The more difficult or responsible the aviators' duty, the greater the requirement that they be free from demonstrable disease. This requirement is exemplified by the stringent health examinations given some special-mission military aircrews and, of course, the astronauts. A situation is attained where individuals selected for some aviation and space operations are not simply healthy in the general sense but, perhaps better stated, are superhealthy. Although the classic patient is comfortable in the predictable terrestrial environment, the aviator must contend with an entirely different, demanding, dynamic, and at times, totally hostile environment.

In the practice of aerospace medicine, we may deal with the normal physiology in an abnormal environment. This reality forces a fundamental change in the physician's approach to her responsibilities toward her patient, the aviator. Health maintenance with minimal therapeutic intervention becomes the sine qua non for the practitioner of aerospace medicine. The specialist will often be required to assist the aviator in competing successfully in the abnormal environment of aviation. This assistance may range from simple tasks such as demonstrating how to ventilate and equilibrate the air pressure of the middle ear or sinus, demonstrating methods to improve tolerance to acceleration (G), and managing potential airsickness to more complex tasks such as human involvement in research to extend performance in this stressful environment. Thus, in classical medicine, one deals with abnormal physiology in a normal environment, whereas in aerospace medicine, one is concerned with normal physiology in an abnormal, or flight, environment.

In its fullest context, the practice of aerospace medicine is multidisciplinary, extending into the fields of basic science: physics, chemistry, mathematics; and the engineering disciplines: aeronautical, mechanical, electrical. Many of the

health care specialties also have contributions to make in assisting the flight surgeon or aeromedical practitioner with responsibilities in aerospace medicine.

Aviation Medicine

As was discussed in Chapter 1, aircrew medical standards were developed in a dynamic process during World War I. The concept that anyone could fly was altered so that only the most perfect human specimens were allowed to fly, then altered again to reflect the physical and psychologic health necessary to successfully meet the realistic, rather than ideal, requirements for functioning in the flight environment. Today, a flying physical examination remains one of the requirements for acquiring a pilot's license, for entering military aviation, or for fulfilling most aircrew duties aboard an aircraft.

In reflecting on those early days, Dr. H. G. Anderson, a medical officer in the Royal Air Force, described some of the factors considered with the physical requirements:

In selecting candidates for the Air Service, what is looked for is the sound constitution, free from organic disease, and a fairly strong physique in order to withstand altitude effects, such as cold, fatigue, and diminished oxygen. It is essential there should be normal hearing and good muscle and equilibration sense. As the aviator is so dependent on his eyesight, too much importance cannot be attached to this part of the examination. But next to vision, and most important of all in obtaining the best aviator, is the question of temperament. Undoubtedly, there is a particular temperament or aptitude for flying, and its distribution is peculiarly interesting, whether looked upon from its racial aspect and ethnological origin or in relation to previous health, life and habits. Unfortunately, this temperament is a difficult matter to estimate clinically, and especially so in the examining room. The ideal aviator must have good judgment, be courageous, and not upset by fear, although conscious of the perils of his work. He must be cool in emergencies, able to make careful and quick decisions and act accordingly. His reaction-times must never be delayed—he must be ever alert, as mental sluggishness in flying spells disaster. . . . With regard to relation of habits in this special aptitude for flying, the latter is found most commonly among those used to playing games and leading an outdoor life. The yachtsman and the horseman, with their finer sense of judgment and "lighter hands," should make the most skillful pilots. . . . Every now and then one meets the type with splendid physique and apparently unshakable courage and finds that he learns to fly indifferently or is unable to learn at all, and again one meets the weedy, pale type learning quickly to fly and turning out to be a first-rate pilot (1).

Once the need for aircrew selection was firmly established, the next task became one of health maintenance. In World War I, each nation with an aviation arm independently learned of the requirements for aircrew health maintenance. Those early aviators were unable to perform and survive if suffering from minor illness, excessively fatigued, medicated, or intoxicated. The combat surgeon did not understand the unforgiving environment in which the aviator frequently found himself. It became necessary to train special physicians to care for the flyer and to give emphasis to the aircrew's health care maintenance. Today, the concept of the squadron flight surgeon is a principal tenet in military aerospace medicine. This concept is further represented in the Federal Aviation Administration's (FAA) health program for air traffic controllers, in the National Aeronautics and Space Administration (NASA), and among many airlines who provide aviation medicine practitioners for the care of the cockpit and cabin crews.

As World War I continued, aircrews became ill or were injured in accidents or combat, thus creating a new question to be answered: when should a disqualified aviator be returned to aircrew duty? Today, this question poses some of the greatest challenges to the specialist. Should an individual be returned to flying following severe head trauma, following mild coronary infarction, following coronary bypass, or after receiving treatment for carcinoma? Should a pilot be disqualified from flying simply because of chronologic age? Pilots see the physician as a controlling element in their careers, and this perception creates the potential for an adversarial relationship. The practitioner must always remain sensitive to this perception and manage it; otherwise, his effectiveness will become compromised.

At the request of the United States Department of Commerce, the United States Army permitted Dr. Lewis Bauer to resign his commission from the medical corps to become the first medical director of the newly created aeronautics branch of the Department of Commerce (Fig. 2.1). This was in November, 1926, and many of the young men who had gained their aviator's wings in World War I were involved in the new industry of commercial aviation (2). Dr. Bauer

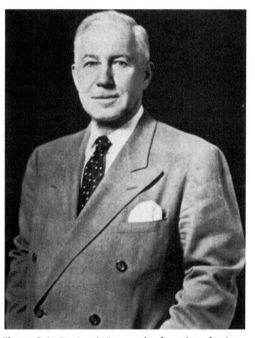

Figure 2.1. Dr. Lewis Bauer, the founder of aviation medicine in the United States (courtesy of the Aerospace Medicine Association).

had two immediate tasks. One was the formulation of physical standards for licensing civilian airmen and the other was to select physicians throughout the country and qualify them to perform these new examinations. From his Army Air Corps experience, Dr. Bauer was familiar with the military's established physical requirements, and from this source he developed an outline of standards to be applied to the nation's civil pilots. As had been the case in the military, civilian physicians with impeccable credentials were not necessarily aware of the unique occupational requirements for civil flying and, thus, had little depth of understanding for the rationale embodied in the physical examination requirements. With a few exceptions, these chosen physicians required further training in aviation medicine. Through these efforts, a second cadre of physicians was created that matched those in the military service.

Further maturing of the specialty of aviation medicine occurred with the extensive growth and advances of aviation during World War II. It was during this period that technology advanced from the biplane to sweptwing, from a few hundred miles an hour to supersonic flight, from the open cockpit to the pressurized cabin, and from the occasional aircraft to huge aerial armadas.

Space Medicine

The evolutionary process of space medicine began in the United States in February, 1949, when the United States Air Force School of Aviation Medicine established a department of Space Medicine (3). This department was established under the direction of the school's commander, General Harry Armstrong. The department was interdisciplinary, with major scientific representation in the medical sciences, astronomy, engineering, and bioclimatology. Once the department of Space Medicine was organized and functioning, Dr. Hubertus Strughold was ap-

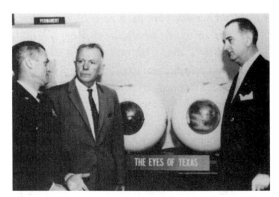

Figure 2.2. Dr. Hubertus Strughold, the father of space medicine, second from the left with General Bensen, a pioneer in aviation and space medicine, and then Senator Lyndon Johnson in front of the "Eyes of Texas," a model used to teach flight surgeons the muscular control of the eye (official United States Air Force photo).

pointed Director (Fig. 2.2). To many, Dr. Strughold is the "Father of Space Medicine." The formation of this new department, so focused on the future, was anticipated by events of the previous year, when a panel was organized by the school to discuss the challenging subject, "Aeromedical Problems of Space Travel."

The dreamers and the skeptics each had their opinion and their definition of space medicine. To help bring order out of chaos, The *Journal of Aviation Medicine*, in 1950, stated in its editorial page: "Space medicine is concerned with the medical problems involved in modes of travel which are potentially capable at least of transporting us beyond the earth's gravitational field: and it is also concerned with special hazards encountered in the upper part of our atmosphere and beyond." The mood was apparently right to dream of the future, for that same year the space medicine branch of the Aviation Medicine Association was established. In 1950, Dr. Strughold presented a paper that was to become a classic, entitled "Where does Space Begin?" which was subsequently published in 1952 as "Atmospheric Equivalence" (4). In this intellectually challenging and stimulating paper, he first proposed the now well-recognized concept that space is not a set boundary but a continuum along which, for various situations, one moves from terrestrial to celestial.

Strughold's first zone of transition occurs at 16 km, where the pressure of the atmosphere is reduced to 87 mm Hg. At this altitude, as a result of water vapor and carbon dioxide offgassing, the astronaut would be unable to draw any air into the lungs, even if 100% oxygen were available. The next transition occurs at 20 km, where the atmospheric pressure drops to 47 mm Hg. Because of the astronaut's body temperature, fluids, including blood, would begin vaporizing, and the astronaut exposed to this atmosphere would experience the same desiccating process as in the farthest reaches of space. Above this altitude, the air is too rarified to be compressed effectively to support a pressurized cabin. Consequently, it is necessary to introduce the closed-cabin environment, or space cabin.

At 30 km, the astronaut moves into the ozone layer produced by the high flux of ultraviolet radiation. The space crewman is now approaching an altitude where he/she must be protected from the ultraviolet light itself. At 100 km, the pilot and craft are subjected to the full impact force of meteorites. At 150 km, the astronaut witnesses the true black void of space because the atmosphere is too thin to scatter visible light, and illumination occurs only from the direct rays of the illuminating object. Beyond 160 km, the craft reaches an orbiting altitude, and the astronaut, for the first time, experiences the weightlessness of space.

With recognition of the new frontier that was being entered, names were changing across the aeronautic world. Aerospace became a common word used in the context of aerospace industry, aerospace technology, and aerospace medicine. The Aero Medical Association became the Aerospace Medical Association, and its journal, the *Journal of Aviation Medicine*, was renamed *Aerospace Medicine*. For the time being, the transition was complete—aviation and space were integrated into aerospace. The transition from aviation to aerospace medicine was more form than function. The principles of practice are the same for both. The stressors to the crew member, whether the pilot or astronaut, have many similarities, as well as occasional significant differences. The appropriately trained practitioner can function effectively in both realms.

RECENT AERONAUTIC DEVELOPMENTS

No single development or technology can describe or explain the transition that has occurred in the past several decades within the aerospace industry. As witnessed repeatedly in history, the requirements of national defense provided the needs that technology strove to satisfy. Major developments occurred in propulsion systems, fuels, aeronautical design, structures, materials, avionics, electronics, and bioscience.

Technology for War

In the mid- and late 1930s much was happening in the world of aviation to prepare for the war to come. The first American four-engine bomber was successfully flown in the summer of 1935 and became known in World War II as the B-17 "Flying Fortress." The aircraft could carry a full bomb load nearly four thousand kilometers at an average speed of 370 kph. Without bombs, it had an altitude capacity in excess of 10,000 m. Because the aircraft was unpressurized, those engaged in aviation medicine initiated major developments in oxygen systems, electrically heated thermal protective clothing, and special garments to protect against antiaircraft artillery. Although the B-17 could fly high, it in no way established an altitude record. An Italian aviator, Colonel Mario Pezzi, climbed over 18,000 m in 1938.

To support high-altitude flight, the engineers and physicians working in aviation medicine developed the novel BLB oxygen mask. The initials stood for the physicians involved with the development: Boothby, Lovelace, and Bulbulian. The mask provided a self-regulated mixture of oxygen, air exhaled from the lungs, and atmospheric air during flights to moderately high altitudes. Another hazard of high-altitude flying was pilot fatigue. Research in this area and concomitant aeromedical problems earned the coveted Collier trophy in 1940 for Boothby, Lovelace, and Armstrong. Much of this earlier research work in support of the expanding aeronautical environment was published by Armstrong in 1939 in his book, *Principles and Practices of Aviation Medicine*, which was the first inclusive text that attempted to bridge the complex and diversified engineering and medical problems encountered in modern flight of the day.

During the same period, Isaac Newton's third law of motion, "To every action there is an opposed and equal reaction," would be applied to an aeronautical propulsion system developed by Frank Whittle. In Germany, Dr. Hans von Ohain labored along similar lines to develop the engine that powered the world's first jet plane. By 1942, this technology was applied to the development of a combat-fighter aircraft, the Messerschmidt ME-262. It was the Whittle engine, which arrived in the United States in 1941, that became the prototype for America's first entry into reaction engine flight. The initial development and testing of America's first jet aircraft created a potential problem. Although test flights were flown in the Mojave Desert in California, it was still possible that some inquiring eyes might see the aircraft on the ramp while it was undergoing maintenance. The absence of a propeller might lead to some unwanted speculation. To avoid the speculation, a large balsam wood propeller was attached around a ring. The ring could be placed over the pointed nose of the airplane whenever it was outside the hangar, thus avoiding potentially embarrassing questions.

The combination of improved aeronautic structures and high-energy power plants made it possible for the airframe to withstand high acceleration, or "G." This G acting on the pilot could exceed the compensating capacity of the cardiovascular system, rendering the pilot unconscious. A Canadian aeromedical researcher, Dr. W.M. Franks, began investigating the problems

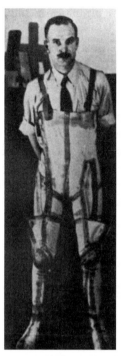

Figure 2.3. Dr. W. M. Franks, a Canadian aeromedical researcher in an early G protection suit of his design (courtesy of the National Air and Space Museum).

of acceleration in flight. Working at the University of Toronto, Dr. Franks developed the first operationally practical anti-G suit to be worn by pilots during combat (Fig. 2.3).

In this initial development, a fluid pressure was applied to the calves, thighs, and abdomen to prevent vascular pooling and enhance adequate return of blood to the heart. This suit successfully raised the G tolerance for the aircrew members who wore it.

With the increasing altitude capability of aircraft, there was the additional requirement for a pressure environment that was comfortable and safe for both crews and passengers. Initial work was begun at the Aeromedical Research Laboratory under the direction of its commander, Dr. Armstrong. With the use of the XC-35 in the late 1930s, the concept of a pressure cabin was proven and was later applied to passenger aircraft with the development of the Boeing 307 Stratoliner.

On the day the United States entered World War II, a flight surgeon made the supreme sacrifice. The first operational squadron of B-17s were being deployed to Hawaii at the time the island was under attack by naval aircraft of the Japanese Imperial Fleet. Aboard one of the flying fortresses was the squadron's new flight surgeon, Lieutenant William R. Schick. His flight medical training had been cut short to permit him to deploy with his squadron to the Pacific. Although most of the B-17s successfully landed in Hawaii despite the ongoing Japanese attack, one plane was shot down and crashed, killing all aboard, including Dr. Schick. He was the first flight surgeon to be killed in combat and would, unfortunately, be joined by many others. In the recent Desert Storm operation, a Pilot-physician was killed in combat—Dr. Thomas F. Koritz.

To conduct the air battles in World War II, over a million military aircraft were constructed and flown by the belligerent forces. In the United States, tens of thousands of aircrewmen were selected to undergo aviation training. This required significant improvements in the medical selection process for aircrew personnel. Many of the techniques and examination procedures developed during the mid-1940s are still used today in the selection of military aircrew personnel. The concept of the squadron-level flight surgeon became fully ingrained into military aviation.

Postwar Aeronautic Developments

The excitement of aviation, which was so infectious during the war, spread into the postwar period. The public had lost its distrust and fear of flying. Large aircraft were now available to enter into civilization air commerce. The reliability of the Douglas DC-3 had been established, and the four-engine DC-4 had been developed, proven, and was ready to enter the civil transportation system. The Lockheed Constellation became the American flagship for a number of airlines engaged in international commerce.

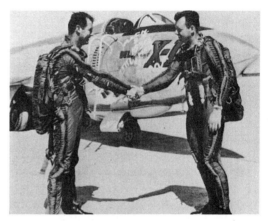

Figure 2.4. The Aeromedical Laboratory's T-1 partial-pressure suit being worn by test pilots in front of the Bell X-1 (courtesy of Bell Aviation).

In October, 1947, accompanied by his flight surgeon, Dr. John Stapp, Captain Charles Yeager was escorted to a waiting B-29, which carried under its wing the Bell X-1. On that day, Captain Yeager would be the first man in the world to accelerate past the shock wave known as the "sound barrier." To protect him from the low-pressure environment of high altitude, Yeager wore the T-1 partial-pressure suit developed by the Aeromedical Laboratory (Fig. 2.4). Thus, with each new milestone in aeronautic development, there often preceded a concomitant development in both technology and aerospace medicine.

Just as Yeager became famous as the first man to break the sound barrier, his flight surgeon, John Paul Stapp, became known as "the fastest man on earth" (Fig. 2.5). In December, 1954, while riding a rocket-propelled sled on a track over 11 km in length, Dr. Stapp attained a ground speed of 1027.93 kph. The braking at the termination of the run was estimated to be 40 times normal earth gravity. The objective of the test was to demonstrate that a properly positioned and restrained astronaut could endure the sudden impact of his spacecraft with the atmosphere upon reentry from space.

Similarly, the high-altitude flight, Man High II, took Dr. David G. Simmons in a 32-hour flight to an altitude of 34,000 m for the purpose

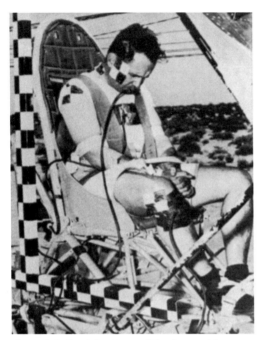

Figure 2.5. Dr. John Stapp, "The Fastest Man on Earth," instrumented and restrained in preparation for a ride on a rocket-propelled sled (official United States Air Force photo).

of assaying the potential hazards from prolonged exposure to cosmic radiation (Fig. 2.6). Both the balloon flight and the sled ride were preludes to man's ventures into space.

Man's Ventures into Space

On the evening of October 4, 1957, the scientists and engineers of the Soviet Union successfully launched into orbit the earth's first artificial satellite. Sputnik I took with it into orbit more than simply a radio beacon; it also marked man's entry into the space age. A month later, on November 3, the Soviet Union launched the first biosatellite. This satellite carried aloft a female dog, Laika, but more significantly, it carried life-support systems to maintain the vital functions of this animal for a week's orbit in space. To monitor her biofunctions, automatic instruments using radiotelemetry signaled vital physiologic data back to earth-based stations.

It was clear that humans would soon be voy-

aging in space. To prepare for the inevitable, the United States selected seven military test pilots to become America's first astronauts. Part of the selection process required an in-depth medical assessment. These extensive examinations were conducted at the Lovelace Foundation in Albuquerque, New Mexico. However, it was not one of these seven astronauts who would first fly into space but the Soviet cosmonaut, Yuri Gagarin (Fig. 2.7).

This first manned flight in space, circumnavigating the globe, was conducted on April 12, 1961, and received worldwide acclaim. A month later an American astronaut, Alan Shepard, flew into space on a suborbital flight that lasted 15 minutes. The first American to make an orbital flight was John Glenn in the Friendship 7 in February, 1962. Supporting all of these manned flights, whether launched in the Soviet Union or in the United States, was an enormous foundation of biomedical research. The technology developed in those first days of manned space flight provides a firm foundation for today's manned space programs. A major challenge to space medicine and bioscience has been the development of the life-support systems for the multicrewed space vehicles and laboratories: Apollo, Soyuz, Skylab, Salyut, Mir and, to a lesser degree, the space shuttle. Just as challenging has been the development of systems permitting cosmonauts and astronauts to engage in extravehicular activity, whether in orbit or, in the case of Apollo, on the lunar surface.

Advances in space have not been without human tragedy for both the United States and the Soviet Union. In January, 1967, a launch pad fire took the lives of the three Apollo astronauts. A re-entry malfunction was fatal to Soviet cosmonauts. On January 28, 1986, at 11:39 A.M. EST, only 73 seconds after lift-off, the world witnessed on television the disintegration of Challenger with the loss of seven astronauts.

Risk analysts have estimated that the odds of a major failure in Shuttle operations is between 1 and 2 per 100 flights. The Aerospace Medicine Specialist must strive to reduce the risk at each

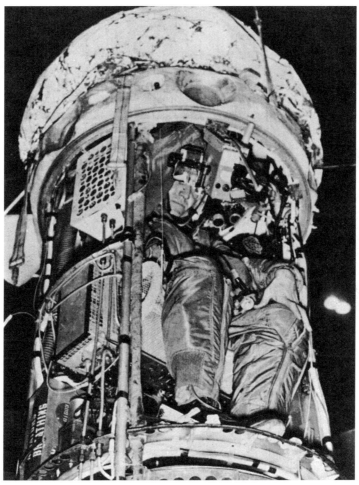

Figure 2.6. Dr. David Simons preparing for his record altitude balloon flight in the Man High II Project (official United States Air Force photo).

stage of manned space activities: research, development and operations.

Civil Aviation

In 1952, the deHavilland Comet introduced commercial jet transportation to the flying public. Two years later, in 1954, a Comet suddenly and inexplicably disintegrated at an altitude of 12 km. Several months later, the accident was repeated, again over the Mediterranean and with no warning, simply a catastrophic, instantaneous failure of the aircraft. In investigating these two accidents, specialists in aviation medicine provided the vital clues for reconstructing the events of these air disasters. The investigations established metal fatigue as the culprit behind the rapid disintegration of the pressurized cabin.

A Harvard University professor, Dr. Ross MacFarland, who pioneered medical support for Pan-American Airways, published his text *Human Factors in Air Transportation* in 1953. This text became a classic in defining the human parameters that must be considered in the construction and operation of aeronautic transportation systems.

The adaptation of defense technology to civil aviation continued with the introduction of the supersonic transport. A joint effort between the British and French governments, the Concorde

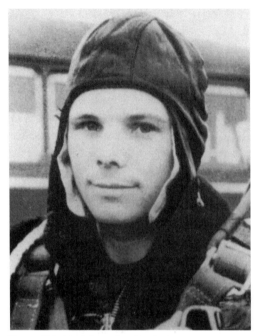

Figure 2.7. Yuri Gagarin, the Soviet cosmonaut who was the first man into space (courtesy of the Soviet Embassy).

was built on the technologies developed for military aircraft. From the beginning, aeromedical advice was sought from specialists in aerospace medicine as the aeronautical and engineering communities began designing and developing the higher- and faster-flying commercial airliner. Designers took into consideration human factors for the cockpit crew, as well as for the passengers in the cabin. Although fraught with political and economic realities, the Anglo-French Concorde established a clear technology capability in addition to proving aeromedical feasibility.

The air transportation system in the United States is an important element in this nation's business and economic community. The aviation industry contributes over $50 billion to the gross national product and employs approximately one million people in a variety of jobs. Close to 80% of the free world civilian transports are manufactured in the United States, and the sale of these aircraft has contributed significantly toward the nation's balance of trade. Today, 90%

of long-distance travel in public carriers occurs on aircraft; domestically, over 450 million passengers will board aircraft in any one year, thus generating in excess of 405 billion revenue-passenger-miles. Internationally, 95% of travel is aboard aircraft. In any one year, approximately 40 million passengers will board international flights, generating over 3 billion revenue-passenger-miles. Currently, over 12 million revenue-cargo-tons are implaned annually.

THE SPECIALTY OF AEROSPACE MEDICINE

In 1947, a motion was referred to the Executive Council of the Aero Medical Association introducing the concept of certification in aviation medicine. In supporting certification, Major General Grow, the Army Surgeon, stated:

The time has come when the Aero Medical Association should adopt standards for certification in aviation medicine and proceed with the formulation with a competent board recognized by the American Medical Association and operating conjointly with the American Medical Association. We should recognize those doctors who have devoted the major portion of their professional careers to aviation, and also protect the airlines and the military services by public standards of proficiency. Certification from such a board would be evidence of recognition by a properly qualified body of an individual doctor's ability to examine flyers and to advise concerning problems in aviation medicine (5).

Since the beginnings of aviation medicine in World War I, over 6000 physicians had by then completed postgraduate training in aviation medicine in both the United States and Canada. In addition to the 2000 medical officers serving with the aviation elements of the Armed Forces of the United States and Canada, there were 1500 medical examiners in civil aviation. Many, through experience, training, and research, had become recognized international experts in the field of aviation medicine.

The Aero Medical Association contacted the American Board of Preventive Medicine and Public Health to see if some arrangements could be worked out for the possible inclusion of aviation medicine in their specialty board process. As these discussions were being conducted, the Air Force medical service established residency training in aviation medicine at a number of its bases and coupled the program with a year of graduate training at Johns Hopkins University School of Public Health and Hygiene. Postgraduate year preceptorships were established under the sponsorship of a number of major United States airlines, and both the Mayo and Lovelace Clinics began planning for fellowships in the specialty.

In 1953, the American Board of Preventive Medicine formally appeared before the American Medical Association Council on Medical Education and Hospitals and spoke in favor of incorporating aviation medicine into their board. The day following this appearance, the council approved the decision to authorize certification in aviation medicine. In November, 1953, the American Board of Preventive Medicine officially certified the first group of physicians in the specialty of aviation medicine. As humankind moved toward the frontiers of space, the name of the specialty became aerospace medicine.

Training in Aerospace Medicine

The physician interested in the specific requirements for becoming a candidate for board certification in aerospace medicine is referred to the current edition of the Directory of Approved Internships and Residencies. In summary, the program of education and training covers 4 postgraduate years. The candidates must have completed 1 year of clinical training, which is usually the first postgraduate year following graduation from medical school or internship. A year of academic training is required with em-

phasis on biostatistics, epidemiology, health care administration, and environmental health. Most frequently, this year culminates in the award of a Master's degree in Public Health. A third year is spent concentrating on the physiologic, environmental, and clinical peculiarities of aerospace medicine. The final year is a practice year in such activities as clinical practice, research, teaching, or additional academic training.

For physicians graduating after 1983, the formalized, structured residency program is the only acceptable route for attaining qualification as a candidate for certification in aerospace medicine. For physicians graduating from medical school prior to 1984, options to the formalized program remain. These equivalencies generally require extensive experience as a practitioner in aviation medicine or previous certification in a specialty that is parallel to aerospace medicine. It is recommended that any physician considering an equivalency route to qualification communicate with the American Board of Preventive Medicine regarding current policy.

Civilian Training

Training in aerospace medicine is available through a number of institutions, both governmental and academic. For the individual interested in aviation medicine as an aeromedical examiner for the FAA, training programs are available in various regions throughout the United States in the form of seminars. In addition, the Civil Aviation Medicine Institute in Oklahoma City, Oklahoma, provides in-resident educational programs of various durations. These educational courses are designed to meet the demanding needs of the civilian practitioner and thus are short, intense, and frequently cover weekends.

For the physician seeking formal residency in the field, a university-based program is available at Wright State University in Dayton, Ohio. It is possible for the total residency program to be conducted at this one institution, beginning with a Master's degree in aerospace medicine and followed by practice opportunities across a broad spectrum of aeromedical interest. The university is located in the hometown of and named for Wilbur and Orville Wright, whose engineering and scientific ingenuity ushered in aviation. The site of the university is only a few kilometers from the farm field where the Wrights conducted much of their development and test flying. The university is also situated in the heart of the nation's major aeronautic research and development complex, the United States Air Force's Wright-Patterson installation. The resident has the full opportunity to make use of the technical libraries and facilities of much of the Air Force complex, including close association with the Harry G. Armstrong Aerospace Medical Research Laboratory.

Graduate educational and training opportunities are available with the National Aeronautics and Space Administration (NASA). Residents, usually at the third-or fourth-year level, are accepted principally at the Johnson Manned Space Center near Houston, Texas, and NASA-Ames in California for training in bioscience and operational space medicine. Because post-graduate training in aerospace medicine is a dynamic process, other institutions can be expected to offer educational, clinical, and research opportunities to residents in the field of aerospace medicine. A Fellowship in Space Medicine is available at the University of Texas—Galveston.

Air Force Programs

As would be expected, the United States Air Force has the largest training program in the field of aerospace medicine (Chapter 21). Each year, hundreds of physicians attend the United States Air Force School of Aerospace Medicine (USAFSAM) to take an 8-to 10-week course in aerospace medicine. The course is designed to train physicians to serve as flight surgeons for operational flying units. The course is normally available only to physicians with federal affiliation in the active or reserve forces of the Department of Defense or physicians in the Coast Guard, NASA, or FAA.

To meet its mission requirements, the Air Force also conducts a residency program in aerospace medicine. Approximately 20 residents per year enter this program after first attending an academic institution to acquire a background in preventive medicine; they then spend 1 or 2 years at USAFSAM or alternate facilities for formal training and research opportunities.

Army Programs

To support the large United States Army aviation program, physicians attend the basic course in Army aviation medicine at the Army helicopter center at Fort Rucker, Alabama. In many ways, the training program parallels that given by the Air Force. Because the Army's requirements for career aerospace medicine specialists are not as large as its sister services, Army specialty training is conducted either with the Air Force or Navy (Chapter 22).

Navy Program

Pensacola Naval Air Station in Pensacola, Florida, has historically been the site of Naval aviation medicine activity (Chapter 23). The initial training of Naval flight surgeons is somewhat longer than in the Army or Air Force because their program includes practical aeronautical training and experience. The limited residency program includes 2 years at Pensacola Aeromedical Center and 1 academic year at a school of public health. No more than five Naval flight surgeons per year receive the opportunity for residency training in aerospace medicine.

Aerospace Medicine Association

One of the major responsibilities of the Aerospace Medicine Association is to provide postgraduate continuing education in the field of aerospace medicine. This is accomplished in three ways. The Aerospace Medicine Association's major effort in continuing education is the sponsorship of the Annual Scientific Meeting held in May of each year at various locations throughout the United States. This intense 4-day program provides scientific sessions, seminars, workshops, and tutorials adequate to meet the needs of all pertinent disciplines: aerospace medicine, bioscience, and the engineering specialties. A second effort of the Association in meeting continuing educational requirements is the publication of its journal, *Aviation, Space, and Environmental Medicine.* The journal contains scientific articles and clinical case reports designed to meet the needs of all specialists in the field. Finally, the Aerospace Medicine Association periodically sponsors regional seminars that address specific topics of interest to the practitioner in aerospace medicine. The seminars provide a forum to present the most current scientific data available in areas of intense interest to the practitioner of aerospace medicine.

PROFESSIONAL OPPORTUNITIES IN AEROSPACE MEDICINE

Historically, the largest employer of physicians trained in aerospace medicine has been the Department of Defense. Within the three branches of the service, approximately 800 flight surgeons are practicing aerospace medicine in a variety of capacities. Many of the greatest professional challenges in the field have been associated with military aviation. With few exceptions, the military aerospace medical specialists and colleagues from other scientific and engineering disciplines defined physiologic hazards and sought the aeromedical solutions. This has been true in the past, is true today, and is expected to remain true in the future.

Unlike their peers in civilian life, the military flight surgeon most often is a crew member flying in the aeronautic system his or her unit supports. This fact ensures that he/she becomes acquainted with the stressors of operational flying. For the foreseeable future, increased responsibility, new challenges, and an expanding role awaits the military flight surgeon.

Positions in both operational space mission support and research are available to the practitioner of aerospace medicine within NASA. The bioscience and aerospace research programs are broad-based and include aeronautical systems, as well as manned space activity. NASA aerospace medical physicians fulfill the classic flight surgeon role for the astronaut corps. This role includes the day-to-day medical support of the astronaut, as well as the more crucial support for actual space flight missions.

The FAA is the other major civil service employer of practitioners of aerospace medicine. Aeromedical personnel are assigned at all levels of the administration's organization and conduct clinical, administrative, and research activities.

A variety of industrial opportunities are available to the aerospace medical practitioner. Major airframe corporations in the United States employ aeromedically trained specialists not only in a clinical corporate role but also in a research and development role. These physicians serve as principal consultants on the development of new life-support systems, human factor solutions to man-machine interaction, and bioscience requirements for new aeronautic systems. The airline industry employs aerospace medical specialists both full-time and as corporation consultants. Several of the major airlines have their own corporate aeromedical departments to support the acute and prospective health care needs of the cockpit and cabin crews. Other companies employ established clinics or private practitioners to provide aeromedical services on a fee-for-service or contractual basis.

Throughout the United States, physicians are engaged in the private practice of aerospace medicine. These clinicians meet the needs and requirements of tens of thousands of private pilots who require periodic health assessments to maintain their aeronautic rating or who require specialty care for a medical condition that could compromise their continued flying.

Since its formation, over 1000 physicians have been certified by the American Board of Preventive Medicine in the specialty field of aerospace medicine. Many of these physicians continue to be actively engaged in various aspects of the field. The Board has certified approximately 7,000 physicians in all fields of preventative medicine. In addition to those physicians engaged in aerospace medicine, there have been 3200 in public health, 700 in general preventive medicine, and 2200 in occupational medicine. Few specialties in medicine provide as many varied opportunities for intellectual growth and professional accomplishment and satisfaction as does aerospace medicine.

Within the United States, all are touched by the aerospace industry. The impact of aviation and space on the social fabric of the nation, on its economy, and even its political structure is scarcely appreciated; however, the impact is predictable when viewed in the context of the past. Much that has been accomplished would have been impossible without the contributions of specialists in aerospace medicine. Challenges remain as new aeronautic systems enter commercial and military service and as sustained manned space operations increase. Aerospace medicine will be expected to meet these challenges.

REFERENCES

1. Anderson HG. The medical and surgical aspects of aviation. London: Oxford University Press, 1919.
2. Engle E, and Lott A.S. Man in flight. Annapolis, Maryland: Leeward Publications, 1979.
3. Peyton G. Fifty years of aerospace medicine. AFSC Historical Publications. Series No. 67–180, Washington, D.C.: Government Printing Office, 1967.
4. Strughold H. Atmospheric space equivalence. J Aviat Med, 1952;25:420, 1952.
5. Benford RJ. Doctors in the sky. Springfield, Illinois: Charles C Thomas, 1955.

Chapter 3

The Future Perspective

George C. Mohr

It is unwise to treat of any medical subject as if it were complete.

Peter Mere Latham

The remarkable upswing in scientific inquiry during the nineteenth and twentieth centuries provided mankind with basic new insights into the natural laws governing the physical environment. Armed with this new knowledge, modern society has systematically developed an interlacing set of technologies enriching the quality of life and providing additional scientific tools to gain even more new knowledge. Consistent with this trend, the exciting advances in aviation occurring since the first powered, piloted flight in 1903 have catapulted modern aviation into the aerospace age. The initial exploration phase of aviation rapidly gave rise in less than half a century to the extensive commercial use of this new capability. Even while the boundaries of aviation technology were continuing to expand unabated, the first orbital space flight with a human on board in 1961 triggered anew the cycle of exploration, expansion, and full utilization, leading once again to new discovery.

Scientific advances provide the starting point for the development of new technology. Scientific investigation is basically a pioneering search for new knowledge. Technology development, on the other hand, focuses on the practical application of new knowledge to provide desired goods or services to the consumer. Transforming scientific knowledge to technology requires the combined contributions of many seemingly distinct disciplines drawn from the fields of science, engineering, and management. During the nineteenth century, the genesis of new technol-

ogy was a slow evolutionary process; however, in the twentieth century, the increasing demand for new goods and services steadily narrowed the interval between a scientific breakthrough and the availability of new technology. This progressive time compression of the technology development cycle is dramatically changing the professional demands placed on the modern technical specialist.

The exponential rise in computing power is one of the most important and pervasive factors likely to shape the technological future of aviation during the next decade. Today's supercomputers are rapidly approaching terra-FLOP capabilities (1,000,000,000,000 floating point operations per second). The continuing cost reductions are making these powerful computing engines available to both industry and academic institutions. Current parallel processing technology is approaching the ultimate speed limits determined by material properties and physical dimensions. The next plateau may well result from new computing architectures radically departing from the von Neumann machines representative of the present generation of computers. Artificial neural network-based software employing photonic computer hardware (photon-based encoding, data transfer and processing) may add true intelligence to the enormous processing speed of today's massively parallel computer designs.

This massive computing power is now enabling a new set of computational science disciplines, supporting empirical investigation with up-front theoretical analysis. Computational chemistry provides a theoretical basis for design of new materials. Examples include high energy density propellants for advanced aerospace propulsion and molecularly tailored composites for the lightweight, high temperature materials needed for next generation aerospace vehicle designs. Computational fluid dynamics is now creating a "numerical wind tunnel" technology able to estimate the three dimensional distribution of pressures, flow velocities and drag forces for a conceptual hypersonic vehicle. Computational physics is revolutionizing our understanding of the energy sources that power global weather systems leading to ever more accurate and timely weather prediction. The newest entry into computational science is computational biology, providing new insights into sensory, cognitive and motor functions. The resulting mathematical models of human information processing, decision-making, and system control performance will enable design of optimal operator-machine interfaces. Current scientific investigation is uncovering the basic cellular processes underlying learning abilities and cognitive performance, unifying the neurochemical and neuroanatomic bodies of knowledge with neurophysiologic models of brain function. This new understanding of biologic mechanisms will have wide-sweeping implications for detection and prevention of disease, selection and training of individuals for specific duties and the design of advanced operator-machine interfaces.

The complexities and range of applications characteristic of today's aerospace technology transcend even the wildest imaginings of the early aviation pioneers. Today's expert can no longer afford the luxury of compartmentalized thinking strictly bounded by classic disciplinary fences. As aerospace technology opens the way to the unconstrained use of both air and space, tomorrow's aerospace physician, in cooperation with scientist and engineering colleagues, will be challenged to contribute collectively to each exciting advance from new concept to new capability as a professional member of the aerospace team. Throughout the rest of this chapter, the nature of some of those advances that may come to be will be explored.

COMMERCIAL AVIATION

Aviation Contributions to the Transportation Industry

Modern transport aircraft provide an increasingly important means of transportation that is not only fast and reliable but also more flexible than most other forms of transportation. It is, therefore, not surprising that the volume of goods and passengers transported by air more than doubled during the decade of the 1980s. Table 3.1 depicts the growth in international and domestic revenue passenger traffic between 1978 and 1988 extrapolated to the year 2000 (1).

In spite of the rapid rise in commercial air traffic, the airspace is still able to support continued growth of the air transport industry though changes are expected to be more evolutionary than in past decades. Increasing deregulation of the industry internationally may result in increasing numbers of scheduled airlines. During the 10 year period from 1978 to 1988, scheduled airlines increased from 236 to 348. The world fleet increased from 6130 to 7300 aircraft. It is anticipated airlines will add 600 to 700 aircraft

Table 3.1.
World International and Domestic Revenue Air Traffic

Year	Passenger-km $\times$ 10^{10}
1978 (Actual)	
Domestic	55.2
International	38.5
Total	93.7
1988 (Actual)	
Domestic	94.0
International	75.6
Total	169.6
2000 (Forecast)	
Domestic	1710.0
International	1740.0
Total	3450.0

a year to the fleet through the year 2000 (1). The continuing globalization of commercial and military industries will create intense competition for existing markets in North America and Europe as well as for new markets in Asia, South America and Africa. To compete successfully, the airline industry will need to offer frequent, reliable and convenient service to all the major cities of the world. For the United States airlines, the airport "hub system" is the weak link with increasingly congested local area airspace and airport congestion. Potential solutions include construction of new airports, expansion of existing facilities and modernization of the air traffic control system (2).

Part of the increase in air traffic congestion will be due to the continued growth in business jet operations, particularly as overseas markets expand. Demand for faster, longer range aircraft is clearly a trend. These aircraft will increasingly compete for the air corridors with the scheduled airlines as well as add to the strain on airport traffic control and ground services. In recent years, airline operators have turned to aircraft with increased load-carrying capacity to remain competitive in the marketplace. This trend is expected to continue, especially as airlines replace the aging airframes in their fleet. The difficulties of boarding or deplaning hundreds of passengers per aircraft will require major changes in airport design to accommodate the high-volume movement of passengers and baggage.

In the United States, the Federal Aviation Agency is responsible for implementing the National Airspace System Plan: a long range endeavor to modernize and upgrade the facilities, equipment, technical work force, policies and procedures for managing air travel within the United States physical airspace with safety and efficiency (3). There are currently over 235,000 active aircraft using the US national airspace relying on over 14,000 air traffic controllers handling more than 180,000 aircraft operations daily. Technological advances in the areas of communications, radar, sensor systems and computer operations are transforming the all-

weather capability of both commercial and general use aircraft alike. This will require the Air Traffic Control System to adopt new technologies to keep pace with the increasing workload. The current National Airspace System Plan is focussing on nine functional areas.

1. Advanced air-ground voice and data communication equipment and frequency management to assure 0.99999 availability.
2. Enhanced interfacility data communication with automatic, high speed message and data packet switching among air route traffic control centers, airport traffic control towers, radar sites and ground-to-air radio sites.
3. Advanced navigation and landing systems including en route navigation, precision landing and visual landing aids.
4. Advanced automated air traffic control system providing air traffic controllers with sophisticated planning and four dimensional traffic monitoring capabilities to detect flight plan conflicts, assign optimal flight altitudes and trajectories and reduce air traffic control delays.
5. Advanced traffic management system to provide air traffic management at the national level, preventing resource overload at hub airports, along popular air corridors or in specific airspace sectors.
6. Advanced flight planning system to provide automation aids for planning the optimal route, cruising altitude, departure time, and destination arrival time, considering weather, flight equipment, aircraft performance and expected traffic density.
7. Surveillance system to provide continuous en route surveillance, air terminal surveillance and airport surface surveillance.
8. Multi-agency advanced weather management system to provide fast, accurate, comprehensive weather information, relying on such state-of-the art radar systems as the Next Generation Weather Radar (NEXRAD) and the Terminal Doppler Weather Radar (TDWR).

9. Maintenance automation system to provide for monitoring and selectively maintaining remote, autonomous subsystems in the air traffic control data acquisition network.

These significant upgrades as they occur will affect virtually all aspects of the aerospace industry, including aircraft development, flight operations and airport design. The human will increasingly assume the role of a semiautonomous executive director, decision-maker, and emergency backup for a host of computer-managed systems in the aircraft and on the ground. This trend has raised basic questions about how best to integrate the human operator with high-technology automated systems to achieve optimal operator-machine system performance and reliability. Finding satisfactory biomedical solutions for these questions promises to be an important challenge for the aeromedical specialists who will support the development and operation of the next generation of air transports.

Technology Projections

The success of the airplane as a transportation vehicle has been due in large part to its speed and ability to interconnect virtually all urban centers worldwide. An equally important consideration is cost-effectiveness. The customer of a transportation system will always be tempted to trade off transportation time and convenience in favor of cost when the economics of the choice are grossly imbalanced. It follows, therefore, that aviation technology must continue to press for reduced cost per ton-mile transported to compete successfully with other transportation options such as truck, train, or ship. Shortly after the invention of powered flight, a French engineer, Louis Brequet, enunciated a principle relating the cruising range of an airplane to its cruise efficiency and fuel fraction. This principle expressed in mathematical form is called the Brequet Range Equation:

$$R = \left[M \times \frac{L}{D} \times I_{sp} \right] \times \left[Ln\left(1 + \frac{WF}{WA} \right) \right]$$

R is the Brequet range factor, usually expressed in nautical miles. The first term defines the cruise efficiency, equal to the product of the aircraft Mach number (M), the lift-to-drag ratio (L/D), and engine specific impulse (I_{sp}) during cruise flight. The second term is equal to the logarithm (Ln) of the quantity 1 plus the ratio of fuel weight (WF) to the combined structural and payload weight of the aircraft (WA). It is clear from examining this equation that flight efficiency increases proportionally with overall improvements in engine design, aerodynamic performance, and cruise speed. Unfortunately, these three factors are not independent across the total speed range encompassing subsonic and supersonic flight regimes. With current technology, the reduced lift-to-drag ratio and engine specific impulse at higher Mach numbers offset theoretical gains in cruise efficiency attributable to supersonic flight. Figure 3.1 illustrates that dramatic increases in cruising range and flight efficiency are not to be expected until flight speed begins to approach hypersonic velocities above Mach 4 (4).

Realistically, many other economic and engineering factors in addition to cruise efficiency influence the cost-effectiveness of an air transport system. The initial capital investment, operating costs, and the revenue-producing load factor also must be considered. Nevertheless, a major challenge for the aircraft designer remains to increase cruise efficiency, and with this goal in mind, aviation technologists will surely continue to push toward hypersonic flight capability.

The United States undertook an ambitious national program in 1986 to develop the materials, aerostructure, propulsion and control technology for a hypersonic crew-operated aerospace vehicle. This National AeroSpace Plane (NASP) program included flight testing of radically new propulsion and materials technologies as well as new designs for power and thermal management and hypersonic flight control. The ultimate objective was to demonstrate the feasibility of an advanced aircraft able to take off and land from

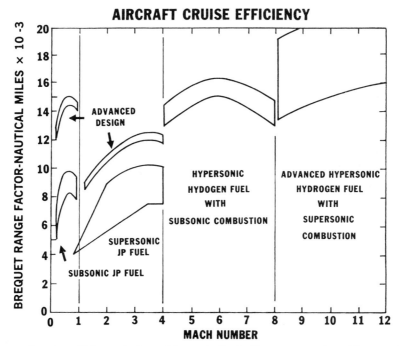

Figure 3.1. Aircraft cruise efficiency. (Adapted from Bisplinghoff RL. Supersonic and hypersonic flight. In: Fourth International Symposium on Bioastronautics and Exploration of Space. Roadman CH Strughold H Mitchell RB, eds. Washington, D.C.: Government Printing Office, 1968;7: 102.)

a conventional runway, cruise at hypersonic velocities and, if desired, go into orbit. A successful outcome of this initiative would open the door for commercial and military exploitation of hypersonic flight operations. Aerospace vehicles of this class capable of cruising at speeds in excess of Mach 10 would theoretically allow access to any point on the earth within 2 hours from any international airport with proper ground services.

Some of the key technology areas that are critically important for achieving practical hypersonic air transportation are identified in Figure 3.2. Of particular importance is the development of advanced materials that exhibit high strength-to-weight ratios, are relatively tolerant to high-temperature conditions, and have a low susceptibility to fatigue failure. Considering future structural design, advanced composites will permit a steady reduction in structural weight, thereby increasing the useful payload. High-temperature

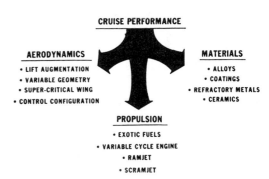

Figure 3.2. Directions of technologic development.

materials, including eutectic alloys, metal matrix composites, and ceramics, will support the development of both heat-resistant airframe components and high-temperature exotic engines able to sustain high-Mach-number flight. Advances in computer-managed avionic systems will soon permit the exploitation of radically new designs for improving aerodynamic and propulsion efficiency. The introduction of advanced avionics integration and systems automation technologies will allow the exploitation of variable-geometry wing design and advanced stability control to optimize L/D (lift-to-drag ratio) over a wide range of airspeeds and altitudes. Rapid advances in computational fluid dynamic modeling will permit accurate prediction of three dimensional pressure and flow distributions for hypersonic vehicles and propulsion systems, considering compressible, real gas behavior. Similarly, the prodigious increase in computational power will support integrated, computer-based propulsion and flight control of the adaptive power and flight management systems required by future high-Mach transports. Many of the pacing technologies are already being realized in the laboratories of various governments and industries. The commercial aviation industry is being provided with an ever-expanding set of technology options for improving the performance of tomorrow's air transport system.

Aeromedical Considerations for Hypersonic Flight

The technology required to develop a practical hypersonic air transportation system will probably become available sometime after the beginning of the twenty-first century. It is important, therefore, to consider how the hypersonic flight environment might affect passenger safety and well-being. Several engineering considerations related to structural and propulsion limitations dictate the airspeed and altitude corridors available to air transports specifically designed for subsonic, supersonic, or hypersonic operations. Figure 3.3 depicts the major design constraints for five classes of air transports. Assuming the propulsion system is air-breathing, the upper boundary of altitude versus airspeed is primarily determined by engine performance. The lower boundary of altitude versus airspeed is driven by sonic boom restrictions for flights below

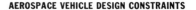

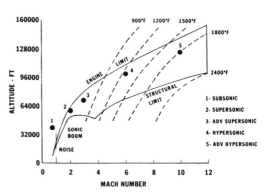

Figure 3.3. Aerospace vehicle design constraints. (Adapted from Bisplinghoff RL. Supersonic and hypersonic flight. In: Fourth International Symposium of Bioastronautics and Exploration of Space. Roadman CH Strughold H Mitchell RB, eds. Washington, D.C.: Government Printing Office, 1968;7: 103.)

15,240 m (50,000 ft) and by structural design requirements for high-Mach-number flight above the 15,240 m (50,000 ft). By extrapolating current technology trends, a nominal cruise altitude and airspeed can be identified that is best for each of the five classes of air transports shown in Figure 3.3. These projected operational environments provide a basis for examining the potential biomedical hazards peculiar to each flight regime.

High-altitude, high-Mach flight potentially exposes the passenger and crew to four types of environmental hazards beyond the risks of subsonic flight at conventional altitudes. First, cabin decompression resulting from a major leak or failure of the pressurization system could seriously incapacitate the passengers and unprotected crew members. Minor leaks are normally compensated for by the pressurization system; however, a major leak, such as would occur with the loss of a window, would cause rapid decompression of the crew and passenger compartment. Figure 3.4 specifies the principal factors determining the cabin decompression rate for a leak rate much larger than the compensatory capacity of the aircraft pressurization system (5). For these conditions, the decompression rate is roughly proportional to the cabin pressure when

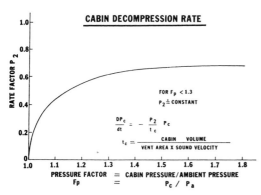

Figure 3.4. Cabin decompression rate. (Adapted from Gillies JA. A textbook of aviation physiology. Oxford: Pergamon Press, 1965.)

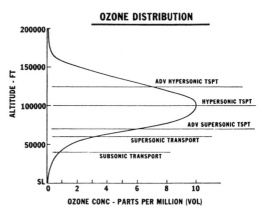

Figure 3.5. Ozone concentration as a function of altitude.

the ratio of cabin pressure to ambient pressure exceeds 1.3. For all such pressure ratios, the time to decompress to 37% (1/e) of the initial cabin pressure is roughly 1.5 times the cabin volume divided by the product of effective leak area times the velocity of sound. This means that for a situation such as a window blowout, the time to decompress to 7620 m (25,000 ft) cabin altitude is largely independent of flight altitude for aircraft operating above 10,668 m (35,000 ft). Characteristically, this decompression time to 7620 m (25,000 ft) will be on the order of 20 to 30 seconds. Within another minute, however, an aircraft flying at 30,480 m (100,000 ft) will continue to decompress to a cabin altitude exceeding the Armstrong Line—the altitude at which the ambient pressure for the unprotected human body attains the equivalent of a vacuum (19.2 km or 63,000 ft). The primary factor driving the seriousness of the decompression hazard at altitudes greater than 10,668 m (35,000 ft) is the time required to descend to 7620 m (25,000 ft) cabin altitude, where passenger supplemental oxygen systems are effective. For a hypersonic transport flying at Mach 6 at 30,480 m (100,000 ft), descent after emergency decompression would expose passengers to cabin altitudes requiring full-pressure suit protection. This clearly being impractical, the solution will require provisions for a true ''space-cabin'' design that will assure a failure-proof pressurization system.

Another hazard peculiar to high-altitude flight is the possible accumulation of toxic ozone levels in the cabin atmosphere. Ozone in the ambient atmosphere is photochemically synthesized from oxygen by the action of 100 to 200 nm ultraviolet light. Ozone is a highly reactive compound that decomposes rapidly when heated in the presence of water vapor. As a result, the ambient ozone concentration varies widely as a function of altitude, latitude, season, and specific weather conditions. Figure 3.5 shows characteristic ozone concentrations as a function of altitude. Typical cruise altitudes for transports of various design are overlaid. Figure 3.6 shows representative data for the predicted and

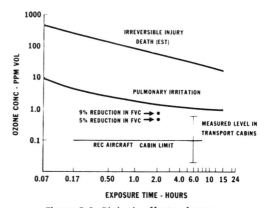

Figure 3.6. Biologic effects of ozone.

observed biologic effects of ozone. Considering the information in these two figures, it is not surprising that passenger complaints are uncommon in conventional subsonic air transport operations. If it were not for the instability of ozone, a more serious problem could be expected as flight altitudes increase. Indeed, suspected ozone-mediated respiratory complaints have been reported for intercontinental subsonic flights above 12,192 m (40,000 ft). Fortunately, however, with increasing altitude, compressive heating of engine-bleed air used for cabin pressurization effectively decomposes much of the ozone in the ambient atmosphere. Moreover, at altitudes compatible with hypersonic flight, the air is so rarefied that sealed cabin pressurization using stored gas supplies will be necessary, eliminating the ozone hazard altogether.

High thermal loading is a third hazard that may be encountered during supersonic or hypersonic fight. Aerodynamic heating can raise the temperature of wing and fuselage surfaces to many hundreds of degrees (See Figure 3.3). Even higher temperatures may occur on the leading edges of wings and tail assemblies as a result of stagnation heating. As was noted before, advances in high-temperature materials technology will be required to assure structural integrity in these hostile thermal environments. Excessive heating of the cabin air may occur not only by conductive heat transfer from the fuselage but also by compressive heating of the engine-bleed air used for cabin pressurization. In the rarefied atmosphere above 15,240 m (50,000 ft), very high pressure ratios are required to maintain the cabin altitude below 1829 m (6000 ft), considered safe and comfortable for passengers and crew. This means that the air exiting the compressor will be very hot and must be cooled before being used to ventilate the cabin. Figure 3.7 illustrates the relationship between flight altitude and compressor exit temperature. Failure of the cabin air-conditioning system for flight regimes above 18,288 m (60,000 ft) would quickly expose passengers and crew to danger-

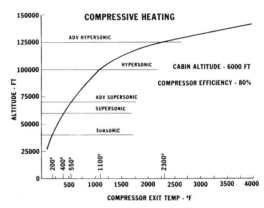

Figure 3.7. Compressive heating. (Adapted from Gillies JA. A textbook of aviation physiology. Oxford: Pergamon Press, 1965.)

ous cabin air temperatures unless the aircraft descended rapidly to lower altitudes.

Cosmic radiation is the fourth environmental hazard posing a threat to passenger and crew safety for flights above 15,240 m (50,000 ft). Energetic particles from solar and galactic origins interact with the earth's atmosphere to produce a complex flux of particulate and electromagnetic radiations that are more intense at high altitude than near the earth's surface. The basic characteristics of primary and secondary cosmic radiation are summarized in Table 3.2.

The atmosphere serves as a highly effective radiation shield, which accounts for the large variation in the radiation intensity at various flight altitudes. A marked latitude dependence is produced by the deflecting effect of the earth's magnetic field on the solar emissions. Figure 3.8 illustrates the characteristic radiation intensities to be expected as a function of altitude and earth latitude (6). A hypersonic transport flying at 30,480 m (100,000 ft) or higher will be exposed to much higher radiation fluxes than a conventional subsonic transport. The duration of time at cruise altitude, however, typically will be much shorter because of the high cruise speeds. Table 3.3 is a comparative analysis of the radiation dose to passengers and crew expected for several types of aircraft. This analysis shows, although the passengers and crew of the hypersonic

Table 3.2.
Primary and Secondary Cosmic Radiation

Type	Altitude	Composition	Variability
Primary	>90,000 m (>295,290 ft)	Protons (85%) Alpha Particles (13%) Heavy Nuclei (2%)	Solar Activity & Latitude: >10000%
Secondary	<19,500 m (<63,980 ft)	Protons Neutrons Pi-mesons Gamma Ray	Altitude: 7000% Latitude: 600% Solar Act.: 75%

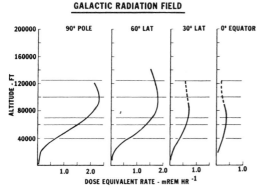

Figure 3.8. Galactic radiation field. (Adapted from Wallace RW Sandhaus CA. Cosmic radiation exposure in subsonic air transport. Aviat Space Environ Med 1978;49(4):610–623.)

transport will be exposed to relatively higher dose rates, the total cumulative dose expected actually will be less than the dose received by the passengers and crew of conventional subsonic transports. It is, therefore, reasonable to conclude that cosmic radiation poses no serious threat to the passengers or crew of a future hypersonic transport.

GENERAL AVIATION

Medical Challenges

Operating an aircraft involves six basic kinds of activity: flight path control, vigilance to avoid other aircraft or obstacles, communication, navigation, aircraft systems operation, and ancillary housekeeping tasks. In the past, the focus of aerospace medical interest was on the medical certification and support of the commercial airline pilot because of the physiologic demands of transmeridian flight, extended flight duty days and growing cognitive workload. Most general aviation aircraft were used for fair weather flying in accordance with visual flight rules. With the growing popularity of privately owned aircraft to support business travel, increasing numbers of general aviation aircraft are being equipped with transponders, altitude recording equipment, and other modern communication and navigation equipment necessary for instrument flight rule operations. New and emerging high-technology avionics systems, now radically changing the pilot-cockpit interface in air transports will, as costs come down, find increasing application in general aviation aircraft. The introduction of multipurpose displays, automated flight management systems, and sophisticated communication navigation systems will change the work load for the general aviation pilot in the same manner it is affecting the work load of the air transport pilot. The future general aviation pilot will undoubtedly fly a far more complex machine than the conventional private aircraft used in the 1970's, routinely flying in controlled airspace, operating in and out of busy urban airports, with fewer restrictions because of weather conditions and flight distance. Although routine piloting tasks will be simplified, pilots will be more dependent on increasingly complex ''black box'' systems. They will need to thoroughly understand the limitations of these systems and be prepared to take control in the event of a system failure. These

Table 3.3.
Comparison of Transport Radiation Exposure

Type of Aircraft	Cruise Time (hours)[a]	Dose Rate (mSv hr^{-1})[b]	Total Dose (mSv)	Dose Ratio
Subsonic	8.4	50	420	1.00
ADV Subsonic	8.4	50	420	1.00
Supersonic	3.8	98	370	0.88
ADV Supersonic	2.5	111	280	0.67
Hypersonic	1.3	121	160	0.38
ADV Hypersonic	0.8	109	90	0.21

[a] Cruise range equals 8000 km.
[b] Flight altitude equals 13,300 m (43,635 ft) between 30° and 60° north latitude.

changes in the character of general aviation will require a concomitant reassessment of aeromedical practices. First, medical qualification standards will need to become more selective. In particular, conditions that might significantly degrade visual functions or increase the risk of in-flight incapacitation will receive increased emphasis. Because the general aviation pilot frequently will be competing with the transport pilot for a safe share of the same airspace, the medical selection and retention standards for both groups can be expected to converge. Second, automated medical data collection, storage, retrieval, and analysis systems will have to be developed. To assure an effective medical standards program suitable to serve an enlarging and increasingly mobile population of flyers, the medical examination, review, and certification process will need to be electronically managed in near realtime. Individual medical findings will be assessed against population norms validated by operational experience data. High-risk cases will be isolated for more intensive evaluation before exceptions are granted. Finally, good human-factors engineering practice will receive greater emphasis during the design and certification of general aviation aircraft. The private aircraft of the future will be equipped to fly faster, farther, and higher, employing today's high-technology systems that will be affordable tomorrow. The designer will need to build in "pilot friendliness and reliability" to assure proficiency levels attainable by the part-time pilot

are sufficient for managing the aircraft safely under both nominal and degraded flight conditions. Even with optimal aircraft design, tomorrow's aeromedical provider will have to be increasingly aware and vigilant about the physiologic and cognitive demands of even the routine flying experience. Disturbed mental states, medications, substandard proficiency, minor illnesses, fatigue, and preoccupation will become matters of critical concern for both the flyer and the physician. In the end, the aeromedical provider serving tomorrow's general aviation community will become far more than a medical examiner. The medical practitioner will, in fact, become a critical partner in the exciting and expanding age of flight.

MILITARY AVIATION

Technology Explosion

The unrelenting demand for increased performance in our first-line combat aircraft has required military aviation research and development to remain on the leading edge of technology. Advances in aircraft performance since World War I have followed the familiar sigmoid curve characteristic of most processes sustained by the investment of economic resources over time. Figure 3.9 illustrates an interesting phenomenon associated with technology-driven systems development. When further progress is inhibited by physical constraints, a

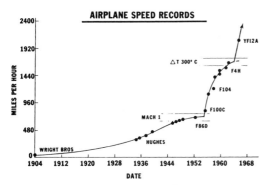

Figure 3.9. Airplane speed records.

technology breakthrough is usually found that permits further rapid advances until the next physical limitation is encountered. The impact of these often unexpected major technology advances makes it difficult to forecast the future with confidence.

Military aviation contributes to national security by assuring global reach and global power. To accomplish this goal, a variety of aircraft and ground-support systems are required, ranging from high-performance fighters to long-range bombers and heavy-lift transports. Whatever the design characteristics of a given aircraft system, certain basic technologies will always bound the achievable performance in the end product. The following is a list of the six key technology areas, with examples of representative technology initiatives that will likely have major impacts on next-generation military aircraft:

Propulsion
    Variable cycle engines
    Ram jet-scram jets
Aerodynamics
    Drag reduction
    Adaptive wing
Flight control
    Digital flight control
    Integrated fire, flight, propulsion control
Structures and materials
    Composites
    High-temperature materials
Avionics

Multispectral sensors
Very high-speed integrated circuits
Weapons
    Precision-guided standoff weapons
    Autonomous weapons

The development of efficient propulsion systems for air vehicles capable of both subsonic and supersonic flight is a major challenge to technology. The three basic components of all jet engines employing rotating elements are the compressor, combustor, and turbine. This "core engine," being a thermodynamic system, is driven by the combustor temperature. Hence, the availability of high-strength, high-temperature materials is crucial to further engine improvements. To increase full efficiency for subsonic, heavy-lift aircraft, engine designers have produced the turbofan engine. This design employs a shaft-driven fan in front of the compressor to increase the momentum of a secondary stream of air bypassing the combustor. The ratio of air mass flow through the fan to the air mass flow through the core engine is defined as the bypass ratio. This parameter profoundly affects both thrust and fuel efficiency. Unfortunately, the best bypass ratio varies widely as a function of airspeed and engine-airframe integration. Research and development efforts may one day produce a variable-cycle engine that can be continuously optimized for all flight conditions over a broad range of airspeeds, altitudes, and thrust demands. Such an engine will require advanced electronic control systems to sense engine status and regulate gas flow, fuel flow, and internal operating pressures.

The next benchmark in advanced air-breathing engine technology will undoubtedly involve the ram jet-scram jet family of propulsion systems, uniquely suitable for powering high supersonic and hypersonic combat aircraft. The ram jet-scram jet is an exceedingly simple heat engine that consists of an inlet, a combustor, and a nozzle. From a thermodynamic standpoint, these engines are extremely efficient, but, unfortunately, operate only after high supersonic airspeeds have already been attained. To exploit ram jet-scram jet propulsion in a combat aircraft, a hybrid engine is required that is designed to operate selectively as a turbojet on takeoff, landing, and acceleration to supersonic cruise, transitioning to a ram jet-scram jet mode during high-Mach-number flight.

Major advances in flight control and aerodynamic design also will be needed to keep pace with aircraft performance requirements. The efficiency of an airfoil is determined by its lift-and-drag characteristics, commonly called L/D. An airfoil optimized for high performance in subsonic regimes will normally not perform well supersonically. A number of advanced technologies are emerging that will reduce the transonic and supersonic L/D penalties while preserving superior subsonic performance. These include relaxed static stability, variable camber wing geometry, conformal weapons storage, and configuration shaping. The practical application of advanced aeromedical designs will be possible, in large part, because of advances in computer-based, digital flight control technology. Through the extensive use of sensors, data busses, and subsystem integration, the combat aircraft of the future will be under real-time computer control, constantly adjusting flight characteristics, propulsion efficiency, and weapons delivery strategies to assure the best combat performance.

To achieve further increases in aircraft speed, maneuverability, and range, advanced structures and materials technology also will be required. New polymers and composite materials promise significant performance gains. Weight savings of as much as 50% will be possible. Moreover, composite materials are readily bonded, thus reducing the requirement for conventional fasteners, which will further improve the inherent fatigue resistance of these new materials. For other applications, advances in high-temperature materials technology will continue to be the pacing factor for the development of advanced engines and high-Mach aircraft. Superalloys, metal matrix composites, ceramics, and refractory metals technologies are expected to push the de-

sign temperature boundary out to 1550° F by the year 2000. Many forecasters believe that avionics will be the dominant technology driving the design of combat aircraft in the future. Through the magic of electromagnetic and electro-optical sensors, the pilot of the future will maintain visual contact with the flight environment both close at hand and beyond unaided visual range unhindered by weather or darkness. The heart of the next-generation avionics system will be a very high-speed microcomputer. Introduction of submicron chip technology, with thousands of elements on a single 1-cm^2 chip able to perform millions of operations per second, will revolutionize aircraft and weapon systems design. Astronomic quantities of information will be gathered, processed, stored, and distributed in real-time. The number of potential applications within the grasp of future aircraft design engineers is almost unlimited. Examples of new technologies on the horizon include integrated communication, navigation, and identification systems linked to overhead satellites; integrated fire, flight, and propulsion control systems designed to deliver standoff, semiautonomous weapons on highly defended targets; automatic target detection, recognition, and tracking systems designed to operate beyond visible range; sophisticated countermeasure and counter-countermeasure systems designed for hostile electromagnetic and electro-optical environments; and advanced cockpit display systems providing three-dimensional, color, pictorial imagery from stored digital data bases and processed sensor data.

Future advances in military aviation technology will not only affect what the aircraft can do but also will affect the role of the pilot and systems operator. The next section will briefly examine some of the possible impacts on the aircrew of these new technologies as they are introduced into operational aircraft.

Aircrew Demands

The demands placed on the pilot of modern combat aircraft have become increasingly complex.

The speed of battle has increased to the point where the pilot is allowed only seconds to assess the situation and take proper action. He is expected to sustain continuous operations under adverse conditions and at night. He must penetrate high-threat environments and strike hardened targets with pinpoint accuracy. These requirements have driven the development of ''high-technology solutions'' that unfortunately have added to the number and difficulty of the pilot's tasks. This increasing complexity threatens to overwhelm the pilot's capacity to cope successfully. For example, one of the front-line United States fighter aircraft has nearly 300 switches per crew member. Similarly, a front-line British fighter has more than 50 cockpit displays (7). When the pilot's cognitive and psychomotor performance capacities are compared with the total task demands of flying a modern combat aircraft, the pilot is near or at the work load saturation point.

Because of this growing complexity of military aviation systems, some forecasters believe the human pilot and systems operator will soon be removed entirely from the cockpit and be replaced by a computer. In fact, computer control is already being applied to manage subsystem functions beyond the bandwidth capacity of the human sensorimotor system. A good example is the digital flight controller used to make the high-frequency control surface adjustments necessary to maintain dynamic stability of a statically unstable aircraft. The human operator, however, still has many attractive features that increase overall weapon systems effectiveness. The following list summarizes the important capabilities of the human operator.

Sensitivity to a Wide Variety of Stimuli
Ability to Detect Unanticipated Events
Ability to Generalize in Complex Situations
Ability to Recognize Patterns in High Noise Environments
Inductive Reasoning
Judgment-based Decision-making
Adaptive Learning

Ability to Gather Information from Secondary Events

The preferred solution to the growing operator work load problem need not be simply removing the pilot from the cockpit. The pilot provides a capability for autonomous problem-solving and executive control that will be difficult to duplicate with anything short of a computer exhibiting high-order artificial intelligence. Such a computer is not likely to be available until well into the twenty-first century. An alternative solution may be found through application of revolutionary new concepts for the design of the operator-machine interface. This operator-system interface is both a physical entity and a dynamic process supporting two-way transfer of information (8). In the most general sense, the interface is composed of four elements: (1) a physical dynamic structure that presents information to the operator and permits the operator to manipulate the system, (2) a set of operator-system interaction processes, (3) a computational subsystem architecture and (4) a set of computational processes performed by the machine. The functional features of an ideal user-friendly system interface would complement natural human abilities by employing holistic information displays, transparent decision aids and intuitively natural control operations. There are several advanced technologies currently under development that will significantly improve the functional effectiveness of next generation operator system interfaces. Some of the most important advances include: (1) scientifically robust interface design methodologies, (2) virtual world technologies and (3) advanced computational support technologies. Application of these technologies will transform the operator-system interface into an ''intelligent partner'' able to recognize operator intent, anticipate performance requirements, adapt to changing situations and maintain a cooperative relationship between the environment, the system and the human decision-maker. With current technology, the pilot has to mentally fuse information derived from a diverse set of unitary sources, reach a decision about a desired change in aircraft or weapons status, and then manipulate several controls in a particular sequence. In the future, through system integration, the pilot will receive processed information that is formatted to convey an accurate situational awareness, together with the available options. The computer-managed aircraft and weapons subsystems will be automatically configured to achieve the proper flight path, activate countermeasures, acquire and track targets, arm and launch weapons, and safely exit the aircraft from the threat area. Although this kind of technology will likely reduce pilot work load, it will also radically change how the aircrew trains, flies, and maintains combat efficiency. Several key crew technology initiatives will be needed to support the next generation of combat aircraft.

CREW TECHNOLOGY DIRECTIONS

Integrated Protection

Aircrew flying a modern combat aircraft are not only exposed to high work load demands, but also must perform effectively in a physiologically hostile environment. The speed, range, maneuverability, and altitude capability of modern aircraft require the pilot to wear a variety of separate personal equipment assemblies. The list of such items keeps increasing with each new system. For example, currently used personal equipment provide protection against head impact, flashblindness, high intensity noise, hypoxia, thermal burn, altitude decompression, cold water immersion, sustained acceleration, and chemical agent exposure. In addition, the pilot is seated and restrained in a powered escape system and surrounded by confining cockpit equipment and fuselage structure. The challenge today is to reverse the trend of layering on protection, which adds to the encumbrances on and discomfort of the crewmember. Continuing research and development are needed to reduce the bulk, weight, and complexity of personal protective equipment through functional integra-

tion, the application of new materials, and use of microelectronics. Alternative protective approaches also must be developed such as engineering the protection into the cockpit rather than placing it on the pilot. Although a shirtsleeve environment may be a long time coming, steady improvement will be essential to keep the pilot both safe and efficient.

Workload Management

Based on observed trends, the overall operator-machine performance required for air combat success will soon outstrip the unaided capabilities of the pilot to perform essential tasks. For example, air-to-ground or air-to-air weapons delivery while maneuvering defensively requires real-time solution of the equations of motion for three independent bodies. Terrain-following and terrain-masking maneuvers in night weather require the fusion of sensed data from several sources and the prediction of three-dimensional flight path trajectories optimized to avoid terrain obstacles while reducing exposure to enemy sensors. To do these tasks at all, a high degree of automation is required. In future systems, automation strategy will become an essential part of the overall design process, when a new technology is being considered. Many factors contribute to pilot work load. Important sources include information saturation, divided attention, time-line compression, high bandwidth control requirements, and small-scale task demands. Many alternative automation strategies for coping with these factors are theoretically possible; however, to choose the best strategy, pilot work load must be measured objectively. Evidence is mounting that work load measurement using a battery of subjective, behavioral, and neurophysiologic tests is practicable. It is probable that a modular, self-contained, microcomputer-controlled test system will soon be available to assess the extent that alternative cockpit designs can reduce work load during combat operations.

Virtual World Technology

When the next generation of combat aircraft enters the inventory, the aircrew will require a vast amount of information derived from off-board sensors carried on space, air, sea and ground-based platforms. The continuous data stream will be fed through a network of data processing nodes yielding highly compressed information that must be critically analyzed, distributed and displayed to the pilot in the cockpit. The timely and efficient management of cockpit information is one of the critical factors affecting situational awareness and aircrew workload. The virtual world technologies hold significant promise for meeting the challenge of effective management of cockpit information. A "virtual world cockpit" is basically a cockpit the crewmember wears (9). A highly specialized helmet system worn by the crewmember incorporates miniature image sources, three dimensional virtual display optics, three dimensional audio display generators, head and eye position sensing elements and a high fidelity voice control interface. Sensor imagery and computer-generated synthetic representations of the three dimensional external world will be displayed in virtual space, stabilized with world coordinates and correlated with the pilot's visual point of regard. Computer-generated "virtual switches" will also be displayed in a convenient sector of the pilot's visual field, operable by pointing a finger or fixating with the eye and issuing a voice command. The holistic fusion of correlated information and the use of intuitive control modes will eliminate present-day cluttered cockpits, markedly reduce workload and assure optimal situational awareness, providing the combat pilot with an unparalleled advantage.

Crew-centered Cockpit Design Methodology

Future cockpits will be designed using a versatile new approach for optimizing the operator system interface. The process begins by identi-fying the functions best performed by the aircrew member contrasted with those functions best automated and assigned to the machine. The procedure involves a formally documented sequence of design and analysis tasks, including mission decomposition, operator-system function allocation, design mechanization, simulation and test and system specification development. For each task a set of standard tools are being developed. Mission decomposition tools include analysis routines for decomposing mission requirements into goal hierarchies, mission time lines and function sets using dynamic model analysis of system performance requirements. Function allocation tools will link critical functions to mission segments using dynamic models of task requirements and information flow across the operator-machine interface. Design mechanization, simulation and test tools will include computer-aided design routines, operator-system performance models and reconfigurable cockpit simulations enabled by rapid electronic prototyping for operator-in-the-loop performance assessment. Final system design specifications will be confirmed through full mission simulation and analysis to confirm the best design from a small set of design options surviving the iterative design process. Since the design process will be largely quantitative and fully documented, design errors will be detected early in the cycle and the corrective changes can be easily analyzed for their overall system performance impact.

Modeling and the Design Process

In the most general sense, a model is an analytic description of an organized system. Because a design engineer is primarily interested in organizing a collection of components to construct a system, it is not surprising that models have found wide-spread application in the design process. The principal goal of operator-machine modeling is to characterize the human in system terms. By capturing human behavior in a form suitable for mathematical manipulation, crew technology models provide an invaluable tool for performing operator-machine analyses and for specifying human factors design points.

Crew technology models are classified into three general categories: physical, physiologic and behavioral models. The models in each category are generally tailored to a common class of problems; however, when necessary, individual models can be cascaded to provide a more global description of human behavior. Physical models include inertial response models useful for the design of personnel seating and restraint systems, especially for development of ejection seats. When an inertial response model is cascaded with a biomechanical model defining bone, joint, and soft tissue properties, the result is an injury prediction model. Such models are used to specify injury limits for ejection seat and crash-impact protection system design. Physiologic response models provide a quantitative description of human tolerance to a variety of aviation stress environments. Models of this type are available to predict the physiologic effects of exposure to thermal extremes, hypoxia, altered atmospheres, vibration, air combat acceleration, aerobic exercise, and, in varying degrees, combinations of these stresses. Physiologic models are particularly useful in supporting personal protective equipment design and in prescribing operational safety limits.

A significant challenge for tomorrow's model builders will be to advance the state of the art in behavioral models predicting psychomotor and cognitive performance. A model is no better than the data base from which it is derived. The critical issue for performance modeling is how to define and measure the constituent variables. Efforts continue to develop performance models describing sensory and perceptual processes, cognitive functions, including decision-making, and motor functions, including discrete and continuous control operations. An ambitious and potentially useful area of current modeling research seeks to predict individual differences in learning ability. The model defines how individuals acquire procedural and declarative knowledge and use short and long term memory to acquire cognitive skills. This modeling product will likely provide a scientifically robust means to select and classify individuals for high technology jobs according to their natural learning abilities. Moreover, the learning abilities model will provide an insightful basis for designing advanced computer based training systems such as artificially intelligent tutoring systems.

Another perspective on how the human operator contributes to operator-machine effectiveness is obtained through work load modeling. The term ''work load'' is difficult to define and has led to considerable confusion in the scientific community. Current evidence, however, suggests that work load is the complex interaction of task demands, coping capacity, coping cost, and criterion performance threshold. This relationship shows that work load is high when the task is difficult, demanding intense effort to achieve the criterion performance required for a successful outcome. Investigations to date support the hypothesis that work load associated with combat operations can be measured and modeled using a battery of subjective, behavioral, and neurophysiologic tests. This is a critical technology that will have a profound effect on future crew technology contributions to military aviation.

As we look to the twenty-first century, the thrust of operator-machine modeling will undoubtedly focus on the development of a general purpose ''software pilot-assistant'' equipped with a high-order artificial intelligence. The software pilot (embodying a mathematical description of the human operator) will be able to assume an ever-broader responsibility for accomplishing those missions that would place human health and well-being in jeopardy. The role of the human in future systems will then focus on defining goals, costs, and criteria for success, as well as disallowed options. Perhaps by that time, armed conflict itself will have become a disallowed option.

THE FUTURE OF HUMANS IN SPACE

Exploration and Preparation

Less than three decades have passed since the first person ventured into space. Humans however, have already learned to live and function in this new environment for periods of up to a year. This is not really surprising because space flight in many ways is a natural extension of high-Mach-number atmospheric flight. The pacing technologies are similar and the life-support requirements for passengers and crew tend to converge as the aircraft designer seriously contemplates hypersonic flight velocities. The nature of flight operations in true space does differ, however, in several important respects from flight operations in the sensible atmosphere. The following list describes some of the unique features of the space flight environment:

Provides an infinitely large maneuvering volume
Is a sparse molecular medium
Supports a mission duration largely independent
   of propulsive energy cost
Obeys the laws of orbital motion
Involves high velocities and global operations
Provides a highly predictable vehicle trajectory
Exhibits a state of microgravity
Permits vehicle/structure size to be large

Humankind is now on the threshold of a new era of space activity that will see extensive commercial and military use of space in the coming decades.

Advances in space propulsion and power are two critically important technologies required to achieve the full potential of orbital operations with crews in space. For the immediate future, barring a breakthrough in fusion power, placing large payloads in earth orbit will depend on chemical rocketry. The two parameters that must be made large to achieve the required heavy-lift capability are the specific impulse and specific thrust of the engine. Specific impulse is directly

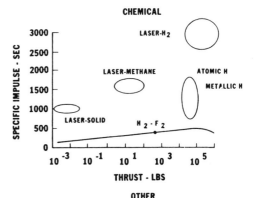

ADVANCED PROPULSION SYSTEMS

Figure 3.10. Advanced propulsion systems.

proportional to the square root of combustion chamber temperature divided by the average molecular weight of the combustion products. Specific thrust increases in a complex manner as the product of combustion chamber temperature and the ratio of combustion chamber pressure to nozzle exit pressure increases. Figure 3.10 illustrates some of the options for future space propulsion. With conventional fuel-oxidizer rocket engines, the low achievable specific impulse is a severe constraint. With more exotic designs, such as a laser-hydrogen propulsion system, the combination of very high working temperatures and very low exhaust particle Z number makes a tenfold increase in specific impulse theoretically possible. With increased propulsion performance, higher achievable payload fractions will make it economically feasible to transport into orbit sufficient material to construct large, permanent space stations.

An ability to generate large amounts of onboard power is the second critical requirement for operating a viable inhabited space station. Space vehicles in current use rely primarily on solar cells, fuel cells, and batteries. Batteries are best suited for supplying emergency power only. Fuel cells serve well as a source of power for life-support systems, communication equipment, and station-keeping services. Unfortunately, the operating life-time of fuel cells will likely remain limited to a few months between major servicing and recharge.

For highly reliable, long-duration power generation, photovoltaic solar cells are extremely attractive. To produce significant power, however, a large array is required. For example, a proposed design for a practical satellite solar power station with a 500-MW capacity requires two 10.4-mile^2 solar collector panels to capture the requisite amount of solar energy. Another approach for generating large quantities of power for long periods of time is to use nuclear reactors. In each case, however, many tons of material must be transported into space to build the power generation station, further underscoring the need for an efficient heavy-lift, earth-to-orbit transportation system.

Colonization and Space Enterprise

Space crew operations to date have been principally concerned with scientific investigation and lunar exploration. Autonomous satellite operations, on the other hand, have been far more extensive and are already providing profitable and essential services to the civil and military sectors. An autonomous satellite is adequate to serve as a weather observatory, navigational or communications relay station, intelligence sensor platform, or even as an automated scientific laboratory. Even so, such satellite systems are not well suited to carry out large-scale space operations such as earth power generation, materials processing, manufacturing, space defense, satellite repair, or complex research and development activities. For these missions, humans will need to live and work in space for extended periods.

The industrialization of space has the potential to provide vast benefits to society. To move toward achieving this goal, a permanent orbiting research and development test center will be needed such as the planned Space Station Freedom. Such a space complex initially will make

possible definitive studies of human pathophysiologic responses to the space environment. Based on these studies, protective countermeasures can be identified to deal effectively with problems such as space asthenia, space sickness, and radiation hazards. Ultimately, space crews will explore the nearby planets with a mission to Mars in current planning. While the benefits to human society are being debated, there can be little doubt the final return on the investment will far exceed any forecast made before the goal is achieved.

Once human physiologic and performance capabilities are fully understood, full-time space test center personnel can devote their efforts to developing the special materials processing, manufacturing, and construction techniques needed to build a profitable space industry. The scientific benefits to be derived from a large space test center occupied by test personnel will unquestionably be significant. Unique research opportunities will accrue in such areas as space physics, astronomic sciences, and earth sciences. The evolution of industry in space will become a major stimulus for developing space-adapted robots with high-order artificial intelligence. It is entirely reasonable to expect that intelligent robots will be used to perform most of the production, maintenance, and repair tasks needed to keep a space factory operating. Examples of space processing and manufacturing activities suitable for robot-managed operations include the production of ultrapure metals, flaw-free crystals, controlled-property alloys, microchips, biologic materials, and metal foam materials. The human operator will be needed, however, to supervise robot reprogramming (education), specialized robot repair and maintenance, and, of course, to intervene when malfunctions occur requiring unprogrammed corrective action.

Once a significant level of space industry is established, the process of space colonization can proceed in earnest. Space mining operations to exploit mineral resources on the moon and from the asteroid belt will become practical. With the availability of both unlimited energy and virtually unlimited space material resources, the space colony could theoretically become largely self-sustaining, without needing to draw on terrestrial resources. In fact, the opposite would be more probable, with the space colony supplying power and manufactured products to the earth community. In this connection, it is not beyond reason to expect the benefits of space industry to affect positively, virtually all of the basic needs of modern society. The following is a list of the areas where space industry can enrich the quality of life:

Energy—solar power
Food production—earth resources
Education—telecommunication
Water supply—earth resources
Natural catastrophe control
    Weather prediction
    Earthquake prediction
Arms control—intelligence gathering
Pollution control—earth resources
Conservation—earth resources
Health—space processing

This chapter contains many speculations on the future of humans in aerospace. How much of this speculation will become reality will only be discovered with the passage of time. The practitioner of the art and science of aerospace medicine, however, should never forget the words of Dr. Latham: "It is unwise to treat of any medical subject as if it were complete."

REFERENCES

1. Ott J. New carrier-government relationships to spur basic changes in world airlines. Aviat Week Space Technol 1990;132(12):108–115.
2. Ott J. Plans to fund new airports stir battle in congress. Aviat Week Space Technol 1990;132(7):132–134.
3. Pozesky MT Mann MK The US air traffic control system architecture. Proc of the IEEE. 1989;77(11):1605–1617.
4. Bisplinghoff RL. Supersonic and hypersonic flight. In: Fourth International Symposium on Bioastronautics and Exploration of Space. Roadman CH Strughold H Mitchell RB. eds. Washington, D.C.: Government Printing Office, 1968;7:95–111.
5. Gillies JA. A textbook of aviation physiology. Oxford: Pergamon Press, 1965.
6. Wallace RW Sandhaus CA. Cosmic radiation exposure in subsonic air transport. Aviat Space Environ Med 1978; 49(4):610–623.
7. Committee on Automation in Combat Aircraft, Air Force Studies Board, Assembly of Engineering NRC Automation in combat aircraft. Washington, D.C.: National Academy Press, 1982.
8. Eggleston R. Adaptive intelligent user interface research. Presented to the USAF Scientific Advisory Board, Biomedical Sciences Panel Nov 90.
9. Green RJ Self HC Ellifritt TS, eds. 50 years of human engineering, history, and cumulative biography of the Fitts Human Engineering Division. 1995;1:38–45.

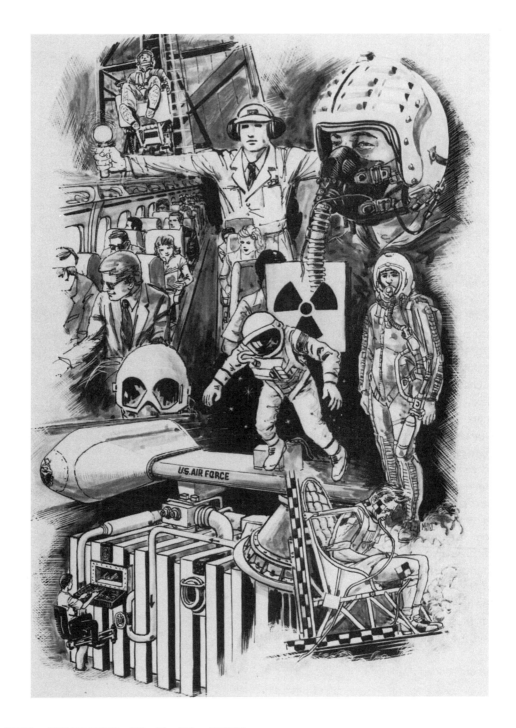

SECTION II

Physiology in the Flight Environment

The challenges to flight in the aerospace environment are many and varied. It is necessary for the aerospace physician to understand the components of that environment, the stresses they induce, and the changes that occur as a result of aerospace flight activity. Humankind was created as a terrestrial being and must be protected as we venture into the aerospace realm.

Our demand for oxygen must be met or hypoxia results. Vital physiological functions require a pressure environment or atmosphere. Our sensory systems are not adapted to rapid changes in acceleration, nor for that matter, to very gradual accelerative alterations. Mechanical forces such as noise, vibration, and impact can degrade the auditory sensory system or severely damage the musculoskeletal system. Thermal stress levels must be controlled within narrow limits, if optimal physical and mental performance is to be maintained. All of these stressors and more may impinge on the aviator or astronaut. Therefore, the operator must be protected as must the passenger and the patient.

Recommended Readings

Adler HF. Dysbarism. Aeromedical Review 1–64. Brooks AFB, TX: USAFSAM, 1964.

Bulhmann AA. Decompression—Decompression sickness. New York: Springer-Verlag, 1984.

Crampton GH. Motion and space sickness. Boca Raton: CRC Press Inc, 1989.

Dove AA, Davis JC. Diving medicine. Philadelphia, PA: W.B. Saunders Co., 1990.

Gillies JA, ed. A textbook of aviation physiology. London: Pergamon Press, Ltd, 1965.

Langham WL, ed. Radiobiological factors in manned space flight. Publication no. 1487. Washington, DC: National Academy of Sciences, 1967.

Mohler SR. G effects on the pilot during aerobatics. Office of Aviation Medicine Report AM-72-28. US Government Printing Office, Washington, DC: Federal Aviation Administration, July, 1972.

National Aeronautics and Space Administration. Biomedical results from Apollo. NASA SP-368, Washington, DC: Government Printing Office, 1975.

National Aeronautics and Space Administration. Biomedical results from Skylab. NASA SP-377, Washington, DC: Government Printing Office, 1977.

Nicogossian AE, Huntoon CL, Pool SL, eds. Space physiology and medicine. 3rd ed. Philadelphia: Lea and Febiger, 1994.

Rivolier J. High altitude deterioration. New York: S Karger Publishers, Inc., 1985.

Schneck DJ. Engineering principles of physiologic function. New York: New York Press, 1990.

Shiraki K, Yousef MK, eds. Man in stressful environment. diving, hyper and hypobaric physiology. Springfield, IL: Charles C. Thomas, 1987.

Shiraki K, Yousef MK, eds. Man in stressful environments. thermal and work physiology. Springfield, IL: Charles C. Thomas, 1987.

West JB, Lahiri SK. High altitude and man. Bethesda, MD: American Physiological Society, 1984.

Chapter 4

The Atmosphere

Roy L. DeHart

The air nimbly and sweetly recommends itself unto our gentle senses.

Shakespeare

Surrounding the celestial body we call Earth is a very thin layer of air. A layer so thin that it extends the radius of this planet by only 2–1000ths (2/1000). However, it is within this envelope where weather occurs and the region that we are so dependent upon for the oxygen we breathe exists. It is also in this envelope of the atmosphere that most aeronautical activities occur.

THE ATMOSPHERE

The atmosphere is a mixture of gases and water. Its composition varies with extreme altitude but remains reasonably consistent at typical flight altitudes from sea level to 60 km (40 miles). The composition of dry air within this altitude range is provided in Table 4.1. The total mass of the atmosphere is 5.6×10^{14} tons (5.1×10^{14} metric tons).

Humidity

There are minor changes in the proportion of gases in the atmosphere if water vapor is a consideration. The amount of water vapor can vary from zero at high altitudes to 4% in tropical regions. A global average of 1% has been agreed to by atmospheric scientists. Ninety percent of this moisture is concentrated within the first 8 km of the atmosphere.

Atmospheric water vapor is referred to as humidity. The amount of water vapor that has been retained in the air is directly related to air temperature; the higher the temperature, the greater the amount of water possible. When the maximum amount of water that can be retained in the air is reached, the air becomes saturated. Saturation can be achieved by either increasing the water vapor or decreasing the temperature.

Temperature

Heat is a form of physical energy. When it is transferred to the atmosphere it increases the temperature of the atmosphere. This transfer occurs by radiation, conduction, and convection. The atmosphere is a heat transferring system affected by the thermal energy from the sun and the earth's gravitational field. As air is heated, it expands, achieving a reduction in its density, and thus it rises. This physical action of the atmosphere is, in part, driven by the effects of uneven heating causing the less dense air to rise and more dense air to sink. This resulting vertical movement of air results in wind and weather.

As one ascends in altitude, there is a steady decrease in the atmospheric temperature. This observed decrease in temperature with increasing altitude is known as the *lapse rate*. Although the rate may vary due to location or local atmospheric conditions, the average rate is 6.5°C per km or 3.5°F per 1000 ft.

The lapse rate is important in aiding the vertical mixture of the air, producing storms and rainfall. However, the lapse rate is only operative at

59

Table 4.1.
The Normal Composition of Clean, Dry Atmospheric Air Near Sea Level

Constituent	Content (%)[a]	Molecular Weight (g)[b]
Nitrogen	78.08	28.0134
Oxygen	20.95	31.9988
Argon	0.93	39.948
Carbon dioxide	0.03	44.00995
Neon	0.0018	20.183
Helium	0.0005	4.0026
Krypton	0.0001	83.80
Xenon	0.000009	131.30
Hydrogen	0.00005	2.01594
Methane	0.0002	16.04303

[a] The numbers will not add up to 100% due to rounding.
[b] Based on the carbon^{12} isotope scale, for which $C^{12} = 12.0000$.

lower altitudes, extending to 8 km at high latitudes and up to 60 km as the equator is approached.

Beyond this boundary level, the temperature becomes stable, then more gradually increases to an approximate altitude of 50 km with little vertical mixing. Temperature again begins to drop through 80 km. As 100 km is reached, the temperature again increases; however, the air density is so thin that heat exchange has little relevance. Even though the temperature can reach 1000 K, this reflects molecular activity or energy, not heat transfer, as a thermometer would register less than 100 degrees Kelvin. These temperature changes with altitude are illustrated in Figure 4.1.

Standard Atmosphere

Because there is actual atmospheric variability in which every parameter is being measured, as well as variability in the techniques being used to make the observation, numerous attempts have been made to define a standard atmosphere. Various organizations both within the United States and internationally have attempted to define for the scientific community this standard atmosphere (1–3). One such definition has been promulgated by the World Meteorological Organization (WMO):

. . .A hypothetical vertical distribution of atmospheric temperature, pressure and density which, by international agreement, is roughly representative of year-round midlatitude conditions. Typical usages are as a basis for pressure altimeter calibrations, aircraft performance calculations, aircraft and rocket design, ballistic tables and meteorological diagrams. The air is assumed to obey the perfect gas law and hydrostatic equation which, taken together, relate temperature, pressure and density with geopotential. Only one standard atmosphere should be specified at a particular time and this standard atmosphere must not be subjected to amendment except at intervals of many years.

Traditionally, units of length have been used to define air pressure based on historic use of the mercury barometer. The rise or fall of the mercury column as measured in millimeters or inches is frequently used to express atmospheric pressure. As this is an indirect way of expressing pressure, it has become more common to discuss atmospheric pressure in terms of force rather than length thus, the millibar (mb). The bar is an engineering term for pressure equal to 1 million dynes per square centimeter.

Observing the daily weather report it becomes apparent that atmospheric pressure varies continuously over a relatively narrow range. The average of these fluctuations, adopted to specific standard conditions of temperature and latitude, is defined as the standard atmosphere (ASA). At a temperature of 15°C at a latitude of 45°, the normal pressure at sea level is given as 1013.2 mb, 29.92 in Hg, or 760 mm Hg (760 torr). Examples of this relationship of pressure to differing terminology are presented in Table 4.2.

In the international aviation industry, the measure of atmospheric pressure is in inches of mercury (in Hg). The altimeter is set for the local barometric pressure to assure that the altimeter accurately reflects the pressure differential between local atmospheric pressure variation and true pressure altitude. At altitudes above 24,000 ft, where ground clearance is usually not a

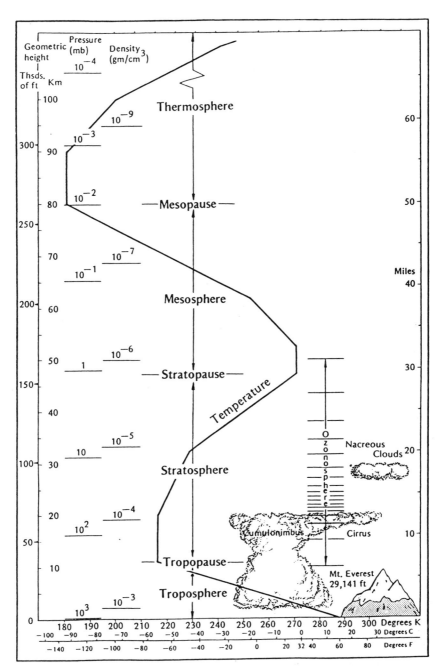

Figure 4.1. Structure of the atmosphere from sea level to 110 km (20 miles). Altitude in meters and feet, temperature at altitude in degrees K and C, pressure (mb) and density (gm/cm³). (U.S. Naval Weather Research Facility).

Table 4.2.
Examples of the Relationship of Pressure to Differing Terminology

Altitude		Pressure				Density
m	ft	mb	in Hg	mm Hg	PSIA	Kg/m^3
Sea Level		1013	29.91	760	14.7	1.225
200	655	989	29.21	742	14.4	1.196
500	1,640	955	28.20	716	13.8	1.154
1000	3,280	899	26.55	674	13.0	1.086
2000	6,560	795	23.48	596	11.5	0.961
5000	16,400	540	15.95	405	7.8	0.653
10,000	32,800	265	7.83	199	3.8	0.321
15,000	49,200	121	3.57	91	1.8	0.147
20,000	65,600	55	0.99	41	0.8	0.066

concern, but aircraft vertical separation is, all altimeters are set at 29.92 in Hg.

Standardized sea level pressure is that exerted by a 760 mm high column of Hg having a density of 13.5951 grams/cm^3 and subject to an acceleration due to gravity of 9.80665 m/sec^2 (g). An increase in altitude will result in a reduction of barometric pressure.

In addition to the effect of altitude on pressure, it should be noted that atmospheric pressure at any given altitude of interest in aviation is not constant, varying with the movement of high- and low-pressure centers, as well as with alterations in the energy absorbed by the atmosphere. This variation, although not particularly great in terms of mean monthly averages at sea level, can range from as low as 955 mb, in the case of an Icelandic low, to as high as 1055 mb, for a Siberian high. At sea level, this 100-mb variation would be equivalent to approximately 853 m (2500 ft). The height increment, due to a 1-mb change in pressure, increases with increasing altitude. This increase is the principle reason for the standard pressure in aircraft flying above certain heights and the adjustment of the altimeter to airfield pressure in the preparation for landing.

Density

The density of a gas is defined as mass per unit volume and in the Standard Atmosphere Table

is expressed in kg/m^3. At sea level, the density is 1.2250 kg/m^3. With increasing altitude, density decreases in an exponential fashion in accordance with the perfect gas law when temperature is held constant. Thus, one would calculate that at approximately 5.5 km, the density would be one-half that at sea level, and at 11 km, the density would be one-quarter that at sea level, and so on. In actual practice, density does not decline this rapidly because the temperature is not constant from ground level up as indicated by the lapse rate and density also varies with the seasons and the location. In calculations using the United States Standard Atmosphere, the density equal to one-half that at sea level is reached at an altitude of approximately 6.65 km (18,000 ft).

STRUCTURE OF THE ATMOSPHERE

The atmospheric structure can be divided into several descriptive systems. The usual system divides the atmosphere into: troposphere, stratosphere, mesosphere, and thermosphere (Figure 4.1) (4).

Troposphere

The troposphere is the region nearest the surface, which has a more or less uniform degree of temperature with altitude. The nominal rate of temperature decrease is 6.5° K/km, but inversions are common. The troposphere, the domain of weather, is in convective equilibrium with the sun-warmed surface of the earth. The tropopause, which occurs at altitudes between 8 and 16 km (higher and colder over the equator), is the domain of high winds and highest cirrus clouds.

Stratosphere

The region next above the troposphere, which has a nominally constant temperature is the stratosphere and is thicker over the poles and thinner, or even nonexistent, over the equator. Maximum atmospheric ozone is found near the stratopause. Rare nacreous clouds are also found near the stratopause. The stratopause approaches 45 km altitude in middle latitudes. Stratospheric temperatures are in the order of arctic winter temperatures.

Mesosphere

The mesosphere is the region of the first temperature maximum. The mesosphere lies above the stratosphere and below the major temperature minimum, which is found near 80 km altitude and constitutes the mesopause. This is a relatively warm region between two cold regions, and the region where most meteors disappear. The mesopause is found at altitudes of from 70 to 85 km. The mesosphere is in radiative equilibrium between ultraviolet ozone heating by the upper fringe of the ozone region and the infrared ozone and carbon dioxide cooling by radiation to space.

Thermosphere

The region of rising temperature is above the major temperature minimum around 80 km. There is no upper altitude limit. This is the domain of the auroras. Temperature rises at the base of the thermosphere are attributed to too infrequent collisions among molecules to maintain thermodynamic equilibrium. The potentially

enormous infrared radiative cooling by carbon dioxide is not actually realized owing to inadequate collisions.

Ozone

Ozone is produced in the upper atmosphere by the photodissociation of molecular oxygen followed by the recombination of atomic oxygen with the oxygen molecule. The ozone rich layer extends from 10 km to 50 km; however, there are no sharp boundaries. The region is so rarefied that if all ozone present was pressed at sea-level pressure, a layer less than one cm or a fraction of an inch thick would form.

The importance of this region is the high absorption rate for ultraviolet energy from the sun. The ozone layer, although a potential problem for cabin pressurization of high altitude aircraft such as the Concorde, forms a protective shield from ultraviolet induced skin damage and DNA disruption on the earth's surface. The aerospace industry's effect on ozone at altitude is further discussed in Chapter 35. The formation of ozone is enhanced at a wavelength of 200 nm (short ultraviolet). It is postulated that even minor declines in the ozone concentration can lead to increases in the incidence of skin cancer.

Auroras

These beautiful, high-altitude light displays occurring near the Polar Regions, result from high energy electron interaction with the very thin upper atmosphere. These phenomenal displays of light perform streamers, rays, arcs, bands, curtains or patches that appear to shimmer and dash across the sky. These are associated with large magnetic storms on the surface of the sun and their incidence and magnitude parallel the sun spot cycle.

THE GAS LAWS

Any consideration of the atmosphere in terms of its physical properties, chemical composition, and physiological suitability requires an understanding of the basic and classic gas laws.

Boyle's Law

Boyle's Law, which has its origin in experiments conducted by Robert Boyle in the 1660s, states that ''... when the temperature remains constant, the volume of a given mass of gas varies inversely as its pressure. . .'' This law applies to all gases and may be expressed as follows:

$$\frac{V_1}{V_2} = \frac{P_2}{P_1}$$

where V_1 is the initial volume; V_2 is the final volume; P_1 is the initial pressure; and P_2 is the final pressure. For example, with a two-fold pressure increase on a gas, there is a resulting decrease by one-half of the original volume.

For physiologic purposes, Boyle's Law can be considered a precise statement of facts. Under high-pressure situations, however, Boyle's Law is only an approximate statement of science as the attraction of the molecules for each other increases the effect of applied pressure and the space occupied by the molecules themselves, which decreases the effective volume.

It follows from Boyle's Law that ''... at constant temperature, the density of a given mass of gas varies directly as its pressure. . .'' This may be expressed as follows:

$$\frac{D_1}{D_2} = \frac{P_1}{P_2}$$

where D_1 is the initial density; D_2 is the final density; P_1 is the initial pressure; and P_2 is the final pressure.

Charles' Law

An additional development in the early formulation of the laws of ideal gases came from the French physicist Charles, who concluded that ''When pressure is constant, the volume of a gas is very nearly proportional to its absolute temperature.'' Charles' Law is expressed as follows:

$$\frac{V_1}{V_2} = \frac{T_1}{T_2}$$

where V_1 is the initial volume; V_2 is the final volume; T_1 is the initial absolute temperature; and T_2 is the final absolute temperature.

The absolute temperature is based on absolute zero, is expressed in Kelvin (K) and is 273°C colder than 0°C. Thus, in our atmosphere, the temperature range is relatively narrow when adjusted for the absolute temperature:

$$K° = C° - 273°$$

Likewise, when pressure is constant, it can be shown that density will vary inversely with temperature. If the volume remains constant, the pressure on the gas varies directly with the absolute temperature. To correct for temperature given in Celsius (Tc):

$$P2 = P1 + \frac{1}{273} TcP_1$$

General Gas Law

Combining Boyle's and Charles' Laws to relate volume to both temperature and pressure results in the following equation:

$$\frac{P_1V_1}{T_1} = \frac{P_2V_2}{T_2}$$

It can be readily seen that if T_1 equals T_2, this is an expression of Boyle's Law. Likewise, if P_1 equals P_2, this is an expression of Charles' Law. Because both pressure and volume increase in proportion to the increase in temperature and these increases are equal, it is possible to express this equation as follows:

$$PV = RT$$

In this general gas equation, R is derived from P_2V_2, where P_2 and T_2 are standard pressure (760 mm Hg) and temperature (273°K) and V_2 is 22.4 L, the volume that a gram molecular weight (mole volume) occupies in the gaseous state under these conditions. More commonly, this equation is written as follows:

$$PV = nRT$$

where n is the number of moles. The typical values for R are as follows:

0.08205 L—atmosphere per degree per mole
82.05 cm^3—atmosphere per degree per mole
62.36 L—mm Hg per degree per mole
8.314 $\times$ 10^7 ergs per degree per mole

Dalton's Law

Dalton's Law deals with the pressure of a mixture of gases and states that ''. . . the total pressure of a gas mixture is the sum of the individual or partial pressures of all the gases in the mixture. . .'' Thus,

$$P = P_1 + P_2 + P_3, \text{ and so forth}$$

where P is the total pressure of the gas mixture and P_1, P_2, and so on are the partial pressures of each gas in the mixture.

The partial pressure of each gas in the mixture is derived by the following equation:

$$P_1 = F_1 \times P$$

where P_1 is the partial pressure of gas 1; F_1 is the fractional concentration of gas 1 in the mixture; and P is the total pressure of the gas mixture.

Henry's Law

Henry's Law deals with the solubility of gases in liquids and states that ''. . . the quantity of gas dissolved in 1 cm^3 of a liquid is proportional to the partial pressure of the gas in contact with the liquid. . . '' The absolute amount of any gas dissolved in liquid under conditions of equilibrium (i.e., the number of gas molecules entering and leaving the liquid per unit of time is equal) is dependent on the solubility of the gas in the liquid and the temperature, as well as the partial pressure of the gas. If a chemical reaction occurs between the gas and the liquid, Henry's Law does not apply.

This relationship of pressure and dissolved gas becomes critical in the aerospace environment when considering absorbed gas in the body and rates of change of ambient pressure. The most frequent clinical example is ''aviator's bends'' (Chapter 7).

BIOSPHERIC PROPERTIES OF THE ATMOSPHERE

The unprotected human can make use of only a small portion of the atmosphere. Without clothes or some heat source for thermal protection, the thermal biosphere for man would end at an altitude of approximately 1000 m; without supplemental oxygen, the respiratory biosphere would extend (for a very small number of people and a short period of time) to the height of Mount Everest, or 8864 m. Without the pressurized aircraft cabin and even with supplemental oxygen, the biosphere would terminate at approximately 12,000 m. Thus, even though the physical aspects of the atmosphere can be described in great detail and over broad ranges, without support equipment the functional limits for man in flight are reached at much lower altitudes.

Oxygen

The percentage composition of oxygen in the earth's atmosphere is virtually constant up to an altitude of about 60 km. The partial pressure (Dalton's Law) of oxygen, however, decreases with altitude as a function of decreasing total barometric pressure. The normal ambient oxygen partial pressure (P_{O_2}) of about 160 mm Hg at sea level is reduced to 80 mm Hg at 5.5 km, 40 mm Hg at 11 km, and so forth. In the alveoli, this reduction with decreasing pressure is of greater significance because of the presence of more or less constant partial pressures of both water vapor (47 mm Hg at the normal body temperature of 37°C) and carbon dioxide (40 mm Hg under normal ventilation conditions). Thus, according to the alveolar gas equation, the alveolar oxygen partial pressure (PAO_2) is about 100 mm Hg at sea level. At 523 mm Hg (3048 m), PAO_2 is around 33 mm Hg. Based on the results of various mountaineering expeditions as well as studies of people native to high-altitude regions of the world, it would appear that the limit for acclimatization or adaptation is in the range of 4572 to 5486 m. This range of total pressure breathing ambient air can, therefore, be considered as the first functional respiratory limit in the biosphere.

Breathing 100% oxygen raises this functional limit somewhat, but at an altitude of 15,240 m, or 87 mm Hg, the combined pressure of water vapor and carbon dioxide in the lung essentially equals the total ambient barometric pressure. Physiologically, then, a point is reached where gas exchange is not possible. This point may be thought of as the dividing line between hypoxia and anoxia.

Pressure

Even if it were possible to provide respiratory support by means of pressure breathing above the 87 mm Hg limit, another functional physiologic limit would be reached at a barometric pressure of 47 mm Hg (19,200 m). At this pressure, the water vapor pressure of our body fluids equals the barometric pressure, and a phenomenon known as ebullism occurs. The manifestations of ebullism include bubble formation in the blood, mucous membranes of the mouth, and the conjunctiva of the eye, as well as a swelling of the skin due to diffuse bubble formation in the tissues. This functional limit can be circum-

vented only with full- or partial-pressure suits or by pressurized cabins.

Both of these solutions have finite limits. The suit solution has an altitude limit in the case of the partial-pressure suit and a time limit for wearing either of the garments. The pressurized cabin has a practical limit of 25 to 30 km due to the power required to compress the rarefied atmosphere at those altitudes, as well as the difficult problem of rejecting the heat generated as a result of such compression.

Space-Equivalent Regions

In 1951, H. Strughold published his classic paper asking the question, "Where does space begin?" (5) In this publication, he pointed out the amazing fact that the larger portion of the earth's atmosphere is equivalent in many respects to space. For people, in their endeavors to move from terra firma into the atmosphere and beyond, there is a transition through regions that become equivalent to space from the physiologic perspective for the human operator.

The first region addresses the need for providing oxygen for respiration as one ascends. At 4 km oxygen may be required for proper mental functioning. As the total air pressure decreases to 87 mm Hg, an altitude of 15 km (45,750 ft), oxygen must be provided under pressure.

The second region addresses the barometric pressure and body fluids. The water vapor pressure of our body fluids at the normal body temperature of 37°C is 47 mm Hg. At or below this pressure in an ambient setting, these fluids "boil." From his early studies of this phenomena in the 1930s, this altitude level of 20 km (61,000 ft) has become known as the Armstrong Line, named for H.G. Armstrong. An altitude has been reached that requires protection of the operator either by pressure suit or pressurized cabin.

Region three necessitates a sealed cabin. At approximately 25 km, the air density has become so thin that compression of this air to physiologic levels in the cabin is technically difficult.

Thus, the solution beyond this altitude is to pressurize and seal the cabin.

At level four, energetic particles introduce a radiation hazard. Above 40 km the atmosphere provides little or no protection from these high energy particles.

Region five introduces the hazard of solar radiation, although it is not anticipated that a human would be freely exposed to ultraviolet energy at these altitudes. Above 45 km there is little remaining protection from the ozone umbrella of the atmosphere.

Region six brings the blackness of space. Because of the thin atmosphere at an altitude of 100 km, light scattering is no longer occurring. Strughold defined this as the transitional zone from atmospheric optics to space optics.

Region seven introduces the "silence of space." Again with the rarefied atmosphere, there is no longer a sufficient density of molecules to promulgate sound. There is neither sound barrier nor sonic boom as we enter the dysacoustic zone above 120 km.

As we continue ascent, the region of 140 km brings us beyond the meteor safe wall which has previously been provided by the atmosphere.

Region nine begins as 150 km (96 miles) is approached. The rarefied air becomes incapable of providing adequate resistance to the vehicle and heating of the structure as well as control via air dynamic force ceases. The craft has passed the aerothermodynamic border of the atmosphere.

Approaching 200 km there is no longer any aerodynamic support to the vehicle. We have long since passed the region where aerodynamic lift and control surfaces effects were significant around the 80 km level known as the Van Karman Line. The craft is now controlled by ballistics and dynamic weightlessness becomes a permanent condition.

As ascent in altitude through the atmosphere occurs, we pass through region after region where systems necessary for space flight are introduced in order to protect the aviator/astronaut.

ACKNOWLEDGMENTS

Segments from the 1st edition's chapter, The Biosphere, authored by BE Welch, are included.

REFERENCES

1. Gleim IN. Aviation weather and weather services. Gainesville, FL: Gleim Publications Inc. 1995.
2. United States Committee on Extension to the Standard Atmosphere: United States Standard Atmosphere. Washington, D.C.: Government Printing Office, 1962.
3. United States Committee on Extension to the Standard Atmosphere: United States Standard Atmosphere Supplement. Washington, D.C.: Government Printing Office, 1966.
4. United States Standard Atmosphere, 1976. Washington, D.C.: Government Printing Office, 1976.
5. Strughold H Harber H Buettner K Harber F. Where does space begin? Functional concepts at the boundaries between atmosphere and space. J Aviation Med, 1951;22: 342–349.

Chapter 5

Respiratory Physiology

Paul J. Sheffield and

Richard D. Heimbach

"Each person is born to one possession which outvalues all his others—his last breath."

Mark Twain, 1897

Respiration is the process by which one exchanges gases with the environment. Its purpose is to trade carbon dioxide for oxygen and to help maintain body temperature and acid-base balance. The cardiopulmonary system provides the mechanism. It is designed to work most efficiently in a narrow range of environmental pressure near sea level. However, productive work has been achieved in a wider range of environments from deep undersea to the lunar surface, made possible by combining life-support systems, training, and human adaptation.

Deviation from the normal atmospheric environment can result in several physiologic problems involving respired gases: hypoxia, oxygen toxicity, carbon dioxide intoxication, hyperventilation, nitrogen narcosis, and decompression sickness.

To understand the physiologic disturbances caused by these and other conditions, one must understand the physiology of respiration under both normal and abnormal environmental conditions.

THE RESPIRATORY PROCESS

Respiration can be divided into two processes. External respiration involves the ventilation of the lungs and the transfer of gases through the pulmonary membranes (alveolar and capillary)

into the blood. Internal respiration is the process of transporting gases to and from the tissues and exchanging gases in the tissues. Gas exchange occurs in the following phases:

1. *Ventilation*—a cyclic process by which inhaled air is drawn into the alveoli and an approximately equal volume of pulmonary gas is exhaled. Some of the important conditions that interfere with the ventilation phase include exposure to reduced barometric pressure while breathing air, breathing gas mixtures with an insufficient oxygen pressure or concentration, pneumonia, atelectasis, and pneumothorax.
2. *Diffusion (lung)*—the process by which oxygen and carbon dioxide pass through the alveolar membrane and capillary walls. Examples of diffusion phase problems are emphysema, pneumonia, near-drowning, and pulmonary oxygen toxicity.
3. *Transportation*—the transfer of gases by the blood between the lungs and the tissues. Transportation problems are produced by anemia, hemorrhage, hemoglobin abnormalities, exposure to carbon monoxide, or restriction of blood flow.
4. *Diffusion (tissues)*—the process by which gases are exchanged between the blood and tissues. Examples of tissue diffusion phase

problems are pH abnormalities and carbon monoxide poisoning.

5. *Utilization*—the chemical reactions within the cells that use oxygen to produce the energy needed to sustain life. This process is inhibited by carbon monoxide, ethyl alcohol, cyanide, and hydrogen sulfide.

A number of physical and physiological conditions exist that interfere with gas exchange in the various phases of respiration and result in tissue hypoxia. These conditions are summarized in Table 5.1.

GAS EXCHANGE BETWEEN THE ATMOSPHERE AND BLOOD IN THE LUNGS

Functional Anatomy

The respiratory structure can be divided into two functional regions—the conductive airways and the gas-exchange region. The conductive airways contain the oral and nasal cavities, pharynx, larynx, trachea, and the first several branches of bronchi. The gas-exchange region contains the terminal bronchioles, respiratory bronchioles, and the alveolar ducts, which are lined with alveoli. Gas contained within the gas-exchange region is called alveolar gas. It is exchanged with blood through the alveolar-capillary membrane, which has a surface area of about 50 to 100 m^2. The gas-exchange region of the lung has a volume of about 2500 ml and contains most of the gas held in the lung.

Because no significant exchange of oxygen and carbon dioxide occurs in the conductive airway, the internal volume of the airway is called the anatomic dead space. The anatomic dead space, in milliliters, for an adult is about equal to the person's ideal weight in pounds. The anatomic dead space varies with sex and age. Measured in a reclining position, the mean anatomic dead space for young women is 104 ml; for young men, 156 ml; and for older men, 180 ml. The anatomic dead space may be reduced in

asthma as a result of bronchial narrowing. It is enlarged by bronchiectasis or emphysema.

From the nasopharynx, air passes through the pharynx, where it is humidified and warmed. The air next enters the larynx and trachea and passes into two branches known as bronchi that distribute the gas to each lung. The bronchi repeatedly subdivide into smaller bronchi until they each reach a diameter of approximately 1 mm. Cartilaginous structures of the walls disappear, and the smaller air passages are called bronchioles. The bronchioles continue to branch until they become alveolar ducts, which lead to the alveolar sacs. The septa that separate the alveoli have an excellent capillary network. Here, the air and blood meet to carry on the process of gas exchange.

In addition to the lung's role in gas exchange and metabolism, it also functions as a biologic barrier between man and the environment. The airways and lung parenchyma prevent the entry of or remove injurious particles so that the lung is sterile as the air reaches the terminal lung units. Filtration begins in the nose, where particles larger than 10 μm and smaller than 0.5 μm are removed. As the airstream changes directions sharply in the nasal pharynx, the majority of the remaining particles of about 10 μm impact on the posterior wall of the pharynx. Particles of 0.1 μm and smaller are deposited mainly as a result of Brownian motion because of their constant bombardment by gas molecules. The epithelial surface of the trachea and bronchi contains mucous-secreting goblet cells and mucous-secreting glands that distribute a layer of mucus over the surface of ciliated cells, which extend out to the terminal bronchiole, or sixteenth generation of airways. This layer of mucus is continuously moved by the action of the underlying cilia from the places of production up through the trachea, where the mucus is then swallowed or expectorated. This system, known as the mucociliary escalator, is the mechanism by which particles deposited on the airway surface down to the size of about 5.0 μm are removed.

Table 5.1.
Conditions That Interfere With Gas Exchange in the Various Phases of Respiration

Phase of Respiration	Condition	Specific Cause	Type of Hypoxia
Ventilation	Reduction in alveolar Po_2	Breathing air at reduced barometric pressure Strangulation/respiratory arrest/laryngospasm Severe asthma Breathholding Hypoventilation Breathing gas mixtures with insufficient Po_2 Malfunctioning oxygen equipment at altitude	Hypoxic hypoxia
	Reduction in gas exchange area	Pneumonia Drowning Atelectasis Emphysema (chronic lung disease) Pneumothorax Pulmonary embolism Congenital heart defects Physiologic shunting	Hypoxic hypoxia
Diffusion	Diffusion barriers	Hyaline membrane disease Pneumonia Drowning	Hypoxic hypoxia
Transportation	Reduction in oxygen-carrying capacity	Anemias Hemorrhage Hemoglobin abnormalities Drugs (sulfanilamides, nitrites) Chemicals (cyanide, carbon monoxide)	Hypemic hypoxia
	Reduction in systemic blood flow	Heart failure Shock Continuous positive pressure breathing Acceleration (G forces) Pulmonary embolism	Stagnant hypoxia
	Reduction in regional or local blood flow	Extremes of environmental temperatures Postural changes (prolonged sitting, bed rest, or weightlessness) Tourniquets (restrictive clothing, straps, and so forth) Hyperventilation Embolism by clots or gas bubbles Cerebral vascular accidents	Stagnant hypoxia
Utilization	Metabolic poisoning or dysfunction	Respiratory enzyme poisoning or degradation Carbon monoxide Cyanide Alcohol	Histotoxic hypoxia

Lungs of older individuals who have worked in dusty trades contain a residue of particles that have been deposited in the lung over several years. Autopsy findings have shown that approximately half of the particles are smaller than 0.5 μm in diameter. Of those that were larger, almost all were between 0.5 and 5.0 μm in diameter. Fibers, for the most part, were observed to be less than 50 μm long and 3 μm in diameter, although occasional fibers were as long as 200 μm. Asbestos fibers up to 300 μm long have been found in alveoli, suggesting that the aerodynamic property of asbestos fibers allows them to orient themselves parallel to the airstream and behave in a manner similar to that of particles of about 1 μm in diameter.

Table 5.2.
Composition of Respired Air at Sea Level

Respiratory Gas	Gas Partial Pressure (mm Hg)				
	O_2	CO_2	N_2	H_2O	Total
Inspired ambient air	159	0.3	595	5.7	760
Tracheal air	149	0.3	563.7	47	760
Expired air	116	32	565	47	760
Alveolar air	100	40	573	47	760
Arterial blood	95	40	573	47	755
Venous blood	40	46	573	47	706
Tissues	40	46	573	47	706
	or less	or more			or less

Composition of Respired Air

The composition of respired air varies at different sites in the respiratory process. Table 5.2 lists the gas tensions in a normal person at rest when air is breathed at sea level. Because gas molecules move by diffusion from a region of higher concentration to a region of lower concentration, the partial-pressure gradients are responsible for the entire gas exchange between the atmosphere, alveoli, blood, and tissues. No active gas-transfer mechanisms exist anywhere in the respiratory process.

At sea level, the atmospheric pressure is approximately 760 mm Hg. Excluding the rare gases of the atmosphere, air is composed principally of nitrogen, oxygen, and a small amount of carbon dioxide. The rare gases, i.e., argon and krypton, appear to have no biologic significance and are included in the values for nitrogen. As air passes through the respiratory tract, it is warmed or cooled, cleansed, and humidified by the mucous membranes. The air is saturated with water vapor by the time it reaches the trachea. At a body temperature of 37°C, water vapor exerts a pressure of 47 mm Hg. Water vapor pressure varies with the existing body temperature. In extremes of body temperature, such as fever and hypothermia, water vapor pressure is considerably altered, as shown in Table 5.3. When calculations are used for gas partial pressures, water vapor must be subtracted from the total pressure. Thus, at sea level, the total pressure of the dry

Table 5.3.
Effect of Body Temperature on Water Vapor Pressure

Body Temperature (°C)	Water Vapor Pressure (P_{H_2O} in mm Hg)
40 Fever	55.3
37 Normal	47.1
35 Hypothermia	42.2
30 Hypothermia	31.8
25 Hypothermia	23.8
20 Hypothermia	17.5

gases in the alveoli is 713 mm Hg (760 mm Hg − 47 mm Hg).

Pulmonary Ventilation

Ventilation is the exchange of gases between the environment and the blood in the lungs. It primarily involves the exchange of oxygen and carbon dioxide. The lung, however, also acts as a reservoir of blood and filters certain toxic materials from the pulmonary circulation such as bubble nuclei, blood thrombi, and biologically active agents like bradykinin and serotonin.

Under normal conditions, respiration is a subconscious process that occurs at a rate of 12 to 20 breaths/min, averaging 16 breaths/min. With some conditions in aerospace operations (i.e., positive pressure breathing, sustained G forces, gastrointestinal tract distention following rapid decompression, and immersion in water to the neck), however, the breathing rate is altered, and one must make a conscious effort to breathe.

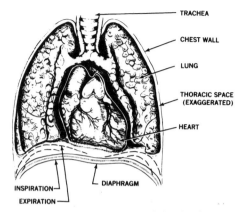

Figure 5.1. Relative positions of the diaphragm during inhalation and exhalation.

Because the lungs communicate freely with outside air and the thorax is a closed cavity, any change in thoracic volume will result in a change in lung volume. Inhalation is accomplished by contracting or lowering the diaphragm and elevating the ribs. When the diaphragm contracts, it becomes flattened and loses its dome-shaped appearance, thus increasing the top-to-bottom dimension of the thorax, as shown in Figure 5.1. Concomitantly, the external intercostal muscles contract, thereby elevating the rib cage and increasing the front-to-back dimension of the thorax. The result is an overall increase in thoracic volume and a drop in intrathoracic pressure (Boyle's Law) in the range of 4 to 9 mm Hg below atmospheric pressure. At sea level, this change would be equal to an intrathoracic pressure of 756 to 751 mm Hg during a normal inhalation. A pressure differential is thus created between the lung interior and ambient air. Because air will move from an area of higher pressure to one of lower pressure, air rushes into the lungs until the intrapulmonic pressure again equals the ambient air pressure. When the lung reaches a certain degree of expansion, specialized stretch receptors provide inhibiting impulses via the vagus nerve to inhibit central respiratory activity (Hering-Breuer reflex). The inspiratory phase of respiration is then complete, and the lung passively recoils to its resting position.

Upon completion of inhalation, the intrapul-

monic pressure is equal to the ambient pressure (760 mm Hg at sea level) and the intrathoracic pressure is about 9 mm Hg below ambient pressure (751 mm Hg at sea level).

During normal respiration, exhalation is largely passive because little muscular activity is required to assist in the process. During normal, quiet exhalation, the inflated lungs return to their original position by virtue of the elastic recoil of the tissue. Simultaneously, the diaphragm relaxes. Because of tissue recoil, the volume within the lung is decreased. Consequently, intrapulmonic pressure increases, producing a momentary pressure differential between the lung and outside air. This time, the greater pressure is within the lung (about 3 mm Hg above atmospheric pressure), and air moves from the lung to the environment.

If the expiratory muscles are needed to exhale, exhalation becomes active. This active exhalation occurs in aerospace operations when one experiences positive pressure breathing (forced, voluntary effort to exhale) or when one must use a straining maneuver during sustained G forces. Under normal conditions, however, inhalation is active and exhalation is passive.

During strenuous exercise, both rib cage and diaphragm activity are coordinated to meet the body's demand for increased lung ventilation. At rest, an individual requires 200 to 250 ml of oxygen per minute; however, this value is increased twenty-fold (5500 ml) during maximal exercise. During vigorous exercise, contracting muscles depress the ribs, force the viscera up against the diaphragm, and move the diaphragm further up into the thorax. By reducing the internal volume of the lung, this action markedly increases the intrapulmonic pressure and allows a greater volume of air to be expired. The consequent increase in the rate and depth of respiration permits greater and more frequent lung ventilation to eliminate carbon dioxide and meet the increased oxygen needs of body tissues.

During heavy exercise, the muscles require about 50 times more oxygen than they need at rest. This increase is achieved by three mechanisms: a sixfold increase in cardiac output, from 5 L/min to 30 L/min; a threefold increase in circulating blood, which is diverted from the spleen and kidneys to the skin and muscles; and a threefold increase in oxygen released from hemoglobin, due to a shift to the right in the oxyhemoglobin dissociation curve.

Lung Measurements

For both physiologic and clinical purposes, the ventilatory function of the lung has been divided into functional volume measurements. These lung volumes are defined as follows:

1. *Tidal volume*—the volume of air inspired and expired with each normal breath (about 500 ml).
2. *Inspiratory reserve volume*—the extra volume of air that can be inspired above the normal tidal volume by a conscious, forceful inspiration (about 3100 ml).
3. *Expiratory reserve volume*—the volume of air that can be expired by a forceful expiration after the end of a normal tidal expiration (about 1200 ml).
4. *Residual volume*—the volume of air in the lungs that cannot be exhaled (about 1200 ml).

Table 5.4 lists the approximate lung volumes in healthy subjects 20 to 30 years of age. Figure

Table 5.4.
Lung Volumes in Healthy Subjects 20 to 30 Years of Age

Functional Measurements	Approximate Values (ml)	
	Males	Females
Tidal volume (TV)	500	450
Inspiratory reserve volume (IRV)	3100	1950
Expiratory reserve volume (ERV)	1200	800
Residual volume (RV)	1200	1000
Inspiratory capacity (IC)	3600	2400
Functional residual capacity (FRC)	2400	1800
Vital capacity (VC)	4800	3200
Total lung capacity (TLC)	6000	4200

Modified from Comroe JH, Jr.: Physiology of Respiration. Chicago: Yearbook Medical Publishers, Inc., 1965.

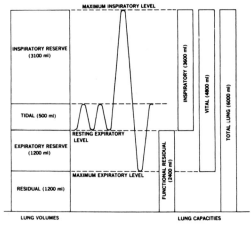

Figure 5.2. Lung measurements.

5.2 shows that the total capacity of the lungs is equal to the sum of the four volumes just defined. The capacities of the lung are important because they represent the functional combinations of these volumes and are defined as follows:

1. *Inspiratory capacity*— the tidal volume plus the inspiratory reserve volume. The amount of air that one can inspire, beginning with the end of a normal expiration and forcibly inspiring to the maximum extent (about 3600 ml).
2. *Functional residual capacity*—the residual volume plus the expiratory reserve volume. The amount of air left in the lungs at the end of a normal expiration (about 2400 ml).
3. *Vital capacity*—the sum of the expiratory reserve volume, the tidal volume, and the inspiratory reserve volume. The amount of air the lungs can hold between the limits of a maximum forceful inspiration and a maximum forceful expiration (about 4800 ml).
4. *Total lung capacity*—the sum of the four lung volumes. The total capacity of the lungs to hold air (about 6000 ml).

With the exception of functional residual capacity, total lung capacity, and residual volume, measurements of all lung volumes and capacities

Table 5.5.
Effect of Inspired Oxygen Concentration on Pulmonary Ventilation

Oxygen Concentration in Inspired Air (%)	Tidal Volume (ml)	Respiratory Rate (breaths/min)	Respiratory Minute Volume (L/min)	Alveolar Ventilation (L/min)
21	500	14	7.0	4.9
18	500	14	7.0	4.9
16	536	14	7.5	5.4
12	536	14	7.5	5.4
10	593	14	8.3	6.2
8	812	16	13.0	10.4
4.2	933	30	28.0	23.2

Modified from Comroe JH, Jr.: Physiology of Respiration. Chicago: Yearbook Medical Publishers, Inc., 1965.

can be made with a spirometer or similar recording device. The values shown above for the lung volumes and capacities are approximations because the values vary with age, sex, height, and weight of the subject. More accurate values may be calculated for individual subjects by using regression formulas that account for these variables.

The amount of air inspired per minute is known as respiratory minute volume. It is normally about 6 to 8 L/min. The maximum breathing capacity, the largest volume of gas that can be moved into and out of the lungs in 1 minute, is about 125 to 170 L/min.

Peak inspiratory flow is an important consideration in the design of oxygen masks and regulators. As a rule of thumb, peak inspiratory flow can be determined by multiplying respiratory minute volume by a factor of 3. Thus, a respiratory minute volume in the working individual of 10 L/min would produce a peak inspiratory flow of 30 L/min.

Response to Lack of Oxygen

Table 5.5 indicates the respiratory response to various oxygen concentrations. There is little change in respiration when hypoxic oxygen concentrations of 12 to 21% are breathed for 8 to 10 minutes. But there is a powerful respiratory response when oxygen concentrations of 4 to 8% are breathed. At an inspired oxygen concentration of 4.2% (equivalent to breathing ambient

air at 11,700 m (38,500 ft)), the respiratory rate doubles and respiratory minute volume increases by a factor of 4.

Exposure to Altitude

Table 5.6 shows the effect of acute exposure to altitude on ventilation. The threshold for increased ventilation is first seen on ascent at about 1500 m (5,000 ft). Ventilatory changes are small until about 3700 m (12,000 ft). Tidal volume progressively increases, but there are relatively small changes in respiratory rate until an altitude is reached where hypoxic stimulation is maximal. At 6700 m (22,000 ft), the respiratory rate increases and minute volume is almost doubled. Hyperventilation reduces the partial pressure of carbon dioxide, Pco_2, causing respiratory alkalosis, and a shift of the oxyhemoglobin dissociation curve to the left, thus allowing more oxygen to bind with hemoglobin for transport to the tissues.

Alveolar Ventilation

It is estimated that at birth an infant's lungs contain about 30 million alveoli. At 8 years of age, this number increases to about 300 million. After this age, the number of alveoli do not increase, but they do continue to increase in size until the individual is mature. The diameter of the alveolus is about 0.1 to 0.4 mm, and the wall thickness is about 0.1 μm.

Table 5.6.
Effect of Acute Exposure to Altitude on Pulmonary Ventilation

Pulmonary Function		Altitude in Meters (Feet)				
	Meters:	Sea Level	3700	5500	6700	7600
	(Feet):	Sea Level	12,000	18,000	22,000	25,000
Minute volume (L/min)		8.5	9.7	11.1	15.3	—
Respiratory Rate (per minute)		12.0	14.0	12.0	15.0	—
Tidal Volume (L)		0.71	0.69	0.92	1.02	—
Alveolar P_{O_2}		103.0	54.3	37.8	32.8	30.4
Alveolar P_{CO_2}		40.0	33.8	30.4	28.4	27.0

Note: The ascent was accomplished at 1400 m/min (4,500 ft/min). The subjects remained at altitude for 30 to 60 minutes. Minute volume and respiratory rate are average values. The tidal volume was calculated.
Adapted from Rahn H, Otis AB. Alveolar air during simulated flights to high altitudes. Am J Physiol 150:202;1947.

Alveoli resemble minute, communicating bubbles of gas in the lung fluid. The pressure (P) exerted by the surface tension of a bubble in a liquid is determined by Laplace's Law, as follows:

$$P = 2T/r$$

where T is the surface tension and r is the bubble radius. As exhalation occurs and the alveolar radius decreases, the alveolus tends to collapse completely. Uncountered, this process would result in atelectasis, and respiration could not continue. To counter this problem, specialized cells lining the alveoli, type II Clara cells, secrete a lipoprotein, dipalmitoyl lecithin, which profoundly lowers the surface tension of the alveolar lining fluid and is known as pulmonary surfactant.

As the volume of an alveolus increases or decreases, so does its surface area. On exhalation there is an increase in the thickness of the surfactant film lining the alveolus. The result is a decrease in the tendency to collapse as the alveolar "bubble" becomes smaller. On inhalation, the surface area of the alveolus increases, which decreases the thickness of the surfactant film on the membrane. This process increases the surface tension and prevents overdistension of the alveolus. Thus, pulmonary surfactant reduces the tendency of small alveoli to empty into large ones

during exhalation and prevents overdistension of the alveoli during inhalation. Its presence decreases the stiffness of the lung, reducing the effort required to ventilate. It also reduces the force that tends to draw fluid from the blood into the lung.

Ventilation of the alveoli occurs primarily by diffusion. Diffusion is rapid and the distance involved so small that complete mixing of gas within an alveolus occurs in less than 1 second. Dead space volume and tidal volume are important factors in determining the amount of alveolar ventilation. At the end of normal expiration, the conducting airway is filled with "alveolar gas" that has a P_{O_2} of 100 mm Hg rather than the 149 mm Hg in fresh air. Using Figure 5.3 for illustrative purposes, one can assume that the anatomic dead space is 150 ml and the volume of the next inspiration (tidal volume) is 500 ml. The alveoli receive 500 ml of gas, but its composition differs from that of fresh air entering the nose. The alveoli first receive the residual 150 ml from the conducting airway, which does not raise alveolar P_{O_2} or lower alveolar P_{CO_2} because it is "alveolar gas." The alveoli then receive 350 ml of fresh air. The remaining 150 ml of fresh air remains in the conducting airway at end-inspiration. Thus, the gas that is expired consists of a mixture of inspired air from the dead space and alveolar air and has a composition that is intermediate between the two.

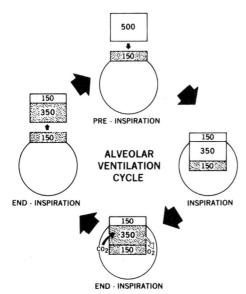

Figure 5.3. Anatomic dead space and alveolar ventilation.

Alveolar-Arterial Gas Exchange

The overall passage of oxygen from the alveolus to the blood involves two distinct steps in a continuous process: physical diffusion through the membrane followed by chemical combination of oxygen with hemoglobin. The amount of oxygen transferred across the alveolar-capillary membrane depends primarily on the oxygen pressure differential. Thus, the efficiency of diffusion is reduced in the presence of a low alveolar oxygen pressure. Furthermore, when the alveolar capillary membrane becomes thickened, as in pulmonary disease, gas exchange is impaired even though alveolar ventilation is normal.

The surface area of the alveolar-capillary membrane is 50 to 100 m^2, 40 times the surface area of the body. Its thickness is 0.1 to 0.5 μm. Resistance to gas diffusion between the lung and the blood is minimized by the large lung surface area and the thinness of the membrane. The network of capillaries around the alveoli is so dense and the capillary segments so short and narrow that there is an almost continuous sheet of blood over the alveolar wall. In the resting adult male, about 140 ml of pulmonary capillary blood is surrounded by approximately 2000 ml of alveolar air. Resistance to flow through the pulmonary bed is so low that the heart can drive 5 to 10 L of blood through the lungs with a driving pressure of less than 15 mm Hg. Pulmonary blood flow ranges from 4 L/min in a resting man to 30 to 40 L/min during heavy exercise.

Figure 5.4 illustrates four pathways used to exchange oxygen and carbon dioxide in the lung. As shown in pathway A, oxygen diffuses through the plasma and into the red blood cell because of a pressure differential of 60 mm Hg. There, hemoglobin rapidly combines with oxygen to form an oxygenated compound called oxyhemoglobin (HbO_2). In the process, an ion of hydrogen (H+) is released. The greater the number of hydrogen ions in a solution, the more acidic the solution becomes. Rapid shifts in acidity are prevented by bicarbonate ions (HCO_3^-). HCO_3^- rapidly diffuses from the blood plasma into the red blood cell and combines with the H+ to form carbonic acid (H_2CO_3). This very weak acid is immediately acted on by a catalytic enzyme known as carbonic anhydrase, which breaks the H_2CO_3 molecule into molecular water and carbon dioxide. The water diffuses out into the plasma. The carbon dioxide, having a higher partial pressure than alveolar air, diffuses into the alveolus.

In pathway B, carbon dioxide is brought from the tissues in a form called carbaminohemoglobin ($HbCO_2$). Because hemoglobin has a stronger affinity for oxygen than carbon dioxide, O_2 replaces CO_2 on the hemoglobin. Like the carbon dioxide released from H_2CO_3, it also diffuses into the alveolus.

In pathway C, plasma protein buffers, which insure a constant plasma pH, tend to release hydrogen ions due to a slight increase in the alkalinity of the plasma. When this occurs, H+ immediately combines with the available HCO_3^- to form H_2CO_3. The H_2CO_3 subsequently breaks down into molecular water and carbon dioxide. This reaction is relatively slow because the catalytic enzyme, carbonic anhydrase, is not present in the plasma to speed the reaction. As in the

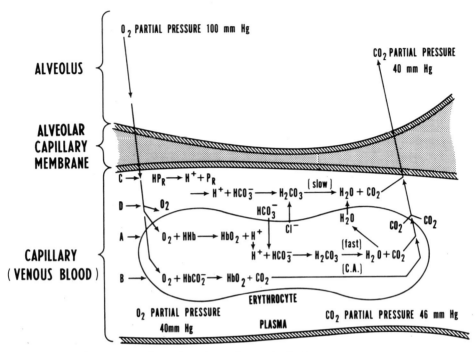

Figure 5.4. Gas exchange in the lungs.

other pathways, the carbon dioxide that is released diffuses into the alveolus because of the partial-pressure gradient. As carbon dioxide is lost, oxygen is gained.

In pathway D, oxygen enters the plasma, where it is transported in physical solution.

TRANSPORT OF GAS BY BLOOD

The red blood cell traverses the alveolus in approximately 0.75 seconds. Thus, gas transfer must occur rapidly. The transfer rate depends on both physical diffusion and the speed of chemical reactions in the blood. After diffusing through the alveolar and capillary membranes, the gas molecule must pass through plasma in the pulmonary capillary, the wall of the red blood cell, and part of the intracellular fluid of the red blood cell before entering into chemical union with hemoglobin.

Several physical factors influence the diffusion rate of a gas: differences in the partial pressure of the gas, solubility of the gas in the fluid,

temperature, and the molecular weight of the gas. Under normal conditions, except for the difference in partial pressure, all of these factors remain constant for a given gas. Thus, the partial pressure of the gas determines the direction and degree of gas exchange. Diffusion, however, is greatly enhanced by four physiologic conditions: (1) the rapid circulatory renewal of blood in the gas-permeable capillaries of the lung and metabolizing tissues, (2) the rapid chemical reactions involving respiratory gases when they enter the blood, (3) the existence of specific enzymes that accelerate oxygen uptake by metabolizing cells and also accelerate the combination of carbon dioxide and water in the blood, and (4) mechanisms to adjust circulation and alveolar ventilation to meet metabolic requirements.

Inert gas (nitrogen), oxygen, and carbon dioxide are transported by the blood by various methods. Nitrogen is transported entirely in physical solution. Only 1.5% of oxygen is transported physically dissolved in the plasma, whereas 98.5% of oxygen is chemically combined with hemoglobin. About 6% of carbon dioxide is transported in physical solution, about 22% is combined with carbamino compounds such as hemoglobin, and about 72% is carried as carbonic acid or bicarbonate ions in the blood buffer system.

Nitrogen

Nitrogen is biologically inert and acts as a diluent gas. Although not involved in any known metabolic activity, it is found in solution in all body tissues and is exchanged at a constant ratio of 1:1 unless there is a pressure change on the body.

The degree to which a gas enters into physical solution in body fluids is directly proportional to the partial pressure of the gas to which the fluid is exposed (Henry's Law). It should be noted that the partial pressure of nitrogen decreases in the alveoli during ascent to altitude (Dalton's Law). Thus, the quantity of nitrogen that dissolves in the plasma for transport throughout the body is reduced on ascent. The reverse of this process occurs during descent, when the partial pressure of nitrogen is less in the plasma than in the alveoli. Henry's Law defines only the relative quantity of gas entering solution as related to gas partial pressures and does not define the absolute amount of gas in physical solution. The absolute amount is determined by the solubility coefficient of the gas in a fluid. Solubility coefficients vary with different fluids and are temperature-dependent.

Nitrogen solubility in plasma at 37°C is 0.0088 ml of N_2/100 ml of plasma/mm Hg P_{AN_2}. It is five times more soluble in fat than in water. When pressure changes occur on the body, nitrogen can produce the adverse effects of decompression sickness.

Oxygen

The solubility of oxygen in plasma at 37°C is 0.0028 ml of O_2/100 ml of plasma/mm Hg P_{AO_2}. The solubility of oxygen in whole blood at 37°C is 0.0031 ml of O_2/100 ml of blood/mm Hg

P_{AO_2}. When air is breathed at sea level, arterial oxygen tension is approximately 95 mm Hg, and the blood transports approximately 0.3 ml of O_2/100 ml of blood. The amount of dissolved oxygen can be increased to 2 ml of O_2/100 ml of blood if 100% oxygen is breathed at sea level. Because solubility is pressure-dependent, the amount of dissolved oxygen is reduced by ascent to altitude and increased by descent below sea level. For example, if oxygen is breathed at 10 m (33 ft) of seawater, a dissolved oxygen content of 4 ml of O_2/100 ml of blood can be achieved.

The oxyhemoglobin dissociation curve forms a typical sigmoid curve (Fig. 5.5). The shape of the curve is ideally suited to meet human physiologic requirements. The oxygen tension normally present in the alveolar gas produces almost complete hemoglobin saturation. On the upper part of the curve, large changes in P_{O_2} have only a slight effect on hemoglobin saturation. This fact is of particular importance to the aviator who ascends to altitude. Conversely, the low P_{O_2} that exists in the tissues serves to enhance oxygen release from hemoglobin. From the slope of the oxyhemoglobin dissociation curve it can be seen that hemoglobin releases abundant oxygen to the tissues with only a small decrease in oxygen tension.

The ability of hemoglobin to combine with oxygen varies with both acidity and oxygen partial pressure. The normal physiologic curve shown in Figure 5.5 is for a pH of 7.40, which corresponds to a P_{CO_2} of 40 mm Hg. The carbon dioxide content of the blood exerts a significant influence on the oxyhemoglobin dissociation curve. An increase in P_{CO_2} shifts the dissociation curve to the right, whereas a decrease in P_{CO_2} shifts the curve to the left. This influence of carbon dioxide is largely a consequence of changes in pH, and similar changes can be produced by other acids. The influence of hydrogen ion concentration on the dissociation curve is known as the Bohr effect.

The influence of carbon dioxide on the oxyhemoglobin dissociation curve is of considerable

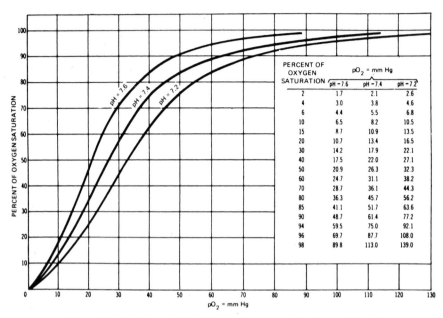

Figure 5.5. Oxyhemoglobin dissociation curves for human blood.

physiologic significance. In the lung, as carbon dioxide is released, the curve is shifted to the left so that, at a given P_{O_2}, more oxygen combines with hemoglobin. In the region of the systematic capillaries, increased tissue acidity shifts the curve to the right, potentiating oxygen offloading. Tissue P_{O_2} is less than the arterial P_{O_2}, resulting in removal first of plasma (nonhemoglobin) oxygen to the tissues by simple diffusion down the pressure gradient. The loss of plasma oxygen decreases plasma P_{O_2}, and oxygen is released from hemoglobin because the association of oxygen with hemoglobin depends on the plasma P_{O_2}. Oxygen diffuses from the hemoglobin to plasma and into the tissues until a pressure gradient no longer exists.

The red blood cell contains high levels of organic phosphate 2,3-diphosphoglyceric acid (2,3- DPG). This compound combines with reduced hemoglobin and decreases the affinity of hemoglobin for oxygen over the middle range of oxygen tensions. The more 2,3-DPG present, the more oxygen will be released at a given oxygen tension. Hypoxia increases the 2,3-DPG in cells and thus increases the oxygen offloading

from hemoglobin when the blood arrives at the tissues.

The oxyhemoglobin dissociation curve also is influenced by temperature. As temperature rises, the curve shifts to the right. The physiologic value of this effect is realized during exercise. As the temperature of the active muscles increases, the release of oxygen to the muscles increases. During cold exposure, when the temperature of the muscles decreases, the curve shifts to the left, and less oxygen is released from hemoglobin.

Carbon Dioxide

The solubility of carbon dioxide in plasma at 37°C is 0.0697 ml of CO_2/100 ml of plasma/mm Hg PA_{CO2}. Although carbon dioxide is about 20 times more soluble than oxygen, only 5 to 6% is carried as dissolved CO_2. Table 5.7 shows the distribution of carbon dioxide in arterial and mixed venous blood of individuals at rest.

Of the 493 ml of carbon dioxide in each liter of arterial blood, 27 ml (5%) is dissolved, 22 ml (5%) is in carbamino compounds, and 444 ml

Table 5.7.
Distribution of Carbon Dioxide in Arterial and Mixed Venous Blood

	ml of CO_2/L of Blood	Percent of Total
Arterial blood		
Total carbon dioxide	492.8	100
As dissolved carbon dioxide	26.9	5
As bicarbonate	443.5	90
As carbamino carbon dioxide	22.4	5
Mixed venous blood		
Total carbon dioxide	533.1	100
As dissolved carbon dioxide	29.1	5
As bicarbonate	472.6	89
As carbamino carbon dioxide	31.4	6
Arteriovenous difference		
Total carbon dioxide	40.3	100
As dissolved carbon dioxide	2.2	6
As bicarbonate	29.1	72
As carbamino carbon dioxide	9.0	22

Data from Lambertsen CJ. Respiration. *In* Medical Physiology. Vol. 2. 14th Ed. Edited by V.B. Mountcastle. St. Louis: CV Mosby Co., 1980.

(90%) is in bicarbonate. In the tissues, 40 ml of CO_2/L of blood is added: 2 ml (6%) stays in solution, 9 ml (22%) forms carbamino compounds, and 29 ml (72%) forms bicarbonate. The pH of the blood drops from 7.40 to 7.37. In the lungs, the processes are reversed, and the 40 ml of carbon dioxide is discharged into the alveoli, for subsequent exhalation into the environment.

GAS EXCHANGE BETWEEN THE BLOOD AND TISSUES

When the red blood cell arrives at the tissue capillaries, it encounters an environment that is different from the one in the lung capillaries. Carbon dioxide leaves the tissues because its partial pressure is higher in the tissues than it is in the blood. As carbon dioxide diffuses from the tissues, oxygen diffuses into the tissues. As shown in Figure 5.6, the reactions that occur at tissue level are the reverse of those in the lungs. In pathway A, the carbon dioxide diffuses through the plasma into the red blood cell, where it rapidly combines with water to produce H_2CO_3, which breaks down into bicarbonate and hydro-

gen ions. The HCO_3^- passes back into the plasma, whereas the H+ is buffered by the red blood cell proteins, particularly hemoglobin. Since reduced hemoglobin is more effective than oxyhemoglobin, oxygen is released from hemoglobin and diffuses from the red blood cell. This process favors the formation of bicarbonate and the uptake of carbon dioxide. To maintain equilibrium of ions, the red blood cell must gain a negative ion in exchange for each HCO_3^- lost. To serve this purpose, the readily available chloride ion diffuses from the plasma into the red blood cell. This process is known as the chloride shift. In pathway B, carbon dioxide displaces oxygen on the hemoglobin to form carbaminohemoglobin. In pathway C, carbon dioxide slowly combines with water in the plasma to produce H_2CO_3, which breaks down into bicarbonate and hydrogen ions. The hydrogen ion is bound by plasma proteins in the blood buffer system. The remaining carbon dioxide is transported in physical solution in pathway D.

TISSUE RESPIRATION

Cellular Metabolism

The physical and chemical processes by which energy is made available for use by the body are called metabolism. The chemical processes that produce energy are known as catabolism. They result in the conversion of either foodstuffs or body tissue into carbon dioxide and water (and sometimes ammonia). Conversely, chemical changes that synthesize materials to be stored as a part of the body are known as anabolism. The energy required for anabolic reactions (such as the formation of protein and body fat) comes only from catabolic reactions. The energy and building blocks for the synthesis of protein and fat are acquired from one of two sources: the digestion of food or the relocation of molecules and energy from some other body tissue.

The chemical energy produced from the process of catabolism is held in the energy-rich phosphate bonds of adenosine triphosphate

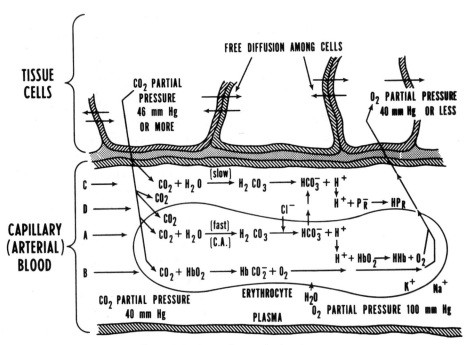

Figure 5.6. Gas exchange in the tissues.

(ATP), which exists in the cytoplasm of the cell. The body converts this chemical energy into useful body functions such as muscle contractions, glandular secretions, chemical synthesis of protein, nerve impulses, urine formation, and body heat. This energy is made available by the hydrolysis of the ATP molecule, which releases a phosphate radical and results in the formation of adenosine diphosphate (ADP). Because the supply of ATP in the cellular cytoplasm is limited, new energy-rich bonds must be continually produced by the oxidation of carbohydrates, lipids, and amino acids. These foodstuffs are degraded in a series of consecutive enzymatic reactions to eventually produce two-carbon acetyl groups of acetyl coenzyme A (CoA). Within the mitochondria of the cell, acetyl CoA is channeled into the Krebs tricarboxylic acid cycle, which is the final common pathway of oxidative catabolism. This process is illustrated in Figure 5.7. Hydrogen atoms, or their equivalent electrons from this process, are then fed into the respiratory chain, a series of electron carriers that transport the electrons to molecular oxygen. This process produces several energy-rich ATP

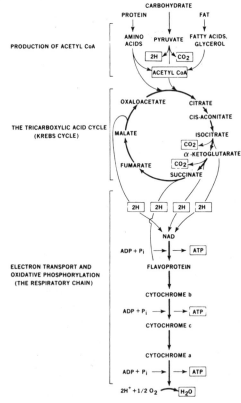

Figure 5.7. Cellular respiration.

molecules by the oxidative phosphorylation of ADP. The production of water in the final step of the chain is catalyzed by an enzyme called cytochrome oxidase. The oxidative phosphorylation process requires a minimum oxygen tension in the mitochondria in the range of about 0.5 to 3 mm Hg. A minimum tissue oxygen value of about 30 mm Hg is required to achieve this level in the mitochondria. As the oxygen tension is increased above these minimum values in the mitochondria, oxidative phosphorylation is unaffected until levels above 250 to 300 mm Hg are reached. Above this value, the rate of oxygen consumption by the mitochondria falls sharply and oxygen toxicity occurs, presumably due to an interruption of the cytochrome oxidase enzyme system.

Tissue Oxygen Requirements

Molecular oxygen must be present in abundance to meet the basic metabolic needs of the cell. About 90% of molecular oxygen consumed by the tissues is involved in the creation of ATP (oxidative phosphorylation); about 9% of oxygen is used to remove hydrogen from amino acids and amines (oxidation), and about 1% is incorporated into complex organic molecules like biogenic amines and hormones (oxygenation). Varying the oxygen tension outside the tissue's normal range can profoundly affect the efficiency with which the enzyme systems catalyze these chemical processes.

The need for maintaining minimal tissue oxygen tension is dramatically demonstrated by measurements in chronic, nonhealing hypoxic wounds. Tissue oxygen levels can be increased in hyperbaric conditions, as compared with normobaric oxygen breathing (Fig. 5.8). Wounds of patients presenting for hyperbaric oxygen (HBO) therapy were repeatedly measured at weekly intervals by implanting a polarographic oxygen electrode in the wound. In a series of 20 patients, all wounds were hypoxic (5 to 20 mm Hg) before HBO treatment was initiated. Daily HBO treatments at 2.4 atmospheres absolute

(ATA) resulted in elevating the wound oxygen tension above 30 mm Hg in all patients in whom healing occurred. Wounds that remained below 30 mm Hg oxygen tension failed to heal. Figure 5.9 shows the baseline transcutaneous oxygen values in four patients treated with hyperbaric oxygen. Two successful cases (healed) had values above 30 mm Hg, and the two unsuccessful cases (non-healing) had values that declined below 30 mm Hg. Figure 5.10 shows the progressively improved wound response to oxygen breathing at 1 ATA for selected weeks of HBO treatment in a problem surgical wound of a high-thigh amputee. A non-healing shrapnel wound to the foot resulted in a number of surgical procedures, failed grafts, and amputations. Hyperbaric oxygen treatment was used to improve the site for grafting. The wound was initially hypoxic with a baseline P_{O_2} of 10–15 mm Hg. By the 19th week, baseline P_{O_2} increased to 30 mm Hg and the wound P_{O_2} response during oxygen breathing indicated improved capillary function. Grafting was successful and the patient was subsequently fitted with a prosthesis.

Hyperbaric oxygen cannot be administered continuously because of its toxic effects (discussed later in this chapter). In addition to the pulmonary and central nervous system effects, cell growth and vascular proliferation are also retarded when oxygen is continuously excessive (Fig. 5.11).

"Normal" Tissue Oxygen Values

"Normal" tissue oxygen tension varies from tissue to tissue and from cell to cell. There is no single "normal" value for all tissues. Instead, there is a series of gradients, the steepness of which varies with arterial oxygen tension, type of tissue, intercapillary distance, and cellular metabolism. Tissue oxygen can be measured by a number of techniques and varies with the type of sensor, e.g., implanted polarographic oxygen electrodes, transcutaneous sensors, tissue tonometry, mass spectrometry, radioactive imaging, and optical methods. The P_{O_2} value

OXYGEN TENSION IN VARIOUS TISSUES DURING INTERMITTENT HYPERBARIC OXYGENATION

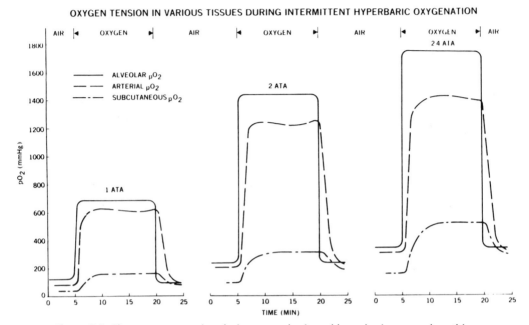

Figure 5.8. Tissue oxygen tension during normobaric and hyperbaric oxygen breathing.

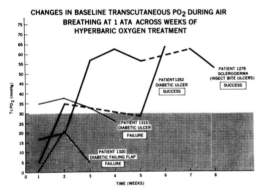

Figure 5.9. Examples of baseline oxygen values in successful (healed) versus unsuccessful (amputees) patients treated with hyperbaric oxygen therapy.

obtained is an indication of the relative abundance of molecular oxygen to support metabolism. Representative tissue oxygen values for arterial blood, venous blood, muscle, subcutaneous tissue, and problem (hypoxic) wounds are shown in Table 5.8.

Respiratory Quotient

The respiratory quotient (RQ) is defined as the ratio of the volume of carbon dioxide expired to the volume of oxygen consumed during the same period. This ratio varies with the chemical composition of the food consumed. The following equations show the oxidative metabolism of carbohydrate (glucose), protein (alanine), and fat (triolein) diets:

glucose: $\qquad C_6 H_{12} O_6$

$$C_6 H_{12} O_6 + 6O_2 \rightarrow 6CO_2 + 6H_2O$$

$$RQ = (6 \text{ Vol. } CO_2) / (6 \text{ Vol.} O_2) = 1.00$$

alanine: $\quad CH_3 CH (NH_2) COOH$

$$2C_3 H_7 O_2 N + 6O_2 \rightarrow (NH_2) CO$$
$$= 5CO_2 + 5H_2O$$

$$RQ = (5 \text{ Vol. } CO_2) / (6 \text{ Vol. } O_2) = 0.83$$

triolein:

$$C_3 H_5 [CH_3 (CH_2)_7 CH = CH (CH_2)_7 COO]_3$$
$$C_{57} H_{104} O_6 + 80O_2 \rightarrow 57CO_2 + 52H_2O$$
$$RQ = (57 \text{ Vol. } CO_2) / (80 \text{ Vol. } O_2) = 0.71$$

Table 5.9 lists the gas exchange, heat production, and respiratory quotients of some commonly ingested materials.

In a resting individual who has eaten a balanced diet and has a cardiac output of about 5.4

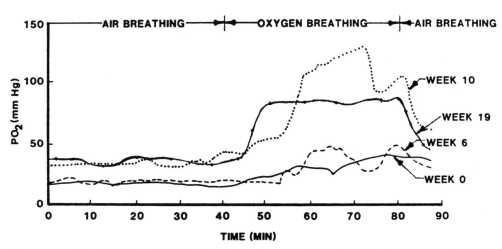

Figure 5.10. Wound response to oxygen breathing for selected weeks of hyperbaric oxygen treatment. Measurements were by implanted polarographic oxygen electrodes. Reprinted by permission of the publisher from: Sheffield PJ. Tissue oxygen measurements with respect to soft-tissue wound healing with normobaric and hyperbaric oxygen. In: Hyperb Oxygen Rev 6(1):18–46. Copyright 1985 by Plenum Publishing.

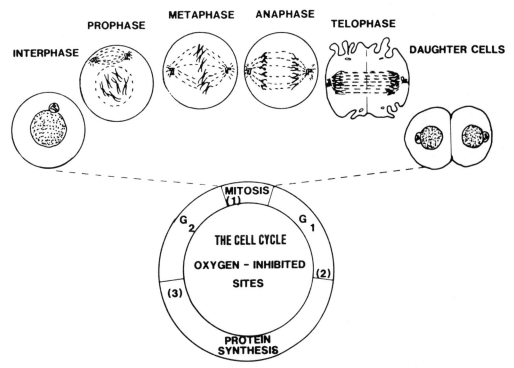

Figure 5.11. The Cell Cycle. The 24-hour cell with markers (numbers in parentheses) indicating the sites of cellular accumulation of oxygen inhibited cells. Reprinted by permission of the publisher from: Sheffield PJ. Tissue Oxygen Measurements. In: Problem wounds: Role of oxygen. Davis JC Hunt TK, eds. New York: Elsevier Science Publishing Co. 1988;3:46.

Table 5.8.
Tissue Oxygen Tension Values for Progressively Increased Inspired Po_2

Experimental Conditions					
Ambient Pressure (ATA)	1.0	1.0	2.0	2.4	3.0
Breathing medium	air	O_2	O_2	O_2	O_2
Ambient Po_2 (mm Hg)	159	760	1520	1824	2280

Representative Tissue Oxygen Tension Values (mm Hg)					
Ideal Alveolar Po_2	104	673	1433	1737	2193
Ideal Arterial Po_2[a]	100	660	1400	1700	2150
Arterial Po_2	—	550 ± 10	1150 ± 25	—	1750 ± 25
Transcutaneous Po_2[b]	69 ± 6	440 ± 95	—	1350 ± 220	—
Venous Po_2[c]	36 ± 4	60 ± 9	101 ± 36	—	—
Muscle Po_2[c]	29 ± 3	59 ± 13	221 ± 72	—	—
Subcutaneous Po_2[c]	37 ± 6	53 ± 10	221 ± 72	—	—
Subcutaneous Po_2[d]	30–50	90–150	200–300	250–500	—
Typical wound Po_2[d]	5–20	200–400	—	1000–1700	—

[a] Blood gas analyzer data from Lamphier EH, Brown IW Jr. The physiologic basis of hyperbaric therapy. In: NRC Committee on Hyperbaric Oxygenation. Fundamentals of hyperbaric medicine. Washington, DC: National Academy of Sciences—Nat. Res. Council, 1966;33–55.

[b] Transcutaneous oxygen data from Workman WT, Sheffield PJ. Continuous transcutaneous oxygen monitoring in smokers under normobaric and hyperbaric oxygen conditions. In: Huch R, Huch A, eds. Continuous transcutaneous blood gas monitoring. New York: Marcel Dekker, 1983;637–644.

[c] Mass spectrometer data from Wells CH, Goodpasture JE, Horrigan DJ, et al. Tissue gas measurements during hyperbaric oxygen exposure. In: Smith G, ed. Proceedings of the Sixth International Congress on Hyperbaric Medicine. Aberdeen: Aberdeen University Press, 1977;118–124.

[d] Implanted polarographic oxygen data from Sheffield PJ. Tissue oxygen measurements with respect to soft-tissue wound healing with normobaric and hyperbaric oxygen. Hyperb Oxygen Rev 1985;6(1):18–46.

Reprinted by permission of the publisher from Sheffield PJ. Tissue oxygen measurements. In: Davis JC, Hunt TK, eds. Problem wounds: Role of Oxygen. New York: Elsevier Science Publishing Co. 1988;3:29.

L/min, the tissues consume about 254 ml of O_2/min (4.7 ml of O_2/100 ml of blood) and produce about 210 ml of carbon dioxide (3.9 ml of CO_2/100 ml of blood (Table 5.10)). Thus, a balanced diet of carbohydrate, protein, and fat produces a respiratory quotient of about 0.83. Unfortunately, determining the respiratory quotient does not furnish exact information about the foodstuff being metabolized. Even when a subject is on a diet consisting of a chemically pure substance, oxidation of that substance to the exclusion of all others does not occur. Apparently, the cells not only oxidize a number of food stuffs concurrently but also convert one compound to another. Thus, the generally accepted concept is that a ''metabolic pool'' exists in which compounds continually enter the pool while others leave it, either to be converted to other molecules or to

Table 5.9.
Gas Exchange and Respiratory Quotients (RQ) For Representative Carbohydrate, Protein, and Fat Compounds

Compound	ml of O_2 Required to Oxidize 1 g	Products of Oxidation of 1g		RQ
		CO_2 (ml)	Heat (kcal)	
Cane sugar	785.5	785.5	3.96	1.00
Protein	956.9	773.8	4.40	0.81
Animal fat	2013.2	1431.1	9.50	0.71

Data adapted from Brobeck JR, Dubois AB: Energy exchange. *In* Medical Physiology. 14th Ed. Edited by V.B. Mountcastle. St. Louis: CV Mosby Co. 1980.

Table 5.10.
Gas Exchange Requirements in Body Tissues

Structure	Mass (kg)	Blood Flow/Min (ml)*	Oxygen Consumed (ml)*	Carbon Dioxide Produced (ml)*	Respiratory Quotient (RQ)
Brain	1.4	750	46.5	46.5	1.00
Heart	0.3	225	29.2	25.0	0.86
Kidney	0.3	1259	17.4	13.9	0.80
Digestive Organs	2.6	1500	50.7	35.4	0.70
Skeletal muscle	31.0	837	49.3	39.6	0.80
Skin	3.6	460	11.8	9.7	0.82
Residual	24.0	380	50.0	40.3	0.81
Whole body	63.2	5411	254.9	210.4	0.83

* Mean value of data collected for 24 hours.
Modified from Lambertsen CJ,: Respiration. *In* Medical physiology. Vol. 2. 14th Ed. Edited by V.B. Mountcastle St. Louis: CV Mosby Co. 1980.

be metabolized to meet the cellular energy requirements.

CONTROL OF PULMONARY VENTILATION

Normal respiratory activity is controlled by complex interactions between the brain, lungs, respiratory muscles, and chemoreceptors. Nerve impulses from each receptor are integrated with others by the respiratory control center.

Neural Control

The respiratory control center is subdivided into the inspiratory center, expiratory center, apneustic center, and pneumotaxic center. These subdivisions are found on both sides of the brain stem. The inspiratory and expiratory centers are in the medulla. The inspiratory centers excite the muscles of inspiration and cause them to contract. The expiratory centers excite the muscles of expiration. When one of these centers is stimulated, the other is automatically inhibited. Oscillation between these two centers is responsible for the respiratory rhythm. In the lower and middle pons are the apneustic centers. Stimulation of the apneustic center causes forceful inspiration but weak expirations. The pneumotaxic centers are in the upper pons. Stimulation of the pneumotaxic center inhibits the apneustic center

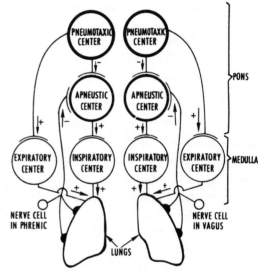

Figure 5.12. The subdivisions of the respiratory center.

and accelerates the rate of breathing. Figure 5.12 illustrates the subdivisions of the respiratory center.

Located in the lungs are many stretch receptors that have a profound effect on the rhythmicity of respiration. When the lungs become stretched, impulses from the stretch receptors excite the vagal nerve endings, inhibit further inspiration, and prevent overdistension of the lungs. The Hering-Breuer reflex is the classical explanation for neural control of respiration. It was discussed earlier in the section entitled

"Pulmonary Ventilation." However, breathing continues in the absence of the Hering-Breuer reflex. If the vagus nerves are severed, the nerve cells of the inspiratory center will discharge impulses to the higher pneumotaxic center (simultaneous with nervous discharge via the phrenic and intercostal nerves). The pneumotaxic center relays a series of impulses to the expiratory center and inhalation is inhibited without the influence of the vagus.

Thus, another possible explanation for neural control of respiration is that cyclic respiratory movements are controlled by the periodic intrinsic activity of the medullary respiratory center. In this concept, inhalation is caused by inspiratory impulses set up within the respiratory center and transmitted via the phrenic and intercostal nerves. During the recovery phase, the impulses are minimized and exhalation occurs. After exhalation, the respiratory center is again excited by cyclic impulses within the center. Another series of impulses are transmitted via the phrenic and intercostal nerves, and inhalation is repeated. In this concept, the Hering-Breuer reflex is responsible for tonically maintaining the proper respiratory center excitability.

In strenuous exercise, oxygen utilization and carbon dioxide formation increase as much as twentyfold. The increased tidal volume and breathing rate, however, increase alveolar ventilation so that blood P_{O_2}, pH, and P_{CO_2} remain within a normal range. At least four different mechanisms may be involved: (1) as the motor cortex transmits impulses to the contracting muscles, it is believed to transmit collateral impulses to excite the respiratory center; (2) movements of the joints excite proprioceptors that transmit excitatory impulses to the respiratory center; (3) increased body temperature is believed to slightly increase respiration; and (4) apparently, a chemoreceptor reflex drive occurs even before arterial oxygen tension has been lowered by exercise.

Breathing 100% oxygen at sea level reduces the hyperpnea at a particular level of exercise. The arterial oxygen content increases by 10%, thereby reducing the degree of muscle anaerobiosis and reducing the fixed acid levels in the blood. In one study, a small decrease in ventilation of an exercising subject was reported within 10 seconds after a single breath of oxygen, which was attributed to the removal of the chemoreceptor contribution to exercise hyperpnea (3).

Voluntary Control

Respiratory movements are under voluntary control. The decision to exert this control and the origin of the nervous impulses that produce it reside within the higher brain centers of the cerebral hemispheres. One can voluntarily breathe fast and deep enough to reduce arterial carbon dioxide tension to half its normal value and completely negate the chemoreceptor control of respiration. Loss of consciousness can result. The voluntary breath holding record (in excess of 13 minutes) was accomplished by combining hyperventilation and 100% oxygen breathing under positive pressure.

Chemical Control

Chemical control is exerted by central chemoreceptors in the respiratory center and peripheral chemoreceptors in the carotid and aortic bodies. The three most important chemical factors are carbon dioxide, hydrogen ions, and oxygen.

The respiratory center is sensitive to arterial carbon dioxide and pH. Carbon dioxide can readily diffuse across the blood-brain barrier and exert its influence on the respiratory center. Questions exist as to whether the respiratory center reacts to carbon dioxide partial pressure or pH. The weight of investigative evidence supports the view that it is pH fluctuation caused by the formation of H_2CO_3 and its subsequent dissociation to $H+$ and HCO_3^- that is of primary importance. Changes in H_2CO_3 are controlled by the net diffusion of carbon dioxide from the blood into the cells of the respiratory center. Because carbon dioxide is one of the end products of metabolism, its presence in the body fluids greatly affects the chemical reactions of the cells. Thus, the tissue P_{CO_2} must be regulated within a narrow tolerance. Stimulation of the respiratory center by fluctuations in carbon dioxide provides a feedback mechanism for the regulation of CO_2 throughout the body. Elevated P_{CO_2} stimulates the respiratory control center to increase alveolar ventilation, thus returning tissue P_{CO_2} to normal. For example, if alveolar P_{CO_2} increases by 3 mm Hg, the respiratory rate increases to 2.5 times normal.

The hydrogen ion concentration appears to have the same basic effect on the respiratory center as does excess carbon dioxide. Excess hydrogen ion concentration increases the activity of the inspiratory center, thus increasing the strength of inspiratory muscle contraction. It also stimulates the expiratory center to increase the force of expiratory muscle contractions, and it excites the apneustic and pneumotaxic centers to enhance both the rate and intensity of the basic respiratory rhythm.

When the arterial carbon dioxide tension drops by as little as 5 mm Hg below normal, the drive to breathe ceases until sufficient carbon dioxide accumulates. Thus, changes in the carbon dioxide tension cause immediate compensatory changes in pulmonary ventilation.

Peripheral chemoreceptors respond to changes in oxygen, carbon dioxide, and pH. The chemoreceptors are located in the bifurcations of the common carotid arteries (carotid bodies) and in the aortic arch (aortic bodies). They are relatively insensitive to changes in carbon dioxide but are highly sensitive to hypoxia. When arterial oxygen tension falls below 45 to 50 mm Hg, the peripheral chemoreceptors stimulate the inspiratory center to increase ventilation. This process also occurs when hydrogen ion concentration is elevated.

The impulses from peripheral chemoreceptors follow two separate routes to the respiratory control center. The carotid body impulses travel to the medulla by the glossopharyngeal nerves, whereas aortic body impulses travel to the medulla by the vagus nerve. Increased hydrogen ion concentration in the arterial blood excites the chemoreceptors and indirectly increases respiratory activity. The direct effects of carbon dioxide and pH on the respiratory center are more powerful than the indirect effects of the peripheral chemoreceptors. Thus, it appears that the chemoreceptors act primarily as an accessory mechanism.

The importance of these bodies is most apparent when the oxygen content of the blood is reduced. The oxygen concentration appears to have little or no direct effect on the respiratory center until the degree of hypoxia is severe enough to directly depress the respiratory center. When the oxygen content of the blood declines, however, impulses from the peripheral chemoreceptors reflexively increase the respiratory activity to provide more oxygen.

Pulmonary ventilation increases two-fold as arterial oxygen tension drops to 38 mm Hg (equivalent to breathing air at 5500 m (18,000 ft)). A further reduction to 35 mm Hg (equivalent to breathing air at nearly 6000 m (20,000 ft)) will increase respiration four to six times, provided carbon dioxide is maintained at its normal level, and is the compensatory mechanism for hypoxia. During periods of severe hypoxia, the reflex drive of the chemoreceptors supersedes the central respiratory center depression and exclusively maintains respiration. Table 5.11 summarizes the chemical control of respiration.

HYPOXIA

". . . The numerous data now enumerated have shown very clearly that the symptoms of decompression are due, not to the lessening of atmospheric pressure, but to the diminuation of the tension of the oxygen which no longer enters the blood, or consequently the tissues, in sufficient quantities to maintain vital combustions at their normal rate."

Paul Bert, 1878.

Table 5.11.
Chemical Control of Respiration

Factor	Central Chemoreceptors (Medulla Ventral Surface)	Peripheral Chemoreceptors (Carotid Bodies)
Carbon dioxide	very sensitive	relatively insensitive
Increased arterial P_{CO_2}	stimulates respiration	reflexly stimulates respiration
Decreased arterial P_{CO_2}	inhibits respiration	—
pH	very sensitive	relatively sensitive
Acidosis	stimulates respiration	reflexly stimulates respiration
Alkalosis	inhibits respiration	—
Oxygen	relatively insensitive	very sensitive
Decreased arterial P_{O_2}	severe hypoxia depresses neural activity	reflexly stimulates respiration (Predominant drive in hypoxia)

The respiratory system has a wide range of flexibility to maintain normal body functions. The respiratory response to the environments to which an individual can be subjected in aerospace operations can have incapacitating results. The most common results are hypoxia, hyperventilation, and hypercapnia.

Hypoxia is a general term that describes the state of oxygen deficiency in the tissues. Hypoxia disrupts the intracellular oxidative process and impairs cellular function. Brain cells with a uniquely high oxygen demand are most susceptible to low oxygen tension. Brain impairment, deterioration of performance, reduced visual function, and unconsciousness occur as a result of hypoxia.

Causes of Hypoxia

Hypoxia from any cause can have serious consequences and can occur at any altitude. Furthermore, hypoxic effects from varying causes are additive. A summary of the causes of hypoxia as they pertain to the various phases of respiration is given in Table 5.1.

Hypoxic Hypoxia

A deficiency in alveolar oxygen exchange is referred to as hypoxic hypoxia. Oxygen deficiency may be due to a reduction in the oxygen partial pressure in inspired air or a reduction in the ef-

fective gas exchange area of the lung. The result is an inadequate oxygen supply to the arterial blood, which, in turn, decreases the amount of oxygen available to the tissues. In aircrews, hypoxic hypoxia usually is caused by exposure to low barometric pressure and is often referred to as altitude hypoxia. Hypoxic hypoxia also can occur in divers who use special gas mixes, if they ascend while breathing a gas with a low oxygen fraction.

Alveolar Oxygen Pressure

The alveolar partial pressure of oxygen is the most critical factor in producing hypoxic hypoxia. It determines the plasma oxygen tension and the degree of oxygen saturation of hemoglobin. Mean alveolar oxygen pressure, P_{AO_2}, can be calculated from the alveolar gas equation, as follows:

$$P_{AO_2} = (P_B - P_{H_2O})\, F_{IO_2} - P_{ACO_2}\left(F_{IO_2} + ((1 - F_{IO_2})/R)\right)$$

where P_B is the ambient barometric pressure; P_{H_2O} is the water vapor at body temperature (47 mm Hg at 37°C); F_{IO_2} is the fraction of inspired oxygen (1.0 for 100% oxygen, 0.21 for air); P_{ACO_2} is the mean alveolar carbon dioxide pressure (40 mm Hg at sea level); and R is the respiratory exchange ratio (RQ) (assumed to be 1.0 for 100% oxygen).

Table 5.12 shows the respiratory gas

Table 5.12.
Respiratory Gas Pressures and Gas Exchange Ratios

Altitude (m)	Altitude (ft)	Pressure (PSIA)	Pressure (mm Hg)	Ambient P_{O_2} (mm Hg)	P_{AO_2} (mm Hg)	P_{ACO_2} (mm Hg)	P_{H_2O} (mm Hg)	Respiratory Exchange Ratio (R)
				Breathing Air				
0	0	14.69	759.97	159.21	103.0	40.0	47.0	0.85
305	1000	14.17	733.04	153.57	98.2	39.4	—	—
610	2000	13.66	706.63	148.04	93.8	39.0	—	—
914	3000	13.17	681.23	142.72	89.5	38.4	—	—
1219	4000	12.69	656.34	137.50	85.1	38.0	—	—
1524	5000	12.23	632.46	132.50	81.0	37.4	47.0	0.87
1829	6000	11.77	609.09	127.60	76.8	37.0	—	—
2134	7000	11.34	586.49	122.87	72.8	36.4	—	—
2438	8000	10.91	564.64	118.29	68.9	36.0	—	—
2743	9000	10.50	543.31	113.82	65.0	35.4	—	—
3048	10,000	10.10	522.73	109.51	61.2	35.0	47.0	0.90
3353	11,000	9.72	502.92	105.36	57.8	34.4	—	—
3658	12,000	9.34	483.36	101.26	54.3	33.8	—	—
3962	13,000	8.99	464.82	97.38	51.0	33.2	—	—
4267	14,000	8.63	446.53	93.55	47.9	32.6	—	—
4572	15,000	8.29	429.01	89.88	45.0	32.0	47.0	0.95
4877	16,000	7.96	411.99	86.31	42.0	31.4	—	—
5182	17,000	7.65	395.73	84.50	40.0	31.0	—	—
5486	18,000	7.34	379.73	79.55	37.8	30.4	—	—
5791	19,000	7.05	364.49	76.36	35.9	30.0	—	—
6096	20,000	6.76	349.50	73.22	34.3	29.4	47.0	1.00
6401	21,000	6.48	335.28	70.24	33.5	29.0	—	—
6706	22,000	6.21	321.31	67.31	32.8	28.4	47.0	1.05
7010	23,000	5.95	307.85	64.49	32.0	28.0	—	—
7315	24,000	5.70	294.89	61.78	31.2	27.4	—	—
7620	25,000	5.46	282.45	59.17	30.4	27.0	47.0	—
				Breathing 100% Oxygen*				
10,058	33,000	3.81	197.10	197.10	109	40	47.0	—
10,973	36,000	3.30	170.94	170.94	85	38	47.0	—
11,887	39,000	2.86	148.08	148.08	64	36	47.0	—
12,192	40,000	2.73	141.22	141.22	—	—	—	—
12,802	42,000	2.48	128.27	128.27	48	33	47.0	—
13,716	45,000	2.15	111.25	111.25	34	30	47.0	—
14,021	46,000	2.05	105.92	105.92	30	29	47.0	—

* Data from Holmstrom FMG. Hypoxia. *In* Aerospace Medicine. Edited by Randall HW. Baltimore: Williams & Wilkins, 1971.[6]

pressures and exchange ratios during exposure to altitude. Values have been measured for air-breathing exposures up to 7600 m (25,000 ft) and for 100% oxygen-breathing exposures up to 14,000 m (46,000 ft). Above these altitudes P_{AO_2} or P_{ACO_2} cannot be measured because unconsciousness occurs so rapidly that steady-state values are not reached. The alveolar gas equation can be used to estimate the values.

Oxyhemoglobin Dissociation Curve

Figure 5.13 compares the oxyhemoglobin saturation at different altitudes. At sea level, a P_{AO_2} of 100 mm Hg results in hemoglobin saturation of 98% (example 1). Ascent to 3000 m (10,000 ft) results in a P_{AO_2} of 60 mm Hg and hemoglobin saturation of 87% (example 2). A healthy person has no difficulty at these altitudes except for a measurable reduction in night vision. With

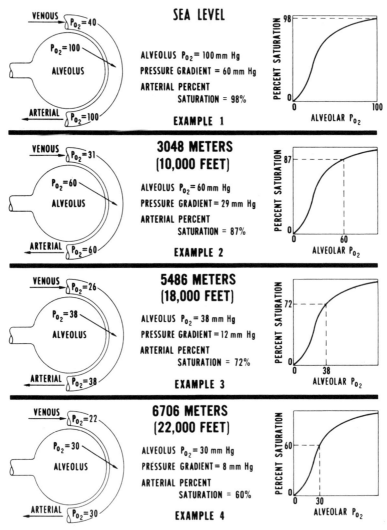

Figure 5.13. Oxyhemoglobin saturation at different altitudes without supplemental oxygen.

a PaO$_2$ of 38 mm Hg and oxyhemoglobin saturation of 72%, symptoms of hypoxia would be experienced within 30 minutes of exposure to 5500 m (18,000 ft) (example 3). Any activity or exercise would reduce this time. Exposure to 6700 m (22,000 ft) results in acute hypoxia, and performance is lost within 5 to 10 minutes (example 4). Exposure to higher altitudes further decreases hemoglobin saturation and shortens the effective performance time (EPT). At altitudes above 7600 m (25,000 ft), PaO$_2$ may actually be lower than the partial pressure of oxygen in the mixed venous blood. This reverses the direction of oxygen flow in the lung, and oxygen diffuses from the blood back into the alveoli. This reduces the arterial oxygen content and, subsequently, oxygen delivery to the brain and other tissues. The onset of hypoxia is more sudden and profound, and the EPT is correspondingly shorter.

Hypemic Hypoxia

Even with normal ventilation and diffusion, cellular hypoxia can occur if the rate of delivery of oxygen does not satisfy metabolic requirements.

An oxygen deficiency due to reduction in the oxygen-carrying capacity of the blood is called hypemic hypoxia.

Oxygen is transported principally by hemoglobin. Hemoglobin has four peptide chains and four hemes. Each heme contains one atom of ferrous iron (Fe^{+2}). Because one molecule of oxygen reacts with one atom of ferrous iron, each hemoglobin molecule reacts reversibly with four oxygen molecules, as follows:

$$Hb_4 + 4O_2 \rightleftharpoons Hb_4(O_2)_4$$

In the hemoglobin molecule, the iron atom remains in the Fe^{+2} state without undergoing a change in valence as oxygen is bound and lost. The iron atom can, however, be oxidized to the Fe^{+3} state by oxidizing agents, such as ferricyanide and sulfa drugs, to produce methemoglobin. If iron is oxidized to Fe^{+3}, it can no longer combine with oxygen.

Carbon monoxide is significant to aircrews because it is present in the exhaust fumes of both conventional and jet engine aircraft, as well as in cigarette smoke. Carbon monoxide combines with hemoglobin about 200 times more readily than does oxygen and displaces oxygen to form carboxyhemoglobin. The normal carboxyhemoglobin level is less than 1% but may increase to 6 or 7% in heavy smokers. Heavy smokers may be less tolerant of increased levels of carbon monoxide in inspired air because of elevated carboxyhemoglobin and nicotine levels, which lower oxygen delivery to the tissues. Oxygen delivery to the skin of smokers is 10% below that of nonsmokers, as shown in Figure 5.14. After smoking a single cigarette, tissue oxygen values are reduced for approximately one hour.

Carboxyhemoglobin levels of 15 to 25% produce headache and nausea. With prolonged exposures, muscular weakness, dizziness, and confusion occur. At levels above 25%, electrocardiographic changes, stupor, and eventual unconsciousness will occur.

Based on the law of mass action, release of carbon monoxide from hemoglobin and from cy-

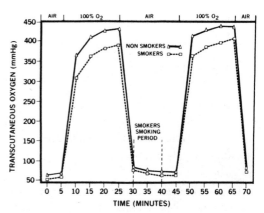

Figure 5.14. Transcutaneous oxygen measurements in smokers and nonsmokers.

tochrome c oxidase can be accelerated by inhaling oxygen. The higher the oxygen pressure, the more rapidly carbon monoxide is eliminated. With hyperbaric oxygen treatment, carbon monoxide is eliminated much more rapidly than with air or oxygen alone. For example, when a carbon monoxide victim breathes fresh air, the half-life of carboxyhemoglobin is 5.5 hours. When breathing 100% oxygen at sea level, the half-life is 1.3 hours, and when breathing 100% oxygen at 3 ATA, the half-life is 23 minutes (7). Hyperbaric oxygen treatment is also used to reduce cerebral edema, and increase oxygen in solution to bypass the CO-bound hemoglobin and deliver oxygen to ischemic tissue.

Stagnant Hypoxia

Any condition that results in a reduction in total cardiac output, pooling of the blood, or restriction of blood flow can result in stagnant hypoxia. Heart failure, shock, continuous positive pressure breathing, and G forces sustained in flight maneuvers create stagnant hypoxia. Local cellular hypoxia can occur as a result of exposure to extreme environmental temperatures, restrictive clothing, or changes in body posture that restrict regional blood flow. Hyperventilation also can cause reduced cerebral blood flow and result in cerebral stagnant hypoxia. Blood clots or gas bubbles (as in decompression sickness) can produce pulmonary emboli and create stagnant hypoxia.

Histotoxic Hypoxia

Metabolic disorders or poisoning of the cytochrome oxidase enzyme system can result in inability of the cell to use molecular oxygen. This condition is called histotoxic (tissue-poisoning) hypoxia.

Unlike hemoglobin, iron atoms in the cytochromes normally undergo reversible changes between Fe^{+2} and Fe^{+3} to serve their role as electron carriers. The oxidized Fe^{+3} form of cytochrome $a + a_3$ complex can accept electrons from the reduced cytochrome c to become the Fe^{+2} form. This is reoxidized by molecular oxygen to the Fe^{+3} form. Only cytochrome a_3 molecules can transfer electrons to molecular oxygen in the final step of cellular respiration. This process is inhibited by carbon monoxide because it competes with oxygen. Ethyl alcohol, cyanide, and hydrogen sulfide also inhibit the cytochrome $a + a_3$ complex and result in histotoxic hypoxia.

Effects of Hypoxia

Hypoxia produces its effects at the cellular level and disrupts normal body functions. Since the highest oxygen requirements are for visual, myocardial, and nervous tissues, these tissues are affected more readily than other tissues.

Respiratory System

One of the first respiratory effects observed in an individual who is becoming hypoxic at altitude is increased depth of breathing. The next effect is increased respiratory rate. These effects are caused by aortic and carotid chemoreceptors, that sense the reduced oxygen pressure of the blood and signal the respiratory center to begin compensatory efforts. An increase in ventilation starts at 1200 m (4,000 ft) but is not significant until the arterial oxygen saturation has decreased to 93% at an altitude of about 2400 m (8,000 ft). A maximum response occurs at 6700 m

(22,000 ft), where the respiratory minute volume is almost doubled. Most of this increase is due to tidal volume rather than to respiratory rate. With the rise in pulmonary ventilation, there is a fall in alveolar carbon dioxide tension and a concomitant increase in the alveolar oxygen tension. The reduction in carbon dioxide decreases hydrogen ion concentration and elevates pH. This change is detected by the chemoreceptors, which reflexly depress respiration. The effects of acute exposure to altitude on pulmonary ventilation are given in Table 5.6.

Cardiovascular System

When oxyhemoglobin saturation declines to 87%, the symptoms of hypoxia become evident. Oxyhemoglobin saturation below 65% is considered critical because the symptoms of hypoxia become severe and consciousness is maintained for only a short time.

Compared with the respiratory and nervous systems, the cardiovascular system is relatively resistant to hypoxia. Cardiovascular responses are reflexive in nature, responding to the hypoxic stimulation of several body structures: the aortic and carotid chemoreceptors, the central nervous system, and the heart. Reflex adjustments act in an integrated fashion to increase heart rate, moderately increase systolic blood pressure, and redistribute blood flow to improve circulation to the brain and heart. The heart rate progressively increases from an altitude of 1200 m (4,000 ft) and reaches a maximum rate at 6700 m (22,000 ft). Table 5.13 shows the effect of altitude on heart rate and arterial oxyhemoglobin saturation.

The increase in cardiac output is significant in that it decreases the arteriovenous (AV) oxygen difference and thus elevates the mean capillary oxygen tension. It should be noted that this occurs because the intracellular utilization of oxygen does not increase with altitude. The fall in oxygen content of arteriovenous blood (AV difference) is related to the cardiac output and the oxygen consumed by the tissues. The AV

Table 5.13.
Effect of Altitude on Heart Rate and Arterial Oxyhemoglobin Saturation

Altitude		Percent of Ground Level Value	
(m)	(ft)	Pulse (at 10 minutes)	Percent of Oxyhemoglobin Saturation (at 3 minutes)
3000	9800	—	87
3700	12,000	114	—
5000	16,400	—	76
5500	18,000	106	—
6100	20,000	124	—
6700	22,000	132	—
7000	23,000	—	71
9000	29,500	—	66

Data from Holmstrom, FMG. Hypoxia. In: Aerospace Medicine. Randall HW, ed. Baltimore: Williams & Wilkins, 1971.

oxygen difference is calculated from the Fick equation, as follows:

$$\text{AV oxygen difference (ml/L)} = \frac{\text{Oxygen consumption (ml/min)}}{\text{Cardiac output (L/min)}}$$

Central Nervous System

The most important alteration in the circulation during altitude exposure occurs in the brain. Upon exposure to altitude, cerebral blood flow decreases due to vasoconstriction secondary to a fall in the arterial carbon dioxide tension. This level is maintained until the arterial P_{O_2} falls to 50 to 60 mm Hg, when hypoxia, a potent vasodilator, overcomes the hypocapneic vasoconstriction and creates an increase in the cerebral blood flow. Because the retina of the eye and the central nervous system have a great requirement for oxygen, they are the first affected by oxygen deficiency. Hypoxia decreases visual and cerebral performance. The effects are in direct proportion to the duration and severity of the exposure. If the oxygen lack becomes acute or is prolonged, cerebral activity ceases and death follows.

Once the local oxygen tension in the mitochondria falls below 1 to 3 mm Hg, the tissue in

that region will convert to anaerobic metabolism and form lactic acid. Thus, the lactic acid test of cerebral tissue is used to determine the cause of death for potential altitude hypoxia victims.

Recognition of the Signs and Symptoms of Hypoxia

The following is an extract of a report filed by Captain R. W. Schroeder in which he discussed his aviation altitude record of 8800 m (29,000 ft) on September 18, 1918:

At 20,000 feet, while still climbing in large circles, my goggles became frosted, making it very difficult for me to watch my instruments. When I reached 25,000 feet I noticed the sun growing very dim. I could hardly hear my motor run, and I felt very hungry. The trend of my thoughts was that it must be getting late. . . I went on talking to myself, and this I felt was a good sign to begin taking oxygen, so I did. I was then over 25,000 feet, and as soon as I started to inhale the oxygen the sun grew bright again, my motor began to exhaust so loud that it seemed something must be wrong with it. I was no longer hungry and the day seemed to be a most beautiful one. . . .

I kept at it until my oxygen gave out, and at that point I noticed my aneroid indicated very nearly 29,000 feet. The thermometer 32° below zero C. and the R.P.M. had dropped from 1600 to 1560. This, considered very good. But the lack of oxygen was affecting me. I was beginning to get cross, and I could not understand why I was only 29,000 feet after climbing for so long a time. I remember that the horizon seemed to be very much out of place, but I felt that I was flying correctly and that I was right and the horizon was wrong.

About this time the motor quit. I was out of gasoline, so I descended in a large spiral. When I had descended to about 20,000 feet I began to feel better. . . .I did not see the ground from the time I went up through the clouds above Dayton, Ohio, until I came down through them again at

4000 feet above Canton, Ohio, over 200 miles from where I started. (8)

Hypoxia Characteristics

Hypoxia is particularly dangerous because its signs and symptoms do not usually cause discomfort or pain. The onset of symptoms is insidious. Individual and daily variances of tolerance occur. The effects of hypoxia begin immediately upon ascent to altitude. Below 3000 m (10,000 ft), the deficiencies are generally so subtle that they normally go unnoticed. Decreases in night vision and drowsiness usually are the only noticeable complaints.

Judgement Impairment

Intellectual impairment is an early sign of hypoxia, making it unlikely that the individual will recognize the disability. Thinking is slow and calculations are unreliable. Fixation, or the tendency to repeat courses of action, is common. Memory is faulty, particularly for events in the immediate past. Judgement is poor, and reaction time is delayed.

Effective Performance Time

Effective performance time (EPT) is defined as the amount of time an individual is able to perform useful flying duties in an environment of inadequate oxygen. EPT is sometimes called time of useful consciousness (TUC). The use of EPT more accurately refers to critical (functional) performance than does TUC. With the loss of effective performance in flight, the individual is no longer capable of taking proper corrective or protective action. Thus, in aerospace operations, the emphasis is on prevention instead of cure. Table 5.14 shows the EPT for healthy, resting individuals at various altitudes.

Individual variations in EPT occur, influenced by individual endurance, experience, physical exertion, and the situation under which exposure has occurred.

Two major factors that markedly reduce EPT are rapid decompression and physical exertion.

Table 5.14.
Effective Performance Time at Altitude

Altitude		Effective Performance Time
(m)	(ft)	
5,500	18,000	20 to 30 min
6,700	22,000	10 min
7,600	25,000	3 to 5 min
8,500	28,000	2.5 to 3 min
9,100	30,000	1 to 2 min
10,700	35,000	0.5 to 1 min
12,200	40,000	15 to 20 sec
13,100	43,000	9 to 12 sec
15,200	50,000	9 to 12 sec

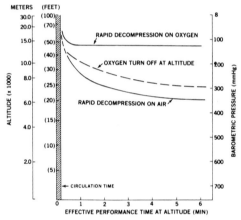

Figure 5.15. Effective performance time (EPT) after rapid decompression.

Upon decompression to altitudes above 10,000 m (33,000 ft), there is an immediate reversal of oxygen flow in the alveoli due to a higher Po_2 within the pulmonary capillaries. This depletes the blood's oxygen reserve and reduces the EPT at rest by up to 50%. Exercise will reduce the EPT considerably. For example, at 7600 m (25,000 ft), a resting individual has an EPT of 3 to 5 minutes, but after performing 10 deep knee bends, EPT will be reduced to about 1 to 1.5 minutes. Figure 5.15 shows the effect of rapid decompression on EPT.

Signs and Symptoms of Hypoxia

The great French physiologist Paul Bert described the first exposures to 23,900 ft conducted in his altitude chamber on March 9, 1874 (9).

"... The two aeronauts went to a pressure of 304 mm of mercury, corresponding to 7300 meters... Nervous phenomena dominated the scene in them; dimness of vision, intellectual indolence were very noticeable in M. Crocen-Spinelli. M. Sivel, who entered the apparatus fasting, began to eat during the decompression; he soon stopped; and as I signed to him through the glass portholes to continue, he replied by a gesture of disgust."

An aviator's defense against incapacitation from altitude hypoxia is to recognize his symptoms and take corrective action to obtain supplemental oxygen. The individual symptoms of hypoxia can be experienced and identified under safe and controlled conditions in a hypobaric (altitude) chamber. Once experienced, these symptoms do not vary dramatically from time to time. However, on occasion, an aviator returning for refresher training in the altitude chamber will report a change in symptoms since the previous exposure. Hypoxia can be classified by either objective signs (i.e., perceived by an observer) or by subjective symptoms (i.e., perceived by the subject). In some cases, a particular response may be noticed by both the subject and the observer. This experience provides the aviator a basis for recognizing hypoxia should it occur in flight.

Objective signs include increased rate and depth of breathing, cyanosis, mental confusion, poor judgement, loss of muscle coordination, slouching, and unconsciousness. Behavioral changes, such as elation or belligerence, may be noted by the hypoxic individual, as well as by the observer.

The subjective symptoms that have been reported include breathlessness, apprehension, headache, dizziness, fatigue, nausea, hot and cold flashes, blurred vision, tunnel vision, tingling, and numbness. Euphoria or anger also might be noted.

Effects on Performance

Hypoxia can be classified by stages of performance decrement. Table 5.15 shows the stages of hypoxia with respect to altitude and oxygen saturation of the blood.

In the indifferent stage, dark adaptation is adversely affected at altitudes as low as 1500 m (5,000 ft), where visual sensitivity at night is reduced by approximately 10%. A 28% reduction in visual sensitivity can occur at 3000 m (10,000 ft), but there are marked individual variations. Performance of new tasks may be impaired. A slight increase in heart rate and pulmonary ventilation occurs.

In the compensatory stage, cardiovascular and respiratory physiologic responses provide some protection against hypoxia. In general, these responses include increases in the respiratory minute volume, cardiac output, heart rate, and blood pressure. The effects of hypoxia on the central nervous system are perceptible after a short period of time. The most important effects of hypoxia at this altitude are drowsiness, decreased judgement and memory, and difficulty with the performance of tasks requiring mental alertness or discrete motor movements.

In the disturbance stage, the physiologic compensatory mechanisms are no longer capable of providing for adequate oxygenation of tissues. Symptoms such as headache, dizziness, somnolence, air hunger, euphoria, and fatigue may develop. Intellectual impairment may prevent the individual from properly assessing the seriousness of the condition. Thinking is slow and unreliable, memory is faulty, motor performance is severely impaired, and critical judgement is lost. The peripheral visual field may gray out to a point where only central vision remains. This is referred to as tunnel vision.

In the critical stage, mental performance deteriorates, and mental confusion or dizziness occurs within a few minutes. Total incapacitation with loss of consciousness rapidly follows with little or no warning.

Factors Influencing Symptoms

The appearance and severity of the signs and symptoms of acute hypoxia are enhanced by several factors: altitude, time spent at altitude, rapid

Table 5.15.
Stages of Hypoxia

Stage	Altitude Breathing Air		Altitude Breathing 100% O_2		Arterial O_2 Saturation (%)
	(M × 1000)	(ft × 1000)	(M × 1000)	(ft × 1000)	
Indifferent	0–3.0	0–10	10.4–11.9	34.0–39.0	98–87
Compensatory	3.0–4.6	10–15	11.9–13.0	39.0–42.5	87–80
Disturbance	4.6–6.1	15–20	13.0–13.7	42.5–44.8	80–65
Critical	6.1–7.0	20–23	13.7–13.9	44.8–45.5	65–60

rate of ascent, physical exertion, extreme environmental temperature, and indulgence in self-imposed stresses such as fatigue, alcohol consumption, tobacco products, certain medications, and inadequate nutrition.

Treatment of Hypoxia

Treatment of hypoxia is to administer 100% oxygen. If respiration has ceased, cardiopulmonary resuscitation with the simultaneous use of 100% oxygen is indicated. The type of hypoxia must be determined and treatment administered accordingly. The following steps are recommended:

1. *Administer supplemental oxygen under pressure.* Providing the aircrew member with adequate supplemental oxygen is the prime consideration in the treatment of hypoxia. Depending on the severity of the condition, 100% oxygen delivered under positive pressure may be required. Consideration must be given to the altitude and cause of the oxygen deficiency. Hypoxia produced by altitude exposure above 12,200 m (40,000 ft) cannot be corrected without the addition of positive pressure breathing (PPB).

2. *Monitor breathing.* After a hypoxic episode, the resulting hyperventilation must be controlled to achieve complete recovery. Maintaining a breathing rate of 12 to 16 breaths/min or slightly lower will aid recovery.

3. *Monitor equipment.* The most frequently reported causes of hypoxia are lack of oxygen discipline and equipment malfunction. Conscientious equipment preflight checks and frequent in-flight monitoring will reduce this hazard. Inspection of oxygen equipment when hypoxia is suspected may detect its cause. Correction of the malfunction will aid in the immediate relief of the hypoxic condition. If treatment for hypoxia does not remedy the situation, oxygen contamination should be considered. Use of an alternate oxygen source, such as the emergency oxygen cylinder or portable assembly, should be considered. Descent should be initiated as soon as possible and the contents of the oxygen system analyzed.

4. *Descend.* Increasing ambient oxygen pressures by descent to lower altitudes, particularly below 3000 m (10,000 ft), is also beneficial. Descent to lower altitude compensates for malfunctioning oxygen equipment that may have caused the hypoxia.

Preventing hypoxia in flying personnel is, to a great extent, a matter of indoctrination. This indoctrination is accomplished by instructing personnel in the proper use and care of oxygen equipment and ensuring that they are aware of their individual symptoms of hypoxia.

Recovery From Hypoxic (Altitude) Hypoxia

Recovery from hypoxia usually occurs within seconds when sufficient oxygen is supplied. Nevertheless, mild symptoms, such as headache or fatigue, may persist after the hypoxic episode. The persistence of symptoms seems to have a higher degree of correlation with the duration of the episode than with its severity.

In some instances following the sudden

administration of oxygen to correct the hypoxic insult, the individual develops a temporary increase in the severity of symptoms, which is known as oxygen paradox. The subject may lose consciousness or develop clonic spasms for a period lasting up to a minute. Usually, this condition is transient and may pass unnoticed. Accompanying symptoms are mental confusion, deterioration of vision, dizziness, and nausea. Initially, the arterial blood pressure falls and the rate of blood flow decreases. The hypotension produced by the sudden restoration of oxygen is probably due to vasodilation, which occurs in the pulmonary vascular bed and is brought about by the direct action of oxygen on the pulmonary vessels. The hypocapnia produced by hypoxia and the decrease in blood pressure, which follows reoxygenation, act together to reduce cerebral blood flow. This reduction in blood flow probably intensifies the cerebral hypoxia for a short period until the cardiovascular effects have passed and the carbon dioxide tension returns to a normal range. Once the P_{CO_2} returns to a normal value, it will stimulate the respiratory center to resume ventilation and resolve the cerebral hypoxia. After a severe hypoxic episode, performance can be impaired for one to two hours.

Prevention of Hypoxia

Hypoxic hypoxia is prevented by ensuring that the individual has sufficient oxygen to maintain a range of alveolar P_{O_2} between 60 and 100 mm Hg. This oxygen level is achieved in aircraft by an oxygen system, cabin pressurization, or a combination of the two.

Cabin Pressurization

In most civilian and military aircraft, hypoxia is prevented by maintaining a cabin altitude below 3000 m (10,000 ft). Supplemental oxygen is required only when cabin pressurization fails. In most military fighter and trainer aircraft, cabin altitude often exceeds this level. The cabin pressurization in such aircraft ordinarily provides a cabin altitude below 7600 m (25,000 ft).

Table 5.16.
Supplemental Oxygen Requirements at Altitude to Maintain Sea Level Air Equivalence

Altitude		Barometric Pressure (mm Hg)	Total Oxygen Requirement (%)
(m)	(ft)		
Sea level		760	21
1524	5000	632	25
3048	10,000	532	31
4572	15,000	429	40
6092	20,000	329	49
7620	25,000	282	62
9144	30,000	225	81
10,363	34,000	187	100

Protection from hypoxia in these aircraft is provided by the combined application of cabin pressurization and supplemental oxygen.

Supplemental Oxygen Requirements

Table 5.16 lists the supplemental oxygen requirements for altitudes up to 10,400 m (34,000 ft) to maintain a physiologic altitude equivalent to sea level. Above this altitude, 100% oxygen must be administered along with positive pressure breathing. Without positive pressure, breathing 100% oxygen at 12,200 m (40,000 ft) would be equivalent to breathing air at 3000 m (10,000 ft).

Night Requirements

Exposure to reduced oxygen tensions at altitudes below 3000 m (10,000 ft) increases dark adaptation time and decreases night vision capability. For this reason, the use of supplemental oxygen may be needed on night flights. One hundred percent oxygen is not required because the object is to maintain the blood oxygen content equivalent to exposures at altitudes of 1500 m (5,000 ft) or below.

Requirement for Pressure Breathing

Although most high performance aircraft are pressurized, there are times when cabin pressure is lost and the occupants are exposed to the reduced pressure at high altitude. To prevent the occurrence of hypoxia above 12,200 m (40,000

Table 5.17.
Pressure Requirements for Exposure Above 10,400 Meters

Altitude		Barometric Pressure (mm Hg)	Calculated P_{AO2}	Additional Oxygen Pressure Required to Provide Equivalent Altitude of	
(m)	(ft)			3000 m[a] (10,000 ft)	Sea Level[b]
10,400	34,000	187	100	None	None
12,200	40,000	141	54	6	46
13,700	45,000	111	24	36	76
15,200	50,000	87	0	60	100
19,800	65,000	43	0	104	144
Space	Space	0	0	147	187

[a] Equivalent altitude of 3000 means P_{AO2} = 60 mm Hg; P_{AO2} = 40 mm Hg: P_{AH2O} = 47 mm Hg; and P total = 147 mm Hg.
[b] Sea level equivalent means P_{AO2} = 100 mm Hg; P_{ACO2} = 40 mm Hg; P_{AH2O} = 47 mm Hg; and P total = 187 mm Hg.

ft) 100% oxygen must be breathed with additional pressure to achieve adequate oxygenation.

It has recently become popular to use one acronym to describe pressure breathing for altitude protection (PBA) to distinguish from the new technique for pressure breathing for high-G protection (PBG). For the purpose of this text, we will use the classic term, positive pressure breathing (PPB). PPB is accomplished with a pressure demand oxygen system. Oxygen regulators are designed to automatically provide positive pressure and 100% oxygen at altitudes above approximately 9100 m (30,000 ft). Table 5.17 shows the positive pressure requirements to prevent hypoxia at altitude. Most oxygen regulators tend to maintain an alveolar oxygen partial pressure of 87 mm Hg, which is equivalent to breathing air at about 1500 m (5,000 ft).

Figure 5.16 illustrates the decrease in hemoglobin saturation with increasing altitude. Percent saturation is plotted against altitude, and the slope of the curve is similar to the standard oxyhemoglobin dissociation curve. In Example 1, the percent saturation, indicated by the dashed line, is roughly equal to that of breathing air at 1500 m (5,000 ft). This percent saturation would remain constant up to 10,400 m (34,000 ft), provided that the oxygen regulator delivers the percentages of oxygen shown in Table 5.17.

Figure 5.16 (Example 2) also illustrates the effect of breathing 100% oxygen at altitudes

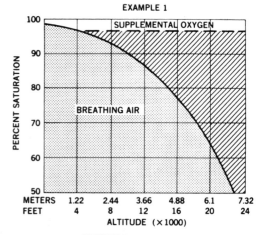

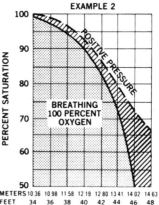

Figure 5.16. Oxyhemoglobin saturation at different altitudes with supplemental oxygen.

above 10,400 m (34,000 ft). When positive pressure is applied to the oxygen, alveolar P_{O_2} increases. The safe ceiling is raised, as reflected by the dashed curve. This level represents the pressure output from an automatic PPB regulator. A limit must be set with regard to the unpressurized flight altitude at which a flyer can operate and function well enough to complete the mission. This altitude limit for sustained flight without a counterpressure garment is approximately 13,100 m (43,000 ft) when using standard equipment that delivers 30 mm Hg pressure. Pressure greater than 30 mm Hg cannot be tolerated for long periods. PPB impedes venous return to the heart and reduces blood flow through the lungs. In the extremities and abdomen, the veins dilate to accommodate the pooled blood, resulting in a rise in venous blood pressure. The subject experiences profound fatigue.

At 36 to 40 mm Hg of PPB which is required at 13,700 m (45,000 ft), pain in the region of the eyes becomes intolerable. Subjects complain of a feeling of congestion in the region of the frontal sinuses. Overdistension may cause pain in the ears and in the posterior pharynx.

At pressures between 60 and 100 mm Hg, lung tissue damage secondary to overexpansion is likely. Loss of consciousness may occur due to decreased cardiac output and pooling of blood in the lower extremities and abdominal vessels.

Technique for Pressure Breathing

During PPB, inhalation is easy and exhalation is difficult. The breathing cycle must be consciously controlled. Practice is required to become accustomed to this reversed breathing pattern. In particular, the tendency to hyperventilate must be avoided. The best technique for PPB is as follows:

1. Establish mental discipline to control the breathing pattern.
2. When inhaling, maintain a conscious tension on the respiratory muscles (the intercostal muscles, diaphragm, and abdominal muscles). Control the expansion of the thorax through muscle tension. As inhalation progresses, steadily decrease muscle tension to allow inflation of the lungs.
3. Pause when the desired lung inflation has occurred.
4. When ready to exhale, positively increase muscle tension for a steady, smooth exhalation.
5. Pause and breathe at a rate slower than normal.

Requirements for Counterpressure Garments

PPB causes distension of the chest and lungs. The lungs are fully inflated at a pressure of 20 mm Hg. Counterpressure to the chest is required when the pressure reaches 60–100 mm Hg. If an aviator is to survive exposures to altitudes above 15,200 m (50,000 ft) for any period of time, additional alveolar P_{O_2} must be provided. Protection is provided by counterpressure garments, commonly called pressure suits. Military directives state that flights above 15,200 m (50,000 ft) are not permissible, regardless of the cabin altitude, unless the aviator is protected by a counterpressure garment.

The purpose of the pressure suit is to protect the aviator from hypoxia. This protection is achieved by applying pressure equally across the body such that a sufficiently low physiologic altitude is maintained so that PPB is not required. For more detailed discussion, see Chapter 6, section on ''Pressure Suits.''

Altitude Acclimatization

Chronic exposure to altitude results in altitude acclimatization, the process by which one becomes more tolerant of an hypoxic environment. The means by which acclimatization is achieved includes the following:

1. Increased respiration and cardiac output due to the hypoxic stimulation of the carotid and aortic bodies.
2. Increased diffusion capacity of the lungs,

probably achieved by a rise in the pulmonary capillary blood volume, increased lung volume, and a rise of the pulmonary arterial pressure.

3. Polycythemia, directly resulting from hypoxic stimulation of red blood cell production by the bone marrow due to an increased release of erythropoietin by the kidney. The increased hemoglobin content improves the capacity of the blood to transport oxygen. The degree of polycythemia is inversely related to the arterial oxygen saturation. This mechanism provides limited benefits within 2 to 3 weeks of exposure.

4. Increased vascularity of tissues, resulting from an increased number and size of capillaries. Like polycythemia, this response requires a long-term exposure to the hypoxic environment.

5. Cellular acclimatization, occurring as the capability of the cells to metabolize oxygen increases in spite of the low oxygen tension. This acclimatization is probably due to changes in the cellular oxidative enzyme systems.

6. Decreased affinity of the hemoglobin for oxygen, resulting from an increased production of 2,3 diphosphoglyceric acid within the red blood cells. The result is a shift of the oxyhemoglobin dissociation curve to the right, which improves the offloading of oxygen to the tissues by as much as 10 to 20% at 4600 m (15,000 ft). At higher altitudes, this decreased affinity for oxygen reduces the uptake of oxygen by hemoglobin in the lungs and has a detrimental effect on tissue metabolism.

7. The renal mechanism compensates for respiratory alkalosis by retaining ammonium ions and excreting large amounts of bicarbonate. Because this is a slow process, it is not detected until over an hour or more and may reach a maximum only after several days.

HYPERVENTILATION

Hyperventilation is of concern because it produces changes in cellular respiration. Although unrelated in cause, the symptoms of hyperventilation and hypoxia are similar and often result in confusion and inappropriate corrective procedures. Despite increased knowledge, training, and improved life-support equipment, both hypoxia and hyperventilation are hazards in flying and diving operations.

Hyperventilation is a condition in which ventilation is abnormally increased. As a result, a loss of carbon dioxide from the lungs occurs, lowering alveolar carbon dioxide tension below normal, a condition known as hypocapnia. The acid-base balance of the blood is disturbed, making it more alkaline, a condition known as alkalosis. Hypocapnia and alkalosis are two important results of hyperventilation.

Causes of Hyperventilation

Hyperventilation in aerospace operations is commonly caused by psychologic stress (fear, anxiety, apprehension, and anger) and environmental stress (hypoxia, pressure breathing, vibration, and heat). Certain drugs also cause or enhance hyperventilation such as salicylates and female sex hormones. In addition, any condition that creates metabolic acidosis will result in hyperventilation.

It is a common practice in diving operations for breathholding divers to voluntarily hyperventilate to extend the breathholding time. Extended breathholding after hyperventilation is an unsafe practice. As the diver descends, lung volume is reduced (Boyle's Law) resulting in increased lung P_{O_2}. Lung P_{CO_2} is elevated initially, but is followed by lowered P_{CO_2} due to reversed gradient because of tissue storage. During the dive, the diver consumes oxygen and produces carbon dioxide. Because alveolar P_{CO_2} increases during compression, CO_2 does not leave the blood to enter the lungs. Arterial CO_2 rises rapidly initially, then is lowered as the tissue stores CO_2. The usual carbon dioxide stimulus to breathe does not occur at depth. As the diver consumes oxygen, arterial P_{O_2} is lowered so that respiration is not stimulated until oxygen drops so low that the breathhold point is reached. As the diver ascends, the lung re-expands and lung P_{CO_2} increases as CO_2 diffuses from the tissues to the lung. Simultaneously, a drop in oxygen partial pressure occurs, causing alveolar oxygen tension to fall to a dangerously low level before the surface is reached. If the diver has remained at depth too long, unconsciousness from hypoxia may occur during the ascent. To avoid unconsciousness on return to surface, trained divers limit their hyperventilation to no more than 3–4 deep breaths, and their breath-hold dive time to 1.5 minutes maximum.

Increased ventilation associated with exercise does not produce hyperventilation because an increase in the carbon dioxide content of the blood is maintained by the increased metabolic activity.

Effects of Hyperventilation

Hypocapnia and alkalosis produced by hyperventilation affect the respiratory (blood buffer system), circulatory (oxyhemoglobin dissociation curve), and central nervous systems.

The Respiratory System

As previously discussed, 90% of the carbon dioxide present in the blood is in the form of carbonic acid or bicarbonate. The overall reaction for bicarbonate formation occurs in two steps, as follows:

$$CO_2 + H_2O \rightleftharpoons H_2CO_3 \rightleftharpoons (H+) + (HCO_3^-)$$

The Law of Mass Action determines the direction in which this reaction proceeds. It is usually driven by the carbon dioxide tension, P_{CO_2}. When the P_{CO_2} increases, the reaction proceeds toward the formation of more bicarbonate and hydrogen atoms (acidosis). When the P_{CO_2} decreases, the reaction reverses to form carbon dioxide and water, at the expense of bicarbonate and hydrogen ions (alkalosis).

Arterial blood normally has a pH (defined as the negative logarithm of the hydrogen ion con-

centration) of about 7.40, a P_{CO_2} of about 40 mm Hg, and a plasma bicarbonate concentration of about 25 mmol/L. When an individual hyperventilates, the excessive elimination of carbon dioxide causes a reduction in hydrogen ion concentration that is too rapid for the blood buffers to replace it. The pH is elevated, and respiratory alkalosis occurs. Because catalytic activity of enzymes is especially sensitive to pH, there is a sharp decline in activity on either side of an optimum pH. Should the pH of the blood fall below 7.0 or rise above 7.8, irreparable damage to cellular respiration will occur. In severe cases, unconsciousness and death occur. In the less severe case, when an individual becomes unconscious, respiration slows sufficiently to allow a buildup of carbon dioxide and correct the alkalosis. Hyperventilation is always a complicating factor when hypoxic hypoxia is encountered because the effects, symptoms, degree of impairment, and EPT are so similar.

The Cardiovascular System

The cardiovascular system effects of hyperventilation are tachycardia, reduced cardiac output, declining blood pressure, and reduced peripheral vascular resistance. Vasoconstriction of the cerebral blood vessels causes a restriction in blood flow to the brain.

The primary cardiovascular effect, however, is the Bohr effect, which causes the oxyhemoglobin dissociation curve to shift upward and to the left. This shift increases the capacity of the blood to onload oxygen in the lungs but restricts offloading of oxygen at the tissue level.

The Central Nervous System

The combined effects of restricted blood flow and oxyhemoglobin binding cause stagnant hypoxia to exist in the central nervous system, which leads to unconsciousness. Hyperventilation also causes increased neuromuscular instability with muscle spasms and tetany when the alveolar P_{CO_2} is reduced to 25 to 30 mm Hg. Tingling usually precedes muscle spasm and tetany. The hands may exhibit carpopedal spasm,

HYPERVENTILATION

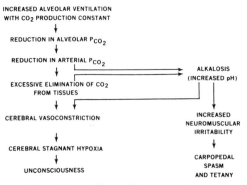

Figure 5.17. Effects of hyperventilation.

a fixation of the hand wherein the fingers are flexed toward the wrist. Figure 5.17 summarizes the effects of hyperventilation.

Recognition of the Signs and Symptoms of Hyperventilation

The signs and symptoms of hyperventilation are easily confused with those of hypoxic hypoxia. Because hyperventilation occurs as an early adaptive mechanism to hypoxia at altitude, it becomes even more difficult to differentiate between the two conditions. The objective signs that are most frequently seen in hyperventilation are increased respiratory rate and depth, muscle twitching and tightness, pallor, cold, clammy skin, muscle spasm, rigidity, and unconsciousness. Symptoms perceived by the subjects include dizziness, lightheadedness, tingling, numbness, visual disturbances, and muscle incoordination.

Table 5.18 compares the symptoms of hyperventilation and hypoxia. It should be noted that the distinguishing differences in these syndromes are few. In hyperventilation, the onset of symptoms is usually gradual, with the presence of a pale, cold, clammy appearance and the development of muscle spasm and tetany. In hypoxia, the onset of symptoms is usually rapid (depending on altitude), with the development of flaccid muscles and cyanosis.

Table 5.18.
Comparison of Hyperventilation and Hypoxic Hypoxia Syndromes

Signs and Symptoms	Hyperventilation	Hypoxia
Onset of symptoms	Gradual	Rapid (altitude-dependent)
Muscle activity	Spasm	Flaccid
Appearance	Pale, clammy	Cyanosis
Tetany	Present	Absent
Breathlessness	X	X
Dizziness	X	X
Dullness and drowsiness	X	X
Euphoria	X	X
Fatigue	X	X
Headache	X	X
Judgement poor	X	X
Lightheadedness	X	X
Memory faulty	X	X
Muscle incoordination	X	X
Numbness	X	X
Performance deterioration	X	X
Respiratory rate increased	X	X
Reaction time delayed	X	X
Tingling	X	X
Unconsciousness	X	X
Vision blurred	X	X

X means that the sign or symptom can occur in either condition.

Treatment of Hyperventilation

The treatment of hyperventilation requires a voluntary reduction in the rate and depth of ventilation. Treatment also may be accomplished by breathing into a bag that collects the exhaled carbon dioxide for rebreathing by the subject. Both breathholding and the use of a rebreathing bag are to be avoided at altitude because of the similarity of the symptoms with those of hypoxia.

Because hypoxia and hyperventilation are so similar and both can incapacitate so quickly, the recommended treatment procedures for aviators correct both problems simultaneously: (1) administer 100% oxygen under pressure; (2) reduce the rate and depth of breathing; (3) check the oxygen equipment to ensure proper functioning; and (4) descend to a lower altitude where hypoxia is unlikely to occur. A tendency to hyperventilate is apparent when one experiences positive pressure breathing. This tendency, however, can be controlled by following the positive pressure breathing procedure previously outlined, particularly if periodically practiced in the hyperbaric chamber.

Prevention of Hyperventilation

To prevent serious emergencies, the crewmembers should be able to recognize both signs and symptoms of hypoxia and hyperventilation. Recognition can only occur by experiencing one's own symptoms and observing signs in others at regular intervals in a controlled environment such as the hypobaric (altitude) chamber.

HYPERCAPNIA

A person at rest will exhale about 0.8 L of carbon dioxide for each liter of oxygen consumed. Thus, in a sealed environment, an individual will gradually deplete the oxygen supply and contaminate the air with carbon dioxide. This problem would arise only if there were a failure of the life-support system that provides the oxygen and eliminates the carbon dioxide. Unlike hypoxia, in which there is a large range of variation before eliciting a respiratory drive, hypercapnia increases respiration with only a slight change in P_{CO_2}.

At sea level, the inspired partial pressure of carbon dioxide is normally less than 1 mm Hg (0.03% of 760 mm Hg). An inspired P_{CO_2} up to 40 mm Hg, about 5% carbon dioxide at sea level, can be tolerated without serious effects. When the inspired P_{CO_2} exceeds 40 mm Hg, a rise of carbon dioxide concentration occurs in the body fluids. Maximum alveolar ventilation occurs when inspired P_{CO_2} reaches about 70 mm Hg. Acidosis is produced by the inability to eliminate carbon dioxide, and the respiratory center is depressed at P_{CO_2} values above 70 mm Hg. Table 5.19 shows the effect of inhalation of carbon dioxide in air at sea level. Individuals exposed to increased carbon dioxide lose consciousness at an inspired P_{CO_2} of 150 mm Hg and die at a P_{CO_2} of 300 mm Hg.

OXYGEN TOXICITY

A common practice in both aerospace and diving operations is to provide artificial atmospheres when air breathing is not practical. Oxygen poisoning can result in either environment if the oxygen tension is maintained at too high a level and breathed for too long a time. Oxygen toxicity is related to the P_{O_2} and not to the percentage of oxygen inspired. The low oxygen partial pressures and short duration of use by flying personnel usually will not cause harm. Long-duration altitude chamber studies with pure oxygen at 250 mm Hg revealed no oxygen toxicity effects on the lung or central nervous system.

The Mercury and Gemini space flights and the pressure suits used for lunar exploration successfully used pure oxygen environments without clinical oxygen toxicity due to the low partial pressures of oxygen maintained. Reduction of red blood cell mass was identified as a physical effect of pure oxygen breathing, largely due to the absence of an inert gas. This problem was corrected by adding small amounts of nitrogen to the breathing mix.

The problem of oxygen toxicity is more significant at sea level and in hyperbaric operations where the partial pressure of oxygen is greatly increased. The toxic effect of oxygen is related to the dose (partial-pressure factor) and the duration of application (time factor). Figure 5.18 illustrates the time/oxygen partial-pressure relationships for both pulmonary and central nervous system toxicity.

Pulmonary Oxygen Toxicity

Prolonged breathing of 60 to 100% oxygen for more than 12 hours at sea level (P_{O_2} of 450 to 760 mm Hg) can irritate the respiratory passage-

Table 5.19.
Effect of Inhalation of Carbon Dioxide in Air at Sea Level on Pulmonary Ventilation

P_{CO_2} (mm Hg)	FI_{CO_2} (%)	Tidal Volume (ml)	Frequency (breaths/min)	Respiratory Minute Volume (L/min)
0.23	0.03	440	16	7
7.6	1.0	500	16	8
15.2	2.0	560	16	9
30.4	4.0	823	17	14
38.0	5.0	1300	20	26
57.8	7.6	2100	28	52
79.0	10.4	2500	35	76

Data from Comroe JH, Jr.: Physiology of Respiration. Chicago: Yearbook Medical Publishers, Inc., 1965.[1]

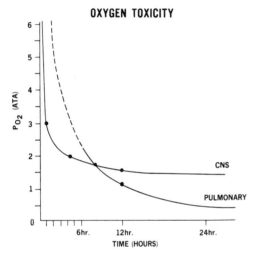

Figure 5.18. Oxygen toxicity time/dose relationship.

ways. Coughing, congestion, sore throat, and substernal soreness are common symptoms, known as the "Lorraine Smith effect." After about 24 hours, decreased vital capacity occurs, followed by serious pulmonary damage: lung irritation, bronchopneumonia, pulmonary edema, and atelectasis. At great oxygen pressures in the hyperbaric environment, pulmonary toxicity can occur much more rapidly, but it is easily prevented by taking intermittent air-breathing periods between each oxygen-breathing exposure. Table 5.20 lists the time to onset of pulmonary oxygen toxicity in eight human studies at various altitudes. In these studies, the most predominant symptom was substernal distress, and the times to onset varied inversely with inspired P_{O_2}.

In animal studies involving prolonged oxygen exposures, severe pulmonary toxicity resulted in the loss of pulmonary surfactant, structural changes, pulmonary edema, extravasation of red blood cells into the airways, massive atelectasis, carbon dioxide retention, acidosis, and death from hypoxia, even in the presence of high inspired P_{O_2}. Once severe pulmonary toxicity occurs, there exists a point of no return: sustaining a high P_{O_2} will produce further pulmonary damage and death, and lowering the P_{O_2} will lead to arterial hypoxemia and death. It is imperative to prevent the damage from reaching this point by controlling the inspired oxygen pressure.

The only known pulmonary toxicity effects in aerospace operations are from the anecdotal reports of substernal awareness and cough after high sustained G maneuvers in fighter aircraft following prolonged oxygen breathing.

Central Nervous System Oxygen Toxicity

Oxygen toxicity of the central nervous system, or the "Paul Bert effect," occurs with exposures to P_{O_2} greater than 2 ATA and is not a problem in aerospace operations. It produces convulsions much like those of grand mal epilepsy. It is of primary concern in hyperbaric chamber operations because 100% oxygen is administered at pressures of up to 2.8 ATA in the treatment of decompression sickness (see Chapter 7). Less serious symptoms related to the central nervous

Table 5.20.
Time to Onset of Pulmonary Oxygen Toxicity Symptoms in Man

Barometric Pressure (mm Hg)	Oxygen Partial Pressure (mm Hg)	Duration of Study (hours)	Time to Onset of Symptoms (hours)	Investigator
760	750	6–7	6–7	Behnke, 1940
760	736	24	14	Comroe, et al., 1945
760	630	57	24	Ohlsson, 1947
760	546	24	24	Comroe, et al., 1945
523	418	168	24–36	Michel, et al., 1960
760	380	24	None	Comroe, et al., 1945
258	242	336	86	Morgan, et al., 1963
190	174	408	216	Welch, et al., 1961

system may precede the convulsion: hypersensitivity, nausea, muscular twitching (particularly facial muscles), fatigue, and muscle incoordination. If such symptoms are recognized in time, the convulsion may be avoided by removing the breathing mask to reduce the inspired oxygen pressure.

The events and signs of an oxygen convulsion are usually the same for each individual. Consciousness is lost when the convulsion starts. Respiration ceases during the tonic convulsive stage, which may last for 1 to 2 minutes. If left unprotected, the convulsing person may sustain physical injuries due to striking hard objects or biting the tongue. Following the convulsion, respiration normally resumes spontaneously, but the victim may remain semiconscious, irrational, and restless for several minutes.

Treatment

If an individual displays any sign of central nervous system oxygen toxicity, the hyperoxic breathing source must be removed quickly. Ambient pressure must never be altered until the convulsion ceases and breathing resumes. Ascent with a closed glottis may lead to fatal air embolism. A padded mouthpiece (never the fingers) can be used to prevent tongue-biting, but this practice is controversial. The victim should be gently restrained to prevent injury from flailing or falling. The victim's head should be turned to one side to prevent aspiration should vomiting occur. If the victim does not resume

normal breathing following the convulsion, the airway should be checked for obstruction and immediate cardiopulmonary resuscitation begun with air.

Victims of central nervous system oxygen toxicity recover promptly and completely when the high oxygen tension is removed. There are no lasting or residual effects, and the victim will be no more susceptible to oxygen toxicity in the future.

Prevention

Breathing 100% oxygen at 2.8 ATA while at complete rest for 30 minutes is an exposure that 98% of subjects can tolerate without signs of oxygen toxicity. As pressure, activity, or exposure time is increased, more individuals will display signs of toxicity. In the treatment of decompression sickness, 100% oxygen is administered to the patient at pressures up to 2.8 ATA for periods up to 285 minutes. To preclude toxicity, intermittent air-breathing is used with the oxygen. If air is breathed for short periods (5 to 10 minutes) between longer oxygen-breathing periods (20 to 30 minutes), the latent period before symptoms occur is safely extended. Pure oxygen is never breathed at pressures greater than 3 ATA. As C.J. Lambertsen has stated: "With more prolonged O_2 exposure, total failure of gas exchange is inevitable. . . and death (occurs) from hypoxia in the presence of and due to the high inspired Po_2.''

REFERENCES

1. Comroe JH Jr. Physiology of Respiration. Chicago: Yearbook Medical Publishers, Inc., 1965.
2. Rahn H, Otis AB. Alveolar air during simulated flights to high altitudes. Am J Physiol 150:202;1947.
3. Lambertsen CJ. Respiration. In: Medical physiology. Vol 2 14th Ed. Mountcastle VB, ed. St.Louis: CV Mosby Co., 1980.
4. Sheffield PJ. Tissue oxygen measurements. In: Problem wounds: role of oxygen. Davis JC, Hunt TK, eds. New York: Elsevier, 1988.
5. Brobeck JR, Dubois AB. Energy exchange. In: Medical physiology. 14th Ed. Mountcastle VB, ed. St. Louis: CV Mosby Co.,1980.
6. Holmstrom FMG. Hypoxia. In: Aerospace medicine. Randall HW, ed. Baltimore: Williams & Wilkins, 1971.
7. Meyers RAM Thom SR. Carbon monoxide and cyanide poisoning. In: Hyperbaric medicine practice. Kindwall EP, ed. Flagstaff AZ: Best Publishing, 1994;343–372.
8. Air Medical Service. War Department: Air Services Division of Military Aeronautics. Washington DC: Government Printing Office, 1919;423–434.
9. Bert P. Barometric pressure: researches in experimental physiology (1878) Hitchcock MA, Hitchcock FA, trans. Columbia OH: College Book Co., 1943.

Chapter 6

Protection in the Pressure Environment: Cabin Pressurization and Oxygen Equipment

Paul J. Sheffield and

Roger L. Stork

"... Certainly Sivel and Croce-Spinelli are not the first aeronauts whose loss science has had to deplore... But here, for the first time we saw two men die in the very bosom of the air, and die while ascending... The first to die in what we call the heavens.

And in a painful jest of fate, they died at the moment when science was furnishing them the means to triumph over the danger to which they fell victims."

Pastor Anthanase Conquel, Jr. 1875 (1)

In 1643, Evangelista Torricelli invented the barometer and first pondered the effects that lowered atmospheric pressures would have on living organisms. Man was not destined to have to deal with these effects until his dream of sustained, controlled flight became a reality in the beginning of the twentieth century. Continual striving for ever-higher flight has brought man face to face with an unchangeable truth: man is trapped within a body biologically adapted to a very narrow range of barometric pressures. In 1939, General Harry G. Armstrong, who later became the United States Air Force Surgeon General, wrote of the need for aircraft designed to pressurize the occupants during high altitude flight (2). It is becoming increasingly apparent that stratosphere, or even substratosphere, flying can never be carried out as a practical routine proce-

dure until there is a change in aircraft design which will maintain a more nearly normal pressure about the occupants.

The first successful pressurized cabin aircraft was the Lockheed XC-35, delivered to the U.S. Army Air Corps in 1939. It was developed to solve the problem of hypoxia. Several depressurizations occurred, some of which caused passengers to be drawn through the failed window or door. Because of repeated door latch failures, Lockheed Aircraft Company developed a "plugged door" that was fitted inside the skin of the aircraft. It could not be blown outwards because it was larger than the aperture.

Today, aircraft and spacecraft are designed to maintain a nearly normal pressure surrounding the occupant, but circumstances can cause a reduction in pressure outside the normal range of human tolerance.

This chapter focuses on the pressurization and oxygen equipment systems that protect aircraft occupants during high-altitude flight. The type of protective equipment is determined by the physiologic needs of the aviator at the peak altitude of exposure, as indicated by the physiologic zones of the pressure environment.

THE PRESSURE ENVIRONMENT

The pressure environment surrounding the earth can be divided into four zones based on physiologic effects: the physiologic zone, the physiologically deficient zone, the space-equivalent zone, and space.

The physiologic zone extends from sea level to approximately 3000 m (10,000 ft), encompassing the pressure area to which we are well adapted. Although middle ear or sinus problems may be experienced during ascent or descent in this zone, most physiologic problems occur outside this zone.

The physiologically deficient zone extends from altitudes of 3000 to 15,200 m (10,000 to 50,000 ft). Decreased barometric pressure reduces the partial pressure of inspired oxygen and causes altitude hypoxia. Protective oxygen equipment is mandatory in this zone. Additional problems may arise from trapped and evolved gases.

Flight between altitudes of 15,200 m and 200 km (50,000 ft and 120 mi) is in the space-equivalent zone. Total pressure progressively decreases from 87 to less than 1 mm Hg. Protection from low pressure is required for travel in this zone. Protection is provided by a sealed cabin or a full-pressure suit.

Altitudes beyond 200 km (120 mi) constitute space. Protection is provided by a sealed cabin or a full-pressure suit. Astronaut candidates earn astronaut status after flight above 80 km (50 mi). United States Air Force Major Robert M. White became the first winged aircraft pilot to be

awarded astronaut status for his X-15 flight to 95 km (59 mi) on July 17, 1962.

Advanced technology has allowed the aircraft industry to develop commercial and military aircraft that far exceed the physiologic tolerance of man. Such advancements include the ever-increasing service ceiling of civilian and military aircraft as well as manned space operations.

In general, the most effective way to prevent physiologic problems is to provide an aircraft pressurization system that limits the occupants' exposure to pressures found in the physiologic zone. In cases when ascent above the physiologic zone is required, protective oxygen equipment must be provided. At altitudes exceeding 15,200 m (50,000 ft), counterpressure garments are required.

AIRCRAFT AND SPACECRAFT PRESSURIZATION

Methods of Pressurization

As shown in Figure 6.1, there are two principal aircraft pressurization schedules: isobaric and isobaric-differential.

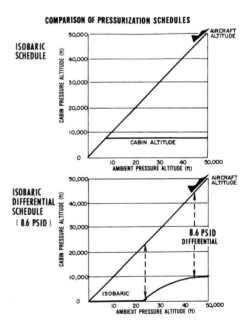

Figure 6.1. Isobaric and isobaric-differential aircraft pressurization schedules.

Isobaric System

Isobaric control maintains a constant cabin pressure as the ambient barometric pressure decreases. Many military and civilian aircraft are equipped with isobaric pressurization systems (e.g., the United States Air Force C-21, the Lockheed L-1011, the Boeing B-747 and the McDonnell Douglas MD 80). Cabin altitudes in these aircraft are maintained at 600 to 2400 m (2,000 to 8,000 ft).

Isobaric-Differential System

Tactical military aircraft are not equipped with isobaric pressurization systems because the added weight would limit the range of the aircraft, and the large pressure differential would increase the danger of a rapid decompression during combat operations. Instead, these aircraft are equipped with an isobaric-differential cabin pressurization system. Aircraft pressurization begins as the aircraft ascends through 1500 m to 2400 m (5,000 to 8,000 ft). The isobaric function controls cabin altitude until a pre-set pressure differential is reached. With continued ascent, the pre-set differential is maintained. Thus, cabin altitude progressively increases as the aircraft ascends. The aircraft featured in Figure 6.1 has an isobaric-differential pressurization system of 8.6 lb/in^2 differential (psid). If the aircraft were flying at 12,200 m (40,000 ft), ambient pressure would be 2.7 psi. Occupants of the aircraft would be exposed to a cabin pressure of 11.3 psi (8.6 psi plus 2.7 psi), a pressure equivalent to 2100 m (7,000 ft) altitude. For example, the United States Air Force C-141 cargo aircraft is equipped with an 8.6 psi isobaric-differential pressurization system. Cabin altitude is maintained at sea level pressure until the aircraft ascends through 6400 m (21,000 ft). Above this level, the system maintains a pressure differential of 8.6 psi up to the service ceiling of the aircraft.

In fighter aircraft, the isobaric-differential pressurization system is set at a lower pressure differential, typically 5 psid. The aircraft is unpressurized to an altitude of 2400 m (8,000 ft), where the isobaric control starts. As the aircraft continues to ascend, cabin pressure is maintained at 2400 m (8,000 ft) until 5 psid is reached. As the flight altitude continues to increase, so does the cabin altitude but at 5 psid.

Advantages of Pressurization

Aircraft must fly at high altitudes for fuel efficiency. Because aircraft pressurization systems are so effective, aviators can participate in high-altitude flight in safety and comfort. Supplemental oxygen equipment usually is not required. In some situations, however, it may be more advantageous for the pilot to use supplemental oxygen: during night flying operations, especially on final approach, emergencies involving loss of pressurization, and emergencies involving the presence of smoke or fumes. Flight rules require one pilot to use oxygen above certain altitudes, usually 13,700 m (45,000 ft), even though the aircraft is pressurized. With aircraft pressurization, the probability of decompression sickness is greatly reduced. Less gas expansion results in fewer gastrointestinal trapped-gas problems. Cabin humidity, temperature, air-flow, and the rate of pressure change can be controlled to acceptable comfort ranges. In multiplace aircraft, passengers and crew are free to move about the cabin unhampered by oxygen masks or special high-altitude support equipment. Thus, fatigue and discomfort are minimized during prolonged passenger flights.

Disadvantages of Pressurization

The primary disadvantage of aircraft pressurization is the possibility of loss of cabin pressure. Should a decompression occur, the occupants of the aircraft are rapidly exposed to the dangers of unpressurized high-altitude flight such as hypoxia, decompression sickness, gastrointestinal gas expansion, and hypothermia. Pressurized flight requires that the aircraft structure must be strengthened to maintain structural integrity. Additional equipment and power requirements are needed to support the aircraft pressurization system. This equipment occupies space, adds weight, and increases fuel costs. The peak performance and payload of the aircraft are decreased because of the added weight, and additional manpower and maintenance costs are involved. In addition, provisions must be made for controlling cabin air contaminants such as smoke, fumes, carbon monoxide, and carbon dioxide. Nonetheless, the advantages of aircraft pressurization far outweigh the disadvantages.

Physical Limitations of Pressurization Systems

A schematic of a typical pressurization system is shown in Figure 6.2. This system depends on air drawn from outside the aircraft being compressed and delivered to the cabin. The altitude limit is about 24,400 m (80,000 ft) on this type of system because of the inability of the compressor system to effectively pressurize the cabin in extremely low-pressure, high-altitude flight.

The mechanical ability of the compressor to provide pressure, ventilation, and air conditioning depends on the pressure ratio, P cabin/P ambient. This ratio is sometimes called the compression ratio and expresses the number of times that the ambient air must be compressed to maintain desired cabin pressure. For example, an aircraft at 14,000 m (46,000 ft) with a cabin altitude of 3000 m (10,000 ft) has a pressure ratio of 5:1 (10 psi to 2 psi). Thus, the air in

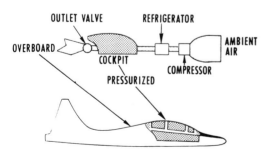

Figure 6.2. The pressurized cabin used in most conventional aircraft.

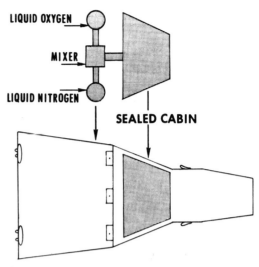

Figure 6.3. The sealed cabin used in spacecraft and shuttlecraft.

the cabin must be compressed to achieve a pressure five times greater than the ambient pressure. As flight altitude increases, the pressure ratio increases dramatically. For instance, an aircraft at 18,300 m (60,000 ft) with a cabin altitude of 3,000 m (10,000 ft) has a pressure ratio of 10:1 (10.1 psi to 1.05 psi).

At very high altitudes, the heat generated in the process of compressing air causes the cabin temperature to rise. For example, an aircraft at 22,900 m (75,000 ft) with a pressure ratio of 20:1 could achieve a cabin air temperature of about 315°C due to adiabatic heating. Thus, a highly efficient cooling system is required for crew survival.

As ascent continues, a point is eventually reached where the density of ambient air is so reduced that it is impossible for the compressor to draw in enough air to pressurize the cabin. Under such conditions, a sealed cabin must be used to maintain an acceptable crew environment. A sealed cabin must be used for sustained flight at altitudes above approximately 24,400 m (85,000 ft). As shown in Figure 6.3, pressurization is attained by the craft carrying its own supply of gases, usually oxygen and nitrogen. These gases are regulated in the proper proportion to provide the required pressure and gaseous environment within the cabin. Spacecraft are equipped with this type of system.

As with all aircraft components, the possibility of a mechanical failure of the system is always present. Failures in aircraft pressurization generally have been due to the failure of canopies, hatches, doors, windows, and their respective seals.

Decompression Rates

The severity and consequences of cabin pressure loss depend on the rate of decompression and the pressure range over which it occurs. Decompressions can be divided into two categories: slow and rapid. A slow loss of cabin pressure can occur when a leak develops in a pressure seal. If unaware of the depressurization, occupants could become incapacitated by hypoxia. A rapid decompression, as will soon become evident, is easily recognized. Three equations have been developed that estimate the time of decompression with varying degrees of accuracy.

Fliegner's equation (3) has been found to be useful as an approximation and is expressed as follows:

$$t = 0.22 \frac{V}{A} \sqrt{\frac{P - B}{B}}$$

where t is the time of decompression in seconds; V is the volume of the pressurized cabin in cubic feet; A is the cross-sectional area of the opening in square inches; P is the initial cabin pressure in psia; and B is the actual flight pressure altitude in psia.

Thus, several physical factors determine the time of decompression:

1. *Volume of the pressurized cabin (V)*—the larger the pressurized cabin, the slower the decompression when all other factors are equal.
2. *Size of the opening (A)*—the larger the opening, the faster the decompression. The principal factor that determines the rate and time

of decompression is the ratio between the volume of the cabin and the cross-sectional area of the opening.
3. *Pressure differential (P-B)*—the initial difference between the pressure within the cabin and the ambient pressure directly influences the rate and severity of the decompression. The greater the differential, the more severe the decompression.
4. *Pressure ratio (P/B)*—the time of decompression depends on the pressure ratio between the cabin and ambient pressures. The greater the pressure ratio, the longer the time of decompression.
5. *Flight pressure altitude (B)*—The physiologic problems that occur following a loss of cabin pressure are directly related to the altitude at which the decompression occurs.

Haber and Clamann (4) developed the general theory of rapid decompression, which offers a more complete analysis of both the decompression time and the process of a rapid decompression (4). In the Haber-Clamann model, the time of decompression depends essentially on two factors. One factor is the relationship between the volume of the cabin and the cross-sectional area of the opening of the cabin. The Haber-Clamann equation defines this relationship as the time-constant of the cabin (t_c) and expresses it as follows:

$$t_c = \frac{V}{AC}$$

where V is the volume of the cabin in cubic feet; A is the area of the opening in square feet; and C is the altitude dependent speed of sound. A value of about 1100 ft/sec can be used for the speed of sound.

The second factor on which the time of decompression depends is a pressure-dependent factor (P_1), a complex function (f) of the ratio (P-B)/P in which P is the cabin pressure before decompression and B is the ambient atmospheric pressure.

Table 6.1.
Pressure-Dependent Factor (P_1) in Decompression[a]

(P/B)	(P_1)	(P/B)	(P_1)
1	0	16	4.9
2	1.7	17	5.0
3	2.3	18	5.1
4	2.6	19	5.2
5	2.9	20	5.3
6	3.2	21	5.4
7	3.5	22	5.5
8	3.8	23	5.6
9	4.0	24	5.6
10	4.1	25	5.7
11	4.3	26	5.7
12	4.5	27	5.8
13	4.6	28	5.8
14	4.7	29	5.9
15	4.8	30	6.0

[a] The relationship between the pressure-dependent factor (P_1) is seen as a ratio of cabin pressure before decompression (P) to cabin pressure at the end of decompression (B). The pressure-dependent factor (P_1) for the total time of decompression (T) of the Haber-Clamann formula is derived from the absolute pressure ratio in the cabin before and after decompression (P/B).

$$P_1 = \frac{f(P - B)}{P}$$

The values for P_1 for any given pressure ratio up to 30 can be obtained from Table 6.1.

The total time of decompression (T) is equal to the product of the time-constant (t_c) and the pressure factor P_1 as follows:

$$T = t_c\, P_1$$

and

$$T = \frac{V}{AC} P_1$$

Thus, the total time of decompression can be estimated if the volume of the cabin, the effective opening area, and the initial and final cabin pressures are known.

Using metric units, Violette's Equation (3) provides another expression of the pressure rela-

tionships during the time of decompression (T) as follows:

$$T = \frac{V}{220A} Cosh^{-1}\frac{P}{B}$$

where V is the cabin volume in m^3, A is the effective orifice in m^2, P is the cabin pressure before decompression, and B is the ambient atmospheric pressure. Decompression rate calculations in Table 6.2 compare the Haber-Clamann, Fliegner and Violette equations.

Physical Characteristics of a Rapid Decompression

Noise
When two air masses collide, a noise is heard that ranges from a "swish" to an explosive sound.

Air Blast
Upon decompression, the rapid rush of air from a pressurized cabin causes the velocity of airflow through the cabin to increase rapidly as the outflow velocity at the orifice approaches the speed of sound. The force of the blast is very high close to the opening. When the decompression occurs, a sudden flow of air can raise flying debris. Loose objects, such as maps, charts, and furnishings, may be blown through the orifice. There have been instances of unrestrained people adjacent to and in the immediate vicinity of the opening being forcefully ejected from the aircraft. Dust and dirt may hamper vision for a short period of time.

Fogging
During a rapid decompression, sudden decreases in temperature and pressure reduce the capacity of air to contain water vapor and fogging may occur. The fog dissipates rapidly in fighter aircraft but considerably slower in aircraft with large cabin volumes.

Table 6.2.
Decompression Rate Calculations For Passenger Aircraft Following Loss of a Window

Factors	Haber-Clamann Formula	Fliegner's Formula	Violette's Formula
Cabin Volume	10,000 ft^3	10,000 ft^3	283 m^3
Area of opening	0.5 ft^2	72 in^2	0.0465 m^2
Time-constant	18.2 sec	—	—
Time of decompression			
From 3,000 ft (13.17 psi) to 25,000 ft (5.46 psi)	34.5 sec	36.3 sec	41.6 sec
From 5,000 ft (12.23 psi) to 40,000 ft (2.72 psi)	50.0 sec	50.4 sec	60.4 sec
From 8,000 ft (10.91 psi) to 45,000 ft (2.15 psi)	52.8 sec	61.7 sec	64.0 sec

Physiologic Effects of Rapid Decompression

The primary physiologic concerns in a rapid decompression are hypoxia, gas expansion, decompression sickness, and hypothermia.

Hypoxia

Of all the physiologic hazards associated with the loss of pressure, hypoxia is the most important. Thus, the most critical need after decompression is oxygen, especially if passengers were not breathing oxygen before the decompression. Rapid reduction of ambient pressure produces a corresponding drop in the partial pressure of oxygen and reduces the alveolar oxygen tension. Following rapid decompression, a significant performance decrement occurs, regardless of altitude. Reduced tolerance to hypoxia after decompression is due to interruption of normal oxygen transport in pulmonary and cardiovascular systems. The alveolar Po_2 falls to a value less than mixed venous Po_2 and reverses the direction of oxygen flow in the lung. This reduces arterial oxygen content and, subsequently, oxygen delivery to the brain and other tissues. Unless supplemental oxygen is acquired within 30 seconds after rapid decompression to 9100 m (30,000 ft), consciousness will be lost. During rapid decompression above 13,700 m (45,000 ft), it is unlikely that there would be enough time to don an oxygen mask.

Under certain flight conditions, it is necessary to wear an oxygen mask securely in place at all times. With the advent of masks that more effectively seal to the face, designers should provide for the relief of over-pressure that can occur during rapid decompression as gas expands in the mask.

Gas Expansion

The physiologic effects of gas expansion resulting from decompression occur primarily in the middle ears, sinuses, gastrointestinal tract and lungs. Chapter 7 (Decompression Sickness and Pulmonary Overpressure Accidents) includes a detailed discussion of these effects.

Decompression Sickness

A principal advantage of pressurized cabins is the protection they afford the aircrew against decompression sickness. In general, decompression sickness does not occur until cabin altitudes above 5500 m (18,000 ft) are reached. The incidence of decompression sickness is small unless the cabin altitude exceeds 7600 m (25,000 ft). As the duration of exposure to the unpressurized environment increases, however, so does the incidence of decompression sickness.

Hypothermia

When decompression occurs, the temperature drops to that of ambient air. Chilling and frostbite could easily occur if proper protective clothing, boots, and gloves were not worn.

Oxygen Equipment

The flyer who is suffering from want of oxygen is far from normal. He may be exhilarated, he may be simply dull and sleepy, or, if he is in a position of danger he may fail to take the measures necessary for the safety of himself and those with him, even when he is well aware of the danger.

. . . [T]he aviator supplied with oxygen while flying is very much more efficient than the same man flying without oxygen, and becomes, therefore, of so much more value as a fighting force. Take, for example, two pilots of equal ability, flying machines being identical in every respect, that man supplied with oxygen will always bring down the other machine because he has retained all his judgement and rapidity of decision and movement unimpaired. He will be able to outmaneuver and outwit his opponent and fire his gun before the other has even made up his mind what to do. Not only that, when he returns to the ground after prolonged flight he will be fresh and able to start out on a new trip, while the man flying without oxygen will be tired out and unable to do any more work that day and possibly the next. The administration of oxygen must of course in no way impair the comfort or the movements of the airman, nor should he have anything further to do while flying, as he already has plenty to look after, in his machine. For this reason the apparatus used must be simple, safe, and entirely automatic; automatic in the sense that while the machine stands on the ground no oxygen is given off, but when it rises in the air the increasing deficiency in the oxygen content of the air is automatically made up for by the delivery of oxygen by the apparatus, without any personal attention from the airman.

This message to the flyer was published in 1919 by the United States War Department (5). Thus, the need for protective oxygen equipment was recognized early in the history of aviation.

Design Requirements

Historically, aircraft oxygen system development paralleled that of aircraft performance. The continuous flow "pipestem" oxygen system

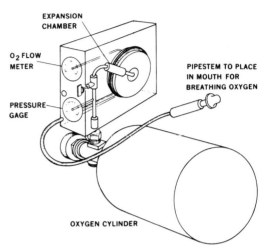

Figure 6.4. The "pipestem" oxygen system used by early aviators.

(Fig. 6.4) was used by early aviators. Protection was limited because of difficulty in maintaining the pipestem between the teeth, inadequate accommodation for nose breathers, and wasted oxygen due to continuous flow. The first practical automatic oxygen delivery system was the Dreyer apparatus (Fig. 6.5), that was designed by Colonel Georges Dreyer for the British Royal Air Force. By 1919, it had been adapted to all United States planes flying to high altitudes (5). The apparatus provided 500 L of gaseous oxygen in two steel bottles at 2200 psi. An aneroid-controlled valve delivered 100% oxygen in increasing quantities during ascent. The india rubber oronasal mask that attached to the flyer's leather helmet also contained a microphone for communication.

General specifications for aircrew breathing gas delivery systems were published by Captain G. B. Obear of the Army Air Service in 1920 (6).

". . . (1) The apparatus at any given altitude should deliver automatically to the aviator sufficient oxygen to supply the deficit at altitude. This is equivalent to bringing the aviator back to sea level physiologically. (2) At all times the aviator should be able to determine the amount of reserve oxygen. (3) The aviator should have some

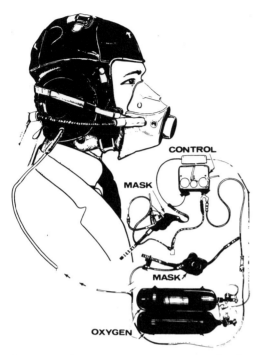

Figure 6.5. The Dreyer oxygen apparatus, the first practical automatic oxygen delivery system.

visible evidence that the oxygen is flowing freely. (4) The instrument should be as small in volume and weight as possible. . . ''

As aircraft performance increased, so did the sophistication of the breathing gas delivery system. The aviator's physiologic requirement must be satisfied under a wide range of conditions, e.g., altitude, acceleration, workload, temperature, and psychological stress. Thus, system testing must occur under simulated operational conditions across the full range of anticipated use. Today there are international standards and agreements that outline the steps to test and man-rate the system. Consensus air standards are published by the Air Standardization Coordinating Committee (ASCC). Standardization Agreements (STANAGs) are published by the North Atlantic Treaty Organization (NATO).

Oxygen Systems

An aircraft oxygen system usually consists of (1) containers for the storage of oxygen either in a gaseous, liquid, or solid state; (2) tubing to direct the flow of oxygen from the source to a metering device or regulator; (3) regulators or metering devices that control the pressure and percentage of oxygen available to the user; and (4) an oronasal or full face mask to deliver oxygen to the user.

Gaseous Oxygen

Aviator's gaseous oxygen is classified as grade A, type I oxygen. Military systems must adhere to military specifications for oxygen that require 99.5% purity by volume and no more than 0.005 mg/L of water vapor at 760 mm Hg and 15°C. Hospital-grade oxygen is not acceptable for use in aviation because of its moisture content. Low water vapor content is critical because the temperature encountered at high altitude would cause freezing and restrict oxygen flow. Gaseous oxygen also must be odorless and free of contaminants, including drying agents. Gaseous oxygen can be delivered either by a low-pressure or high-pressure system.

The storage system for a low-pressure gaseous oxygen system usually consists of light-weight, nonshatterable cylinders, which are color-coded yellow. When fully charged, these cylinders can hold 450 psi. Under normal conditions, they are considered full at a range of 400 to 450 psi. The major limitation of the low-pressure system is its small volume. The system is considered empty at pressures below 100 psi. Should the pressure drop below 50 psi, the system must be purged to prevent a buildup of moisture.

For emergency use, most commercial aircraft rely on high-pressure gas cylinders. Most fighter, bomber, and training aircraft use high-pressure oxygen as a backup breathing system. High-pressure oxygen is contained in nonshatterable cylinders filled to a pressure of 1800 to 2200 psi. Cylinders of this type are color-coded green, are heavy, and have the advantage of storing large amounts of oxygen in a small space.

Liquid Oxygen

Aviator's liquid oxygen (LOX) is classified as grade B, type II. Military specifications require

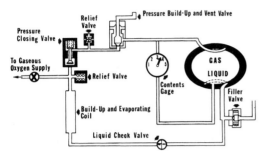

Figure 6.6. Liquid oxygen converter flow diagram.

99.5% purity and no more than 0.005 mg/L of water vapor at 760 mm Hg and 15°C. The boiling point of LOX is -182.8°C, and its expansion ratio is 1 to 850 ± 10 L at 760 mm Hg and 21.1°C. Thus, 1 L of liquid oxygen provides 840 to 860 L of gaseous oxygen. Liquid oxygen is produced from compressing and cooling ordinary filtered air. The liquid air produced is then warmed slowly to -195.6°C, at which point nitrogen vaporizes, leaving liquid oxygen. The entire process is repeated several times to ensure the production of nearly pure liquid oxygen. Gaseous oxygen is then produced by allowing the liquid to evaporate.

Military fighter and training aircraft usually operate with an oxygen converter pressure of 70 to 90 psi. Multiplace aircraft routinely maintain a converter pressure of 300 psi. This higher pressure is necessitated by the increased number of crew and passenger positions and by the need for a readily available oxygen source for recharging portable oxygen cylinders.

For the majority of aircraft in use today, the LOX system is superior to the gaseous oxygen system. The oxygen capacity of a single 25-L converter is equal to about 105 6.9-ft^3 bottles of high-pressure gaseous oxygen. Liquid oxygen has about a 3.5 to 1 weight advantage over a gaseous oxygen system and an 8 to 1 advantage in terms of space saved. A typical liquid oxygen converter flow diagram is shown in Figure 6.6.

Solid Chemical Production of Oxygen

Chemical generation of oxygen offers several advantages over gaseous systems: self-contain-

ment, easy storage, simple flow regulation, and a 20-year shelf life. Once activated, however, the generator continues to produce oxygen until the chemical agent is depleted.

Presently, chemical combinations, or solid-state oxygen systems, are limited to emergency use by passengers in military and civilian aircraft. The system consists of a continuous flow breathing mask with lanyards connected to actuating pins of a sodium chlorate candle or some similar oxygen-producing device. Upon removal of the mask and actuation of the pins, a chemical reaction is initiated. One such candle utilizes the following chemical reaction:

$$NaClO_3 + Fe \rightarrow FeO + NaCl + O_2$$

To begin the chemical process, heat is provided to an iron-enriched area by the percussion cap, or friction igniter. When the temperature of the reaction rises above 250°C, the process is self-supporting, and the reaction proceeds down the length of the candle. The amount of oxygen produced depends on the size and burning rate of the candle. The sodium chlorate candle shown in Figure 6.7 is typical.

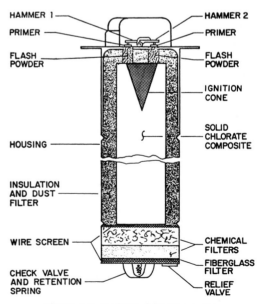

Figure 6.7. Sodium chlorate candle.

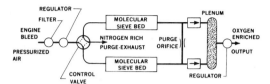

Figure 6.8. Molecular sieve oxygen generator.

Onboard Oxygen Generation System (OBOGS)

The concept of producing oxygen in flight has long been attractive. The OBOGS concept offers the benefits of increased operational safety and reduced logistic support of the oxygen system. Several OBOGS systems have been examined (e.g., electrochemical concentration, fluomine chemical absorption, molecular sieve, and permeable membrane systems). Molecular sieve oxygen concentration was selected as the system of choice.

Molecular Sieve

Oxygen can be produced for aircrews by a molecular sieve (Fig. 6.8). This system uses pressurized air from a stage of the turbine engine compressor that is distributed to alternating molecular sieve beds. Each molecular sieve contains crystalline aluminosilicate compounds called zeolites. As pressurized air is passed through the bed, the mixture is separated into its components. The oxygen-enriched portion is then separated out and temporarily stored in a plenum. From the plenum, oxygen is then provided to the breathing regulator. The major disadvantage of this system is the presence of impurities. At best, the operational units can only provide up to 95% oxygen, with 5% argon present. Recent laboratory developments using carbon molecular seives produced greater than 99% oxygen.

Oxygen Contaminants

Control of contaminants has been a concern since the first oxygen system was developed for high altitude balloon flights in the 1870s. M.

Limousin, a distinguished French pharmacist, provided the oxygen system for the balloon, Zenith. On April 15, 1875, two of the balloon's three aeronauts died from hypoxia at an altitude of about 8600 m (28,200 ft).

"... To neutralize as much as possible the detestable smell which the greased goldbeaters' skin (ox stomach) gave the gaseous mixture, I put in for each balloonist very small wash bottles provided with a curved tube furnished with rubber so that they could be held in the mouth like a pipe, leaving the hands free to put down observations in a notebook. With this arrangement the gas, passing through water flavored with benzoin, reached the lungs fresh and perfumed..."
(1)

Generally speaking, breathing gas contaminants are divided into five types: solid inert contaminants, dissolved inert contaminants, toxic substances, odor-producing contaminants, and combustible contaminants. Solid inert contaminants are small, insoluble particles that do not react with liquid oxygen. These particles range from rust and metal fragments to frozen carbon dioxide and ice. Nitrogen and argon are considered dissolved inert contaminants. They are unreactive and are soluble in liquid oxygen. Toxic substances usually are found in such low concentrations that they rarely present a problem. Odor-causing contaminants are of great concern, and their presence must be kept as low as possible. Even though they may be nontoxic, they can lead to nausea, anxiety, and decreased performance. Examples of combustible contaminants are methane, ethane, acetylene, and ethylene.

Several sources of contamination are possible for aviator's breathing oxygen. In the production of liquid oxygen, the air used contains 78.03% nitrogen, 20.99% oxygen, and 0.94% argon by volume. The remaining 0.04% is a composite of carbon dioxide, helium, neon, krypton, xenon, and various hydrocarbons such as methane and acetylene. Carbon monoxide, hydrogen sulfide, hydrogen cyanide, nitrous oxides, and ammonia also are found in trace amounts. In addition to trace gaseous contaminants, solid particles can be introduced by worn valves, pumps, and filters. Refrigerants and solvents used in the oxygen production plant can also be found. Furthermore, contaminants can be introduced during the transfer of liquid oxygen to storage facilities. When supply hoses are initially connected, atmospheric contaminants may be present and could be carried into the converter via the moving liquid. Contaminants may enter the disconnected transfer hose and enter the system in the next recharging cycle. All of these possible contaminants must be vigorously controlled to protect the aviator.

Oxygen Regulators

The type of regulator used determines the overall capability of the oxygen delivery system. Three basic oxygen delivery systems are used in aircraft: continuous flow, diluter demand, and pressure demand.

Continuous-Flow Oxygen Systems

Although the continuous-flow oxygen system is no longer widely used in military aircraft, it is available in many civilian aircraft. Continuous-flow oxygen systems provide protection for passengers up to an operational altitude of 7600 m (25,000 ft). It provides an emergency ''get-me-down'' capability for altitudes up to 9100 m (30,000 ft). The regulators used in this system provide a continuous flow of 100% oxygen. The three major types of regulators are manual, automatic, and automatic with manual override.

Manual continuous-flow oxygen regulators can be adjusted to meet user requirements according to the altitude of exposure. The regulator valve is calibrated in thousands of feet and is adjusted to reflect that altitude. The primary function of the regulator is to reduce the inlet pressure to a reasonable range and to provide a flow to the breathing mask.

Automatic continuous-flow oxygen regulators are used in both military and civilian air-craft. As the altitude increases, the flow of oxygen gradually increases through the action of the aneroid.

Automatic oxygen regulators with manual override offer a major advantage over other automatic continuous-flow regulators because in an emergency situation, an extra flow of oxygen can be obtained. This type of regulator would include a pressure guage and a manual override selector. When the user inserts the breathing mask connector, an aneroid automatically delivers 100% oxygen at the correct flow rate. When additional oxygen is required, the manual override can be operated on three different settings to provide increased flow.

Diluter-Demand Oxygen Systems

When operational altitude increased above 7600 m (25,000 ft), it became evident that continuous-flow oxygen systems could not provide the required physiologic protection. This requirement resulted in the development of diluter-demand system, which allows oxygen to flow only on inspiration. The diluter feature mixes ambient air with oxygen to achieve a gradual increase in oxygen percentage as altitude increases, until 10,400 m (34,000 ft) is reached, where the regulator provides 100% oxygen. This system has an operational altitude ceiling of 10,700 m (35,000 ft) and an emergency ceiling of 12,200 m (40,000 ft).

Pressure-Demand Oxygen Systems

High-performance aircraft routinely fly above 12,200 m (40,000 ft) altitude. At these altitudes, even when 100% oxygen is breathed, the oxygen content of the blood is decreased below normal levels, unless positive pressure breathing is also applied. This can be achieved by a pressure-demand oxygen system. The range of pressure is limited due to the susceptibility of lungs to damage from elevated pressures. Nonetheless, it is adequate for routine operational ceilings of 13,100 m (43,000 ft), with an emergency ceiling of up to 15,200 m (50,000 ft) for short periods of time. The regulators used in this system are

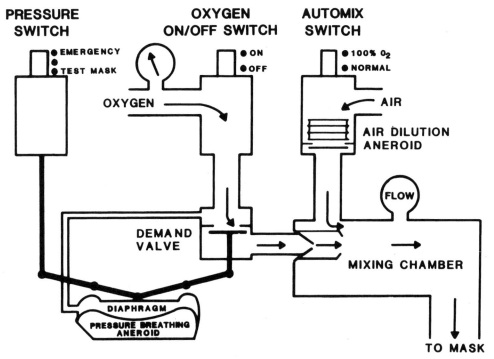

Figure 6.9. Schematic of Automatic Pressure Demand Oxygen Regulator.

slightly different from those used in diluter-demand systems, but they function in the same manner until the positive pressure portion is activated.

Automatic Pressure-Demand Oxygen Regulator

The automatic pressure-demand oxygen regulator (Fig. 6.9) has an aneroid that automatically provides the prescribed oxygen and positive pressure at a given altitude. The regulator functions exactly as a diluter-demand regulator when the normal setting on the oxygen dilution (automix) is selected. On the normal setting at sea level, the regulator's ambient air port is open so that air is provided to the user. As altitude increases, an aneroid senses the change in barometric pressure and gradually closes the ambient air port, thereby increasing the fraction of oxygen. As the user approaches 10,000 m (34,000 ft) the aneroid completely closes the ambient air port and 100% oxygen is delivered to the user. At 8,500 to 11,600 m (28,000 to 38,000 ft), de-

pending on the type of regulator, oxygen is provided to the user under continuous positive pressure. When the oxygen automix is set to 100% oxygen, the ambient air port is closed and 100% oxygen is delivered to the user, regardless of altitude. With the use of positive pressure breathing for $+G_z$ acceleration protection (PBG), oxygen regulators have been developed to automatically deliver PBG at preset aircraft acceleration levels.

Mask-Mounted Pressure-Demand Oxygen Regulator

Small pressure-demand oxygen regulators have been incorporated into quick-don masks used by transport crews in aircraft like the C-12 and C-21. The regulator uses a two- or three-position control knob or lever to select between "normal," "100% oxygen," or "emergency." In the "normal" setting, automatic dilution of oxygen occurs. In the "emergency" setting, the regulator delivers 100% oxygen plus a slight positive pressure (Fig. 6.10).

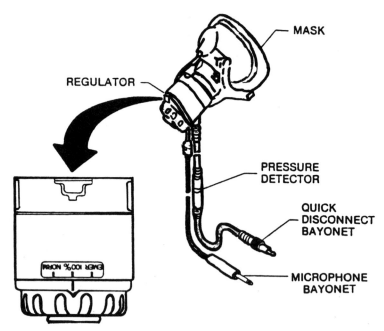

REGULATOR —

MASK

PRESSURE DETECTOR

QUICK DISCONNECT BAYONET

MICROPHONE BAYONET

Figure 6.10. Mask Mounted Pressure Demand Regulator.

Chest-Mounted Pressure-Demand Oxygen Regulator

This small pressure-demand oxygen regulator is designed to fit in the dovetail mounting block of the parachute harness or shoulder strap of the restraint system. Cabin air is automatically mixed with 100% oxygen based on cabin altitude. A manual control knob allows the user to select either 100% oxygen or an emergency pressure setting. It automatically delivers 100% oxygen at 9100 m (30,000 ft) and positive pressure at 10,700 m (35,000 ft). This regulator has an operational ceiling of 13,100 m (43,000 ft) and an emergency limit of 15,200 m (50,000 ft). It also has an antisuffocation device that warns the user if he has become disconnected from the system.

Portable Oxygen Systems

Portable oxygen assemblies are used by crew members who need to move about the cabin unincumbered by long oxygen supply hoses. Portable oxygen systems are also used during emergency escape from the aircraft. Both high and low pressure systems are used.

Pressure-Demand Portable Assembly

The pressure-demand portable assembly consists of a low-pressure gaseous cylinder coupled with a pressure-demand regulator. The system is charged to 425 ± 25 psi and provides 100% oxygen up to 9100 m (30,000 ft). At higher altitudes, the pressure control valve can be operated manually to achieve positive pressure breathing.

High-Pressure Portable Systems

Although not widely used, the high-pressure portable systems are found on some military and civilian aircraft. The system consists of a 1800 to 2200 psi high-pressure cylinder, diluter-demand regulator, oxygen pressure gauge, and flow indicator. At 7600 m (25,000 ft) the system provides the user with about 50 minutes of oxygen in the NORMAL setting and about 40 minutes of oxygen on the 100% setting.

Emergency Oxygen Cylinders

Portable oxygen systems are used as an emergency source of oxygen during primary system failure, system depletion, or for egress from the aircraft. The assembly is charged at 1800 to 2200 psi and provides approximately 8 to 10 minutes of oxygen supply. This is enough oxygen to eject from an aircraft and descend in a parachute from an altitude of 15,200 m (50,000 ft). The system can be activated manually by pulling the ball handle, or ''green apple.'' It is automatically activated during an ejection sequence.

On some military transport aircraft, the emergency oxygen cylinder is used in a passenger oxygen kit (POK). In this configuration, it is provided with a continuous flow mask (Dixie Cup) for use by passengers in the event of aircraft decompression.

Oxygen Masks

One of the most critical features in the oxygen supply system is the breathing mask. Significant reductions in oxygen delivery occur with an improperly fitted or poorly designed mask.

Continuous-Flow Masks

A multitude of masks can be used on a continuous-flow system. Most of them work on the same general principle: oxygen enters the mask from a reservoir bag, and with each inhalation from the reservoir bag, oxygen is replaced. Most of these masks mix 100% oxygen with ambient air. The most common example of a continuous-flow mask is found in commercial passenger aircraft (Fig. 6.11). These masks are usually stored in the overhead bin or in the seat back facing each passenger.

Pressure-Demand Masks

Unlike diluter-demand masks, the pressure-demand masks have the capability to hold positive pressure. A face seal allows the mask to form a pressure seal. The mask contains an inhalation/exhalation valve that allows oxygen to enter the mask upon inhalation and holds the positive pressure until exhalation pressure overrides the regulator pressure.

Pressure-Breathing Oxygen Mask

Initial pressure-breathing oxygen mask designs were distinctive because they incorporated a rigid exoskeleton in addition to the face form. They included a combined inhalation/exhalation valve, microphone, and associated mask attach-

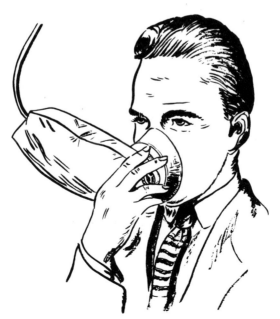

Figure 6.11. Passenger Oxygen mask with reservoir bag.

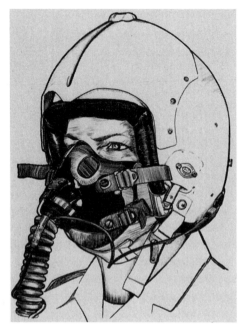

Figure 6.12. Typical pressure-breathing oxygen mask.

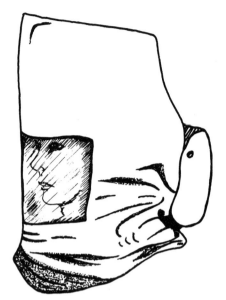

Figure 6.13. Emergency escape breathing device.

ment assembly. The exhalation valve allows exhalation to take place when the internal mask pressure exceeds the pressure being supplied to the mask by about 1 mm Hg. Figure 6.12 is a typical pressure-breathing oxygen mask.

Quick-Don Pressure-Demand Mask Assembly

The quick-don pressure-demand assembly utilizes the standard pressure-breathing oxygen mask but adds a quick-donning harness. This system is used in multiplace aircraft where the routine use of oxygen equipment is not required. Should an emergency arise, the crew can put on the oxygen mask in a minimum amount of time, unencumbered by the need for a flight helmet.

Emergency Escape Breathing Device (EEBD)

The EEBD provides respiratory and eye protection to the user in oxygen-deficient, smoke-laden, or other toxic atmospheres (Fig. 6.13). This device consists of a loose-fitting hood with a neck seal. Unlike a face-piece or mouthbit de-

sign, use of the hood permits oral communication without compromising protection. Originally designed for use on board naval vessels, the EEBD is intended for one-time use and is not rechargeable. A 15-minute supply of oxygen is furnished by a solid-state chemical oxygen generator, attached to the hood behind the neck.

Civil and Commercial Aircraft Crew and Passenger Oxygen Systems

Pressurized or unpressurized aircraft that routinely fly at altitudes greater than 3000 m (10,000 ft) usually have a permanently installed oxygen system. Light aircraft that fly below 3000 m (10,000 ft) usually have portable oxygen equipment. Because of the restricted size and weight of the portable system, the duration of the oxygen supply is limited.

In general and commercial aviation, there has been a dramatic increase in the number of aircraft (Table 6.3) requiring supplemental oxygen systems for flights in the range of 3700 to 15,200 m (12,000 to 50,000 ft). These aircraft are equipped with the least expensive oxygen systems available that meet minimum physiologic needs, usually a continuous-flow system.

Table 6.3.
Commercial Aircraft Oxygen Systems

Oxygen Equipment	Number of Outlets	Capacity-Cubic feet	Capacity-Liters	Hours Duration (One User)	Altitude Ceiling (above MSL) Meters
Puritan-Bennett					
2P 202	2	11	311	1.7	6700
2P 202	2	15	424.5	2.4	6700
2P 202	2	22	623	3.4	6700
2P 204	4	22	623	3.4	6700
2P 204	4	38	1025	5.9	6700
2P 400	4	22	623	3.86	6100
Scott Aviation					
Mark I	1	11	311	3.13	5000
Mark II	1	22	623	6.2	5000
Mark III	2	22	623	5.0	5800
Rajay Sky Ox					
Sk 9–20	2	20	566	6.2	6100
Sk 10–20	4	20	566	6.2	6100
Sk 9–35	2	35	990	7.5	6100
Sk 10–35	4	35	990	7.5	6100
Sk 9–50	2	50	1415	10.7	6100
Sk 10–50	4	50	1415	10.7	6100
Fluid Power					
Model 2500	2	10.6	300	2	7600

Data modified from Silitch MF. Oxygen to go. AOPA Pilot, January, 1981.

The solid chemical generation of oxygen is being used increasingly in private aircraft, general aviation, and commercial jumbo jets. Portable units are used primarily in private aircraft, whereas permanent units are used in commercial aircraft. The location of these units varies. In the Lockheed L-1011, the units are overhead; in the Airbus Industries A-300B, the units are located in the back of the passenger seat; and in the McDonnell-Douglas DC-10, the units may be in other locations. Each oxygen-generating unit is activated when the mask is removed from its housing or is pulled toward the face. Either action will activate a spring-loaded firing mechanism and initiate the flow of oxygen. Some units are activated by an electrical squib instead of a mechanical percussion mechanism. Masks are presented to the user when cabin altitude ascends to 4300 $\pm$ 150 m (14,000 $\pm$ 500 ft).

Some commercial air carriers use high-pressure reduction regulators and automatic aneroids set for 4300 m (14,000 ft). Upon automatic activation, oxygen pressure in the lines opens the don latch in the mask housing compartment. Oxygen flow to the mask is initiated by removal of the mask from the compartment and pulling on the supply hose to disconnect a pin. Depending on the altitude, an aneroid determines the liter flow per minute.

These continuous flow systems generally use a rebreather mask or a phase sequential type mask. Rebreather masks dilute 100% oxygen with air in the rebreather bag. Further mixing takes place upon inhalation through air inlet holes in the face piece. During exhalation, some of the air is forced back into the rebreather bag and the oxygen concentration never reaches 100%, limiting its effectiveness to about 7600 m (25,000 ft). The rebreather mask is a low-cost, universal-fit mask, but it offers only minimal hypoxia protection. Carbon dioxide can accumulate in the rebreather bag, and the mask offers no protection against the inhalation of smoke or fumes.

The phase sequential mask also has a reservoir bag, but there is a check valve between the reservoir bag and the mask. Upon inhalation, the user is provided 100% oxygen from the reservoir bag. During exhalation, the flow of oxygen fills the bag. The check valve prevents exhaled air from entering the reservoir bag, thus assuring 100% oxygen concentration for inhalation. These masks are effective up to 10,700 m (35,000 ft) and are approved for air carrier passenger use up to 12,200 m (40,000 ft). The mask is expensive and has an inadequate suspension system, but it is effective.

Pressure Suits

". . . In five minutes he was at the equivalent of 26,000 ft. In 30 minutes he was at 80,000 ft. and in 50 minutes he was at 90,000 ft. After a few minutes he was brought down none the worse for the experiment."

The above quotation came from Professor J.S. Haldane on November 27, 1933, as he described the first successful test of a high-altitude pressure suit that he had built as a modified diving suit (7).

In 1934, Wiley Post made the world's first flight in a pressure suit. He flew approximately 25 hours on several flights up to 14,900 m (49,000 ft) in the pressure suit he designed to aid him in an attempt to break the transcontinental speed record. Although he set no records, these flights set the stage for the development of a variety of counterpressure garments and pressure suit assemblies designed to protect aviators during high-altitude and space flight.

The purpose of the counterpressure garment is as follows:

1. To protect against hypoxic hypoxia.
2. To prevent rupture of the lungs under high positive pressure breathing. The possibility of lung damage is greatly increased with breathing pressures of 60 to 100 mm Hg.
3. To prevent the undesirable effects of pressure

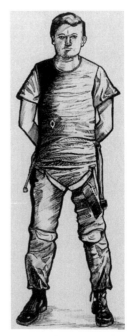

Figure 6.14. British jerkin and anti-G suit.

breathing (See Chapter 5). It is undesirable to apply more than 40 mm Hg positive breathing pressure without counterpressure.

For brief exposures of approximately 1 minute at a maximum altitude of 21,300 m (70,000 ft), "get-me-down" counterpressure garments such as the British pressure jerkin (Fig. 6.14) can be used. For prolonged exposures, either a partial-pressure suit (Fig. 6.15) or a full-pressure suit (Fig. 6.16) is required.

In 1947, the United States Air Force was asked to develop a practical, operational, partial-pressure suit system, while the United States Navy was assigned the task of developing the full-pressure suit. Since that time, many designs from various countries have been developed, but they can all be categorized according to these three basic types of protective systems.

Get-Me-Down Systems

A get-me-down counterpressure garment is used to protect the pilot from unconsciousness due to

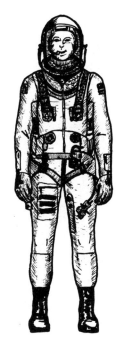

Figure 6.15. NASA launch-entry partial-pressure suit.

hypoxia. These systems usually provide less than one minute of protection at the peak altitude and require descent to 12,200 m (40,000 ft) within one to three minutes (8). Key components of get-me-down systems are a pressure demand mask, a torso vest, and an anti-G suit. The pressure breathing mask may be required to deliver pressures in excess of 60 to 100 mm Hg in order to maintain adequate alveolar oxygen pressure. A torso vest or jerkin (Fig. 6.14) provides chest counterpressure to balance the high breathing pressure. An anti-G suit usually inflated at a ratio of 3 to 4 times breathing pressure, reduces the pooling of blood in the abdomen and legs that would otherwise result from sustained pressure breathing and torso counter-pressure. At the moment of decompression, any part of the body lacking counterpressure protection will be subjected to hemodynamic disturbances (e.g., blood pooling, swelling due to separation of gas from tissue, and peripheral vasoconstriction due to cold). Since get-me-down systems do not protect against decompression sickness or cold temperatures, these physiological concerns will limit

their use. The major shortfall, however, is the short duration of protection that necessitates immediate descent following rapid decompression.

Partial-Pressure Suit

The partial-pressure suit is form-fitted by adjusting laces on the sleeves, chest, back, and legs of the suit. The suit contains a torso bladder that covers the wearer completely except for the arms and lower legs. Bladders on the suit exterior, called capstans, extend down the back and along the arms and legs. The capstans are attached to the suit by means of crossing tapes sewn to the suit in a figure eight such that when the capstans inflate, the fabric of the suit is drawn tight against the body of the wearer. When inflated, the capstan pressure must be five times the desired counterpressure. For example, should the user require a breathing pressure of 100 mm Hg (approximately 2 psi), the suit must be balanced by 2 psi of counterpressure; thus, 10 psi must be supplied to the capstan. A dual function regulator in the seat of the aircraft provides the needed oxygen breathing pressure and capstan pressure.

A full-pressure suit helmet is worn with the partial pressure suit for reasons of comfort. It is sealed at the neck to provide breathing oxygen and increased pressure to the entire head. The overall objective is to supply the proper amount of counterpressure to balance the breathing pressure required to prevent hypoxia at a given altitude. An example is the launch entry suit (Fig. 6.15), a partial-pressure suit used during launch and re-entry in the space transportation system (NASA shuttle). The launch entry suit consists of a helmet and counterpressure/antiexposure suit that is integrated into one unit. It is designed to sustain the crewmember at or below 30,500 m (100,000 ft) altitude for a period of 30 minutes. The lower extremity bladder system can independently provide gravity protection.

Full-Pressure Suits

The full-pressure suit is designed to provide a safe environment or counterpressure by surrounding the entire body with a pressurized gas envelope. These suits allow mobility, comfort, and protection of the user.

In normal operational U-2 and TR-1 missions, a 3.5 psi full-pressure suit is unpressurized when the aviator is exposed to altitudes below 10,700 m (35,000 ft). If this altitude is exceeded by aircraft ascent or loss of pressurization, the suit-mounted controller automatically inflates the suit to a given pressure, which, when added to the atmospheric pressure at that altitude, will equal 3.5 psi. Thus, the aviator wearing a 3.5 psi full-pressure suit is never exposed to a pressure altitude greater than 10,700 m (35,000 ft) regardless of aircraft altitude. Oxygen for breathing is supplied under a slight positive pressure directly to the helmet oronasal breathing cavity, which is separated from the rear of the helmet by a close-fitting face barrier. The slight positive pressure is necessary to help prevent carbon dioxide from accumulating in the front of the helmet and to prevent the user from experiencing negative breathing pressures.

Because the suit is airtight, body heat can become a severe problem. As a result, a suit ventilation system is provided to pick up body heat and moisture. Thermal regulation in some designs is achieved by a flow of air, whereas other designs use circulating fluids in the tubing network woven in the undergarment. To maintain fluid balance, the aviator can ingest liquids through a small orifice in the helmet shell. An example of a full-pressure suit is the one used to explore the lunar surface (Fig. 6.16).

SUMMARY

Humans, indeed, perform well in a very narrow range of barometric pressures. As discussed in Chapter 5, hypoxic (altitude) hypoxia is prevented by maintaining an alveolar oxygen tension range of between 60 and 100 mm Hg. Dur-

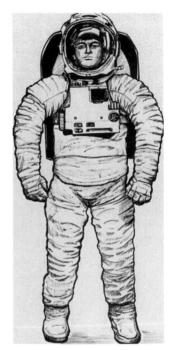

Figure 6.16. ILC Dover full-pressure suit used to explore the lunar surface.

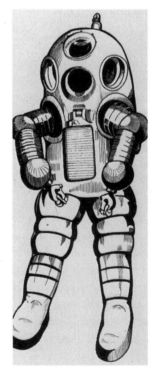

Figure 6.17. Jims suit used to explore the ocean depths.

ing high-altitude flight, the logical way to provide this level of alveolar oxygenation is to use supplemental oxygen, to maintain effective cabin pressurization, or to combine the two. In many aircraft, cabin altitude is maintained below 3000 m (10,000 ft), and supplemental oxygen equipment is readily available for all occupants should the cabin pressurization system fail. In fighter-type aircraft, cabin altitude often exceeds 3000 m (10,000 ft) up to a maximum altitude of 7600 m (25,000 ft), requiring continuous use of oxygen equipment to prevent hypoxia. To prevent hypoxia at cabin altitudes above 3000 m (10,000 ft), supplemental oxygen must be used. Above 10,400 m (34,000 ft), it is necessary to breathe 100% oxygen under increasingly higher pressures. As one continues to ascend, a point is reached at about 15,200 m (50,000 ft) where the oxygen is driven into the lungs under such force that lung damage will occur unless external counterpressure is applied against the chest. Equipped with proper counterpressure garments and life-support units, man has been able to perform effectively in the extreme pressure envi-

ronments extending from a complete vacuum on the lunar surface (Fig. 6.16) to an excess of 40 atm of pressure on the ocean floor (Fig. 6.17).

REFERENCES

1. Bert P. Barometric pressure, researches in experimental physiology (1878). Hitchcock MA Hitchcock FA. Columbus, OH: College Book Company, 1943; 969–972.
2. Armstrong HG, ed. Principles and practice of aviation medicine. Baltimore: Williams & Wilkins Co., 1939.
3. Fryer DI. Failure of the pressure cabin. In: Gillies JA, ed. Textbook of aviation physiology. New York: Pergamon Press, 1965;187–206.
4. Haber F Clamman HG. Physics and engineering of rapid decompression. Project No 21-1201-0008 Report 3, AD 20–374. Randolph Field, TX: USAF School of Aviation Medicine, 1953;1–29.
5. Air Medical Service. War Department: Air Services Division of Military Aeronautics. Washington, D.C.: Government Printing Office, 1919; 423–434.
6. Silitch MF. Oxygen to go. AOPA Pilot, 1981;24(1): 53–61.
7. Wilson CL. Emergency pressurization of aerospace crews. In: Randell HW, ed. Aerospace medicine. 2nd Ed. Baltimore: Williams & Wilkins Co., 1971.
8. Sharp GR. The pressure cabin. In: Dhenin G Ernsting J. Aviation medicine. London: Tri-Med Books Ltd., 1978; 151–175.

Chapter 7

Decompression Sickness and Pulmonary Overpressure Accidents

Richard D. Heimbach,

Paul J. Sheffield

I shall add on this occasion . . . what may seem somewhat strange,
what I once observed in a Viper . . . in our Exhausted Receiver,
namely that it had manifestly a conspicuous Bubble moving to and
fro in the waterish humour of one of its Eyes.

Sir Robert Boyle, 1670

Pathologic effects can follow a significant reduction in the ambient pressure to which an individual is exposed. These effects are of two types: direct and indirect. Direct effects are the consequence of the expansion of gas within the body cavities that do not have open communication with the ambient environment. For example, breath-holding during pressure change can cause pulmonary overpressure and result in cerebral air embolism. Indirect effects result from the evolution of gas, which was previously dissolved in tissue fluids, when a pressure reduction occurs. This latter condition is most commonly referred to as decompression sickness. There is a current move to group both cerebral air embolisms and decompression sickness into a single category of decompression illness. For the purpose of this text, we will apply the terms separately.

DECOMPRESSION SICKNESS

The first identifiable human cases of decompression sickness were reported in 1841 by M.

Triger, a French mining engineer, who noticed symptoms of pain and muscle cramps in coal miners who had been working in an air-pressurized mine shaft. The disease was first scientifically described in 1854 by two French physicians, B. Pol and T. J. J. Watelle, who presented a discussion with many case histories. Because the syndrome was first encountered as a result of hyperbaric exposure, the disorders are described principally using diving and caisson terminology.

Caisson Terminology

Because caisson, or tunnel, workers were the first to suffer from the syndrome now known as decompression sickness, the early terminology describing this disorder was related to that occupation, hence, the names caisson disease and compressed-air illness. The terms related to specific symptoms were devised by the caisson workers themselves. Bends was used to describe the pain in the bowels or lower extremities that caused the victim to assume a stooping posture. Chokes was the term used for victims suffering from dyspnea and a peculiar choking sensation. Other terms used by these workers included staggers (vertigo), prickles (skin sensations), and fits (convulsions).

Diving Terminology

Exhaustion and decompression sickness were common among early divers, particularly when they performed work at depths greater than 21 m (65 ft). In 1869, the French physician L. R. de Mericourt published the first comprehensive medical report on diver's decompression sickness. The divers themselves added such terms as diver's bends, diver's paralysis, diver's palsy, and diver's itch to describe their symptoms. When French physiologist Paul Bert formulated the bubble theory of compressed air illness in his 1878 classic work, *Barometric Pressure*, he provided convincing evidence for the use of recompression to treat the disorder.

Aviation Terminology

As early as 1917, Yandell and Henderson predicted the possibility of decompression sickness in aviators. In the 1930s, when balloon and aircraft altitude records were set above 15,240 m (50,000 ft) altitude decompression sickness became a common occurrence. Before 1959, among the 743 serious (type II) cases of this disorder, at least 18 aviators died from altitude decompression sickness. Variations in terminology used to describe the disorder reflected an uncertainty about its cause(s): high-altitude diver's disease, high-altitude caisson's disease, dysbarism, and aerobullosis. The term decompression sickness came from the American translation of a German term introduced by Benzinger and Hornberger in 1941. Except for the older term caisson disease, the term decompression sickness has best withstood the test of time and is now widely used to describe the disorder.

The term altitude decompression sickness is now commonly used with reference to cases induced by exposure to pressures less than sea level equivalent.

THEORETICAL CONSIDERATIONS

The mechanisms involved in both altitude and diving decompression sickness are identical. Therefore, this discussion will deal primarily with the theoretical aspects of decompression sickness resulting from hyperbaric exposures. The precise causes of decompression sickness are not clearly understood. Although the conditions required to produce decompression sickness and the factors influencing bubble formation and growth are known, research continues as to the relative importance of such factors as intracellular bubble formation and the release of humoral agents from the tissues by expanding gas, blood sludging, intra-capillary bubble formation, and venous bubbles.

Factors Influencing Bubble Formation

Bubble Nuclei

Differential pressures between 100 and 1000 atmospheres absolute (ATA) are required for bubbles to form spontaneously in physical systems. Therefore, even in body fluids supersaturated with nitrogen, bubbles will not form unless bubble nuclei already exist. Bubble nuclei can be produced in areas of negative hydrostatic pressures by muscle shear forces or turbulent blood flow found at points of vessel constriction or bifurcation. Negative pressures also may exist at hydrophobic surfaces of cells or blood vessel walls. Although large microbubbles have been demonstrated in decompressed experimental animals, the actual sites for bubble formation or the sites of bubble nuclei production have not been demonstrated. Bubbles have been observed in veins, arteries, lymphatic vessels, and tissue spaces. Exactly what each compartment contributes to the syndrome of decompression sickness is difficult to interpret.

Supersaturation

During decompression from any atmospheric pressure, some quantity of inert gas in the tissues must diffuse into the blood, travel to the lungs, and leave the body in the expired air because the quantity of inert gas that can remain dissolved in tissue is directly proportional to the absolute ambient pressure. During ascent, the reduction in barometric pressure creates a condition whereby the tissue inert gas tension (P_{N_2}) is greater than the total barometric pressure (P_B). This condition is called supersaturation. Thus, if the decompression exceeds some critical rate for a given tissue, that tissue will not unload the inert gas rapidly enough and will become supersaturated.

Critical Supersaturation

Apparently, a level of supersaturation is reached that the body can tolerate without causing the inert gas to come out of solution to form bubbles. Once the critical supersaturation ratio is reached, however, bubbles develop that can lead to decompression sickness. The English physiologist J. S. Haldane first described the concept of critical supersaturation in 1906. Haldane was commissioned by the British Admiralty to investigate and devise safe decompression procedures for Royal Navy divers, and his work demonstrated that humans could be exposed to hyperbaric pressures and subsequently decompressed without suffering decompression sickness as long as the total pressure reduction was no greater than 50%. No current decompression schedules use Haldane's 2-to-1 rule, but it is discussed here to show a mathematical concept. If Haldane's 2-to-1 relationship of allowable total pressure change is converted to a P_{N_2}-to-P_B relationship, the critical supersaturation ratio (R) would be

$$\frac{P_{N_2}}{P_B}$$

For example,

$$R = \frac{P_{N_2} \text{ at 2 ATA}}{P_B \text{ at 1 ATA}} \tag{1}$$

$$R = \frac{(2)(0.79)}{1} = \frac{1.58}{1} = 1.58/1$$

In fact, there are apparently a number of critical supersaturation ratios for the various mathematical compartments, representing different tissues.

A person living at sea level and breathing atmospheric air will have a dissolved P_{N_2} of 573 mm Hg in all body tissues and fluids, assuming that P_B equals 760 mm Hg; PA_{O_2} equals 100 mm Hg; PA_{CO_2} equals 40 mm Hg; and PA_{H_2O} equals 47 mm Hg. If that person is rapidly decompressed to altitude, a state of supersaturation will be produced when an altitude is reached where the total barometric pressure is less than 573 mm Hg, a condition that occurs at an altitude of 2290 m (7,500 ft). Thus, the altitude threshold above which an individual living at sea level would encounter supersaturation upon rapid decompression is 2290 m (7,500 ft).

The lowest altitude where a sea-level acclimatized person has encountered symptoms of decompression sickness is approximately 5490 m (18,000 ft). The degree of supersaturation at this altitude can be expressed as a ratio, as follows:

$$R = P_{N_2}/P_B \tag{2}$$

If the tissue P_{N_2} equals 573 mm Hg and P_B equals 372 mm Hg, then R equals 573/372, or 1.54. This value approaches the critical supersaturation ratio expressed by Haldane. The incidence of altitude decompression sickness increases markedly above 7620 m (25,000 ft), where the supersaturation ratio is 2.03.

Symptoms can occur at much lower altitudes when "flying after diving." Many cases of decompression sickness have been documented in divers who fly too soon after surfacing. Altitudes as low as 1520 to 2290 m (5,000 to 7,500 ft) may be all that is necessary to induce bubble formation in a diver who has made a safe decompression to the surface. The problem involves the higher tissue P_{N_2} that exists after diving. The Divers Alert Network at Duke University has documented several cases in which divers have developed bends during and after flying in a commercial aircraft. The Undersea and Hyperbaric Medical Society's recommended surface interval between diving and flying ranges from 12–24 hours depending upon the type and frequency of diving (1).

Factors Influencing Bubble Growth

Gaseous Composition

Nitrogen, or another inert gas, is generally considered to be the primary gas involved in symptomatic bubbles. If nitrogen were the only gas initially present in the newly formed bubble, an immediate gradient would be established for the diffusion of other gases into the bubble. Hence, a bubble will quickly have a gaseous composition identical to the gaseous composition present in the surrounding tissues or fluids. When bubbles are produced upon decompression from hyperbaric conditions, gases other than nitrogen represent only a small percentage of the total gas composition of the bubble. The role of other gases may be more significant in bubbles formed at altitude because they represent a much larger percentage of the total pressure within the bubble.

Hydrostatic Pressure

The tendency for gases to leave solution and enlarge a seed bubble can be expressed by the following equation:

$$\Delta P = t - Pab \qquad (3)$$

where ΔP is the differential pressure, or tendency for the gas to leave the liquid phase, in dynes/cm^2; t is the total tension of the gas in the medium, in dynes/cm^2; and Pab is the absolute pressure (that is, the total barometric pressure on the body plus the hydrostatic pressure).

Within an artery at sea level, t equals 760 mm Hg. The absolute pressure, Pab, is 760 mm Hg plus the mean arterial blood pressure (100 mm Hg), or 860 mm Hg. Therefore,

$$\Delta P = 760 - (760 + 100)$$
$$\Delta P = -100 \text{ mm Hg} \qquad (4)$$

When the value of ΔP is negative, there is no tendency toward bubble formation or growth. If the value for ΔP becomes zero or positive, bubble formation or growth is likely to occur.

Within a great vein at sea level, P_{O_2} equals 40 mm Hg, P_{CO_2} equals 46 mm Hg, and P_{H_2O} equals 47 mm Hg; thus, t equals 706 mm Hg. Absolute pressure, Pab, is 760 mm Hg plus the mean venous pressure (which in the great veins in the chest may be 0 mm Hg). Therefore,

$$\Delta P = 706 - (760 + 0)$$
$$\Delta P = -54 \text{ mm Hg} \qquad (5)$$

By suddenly exposing a person to an altitude of 5490 m (18,000 ft) without time for equilibration at the new pressure, venous ΔP would have a large positive value:

$$\Delta P = 706 - (380 + 0)$$
$$\Delta P = +326 \text{ mm Hg} \qquad (6)$$

The value for t in the above equation also can be increased in local areas by high levels of carbon dioxide production. Hence, in muscular exercise, a high local P_{CO_2} associated with a reduction in barometric pressure, P_B, causes higher positive values of ΔP than with a reduction in P_B alone. Further, because of the high solubility and rapid diffusion of carbon dioxide, locally high levels of this gas would produce the rapid growth of bubbles.

Hydrostatic pressure is, therefore, considered to be a force opposing bubble formation or bubble growth and includes not only blood pressure and cerebrospinal fluid pressure but local tissue pressure (or turgor), which varies directly with blood flow.

Boyle's Law Effects

Once a bubble is formed, its size will increase if the total pressure is decreased. During hyperbaric therapy, bubble size is reduced during compression. The surface tension of a bubble is inversely related to bubble size and opposes bubble growth. Thus, as total pressure is increased, the surface tension opposing bubble growth also is increased. Once a critically small bubble size is achieved, the surface tension is so great that the bubble can no longer exist. The bubble collapses, and its gases are dissolved.

Pathophysiology of Bubbles

Gas bubbles that form in body tissue and blood have two effects. The first is the direct mechanical effect of bubbles, which distort and disrupt tissue. This effect causes pain and blocks circulation, causing ischemia and possible infarction.

The second effect results from biochemical changes occurring at the blood-bubble interface. Platelet aggregation occurs, with the release of vasoactive substances such as serotonin and epinephrine leading to vasoconstriction. The release of platelet factor 3 accelerates clotting and leads to further circulatory embarrassment. Blood viscosity increases, with a concomitant rise in capillary flow resistance and capillary pressure. This effect, coupled with an hypoxic loss of capillary wall integrity, leads to large shifts of fluid from the intravascular to the extravascular space and a further hemoconcentration. The bubble effects in decompression sickness are shown in Figure 7.1.

PROTECTION AND PREDISPOSING FACTORS

Protection against decompression sickness is based on controlling the tissue nitrogen-to-ambient pressure ratio (P_{N2}/P_B). When an inert gas, such as nitrogen, is breathed, the tension of the

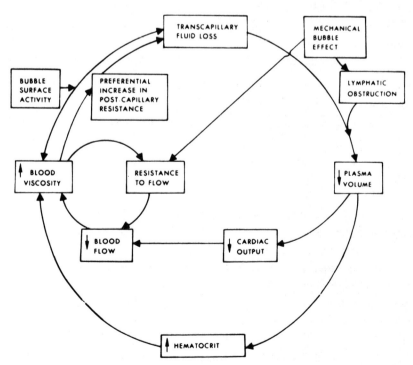

Figure 7.1. Bubble effects in decompression sickness.

gas dissolved in tissue fluids increases until equilibrium with the partial pressure of the gas in the respired medium is reached. With pressure reduction (decompression), supersaturation can occur. Some degree of supersaturation can be tolerated. The critical P_{N_2}/P_B ratio differs for each body tissue. When the safe limits of decompression are exceeded, gas separates from solution in the blood and other tissues. This process is the initiating event for decompression sickness. For diving, safe decompression limits vary with time and the depth of the dive and are published as decompression tables in a variety of diving manuals, one of which is the United States Navy Diving Manual (2).

Even though the diver follows the decompression tables to safely decompress at sea level, the supersaturation limits can be exceeded if the diver continues to ascend to altitude; for example, the individual who flies immediately following a scuba dive. Similarly, an individual whose body tissues are in equilibrium at sea level achieves a condition of supersaturation during decompression to altitude. Like the diver who exceeds the safe decompression limits, the aviator also can ascend to altitudes, usually above 5490 m (18,000 ft), where gas will separate from solution to create bubbles that result in decompression sickness.

The aviator is protected from decompression sickness in two ways: aircraft pressurization and denitrogenation. Aircraft pressurization is a method of maintaining the aircraft cabin pressure and, therefore, the physiologic altitude to which the aviator is exposed, at a considerably lower pressure altitude than the actual altitude at which the aircraft is flying. With adequate aircraft pressurization, the individual is not exposed to reduced barometric pressures where bubbles can form. Protection from decompression sickness exists because the P_{N_2}/P_B ratio remains below a critical threshold as the value of P_B remains high.

Denitrogenation is a method by which one breathes 100% oxygen for the purpose of eliminating nitrogen from the body before going to altitude. This method is used to protect the individual who must ascend to high altitudes that can produce decompression sickness. With 100% oxygen breathing, oxygen replaces other tissue-dissolved gases, including nitrogen. Thus, the amount of nitrogen in each body tissue is reduced before ambient pressure reduction occurs. Again, the P_{N_2}/P_B ratio remains below a critical threshold because the value for P_{N_2} is reduced.

For example, an aviator rapidly ascends from sea level (P_B = 760 mm Hg) to 5490 m (18,000 ft) (P_B = 380 mm Hg). The aircraft pressurization system maintains pressure in the cabin at 2440 m (8,000 ft) (P_B = 565 mm Hg). Assuming that all tissues are saturated at sea level (P_{N_2} = 573 mm Hg) and that offgassing occurring during the rapid ascent is insignificant, the P_{N_2}/P_B ratio would be 1.01:

$$\frac{P_{N_2}}{P_B} = \frac{573 \text{ mm Hg}}{565 \text{ mm Hg}} = 1.01 \qquad (7)$$

If the aircraft were not pressurized the P_{N_2}/P_B ratio would be 1.51:

$$\frac{P_{N_2}}{P_B} = \frac{573 \text{ mm Hg}}{380 \text{ mm Hg}} = 1.51 \qquad (8)$$

If unpressurized flight occurred to 9140 m (30,000 ft) (P_B = 226 mm Hg) the P_{N_2}/P_B ratio would be 2.54:

$$\frac{P_{N_2}}{P_B} = \frac{573 \text{ mm Hg}}{226 \text{ mm Hg}} = 2.54 \qquad (9)$$

If before unpressurized flight to 9140 m (30,000 ft) the aviator had denitrogenated at sea level such that one half of the total nitrogen was eliminated from his body and state of equilibrium was reached for all body tissues, the P_{N_2}/P_B ratio would be 1.27:

$$\frac{P_{N_2}}{P_B} = \frac{287 \text{ mm Hg}}{226 \text{ mm Hg}} = 1.27 \qquad (10)$$

The process of denitrogenation is very effective in eliminating nitrogen from the body. When 100% oxygen is breathed using a tightly fitted mask, an alveolar nitrogen pressure of nearly zero is established and a marked pressure differential (about 573 mm Hg) between the alveoli and body tissues results. Nitrogen rapidly diffuses from the tissues into the blood, where it is transported to the lung and is exhaled. The amount of nitrogen eliminated is time-dependent.

Figure 7.2 shows the total amount of nitrogen washed out of the body by denitrogenation. Assuming that the average person contains 1200 cm^3 of dissolved nitrogen, slightly more than 350 cm^3 can be eliminated by prebreathing 100% oxygen for 30 minutes. Denitrogenation prior to initiating ascent to altitude significantly reduces the incidence of altitude decompression sickness. Once begun, denitrogenation should not be interrupted. Air-breathing interruptions of only a few minutes greatly decrease the efficacy of denitrogenation in the prevention of decompression sickness. If such an interruption is unavoidable, the only safe course of action is to begin denitrogenation again from time zero.

Denitrogenation eliminates nitrogen from various tissues at different rates. These rates are dependent on the solubility of nitrogen in specific tissues but, more importantly, also on the circulatory perfusion of the tissues. Thus, all body tissues come into equilibrium with each other and with respired gas at different times. As a practical matter, then, with altitude exposure (pressure reduction), the P_{N_2}/P_B ratio of certain tissues may exceed the critical value for bubble formation while the P_{N_2}/P_B ratio of other tissues remains within a safe range. This fact may partially explain why signs and symptoms of decompression sickness occur at characteristic locations in the body.

Attempts have been made to correlate the incidence of both diving-induced and altitude-induced decompression sickness with various physical and physiological factors. Some of these factors influence group susceptibility to decompression sickness, although none can be used to predict individual susceptibility. The association of these factors with decompression sickness is summarized in the next sections.

Altitude Attained

No reliable evidence exists for the occurrence of decompression sickness with altitude exposures of less than 5490 m (18,000 ft) unless there was a recent (within 24 hours) previous exposure to compressed gas breathing (e.g., scuba diving or hyperbaric exposure). With increasing altitude, the incidence of decompression sickness increases, as does the ratio of severe to mild cases. Exposures to altitudes of 7930 to 14,400 m (26,000–47,500 ft) for times varying from approximately 30 minutes to 3 hours will result in a 1.5% incidence of decompression sickness. The severity of the cases will increase with increasing altitude.

In a review of 145 cases of altitude-induced decompression sickness necessitating treatment, Davis and colleagues (3) reported that 13% of these cases occurred with altitude exposures of 7620 m (25,000 ft) or below and 79% occurred with exposures of 9140 m (30,000 ft) or greater.

Duration of Exposure

At all altitudes above 5490 m (18,000 ft), the longer the duration of exposure, the greater the incidence of decompression sickness.

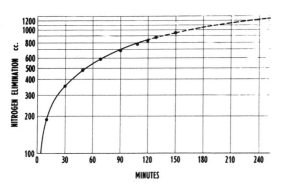

Figure 7.2. Nitrogen elimination curve.

Temperature

No correlation exists between the frequency of decompression sickness and the ambient temperature in the range of 21.1 to 34.3°C. At an ambient temperature of -23.3°C, however, the incidence of decompression sickness is twice that at 21.1°C, with a larger ratio of serious cases to mild cases.

Previous Exposures to Altitude

A second exposure to an altitude greater than 5490 m (18,000 ft) following an exposure to such an altitude in the preceding 3 hours will greatly increase the chance of decompression sickness occurring, even if the first exposure was asymptomatic. A recurrence of symptoms is almost certain if the first exposure is symptomatic.

A 2-hour exposure to an altitude of 7620 m (25,000 ft) followed in 18 hours by a rapid decompression from 2440 to 6700 m (8,000 to 22,000 ft) will result in detectable Doppler bubble signals over the pulmonary artery. In addition, the incidence of decompression sickness following the rapid decompression will be twice that following the initial altitude exposure.

Repeated daily exposures to altitude have been variously reported as increasing susceptibility, having no effect on susceptibility, and even decreasing susceptibility to decompression sickness. Of special interest is the series of cases reported by Davis and colleagues (3), in which the incidence of decompression sickness in inside attendants undergoing two to four altitude exposures per week accompanying students in altitude chamber training was three times greater than the incidence in students.

Flying Following Diving

If an individual breathes a gas at pressures greater than sea level before altitude exposure, his susceptibility to decompression sickness will significantly increase. Retrospective case reviews as well as prospective animal and human

investigations have resulted in a number of recommendations by various agencies as to the sea level surface interval necessary to safely fly after diving. The Undersea and Hyperbaric Medical Society reviewed this material and recommended the following (1):

Dive Schedule	Minimum Surface Interval
1. No-decompression dives	
a. Less than 2 hours accumulated dive time in the 48 hours preceding surfacing from the last dive	12 hours
b. Multiday, unlimited diving	24 hours
2. Dives requiring decompression stops (but not including saturation dives).	24–48 hours

Saturation diving presents complex problems and is beyond the scope of this chapter. The interested reader is referred to the specialized literature on the subject.

Age

A rather striking increase in the incidence of decompression sickness occurs with increasing age. This increase occurs in both compressed air workers and aviators, with a threefold increase in incidence between the 19- to 25-year-old and 40- to 45-year-old age groups. The mechanism underlying this phenomenon is not understood but may result from changes in circulation due to aging.

Gender

Much controversy exists regarding the possible differences in susceptibility to decompression sickness between men and women. The scientific resolution of this question has been hampered by emotional and political factors, and, unfortunately, studies are limited. It is the clinical judgment of those most experienced in the treatment of decompression sickness, however, that women present more problems in the clinical management of this disorder than do men.

Exercise

The association between physical exertion and decompression sickness has been well established. During World War II, altitude chambers were used to select out bends-prone individuals from American aircrews. The subjects were taken to an altitude of 12,190 m (40,000 ft) and exercised until one half of them developed bends. The remaining bends resistant subjects were assigned to high altitude, unpressurized bomber missions. The effect of exercise on the incidence of decompression sickness is equivalent to increasing the exposure altitude 915 to 1520 m (3,000 to 5,000 ft).

Injury

No convincing evidence exists to associate previous injury with decompression sickness. Based on theoretical considerations, however, it is thought that during the acute stages of an injury to a joint, that joint may have increased susceptibility to bends because of perfusion changes associated with the injury and/or healing mechanisms.

Body Build

For a long time, a basic tenet of diving and aerospace medicine (almost a religious dogma) has been that obesity increases the susceptibility to decompression sickness. Although it seems prudent to continue to accept this principle because of other known adverse effects of obesity, no scientific validation exists.

Other Factors

No definitive results have come from investigations of possible correlations between de-

compression sickness and such factors as physical fitness, hypoxia, and diet.

MANIFESTATIONS OF DECOMPRESSION SICKNESS

In decompression sickness, bubbles can form in all parts of the body. Various target organs, however, seem to be affected most readily, and the effects on these anatomic locations account for the signs and symptoms seen. The pathophysiology of bubbles was discussed earlier in the section so named. In this section, the clinical manifestations of bubble formation and the classic syndromes of decompression sickness will be described.

Bends

The bends, manifested by pain only, is seen in 65 to 70% of the cases of altitude induced decompression sickness. It tends to be localized in and around the large joints of the body. Smaller joints, such as interphalangeal areas, sometimes may be affected, particularly if these joints underwent significant active motion during altitude exposure.

Bends pain is deep and aching in character and ranges from very mild (joint awareness) to so severe that the patient does not wish to move the affected joint. Active and passive motion of the joint tends to aggravate the discomfort, whereas local pressure, such as with an inflated blood pressure cuff, tends to relieve the pain temporarily.

The pain may occur during the altitude exposure, on descent, shortly after descent, or, in some cases, only become manifest many hours after descent. In most cases, bends occurring at altitude will be relieved by descent because of the increase in barometric pressure. In some cases, bends relieved by returning to ground level will recur at ground level. In these cases, as well as those cases where pain is not relieved by descent, hyperbaric oxygen therapy is the definitive form of treatment.

Chokes

The syndrome called chokes is rare in both diving and aviation, accounting for less than 2% of decompression sickness cases. This condition is a life-threatening disorder, however. The mechanism of chokes is multiple pulmonary gas emboli. The characteristic clinical picture consists of substernal chest pain, dyspnea, and a dry nonproductive cough. In most cases, the pain is made worse on inhalation. Patients with chokes feel generally and severely ill. Altitude-induced chokes will invariably progress to collapse of the individual if the altitude is maintained. The aviator whose symptoms are not completely relieved by descent to ground level must be treated in a hyperbaric chamber as quickly as possible. This treatment also is required for chokes secondary to decompression following diving.

Neurologic Decompression Sickness

Neurologic decompression sickness presents a clinical picture with signs and symptoms referable to the nervous system. It has become apparent that one should probably limit the term neurologic decompression sickness to those cases in which there is involvement of the central nervous system. Peripheral nerve involvement with mild paresthesia is commonly associated with bends and does not increase the gravity of the disorder from a prognostic point of view. Central nervous system involvement, however, can herald significant and permanent neurological deficits, particularly if aggressive and proper treatment is not instituted promptly.

Central nervous system involvement occurs in 5 to 7% of cases of decompression sickness, either from diving or altitude exposure. In cases of altitude decompression sickness where symptoms are not relieved totally by descent, however, the central nervous system is involved in 35 to 50% of the cases.

Neurologic decompression sickness presents in one of two forms: a spinal cord form and a brain form. The spinal cord form is seen almost exclusively following diving and is extremely rare following altitude exposure. The brain form of the disorder is more commonly seen following altitude exposure and is uncommon but not rare following diving exposure. The reasons for the variance in the incidence of brain and spinal cord neurologic decompression sickness in diving and altitude exposure have not yet been elucidated. The clinical manifestations of the two forms of this disorder will be discussed separately.

Spinal Cord Decompression Sickness

In many cases, the first symptom of spinal cord decompression sickness is the insidious onset of numbness or paresthesia of the feet. The sensory deficit spreads upward, accompanied by an ascending weakness or paralysis to the level of the spinal lesion. Other cases begin with girdling abdominal or thoracic pain, which precedes the onset of sensory and motor deficits. Within 30 minutes of onset, the entire clinical picture of a partial or complete transverse spinal cord lesion is manifest.

The lesion in spinal cord decompression sickness has been well documented as bubbles formed in or embolized to the paraspinal venous plexus. Poorly collateralized segmental venous drainage of the spinal cord and normally sluggish blood flow through the paraspinal venous plexus can result quickly in mechanical blockage of venous drainage by bubbles and solid elements formed at the blood-bubble interface. This blockage, in turn, results in a congestive, or "red," infarct of the spinal cord.

Brain Form of Decompression Sickness

In most cases, the clinical picture of a patient suffering from the brain form of decompression sickness is one of spotty sensory and motor signs and symptoms not attributable to a single brain locus. Headache, at times of a migrainous nature, is commonly present. Visual disturbances, consisting of scotomas, tunnel vision, diplopia, or blurring, are common. At times, extreme fatigue or personality changes that range from emotional lability to a significantly flattened affect are the presenting symptoms.

For the physician not acquainted with the clinical picture of multiple brain lesions, the diagnosis can be very difficult. A number of these patients have been misdiagnosed as hysterical and have progressed to vasomotor collapse because proper and immediate definitive treatment was not rendered.

Circulatory Manifestations

Generally, circulatory impairment is manifested as shock following the development of chokes, severe bends, or severe neurologic impairment (secondary collapse). Circulatory collapse without other symptoms preceding the development of shock (primary collapse) occurs rarely. So-called postdecompression collapse following altitude exposure, with the shock state occurring after descent to the ground level, has been described as a separate type of circulatory impairment. It probably is not separate but rather represents delay in onset as sometimes seen with other types of altitude decompression sickness.

Possible mechanisms of circulatory collapse include direct involvement of the vasomotor regulatory center or massive blood vessel endothelial damage by bubbles, with a subsequent loss of intravascular volume. Extreme hemoconcentration has been documented in many cases, with hematocrits up to 70%.

Circulatory collapse is marked by its lack of response to fluid replacement, which is similar to the lack of response commonly seen in cases of severe head injury that results in a central sympathectomy.

Minor Manifestations

Skin bends is a disorder that may present as pruritus or formication only. The sensation generally passes within 20 to 30 minutes, and no treatment is necessary. Skin bends, however, may occur with the appearance of mottled or marbled skin lesions. The appearance of these lesions is

evidence of a neurocirculatory effect of bubbles within the body. Up to 10% of patients with such skin lesions will experience circulatory collapse if untreated.

Pitting edema, if seen alone, is considered a minor manifestation of decompression sickness in that it will resolve spontaneously without sequelae. Pitting edema is thought to arise from lymphatic blockage by bubbles. It rarely results from altitude exposure.

Chronic Effects

Aseptic bone necrosis is a debilitating condition, common among divers and caisson workers but has only been well documented in three cases following altitude exposure. Areas of bone infarction, if located in juxta-articular locations, rapidly lead to erosion of overlying cartilage and severe osteoarthritis. The shoulders, knees, and hips are the only joints affected. Early lesions are asymptomatic and are only found on radiographic surveys. The exact relationship between aseptic bone necrosis and episodes of bends is unknown. The disease is seen when compressed air exposure occurs on a regular and frequent basis and is seldom seen in less than 1 year after beginning such exposures.

Permanent neurologic deficits result from spinal cord decompression sickness and are most feared by divers. Even with proper and rapid treatment, approximately 15% of patients who have suffered spinal cord decompression sickness will manifest some degree of permanent neurologic deficit from minor sensory and motor losses to complete paraplegia.

DIAGNOSIS AND MANAGEMENT OF DECOMPRESSION SICKNESS

Decompression sickness rarely occurs unless one of the following conditions exists:

1. A diver surfaces following a dive deeper than 10 m (33 ft) of sea water. In most cases, the diver will have failed to follow recognized

single or repetitive dive decompression schedules.

2. Exposure to altitude greater than 5490 m (18,000 ft). In most instances, decompression sickness will not occur (without preceding exposure to compressed gas breathing) at altitudes below 7620 m (25,000 ft) although a few cases have been documented at altitudes of 5640 m (18,500 ft).

3. Exposure to altitude shortly following exposure to compressed gas breathing (e.g., scuba diving or hyperbaric chamber exposure). Decompression sickness has occurred while flying in pressurized aircraft at a cabin altitude as low as 1370 m (4,500 ft) following scuba diving in the preceding 3 hours.

The following procedures should be followed in all cases of decompression sickness (including bends pain only) persisting after a dive or after a flight:

1. One hundred percent oxygen should be administered using a well-fitted aviator's mask or anesthesia mask.

2. If a hyperbaric chamber is on site, the patient should be immediately treated according to the proper Treatment Table. No observation period is warranted at ground level.

3. If there is no on-site hyperbaric chamber, arrangements should be made to immediately transport the patient to the nearest hyperbaric facility capable of administering proper treatment. The patient should be kept on 100% oxygen by mask while awaiting and during transportation to the chamber. If the patient has bends pain only, the symptoms of which clear completely without recurrence while awaiting transport, movement to hyperbaric chamber can be cancelled.

4. If bends pain is relieved while awaiting transport but recurs, the patient should be transported to the hyperbaric chamber and treated even if symptoms are relieved again after recurrence.

5. Any patient with signs or symptoms of neuro-

logic decompression sickness, chokes, or circulatory collapse should be immediately transported to the nearest hyperbaric chamber for treatment, regardless of whether the symptoms persist.

6. Transportation must be at or near the ground-level barometric pressure of the site at which the patient embarks. Aircraft used for the movement of these patients must possess this pressurization capability. In no case should the cabin pressure altitude be more than 305 m (1,000 ft) higher than the pressure altitude at the point of embarkation. If at all possible, it is best to avoid moving patients to a hyperbaric chamber located at a pressure altitude greater than 1070 m (3,500 ft) higher than the point of embarkation.

7. Return to flying no earlier than 72 hours after resolution of pain-only bends.

The diagnostic and treatment decision points described above are summarized in Figure 7.3.

HYPERBARIC THERAPY FOR DECOMPRESSION SICKNESS

Physiologic Basis of Hyperbaric Therapy

Hyperbaric therapy is achieved by applying two physical factors related to the pressure environment. The first factor is the mechanical compression of gas-filled entities such as bubbles. The second factor is the elevation of the partial pressure of inspired gases and the subsequent increase in the amount of the various gases that enter into physical solution in body fluids. The use of hyperbaric oxygen therapy for treating decompression sickness results in bubble size reduction, a positive nitrogen gradient to reduce the size of bubbles and resolve them, perfusion of ischemic tissues, and correction of local tissue hypoxia.

As an individual is exposed to a change in barometric pressure, a bubble deep within the body tissues responds to the pressure change. During compression, the surrounding barometric

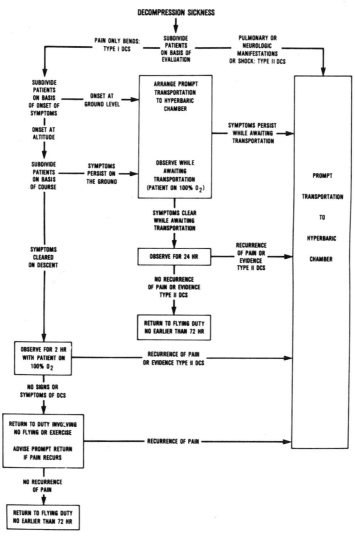

Figure 7.3. Diagnostic and treatment decision points for decompression sickness.

pressure is increased, producing a reduction in bubble volume in accordance with Boyle's Law. Figure 7.4 presents the expected decrease in bubble volume and diameter as a function of the total pressure applied. Figure 7.5 compares the expected decrease in bubble size of a bubble formed at sea level with those formed at altitudes of 5490 and 11,600 m (18,000 and 38,000 ft). During compression, the bubble becomes smaller and the surface tension increases. Below a certain critical diameter, the surface tension becomes so great that the bubble collapses and the gas within it dissolves.

Applying hyperbaric pressure in treating decompression sickness will, therefore, either eliminate the bubbles entirely or reduce their size to a significant extent. The amount of size reduction will depend on the absolute bubble size at the onset of therapy. Even though some bubbles may not be eliminated completely by the initial application of pressure, their reduction in size aids in partially restoring circulation in the case of intravascular bubbles and reducing the mechanical effects of extravascular bubbles.

Bubbles that are too big to resolve upon the initial application of pressure will continue to

DEPTH IN FEET	PRESSURE IN ATA	RELATIVE VOLUME (PERCENT)	RELATIVE DIAMETER (PERCENT)
0	1	100	100
33	2	50	79.3
66	3	33.3	69.3
99	4	25	63
132	5	20	58.5
165	6	16.6	55
297	10	10	46.2

Figure 7.4. Bubble volume and diameter relationships.

decrease in size with the time spent at increased pressure. This gradual decrease in size is due to the diffusion of gases from the bubble to the surrounding tissues and fluids. Diffusion of gases from the bubble occurs because the partial pressure of gases within the bubble increases when the volume is reduced during compression. The elevated partial pressure of gases inside the bubble creates a gradient favorable for gas elimination from the bubble, as presented in Figure 7.6. Figure 7.6 also shows that if the individual breathes air, the favorable gradient will lessen with time as the surrounding tissues and fluids approach equilibrium at the new nitrogen partial pressure. Thus, the bubble will be resolved more rapidly if the individual breathes 100% oxygen because a favorable gradient for nitrogen elimination from a bubble will improve with time, and the bubble will more rapidly diminish in size. During hyperbaric therapy, the patient intermittently breathes 100% oxygen at increased pressure. Breathing 100% oxygen provides an increased gradient for eliminating nitrogen from evolved bubbles and aids in their resorption. The increased gradient also speeds the

elimination of nitrogen from supersaturated tissues and thus helps prevent further bubble formation. Therefore, if a sufficient time is spent at depth, all bubbles will resolve.

Hyperbaric oxygenation results in increased oxygen tension in the capillaries surrounding ischemic tissue. The increased oxygen tension extends the oxygen diffusion distance from functioning capillaries and corrects the local tissue hypoxia. Overcoming the tissue hypoxia tends to disrupt the vicious cycle of hypoxia-induced tissue damage that causes tissue edema and interferes with circulation and oxygenation.

Figure 7.7 shows the level of tissue P_{O_2} that can be achieved in ischemic tissue during 100% oxygen breathing at 1 ATA and 2.4 ATA. These data were collected by Sheffield and Dunn (4) using a polarographic oxygen electrode implanted in an ischemic, hypoxic, nonhealing wound and are shown to illustrate that tissue P_{O_2} can be elevated in areas with poorly functioning capillaries when hyperbaric oxygenation is applied. In this case, the baseline wound oxygen tension during air breathing at 1 ATA was 20 mm Hg, compared with 30–40 mm Hg in healthy skin. Wound oxygen tension increased to 200–300 mm Hg during 100% oxygen

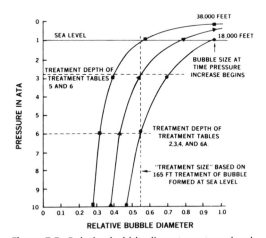

Figure 7.5. Relative bubble diameters at sea level, 5490 m, and 11,600 m. The treatment tables referred to in this figure are the standard United States Navy Treatment Tables. See Table 7.1 and Figures 7.8, 7.9, 7.13, and 7.14 for more information on these tables.

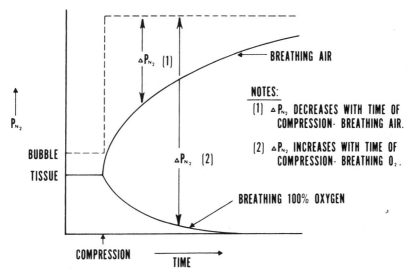

Figure 7.6. Bubble nitrogen gradients when breathing air versus pure oxygen.

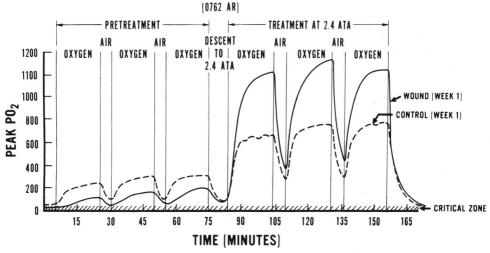

Figure 7.7. Tissue oxygen tension after 1 week of hyperbaric oxygenation (HBO) for a nonhealing surgical wound.

breathing at 1 atmosphere absolute (atm abs) and above 1,000 mm Hg during 100% oxygen breathing at 2.4 (atm abs). It should be noted that the higher tissue oxygen tensions achieved under hyperbaric conditions result in an increased oxygen diffusion distance. This phenomenon is especially important when one considers the need to deliver oxygen to an area in which flow through several capillaries may be disrupted due to bubbles or sludging.

Treatment of Altitude Decompression Sickness

Although most cases of decompression sickness occurring at altitude will be completely relieved by descent to ground level, approximately 2% of cases will persist. In addition, a significant number of patients will experience the initial onset of symptoms of decompression sickness after descent, so-called ''delayed cases.''

Prior to 1959, over 17,000 cases of altitude-induced decompression sickness were documented. Of these cases, 743 were reported as serious, including 17 fatalities. Davis and colleagues (3), commenting on a review of these 17 fatalities, made the following observations. All died in irreversible shock that was unresponsive to fluid replacement and drug therapy. Almost all cases began as simple bends pain, neurologic manifestations, or chokes, which only after several hours progressed to circulatory collapse and death. It should be noted that none of the 17 fatalities were treated by hyperbaric therapy. In their review of 145 cases of altitude decompression sickness treated in hyperbaric chambers, these same authors emphasized that shock was the initial clinical picture in only one case, whereas seven other cases began with other manifestations and progressed to shock. In this series of patients, no fatalities occurred among those who were treated in hyperbaric chambers (3). Since 1959 when hyperbaric oxygen therapy was implemented for this disorder, only one aviator is known to have died from altitude decompression sickness. Death was attributed to the severe exposure in unpressurized flight and long delay before hyperbaric treatment.

As early as 1945, Behnke (5) advocated the use of compression therapy to treat cases of altitude decompression sickness that did not resolve upon descent to ground level. It was not until 1959 that a United States Air Force aviator was successfully treated by compression (6). In 1963, Downey and colleagues (7), using a human serum in vitro model, demonstrated the persistence, at ground level, of bubbles formed at altitude. Upon compression to pressures greater than sea level, the bubbles cleared. In vivo confirmation of Downey's work was reported by Leverett and colleagues in 1963 (8).

Much of the present-day understanding of bubble behavior and effects with changing pressures is based on that work. Present-day standards of care mandate immediate hyperbaric therapy for all cases of altitude decompression sickness persisting or recurring after descent to ground level.

Treatment Procedures

Once the diagnosis of decompression sickness has been made, hyperbaric therapy is required. It is never acceptable to continue observation of a patient with signs or symptoms of decompression sickness. The use of oxygen at 1 ATA for such patients should be restricted to the period of initial observation and examination, the time required for transportation to a hyperbaric chamber, and the time required to prepare the hyperbaric facility for use. Oxygen at 1 ATA is not a substitute for hyperbaric therapy.

Although a number of treatment tables are used successfully throughout the world, the United States Navy Treatment Tables are considered authoritative for treating decompression sickness in this country. Standard Navy Treatment Tables 1, 2, 3, and 4 are shown in Table 7.1. Because of the poor success rate of these air treatment tables before 1964, Goodman and Workman (9) developed the oxygen treatment tables now labeled as Tables 5 and 6. The oxygen treatment tables were adopted by the Navy in 1967 and have proved to be highly effective in treating decompression sickness. Treatment Table 5, as modified by the United States Air Force (USAF), is shown in Figure 7.8. The outlined treatment is 135 minutes in length and is designed for the treatment of bends pain only. Treatment Table 5 can be used for bends if the patient responds completely within 10 minutes of breathing oxygen at 60 fsw (18 m). If the symptoms do not disappear within 10 minutes, the patient is committed to Treatment Table 6. The high recurrence of symptoms after use of Treatment Table 5 has caused it to fall in disfavor, with a preference for Table 6 for the treatment of all cases of bends pain only.

Table 7.1.
Standard United States Navy Treatment Tables 1, 2, 3, and 4

Stops	Table 1	Table 2	Table 3	Table 4
Feet of Seawater	Time at Stop (minutes)	Time at Stop (minutes)	Time at Stop (minutes)	Time at Stop (minutes)
165	—	30 (air)	30 (air)	30–120 (air)
140	—	12 (air)	12 (air)	30 (air)
120	—	12 (air)	12 (air)	30 (air)
100	30 (air)	12 (air)	12 (air)	30 (air)
80	12 (air)	12 (air)	12 (air)	30 (air)
60	30 (oxygen)	30 (oxygen)	30 (oxygen)	360 (air)
50	30 (oxygen)	30 (oxygen)	30 (oxygen)	360 (air)
40	30 (oxygen)	30 (oxygen)	30 (oxygen)	360 (air)
30		60 (oxygen)	720 (air)	660 (air)
				60 (oxygen)
20			120 (air)	60 (air)
				60 (oxygen)
10			120 (air)	60 (air)
				60 (oxygen)
	5 minute ascent on oxygen	5 minute ascent on oxygen	1 minute ascent on air	1 minute ascent on air
Surface	↓	↓	↓	↓

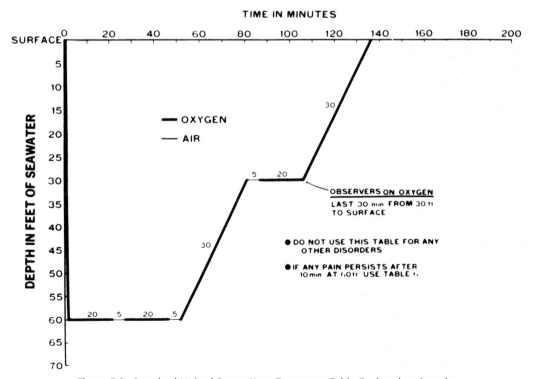

Figure 7.8. Standard United States Navy Treatment Table 5—bends pain only.

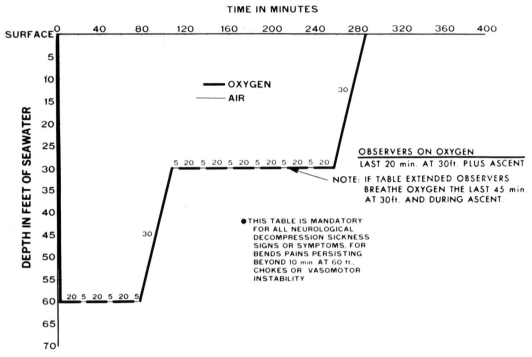

Figure 7.9. Standard United States Navy Treatment Table 6—decompression sickness.

Treatment Table 6, as modified by the USAF, is shown in Figure 7.9. It is reserved for cases involving the central nervous system or cardiopulmonary systems and for recurrences of previously treated decompression sickness. Treatment Table 6 also is used to treat bends pain cases that are not relieved within 10 minutes on 100% oxygen at 60 fsw (18 m). U.S. Navy Treatment Table 7, shown in Figure 7.10 is only used in life threatening situations when other treatment tables have failed to resolve symptoms of serous (type II) decompression sickness or cerebral gas embolism. Since patients treated on Table 7 will be in the hyperbaric chamber for at least 48 hours, this treatment should only be undertaken when all medical and non-medical care of the patient can be provided in the chamber for this period of time. Decision points for the treatment of decompression sickness are shown in Figures 7.11 and 7.12.

Where long delays between onset and treatment occur, the manifestations of decompression sickness become more serious. They seem to be aggravated by the development of secondary edema and vascular obstruction or impairment from thrombosis. Hyperbaric oxygenation in such circumstances probably provides more benefit than does the mechanical compression of bubbles.

General considerations in the use of the decompression sickness treatment tables are as follows:

1. Follow the treatment tables accurately.
2. Use qualified medical attendants inside the chamber at all times.
3. Maintain the normal ascent and descent rates.
4. Examine the patient thoroughly at the depth of relief or treatment depth.
5. Treat an unconscious patient for air embolism or serious decompression sickness unless the possibility of such a condition can be ruled out.

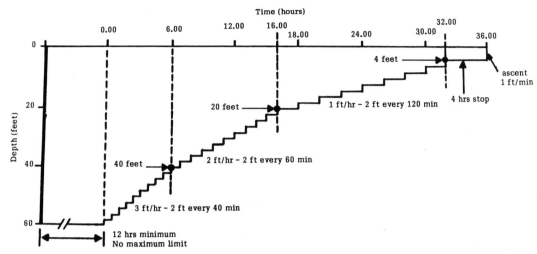

Figure 7.10. Treatment Table 7.
1. Used for treatment of unresolved life threatening symptoms after initial treatment on Table 6, 6A, or 4.
2. Use only under the direction of or in the consultation with a Diving Medical Officer.
3. Table begins upon arrival at 60 feet. Arrival at 60 feet accomplished by initial treatment on Table 6, 6A or 4. If initial treatment has progressed to a depth shallower than 60 feet, compress to 60 feet at 25 ft/min to begin Table 7.
4. Maximum duration at 60 feet unlimited. Remain at 60 feet a minimum of 12 hours unless over-riding circumstances dictate earlier decompression.
5. Patient begins oxygen breathing periods at 60 feet. Inside attendant need breathe only chamber atmosphere throughout. If oxygen breathing is interrupted no lengthening of the table is required.
6. Minimum chamber O_2 concentration 19%. Maximum CO_2 concentration 1.5% SEV (12 mm Hg). Maximum chamber internal temperature 85°F.
7. Decompression starts with a 2 foot upward excursion from 60 to 58 feet. Decompress with stops every 2 feet for times shown in profile above. Ascent time between stops approximately 30 sec. Stop time begins with ascent from deeper to next shallower step. Stop at 4 feet for 4 hours and then ascend to the surface at 1 ft/min.
8. Ensure chamber life support requirements can be met before committing to a Treatment Table 7.

6. Use the air tables only if oxygen cannot be used.
7. Watch for oxygen toxicity.
8. Remove the oxygen mask if oxygen convulsion occurs and protect the patient from flailing injury.
9. Maintain oxygen usage within the time and depth limits.
10. Check the patient's status before and after coming to each stop and periodically during long stops.
11. Wake patient if asleep through changes of depth for more than 1 hour at a time at any stop (symptoms can develop or recur during sleep).

12. Observe the patient for at least 6 hours after the treatment for a recurrence of symptoms.
13. Maintain accurate timekeeping and recording.
14. Maintain a well-stocked medical kit.

Patient Condition Worsens

The following is a list of considerations if the patient's condition worsens:

1. Stop the ascent if the patient's condition is worsening.
2. Treat the patient as a recurrence during treatment.
3. Use Table 4 or Table 7 if needed.

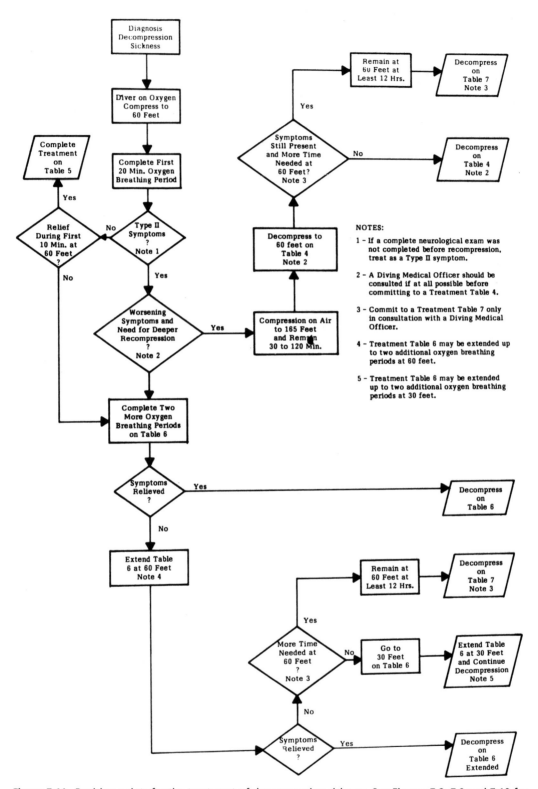

Figure 7.11. Decision points for the treatment of decompression sickness. See Figures 7.8, 7.9 and 7.10 for Standard United States Treatment Tables 5, 6 and 7. See Table 7.1 for Standard United States, Treatment Table 4.

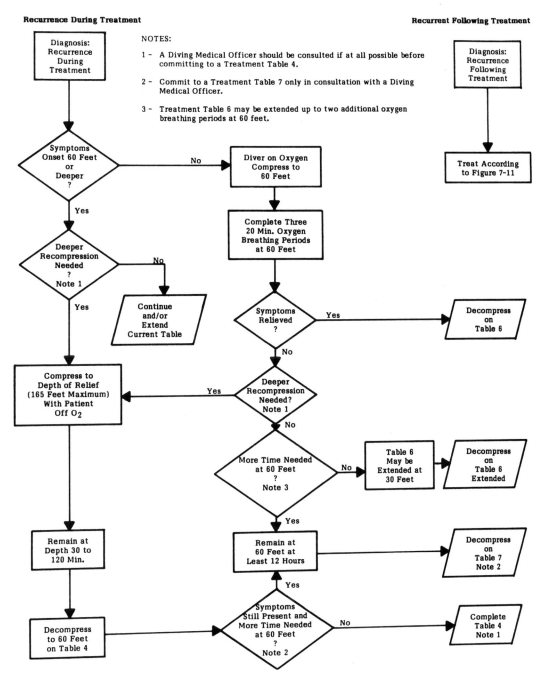

Figure 7.12. Decision points for the treatment of recurrent symptoms of decompression sickness. See Figure 7.11.

Recurrence of Symptoms During Treatment

The following is a list of considerations in the event of a recurrence of symptoms during treatment:

1. Recompress to 60 fsw (18 m) and treat on Table 6 with extensions as needed.
2. Start intravenous infusion of crystalloid solution.
3. Start the following dexamethasone schedule: 20 mg intravenously immediately, then 4 mg every 6 hours intramuscularly.

Recurrence of Symptoms Following Treatment

The following is a list of considerations in the event of a recurrence of symptoms after treatment:

1. Recompress to 60 fsw (18 m) and use Table 6.
2. Repeat Table 6 if the patient becomes worse after initial treatment. In neurologic cases, continue daily hyperbaric oxygen on Table 6 for as long as improvement occurs, or until the patient's condition plateaus. This does not usually require more than 5–8 treatments.
3. Use Table 7 if needed.

Using Oxygen

The following is a list of considerations for using oxygen:

1. Use oxygen as permitted by the treatment tables. Halt the use of oxygen only if the patient tolerates the oxygen poorly or if it is unsafe to use in the chamber.
2. Take all precautions against fire.
3. Attend the patient carefully, being alert for the symptoms of oxygen toxicity.

Inside Observers

The following is a list of considerations for inside observers:

1. The team members should be qualified to serve as inside medical attendants during treatment. A patient should never be left alone in the chamber.
2. The inside medical attendant should be alert for any change in the condition of the patient, especially during oxygen breathing.
3. The inside medical attendant who has been with a patient throughout treatment should breathe oxygen, as follows:
   a. On Table 1, breathe oxygen at 40 ft (12 m) for 30 minutes.
   b. On Table 2, breathe oxygen at 30 ft (9 m) for 1 hour.
   c. On Table 3 or 4, breathe oxygen the last 30 minutes at 40 ft (12 m) and the last hour each at 30 ft (9 m), 20 ft (6 m) and 10 ft (3 m).
   d. On Tables 5 and 6, breathe oxygen during the last 30 minutes of treatment, that is, on ascent from 30 ft (9 m) to the surface.
   e. On Table 6, which has been lengthened, breathe oxygen during the last 45 minutes at 30 ft (9 m) and during the 30-minute ascent to the surface.

Anyone entering or leaving the chamber before completing the treatment should be decompressed according to the standard Navy air or oxygen decompression tables.

Outside attendants should specify and control the decompression of anyone leaving the chamber. A physician outside the chamber must review recommendations concerning the treatment or decompression made by those, including physicians, inside the chamber.

Most Frequent Errors Related to Treatment

The following is a list of the most frequent errors related to treatment:

1. Failure of the patient to report symptoms early.
2. Failure to treat doubtful cases.
3. Failure to treat promptly.
4. Failure to treat adequately.

5. Failure to recognize serious symptoms.
6. Failure to keep the patient near the chamber after treatment.
7. Failure to ensure that personnel inside the chamber avoid cramped positions that might interfere with circulation.

Adjuvants to Hyperbaric Therapy

Hyperbaric therapy is the only definitive treatment for decompression sickness. Secondary effects resulting from biochemical events at the blood-bubble interface or damage to vessel endothelia, however, must be treated appropriately. In serious cases of decompression sickness, a marked loss of intravascular volume can occur by transudation of plasma across damaged capillary walls. Hemoconcentration producing malperfusion of tissue and sludging of red blood cells should be avoided or corrected by the prompt and adequate administration of intravenous Ringer's lactate or normal saline solution. In some cases, up to 1 L/hr of intravenous crystalloid solution will be necessary to correct the hemoconcentration. Frequent checks of urinary output are the best guide to the adequacy of the intravenous fluid therapy. Urinary output should be maintained at 1 to 2 ml/kg/hr. Dexamethasone, 20 mg intravenously followed by 4 mg intramuscularly every 6 hours, may be useful in the prevention or treatment of central nervous system edema. In cases of neurologic decompression sickness affecting the spinal cord, an indwelling urinary catheter should be placed because these patients most commonly develop a neurogenic bladder.

Cases of decompression sickness following diving do not result in near-drowning as frequently as do cases of cerebral air embolism; nevertheless, the possibility of near-drowning must be evaluated and treatment begun when warranted. In such cases, intensive pulmonary care is mandatory. Endotracheal intubation, assisted ventilation, and correction of acidosis by the frequent and adequate intravenous administration of bicarbonate may be necessary.

None of the above procedures should delay movement of the patient to a hyperbaric chamber except when necessary as immediate life-sustaining measures. It is just as important, however, to institute or continue such procedures after hyperbaric therapy is begun as part of the overall intensive care management of serious cases.

DIRECT EFFECTS OF PRESSURE CHANGE

Gas contained within body cavities is saturated with water vapor, the partial pressure of which is related to body temperature. Because body temperature is relatively constant (37°C), the partial pressure of the water vapor is also constant at 47 mm Hg. In determining the mechanical effect of gas expansion, one must account for the noncompressibility of water vapor, which causes wet gases to respond to pressure changes differently than dry gases. Thus, the following relationship can be expressed as Boyle's Law with reference to wet gas:

$$V_i(P_i - P_{H_2O}) = V_f(P_f - P_{H_2O}) \quad (11)$$

where V_i is the initial volume of the gas; V_f is the final volume of the gas; P_i is the initial pressure of the gas in the cavity in mm Hg; P_f is the final pressure of the gas in the cavity in mm Hg; and P_{H_2O} is the partial pressure of water vapor (47 mm Hg at 37°C). Over a given pressure reduction, wet gas will expand to a greater degree than dry gas. The relative gas expansion is a ratio of the final volume of the gas (V_f) to the initial volume (V_i) of the gas and is expressed in the following equation:

Relative gas expansion

$$= \frac{V_f}{V_i} = \frac{P_i - P_{H_2O}}{P_f - P_{H_2O}} = \frac{(P_i - 47)}{(P_f - 47)} \quad (12)$$

Figure 7.13 illustrates the increased volume of wet gases at a given pressure over that of a dry gas.

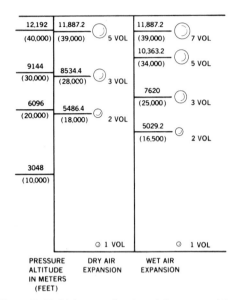

PRESSURE ALTITUDE IN METERS (FEET)   DRY AIR EXPANSION   WET AIR EXPANSION

Figure 7.13. Volumes of wet and dry gases with varying pressures.

When one experiences a change in ambient pressure, a pressure differential is established between gas-containing body cavities and the external environment. To the extent that gas can move between body cavities and the external environment, this pressure differential will be relieved. It also can be relieved by a change in the volume of the body cavity (compliance). When the pressure differential is not relieved, pathologic effects on involved tissues are likely to occur. The magnitude of the pathologic effects is related to the ratio of the pressure of the gas within the affected body cavity to the ambient pressure and not to the absolute value of the pressure differential. This is predictable from examining the pressure-volume relationships of Boyle's Law. Therefore, divers, for example, experience more difficulties with the mechanical effects of pressure change when descending from sea level to 33 fsw (10 msw) (equations 13 and 14), than they do when descending from 99 to 132 fsw (30 to 40 msw) (equations 15 and 16). Note that the pressure differential is identical for both circumstances, but the pressure ratio is considerably different.

Pressure differential:

$$P_f - P_i = 1520 \text{ mm Hg} - 760 \text{ mm Hg}$$
$$= 760 \text{ mm Hg} \qquad (13)$$

Pressure ratio,

$$\frac{P_f}{P_i} = \frac{1520 \text{ mm Hg}}{760 \text{ mm Hg}} = 2 \qquad (14)$$

Pressure differential:

$$P_f - P_i = 3800 \text{ mm Hg} - 3040 \text{ mm Hg}$$
$$= 760 \text{ mm Hg} \qquad (15)$$

Pressure ratio,

$$\frac{P_f}{P_i} = \frac{3800 \text{ mm Hg}}{3040 \text{ mm Hg}} = 1.25 \qquad (16)$$

Medically significant pressure changes occur in both flying and diving. There is a marked difference, however, between these two operations with respect to the magnitude and rate of the pressure changes. An aviator descending to sea level from 7620 m at 1520 m/min (25,000 ft at 5,000 ft/min) will experience a total pressure change of 478 mm Hg at a rate of 2.3 mm Hg/sec. A diver descending from sea level to 165 fsw (50 msw) at a rate of 60 ft/min (18 m/min) will experience a total pressure change of 3800 mm Hg at a rate of 23 mm Hg/sec.

In general, one can successfully cope with the changes in barometric pressures that occur within the flying or diving envelopes. As long as the pressure in the various body cavities can equalize with the ambient pressure, one can withstand tremendous pressure changes. For example, meaningful work has been performed by aviators at pressures equivalent to 0.1 atm abs (15,240 m or 59,000 ft) and by divers at pressures equivalent to 69 atm abs (686 m or 2250 ft).

If equalization of pressure is not attained, difficulties ranging from mild discomfort to severe pain, tissue damage, and complete incapacitation will be experienced. The areas of primary concern are the lungs, middle and inner ear, paranasal sinuses, teeth, and the gastrointestinal tract.

The Lungs

Unless air is continually exchanged between the lungs and the outside environment during changes in ambient pressure, severe pathologic disorders can result from the effects of Boyle's Law. Airflow during pressure change will not occur with voluntary breathholding or the apneic phase of tonoclonic seizure.

Consider the potential problem of a breathholding descent during diving. The average total lung capacity is 5800 cm^3. The residual volume (i.e., the volume to which the lungs can be reduced with forceful expiration) is 1200 cm^3. If the air volume within the lungs is reduced below 1200 cm^3, the actual lung volume will decrease no further due to the elastic and fibrous skeletal structure of the lung tissue. The volume deficit is made up by the leakage of plasma and whole blood into the lungs. This is the classic description of the pathologic condition called "lung squeeze" and is more common in breathholding diving than in descent from altitude. To achieve lung squeeze, the air volume within the lungs must be reduced to about 20% of the original volume. To achieve this on descent from altitude, an aviator would have to make a breathholding descent from 11,890 m (39,000 ft) to sea level. A breathholding dive to 132 fsw, however, will result in such a fivefold decrease in the original lung volume. Such a dive is well within the capabilities of many expert divers.

In compressed-gas diving, respirable gas is supplied to the diver from the surface, from a diving bell or hyperbaric chamber, or from a self-contained underwater breathing apparatus (scuba). The gas may be supplied through regulators designed to match intrapulmonary gas pressure to the surrounding ambient pressure. The compressed-gas-supplied diver avoids lung squeeze on descent but runs an added risk on ascent. During ascent to the surface, the diver must continually equilibrate the intrapulmonary pressure to the surrounding pressure. This equilibration is usually accomplished by releasing gas from the lungs by normal breathing or, in the event of the loss of gas supply at depth, by slow continual exhalation on ascent. Failure to do so results in intrapulmonary gas expansion according to Boyle's Law and, after the elastic limit of the thorax is reached, a relative rise of intra-alveolar pressure. A rise in intra-alveolar pressure of 50 to 100 mm Hg above ambient pressure is sufficient to force gas into extra-alveolar compartments, resulting in one or more of the clinical conditions grouped under the term pulmonary overpressure accidents.

Pressure differentials sufficient to cause a pulmonary overpressure accident in the compressed-gas-supplied diver can occur on ascents as shallow as from 2 m (7 ft) to the surface. Moreover, a pulmonary overpressure accident is a distinct risk to an aviator whose aircraft suffers a sudden loss of cabin pressure at high altitude.

Autopsies of fatalities following pulmonary overpressure accidents have demonstrated extra-alveolar gas in essentially every tissue examined. Following such an accident, however, the clinical picture seen will be that of arterial gas embolism, mediastinal and subcutaneous emphysema, and/or pneumothorax. The latter two manifestations are recognized by physical and radiographic examination and are managed by conventional measures. The manifestations of arterial gas embolism have an immediate onset following the rapid pressure reduction and may include loss of consciousness, local or generalized seizures, visual field loss or blindness, weakness, paralysis, hypoesthesia, or confusion. A patient presenting with any of these signs or symptoms within 15 minutes following exposure to a rapid pressure reduction must be assumed to have suffered an arterial gas embolism and be treated for such.

Predisposing Factors

In addition to breathholding during ascent, pulmonary overpressure accidents also can occur as a consequence of preexisting disease that limits the egress of gas from the lungs. Thus, the risk is increased by asthma, chronic bronchitis, air-containing pulmonary cysts, and other obstructive airway disease. Some pulmonary overpressure accidents have occurred without demonstrable cause in patients who exhaled during ascent and had no subsequent lung disorders. In these cases, local pulmonary air trapping is thought to have occurred by redundant tissue, mucous plugs, or similar mechanisms establishing a one-way valve in a small air passage, which allowed gas to pass during compression but not during decompression.

An increasing number of cases of gas embolism are caused by the introduction of air or other gas into the arterial or venous system during surgical procedures or following the establishment of indwelling arterial catheters. With the increasing use of indwelling catheters and surgical procedures involving invasion of the cardiovascular system, the number of gas embolism cases also has increased. Stoney and colleagues (10) have estimated that the accidental introduction of air through arterial lines occurs in more than 1 in 1000 cases.

Diagnosis

The most difficult differential diagnosis is between gas embolism and neurologic decompression sickness when decompression is involved. This diagnosis is important because of the need to select a proper treatment table. The key factor in reaching a proper diagnosis is the time before the onset of symptoms. The onset is immediate with gas embolism, with symptoms usually occurring within 1 to 2 minutes of reaching the surface. This fact is of critical importance if the person is diving alone because drowning may obscure the underlying gas embolism.

The symptoms and signs elicited in a USAF series of 13 patients treated for gas embolism as a result of recreational scuba diving are listed in Table 7.2. The most common presenting sign was coma, noted in 70% of patients, followed by paralysis, which occurred in 54% of patients. These signs may clear rapidly, and, by the time

Table 7.2.
Signs and Symptoms in Scuba Related Gas Embolism—13 Cases

Sign/Symptom	Number of Cases	Percent
Loss of consciousness	9	70
Loss of movement–extremity	7	54
Seizure	5	38
Loss of sensation–extremity	4	31
Vertigo	4	31
Mediastinal emphysema	3	23
Nausea and vomiting	3	23
Chest pain (unilateral)	2	15
Subcutaneous emphysema	2	15
Aphasia	1	8
Blindness	1	8
"Spaced-out" aura	1	8

the patient is first seen by a physician, the clinical picture may be quite similar to a mild stroke or transient ischemic attack. This should not, however, interfere with the diagnosis of a probable gas embolism if the patient has been exposed to a rapid pressure change.

The diagnosis of a surgical gas embolism should be considered in any patient with indwelling arterial or venous lines (particularly a central line). The sudden onset of seizure or coma is frequently the presenting sign. Venous gas embolism is more common and much less of a problem due to the well-known microfiltration capability of the lung. Nonetheless, it may present as a systemic embolism in the presence of a patent foramen ovale with right to left shunting.

In surgical cases, general anesthesia may mask the unusual symptoms; however, failure of the patient to awaken normally or the presentation of an unexplained neurologic deficit should alert one to the diagnosis of possible intraoperative gas embolism. A brief neurologic examination may reveal a myriad of central nervous system findings depending on the location of the gas. Funduscopic examination may reveal arteriolar bubbles in some instances. Computerized tomographic (CT) scanning of the head may be used diagnostically when it is immediately available.

In the diagnosis and treatment of gas embolism, time is of the essence. Although some patients survive a delay of up to 24 hours the experience of treatment facilities, with a mortality range of 20–25%, indicates that time from embolus to treatment is a most important factor.

Treatment

To provide effective therapy for gas embolism, it is important to remember the basic difference between decompression sickness (air or gas bubbles evolving from solution) and gas embolism (gas bubbles that enter the arterial or venous circulation directly). Although the manifestations of decompression sickness are diverse, they are rarely fatal when treated by proper hyperbaric therapy within hours to days of occurrence. Conversely, the onset of gas embolism is sudden, dramatic, and life-threatening. Bubbles obstruct the systematic or pulmonary arterial circulation. As decompression continues, they expand to produce local endothelial cell damage and herniation into the vessel walls. In addition, plasma proteins react to the invading bubbles by denaturization and attachment to the bubble wall. Activation and agglutination of platelets to the bubbles occur, with release of very potent vasoactive amines and prostaglandins, which produce immediate hypoxia symptoms that may appear as neurologic deficits.

The rationale for hyperbaric therapy for decompression sickness also applies to the management of gas embolism: mechanical compression of bubbles and hyperbaric oxygenation of tissues. Because of the massive amounts of air that are often introduced into the cerebral circulation of gas embolism victims, it is usually necessary to mechanically compress the entrapped air maximally. The volume of air can be reduced by 83% by compressing to 6 atm abs (50 msw or 165 fsw) (see Figure 7.4). The volume is further reduced by placing the victim in the Trendelenburg (30° head-low) position. This position increases cerebral hydrostatic pressure and, in some cases, forces small bubbles from the arterial circulation across the cerebral capillary bed into the venous circulation, where it produces less potential harm to the victim. It must be emphasized that 100% oxygen breathing cannot be administered at 6 atm abs due to the extremely short time to central nervous system oxygen toxicity. Convulsive seizures would occur in less than 5 minutes. Elevated oxygen percentages, however, can be administered in the form of 50/50 Nitrox (a mixture of 50% oxygen and 50% nitrogen). This mixture will assist in correcting tissue hypoxia and ischemia because of the improved oxygen diffusion distance.

When it has been determined that maximum benefit has been attained from the mechanical compression of the entrapped air, the patient must be brought to shallower depths so that 100% oxygen can be administered. Because of the advantages of treating with 100% oxygen, the United States Navy Diving Manual suggests initial compression to 2.8 atm abs (18 msw or 60 fsw) for one 20 minute oxygen breathing period before making the decision on whether to pressurize to 6 atm abs (50 msw or 165 fsw) (2).

A summary of the decision points in the treatment of gas embolism is presented in Figure 7.14. Hyperbaric therapy is the only definitive treatment for arterial gas embolism. All other methods are adjunctive in nature. As soon as the diagnosis is made, the patient should be placed in the chamber and rapidly compressed with air to 2.8 atm abs. The patient is placed on 100% oxygen for a 20 minute breathing period. If symptoms stabilize or improve, treatment continues on Table 6 (Figure 7.9). If symptoms worsen, the patient is compressed to 6 atm abs and treatment continues on Table 6A (Fig. 7.15), or on the modified Treatment Table 6A shown in Figure 7.16.

Variation from the standard Table 6A is potentially harmful to both the patient and inside observers and should not be done without prior consultation with experts in diving medicine.

Adjunctive measures that should be used are intravenous fluids and steroids in pharmacologic doses. Hemoconcentration is frequently seen in gas embolism and may be related to tissue

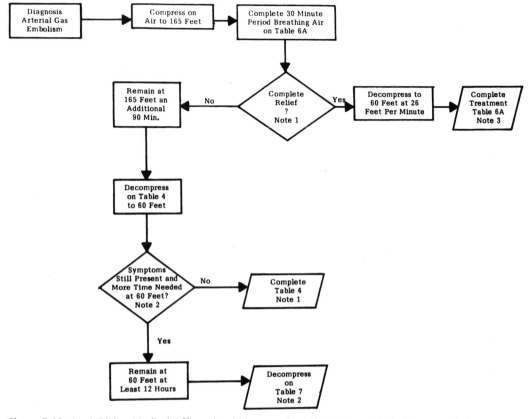

Figure 7.14. 1—A Diving Medical Officer should be consulted if at all possible before committing to a Treatment Table 4.
2—Commit to a Treatment Table 7 only in consultation with a Diving Medical Officer.
3—Treatment Table 6A may be extended if necessary at 60 and/or 30 feet (Fig. 7.12).

hypoxia and edema. Divers are also commonly dehydrated secondary to pressure diuresis and lack of normal oral fluid intake. Vigorous hydration is important to minimize sludging and obstruction of microvascular blood flow caused by the elevated hematocrit. Balanced saline solution (Ringer's lactate) or isotonic saline without dextrose should be administered intravenously at the rate of 1 L/hr until the patient voids or is catheterized for at least 500 ml. Sugar (glucose) is specifically not given to prevent further dehydration secondary to glycosuria and a resultant osmotic diuresis. Once adequate hydration is achieved, the rate is slowed to 150 to 200 ml/hr for the remainder of the treatment.

As soon as possible, dexamethasone is admin-istered intravenously in a dose of 20 mg followed by 4 mg intramuscularly every 6 hours for 24 to 48 hours. There is no supportive evidence for the idea that steroids may increase an individual's susceptibility to oxygen toxicity. Anticoagulant or antiplatelet medications are not currently recommended for treating gas embolism.

Transport of Patients

One hundred percent oxygen should be started as soon as possible, using a tightly fitted aviator's or anesthesia-type mask. The patient should be placed in a recumbent position while awaiting and during transport to the hyperbaric chamber. If transport is required, it is of utmost

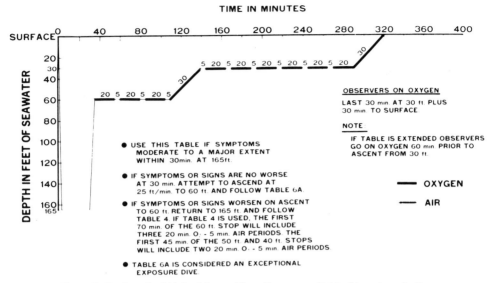

Figure 7.15. Standard United States Navy Treatment Table 6A—air embolism.

importance to maintain near sea-level pressure. The use of "low-flying" helicopters is contraindicated if ground transportation is available. Even slight decreases in pressure cause bubble enlargement and may significantly alter the clinical course of the patient.

During transport, intravenous fluids should be administered using balanced saline solutions or normal saline. Patients suffering from the more serious forms of decompression sickness or from cerebral gas embolism should be accompanied during transport by personnel capable of giving respiratory and cardiac life-support care.

Immediate hyperbaric therapy is essential. Good response, however, has been seen in some cases after long delays before reaching the chamber. This makes it mandatory to give the patient the benefit of a trial of compression and hyperbaric oxygen even in the late case. Of course, every minute that elapses before the start of compression makes the prognosis more guarded.

Return to Flying Duties

A decision as to when and if to return a person to flying duties following a cerebral gas embolism is complex. Consideration must be given to the circumstances under which the gas embolism occurred and the presence or absence of underlying pulmonary pathology (as predictors of recurrence) as well as evidence for residual neurological pathology. A rational approach is to consider a cerebral gas embolism a head injury. The patient evaluation strategies following head injuries used by the appropriate regulating agencies (Federal Aviation Administration or military authorities) then provide a basis for decisions on return to flying duties. In no case, however, should a patient return to such duties earlier than

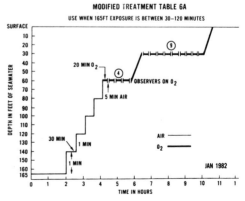

Figure 7.16. Standard United States Navy Treatment Table 6A (modified)—air embolism.

3 weeks following such an incident to assure complete pulmonary healing has occurred.

Other Gas-Containing Cavities

Direct effects of pressure change on the ear, paranasal sinuses, and teeth are described in Chapter 17, Otolaryngology in Aerospace Medicine. This section addresses these effects on the gastrointestinal system and on medical equipment.

The Gastrointestinal Tract

Gas is normally contained in the stomach and the large bowel. As previously discussed, wet gases expand to a greater extent than do dry gases. Expansion within the closed confines of the gastrointestinal tract during ascent can cause stretching of the enclosing organ and produce abdominal pain. In addition to pain, respiration also can be compromised by gas expansion, forcing the diaphragm upward. If pain is allowed to proceed and relief is not obtained by belching or the passing of flatus, flight operations will be jeopardized. Severe pain may cause a vasovagal reaction with hypotension, tachycardia, and fainting. The best treatment of gastrointestinal tract discomfort due to gas expansion is the avoidance of gas-producing foods. Chewing gum may promote air swallowing and should be avoided at least during ascent. The crewmember should be instructed to pass gas when discomfort occurs. Abdominal massage and physical activity may promote the passage of gas. If this is unsuccessful, a descent should be initiated to an altitude at which comfort is achieved.

Effects of Pressure Change on Medical Equipment

Varying volumes of gas may be trapped in medical equipment being used in the aerospace or hyperbaric environment. Examples of such equipment include drip chambers for intravenous fluids, endotracheal cuffs, water traps used with chest tubes, and sphygmomanometer cuffs.

During ascent, an unvented sphygmomanometer cuff will inflate and tighten around a patient's arm. If air is used to inflate an endotracheal cuff, significant ambient pressure reductions, particularly as seen with ascents from hyperbaric environments, can cause tracheal mucosal sloughing if allowed to persist. A wise precaution is to inflate endotracheal cuffs with normal saline rather than air in such environments. Water levels in water traps should be checked often or opened to ambient pressure when significant changes in pressure occur. The air space in intravenous line drip chambers will decrease in volume with increased pressure in hyperbaric chambers. Additional air will have to be added to the drip chamber to monitor the drip rate. On ascent, the volume of air will increase, and if added air is not replaced with fluid, intravenous air will inadvertently be administered.

The possible effects of changes in pressure on all medical equipment should be considered before such equipment is used either in a hyperbaric chamber or in flight. When possible, the equipment should be functionally tested in the pressure environment in which it is to be used before it is used with patients.

The quest to fly ever higher and dive even deeper has expanded man's pressure environmental envelope well beyond that to which he is physiologically adapted. Pathologic changes resulting from exposure to these environments have defined new sets of clinical syndromes specifically related causally to pressure changes. Studies of the pathophysiology underlying these syndromes have unmasked two separate categories of disorders: indirect effects of pressure change resulting from the evolution of gas from solution and direct effects of pressure change on gas-containing body cavities. In addition, it is now recognized that the pressure environment represents a physiologic continuum from the increased pressures encountered by divers to the decreased pressures encountered by aviators and astronauts. This continuum is dramatically exemplified by the diver who surfaces safely only to experience decompression sickness a few hours later while flying at low altitude.

As we have learned more about the physiologic changes that occur with changes in pressure, we have been able to develop rational treatment methods to cope with the medical disorders they bring about. Thus, hyperbaric therapy, with specific treatment profiles for mild and severe decompression sickness and for gas embolism, has lessened mortality and the incidence of permanent residual deficits. Adjuvants to hyperbaric therapy are increasing our ability to deal with these disorders. Further refinements in therapeutic techniques are necessary, however, as evidenced by a 15% failure rate in the treatment of serious forms of decompression sickness and cerebral gas embolism.

Advances in technology have allowed for the development of systems capable of transporting man into increasingly more severe pressure environments. Similar technologic advances have made possible the development of the life-support equipment necessary to prevent the pathophysiologic consequences of exposure to these environments. Unfortunately, the development of practical, effective life-support systems tends to lag behind the development of transport systems. Historically, this lag resulted from a lack of knowledge about the physiologic consequences of exposure to hostile environments. Today, however, these consequences are much more predictable. The effective and safe use of advanced flying and diving systems depends on parallel developments in biotechnology. The compatible marriage of man to machine presents an ongoing challenge now and in the foreseeable future.

REFERENCES

1. Sheffield PJ. Flying after diving guidelines: a review. Aviat Space Environ Med 1990;61:1130–1138.
2. Naval Sea Systems Command. United States Navy diving manual. Vol I. Flagstaff, AZ: Best Publishing, 1993.
3. Davis JC, Sheffield PJ, Schuknecht L, et al. Altitude decompression sickness: Hyperbaric therapy results in 145 cases. Aviat Space Environ Med 1977;48:722.
4. Sheffield PJ, Dunn JM. Continuous monitoring of tissue oxygen tension during hyperbaric oxygen therapy—a preliminary report. Proceedings of the Sixth International Congress of Hyperbaric Medicine. G. Smith, ed. Aberdeen, Scotland: Aberdeen University Press, 1979.
5. Behnke AR. Decompression sickness incident to deep sea diving and high altitude ascent. Medicine 1945;24: 381.
6. Donnell AM Jr., Morgan CP. Successful use of the recompression chamber in severe decompression sickness with neurocirculatory collapse. Aerospace Med 1960; 31:1004.
7. Downey VM, Worley TW, Hackworth R, et al. Studies on bubbles in human serum under increased and decreased atmospheric pressures. Aerospace Med 1963; 35:116.
8. Leverett SD, Bitter HL, McIver RG. Studies in decompression sickness: Circulatory and respiratory changes associated with decompression sickness in anesthetized dogs. SAM-TDR-63-7, United States Air Force School of Aerospace Medicine, Brooks Air Force Base, TX, 1963.
9. Goodman MW, Workman RD. Minimal-recompression oxygen-breathing approach to treatment of decompression sickness in divers and aviators. Research Report 8-65, United States Navy Experimental Diving Unit, Washington, D.C.: Government Printing Office, 1965.
10. Stoney WS, Alford WC Jr., Burrus GR, et al. Air embolism and other accidents using pump oxygenators. Ann Thorac Surg 1980;29:336.

RECOMMENDED READING

Bennett PB, Elliott DH, eds. The physiology and medicine of diving and compressed air work. 2nd ed. Baltimore: Williams & Wilkins, 1975.

Davis JC, Hunt TK, eds. Hyperbaric oxygen therapy. Bethesda, MD: Undersea Medical Society, 1977.

Fryer DI. Subatmospheric decompression sickness in man. Slough, England: Technovision Services. The Advisory Group for Aerospace Research and Development, NATO, 1969.

Adler, HF. Dysbarism. Aeromedical Review 1–64.: United States Air Force School of Aerospace Medicine, Brooks Air Force Base, TX, 1964.

Philp, RB. A review of blood changes associated with compression-decompression relationship to decompression sickness. Undersea Biomed Res 1974;1:117.

Gray JS, Mahady SCF, Masland RL. Studies on altitude decompression sickness III. The effects of denitrogenation. J Aviat Med 1946;17:606.

Cooke JP. Denitrogenation interruptions with air. Aviat Space Environ Med 1976;47:1205.

Kindwall EP, ed. Hyperbaric medicine practice. Flagstaff, AZ: Best Publishing, 1994.

Chapter 8

Biodynamics: Transient Acceleration

James W. Brinkley

James H. Raddin, Jr.

Real science exists, then, only from the moment when a phenomenon is accurately defined as to its nature and rigorously determined in relation to its material conditions, that is, when its law is known. Before that, we have only groping and empiricism.

Claude Bernard

From the dawn of time, people have had a problem with transient acceleration. Pedestrian existence was fraught with a wide range of hazards, from falls onto hard surfaces to hard surfaces falling. The equestrian age led to new respect for the low but sturdy tree limb. Surface vehicles increased the potential for relative velocities and their rapid diminishment. The greatest relative velocities could always be produced through the use of two such vehicles. The advent of powered flight provided the potential for establishing even larger relative velocities between people and their accustomed environment. Well-laid plans have usually been made to allow the gradual elimination of these velocities and a benign termination of the experience. This chapter recognizes the inadequacy of some of those plans.

HISTORY OF THE SCIENCE

In 1908, when people had little experience in powered flight, United States Army Lieutenant Frank Selfridge died of injuries sustained in the crash of the airplane in which he was riding. The pilot, Orville Wright, also was injured. Attention

was drawn to the problem of minimizing the adverse effects of sudden changes in velocity. At first, little was done. After all, aviation presented a multiplicity of challenges that were encountered on every flight. Crashes did not occur with each flight, and if you planned to crash, some would suggest that you shouldn't go up. Eventually, the necessity for transitory acceleration protection became more clearly recognized.

The seat belt was probably introduced in 1910. Its initial function was simply to hold the occupant in the seat during vibration, turbulence, or maneuvers. The seat belt, however, was eventually refined to act as an impact protection devise. A double shoulder harness was added to the belt in 1939.

The protective helmet was adapted from sports following Selfridge's accident but did not come into general military use until much later. Early helmet tests were performed by volunteer subjects who dashed their heads against stone walls and then described the experience. Refinements, such as accelerator measurement and a heavy pendulum for controlled impacts, were added later.

Rigid parachutes apparently were used to jump from high places by the Chinese around 1100. The parachute, as an alternate means of descending from flight, dates to around 1793 for descent from a balloon and as early as 1912 for descent from a Benoise aircraft. The 1912 jump was made over Jefferson Barracks, St. Louis, Missouri. The parachutist, Captain Albert Berry, jumped from the landing gear axle. The weight of his falling body pulled the parachute from a metal container mounted above the axle. As aircraft speeds increased and the motion of the aircraft became more violent when control was lost, bailing out over the side became more and more difficult. Some mechanism was, therefore, sought to facilitate escape from a disabled aircraft.

The work on ejection seats was done by the Germans, Swedish, British, and Americans during and after World War II. The primary stimulus for most early developments was the use of centered, aftmounted pusher propellers. The Swedish conducted dummy ejections from a B-3 bomber using compressed air in January, 1942 and from a B-17 using a ballistic catapult in February, 1944. The Germans apparently had an operational ejection seat in the Heinkel 162 in 1944. The first Swedish emergency ejection took place on July 29, 1946 from a J-21A with a pusher propeller, saving the life of the pilot. Sir James Martin conducted the British developments, achieving an experimental ejection of a volunteer subject on July 24, 1946 from a modified Meteor III. The first British emergency ejection took place on May 30, 1949 from a prototype flying wing. United States researchers at Wright-Patterson AFB, Dayton, Ohio, conducted an experimental airborne ejection in August, 1946. The first emergency ejection in the United States Air Force took place on August 29, 1949 from an F-86.

Developments in protecting humans from the adverse effects of transient acceleration have been pursued along many lines. Definition of the ability to withstand brief acceleration has proceeded hand-in-hand with the search for more efficient and less injurious ways to apply the forces necessary to produce it. Vehicle designers have improved structural designs to decrease the potential for collapse or intrusions into the occupant's living space. The means have been devised to provide supplemental protection when the need arises and to adapt the performance of the protection system to the challenge being encountered.

At the same time, advances in aerospace technology and new applications of existing technology have been accompanied by the potential for more severe acceleration environments. Moderate- and high-speed flight at very low altitude has decreased the time and distance available to accomplish ejection initiation and recovery prior to ground impact. High-speed flight at high altitude has compounded the problems of vehicle clearance during emergency egress, windblast, and parachute opening shock, as well as the necessity for simultaneous protection from other environmental extremes. Space operations may well require orbital vehicle escape systems, which will experience even greater environmental extremes, including those of atmospheric reentry.

The impact protection field is diverse, challenging, and complex. Certain fundamental underpinnings, however, provide the basis for understanding the specific techniques and applications.

DEFINITIONS AND BASIC PHYSICAL RELATIONSHIPS

Acceleration

Acceleration takes place whenever the velocity of an object changes, either in magnitude or direction. Acceleration is a vector quantity. This means that it has a direction or orientation, as well as magnitude or size. Whenever the magnitude is expressed, the direction also must be specified before the acceleration can be considered to be defined. Acceleration magnitude is expressed in terms of velocity units per unit of time. For example, if velocity magnitude is expressed in meters per second, acceleration magnitude would be expressed in meters per second per second or meters per second squared. For convenience, transitory and sustained accelerations in aerospace applications are frequently expressed in terms of ''g.'' One g is the magnitude of the acceleration of an object when it is dropped in a vacuum at the earth's surface. The value is approximately 9.8 m/sec^2. Substantial confusion has resulted from the erroneous practice of using g as a unit of force instead of or as well as acceleration. Meters per second squared and g are always and only units of acceleration magnitude. Another source of confusion is the use of the term deceleration, as if it were physically distinct from acceleration. When used, deceleration simply refers to acceleration that tends to reduce an established velocity.

Impact Acceleration

Impact acceleration is defined as a short-term or transient acceleration that is not sustained long enough to result in a significant unchanging or steady-state component in the mechanical response by the accelerated body. Longer duration accelerations are called sustained accelerations and are treated in Chapter 9. Implicit in this response definition of impact is the requirement for an acceleration magnitude sufficiently high for some observable transitory mechanical response to occur. The accelerated body must be compressed, rearranged, or otherwise mechanically affected in an impact acceleration. A further implication of this is that various parts of the impacted body will experience somewhat different accelerations in response to impact. Sustained acceleration eventually tends to produce substantially similar acceleration responses in all the body parts.

Attempts have been made to define impact accelerations in terms of duration. For example, acceleration events having durations less than 1 or 2 seconds have been defined as impacts by various authors. The transitory versus steady-state response definition proposed in this chapter, however, will have different ranges of duration for different accelerated bodies, depending on the frequency response of the body. A fixed time duration definition is, therefore, not generally applicable over the range of acceleration profiles and accelerated bodies that are of interest in aerospace medicine. Instead, the response and the resulting stress determine the category.

Sustained acceleration protection is applied in those situations in which the stresses are primarily physiologic and sustained. Impact acceleration protection is applied in those situations in which the stresses are primarily mechanical and transitory. Extensive overlap occurs in the two forms of acceleration. Physiologic disruptions, such as unconsciousness, may be produced by impact or by sustained acceleration, but the mechanism in impact is traumatic instead of hemodynamic. Ideally, the techniques of impact protection should blend into and complement the techniques of sustained acceleration protection, just as the actual acceleration stresses often overlap the two definitions.

Coordinate Systems

The direction and magnitude of an object's velocity must always be measured with respect to some other points that establish a reference frame. For example, an aircraft flying in formation may have a low velocity with respect to a wingman and a relatively high velocity with respect to a control tower. The velocity of an object, which is a vector quantity, is simply the time rate of change of the object's position vector in the chosen reference frame. Similarly, the acceleration of an object, also a vector quantity, is simply the time rate of change of the object's velocity vector in the chosen reference frame. Velocity and acceleration values measured with respect to one reference frame are identical to those measured in another reference frame if, and only if, there is no relative motion between the reference frames. Acceleration will still be the same even when one frame is translating at constant velocity with respect to the other frame. In general, the velocity and acceleration values to be observed with respect to one frame can be computed from the values observed with respect to another frame if the relative motions between the two frames are well described.

The reason all of this is important in a discussion of impact is that experimental measurements and real-world situations frequently may be misinterpreted if the reference frames are not clearly understood. For example, a fixed motion picture camera on an impact test sled will measure the motion of a subject with respect to the sled, but the sled will generally be moving and accelerating with respect to the earth. Linear accelerometers mounted to the subject are sometimes used to deduce acceleration with respect to the earth. Rotation of the subject, and thus the accelerometers, however, can make this determination difficult at best and often impossible. Comparison of impact response data derived from a sled-fixed camera with data derived from a subject-fixed accelerometer will require additional measures of sled and subject motions, including rotations.

Reference frames used in describing impact accelerations vary with the vehicle and the measurement systems involved. For human exposures, however, it has been convenient at least to express head and chest accelerations with respect to an earth-fixed frame which rotates with the body part. A convention has been established to define an orthogonal, mutually perpendicular set of three axes for the head and chest. In a forward-facing, erect position, the x-axis is oriented front to back or perpendicular to a coronal plane, the y-axis is oriented laterally or perpendicular to a sagittal plane, and the z-axis is oriented vertically or perpendicular to a horizontal plane. These axes are shown in Figure 8.1. Some attempts have been made to define these axes very precisely using radiographic landmarks, but the practical utility of these approaches has not been established because anatomic variations tend to nullify the presumed increase in accuracy. Approximate definitions have been ade-

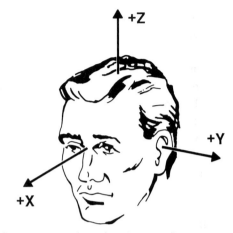

Figure 8.1. Head acceleration coordinate system.

quate for most purposes. Other groups have defined anatomic coordinate systems for other body parts such as the pelvis, hand, and foot, but these have not found wide practical application in aerospace medicine.

Confusion has resulted from the definition of the positive directions for the acceleration axes defined above. As shown in Figure 8.1, +x is anterior, +z is cephalad, and +y is to the left by recent agreement of the International Standards Organization. This leads to a so-called right-handed system where +x is along the right index finger, +y is along the right middle finger held at a right angle, and +z is along the thumb, when it is held at a right angle to the other two. Until recently, a left-handed convention for acceleration has been used with the sign of the y axis reversed from the right-handed system. The left-handed convention resulted from an early approach that defined a right-handed system for reaction forces. Since the reaction forces are positive in the directions opposite to the accelerations, the new acceleration convention leads to a left-handed system for the reaction forces. If you don't believe that, turn a right-handed glove inside out and try it on the left hand.

An acceleration that tends to increase the forward velocity of the head and/or torso, then, is +x acceleration. Equivalently, +x acceleration may also decrease the rearward velocity of these structures. Reaction forces commonly have been used to visualize these motions. With this technique, +x acceleration becomes eyeballs-in acceleration. This works well and accommodates both increasing forward velocity and decreasing rearward velocity because it is easy to imagine which way you accelerate to push your eyeballs in. One still must, however, remember the sign change associated with eyeballs-in (−x reaction) for +x acceleration. Similarly, +z is eyeballs-down and +y is eyeballs-right.

Acceleration and Force

Perhaps the most basic tenet of physics is the Newtonian relationship between acceleration and force:

$$F = m \, a \qquad (1)$$

A net force (F) on a mass (m) will produce an acceleration (a) in the same direction as the force. Equivalently, the velocity of a mass cannot be altered, either in direction or magnitude, without application of a force to produce the change. Acceleration can be calculated by multiple, timed observations of position, and force can be measured by the use of a spring scale, but aggregate mass is deduced from Equation 1. Force may be applied mechanically, gravitationally, electrostatically, or magnetically. Mechanical force application is most common in impact situations and requires physical contact between the accelerated object and some object that applies the accelerating force. Force application, by any means, is always a mutual experience for at least two objects. When a hammer applies force to a nail, the nail applies an equal and opposite force to the hammer. An ejection seat applies force to the occupant, but the occupant applies an equal and opposite force to the seat. The force applied to the seat has been termed a reaction force. It can be seen that accelerated bodies apply reaction forces in a direction opposite to the direction of the acceleration. This is a consequence of the accelerating force being applied in the direction of acceleration. In this chapter, impact always will be an acceleration expressed in g or meters per second squared. It always will be produced by a force in the direction of acceleration expressed in newtons (kilogram-meters per second squared). It will be seen that force units are simply the product of mass units and acceleration units, which is to be expected from Equation 1. Thus, the commonly used term, g-forces, is a misnomer.

Translational and Angular Motion

Motion can be described in a displacement sense, such as for a piston with respect to a cylinder, or a rotational sense, such as a drive shaft with respect to an engine. Many displacements have an angular quality to them even when no true rotation or spinning is taking place. This occurs whenever the motion is not precisely along the radius or line connecting the object's center of mass to the chosen reference point. It is called orbital motion because none of the displacement motion of an object in a perfect circular orbit is along a radius drawn to the center of the circle. In general, motions must be characterized by three components: rotation, called spin, displacement perpendicular to the reference radius, called orbital, and displacement along the reference radius, called central. The first two are angular motions. The last two are translational motions because they always involve motion of the center of the mass. It should be observed that the angular and translational definitions overlap and both apply to orbital motions. Forces applied to an object may be resolved into components along the radial reference line and perpendicular to it. The perpendicular component, multiplied by the length of the radius, is a measure of the angular force, or torque. If the chosen reference point is the center of mass of the object, the torque is a measure of a tendency to change its spin motion. The other component, radial to the center of mass, is a measure of the tendency to change its translational motion. If the chosen reference point is other than the center of mass, the force component radial to the center of mass can be further resolved into a component radial to the outside reference point and a component perpendicular to it. The perpendicular component, multiplied by the radius, is a torque with respect to the reference point and measures the tendency of the force to change the orbital motion with respect to the reference point. The radial component of the force measures the tendency to change the central motion with respect to the reference point and is termed a central force.

In general, motions of objects undergoing impact accelerations include spin, orbital, and central components with respect to commonly used frames of reference. Furthermore, the chosen reference frames frequently are accelerating and rotating during the events, leading to relatively involved computations, to arrive at comparable, comprehensible, and relevant descriptions of the forces and motions involved.

Velocity Change and Momentum

Balanced forces on an object, yielding a net force of zero, do not cause acceleration, and, therefore, no velocity change takes place. Impact, being an acceleration, requires a nonzero net force application to the impacted or accelerated object. The characteristics of the force, the means of application, and the characteristics of the impacted object taken together determine the response. Impacts, in order to create a problem for human subjects, must be sustained long enough to produce some significant velocity change. Automobile crashes at 1 km/hr are not really crashes.

In situations of interest for human occupants of aerospace vehicles, impact conditions tend to be defined by velocity changes or, equivalently, by acceleration histories as a function of time instead of by applied forces. In fact, the definition is often provided by giving vehicle accelerations and/or velocities because the forces imposed on the human occupant are difficult to describe, involving curving, yielding contact surfaces for the human body and for the restraints and supports. The problem is avoided by defining a collision situation between the occupant and his or her own vehicle. The situation may arise from a prior collision of the vehicle with something else, such as the ground, in which the vehicle velocity is rapidly changed, or it may arise from a sudden velocity change to which the occupant must accommodate, such as that imparted to an ejection seat. In any case, the velocity change of the vehicle is specified, and the occupant's behavior in the resulting collision with his or her vehicle is observed.

This is where momentum comes in. Momentum is simply a measure of the authority one has in conducting the business of collisions. Newton expressed it as follows:

$$p = m v \qquad (2)$$

Momentum (p) equals mass (m) times velocity (v). It makes sense intuitively, too. If one has great mass, one has great authority. If one has great speed, one has great authority. If one has both great mass and great speed, one's great authority is multiplied. Momentum also is a vector quantity, with its direction determined by the velocity vector.

In many cases, the total momentum of colliding bodies is virtually unchanged, as in the contact between two billiard balls. In aerospace vehicle collisions, either the vehicle isn't affected much by the occupant or, if it is, the defined velocity change of the vehicle already includes the occupant's effects on it. In such cases, the occupant's momentum, or authority in future collisions, is changed. The currency for transacting changes in authority is called kinetic energy, or work.

$$E = 1/2 \, m \, v^2 \qquad (3)$$

Kinetic energy (E) equals $\frac{1}{2}$ mass (m) times velocity squared (v^2).

$$W = Fx \qquad (4)$$

Work (W) equals force (F) times the distance through which the force acts (x). Units of work and energy are both kilogram-meters squared per second squared or newton-meters. Work and energy are, therefore, equivalent. Neither is a vector quantity. Comparing Equations 2 and 3 demonstrates that velocity is more important than mass in determining energy, whereas mass and velocity are equivalent in determining momentum. Less apparent is the observation that, whereas energy is a measure of the effect of force over distance (Equation 4), momentum is a measure of the effect of force over time (Equation 2, with the understanding that velocity is acceleration times time and with a good recall of Equation 1).

$$p = m\,v = m\,a\,t = F\,t \qquad (5)$$

Equations 4 and 5 are only true for constant forces. If the forces vary with distance or time, each little distance or time increment must be multiplied by the effective force during that time and the resulting products summed up. This process will be recognized as integration. Momentum transfer becomes the integral of net force with respect to time, whereas work is the integral of net force with respect to distance. Because the relationship between distance and time is velocity, work is a function of force, velocity, and time, whereas momentum is related simply to force and time.

These concepts are presented primarily to establish a basis for an appreciation of the impact event. Specifically, peak acceleration is clearly not of significance unless it is sustained for an adequate time to lead to an appreciable velocity change. In addition, the energy transfer associated with an acceleration pulse of a given duration is greater for objects moving at higher velocity in the direction of the acceleration. Because energy or work is required to produce mechanical damage, this consideration is of no small importance but not particularly obvious without recourse to the basic equations. At least it should be apparent that peak vehicle accelera-

tion in g does not satisfactorily describe an impact event. Instead, at the minimum, the acceleration history prior to the event, the acceleration pulse shape, magnitude, direction, and duration from which velocity change can be computed, the characteristics of the impacted subject, and the nature of the subject's contacts and attachments to the vehicle must be specified.

Angular Momentum and Torque

Angular motion can be described using a quantity analogous to linear momentum. Because there are two kinds of angular motion, two terms are in the description. Orbital motion leads to a momentum based on mass, the radius or distance to the reference point, and the velocity perpendicular to the radius. For pure, circular orbital motion about a fixed reference point, the velocity is always perpendicular to the radius. Spin motion provides the second term and is described by the moment of inertia and the angular velocity, where the moment of inertia is simply a measure of the mass and its distribution with respect to the axis of rotation of interest. Mass concentrations located well off this axis are far more significant than mass near the axis. In fact, each piece of mass is multiplied by the square of its distance from the axis of rotation to arrive at the moment of inertia, which has units of kilogram-meters squared. Angular velocity is in radians per second, where radians do not count as units because they are not mass, length, or time. The complete angular momentum definition, then, is as follows:

$$L = I\omega + mrv_{\perp} \qquad (6)$$

Angular momentum (L) equals moment of inertia (I) times angular velocity (ω) plus mass (m) times radius (r) times velocity perpendicular to that radius ($v_{\perp}$). The units of each term are kilogram-meters squared per second squared, or newton-meters, just like linear momentum. Changing angular momentum requires an expenditure of energy, just as for the linear case.

Changes require the application of torque, as previously defined. Angular momentum is a vector quantity and requires torque to change its direction as well as its magnitude. In impact events, linear momentum is frequently converted to angular momentum before being dissipated. The required torque to make the conversion derives from motion of body structures around more centrally located anchor points.

Stress-Strain

So far, relationships have been discussed which have been applied to and illustrated with rigid bodies. A rigid body is an imaginary nondeformable solid that can be completely described by its shape, mass distribution, position, orientation, and motion. It never breaks, bends, or distorts and, therefore, does not exist. Things that do exist also move under the influence of forces, but they can and do break, bend, and otherwise distort, thus making their physical description more difficult. The approach that has been taken conceptually involves the treatment of each tiny segment of the object as a rigid body, so that the summation of the behavior of the parts describes the behavior of the whole. This concept is called continuum mechanics because objects are described as continuous aggregates of tiny rigid bodies held together in various ways. In practice, since the forces cannot be measured for each little part, gross observations are made of forces and motions and the infinitesimal values deduced for purposes of description.

An example should help. In Figure 8.2, a and b show loadings of an imaginary rigid bar in tension. The situations are well described by the tension forces, as noted. Any weight could be used with easily calculable results. Similar loadings of real bars in tension are shown in c and d of Figure 8.2; if the bars don't break, the tension force descriptions are identical to those of Figure 8.2b, but the description here is inadequate. It is clear that, if the bar material is identical, the situation is more stressful for the thin bar than for the fat one. The stressfulness of the situ-

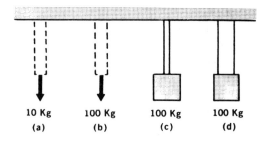

(a) 10 Kg TENSION FORCE APPLIED TO IDEALIZED BAR,

(b) 100 Kg TENSION FORCE APPLIED TO IDEALIZED BAR,

(c) FORCE APPLIED AS IN (b) TO A SMALL CROSS-SECTION BAR,

(d) FORCE APPLIED AS IN (b) TO A LARGE CROSS-SECTION BAR .

Figure 8.2. Model of stress and strain.

ation must be evaluated when real materials are used. This has been formalized as follows:

$$\sigma = \frac{F}{A} \qquad (7)$$

Stress (σ) equals force (F) divided by the cross-sectional area (A). This equation works rather well because the force on each little cross-sectional portion of the bar can be deduced if its area is defined. For the same total force, overall stress will be greater for small cross-sectional areas and lesser for large cross-sectional areas. Computing the stress for c and d in Figure 8.2 gives a more complete description of what is happening to the real material.

Stress is expressed in units of newtons per square meter or pascals. Stress also can be applied to surfaces using the same formulation (Equation 7). In fact, a stress vector can be defined incorporating the directional characteristics of the force. For example, hydrostatic pressure on a surface is a stress of force per area and is always directed perpendicularly to the surface.

Stress is actually independent of material characteristics. The material characteristics, however, determine what an object will do when subjected to stress. Any stress will produce some sign of strain in real materials. The type of strain varies with the type of stress and the material characteristics. Stress that is perpendicular to each tiny cross-sectional area is called normal stress and tends to produce compression or elongation. Stress that is parallel to each tiny cross-sectional area is called shear stress and tends to produce bending, twist, or similar distortion. Material characteristics also play a part. Some materials have good strength in compression but are poor in shear. A stack of blocks and water are two examples. Other materials have good strength in tension but are lousy in compression. Rope is an example. Often, materials convert one kind of external stress into other kinds of internal stress because of their internal structures and the interaction of their internal forces during deformation or strain. Compression of a structural member may produce significant shear stresses internally. The various types of strain responses to stress are formalized in dimensionless units expressing either a ratio of the change of length or a trigonometric function of the distortion angle associated with bending or twist.

For many materials, the relationship between a particular stress and the resulting strain can be rather simply expressed, as long as the stress is held within a limited range, obviously below the breaking point. In this so-called linear range, certain materials may act like springs, for example, and have a strain that is proportional to the stress, like a spring's displacement is proportional to the applied force. A real spring, however, loaded with a given constant force for a long time, will have a displacement that slowly continues to creep along slightly, almost as if the spring were relaxing under the persistent load. This behavior of initial compression or tension with a further tendency to creep or relax can be modeled by a combination of strain displacement and strain velocity, each proportional to stress, which is called a viscoelastic model (elastic for spring and visco for the flow of viscous fluids). Interestingly enough, these two characteristics can be used to describe the behavior of most materials in their linear range. Some are more like springs, whereas other materials are more like very viscous fluids, such as glycerine, less viscous fluids, such as water, or even less viscous fluids, such as air. Fluids also may

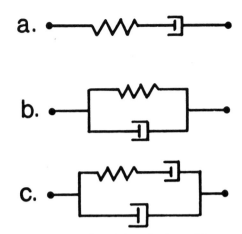

Figure 8.3. Examples of viscoelastic models. spring: Force proportional to displacement. Damper: Force proportional to velocity.
⎼⌇⌇⌇⌇⌇ Spring
⎼▢⎼ Damper

be compressible or incompressible, which determines their utility as springs.

A few simple viscoelastic models are shown in Figure 8.3. Such models can be used to describe the behavior of materials subjected to stress, including such phenomena as strain rate dependence or frequency response and hysteresis, which is the tendency of strain characteristics to vary from the loading phase to the unloading phase. They do not describe the behavior of materials in their nonlinear range, at or near the breaking or yield points.

In situations of interest in impact protection, normal and shear stresses on the human body are directly produced at points of force application, indirect internal stresses are induced at other locations within the body, and gross center of mass accelerations occur. The resulting strains are tolerable when the situations are controlled to assure that yield points are not reached for structures of significance. The techniques available to provide this control will be discussed in this chapter.

Rate Dependency and Frequency Response

The response of a mechanical system to an accelerating force depends not only on the magnitude, direction, and duration of the applied force but also on the rate at which the force builds up. If force is applied slowly, acceleration builds up slowly, can be accommodated, and is called sustained acceleration. If force is applied rapidly, acceleration builds up too rapidly for the mechanical system to track it and a transient or impact response occurs, which differs considerably form the steady-state response that would have resulted if the same force had been applied slowly. The interesting thing about all this is that slow application for one system is fast for another. In fact, slow application for an adequately restrained system may be too fast for the same system inadequately restrained. The ability of a system to track accelerating forces of varying application rates is described by its frequency response.

Frequency response is so named because the application of smoothly alternating or sinusoidal forces or vibration of varying frequencies allows the measurement of responses that reveal the system's tracking ability. A system's tracking ability can be measured by how well it follows the magnitude of an applied vibration's displacement and by how well it tracks the timing or phase of the applied vibration. Systems which track both amplitude and phase faithfully are called ''well coupled'' systems. Systems which resist velocity are called ''damped systems,'' with the degree of damping determined by the degree of velocity resistance. Determination of frequency response under differing restraint conditions can serve as an evaluation of their relative effectiveness in the face of different kinds of challenges.

A significant characteristic of some mechanical systems is their natural tendency to respond to a nonsinusoidal, brief force application with a sinusoidal mechanical response at a fixed frequency. A familiar example is the tuning fork. A system's mechanical response is called its natural frequency, or its resonant frequency. If a system is subjected to sustained vibration at its natural frequency, it will respond at that frequency with increasing amplitude until restric-

tion or mechanical failure is reached. The human body has natural frequencies not only for its gross structural elements, such as arms and legs, but also for various substructures such as internal organs. This fact may not seem particularly important since we are talking about impact and not vibration. Even the waveform of a limited duration impact pulse, however, can be described in mathematical terms involving a sum of various frequencies. It also has physical effects consistent with its frequency description and the frequency response of the system. For example, particular impact pulses can have more drastic effects on particular structures or substructures if there is a high power content in the impact pulse at the applicable natural frequency of the structure. This statement may sound somewhat odd, but you have probably subconsciously used this principle more than once. For example, why do you think some thumps on a tuning fork have more impressive effects than others? Have you noticed that a softer thumping surface works better for low-pitched forks? The softer surface slows the rate of force application and, therefore, lowers the frequency spectrum of the force pulse to better match the natural frequency of the fork.

Aerodynamics

Aerodynamics concerns itself with the flow of fluids around objects. This is of interest when situations such as high-speed ejection allow such flow to impose large forces, which result in transitory accelerations of the human body and its parts.

Aerodynamic forces are defined relative to the flight path. Forces perpendicular to the flight path, including side forces, are called lift. Forces along the flight path are called drag. Those forces tending to simply change the angle of the body as it moves along its flight path are called moments. On a wing, for example, the desired lift, or net upward force, derives both from an increase in pressure below the wing and from a decrease in pressure above the wing. One simplified way of thinking about the source of these forces begins with the observation that, with certain assumptions, energy of the flow in a steady state must be constant when no work is being done. That energy is determined by the sum of pressure energy, thermal energy, and speed energy. It follows, then, that when constant-temperature air moves faster over the top of a wing because of the wing's shape, the pressure must decrease for the energy to remain constant. The difference in pressure above and below the wing produces lift.

Two sources of drag force are similar to the lift situation. The most commonly quoted drag component is due to the pushing of the object from the front by the force of the moving wind. Aerodynamicists call this dynamic pressure, q, and point out that it is proportional to air density and the square of the velocity among other factors, such as air viscosity and elasticity. The drag force produced on a body by a given level of dynamic pressure is determined by its area, shape, and orientation. A less well-understood drag component is due to the sucking of the object from behind by the decreased pressure produced in its wake. This component can be quite significant. If a complete vacuum were to be produced in a wake at sea level, the available wake drag would be over 0.98 kg/cm_2. That would be equivalent to the dynamic pressure, or pushing drag, imposed at an indicated airspeed of about 800 knots. Finally, a third drag component, not related to the lift analogy, is due to the surface friction of the air flowing around the object. This component also can be quite significant, depending on the roughness of the surface and the flow properties near the surface. Similar drag concepts apply to the motion through a body of water. However, the total drag on a body moving through water is substantially greater than that for a body moving through air at the same speed.

This area is complex, and aerodynamic descriptions frequently tend to be experimentally determined, even for smooth, simple, well-defined geometric structures in steady-state flow. Ejection seats and human arms are irregular, complex, and poorly defined, making them even less amenable to precise modeling for flow with

rapidly changing speed. Some observations of relationships can nevertheless be made. Consider, for example, a coasting car with an initial speed of 100 km/hr. The car will be retarded by rolling friction and by aerodynamic drag and will decelerate at a rate determined by its mass and the retarding force (a = F/m). If the occupant extends an arm from the window, the arm will be forced back relative to the window unless without active resistance because the aerodynamic drag force relative to the arm's mass is greater than the aerodynamic drag and rolling friction force relative to the gross vehicle mass. The arm, therefore, decelerates at a greater rate.

The same situation exists for an unrestrained extremity protruding from a crewmember/ejection seat unit catapulted into a high-speed windstream. Limb flailing is produced by an inequality between the ratios of aerodynamic drag and mass for the flailing member, as compared to the overall occupant/seat unit. Injury can result simply from the differences in acceleration of the occupant's torso and flailing body parts. The flailing part also may strike a surface such as the seat edge, equalizing the velocities but producing injury in the process.

Application of Force

Penetrating Impact

Impact accelerations are produced by the sudden mechanical application of force requiring direct contact between an impacting object and the impacted structure. If the area over which the force is applied is small and/or if the impacted structure is fragile, the contact force may be sufficient to produce penetration into the impacted structure. Bullet wounds provide a typical example. If the impacting bullet passes completely through the impacted body part, the momentum transfer may be considerably less than would have occurred if the impacting object lodged within the impacted structure. The amount of the difference depends on the penetrating object's residual velocity after passing through. Damage to the impacted structure from penetrating impact is typically determined more by the direct trauma associated with the penetration and less by the gross impact accelerations imposed on the involved body part. Therefore, the subject of penetrating impact will not be pursued further in this chapter.

Blunt Impact

The remaining impact force applications can be considered nonpenetrating impact, or blunt impact. This type of impact is the typical means of force application for restrained occupants of aerospace vehicles. The term, however, is most commonly applied to the more limited situation in which only a portion of the body is accelerated with respect to the rest of the body by localized, nonpenetrating force application. An example would be an aircraft birdstrike in which the bird shatters the windscreen and strikes the helmeted head of the pilot. Although penetration of the head may not occur, significant internal structural damage is still possible. These impacts are clearly of interest in aerospace medicine.

Whole-Body Acceleration

The primary concern of this chapter is with those nonpenetrating impact situations in which significant accelerations are imposed on the center of mass of a human being. The forces are typically applied bluntly by means of seat surfaces, restraints, distributed windblast force, or some combination of these factors. Typical localized blunt impact to inadequately restrained body parts also may ensue as a result of relative motions such as that of the head or extremities with respect to the torso. In these cases, the body part may strike a fixed surface such as the instrument panel or seat. Whole-body acceleration, then, involves generalized blunt impact and may secondarily include localized blunt impact.

IMPACT RESPONSE AND INJURY MECHANISMS

Subject Response

Mechanical Response

The human body responds to applied forces by a combination of acceleration and strain. Accelerations are force-dependent and are determined by the ratio of force to mass. Strains or deformations are stress-dependent and are determined by the ratio of force to area and by the viscoelastic characteristics of the material. The trick is to apply adequate accelerations over the appropriate times to produce the required velocity change while minimizing strain. Strain is associated with injury.

Descriptions of impact response usually concentrate on the displacements of the subject with respect to the vehicle and the accelerations of the subject with respect to an external fixed reference. Displacements with respect to the vehicle can be good or bad, depending on whether they increase or decrease the subject's accelerations with respect to an external fixed reference. They may increase accelerations in two ways. One way is by allowing the subject to strike a portion of the vehicle not designed for restraint. Impact of a subject's head with an instrument panel is a good example. This leads to increased head accelerations during the collision. Elastic collisions not only stop the closing velocity but require more of the same acceleration to produce a separation velocity in the other direction. In other words, elastic collisions are bounces. They can involve nearly twice the momentum and energy transfer associated with inelastic collisions, which are nonbounce, or hit-and-stick collisions.

A second way in which displacements can increase accelerations can be seen by considering what occurs in a head-on vehicle crash into a fixed structure. The vehicle's initial velocity is rapidly decreased to zero relative to the structure if the collision is inelastic. If the vehicle and the structure were idealized rigid bodies, the velocity change would occur instantaneously and the acceleration would be infinite. In the real world, however, the vehicle and the fixed structure usually deform to some extent, allowing finite acceleration over some small time interval to produce the required velocity change. Clearly, for a given velocity change, shorter stopping distances require stopping times and, therefore, higher accelerations.

In our vehicle crash, assume the occupant to be perfectly restrained to the vehicle from the bottom of the neck to the tips of the toes. Only the head and neck protrude from this otherwise perfect restraint system. Further, assume that vehicle acceleration in the crash is high but not infinite, of a duration that is short but not zero, such as a 25-m/sec velocity change in 1 m. In the crash, then, the occupant's body experiences acceleration identical to that of the vehicle. The head, however, does not. Some would say that the head is thrown forward. In point of fact, the head continues forward with the same velocity it had at the instant of impact, until some force acts to cause an acceleration. In this case, that force is provided by the neck, which is placed in tension as the head tries to keep going. In the upright position, the neck is initially well aligned to produce vertical forces on the head, but our crash requires horizontal force. From the neck, this force is initially off-axis with respect to the head's center of mass. Such off-axis forces are called torques and produce rotations. The head, therefore, is rotated to better align the center of mass with the required horizontal neck tension. This process takes time, during which the head continues forward with respect to the rest of the body. In fact, a velocity difference is built up between head and body because the body, in the early stages of the crash, does a much better job of stopping. In this case, the head will have to undergo much of the velocity change in less time than the body because the head starts late. Higher acceleration is required for the head simply as a result of the head displacement relative to the vehicle. Even worse, since necks have some springiness to them, the head not only moves forward and comes to a stop, but also pitches back again at the end. The result is similar to the case of an elastic collision, even without hitting anything, and implies a greater total velocity change for the head and, of course, more acceleration.

As mentioned earlier, however, some displacements of the subject with respect to the vehicle can be good. Such displacements may be produced to attenuate the effects of vibration or modest impacts. Consider our vehicle occupant perfectly restrained to the vehicle with metal seats and no springs or shock absorbers. A ride down a rough road would be most unpleasant. For this reason, some means of viscoelastic displacement of the occupant is built into most human restraint systems to allow much vibration and many sharp spike impacts to be minimized, particularly when little if any overall velocity change is required. Great care must be taken in the design of such systems to define the range of acceleration challenges that will be imposed. Otherwise, the displacement system can make things worse by bottoming out. The bone-jarring crunch at the bottom of a really deep pothole testifies to the limitations of automobile springs and shock absorbers. Similar limitations apply to any aerospace impact attenuation system.

The goal of restraint system design, then, is to match the characteristics of the restraint system to both the mechanical response to human occupants and the potential accelerations that may be encountered. The matching criteria are maximum isolation from the vehicle during short-term events and minimum isolation from the vehicle during significant transitory accelerations that produce appreciable velocity changes. The contradictory nature of these criteria makes restraint system design a challenging task.

Biologic Response

When the human body or its parts are subjected to strain and acceleration, events may occur that are of structural and physiologic significance. These events may not be easily discernible through observation of the overt mechanical response. The most apparent effects are probably strains at points of stress application. These may include lacerations, contusions, joint injuries, and fractures. Acceleration of the body or its parts also may indirectly produce strains at points distant from direct stress applications. Examples are fractures of the spine during ejection acceleration and transection of the aorta during a forward-facing, head-on crash. Such strains result from internal structural loading or from differential acceleration of internal body parts that are attached to one another or are free to collide. Some of these effects may be subtle. For example, retinal or other hemorrhage may occur as a result of hydrodynamic blood surges or motion of a blood vessel with respect to the retina.

If each particle of the human body could be uniformly accelerated with respect to each adjacent particle, velocity changes could be accomplished without untoward physiologic response or injury. If there is no difference between the acceleration of each particle, there is no change in the respective positions of the particles. Thus, the deflections that cause mechanical failure of body tissues or stimulate adverse physiologic responses would not occur. This is a fundamental principle in understanding the mechanisms of injuries that result from transient acceleration and the approaches that are used to provide protection for the human body.

In their daily activities, people tend to minimize the deflections that might cause injury or discomfort by controlling the accelerations acting on their bodies. They accomplish this by the control of their body position, design of vehicles, and avoidance of collisions. When large velocity changes must be accomplished, the body is accelerated and decelerated gradually. A practical mechanical method to achieve simultaneous, uniform acceleration of each body particle has not been found when a relatively large velocity change must be accomplished in a short period of time. Such methods, unfortunately, remain in the domain of science fiction.

When a large acceleration is unavoidable, several methods are used to provide protection. The first is to minimize the applied acceleration as much as possible. For example, the magnitude of the acceleration may be reduced by redistributing the velocity change over a longer period of time. The second method is to restrict the motion of the major body segments to reduce the relative displacements of the body segments

and their internal organs. This method is most commonly accomplished by restraining the body segments to a supporting structure such as a vehicle seat.

The effectiveness of a transient acceleration protection system is evaluated in terms of how well it prevents injuries. The injuries may result from high-contact pressures under the restraints, impact of the body segments with the vehicle structure, or whole-body acceleration, such as in spinal fractures incurred during the use of an ejection seat. In each case, the conditions of loading of the affected body element and the properties of the element, that is, its load-carrying viscoelastic characteristics and failure limits, determine the injury potential for any given set of acceleration conditions.

Injury Mechanisms

Human tolerance to transitory acceleration is defined in various ways. Under given conditions, it may be considered to be a maximum acceleration exposure level that generally does not result in significant injury or death. A given level, however, may result in no injury for one subject and death for another, so this definition is vague at best. Two observations explain its lack of precision. One observation is that resistance to injury varies from specimen to specimen, implying that a range of tolerance must be expected. The second observation, that the description of vehicle acceleration does not define the proximate cause of specific injuries, is more important. The end point of death or significant injury may be reached through various kinds of effects on different organs, structures, or systems. Therefore, before an assessment of the range of injury resistance or strength can be made, the way or ways must be defined in which the vehicle acceleration leads to imposition of the proximate cause of potential injuries. Defining the steps along the path from vehicle acceleration to localized stress is the process of defining the injury mechanism.

Injury mechanisms are usually difficult to

work out in detail because force and stress measurements are increasingly difficult to make at the various steps beyond the vehicle acceleration stage. Many forces and stresses are internal to the subject. Compounding the force measurement problem are difficulties in defining or measuring the effective mass of body segments and the effective internal musculoskeletal and soft tissue forces. Experimental data are often in the form of kinematic descriptions that only define motions, without regard to force or mass. Kinetic descriptions would be far more useful from a protection viewpoint, because they would include the relation of the motion of masses to the forces acting on them to allow a more rational definition of protective interventions in the process, since the required protective forces and their own resulting stresses could be better assessed.

Precise injury mechanisms should meet the following criteria: (1) the load transmission path from seat structure and restraints to the point of injury should be clearly defined; (2) the defined load transmission path should be in accordance with physical principles by taking into account the origins of the loads, the motions of the transmitting structure under loading, and the capability of the transmitting structure to carry the presumed loads; and (3) the transmitted load should produce sufficient stress at the appropriate point to account for the injury. Even when these criteria are met, the proposed mechanism remains hypothetic. Verification often requires measurements that are inaccessible in conjunction with experiments that would be ethically inappropriate. Instead, proposed mechanisms generally achieve the status of working hypotheses on the basis of convincing argument, calculations with models, experimentation with human surrogates, and/or usefulness in devising successful protection schemes. The success of a protection concept, advanced on the basis of the presumed validity of a proposed mechanism, can still be misleading because alternate mechanisms also may be interrupted by a given protective intervention.

In the face of such difficulties, proposed mechanisms are often deficient. In the extreme, an alleged mechanism may simply identify a hyperflexion or similar injury mode and indicate that it is caused by vehicle acceleration. The result of such deficiencies in our knowledge of mechanisms is that adequate protection concepts become more difficult to define. To illustrate the problem, three injury types will be briefly examined with emphasis on the difficulties in defining precise mechanisms.

Concussion Resulting from Impact

The difficulty in defining the injury mechanism of concussion resulting from impact has historically been associated not so much with describing applied forces or load transmission paths. Instead, the trouble is encountered in defining the injury itself and its proximate cause. Concussion has been variously defined as usually requiring the traumatic loss of consciousness and/or post-traumatic disturbance of thought process or memory, usually without demonstrable gross anatomic damage to the brain. The last criterion is difficult to assure without post-mortem examination and is often ignored or separately described when data allow. The cause of concussion is even less clear. Various hypotheses have been advanced, generally concentrating on the brain stem and the reticular activating system. The necessary and sufficient localized stress has been considered to be direct translational acceleration, pitch axis rotational velocity and displacement producing a pinching of the brain stem, or a variety of generalized traumatic effects at the cellular level produced by brain oscillations, fluid waves in the cerebrospinal fluid or brain stem tissue, resonance cavitation, vascular hemodynamic wave propagation, or other effects. One or more injury mechanisms may be proposed to produce each of the localized stresses as a result of a given impact event. In all likelihood, alterations in thought process can be produced by several of these stresses individually and in various combinations. The relative importance of the various causes in typical situations of interest in aerospace medicine is not clear. Current mechanisms are, therefore, deficient. From what we know, however, it appears prudent to minimize both head motions relative to the body and peak head accelerations.

Vertebral Fracture Resulting from Ejection

The difficulty in defining the injury mechanism of vertebral fracture resulting from ejection has not so much been in describing the injury and the required localized stress or even in defining the applied forces. Instead, the trouble is encountered in sorting out the stresses in the load transmission path, particularly with superimposed motions. The force imposed on a given vertebral body during upward ejection ultimately depends on the acceleration experienced by the vertebral body immediately below it and the time-varying effective mass above it, which must be supported or accelerated. Of course, the dynamic behavior of this force is further modified by the characteristics of the intervertebral disk and other associated connective and soft tissue. The importance of the effective supported mass may be appreciated by imagining an ejection of the lower portion of a human, the most superior point of which is the isolated, exposed first lumbar vertebra. The force imposed on the inferior face of this vertebral body could then be well approximated by the acceleration of the second lumbar vertebra multiplied by the mass of the first, neglecting gravity and the intervertebral disk. If more mass were to be attached to this preparation by stacking it on top of the vertebral body, the force would be increased accordingly.

In reality, the effective mass above a given vertebral body varies with the availability of alternate load paths. The arms, for example, may be supported and thus accelerated partially by contact with the anterior thighs or the seat structure. The time-varying remainder of the upper extremity's mass is accelerated by forces transmitted through the lower spine. Even these forces have alternate paths around portions of the upper spine. This derives from the fact that

the bony articulation of the arm with the spine is not a simple, rigid, structural load path. Try working your way from arm to spine by following the bones. The humerus articulates with the scapula through a ball-and-socket joint held together by muscular attachments and a fibrous capsule. The scapula connects to the clavicle through a laterally placed fibrous attachment. The medial clavicle connects to the upper portion of the sternum in a similar fashion. Finally, most of the ribs connect to the sternum through fibrocartilaginous attachments of varying rigidity, and these ribs can be followed around to the spine. This connection is tenuous. Soft tissue-mediated load paths can be more significant than the strictly bony ones. They usually are variable and hard to trace.

In addition, the stress imposed by a given force varies dramatically with spinal orientation. Flexion or extension during the event can convert compression stress to tension or produce compression and tension stress on different portions of the same vertebral body. Measurement difficulties are profound. Surfaces are sufficiently complex so that simplifications necessary for modeling may obscure significant effects. Tissue behavior under stress is also poorly understood at high strain rates. Current understanding of injury mechanisms is, therefore, imprecise. From a protection point of view, however, minimizing relative motions certainly would make things more predictable, and the provision of alternate load paths around the spine would be reasonable under almost any set of assumptions.

Upper Extremity Injury Resulting from Windblast

The initial difficulty in defining the injury mechanism of upper extremity injury resulting from windblast has not been in describing the required localized stress or the load transmission path but in sorting out initial applied forces. Once the extremity is flailing around the side of the ejection seat, the forces of contact with the seat structure or forced motion beyond joint limitations are primarily of academic interest. The mechanism of injury begins with dislodgement of the extremity from a normal position. Therefore, research efforts have focused on the measurement of the forces and torques that cause dislodgement. Wind tunnel tests have been performed to measure these parameters using volunteer subjects at low airspeeds and rigid models of the human body at higher speeds.

The forces and torques acting to dislodge each body segment are a function of the flow field surrounding the segment and the aerodynamic characteristics of the segment. Unfortunately, the flow field around a segment is significantly influenced by the presence of nearby objects, and the aerodynamic characteristics are significantly influenced by individual variations, personal equipment, and body position. The aerodynamic forces and torques acting on a body segment of the seat occupant are, therefore, complex time functions. They are modified by the flow field changes caused by the aircraft fuselage, the ejection seat, and even the proximity of other body segments (1). They vary from subject to subject and with orientation or voluntary muscle action. The difficulty of determining the direction and magnitude of these aerodynamic forces is further compounded by the typical lack of angular stability of the ejecting seat with respect to the incident wind and the presence of other forces, such as those generated by the ejection catapult and deployment of a drogue parachute to decelerate the seat more rapidly.

When these complexities are considered, the definition of a specific injury mechanism is usually no more than hypothetic. What does appear clear is that protective interventions should be applied as early in the event as possible and that seat angular stabilization techniques should be used to limit the direction and improve predictability of the aerodynamic and inertial forces.

IMPACT PROTECTION SYSTEMS

Range of Challenge

Transient accelerations that present an injury hazard occur inadvertently, as in vehicular crash,

and by design, as in the case of spacecraft landings or aircraft emergency escape system performance. Whether inadvertent or deliberate, the acceleration magnitude, direction, and pulse shape are commonly quite variable. In most instances, if protective provisions are present, they are spartan. The reasons for this condition are clear. First, it is the nature of humans to believe that accidents will only happen to others. For this reason, it seems foolish to endure the additional inconvenience and cost of protection. The rationalizations cited are often elaborate and presented with considerable zeal and include references to the abridgement of individual freedoms. Second, when transient accelerations are an inherent feature of a system design, the system is usually a spacecraft or aircraft system where the weight of the protection system involves costs in the size of the launch system or range and performance of the aircraft. The challenge to the designer of protection equipment is immense.

The development of vehicular crash protection equipment is perhaps the most well-known challenge. The crash environment experienced in aviation accidents is quite difficult to predict. In commercial, military, and general aviation, primary emphasis is given to protection against acceleration vectors acting in the x-axis, although y-axis and z-axis accelerations may be very high. Commercial airline passenger seats and restraints are usually designed to withstand x-axis crash accelerations up to 9 g although recent federal regulations will require seats to withstand 16 g. Crew seats and rear facing passenger seats in military transport aircraft are usually designed to 16-g crash conditions. The stiffer structures of military fighter aircraft provide less attenuation of crash loads, and, therefore, the seats are usually designed to withstand up to 40 g in the x-axis.

The most comprehensive description of crash environments has been assembled to provide design criteria to improve the crashworthiness of military helicopters (2). These data describe the crash conditions in probabilistic terms for impact velocity, acceleration vector direction, and pulse shape.

The acceleration environment encountered during emergency escape from spacecraft or military aircraft is the most diverse and complex challenge to the designer. The escaping crewmember is first exposed to a high acceleration directed parallel to the spinal column to catapult the seat and occupant from the cockpit. The acceleration magnitude may be 10 to more than 20 g, depending on the type of ejection seat design, the mass of the occupant, the pre-ignition temperature of the catapult propellant, and the normal variance in propellant performance. The catapult may produce a velocity ranging from 13 to 18 m/sec. As the seat separates from the aircraft, a rocket is ignited to develop additional velocity to assure clearance of the aircraft vertical stabilizer at high speed and to provide adequate trajectory height for parachute opening at low altitude. The rocket is aligned to apply its force vector through the expected center of gravity of the seat and occupant. When the rocket is mounted on the back of the seat, the rocket nozzle is aligned to produce a +x-axis acceleration component as well as a +z-axis acceleration.

At higher airspeeds, the effect of the +x-axis acceleration component of the rocket thrust becomes relatively small, as the effect of the aerodynamic pressure of the windstream becomes higher. The aerodynamic force increases as the square of the wind velocity. Therefore, at high airspeeds, the primary acceleration component acting on the seat occupant is the aerodynamic deceleration acting, at least initially, in the −x-axis. When the ejection airspeed is in the range of 500 to 600 knots, sea level equivalent, the aerodynamic deceleration level may be as high as 30 to 40 g for typical body and seat drag coefficients.

Once the velocity of the crewmember has been reduced to a safe parachute deployment speed of approximately 250 knots for conventional systems, the crewmember is exposed to another acceleration pulse known as parachute opening shock. This acceleration is created by the large drag force developed as the parachute canopy fills with air. The pulse is of relatively long duration, on the order of 1 to 2 seconds at 300 m, and may range in peak value from 10 to 20 g under ideal conditions. The acceleration magnitude is a function of the deployment velocity, air density, deployment orientation of the parachute canopy and lines, mass of the parachutist, and several other variables.

After completion of the parachute opening sequence and descent to the earth's surface, the ejectee is greeted by a final acceleration on ground impact. A military parachute will lower the parachutist to the earth at a velocity of approximately 6.4 m/sec. The landing impact is equivalent to that experienced after a jump from a height of 2.1 m. The resulting impact forces are a function of the effectiveness of the parachutist's fall technique, that is, the ability to use legs as impact attenuators, and the direction and velocity of horizontal drift.

Range of Human Impact Tolerance

The primary factors that determine human tolerance to transient acceleration exposures are the direction, magnitude, and time history of the acceleration, the distribution of force to the human body, and the physical state of the body. The variance and complexity of the acceleration environments encountered in aerospace design problems are generally well understood qualitatively, although too frequently not adequately quantified. Understanding the sources of variances associated with the human factors is also important.

The distribution of force to the human body is a function of the method of body support and restraint. The method that is used may have a very powerful effect on the tolerability of a specific set of acceleration conditions. For example, an individual restrained by a lap belt during a high-speed automobile crash has a much greater chance of survival than an individual without any restraint. Furthermore, an individual restrained by a lap belt and two shoulder straps can survive greater impacts than would be sur-

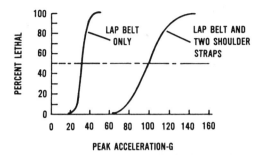

Figure 8.4. Probability of lethal injury estimated from impact tests of baboons restrained by lap belt or lap belt and two shoulder straps.

vivable with a lap belt alone. This relationship is illustrated by data collected with these two restraints, as shown in Figure 8.4 (3,4). The data, which were obtained in tests with baboons, show the very large difference between the mean lethal acceleration levels and the differences in the statistical variance for each restraint system.

The population to be protected is a key factor in the variance of acceleration tolerance. It is reasonable to expect that the variance will be greater in the general population than in a subset composed of military aviators. The factors that contribute to the variance in the tolerance of a given individual to a specific transient acceleration are primarily those that influence the physical state of the individual. These include age, size, body habitus or proportion, level of physical conditioning, and freedom from anatomic variations predisposing to injury. The extent to which each of the sources of variance contributes to the overall variation in an individual's capacity to withstand acceleration is currently not well defined. The general effects of factors such as age, however, are seen in laboratory tests of cadaver tissues, as well as experience with military aircraft escape systems.

Variation of the strength of materials under mechanical loading is not a problem that is unique to biologic materials. Large variability in the breaking strength of materials, components, and entire systems is recognized in most engineering design applications. For example, the mechanical properties of metal structural ele-

ments specified in engineering handbooks are usually based on minimum typical properties. In at least 99% of the samples of the element, the properties, such as tensile strength, are expected to exceed the minimum values. Other factors, such as material temperature, sensitivity to repeated loading, and service life, must be taken into consideration when these factors exceed the bounds of the original test conditions. In some cases, as in the case of human acceleration tolerance, it is not practical to quantify the effects of each of these factors in any detail. Therefore, a factor of safety is selected and added to the mechanical properties to assure a safe design. This same technical approach is appropriate for the specification of biologic material properties and the design of protection equipment.

Design Strategy

The design of protective equipment for aerospace applications must adhere to the same engineering principles that are applied to other components of vehicle design. The weight of the equipment must be minimized and, therefore, overdesign cannot be tolerated. On the other hand, underdesign could result in serious injuries that have major operational, humanitarian, and product liability implications.

The design process used to develop and evaluate protective equipment must include a comprehensive assessment of the severity of the acceleration environment, the characteristics of the personnel to be protected, and the normal mobility, performance, and comfort requirements for these personnel. This assessment is necessary to provide an objective basis for the selection of protection approaches and evaluation of the risks and benefits associated with these approaches.

Restraint Systems

The effectiveness of a restraint system depends on (1) how well the restraint configuration can transmit loads between the seat or vehicle structure and the occupant; (2) the ability of the restraint to control the motion of the restrained anatomic segments; (3) the restraint contact pressure; and (4) the load-carrying capability of the restrained anatomic segments. These factors are controlled by the choice of restraint material properties, restraint tie-down locations, belt area and flexibility, and anatomic-bearing areas. These choices are governed by the anticipated acceleration conditions, surrounding vehicle structure, space for body movement, encumbrance of occupant, and acceptance of risk, weight, and cost.

The first and most common restraint used in aerospace applications, the lap belt, provides a relatively low level of impact protection. The restraint loads are intended to be carried through the pelvis, and existing tolerance data are based on that presumption. Unfortunately, if the belt is improperly tightened or positioned or the acceleration vector is oriented to cause rotation of the pelvis, the belt will slip over the iliac crest and against the abdomen, causing the belt loads to be applied against the lumbar spine with the abdominal organs interposed.

When the lap belt is the only restraint, the most common injuries are caused by the impact of body extremities with the vehicle. Figure 8.5 shows the strike envelopes of body extremities during forward-facing impact with lap belt and

lap belt-double shoulder strap restraint configurations (2). The reduction of the strike envelope obtained through the use of two shoulder straps is demonstrated in this illustration. Shoulder straps may also reduce the strike envelope for sideward and vertical impacts (2). The use of shoulder straps also improves human tolerance to acceleration in any direction by increasing the restraint-bearing area, increasing the load paths into the torso mass, and reducing the relative motion between body parts. Where high upward acceleration components are anticipated, shoulder straps may help maintain the initial alignment of the load-carrying spinal vertebrae.

Despite the aforementioned advantages of shoulder straps, the tension loads in these straps create a potentially serious problem if the straps are attached to the center of the lap belt, as they are in most military harness configurations. These strap loads, developed under forward-facing impact conditions, lift the lap belt over the iliac crests of the pelvis, allowing the belt to bear on the abdomen and the inferior costal margin. This problem has been observed in human tests at acceleration levels as low as 10 g with a velocity change of 5.5 m/sec. Stapp (5) reported that test subjects reached the threshold of voluntary tolerance with this restraint configuration at 17 g for impact velocities greater than 30 m/sec. All of the tests conducted by Stapp at higher acceleration were accomplished using a pair of crotch straps devised to carry the tension loads of the shoulder straps into the pelvis and seat structure. Each strap was attached to an adjacent rear corner of the seat and to the lap belt buckle, forming an inverted V. More contemporary restraint harnesses use a single strap that connects the lap belt buckle and the front central portion of the seat. The single crotch-strap installation is simpler and provides better restraint during vertical vibration, but its effectiveness has not been demonstrated at the high acceleration levels explored by Stapp.

In view of the large influence the restraint system has on the tolerability of impact, the restraint configuration must be considered when

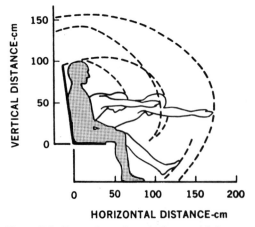

Figure 8.5. Extremity strike envelopes with lap belt and belt-shoulder straps restraint configurations.

interpreting human test results and their operational implications. For example, Stapp successfully demonstrated that humans are capable of tolerating very severe transient acceleration exposures. Acceleration levels up to 45.4 g, with a rise time of 0.11 seconds and a velocity change of approximately 56 m/sec, were endured in a forward-facing body position (5). The restraint system, however, was not a conventional military harness. The configuration was composed of 7.6-cm wide webbing and included a lap belt, two shoulder straps, inverted V crotch straps, and a strap that encircled the subject's chest at axillary height. The bearing area of the restraint was reported to be 553 cm^2. A conventional military harness, composed of two 4.5-cm wide shoulder straps and a 7.6-cm wide lap belt, has a bearing area of approximately 330 cm^2 and does not provide the effective coupling of the various parts of the torso that the Stapp configuration provided. Unfortunately, a harness configuration of the type Stapp used has not been practical in aerospace applications because of its multiple release points and the restriction of the occupant's mobility.

Efforts to develop a restraint system that will provide a high bearing area and better control of body segment motion during impact have been numerous, but the most innovative efforts have focused on the use of inflatable bags. This approach provides a restraint that does not encumber the vehicle occupant until the impact occurs. When predetermined acceleration levels are sensed on the vehicle structure, the bag restraint is inflated by compressed gas, pyrotechnic gas generators, or a combination of the two systems. In automotive applications, the inflatable bags are constructed of a porous material to control the forces transmitted to the occupant by allowing the gas to vent through the cloth during impact loading. Inflatable restraints considered for aircraft escape system applications have so far been designed only to provide additional body restraint and support to supplement existing harness configurations. Furthermore, because of the time available early in the escape sequences,

they do not require the fast inflation capability of the automotive restraint.

Body Support Systems

Many aerospace designers have proposed that the ideal body support system is a rigid, individually contoured couch. This approach ensures that each external body segment will be simultaneously accelerated and that the support pressure exerted on the body surfaces will be minimized. Designs of this type have been found to be very effective in laboratory impact, vibration, and centrifuge tests. The rigid contour approach was used in the Project Mercury astronaut couch design and in the design of the seat and seatback used in Project Gemini. The disadvantages of the approach are the high cost of individual fitting and the discomfort of the rigid contour after a relatively short occupancy because only one body position matches the contour.

Attempts to circumvent the disadvantages of the rigid couch design have included the design of net couches. These designs provide relief from the comfort problems and high manufacturing costs of the rigid contour couches. Thus far, net body support systems have been found to be very effective in sustained acceleration but have not provided good protection in either vibration or impact. The problem has been related to the elasticity of the net material. In both vibration and impact tests, the net body suspension system tended to resonate at or near the major resonances of the body segments, and the motion of the body segments was not harmonious. The motion of each body segment was not in time phase with the motion of the other body segments.

The most successful body support systems that have aerospace vehicle applications have (1) slight contouring to control body position; (2) dimensions that accommodate large variations in body size; (3) relatively rigid, lightweight sheet metal structures; (4) padding to provide isolation from small-amplitude, high-frequency impacts and vibration; and (5) minimal cushioning of the seat to reduce flight fatigue without major degradation in impact protection. Armrests are often provided to increase comfort. If the armrests are properly positioned, they permit the mass of the arms to act through the armrest structure rather than through the spine during + z acceleration.

Impact Attenuation

The forces imposed on a vehicle occupant during a crash or other transient acceleration of the vehicle are influenced to a significant degree by the mechanical properties of the materials between the occupant and the source of the accelerating force. Unless these interposed materials in the vehicle structure or the body support and restraint system are nondeformable, they will alter the magnitude and time phase of the forces that the occupant will experience. At first glance, this characteristic appears to be intuitively desirable. One might expect that deformable materials and structures, like soft cushions, should always protect an individual during an impact. Unfortunately, this intuition may lead to a faulty if not injurious conclusion.

Materials positioned between the occupant and the acceleration source can amplify the acceleration to which the occupant will eventually be exposed in a number of ways. First, the materials may store energy during the impact and then release it in rebound. Thus, the occupant is exposed to a larger velocity change than the vehicle. This condition occurs when vehicle structure or body support and restraint system deformations are elastic. Second, these deformations may delay the acceleration of the occupant and create a large velocity difference between the occupant and the vehicle. Of course, the occupant acceleration must subsequently exceed the vehicle acceleration to eliminate the velocity difference. An ejection seat cushion is a common component that can cause this second problem by virtue of the cushion material stiffness and the distance it creates between the seat structure and the seat occupant. During ejection, the

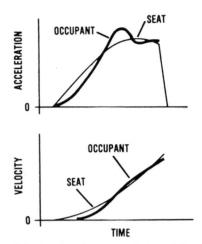

Figure 8.6. Acceleration and velocity of ejection seat and occupant; the acceleration of the occupant is delayed by the soft-seat cushion.

seat will develop a higher velocity as it compresses the seat cushion, as shown in Figure 8.6. Once the seat cushion has been fully compressed, the occupant is then accelerated to the higher velocity of the seat and often beyond.

Impact attenuation is accomplished when the forces transmitted between the acceleration source and the occupant can be limited to less than the levels that would be experienced if the occupant were rigidly coupled to the source. The acceleration being transmitted to a vehicle occupant may be attenuated by vehicle structural deformation, impact attenuation devices mounted between the seat and the vehicle, body support and restraint materials, and impact-attenuating materials mounted on the body such as in a flight helmet.

Attenuation of acceleration as it is transmitted through a vehicle structure, without failure of the structure, may occur because of the relatively low stiffness of the structure and its friction damping. Therefore, the high-frequency components of the acceleration cannot be transmitted through the low-frequency structure without being attenuated. This method is used in the design of automotive suspension systems. Automobile springs are selected so that the stiffness of the springs and the mass of the automobile body and occupants create a low-frequency mechanical system. Sharp impacts that occur along the roadway are attenuated into low-frequency, low-amplitude motion of the automobile body by the suspension system. Shock absorbers, which are viscous dampers, prevent the body from continued oscillation after the initial response.

In a vehicular crash, acceleration is attenuated by the collapse of structural members, but the occupied area of the vehicle must remain intact. The attenuation that is provided by structural collapse is a major factor in both aircraft and automotive crash protection because relatively large attenuation distances are available. Unfortunately, the acceleration-limiting capability of an aircraft structure is not well controlled by design or adequately predictable by experimental results or numeric methods. For this reason, vehicles at high risk of crashing, such as some military helicopters, use seat-mounted impact attenuation devices to provide the final stage of acceleration limiting. These devices are intended to attenuate the imposed acceleration of the vehicle, as shown in Figure 8.7. This illustration shows how the attenuation device acts to limit the acceleration of the seat and occupant by providing additional stopping distance. Energy storage and rebound is usually avoided by using viscous or friction damping or permanently deforming materials such as metal tubes or bands. The performance of impact-attenuation devices, however, is limited by the amount of stroke distance that is available. If the impact velocity exceeds the capability of the attenuation device, the stroke limit will be reached before the seat and occupant velocity are equal to the vehicle velocity. When this point is reached, the phenomenon referred to as bottoming occurs, and the acceleration of the seat and occupant will increase until the velocity of the vehicle is reached, as shown in Figure 8.8.

Commonly used impact-attenuation devices also may have other properties that limit their usefulness. These devices are often force-limiting mechanisms, and, therefore, their perfor-

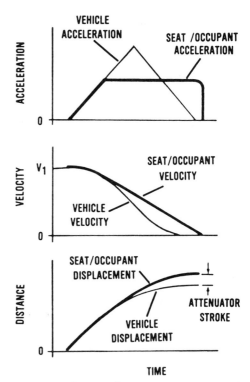

Figure 8.7. Influence of impact attenuator on vehicle seat occupant acceleration, velocity, and displacement.

mance is predictable on the basis of occupant mass only if the seat and occupant are rigid masses or if the vehicle acceleration is applied slowly enough to avoid causing amplification of the occupant's acceleration response. If the time of the application, which is referred to as rise time, t_r, is too short and the mass of the seat is relatively low, the acceleration of the occupant may influence attenuator performance. Even if this condition is avoided, force-limiting attenuator performance will still vary as a function of variations in subject weight.

The degree of impact attenuation that can be provided by the body support and restraint system or padding that might be worn by an individual is limited by the small displacements that are available. The padding of body support structures is usually selected to provide some comfort and to attenuate structural vibrations and low-energy, high-frequency impacts. Re-

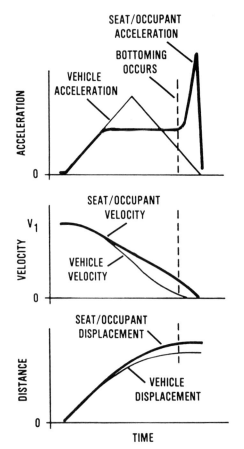

Figure 8.8. The effects of bottoming of an impact attenuator on seat and occupant acceleration, velocity, and displacement.

straint systems usually restrict the movement of the occupant to prevent the occupant's impact with surrounding structures. Attempts to provide impact-attenuating harnesses have so far been unsuccessful because designers have found it impractical to match the mechanical performance of the harness components' dynamic response characteristics to body segments for a large population. Therefore, the severity of impact injuries may be reduced in one anatomic area but increased in another.

MODELING IMPACT RESPONSE

System Dynamics

A fundamental understanding of the impact-response characteristics of mechanical systems is a prerequisite for the meaningful analysis and interpretation of the impact responses of the human body and the influence of protection system designs. The dynamic responses of mechanical systems, whether these systems are steel beams, rubber tires, bones, or muscle, are governed by Newtonian mechanics and can be described in terms of mechanical analogies. These analogies are usually expressed in terms of abstract mathematical equations, but for most individuals the use of more familiar physical models is necessary for the visualization of the analogy and understanding of its implications.

The physical models used to gain understanding of the principles of dynamic mechanical systems in this chapter are lumped parameter models. They are composed of elements such as springs, masses, and dampers, where each element represents only one mechanical property. In other words, the mass is a pure mass without elasticity or damping, whereas the spring and damper are massless. All of the elasticity of the modeled system is represented by the spring, and all the damping is represented by the damper. The lumped parameter model may be a single-degree-of-freedom system with one mass and one spring, where the position of the mass can be defined by a single coordinate, or a multidegree-of-freedom system composed of many masses, springs, and dampers.

The stiffness of the spring, k, is defined by the following equation:

$$k = F/x \qquad (8)$$

where F is the force required to deflect the spring a distance of x. The units of k are newtons per meter. The damper may represent several sources of friction in the mechanical system, but the damping that is most common to biologic systems is viscous damping, which is defined by the following equation:

$$c = F/\dot{x} \qquad (9)$$

where F is the force required to move the mass

at a velocity of $\dot{x}$. The units of the damping coefficient, c, are newton-seconds per meter. The velocity is designated in Newton's notation for a time derivative, as follows:

$$\text{velocity} = \dot{x} = dx/dt \text{ and}$$

$$\text{acceleration} = \ddot{x} = d^2x/dt^2 \quad (10)$$

The equation of motion for a simple system composed of a single mass and spring describes the forces that act on the system. These include a spring force, kx, an external force-time function, f(t), and the inertial reaction force $m\ddot{x}$, as follows:

$$F = -kx + f(t) + (-m\ddot{x}) = 0 \quad (11)$$

where the internal forces act in opposition to the external force and are, therefore, also functions of time.

The dynamic response characteristics of the physical model can be studied mathematically or empirically by observing the response of the model to various excitations. For the sake of simplicity, the mathematics have been minimized, and the response characteristics of the model will be demonstrated graphically. A more thorough treatment of this subject is available elsewhere (6,7).

Because it is usual to specify human tolerance to transient acceleration in terms of acceleration measured at the input point to the human body, the response of the system to excitations at the base will be illustrated. The equation of motion in this case is as follows:

$$\ddot{y} = \ddot{x} + (kx/m) \quad (12)$$

If an acceleration $\ddot{y}$ is instantaneously applied to the base of the spring-mass system to produce a constant continuing acceleration of the base, referred to as a step function, the system will

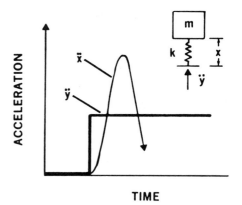

Figure 8.9. Response of spring and mass system to step function acceleration.

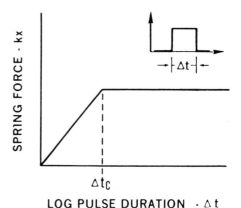

Figure 8.10. Force response of a dynamic system to rectangular base accelerations of varying duration.

respond as shown in Figure 8.9. The peak acceleration of the mass, m, will be twice the acceleration of the base, and the spring force (kx) will be twice as great as would be experienced if the spring were a rigid member.

By measuring the force in the spring of the system as it is exposed to a series of rectangular waveform accelerations applied at the base, the relationship between the acceleration duration and the dynamic response of the system can be seen, as shown in Figure 8.10. The peak spring force increases as the base acceleration pulse duration increases, up to a peak force. It then continues at that level for longer pulse durations. This same experiment can be performed for

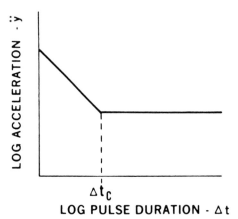

Figure 8.11. Acceleration tolerance of a system with a known spring deflection tolerance.

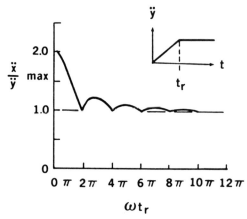

Figure 8.12. Effect of rise time (t_r) on the peak acceleration of a mass ($\ddot{x}$).

other wave-forms and similar results obtained. The peak force is reached at a critical acceleration pulse duration, Δt_c. The value of Δt_c depends on the natural frequency of the system ω, as follows:

$$\Delta t_c = 2/\omega \qquad (13)$$

where $\omega = \sqrt{(k/m)}$. If the acceleration pulse duration is less than Δt_c, neither the duration nor the magnitude of the acceleration are individually sufficient to determine the response of the system. The critical factor is their product, which is simply the velocity change associated with the acceleration pulse. If the acceleration pulse is longer than Δt_c, the peak force in the system is related to the peak input acceleration. When the duration of the input pulse is near Δt_c, the peak force is actually a complex function of the velocity change and the acceleration magnitude.

At some force level, the spring of the system that is represented by the mechanical model will reach a point of deflection where it will fail. By knowing the relationship between the acceleration input and the failure force level, the acceleration tolerance of the system can be specified, as shown in   Figure 8.11. This graph shows that for Δt less than Δt_c, the system can be exposed to increasing acceleration magnitudes

as the duration of the acceleration pulse decreases.

When the acceleration pulse is longer than Δt_c, the response of the dynamic system is also a function of the rise time, t_r, of the acceleration. The acceleration waveform we have studied thus far has had a rise time of zero. If the rise time of the acceleration transmitted to the base of the spring-mass system increases, the deflection of the spring will decrease and the acceleration of the mass will decrease. The theoretical relationship between the acceleration input rise time and the ratio of the acceleration of the mass to the acceleration input to the base of the system is shown in Figure 8.12 (7). For practical purposes, it may be assumed that the acceleration pulse has zero rise time if $t_r < 1/\omega$. The difference between the acceleration input magnitude and the resulting acceleration of the dynamic system can be ignored if $t_r > 10/\omega$.

Because damping exists to some degree in all real physical systems, its influence must be considered in the mechanical model. The equation of motion of the single-degree-of-freedom model with damping is as follows:

$$F = (-kx) - (c\dot{x}) + (f(t)) + (-m\ddot{x}) = 0$$

or

$$m\ddot{x} + c\dot{x} + kx = f(t) \qquad (14)$$

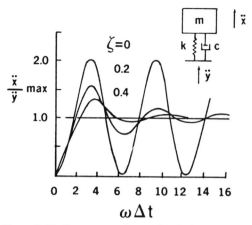

Figure 8.13. Responses of a mechanical system with varying levels of viscous damping to step function base acceleration.

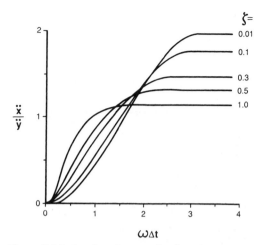

Figure 8.14. Acceleration amplitude ratio as a function of base acceleration pulse duration for selected damping coefficient ratios.

The influence of viscous damping on a spring-mass-damper system subjected to a rectangular-shaped acceleration pulse applied at the base is illustrated in Figure 8.13. The degree of damping is expressed in terms of the damping coefficient ratio, ζ, expressed in terms of the actual damping coefficient, c, and the critical damping coefficient, c_c, as follows:

$$\zeta = (c/c_c) = c/2m\omega \qquad (15)$$

The critical damping coefficient is the value of damping that is just adequate to allow the mass of the system to return from a displaced position to its initial position without oscillation. Figure 8.13 shows that as the damping coefficient ratio increases, the amplitude of the damped system's response decreases with each oscillation and the amplitude of the response also decreases. The deflection of the system or strain in the spring is no longer proportional to the total force as in the case of the undamped system because the damping force now contributes to the total force. A mechanical system with damping can tolerate higher impact acceleration levels before the deflection of the spring reaches the failure level. The relationship between the damping coefficient ratio and the amplification of an input ac-

celeration pulse with rectangular waveform is shown in Figure 8.14.

Human Mechanical Response

Early investigators of human tolerance to transient acceleration recognized the importance of theoretical models in the analysis of experimental findings and in the guidance of further investigations. Kornhauser and Gold (8) proposed and then demonstrated by impact tests with mice that animals exhibit the same impact response characteristics as mechanical systems in terms of their sensitivity to injury. The data from impact tests of 329 mice conducted to determine lethal dose levels could be described in terms of critical velocity change or acceleration level. The relationship that was demonstrated between the acceleration-time function and its lethality implied that the lethality rate corresponded to a critical maximum deflection or strain in a single-degree-of-freedom model. This important finding has been substantiated by other investigators for other animal species. It is important to recognize, however, that the implied model predicts a first-order effect only, that is, lethal dose. It does not predict the exact mode of lethal injury.

Lethal dose sensitivity curves may become

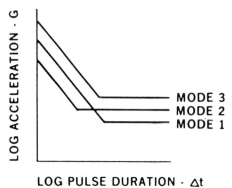

LOG PULSE DURATION · Δt

Figure 8.15. Impact injury limit curves for three modes of injury. (Adapted from Stech EL, Payne PR. Dynamic models of the human body. AMRL-TR-66–157, Aerospace Medical Research Laboratory, Wright-Patterson Air Force Base, Ohio, 1965.)

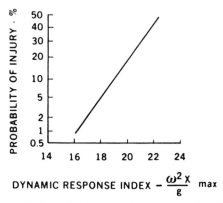

DYNAMIC RESPONSE INDEX $-\dfrac{\omega^2 x}{g}$ max

Figure 8.16. Probability of spinal compression fracture as a function of the dynamic response index.

more complex if the mode of injury is considered. The complexity occurs when more than one mode of injury exists, as shown in Figure 8.15 (9). This situation is likely because any complex biologic system will have a large number of potential injury modes. Most of the injury modes, however, will have no practical significance because the lethal dose will be determined by one or several that occur at lower stress levels due to their lower critical strain limits or their closer relationship to the stress input.

The potential for a complex, multimode injury curve can be conceptualized by considering a case in which a human would be accelerated by a force acting from back to chest. In this case, laboratory experience and observations of accident trauma suggest that the injury limit in the short-duration impulse region of the tolerance curve, where velocity change is the limiting factor, would be head injury. In the longer-duration impact region of the tolerance curve, injuries to the internal organs, such as the heart, liver, or spleen, would be more probable. In this case, it would be reasonable to describe the injury tolerance curve by two or more dynamic models in a parallel arrangement, that is, where there is no interaction between the motion of the models.

In many cases, however, a simple, single-degree-of-freedom model may be adequate. This model is generally feasible if there is one injury mode, the direction of impact is controlled, and the exact location and severity of the injury are not important. In ejection seat design, such a model has been used to predict the probability of vertebral fractures in the lower spine (10). This model is commonly used to evaluate the acceptability of ejection catapult designs and to analyze acceleration data collected during tests of escape systems. In these applications, the mathematical analog of this model is used to calculate the maximum deflection of the model in response to the total acceleration-time history. The maximum deflection value is then related to the probability of injury. The relationship that has been used is shown in Figure 8.16 (11). The output of the model is expressed in terms of the Dynamic Response Index values, which have correlated well with United States Air Force operational ejection spinal injuries (11).

The use of a dynamic model to evaluate the probability of spinal injury provides advantages over the method described earlier in the chapter. This method consists of a description of the acceleration-time history in terms of two or three limiting parameters. The usual limiting parameters were the rate of onset, that is, the slope of the rising portion of the acceleration-time history, and peak acceleration. In some applications, the duration of the acceleration pulse was also considered. This method was based on empiric evidence collected during the development and use of ejection catapults. The method was flawed in many respects. First, it was based on the false premise that there is an absolute limit beyond which injury will occur. Second, it assumed that there is a critical rate of onset that would cause injury. It did not recognize that there is a trade-off between the rate of onset and peak acceleration. Third, the method could not be used to evaluate complex acceleration waveforms. Therefore, it became obsolete when attempts were made to apply the method to problems such as space vehicle landing impact and more advanced aircraft escape system accelerations where complex waveforms are common. Fourth, the method did not provide a means of evaluating the influence of other factors such as the viscoelastic properties of ejection seat cushions.

A major advantage of dynamic models is that they are helpful in understanding the influences of the seat structure, cushion materials, restraint, or impact attenuation devices in modifying the acceleration transmitted to the human body (7). Although the models of the protective system and the human body may be relatively complex, the fundamental principles of protection system dynamics can be illustrated by the use of simple mechanical elements, as shown in Figure 8.17. The input to this model is the acceleration of the vehicle structure, which in most cases is the acceleration of the seat structure. The mass of the protection system or body support cushioning material is normally quite small in relation to the human occupant. For this analysis, it can be assumed that the body support and restraint material is sufficient to prevent injury due to nonuniform motion of the body segments and that the contact pressures will not cause injury.

If the restraint or body support material is very soft in contrast to the effective lumped stiffness of the human body model, the protection system will attenuate impulsive accelerations within the limits of its deflection capability, x_{max}. If the acceleration pulse duration is long enough to exceed x_{max}, however, the occupant will bottom

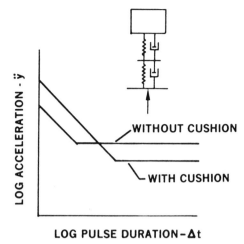

Figure 8.17. Influence of cushion material dynamic response properties on acceleration tolerance of a system with a known spring deflection tolerance.

out and will experience much higher acceleration than he or she would without the protection system. This general relationship is shown in Figure 8.17 for the human body model supported by a soft cushion and exposed to rectangular waveform acceleration inputs.

This simple analysis illustrates the importance of understanding the relationships among the spectrum of the acceleration pulses that might be encountered, the mechanics of the protection system, and the dynamic response properties of the human. It also serves as a warning that a protection system might appear acceptable under laboratory test conditions but prove unacceptable under more severe operational conditions. Restraint materials are commonly tested under static loads, where the influence of system dynamic response is ignored. They also are evaluated under very short-duration impulse loading, where the acceleration level may be the same as the operational condition but where the energy level is too low to produce the operational dynamic response (i.e., restraint strap tension). Tests using static or impulsive loads are acceptable only when these tests can be related to the operational loading conditions. If extrapolation is required, the dynamic response properties of the restraint occupant and the restraint system must be known. Therefore, test conditions should stimulate the anticipated operational environment as closely as possible. Where feasible, the restraint system should be tested with volunteer subjects at subinjury levels and then evaluated with anthropomorphic dummies at the design limits.

EXPERIMENTAL IMPACT

Facilities

Impact tests to measure human responses and to evaluate protection equipment have been accomplished using a wide variety of methods. Pioneering work to establish performance limits for ejection seat catapults was conducted by ejecting prototype seats up extended ejection rails. The test subjects were often the engineers and scientists associated with the escape system development. Catapult acceleration limits were established when the subjects reached their voluntary tolerance levels or were injured. The escape system was ultimately demonstrated by an in-flight ejection, first with anthropomorphic dummies as occupants and then with experimental test parachutists. This approach was used by the United States Air Force for nearly two decades.

The need to establish aeromedical design criteria for aircrew restraint systems for crash protection motivated a fundamental change in method. Experiments were begun at Muroc, California, using a sled propelled along a rail track by rockets. The seat and restraint system designs were evaluated, and the limits of human impact tolerance were explored by rapidly decelerating the sled with friction brakes (5). These experiments were eventually extended to study the effects of transient deceleration and windblast associated with ejection from high-speed aircraft. These later tests were performed on rocket sled facilities at China Lake, California, and Holloman Air Force Base in New Mexico (12). Deceleration was achieved by water brake scoops.

Facilities that can provide more precise control of the impact test conditions have been developed as the experimental efforts in this area matured beyond the initial field test approach. The facilities now used for impact experiments include (1) relatively simple towers that are used to drop test carriages onto decelerators such as metal-deforming devices or hydraulic cylinders; (2) horizontal tracks with various propulsion systems that are used to propel test carriages into decelerators; and (3) high-pressure gas actuators that are used to accelerate a test carriage along either vertical or horizontal rails. The gas-operated actuator facilities offer the greatest degree of impact control and reproducibility because initial conditions prior to the impact can be easily controlled.

Comparison of test data collected from different impact facilities is difficult and must be done cautiously. Factors such as body support and restraint system configuration, restraint pretension, subject bracing, and similarity of the entire acceleration waveform must be considered. The conditions that exist prior to the impact are also critical. For example, the early research to explore human tolerance to $-x$-axis impact was accomplished using deceleration facilities. After accelerating the test sled to a desired velocity by use of a rocket or pyrotechnic catapult, the sled would then coast along the facility track until the deceleration mechanism was contacted. During the coasting phase, however, the test subject would be exposed to a deceleration due to sliding friction and aerodynamic drag. The level of deceleration generally exceeded 1.5 g, and the planned impact pulse sometimes was preceded by coasting deceleration as high as 15 g.

The deceleration level experienced during the sled-coast phase of contemporary horizontal deceleration facilities is about 0.3 g. Impact facilities that are designed to accelerate the sled and subject from a standing start impose no acceleration or velocity prior to the impact event. Recent experimental investigations with animal and human subjects have demonstrated that these preimpact conditions have significant measurable influence in the subject's responses and tolerance to the subsequent impact (13).

These investigations have led to the concept of dynamic preload. Dynamic preload is defined as an imposed acceleration preceding, continuous with, and in the same direction as a subsequent impact. It should not be confused with static load conditions, such as pretension of the restraint, or subject bracing. The experimental investigations of dynamic preload have shown that volunteer subjects perceive their response to impact imposed by an accelerator to be more severe than their response to a comparable decelerator impact preceded by 0.25 g deceleration. Objective measures of the impact response, such as body segment accelerations and restraint loads, provide evidence that confirmed the subjective findings. Furthermore, tests conducted on a decelerator to compare measured forces and body segment accelerations in matched impacts preceded by 0.25 or 0.62 g preload showed that this increase in the dynamic preload will further decrease the measured subject responses.

The explanation for the response differences observed when the dynamic conditions preceding an impact are varied can be understood in part by recalling the properties of accelerated viscoelastic systems. In the case of the accelerated human body, in spite of restraint pretensioning and muscular bracing, many anatomic structures are poorly supported. The head, arms, legs, and various soft tissue masses and internal organs often must undergo some relative displacement before effective acceleration forces can be applied through joints, attachments, or direct contact with other supporting structures. The relative displacement of the lagging segment is a functional dead space. This phenomenon delays the acceleration of the lagging segments. Because of the developing velocity difference, however, the lagging segments will eventually experience a higher acceleration to catch up with the more efficiently accelerated portions of the body. The introduction of dynamic preload presumably acts to decrease the

effective dead space and, therefore, the severity of the overall acceleration response.

Instrumentation

The results of the earliest impact tests with human subjects were assessed by simply asking, "How did that feel?" Subjective responses are still an important aspect of experimental findings. Objective measurements of mechanical responses and physiologic changes, however, are potentially more reliable experimental indicators of the stressfulness of an impact or the effectiveness of a protective technique. The basic problem is to determine what to measure, how to make the measurement, and how accurately the measurement must be made.

From the point of view of experimental impact mechanics, it would be desirable to measure the acceleration, velocity, and displacement of all the human body segments and internal organs as well as the test vehicle during each test. Furthermore, if possible, it would be useful to know what forces produced the observed body segment and organ motions and to determine how these forces may be controlled by various body support and restraint structures. From the point of view of the physician concerned about injury potential, it also would be desirable to relate these motions and forces to tissue deformation or damage and to any changes that may occur in physiologic processes such as cardiac electrical activity. From a practical point of view, however, it is not feasible to measure all of these quantities during an impact test. Certainly, in tests with volunteer subjects, the measurement of internal organ movement is fraught with difficulties and hazards that make it impossible with current techniques.

The researcher must choose those measurements that are necessary and feasible and that will not cause untoward effects on the impact response or protective technique being studied. The physical measurements are usually made using electronic devices such as linear accelerometers, angular rate gyros, or force transducers.

High-speed motion picture cameras also are used in conjunction with reference targets mounted on observable body segments.

The researcher and those reviewing impact test results within the literature must understand the limitations of the measurements in terms such as resolution, linearity, dynamic range, repeatability, and frequency response. A systematic approach to the choice of accuracy is also vital and involves more than a determination of the error from the true value. An inconsistent set of measurements, in which high accuracy in one measurement is wasted because of its use in a calculation with a low accuracy measurement, may result from the lack of error analysis during the experimental design. Because this factor may be neglected by some researchers, caution is advised in interpreting the results of tests in which the instrumentation and its accuracy are not adequately described.

The electronic devices used to measure impact responses are electromechanical transducers that convert a mechanical response within the instrument into an electrical signal proportional to that response. Generally, the devices may be analyzed mathematically using spring-mass-damper models. Load cells are examples. They are basically rather stiff springs that deflect in proportion to the applied load. The small deflections are converted to an electrical potential by an element called a strain gauge that is attached to the spring. Although such a devise may be quite accurate under single-axis loads, it may produce erroneous results if bending or off-axis loads are present. Therefore, it must be calibrated in a configuration representative of the experimental application.

The equipment used to process the outputs of the transducers also may be described in terms of a mathematical model of its response. It is critical to assess frequency response characteristics of these devices, particularly when the measurements are recorded as discrete samples over time. Primary frequencies of interest in measuring human impact responses depend upon the frequency response properties of the body or body segment being investigated. For example, the impact response of the thorax occurs at a frequency around 20 H_z while the skull may respond at a frequency of approximately 100 H_z. The frequency response of the instrumentation system should generally exceed the maximum human response frequency that will be measured by a factor of five. The limits commonly selected are 100 H_z to 200 H_z to measure whole body response.

Acceleration measurement is generally made with small, light, linear accelerometers. The simplest model of such a device is a mass, constrained to move in one direction, that is attached to its case by a spring. The electrical output of the accelerometer is proportional to the deflection of the spring and thus is actually a measure of force. For example, the accelerometer cannot distinguish between gravitational force at rest and the internal force produced during a 1-g acceleration. Furthermore, an accelerometer cannot distinguish between internal force produced by simple translational acceleration of the case and that produced by the rotational motion of the case. As a result, the output of the accelerometer cannot simply be integrated once to produce a measure of velocity and again to yield displacement, unless the acceleration is purely translational and the orientation with respect to the earth is known. Gyroscopic sensors provide more direct measurement of rotational accelerations that can be achieved even with arrays of linear accelerometers. Finally, acceleration data of any kind, when integrated, will produce velocity or position information with errors that increase with time.

To solve the problem of measuring displacement, most researchers have turned to photographic instrumentation. Displacement may be estimated from a series of photographs obtained from high-speed motion picture cameras. Here again, however, the same principles that apply to other forms of data collected and processing must be understood. Resolution and dynamic range are usually limited by the film grain size, frame coverage, and the relative size of the target. The frequency response is limited by the film frame rate and resolution.

Future applications should allow the use of optimal estimation theory to obtain the best estimates for the parameters of interest using the available data sources. Such techniques, exemplified by Kalman filtering, are extensively used in similar applications in inertial guidance. New transducers and electro-optical systems also may provide improved data.

Human Impact Test Results

Thousands of impact tests with human subjects are documented in the research literature. Direct comparisons among the results of these tests are usually difficult because of the differences in acceleration conditions, restraints, instrumentation, subjects, and experimental procedures. An approximate understanding of tolerable conditions in a specific application, however, often can be gained by carefully choosing from among the previous test results. Summaries of substantial portions of the historical database are available and can serve as useful guides to the literature (14,15). Whenever possible, the original test documentation for the chosen cases should be reviewed to verify that the test conditions assure relevance of the data to the intended application.

Perhaps the most dramatic human impact test experience was gained by Stapp (5), who conducted and often participated in rocket sled experiments. The highest acceleration exposure in this series, a 45.4-g deceleration with a velocity change of 56 m/sec, was experienced by Stapp in a forward-facing seat ($-$x-axis). This test involved significant dynamic preload, specially designed restraints, and the preimpact flexion of the neck. It resulted in retinal hemorrhage, but the post-test symptoms were less severe than in earlier tests in this series, in which the peak acceleration was above 38 g. The most severe effects were observed in a test at 38.6 g, in which the subject experienced definite symptoms of shock, several episodes of syncope, and was found to have albuminuria for 6 hours after the

test. The greater severity of the 38-g exposures was attributed to the difference in the rate of onset of the acceleration waveforms. The rate of onset of the 45-g test was 493 g/sec ($t_r = 0.11$ seconds), whereas the rate of onset for the 38-g tests was 1100 g/sec or greater ($t_r = 0.035$ seconds). The limits of human tolerance in the $-$x-axis are much lower when the restraint system is less adequate, as previously discussed.

A restraining surface, such as a seatback in place of straps, and the structural arrangement of the human anatomy has allowed tolerance of very high onset rates when the acceleration vector was oriented in the $+$x-axis. Beeding and Mosley (16) exposed a subject to a peak acceleration of 40.4 g with a velocity change of 14.8 m/sec and rate of onset of 2139 g/sec ($t_r = 0.022$ seconds) on the Daisy decelerator at Holloman Air Force Base. Special restraints and a lower level of dynamic preload were involved. Symptoms of shock, including loss of consciousness after the test, also were experienced.

The limiting factor in $+$z-axis human impact is vertebral fracture. Early investigators observed vertebral fractures during laboratory ejection seat tests and estimated that acceleration levels of 18 to 20 g with a velocity change of up to 17.5 m/sec could be tolerated without injury. Operational experience with United States Air Force ejection seats has shown that these estimates were reasonable. For example, review of 175 ejections accomplished from four aircraft using catapults producing peak acceleration levels ranging from 17.5 to 18.4 g with velocities of 15.2 to 25.9 m/sec showed that vertebral compression factors resulted from 7% of these ejections. The time to the peak acceleration produced by these catapults ranged from 0.1 to 0.18 seconds. The restraint system, which was identical for each of the seats, consisted of a lap belt and two shoulder straps. When the $+$z-axis accelerative forces are applied through a torso harness system, as in parachute opening shock, it appears that somewhat higher levels may be tolerable, although this has not been well defined.

Spinal fracture is also probably the limiting

factor for acceleration applied in the − z-axis when the force is compressive, as in a head-first water impact. In a downward ejection seat, the − z-force is applied partly in traction, through the pelvis by the lap belt, and partly in compression, by the restraint harness shoulder straps. Under these conditions, volunteers have routinely tolerated half-sinewave acceleration profiles up to 10 g with times to peak acceleration ranging from 0.017 to 0.114 sec and velocity change from 1.5 to 15.4 m/sec respectively (17). More elaborate restraint and body support have permitted even higher − z-axis acceleration levels to be endured. Subjects restrained to a rigid couch by two shoulder straps, cross-chest strap, lap belt, crotch strap, and leg straps were exposed to peak accelerations up to 18.5 g with a velocity change of 5.94 m/sec (18).

Human responses to acceleration in the − z-axis provide a noteworthy example of the differences between the effects of sustained and impact acceleration. The acceleration limits for seated subjects, conventionally restrained, exposed to sustained acceleration in the − z-axis are less than half of the impact exposure levels. The sustained acceleration exposures are limited by head pain and red out, which are not observed in shorter duration impact exposures.

The severity of sideward impact is approximately equivalent in either direction given symmetric restraints and supports because the human body is fairly symmetric about the midsagittal plane. Volunteer subjects have been exposed to sideward impact up to 9.95 g with a velocity change of 4.6 m/sec when the subjects were restrained only by a lap belt (19). These experiments were stopped because of the investigator's concern about lateral torso flexion of up to 30°. When a lap belt and two shoulder strap configuration were used, acceleration peaks up to 11.7 g with a velocity change of 4.5 m/sec were tolerated without irreversible injury (20). The limiting factor was transient bradycardia and syncope, apparently related to impingement of the shoulder strap on the carotid body. Adding flat metal plates to support the head, torso, and

legs has permitted ± y-axis impact exposures up to 23.1 g with an onset rate of 1210 g/sec (t_r = 0.04 seconds) and velocity change of 8.4 m/sec. The subject's complaints and physiologic responses to these test conditions suggested that subjective or objective tolerance had not been reached.

Experimental efforts to determine human exposure limits for impact directions involving more than one cardinal axis are limited to research conducted to evaluate a narrow range of impact conditions and a body support and restraint system proposed for a specific space vehicle. These experiments were conducted using a vertical declaration tower, where the dynamic preload is the near-weightless condition of free fall, and a horizontal deceleration track with a dynamic preload of approximately 0.3 g. Seven impact vector directions were explored on the vertical decelerator using six acceleration profiles (21). Peak accelerations measured on the rigid seat ranged from 23.0 to 26.6 g, with impact velocities of 8.0 to 8.6 m/sec and rates of onset of 980 to 1380 g/sec. These seven impact vectors were among 24 orientations explored on the horizontal decelerator in a series of 288 tests with volunteer subjects (22). Maximum accelerations measured on the sled ranged from 11.1 g for the − z-axis to 30.7 g when the acceleration vector was acting from chest to back (− x-axis) and 45° left. Impact velocities were varied up to 13.7 m/sec. None of these tests exceeded voluntary tolerance, but transitory postimpact bradycardia was a consistent finding for those impact vectors in which a component of the acceleration vector acted in the − z-axis. Multiple potentiating interactions prevent simple superposition of the effects observed in the component cardinal axes. New limiting factors may be involved with acceleration directions that allow different injury mechanisms than are present along the cardinal axis.

Surrogate Tests

Tests with anthropomorphic dummies, cadavers, and animals afford the opportunities to test to impact levels that would be intolerable for human subjects and to make precise and sometimes invasive measurements that would be difficult or impossible with living humans. The difficulties in applying these data are formidable, however, because the errors that are introduced in making the transition from surrogate data to living humans are frequently very large. Tests defining the physical properties of isolated tissue preparations may be particularly misleading because of such factors as donor characteristics, postmortem changes, absence of excised supporting tissue, loss of physiologic responsiveness, unrealistic force application, and inadequate strain rates.

The most reliable data always will be derived from tests of fully representative subjects under fully representative conditions. The usual problem is to draw the best conclusions from a combination of tests involving living human subjects under less than representative conditions and tests involving less than representative surrogates exposed to actual anticipated impacts.

DIRECTIONS IN IMPACT PROTECTION

Impact protection research promises continued improvements in our knowledge of how to accelerate people safely. Existing techniques will be refined. New techniques will be exploited. This chapter has presented a systematic overview of the fundamental physical and mathematical principles that form the basis for current practice in this important part of aerospace medicine. It also can be said with certainty that the same principles will be the basis for our future advancements.

Two tools of the trade deserve attention as we look to the future. The first of these is the mathematical model. Models have been used extensively in impact research and in this chapter. They will be more useful in the future. Models may be descriptive or predictive. Descriptive models are equivalent to fitting a deterministic curve to empiric data. They are useful as a mathematical shorthand to describe findings and

also may facilitate our understanding of the physical processes involved. Predictive models are descriptive models that may be used to extend our knowledge beyond what we have observed. Descriptive models are usually examples of the application of inductive reasoning in that they utilize specific findings to formulate general descriptions. The use of predictive models is an example of deductive reasoning in that general descriptions are applied to the prediction of specific untested results. Descriptive models can be, in a sense, validated by repeated observations with comparison to the hypothesized general description. They can even be used for interpolation between two tested conditions. A model used to predict or extrapolate cannot be validated by testing, however, for later use beyond tested regions. Each prediction in a new area must be verified by observation. It is imperative that models be used appropriately in the conduct of impact research. Descriptive models are necessary if we are to understand our data. Predictive models are helpful in devising new techniques and predicting their utility, but the predictions must be verified.

This brings us to the second tool of the trade, namely, human testing. If the fielding of untried techniques is to be avoided, human testing will continue to be a necessity. Particularly in impact research, it must be borne in mind that anthropomorphic dummies are simply mechanical manifestations of mathematical models. They are, therefore, subject to the limitations just described for such models. Animal surrogates and human cadavers are analogs with complex differences from the living human that are difficult to fully appreciate. These differences may, therefore, be the basis for erroneous conclusions from tests with surrogates. Particularly when the goal is to develop a protective system that does not injure the populations in which it is applied, it should be possible to responsibly and ethically design safe verification testing of proposed techniques with a carefully selected population of volunteers.

Impact protection techniques will improve as

research provides the necessary basis for their refinement. Techniques of interest in aerospace medicine will continue to be divided into two basic approaches. One approach involves the protection of occupants of a vehicle subjected to impact. The second approach involves protection of an occupant who escapes from a vehicle, presumably prior to an anticipated impact.

Occupant impact protection places significant demands on the vehicle designer to provide an intrusion-free compartment for the occupant during vehicle impact. Survivable impact conditions are defined by the limiting factor in available occupant protection techniques. In many current applications, the vehicle compartment deficiencies are the limiting factors in survival. As vehicle design improves, however, new occupant protection approaches may be required to take full advantage of the improvements. In a vehicle crash, the basic tenet is to strike an optimum balance between two contradictory requirements on occupant displacement. In one sense, occupant displacement within the vehicle should be minimized to avoid secondary impacts with vehicle structures and to avoid the acceleration amplifications associated with dead space and bottoming. This is the rationale for restraints such as lap belts. In another sense, however, occupant displacement within the vehicle allows more time for the occupant to accomplish the required velocity change and, in turn, allows the controlled application of lower acceleration over a longer period than would have been the case without displacement. This is the rationale for stroking seats in some helicopters. Future applications may allow significant gains by exploiting dynamic preload in occupant protection. This technique would involve anticipatory acceleration of the occupant by a counterstroking seat, triggered by a reliable crash sensor, that would initiate the velocity change prior to the impact. Other novel techniques may become available in the areas of restraint, individual protection such as helmets, postcrash environmental protection against fire, and assisted postcrash egress. These developments should find broad application beyond the sphere of aerospace medicine in related endeavors such as automobile passenger protection.

The second impact protection approach involves escape systems. Current techniques employ ejection seats or separable crewstation escape modules, each with its own set of advantages and disadvantages. The open seat allows rapid parachute deployment but offers poor protection at high speed, even with current limb restraint techniques. The module provides extraordinary windblast protection at high speed but requires relatively long times for deceleration and parachute deployment. As a result, low-altitude escape attempts may be compromised, particularly with significant aircraft sink rates. Both systems may produce significant morbidity during escape, parachute opening, and at ground impact after parachute descent. Likely future directions in escape systems will involve the exploitation of the strong points of each system while addressing some of the other sources of injury as well. The resulting systems may involve some attributes of previous individual capsule systems. New techniques and materials should allow effective encapsulation of a seat occupant during the early stages of ejection. Other approaches that should see application involve decision-making functions to tailor the escape to the prevailing conditions by utilizing dynamic preload, variable thrust catapults, alternative escape path choices, and trajectory control. To ensure that expanded escape capabilities are utilized despite short decision times and severe aircraft accelerations that may be imposed, it is likely that assisted escape initiation techniques will be developed to provide alerting, warning, and, in extreme cases, automatic initiation. Systems will subserve multiple functions so that, for example, g-suits, wind-blast protection, parachute landing protection, flotation, and antiexposure suits may be integrated into one basic device. Escape systems will require such efficiency and innovation to meet the challenge of increasingly severe escape conditions, from high-speed, low-level ejection to orbital escape.

These and other protective techniques will be necessary to allow humans to confidently venture forth in the flying machines of the future and accomplish the various tasks set before them. The required techniques will be as novel as the vehicles, missions, and conditions that demand them. The reassuring observation remains than an appreciation for the utilitarian framework of first principles still provides the best means to their achievement.

REFERENCES

1. Newhouse HL, Payne PR, Brown JP. Wind tunnel measurements of total force and extremity flail potential forces on a crew member in close proximity to a cockpit. AMRL-TR-79-110, Aerospace Medical Research Laboratory, Wright-Patterson Air Force Base, OH: Dec 1980
2. Zimmermann RE, Merritt NA. Aircraft Crash Survival Design Guide. Vol.II USAAVCOM TR 89-D.22B. Aviation Applied Technology Directorate, United States Army Aviation Research and Technology Activity, Fort Eustis, Virginia: Dec 1989
3. Clark TD, Sprouffske JF, Trout EM, et al. Baboon tolerance to linear declaration ($-G_x$): lap belt restraint. In: Proceedings of the Fourteenth Stapp Car Crash Conference. New York: Society of Automotive Engineers, Inc., 1970, 279–298.
4. Clark TD, Sprouffske JF, Trout EM, et al.: Impact tolerance and resulting injury in the baboon: Air Force shoulder harness-lap belt restraint. In: Proceedings of the Sixteenth Stapp Car Crash Conference. New York: Society of Automotive Engineers, Inc. 1972, 365–411.
5. Stapp JP. Human exposures to linear deceleration. Part 2. The forward-facing position and the development of a crash harness. Air Force Technical Report 5915, Aero Medical Laboratory, Wright Air Development Center, Wright-Patterson Air Force Base, Ohio, 1951.
6. Harris CM, ed. Shock and vibration handbook. 3rd ed. New York: McGraw-Hill Book Co., 1987.
7. Payne PR. The dynamics of human restraint systems. In: Impact acceleration stress. Washington, D.C.: National Academy of Sciences, National Research Council Publication 977, 1962;195–257.
8. Kornhauser M, Gold A. Application of the impact sensitivity method to animate structures. In: Impact Acceleration Stress. Washington, D.C., National Academy of Sciences, National Research Council Publication 977, 1962;333–344.
9. Stech EL, Payne PR. Dynamic models of the human body. AMRL-TR-66-157. Aerospace Medical Research Laboratory, Wright-Patterson Air Force Base, Ohio, 1965.
10. Payne PR. Personnel restraint and support system dynamics. AMRL-TR-65-127, Aerospace Medical Research Laboratory, Wright-Patterson Air Force Base, Ohio, 1965.
11. Brinkley JW, Shaffer JT. Dynamic simulation techniques for the design of escape systems: Current applications and future Air Force requirements. In: Biodynamic models and their applications. AMRL-TR-71-29-2, Aerospace Medical Research Laboratory, Wright-Patterson Air Force Base, Ohio, 1971.
12. Hanrahan JS, Bushnell D. Space biology: the human factors in space flight. New York: Basic Books, Inc., 1960.
13. Hearon BF, Raddin JH Jr., Brinkley JW. Evidence for the utilization of dynamic preload in impact injury prevention. AMRL-TR-82-6, Aerospace Medical Research Laboratory, Wright-Patterson Air Force Base, Ohio, 1982.
14. Von Gierke HE, Brinkley JW. Impact accelerations. In: Foundations of space biology and medicine. Calvin J, Gazenko OG, eds. Joint USA/USSR Publication. Washington, D.C.: National Aeronautics and Space Administration, 1975;2:1(6):214–246.
15. Snyder RG. Impact. In: Bioastronautics data book. Parker JF Jr., Weds VR. NASA SP-3006, Washington, D.C.: National Aeronautics and Space Administration, 1973;221–295.
16. Beeding EL Jr., Mosley JD. Human tolerance to ultra-high G forces. AFMDC-TN-60-2, Aeromedical Field Laboratory, Air Force Missile Development Center, Holloman Air Force Base, New Mexico, Jan., 1960.
17. Brinkley JW, Specker LJ, Mosher SE. Development of acceleration exposure limits for advanced escape systems. In: Implications of advanced technologies for air and spacecraft escape. AGARD-CP-472, Advisory Group for Aerospace Research and Development, North Atlantic Treaty Organization, Neuilly Sur Seine, France, April 1989.
18. Shulman M, Critz GT, Highly FM, et al. Determination of human tolerance to negative impact acceleration. NAEC-ACEL-510, US Naval Air Engineering Center, Philadelphia, Nov 1963
19. Zaborowski AV. Human tolerance to lateral impact with lap belt only. In: Proceedings of the eighth Stapp Car Crash and Field Demonstration Conference. Detroit: Wayne State University Press, 1966, 34–71.
20. Zaborowski AV. Lateral impact studies: Lap belt-shoulder harness investigation. In: The Ninth Stapp Car Crash Proceedings. Minneapolis, MN: University of Minnesota, 1966;93–127.
21. Weis EB Jr., Clark NP, Brinkley JW. Human response to several impact acceleration orientations and patterns. Aerospace Med 1963;34(12):1122–1129.
22. Brown WK, Rothstein JD, Foster P. Human response to predicted Apollo landing impacts in selected body orientations. Aerospace Med 1966;37(4):394–398.

Chapter 9

Biodynamics: Sustained Acceleration

Russell R. Burton,

James E. Whinnery

This chapter is primarily concerned with the aeromedical consequences of sustained acceleration forces (G) on humans. To accomplish this goal, the physiology of sustained G will be presented as it relates to aeromedical problems. Modern high-performance aircraft can, within one second, develop 7 to 9 G that can be sustained for several minutes—G levels that produce significant physiologic changes that limit human tolerance to this environment. Therefore, a clear differential between pathologic and physiologic effects is not always achieved; we sometimes do not know if a pathologic process occurs during high sustained-G (HSG) exposures or if the normal limit of physiologic tolerance has been reached.

Acceleration is a unique environment in that it is pervasive, acting directly and continuously upon the body during all G exposures making protection against it literally impossible. We can protect pilots against other potentially hazardous aerospace environments such as hypobaria, thermal extremes, and ionizing radiation, but we cannot yet fully protect pilots against G. True, tolerances are increased to high G levels with so called "G protective" methods, i.e., anti-G suits, anti-G straining maneuvers (AGSM), positive pressure breathing during G (PBG), and body reclining systems but the entire G force still continues to affect all of the body and its contents. In reality, "protective methods" have simply increased the level of G hazard. This fact is not trivial for flight surgeons, since they must be aware that some aspects of the physiology and anatomy of aircrew of high performance air-

craft are significantly altered during every aerial combat maneuver (ACM).

For comparison, aircrew that fly at an altitude of 40,000 ft all day are not exposed to those levels of hypoxia and hypobaria, but aircrew that conduct high-G maneuvers all day have, in fact, been exposed to those high-G levels and, therefore, its physiologic and potential pathologic consequences all day.

HISTORICAL REVIEW

Our understanding of the aeromedical aspects of acceleration is perhaps best appreciated by reviewing the rich and unexpectedly long history of its development. Its history is rather unique among environmental physiologies; it began, not because of a need to understand its potentially hazardous effects on the human, but because of professional curiosity raised in those who observed the profound symptomatology that results from "centrifugation."

The first documented account of a person having a noticeable physiologic effect from exposure to sustained acceleration was described by Charles Darwin's grandfather, Erasmus Darwin, in the late 1700s. He had heard of a man going to sleep while spun atop a stone wheel used to mill corn.

Centrifuges began to appear in the 1800s and were primarily used to produce acceleration for treating mental illness and circulatory disorders. As early as the mid-1800s, the effects of acceleration on respiration, heart rate, and blood distribution were well known by physicians who frequently used themselves as experimental subjects.

In 1903, the year that the Wright brothers first successfully flew their airplane at Kitty Hawk, a captive flying machine built for amusement accidentally caused its engineer to lose consciousness at about 7 G. This accident appears to be the first documented case of the G-loss of consciousness (G-LOC) that concerns today's fighter pilots.

In World War I, pilots reported "fainting" during aerial maneuvers and recovering 20 sec later without apparent aftereffects. This condition of "fainting in the air" was compared by those who had experienced it to the early stages of an anesthetic. Some aircraft mishaps occurred because of this condition that was obviously G-LOC (1).

These reports prompted Drs. A. Broca and P. Garsaux to conduct experiments with dogs using a 6 m diameter centrifuge in France in 1918. They concluded from their studies exposing dogs to up to 98 G for 5 min, that human death from flight was not directly caused by G. But they were concerned about a "decrease of nervous reaction" they had observed which probably describes the G-LOC condition which is of concern today.

In the early 1920s, pilots in air races in the United States often reported "blackout" and G-LOC. Jimmy Doolittle began to systematically study acceleration-induced blackout, earning a Master's Degree in aeronautics on this subject, and was probably the first to describe G-LOC as resulting from decreased central nervous system blood flow.

The first successful human-use experimental centrifuge was built in Germany in 1933. In studies with subjects seated in various positions relative to the G vector that measured G tolerances, scientists described G-LOC and blackout and identified the occurrence of minute cutaneous hemorrhages (petechiasis). Their research concluded that G protection was required for pilots flying above 6 G and for that need, designed an automatic, reclining (swivel-type) seat.

The first U.S. human-use centrifuge was built circa 1938 at Wright Field, Dayton, Ohio. The research conducted on this centrifuge by Armstrong and Heim was reported in the first medical/physiologic review published in the U.S., "The Effect of Acceleration on the Living Organism (2)." This article, written in 1938, is still an excellent review of the principal aeromedical consequences of sustained G.

During World War II, six "high performance" human-use centrifuges were built by the Allies—four in the U.S. ((1) U.S. Army Aeromedical Laboratory, Wright Field, Ohio; (2) University of Southern California, Los Angeles, California; (3) Naval Air Station, Pensacola, Florida; and (4) Mayo Aeromedical Unit, Rochester, Minnesota), one each in Canada (Royal Canadian Air Force Accelerator Unit, Toronto, Canada) and Australia (Royal Australian Air Force, Flying Personnel Research Unit, Sydney University, Australia)—to support research in developing methods to protect pilots from the "dreaded blackout," thereby, increasing the operational performance of allied fighter planes. This research provided: a) the development of several different types of anti-G suits and valves; b) a type of AGSM, then called the M-1 maneuver that was taught to pilots to increase G tolerance; and c) increased understanding of the medical and physiologic consequences of exposures to higher levels of sustained accelerations.

The introduction of modern fighter aircraft in the 1970s (F-15, F-16, F-18) capable of sustaining much higher G caused a resurgence of acceleration research that produced numerous advances in G protection; e.g., improved anti-G suits and valves, physical conditioning programs that increase G tolerance, AGSM training in the centrifuge, and assisted PBG. In addition, an increased understanding of the medical and physiologic aspects of higher levels (up to 9 G) of sustained G exposures on the human has emerged from these studies over the last two decades. This research was primarily conducted in the U.S. and Britain using centrifuges built after World War II; i.e., the U.K. centrifuge at the RAF Institute of Aviation Medicine (RAF/IAM), Farnborough, England, the U.S. Navy centrifuge located at the Naval Air Warfare Center, Warminster, Pennsylvania; and two U.S. Air Force (USAF) centrifuges in the Armstrong Laboratory—one at Wright-Patterson AFB, Ohio and the other at Brooks AFB, Texas.

PHYSICAL PRINCIPLES

Acceleration (a) forces that are sustained for several seconds to minutes are developed during rapid inside turns used in aerial combat maneuvers (ACM) with modern high performance aircraft. ACM's generate centripetal acceleration that results in centrifugal (inertial type) forces that, for all practical purposes, can be duplicated in a centrifuge. This centrifuge capability provides acceleration research, to be conducted in a laboratory under safe and controlled conditions, with operational relevance.

These forces of acceleration are described by Newton's three laws of motion. The first describes inertia, stating that a body remains at rest or in a uniform motion in a straight line unless acted upon by a force. In order to overcome inertia, a force (F) is required, the result of which, is proportionate to the acceleration applied and the "size" of its mass (m); i.e., F = mass (m) × acceleration (a)—Newton's second law of motion. The third law states that for every action (acceleration *centripetal* force) there is an equal and opposite reaction (inertial *centrifugal* force).

Acceleration from a centrifuge, by constantly changing the direction of a mass, is quantified relative to the acceleration produced by the forces of Earth's gravity. This method is convenient and consistent with physical principles because the force of a mass produced by gravity is identical to the acceleration force of a mass produced on a centrifuge as stated by Mach and Einstein with their "Principle of Equivalence." The causes of gravity as it affects the body and those of inertia are not well understood. The acceleration produced by earth's gravity has been measured and is known as earth's gravitational

constant—9.81 m/sec^2. To measure the *centripetal* acceleration (a) produced by a centrifuge, as it relates to the gravitational constant, the following equation is used:

$$a = r\overline{\omega}^2 \qquad (1)$$

Where:
$\overline{\omega}$ = radians per sec[a]
r = centrifuge radius (m)

Mass (M) is a fundamental property of matter that is accelerated (a) proportional to the force applied upon it: M = F/a or F = ma. Using D'Alemberian Analysis (as opposed to Newtonian Analysis)[b] of inertial forces on the gravitational system, particularly useful to biologists, the weight (W) of an object is proportional to its mass (M) where:

$$W = k\ Ma \qquad (2)$$

In the gravitational system k is the reciprocal of Earth's gravity, l/g, so W = M (a/g). A modified form of this equation is particularly useful to biologists as applied in the following form:

$$W/M = a/g = G \qquad (3)$$

Where:
g = 9.81 m/sec^2 (gravitational constant)

G therefore is a dimensionless unit which represents an accelerative or centrifugal force or, if restrained, an inertial force, and is expressed in multiples of Earth's gravity.

Weight (w) is a measure of inertial mass (ma)

---

[a] Radian degree tables are available; but for simple calculations, 360° equals 6.28 radians. Therefore, a 6.2-m radius centrifuge that is rotating at 24 rpm is moving at 150.7 radians per minute (6.28 × 24 = 150.7) or 2.51 radians per second (150.7/60 = 2.51). Using Equation 1 to calculate "a": (2.51)2 = 6.3 × 6.2 = 39.1/9.81 = 4, which produces 4 g of force if mass (m) is kept constant; i.e., g = ma and the inertial force is G = ma.

[b] In D'Alembertian analysis, the centrifugal force becomes the fictitious force, an inertial force, which balances the centrifugal force to achieve equilibrium (30).

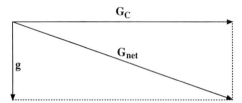

Figure 9.1. Relationship of the force of gravity (g) and the inertial force (G_c) of the centrifuge to the resultant G_{net} force.

that is restrained. The inertial force caused by gravity on a mass that is motionless is called gravitational mass where the mass (at 1 g) equals weight (m = w). When a mass is accelerated, the resulting inertial force (G) (using Eqs. 1, 2, and 3) is measured (for simplicity) in units of earth's gravity; e.g., at 2 G the weight of an individual is twice that of its gravitational mass (or weight on earth as 1 g^c). But the centrifuge inertial mass (weight) computation becomes more complex because the force of gravity $(g)^c$ is pervasive and, while at lower G levels, its influence is significant enough that it must be accounted for in the G environment. This calculation follows using the Pythagorean theorem (Fig. 9.1). Using the example of a 2 G inertial force produced by the centrifuge the net G is $\sqrt{2^2 + 1^2} = \sqrt{5}$ or 2.24 G in a direction (G_{net}) as shown in Figure 9.1. A person with a mass (or "weight") of 75kg at 1g (earth's gravity) will now weigh 75 × 2.24 or 168 kg. A net G vector is rapidly and automatically established by the gondola of the centrifuge as it swings freely outward (one degree of freedom), maintaining a constant rotational rate. At high-G levels, the effect of gravity on G_{net} becomes negligible for most research purposes.

The rotational rate of the centrifuge is changed, as during starting and stopping, by applying a tangential acceleration that creates an inertial tangential force in the opposite direction. This force occurs only during a change in G, as in the beginning and ending of a sustained G

exposure, therefore its minimal physiologic effects are ignored by acceleration physiologists. However, the responses of the vestibular system are not easily ignored, producing brief episodes of disorientation that may, for the first few G exposures, produce motion sickness. As with most physiologic systems, adaptation occurs with repeated exposures on the centrifuge and motion sickness subsides, but the disorienting sensation may persist.

Angular motions of the gondola about the three major axes are designated "rotation" and are defined:

1. Pitch: rotation of the gondola about its lateral axis. Pitch is designated (+), for pitch nose up; and (−), for pitch nose down.
2. Roll: rotation of the gondola about its longitudinal axis. Roll is designated (+), for clockwise; or (−), for counterclockwise, facing the direction of centrifuge revolution.
3. Yaw: rotation of the gondola about its vertical axis. Yaw is designated (+), for nose right; and (−), for nose left, facing the direction of centrifuge revolution.

Axial System Nomenclature

Physiologic studies of sustained acceleration require a standardized method for identifying the position of the subject relative to the G vector. Therefore, an acceleration and inertial force axial nomenclature has been developed that relates to the three major spatial axes of a body. Understanding this nomenclature is particularly important in human and animal physiologic research because the position of the body within the G field frequently dictates physiologic responses and limitations that can establish human tolerances to this environment. For example, the human flies aircraft and the space shuttle (upon reentry) seated upright maintaining a significant portion of their longitudinal axis parallel to increased G_{net} that makes them physiologically vulnerable to the G. To explain further, in the human at one end of this axis is the brain, a

---

[c] The use of "g" to denote the force of gravity and the centripetal force is standard.

vital organ that is particularly susceptible to a reduction in blood flow. This location is precarious during increased G since arterial blood flow within the body is a function of the pressure generated by the heart that is located a significant distance "below" the head in the normally seated person. In this position, the hydrostatic pressure (P_H) developed by the inertial response of the blood within the vascular system, will oppose the systemic arterial pressure (P_a) of the heart, 100 to 120 mmHg. As G increases, this P_H increases directly with the change in G level:

$$P_H = hdG \qquad (4)$$

Where:

h = blood column height (distance between the heart and head that in the human is about 320 mm)

d = blood specific density that remains constant at about 1; and

G = inertial force in G units; i.e., at 4 G (4 times earth's gravitational force) the P_H is four times greater than at 1 G (amounting to about 100 mmHg)

At 4 G, 100 mmHg of P_H = 100 mm Hg of P_a, that significantly reduces blood flow to the brain. If the longitudinal axis of the body relative to the G vector is reduced, h is less, as is P_H, so that with the same P_a (100 to 120 mm Hg), G tolerance is increased. These relationships between P_a and P_H clearly establish the bases for G-level tolerances forming the physical basis for Equation 9 and will be discussed in more detail in the section entitled $+Gz$ Tolerances (3).

The body's physical relationship (position) to the G vector is identified using the axial system of nomenclature that is the established standard for acceleration physiologists. The three major axes are longitudinal, lateral, and horizontal. Longitudinal (vertical) is denoted z; lateral (right/left) is y; and horizontal (supine/prone) is x. The direction of the *centripetal* acceleration force (g) along each of these axes is denoted by a (+) or (−); e.g., $+g_z$ is headward acceleration

Table 9.1.
Nomenclature for Inertial Resultant of Body Acceleration

Linear Acceleration	Physiological	Inertial Reaction
Forward $+g_x$	[a,b]Transverse A-P G Supine G Chest to back	$+G_x$
Backward $-g_x$	Transverse P-A G, Prone G Back to chest G	$-G_x$
Headward $+g_z$	Positve G, Toward feet	$+G_z$
Footward $-g_z$	Negative G, Toward head	$-G_z$
To left $+g_y$	Right lateral G	$+G_y$
To right $-g_y$	Left lateral G	$-G_y$

[a] Uppercase G, unit to express inertial resultant to whole body acceleration in multiples of magnitude of the Earth's gravity.
[b] A-P = anterior-posterior; P-A = posterior-anterior

force, $-g_z$ is footward; $+g_y$ is leftward, $-g_y$ is rightward; and $+g_x$ is forward, $-g_x$ is backward. Of course, the inertial centrifugal forces (G) are opposite the acceleration forces (g) thusly designated by the same directional symbology; e.g., $+g_z$ (headward acceleration) produces $+G_z$ (inertial force) that is directed footward (Table 9.1).

A simple method to remember the nomenclature of this axial system is to place your right hand in front of you with the thumb pointed up, index finger pointed directly forward, and middle finger pointed toward the left so that each finger is perpendicular to the other two. The lower two fingers remain folded against the palm of the hand. Now, each of the three pointing fingers indicates a "positive" direction (axis) of the centripetal acceleration forces: (a) the thumb points to the head, or headward acceleration ($+g_z$); the index finger points back to front, or forward acceleration ($+g_x$); and the middle finger points to left, or leftward acceleration ($+g_y$). Of course, acceleration physiologists are interested in the inertial force (G) direction; therefore, simply reverse the direction of each acceleration force maintaining the same nomenclature.

HUMAN-USE CENTRIFUGES

At the present time the United States Government operates four human-use centrifuges primarily for experimentation and one centrifuge for G training. These centrifuges are located at the Armstrong Laboratory, Brooks AFB (San Antonio, TX), Wright-Patterson AFB (near Dayton, OH), Naval Air Warfare Center (Warminster, near Philadelphia, PA), and NASA at Ames Research Center (South of San Francisco, Sunnyvale, CA). The USAF training centrifuge is located at Holloman AFB, NM. The U.S. Navy aviator training is located at a training centrifuge facility at Lemoore NAS, CA. There are at least 20 research-training human-use centrifuges in foreign countries (4).

Centrifuge Description

The structure of centrifuges for human experimentation and training are similar, but their operation varies considerably. Every centrifuge has a center spindle connected to the drive system about which it rotates. Extending from the center is a rigid arm that has an enclosed compartment at its distal end, called the gondola, that contains the subject. The arms of centrifuges range from about 15 ft (4.6 m) to 50 ft (15.2 m) in currently

operating centrifuges. The minimum length is usually limited by the high rotational rate that can cause a high Coriolis force that has disorienting effects on subjects, particularly when they rotate their head. The maximum length is limited by the torque required of the drive system to accelerate the arm. Ironically, the Naval Air Warfare Center (NAWC) centrifuge with the longest arm (15.2 m) also has the highest G-onset rate of approximately 10 G/sec. This uniquely advanced centrifuge has actively controlled dual gimballing with altitude, thermal and vibration capabilities.

Because torque requirements limit the centrifuge radius, a track-type centrifuge that operates without an arm with a radius of 250 to 300 ft (91.4 m) has been proposed. Not only does the long radius reduce the potential Coriolis effects with head movements but because it doesn't have an arm, unique operational characteristics are possible that would provide aerial combat maneuvers that closely approximate those of different types of advanced fighter aircraft. It should be understood, however, that a reduction in the Coriolis force with an increase in radius length of a centrifuge is not a simple linear function; e.g., increasing the radius 50% from 6 to 9 m reduces the Coriolis force by only 18 percent.

The Armstrong Laboratory human-use centri-

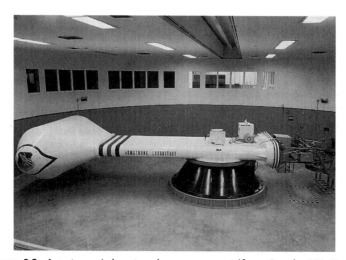

Figure 9.2. Armstrong Laboratory human-use centrifuge, Brooks AFB, Texas.

fuge at Brooks AFB, Texas is shown in Fig. 9.2. This centrifuge with a 20 ft radius arm and 6 G/sec onset rate, has a passive orienting one degree of freedom gondola.

Performance Characteristics

The two major performance characteristics of a human-use centrifuge are the maximum level of G and its onset rate. The onset rate is usually expressed simply as the rate (per sec) of change of the G vector within the gondola (e.g., 6 G per sec onset rate). However, because of the inertia of the system at the beginning of the onset of acceleration and the momentum of the gondola at the end of this onset, the G onset rate is not a linear function, but rather one that is sigmoidal (*S*-shaped). High-G onset capability is an important consideration because high performance aircraft can produce very-high-G onset rates (i.e., >10 G/sec is possible) during ACM. In order to accomplish the highest G onset rate possible with the limited drive-system power that is available, the centrifuge is accelerated slowly to a constant low G level called ''base G'' before the initiation of the high-G onset maneuver. This approach reduces the torque requirements for the drive system.

There are two types of gondola angular controls. The simplest is passive or inertial control; i.e., the gondola mounted on bearings at both ends freely rotates in the roll axis. The other method, active control, uses gondola drive motors with computerized controls to solve the acceleration vector equations so that the G_{net} vector is more closely maintained, thereby reducing the adverse effects of tangential G forces. Such systems use separate drive systems for each of the axes to be controlled. One of the operational support benefits of the active control method is dynamic flight simulation. The Naval Air Warfare Center and the Armstrong Laboratory at Wright-Patterson AFB, Ohio centrifuges have this capability.

The controls of the operations of the centrifuge—G level and G onset rates—are of two types; i.e., closed-loop or open-loop. The closed-

loop control allows the subject to operate the centrifuge, usually using an aircraft-type control stick for operational simulation. The open-loop system provides separate control by personnel operating the centrifuge. In this configuration, the subject's only direct control is to stop the centrifuge. However, the subject is made aware of the type of G profile to expect and when it is about to begin. Visual tracking systems are frequently used during centrifuge studies. They are particularly useful in the closed-loop mode of operation for performance studies that simulate aerial combat. A more detailed description of the operational characteristics of human-use centrifuges in general and specifically for all U.S. and NATO centrifuges is available (4).

Research Instrumentation Requirements

A sophisticated research centrifuge facility requires medical and physiological instrumentation as complex as is found in any modern laboratory. This instrumentation must be completely stabilized before the exposure is begun since any changes or manipulations will require remote control. This situation presents a significant increase in the complexity of experiments conducted using centrifuges. Both invasive and noninvasive instrumentation are frequently employed using relatively small instruments with low-level signals that originate in the gondola. Consequently, to reduce the noise level, adequate data transmission usually requires high-quality slip rings. Telemetry without slip ring induced noise is now only sparingly used because of technical complexities, but may become more useful in the future.

CARDIOVASCULAR RESPONSE TO $+G_Z$

A functioning cardiovascular system that sustains major physiologic activities is at considerable risk during increased G; i.e., it provides the physiologic bases for human $+G_z$ tolerance. Because of its importance and vulnerability, it receives the most research attention (by far) of

Table 9.2.
Effect of 20–40 Seconds at 2, 3, and 4 G on Several Physiologic Parameters[a]

Parameter	+2 G$_z$	+3 G$_z$	+4 G$_z$
Cardiac output (L/min/m^2)	−7/7	−18/−12	−22/−18
Heart rate (bpm)	14/23	35/26	56/45
Stroke index (ml/stroke/m^2)	−24/−9	−37/−30	−49/−43
Pa (mean)[b] (mmHg)	9/25	21/36	27/44
Vascular resistance (dynes s cm^{-5})	17/17	41/53	59/74
S$_a$O$_2$ (%)	−0.5/−3	−2.5/−4	−4/−8

[a] First value is % change from 1 G control of six subjects without anti-G suit inflation. The second value is with inflated anti-G suit (7).
[b] Heart

acceleration physiologists. It also serves the function of the "miner's canary" for subjects during G exposures by monitoring heart rate and rhythm with the electrocardiograph (ECG). An ECG is required for all human G exposures involving research. Consequently with a "normal" ECG and if consciousness is maintained during G exposures, then it is assumed that all physiologic functions are performing adequately.

The physiologic effects *per se* of HSG on the human that are above "natural" G tolerance levels are difficult to ascertain since protective methods are required to increase G tolerance. These methods inherently (as expected) cause physiologic effects that become difficult to separate from the specific effects of increased G; e.g., note the anti-G suit effect in Table 9.2. Therefore only physiologic responses that occur below human G-tolerance levels (i.e., 4 G and less) can be attributable solely to increased G. Indeed, in this chapter, most physiologic parameters reported for humans are at high G levels where multiple G-protection methods are used that result in a complex combination of effects.

Heart Rate

Heart rate increases before the onset of G because of anticipation of the upcoming event. The magnitude of the pre-G increase in heart rate in centrifuge studies is directly dependent on the

anticipated level and duration of the G (5) (Table 9.3). Heart rates during G exposure increase directly with the +G$_z$ level reaching a maximum during sustained G within a few seconds of exposure (6). Heart rate responses to +G$_z$ vary considerably between subjects. It is generally agreed that the heart rate responds to G exposures from three separate sources: (1) Accelerative force effect that is primary for low G levels; (2) physical work of the anti-G straining maneuver, AGSM (to be discussed later in this chapter under "Protection Against +G$_z$") that is used at high G exposures; and (3) general psychophysiologic stress syndrome that accompanies all increased G exposures. The accelerative force effect on heart rate is primarily a response to the baroceptor cardiovascular compensatory reflex to a reduced arterial blood pressure (P$_a$) at the

Table 9.3.
Heart Rates at Various Levels of Sustained +G$_z$ Acceleration (5)

G Level	Number of Subjects	Preacceleration[a] (beats/min)	Peak Acceleration (beats/min)
3	14	92 ± 3	109 ± 3
5	14	93 ± 3	125 ± 4
6	13	98 ± 3	142 ± 4
6.5	14	104 ± 3	153 ± 3
7.0	7	100 ± 9	159 ± 4
7.5	11	113 ± 3	162 ± 4
8.0	10	103 ± 4	156 ± 5
8.5	12	112 ± 4	162 ± 6
9.0	9	116 ± 6	167 ± 4

[a] Mean ± standard error

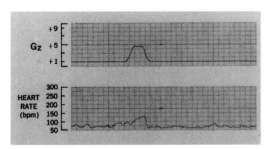

Figure 9.3. Heart rate response with exposure to a 15 second rapid-onset ($+1$ G_z/sec onset rate) to $+4.5$ G_z.

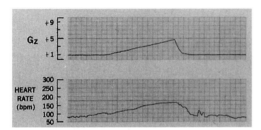

Figure 9.4. Heart rate response with exposure to a gradual-onset (0.067 G_z/sec onset rate) to $+4.5$ G_z.

site of the carotid sinus and the decrease in cardiac output (see following section). The stress effect is a general physiologic response to a stressor (the G) mediated by the sympathetics (i.e., fight on flight reaction). The typical heart rate responses before, during, and after rapid-onset and slow-onset exposures to $+4.5$ G_z are shown in Figures 9.3 and 9.4, respectively. The rate at which the maximum heart rate is reached for the same G level is dependent on the G onset rate and the duration of the G exposure. High sustained G exposures usually induce a maximum heart rate of about 170 bpm (Table 9.3). On rare occasions, heart rates will exceed 200 bpm—usually a medical criterion for terminating a centrifuge exposure. During long exposures to sustained G, heart rate usually increases further near the end of the exposure with the onset of fatigue.

Occasionally, a paradoxic decrease in heart rate may occur during HSG. This phenomenon has been termed high-G bradycardia. Although several mechanisms may be operative, the most reasonable explanation for this phenomenon is that P_a increases at the carotid sinus because of effective anti-G methods that stimulate a reflex reduction in heart rate. However, for safety reasons, an individual being exposed to HSG on the centrifuge with the onset of bradycardia should be stopped because the possibility of cardiac decompensation exists.

Cardiac Output

Cardiac output is the product of stroke volume and heart rate. Increased heart rate at increased G levels signifies a reduction in stroke volume. Stroke volume is directly related to venous return. Before the onset of G, increased heart rate will increase cardiac output that is a common anticipatory physiologic response to most environmental stressors. However, increased intravascular hydrostatic pressures, within the venous system below the heart with increased G, significantly reduces venous return. With a reduction in stroke volume, heart rate increases to maintain adequate cardiac output. As G levels increase and in spite of an increased heart rate, cardiac output decreases because of the reduced stroke volume (7) (Table 9.2). As noted earlier, as the human is exposed to higher G levels, artificial methods are used to increase G tolerance by increasing venous return. The principal method using muscular tensing must be artificially supplemented with the anti-G suit that increases vascular resistance by applying pressure at places below the heart to assist venous return. In turn, cardiac output is maintained at an adequate level to support P_a and blood flow to the head. Comparative physiologic effects of the anti-G suit are shown in Table 9.2.

Regional distribution of cardiac output has been measured in baboons at HSG using microsphere techniques (8). G tolerances are considerably higher in the baboon than in the human because of the shorter eye-heart vertical distance (Eq. 4)—changes measured in baboons are probably not as great as in the human for the

Table 9.4.
Regional Distribution of Cardiac Output in the Baboon (8) with Inflated Anti-G Suit

Parameters	Baseline	During +5 G_z	During +7 G_z
Left ventricle (heart)	363 ± 58[a]	546 ± 69	405 ± 68
Left kidney	472 ± 99	173 ± 60	230 ± 89
Liver	64 ± 11	47 ± 14	31 ± 13
Spleen	234 ± 67	29 ± 11	27 ± 16
Pancreas	237 ± 47	48 ± 13	37 ± 19
Stomach	45 ± 13	12 ± 4	13 ± 5
Diaphragm	52 ± 20	42 ± 17	42 ± 24
Aorta	5 ± 2	6 ± 3	5 ± 2
Muscle	8 ± 3	10 ± 5	7 ± 5
Skin	3 ± 0.5	3 ± 1	2 ± 0.4
Brain			
Cerebrum			
White	29 ± 8	40 ± 11	27 ± 7
Gray	75 ± 16	94 ± 12	50 ± 9
Cerebellum			
White	51 ± 7	65 ± 15	49 ± 12
Gray	51 ± 5	77 ± 10	56 ± 10
Pons	53 ± 6	82 ± 15	60 ± 13
Medulla	47 ± 7	72 ± 18	55 ± 12
Pituitary	106 ± 30	89 ± 33	74 ± 26
Retina	573 ± 163	304 ± 87	223 ± 74

[a] Means ± S.E.

same levels of HSG. Therefore, only the qualitative aspects of these baboon data can be related to the human. A summary of the results are shown in Table 9.4. Although a reduction in cardiac output occurs during HSG, redistribution of blood flow to critical organs, such as the heart and brain, maintain their blood supply. Organs most profoundly affected by HSG to the levels shown are those in the splanchnic region and the eye.

Coronary Circulation

Early electrophysiologic studies in humans exposed to relatively low levels of $+G_z$ suggested the existence of myocardia ischemia/anoxia. These findings plus myocardial pathologies found in experimental animals exposed to HSG caused considerable anxiety about the possibility of inadequate coronary circulation in humans during $+G_z$. However, a recent review of nine coronary-blood-flow studies in animals exposed to $+G_z$, extrapolated blood flow values to the coronary arteries of humans; the review concluded that with the aortic pressure found during moderate G levels where consciousness is maintained by humans (<100 mmHg perfusion pressure), endocardial/epicardial blood flow ratios remain at 1 or above, levels adequate for preventing myocardial ischemia. However, heart muscle perfusion at high G ($+7 G_z$ in swine that is similar to the humans) requires 300 to 500 ml/min/100 gm of tissue that equates to 50% to 75% of an individual's coronary blood reserve. Any significant reduction in this coronary reserve, such as with coronary artery disease, could result in myocardial ischemia with an adverse alteration of cardiac hemodynamic and electrophysiologic function (9).

Electrocardiographic Changes

The electrocardiogram (ECG) is an extremely useful tool for measuring the stress response to acceleration and for evaluating potential pathologic changes resulting from higher and higher $+G_z$ levels. It is also a noninvasive tool to further understand the physiologic response mechanisms to G and for comparison with treadmill exercise testing, both of which result in dynamic ECG changes. The additional volume shifts, cardiac displacement and distension, and reflex compensations make $+G_z$ exposure uniquely complex.

Lead System

The major requirement for recording the electrocardiographic response to $+G_z$ exposure is to obtain a noise-free tracing even during rapid-onset runs and offset of high G. The majority of HSG runs also involve a very vigorous AGSM which adds additional noise and artifacts.

Satisfactory tracings have been obtained using a lead system consisting of two mutually perpendicular leads (sternal and biaxillary). This system has provided adequate monitoring of rate, rhythm and conduction disturbances in a

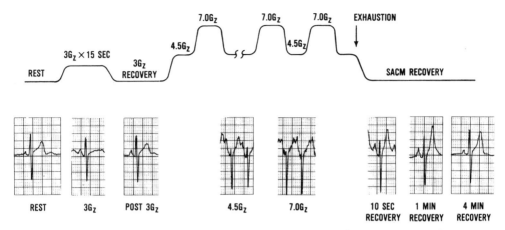

Figure 9.5. Sample electrocardiographic P, QRS, and T-wave changes before, during, and after exposure to +3 G$_z$ followed by a +4.5 to +7.0 G$_z$ simulated aerial combat maneuver (SACM) profile.

diversity of individuals. Although other leads may be used for special purposes and perhaps different leads might be useful for pure diagnostic purposes, for routine monitoring this system is a stable, rapidly attached system.

Many studies have documented the various electrocardiographic changes resulting from G exposure. The majority of these reports have been most interested in documenting the presence or absence of ischemic changes in the ST segment and T-waves.

P-Wave

The changes observed in the P-wave generally reflect changes in atrial depolarization. Observations during exhaustive HSG or simulated aerial combat maneuvers (SACM) verified an increased amplitude and duration of the P-wave. The time course of P-wave changes during a 3 G run followed by a 4.5 to 7 G SACM to exhaustion is shown in Figures 9.5 and 9.6. P-wave changes returned to control levels 3 minutes after the G exposure. P-wave morphologic changes, characteristic of ectopic atrial rhythm and chaotic atrial rhythm, are covered in the sections on rhythm disturbances. During very stressful runs, the P-wave frequently merges into the preceding T-wave. Frequently post-G-exposure, the P-wave disappears completely as a re-

sult of excessive vagal inhibition of the sinoatrial pacemaker.

QRS Complex

Respiration, cardiac movement (displacement, distortion, and rotation), and altered ventricular function can alter QRS amplitude and configuration. The QRS response of normal individuals to +G$_z$ is such that the overall amplitude does not significantly change (Fig. 9.6). Depending on the lead, if the R-wave decreases in amplitude, a reciprocal deepening of the S-wave occurs. These changes probably signify a rotation of the electrical axis of the heart. Similar changes are, however, observed during other forms of stress (e.g., treadmill exercise). Other factors, therefore, may be additive, including decreased end-systolic and end-diastolic volumes as compared with rest, increased end-diastolic and end-systolic pressures as compared with rest, increased catecholamines, and electrolyte disturbances. Which of these mechanisms (position, volume, catecholamines, electrolyte disturbance, or pressure) have the major influence on QRS amplitude and configuration are unknown.

T-Wave

ST segment and T-wave changes have received the most attention by acceleration cardiol-

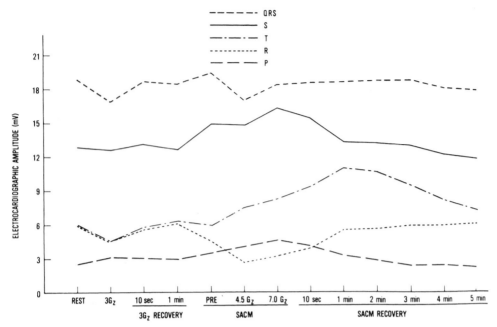

Figure 9.6. P, R, S, T, and QRS amplitude alterations to the $+G_z$ exposures shown in Figure 9.5. Note that at 5 minutes post-SACM, all wave changes have returned to baseline except that T-wave amplitude remains increased.

ogists because of their traditional clinical association with myocardial ischemia or other disorders. Accurate assessment of ST segment changes are hampered by frequently occurring artifacts. Yet, reported ST segment changes suggestive of myocardial ischemia are very infrequent. Individuals with a marked ST segment depression during or after G exposure should be suspected of having ischemic heart disease until proven otherwise. On the other hand, T-wave changes are very frequent. Early in the course of $+G_z$, there is a decrease in T-wave amplitude, sometimes with flattening, diphasic or inverted T-waves, but these changes usually disappear later in the run. The characteristic response observed during a SACM is shown in Figures 9.5 and 9.6.

Post-acceleration T-wave changes following HSG and in particular strenuous SACM, consistently result in large, peaked T-waves. These changes are maximal between 1 and 2 minutes after G and slowly return to normal. Even 5 minutes after G, the T-wave may not be completely recovered. Similar changes occur during and

after treadmill exercise. The exercise-induced changes in T-wave amplitude, especially in endurance-trained individuals and young adults post-exercise, may be due to an increase in stroke volume that corresponds to an increased rate of decline in heart rate after exercise. The tall, peaked T-waves also are suggestive of the "tented T-waves" seen in association with hyperkalemia. Serum potassium is statistically significantly elevated after G; however, the magnitude of the change is small. The rate of change of electrolytes or other metabolites may be more important than the absolute magnitude of the change. Catecholamines have also been associated with the T-wave changes both during and after G. It has been suggested that different responses to norepinephrine and epinephrine cause the observed early and late T-wave changes.

Benign Rhythm Disturbances

Lamb summarized the importance of cardiac rhythm disturbances in relation to the aeromedical environment (10):

Table 9.5.
Major Dysrhythmogenic Stressors[a]

Psychologic Stressors	Physiologic Stressors	Environmental Stressors
Anxiety	Exercise	Altitude
Fear	Respiratory alterations	Acceleration
Task overload	Mechanical distension or distortion	Temperature
Pain	Fatigue	Vibration
	Hormonal alterations	Noise
	Autonomic imbalance	
	Electrolyte alterations	
	Blood flow alterations	

[a] These stressors are listed arbitrarily and many are interrelated. These stressors are dysrhythmogenic in a nonaviation environment. In the aviation environment, many of these stressors are combined.

"Cardiac arrhythmias are frequently the result of hypoxia and G forces and many of them may initiate syncopal episodes. Thus, they constitute a major segment of cardiac problems in flying populations. Cardiac arrhythmias are actually changes in the electrical mechanism of the heart and changes in cardiac rhythm which affect cardiac dynamics. They are not simply electrocardiographic findings. The electrocardiogram merely enables one to detect the changes in the dynamics that are occurring in the heart."

The electrocardiogram is like a window into both pathologic and physiologic processes that affect the heart. The in-flight aerial combat or aerobatic environment is one where multistressors with numerous factors occur simultaneously. These factors, even when they occur alone, are known to be dysrhythmogenic. The major dysrhythmogenic stressors are listed in Table 9.5. Although listed separately, many are interrelated and interactive. So, it would be surprising if dysrhythmias were not observed during G. The aeromedical problem is the determination of which of the dysrhythmias may be clinically significant, and which ones represent normal responses to the $+G_z$ environment. It is also important to define which dysrhythmias may reflect altered physiology and can significantly affect G tolerance.

A number of qualitative descriptions of the number and type of dysrhythmias that result from specific G exposures have been reported. Although it would seem that the occurrence of dysrhythmias during G is variable, it is evident that, to accurately compare the frequency of occurrence, only similar populations being exposed to similar levels and durations of G under comparable environmental conditions are appropriate. The assurance of no pathologic changes resulting from G exposure is costly and time-consuming. For this reason, electrocardiographically monitored HSG runs will likely proceed before other techniques can be developed to monitor this dynamic environment.

Over a consecutive 3-year period at the Armstrong Laboratory, the electrocardiographic responses to a multitude of G exposures were tabulated to determine the spectrum of changes that would occur in a healthy asymptomatic male population. All of the 544 subjects had successfully passed complete aeromedical evaluations before riding the centrifuge, were asymptomatic, and were considered healthy. The results are shown in Table 9.6. It is evident that a variety of rhythm disturbances and other electrocardiographic findings occur as a result of G exposures.

The electrocardiographic responses of 378 fighter aircrew exposed to the standard centrifuge high-G training profiles (maximum level $+9$ G_z) were analyzed at the NAWC. The results are shown in Table 9.7. Once again it is evident that high G-exposures requiring near maximal AGSMs are dysrhythmogenic. None of the electrocardiographic changes listed was symptomatic or compromised G tolerance. Only 7% of the aircrew completed centrifuge training without any rhythm disturbance whatsoever. From a clinical perspective, the more significant dysrhythmias, such as ventricular and supraventricular tachycardia, were short, self-limited runs of 3 to 6 beats. If we combine these two tachycardias with the advanced ventricular ectopy (multiformed PVCs, bigeminal PVCs, and paired PVCs) into a single group of what might

Table 9.6.
Three-Year History of Acceleration-Induced Dysrhythmias at the Armstrong Laboratory
(Brooks Air Force Base, Texas)[a]

Rank	Occurrences	Dysrhythmia Description
1	1566	Sinus arrhythmia (rate varying >25 beats/min between successive beats) (SA)
2	1073	Premature ventricular contractions (PVC)
3	768	Premature atrial contractions (PAC)
4	546	Sinus bradycardia (rate <60 beats/min) (SB)
5	372	Ectopic atrial rhythm (EAR)
6	272	Premature junctional contractions (PJC)
7	171	PVCs with bigeminy/trigeminy (BPVC)
8	126	Multiformed PVCs (MPVC)
9	104	AV dissociation (AVD)
9	104	Paired PVCs (PPVC)

[a] Data from 544 subjects during 9831 $+G_z$ centrifuge exposures

Table 9.7.
The Most Frequent Electrocardiographic Rate and Rhythm Changes Occurring in 378 Consecutive Fighter Aircrew Undergoing Centrifuge G-Training at the Naval Air Warfare Center

Rank	ECG Change	Number of Aircrew with Change	% of Total Aircrew with Change
1	PAC	302	80%
2	PVC	263	62%
3	SA	114	30%
4	PPAC	85	22%
5	PPVC	79	21%
6	EAR	48	13%
7	MPVC	36	10%
8	BPVC	35	10%
9	SB	35	10%
10	SVT	31	8%
11	VT	18	5%

be considered significant dysrhythmias, then 38% of the aircrew had at least one episode during their centrifuge training. The only rhythm disturbance that compromised G tolerance was marked bradycardia with atrioventricular dissociation that occurred post G and because of presyncopal symptoms prevented completion of all training profiles. From an aeromedical standpoint, therefore, in these healthy aircrew the most "significant" rhythm disturbances are those that compromise tolerance and appear to be those most likely associated with excess parasympathetic tone. Based on the relative frequent

occurrence of what might be considered clinically significant dysrhythmias in these flight qualified aviators, it would appear unlikely that they are reflective of pre-existing cardiac disease. Most likely, they reflect a normal response to the rigors of the high-G environment. Aeromedical standards should reflect the responses that do occur during G exposures without excessive disqualification of fully trained fighter crew.

These results unquestionably demonstrate the dysrhythmogenic nature of G. The time of occurrence of dysrhythmias varies; i.e., certain dysrhythmias occur during G and others occur in the post-G period (Table 9.8). The most frequent cause of dysrhythmia distribution is probably autonomic imbalance, with a sympathetic predominance before and during G and parasympathetic predominance in the post G period.

It is likely that disparity in previous observations on the presence or absence of dysrhythmias, especially premature ventricular contractions (PVCs) is related to the comparison of different levels, durations and types of G exposures. The Armstrong Laboratory experience is heavily weighted toward HSG and SACMs that produce maximal heart rates. An increase in ectopy with increasing heart rate is to be expected. Indeed, these types of G exposures have proven to be the most dysrhythmogenic as shown in Figure 9.7—the number of occurrences of PVCs

Table 9.8.
Time of Occurrence of Frequent Dysrhythmias Associated with + G_z Centrifugation

Dysrhythmia	Time of Occurrence*			
	Pre-G	During G	Post-G	All of the Time
Premature ventricular contraction (PVC)	5	65	27	3
Premature atrial contraction (PAC)	5	61	31	3
Premature junctional contraction (PJC)	9	63	22	6
PVC with bigeminy	9	60	21	10
Multiformed PVCs	1	74	25	0
Paired PVCs	9	71	20	0
Sinus arrhythmia	2	4	94	0
Sinus bradycardia	5	8	87	0
Ectopic atrial rhythm	6	5	89	0
AV dissociation	2	7	91	0

* Given as a percentage of the total number of occurrences of each dysrhythmia

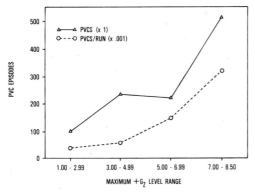

Figure 9.7. Plot of the number of premature ventricular contractions (PVCs) and PVCs/run with + G_z level.

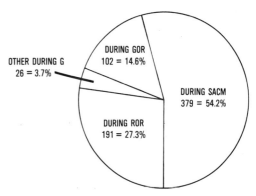

Figure 9.8. Percentage of premature ventricular contractions (PVCs) with various types of + G_z exposure (rapid-onset = ROR, gradual-onset = GOR; SACM = simulated aerial combat maneuver).

increase with the level of G. If the number of PVCs is normalized with the number of runs (within each G range), there is an exponential increase in ectopy as G increases. Further analysis verifies the frequency of occurrence correlation with the magnitude of the G-induced stress. As shown in Figure 9.8, 54.2% of the PVCs occurred during SACM, whereas only 16.5% of the total runs were SACMs. Because SACMs more closely represent in-flight ACM, it follows that high-G maneuvers must have the maximum combinations of factors that cause dysrhythmias. In asymptomatic healthy individuals with normal clinical evaluations, the entire spectrum of these dysrhythmias is probably benign. Even the

more ominous ectopy, such as short runs of non-sustained ventricular tachycardia associated with G, is not necessarily an indication of pathology or pathologic change, but rather a physiologic response to an extremely stressful environment.

Incapacitating Rhythm Disturbances

Specific dysrhythmias do have aeromedical significance. These can potentially result in sudden incapacitation or at least lower G tolerance. Included in this group are sinus arrest with attendant asystole, atrioventricular dissociation

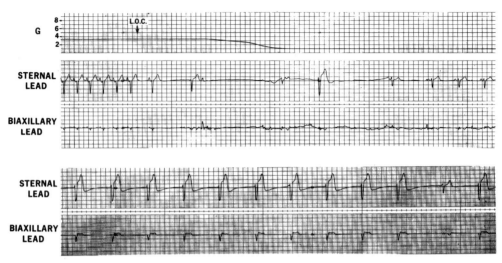

Figure 9.9. Sinus arrest coincident with a $+G_z$-induced loss of consciousness. The recovery rhythm illustrated in the lower tracing was by a slow idioventricular pacemaker.

during G, and supraventricular/ventricular tachycardia.

Prolonged sinus arrest with failure of lower pacemakers to pick up the rhythm is very serious in the aerospace environment. The resultant loss of cardiac output can result in a loss of consciousness (as in a Stokes-Adams attack) or, if coincident with G-LOC, it can increase the incapacitation time. An example of the latter instance is shown in Figure 9.9. In this example, the absolute incapacitation time was approximately 30 sec, compared with the 12 sec average incapacitation usually observed. The most frequent cause of this disturbance in rhythm is thought to be very strong parasympathetic (vagal) tone. This vagal tone can occur: a) Due to a vigorous AGSM or b) immediately post G when the baroreceptors receive an unusually strong stimulation. There is some indication that certain individuals may be particularly sensitive to this problem. These individuals may have a very high vagal tone usually associated, for example, with extreme endurance training. High G-bradycardia should also be considered as detrimental to maintaining normal G tolerance.

Atrioventricular (AV) dissociation, a loss of coordinated atrial and ventricular function, has been observed to decrease G tolerance during SACM. An appropriately timed atrial systole is important for making the final contribution to ventricular filling and to assure crisp closure (without regurgitation) of the AV valves. An example of AV dissociation is shown in Figure 9.10 during a 4.5 to 7 G SACM. The individual was able to tolerate this G profile with appropriate atrial function, but was unable to tolerate 7 G with AV dissociation. As previously suggested, the importance of atrial function may be apparent only during maximal stress as is seen clinically in an extremely ill individual when any decrement in cardiac output cannot be tolerated. The loss of atrial function could result in a P_a loss of as much as 30 mmHg (approximately 1 G of tolerance), a sufficient decrement to go from minimal grayout to blackout, or loss of consciousness.

Any tachydysrhythmia that occurs at a sufficient rate to compromise cardiac output, may be detrimental to G tolerance. To compromise cardiac output, the tachydysrhythmia must be sustained. Short bursts of ventricular tachycardia usually do not compromise heart function. Indeed these short, three- to six-beat episodes may occur in completely healthy individuals exposed to G. Although there is a possibility that this type of dysrhythmia could degenerate into the

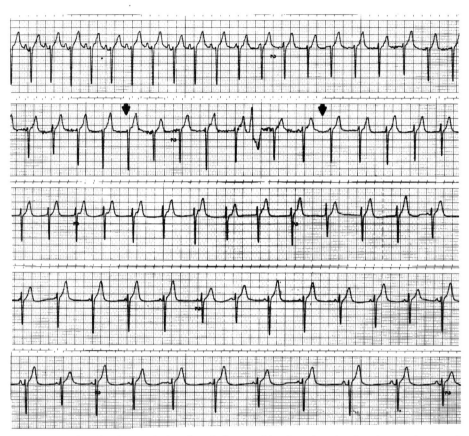

Figure 9.10. $+G_z$-induced atrioventricular dissociation resulting in reduced $+G_z$ tolerance in an endurance-trained subject. The tracing is a continuous electrocardiogram starting with the subject at $+4.5\ G_z$. The AV dissociation occurs as the subject starts up to $+7.0\ G_z$. The first arrow represents the attainment of $+7.0$ G_z. The subject had a complete blackout (second arrow) within 4 to 5 sec at $+7.0\ G_z$ and was returned to $+1.0\ G_z$. AV dissociation with a variable P-wave configuration persists into the recovery period. The subject was able to tolerate $+4.5\ G_z$ but not $+7.0\ G_z$ with AV dissociation.

more severe ventricular fibrillation, it has not been documented in acceleration studies with healthy individuals. G-induced ventricular tachycardia in flight has also been documented in individuals with mitral valve prolapse. Although only limited information is available for women, similar significant dysrhythmias have been observed. There is no apparent difference in the electrocardiographic response of men and women based on existing information.

Dysrhythmogenesis of G Acceleration

A comparison of the frequency and type of dysrhythmias induced by G, compared with other types of stressors, has not been thoroughly investigated. When the frequency of dysrhythmias before, during, and after treadmill exercise was compared with G exposure, a significant increase in the frequency of G induced dysrhythmias was found in a group of healthy males—when maximum-stress G exposure was compared with maximal treadmill exercise and 24-hour Holter monitoring. In male aircrew undergoing aeromedical evaluation, even with submaximal G stress, an equal frequency of rhythm disturbances was found, compared with maximal treadmill exercise stress.

Finally, it is important to make comparisons of G-induced dysrhythmias among similar populations. The centrifuge experiences at the Armstrong Laboratory and the Naval Air Warfare Center have shown that the frequency of G-induced dysrhythmias is, among other things, age-dependent, but age is probably only one of many variables in the susceptibility to G-induced dysrhythmias in healthy individuals.

PULMONARY FUNCTION

The mammalian lung is the site of ventilation in support of gas exchange with the environment and is inherently a compliant structure. Because of this compliance, low-intensity acceleration exposures will significantly affect the physical/mechanical properties of the lung, altering its homeostasis. However, in spite of these G physiologic effects on the lung, respiration has not been shown to limit G tolerance in the acceleration laboratory. Consequently, respiration during G, even though gas exchange in the lung is significantly impaired, apparently supports the aerobic requirements of the body. To some extent, this adaptability is managed because the major physiologic demands during HSG (principally energy demands of the physical aspects of the AGSM that are limiting), are anaerobic with physiologic limitations caused by fatigue because of reduced blood flow and lactic acid accumulation in the muscles.

Nonetheless, knowing about the effects of $+G_z$ on pulmonary physiology is necessary to a comprehensive understanding of the physiology of G. Pulmonary function and its related activities are particularly important in the operational aspects of aviation because: (a) Significant reductions in pulmonary gas exchange that reduce PaO_2 occur during sustained HSG (even while breathing enriched oxygen mixtures); (b) the AGSM has a breathing component; (c) the anti-G suit adversely affects pulmonary gas exchange (Table 9.2); and (d) positive pressure breathing is now used in anti-G systems. Of particular interest to flight surgeons is the occurrence of an important pathologic lung condition called acceleration atelectasis (or aeroatelec-

tasis) during G exposure under certain conditions. An in-depth review on the effects of G on respiration is available (11).

Lung Compliance and Work of Breathing

As G increases in seated individuals who are not using an anti-G suit, the diaphragm is displaced downward primarily increasing the functional reserve capacity by 450 ml and tidal volume by 150 ml at 5 G. Because of greater thoracic wall stiffness and a reflex increase in abdominal wall tension that increases abdominal pressures and resists full descent of the diaphragm, a reduction of 10% in vital capacity occurs at 5 G because of a reduced inspiratory capacity (11).

Compliance during acceleration decreases at a rate of about 15% per G as the lung stretches and increases its resistance to a change in volume (ml) with changing pressures (cm H_2O).

$$\text{Compliance (ml} \div \text{cm } H_2O) = 167 - 24 (G-1) \quad (5)$$

A reduced compliance increases the work of respiration, which is proportional to increased G. The work of breathing at 3 G increases with a doubling of the ''elastic'' component and with an increased respiratory frequency. The reason for this increase in lung ventilation is not known, but may be related to poor blood perfusion in the brain. Consequently, a total increase of 55% in the work of breathing occurs at 3 G.

Regional Lung Volumes and Ventilation (V̇)

When pulmonary hydrostatic pressure increases, it drives the blood towards the base of the lung. This movement of blood within the lung displaces the air towards the apex that produces a gradient of pleural pressures along the longitudinal axis of the lung. These pleural pressures of inspiration increase at the base of the lung from -7 mmHg at 0 G to -2 mmHg at 1 G and

+ 18 mmHg at 5 G. Pleural pressures at the apex of the lung change in the opposite direction from −7 mmHg at 0 G to −12 mmHg at 1 G and −32 mmHg at 5 G.

During acceleration, the alveolae, because of the vast differential in specific density between blood and air (1 : 1000), expand at the top of the lung with those at the base of the lung—where the majority of blood has moved—becoming much smaller; i.e., some even collapse (6). The functional capabilities of these alveolae in different regions of the lung have instigated the concept by physiologists of regional lung volumes. In weightlessness, blood has no weight; therefore, regional lung volumes theoretically should not exist. At 1 G, regional lung volumes begin to appear. At the beginning of inspiration, alveolae located near the top of the lung are ventilated. As the inspiration continues, alveolae located lower in the lung begin to open, progressing in this manner, until at the end of inspiration, all alveolae are experiencing gas exchange with the environment. During expiration, the alveolae at the base of the lung close first (at closure volumes), but remain open longer than expected because of the phenomenon of lung hysteresis. As G levels increase, regional lung volumes become more distinct. During higher G levels, when alveolae at the base of the lung with more than adequate perfusion never become ventilated, functional lung volumes are reduced. On the other hand, alveolae that are best ventilated at the lung apex are not perfused with blood (ventilation-perfusion mismatch). Both conditions prevent gas exchange in those regions; they will be discussed in more detail later in this section.

Lung Perfusion

As hydrostatic pressures increase during increased G, lung perfusion (Q) is redistributed toward the base of the lung. Significant redistribution occurs at relatively low G levels—at 3

G, lung perfusion begins at the mid region of the lung.

The relationship of blood flow in the lung under increasing G can be theoretically determined using the following hydrostatic pressure equation (Eq. 6):

$$h = (P_a - P_A)/d \cdot G \qquad (6)$$

where:
P_a = pulmonary arterial pressure (mmHg)
P_A = alveolae pressure (mmHg)
h = height of the lung perfused (mm)
d,G = see Eq. 4

Equation 6 is a hyperbolic function showing less relative effect on the height of lung perfused as G increases—a large effect at 1 to 2 G, one-third as great a change at 2 to 3 G, and only one-sixth as great a change between 3 and 4 G.

Ventilation-Perfusion Relationship

During increased G, ventilation increases towards the apex of the lung, whereas, perfusion increases at the base of the lung. This regional redistribution of blood and air in the lung in opposite directions creates major differences in the $\dot{V}/\dot{Q}$ ratios in lung regions. At the top of the lung, the $\dot{V}/\dot{Q}$ is infinite because perfusion is zero, and at the base of the lung, $\dot{V}/\dot{Q}$ is zero—no ventilation can occur.

This condition that occurs during increased G is explained by hypothetically dividing the lung into five functional regions as shown in Figure 9.11.

Region I at the apex of the lung has maximum lung volumes without lung perfusion $\dot{V}/\dot{Q} = \infty$; consequently, gas exchange with blood does not occur.

Region II is near midlung, where ventilation and perfusion are matched equally with $\dot{V}/\dot{Q} = 1:1$. The alveolus shown is perfused and ventilated during the entire breathing cycle. Increased P_{IO_2} will increase P_{aO_2}.

ANATOMIC CONDITION	↑P_{IO_2} EFFECT	PHYSIOLOGIC EFFECTS	P_{AO_2} P_{ACO_2}	REGION
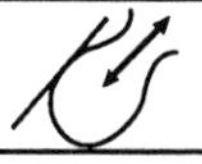 *[diagram]*	O	$\dot{Q}=0$ $\dot{V}/\dot{Q} = \infty$	150:0	I
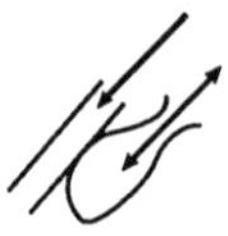 *[diagram]*	$P_{aO_2}\downarrow$	ADEQUATE $\dot{Q}$ ADEQUATE $\dot{V}$ $\dot{V}/\dot{Q} = 1$ NO ALVEOLI CLOSURES	100:40	II
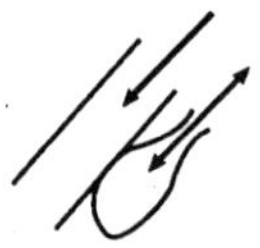 *[diagram]*	$P_{aO_2}\downarrow$	ADEQUATE $\dot{Q}$ ADEQUATE $\dot{V}$ $\dot{V}/\dot{Q} = <1$ ALVEOLI CLOSURES DURING BREATHING PHYSIOLOGIC SHUNTING	80:40	III
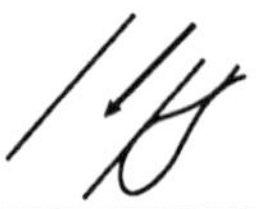 *[diagram]*	O	ADEQUATE $\dot{Q}$ $\dot{V} = 0$ ALVEOLI NEVER OPEN ANATOMIC SHUNTING	40:45	IV
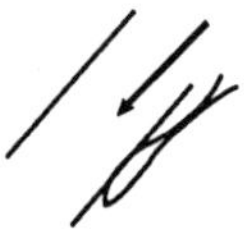 *[diagram]*	CONDITION ↑	ADEQUATE $\dot{Q}$ $\dot{V} = 0$ ALVEOLI COLLAPSE ANATOMIC SHUNTING PATHOLOGIC STATE	0:0	V

Figure 9.11. The lung is divided into 5 regions depending upon its ventilation/perfusion states.

Region III occurs near the base, with excessive perfusion and alveolar ventilation only near the end of inspiration and the beginning of expiration. Increased P_{IO_2} will increase P_{aO_2}, but less effectively than in Region II because there is a shorter period of time for gas exchange.

Region IV at the base of the lung is without ventilation, but there is some gas exchange with residual gas in the alveolae. However, increased P_{IO_2} will not affect P_{aO_2}—the $\dot{V}/\dot{Q}$ ratio is zero.

Region V may occur in the lower area of Region IV as alveolae collapse, causing atelectasis. This condition is discussed later in this chapter in the section entitled "Acceleration-Associated Pathologic Changes."

Inequalities in $\dot{V}/\dot{Q}$ also cause variations in P_{AO_2} and P_{ACO_2}. The $P_{AO_2}:P_{ACO_2}$ ratio at 1 G is approximately 100:40 with a ratio of 150:0 at the apex and 40:45 (characteristic of venous blood) at the base of the lung.

Lung Gas Exchange

The effects on gas exchange in the lung during 1 minute at 3 G in the same subjects breathing air without an anti-G suit, and at 5 G and 7 G in subjects wearing an anti-G suit are compared with these subjects at 1 G in Table 9.9.

The most prominent G effect on gas exchange in the lung is the increase in gas pressure gradients for both CO_2 and O_2 between the blood and alveolae. As functional regions become more diverse during the increase in G, increases in the O_2 gradient $(P_A - P_a)$ and the CO_2 gradient $(P_a - P_A)$ occur. These ever increasing pressure gradients with increasing G (that exist even at 1 G) are caused by $\dot{V}/\dot{Q}$ variations in the lung (Fig. 9.12). The unperfused, but ventilated, alveolae increase the physiologic dead space (DS). Additionally, the increase in lung ventilation, shown as breathing rate (f) and tidal volume

Table 9.9.
Effect of 1-Minute Exposures on Lung Gas Exchange Parameters (Subjects are Breathing Air) (6)

	Without Anti-G Suit		With Anti-G Suit	
	1 G	3 G	5 G	7 G
P_{aO_2}	91.6	84.7	60.2	50.1
P_{aCO_2}	35.0	32.0	32.1	33.2
P_{AO_2}	101.3	112.8	114.8	116.3
P_{ACO_2}	33.6	27.3	20.2	15.8
pH_a	7.422	7.422	7.444	7.418
f	18.6	23.4	32.6	38.9
DS	0.200	0.307	0.579	0.551
DS/TV	0.35	0.38	0.52	0.52
TV	0.68	0.93	1.20	1.13

f = breathing rate/min; DS = dead space; TV = tidal volume

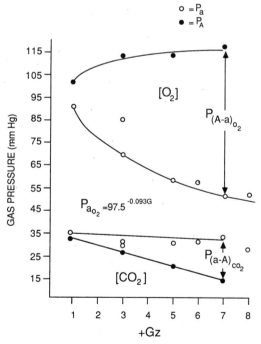

Figure 9.12. Alveolae (P_A)—Arterial pressure (P_a) O_2 gradients and P_a-P_{ACO_2} gradients increase with increasing G levels. Reprinted with permission from Burton RR, Smith AH. Adaptation to acceleration environments. Fregly MJ, Blattis CM, eds. In: Handbook of physiology: environmental physiology. IV. the gravitational environment. New York: Oxford University Press, 1996; 943–970.

(TV), that occurs during G, increases P_{AO_2} (end-tidal) and reduces P_{ACO_2} (end-tidal).

At 5 G and above, lung ventilation is increased voluntarily because of the requirement to do an AGSM, which has a breathing component that must be repeated every 3 to 4 seconds (see section on protection against $+G_z$). However, even at 3 G where the AGSM is not used, an increase in lung ventilation occurs that reflects poor blood perfusion in the brain's respiratory center that increases tissue P_{CO_2} and H^+.

Venous blood passing through the lung without contacting ventilated alveolae is called a right-to-left shunt. The amount of the right-to-left shunt in the lung is calculated as a percentage of the differential in gas pressures between the alveolae and the blood for either CO_2 or O_2. Calculate the percentage by using the data shown in Table 9.9, the shunt at 7 G using O_2 data $[(P_A—P_a)—P_A] \times 100 = 57\%$, and CO_2 data $[(P_a—P_A)—P_a] \times 100 = 52\%$; i.e., approximately 50% of the blood in the lung is not exchanging gas with the alveolae.

Arterial oxygen tension (P_{aO_2}) decreases exponentially as a function of increasing G level (5):

$$P_{aO_2} = 97.5e^{-0.093G} \qquad (7)$$

Where:

P_{aO_2} = arterial oxygen tension (mmHg)

G = level of sustained $+G_z$

Conversely, P_{aCO_2} does not decrease (follow the P_{ACO_2}), but remains relatively constant as the G level increases up to 8 G. There are two reasons for this seeming paradox: (a) increase in lung DS (more than doubling from 1 to 7 G) and (b) a phenomenon known as venous admixture resulting from the right-to-left shunt previously described. A relatively constant P_{aCO_2} allows AGSM-associated hyperventilation without the physiologic problems of a reduction in P_{aCO_2}; i.e., a decrease in cerebral blood flow with vasoconstriction and possible loss of consciousness.

Table 9.10.
Effect of Breathing 100% Oxygen on Alveolae-Blood Gas Gradients at 1 G and 5 G (6)

	At 1 G		At 5 G	
	On Air	On O_2**	On Air	On O_2**
P_{AO_2}	101	663	115	660
P_{aO_2}	92	616	60	570
$(A-a)O_2$	9	47	55	90
% physiologic shunt*	9	8	48	14

* $[(P_A-P_a)-P_A] \times 100$
** 100% P_IO_2

Increased P_{IO_2} reduces, but does not eliminate, the effect of the right-to-left shunt on gas exchange. At 5 G, the use of 100% oxygen reduces the effect of shunting from 48% (breathing air) to 14% (breathing 100% O_2)—calculated using data of Table 9.10. However, there are pathophysiologic problems associated with breathing 100% O_2 because it contributes to acceleration atelectasis. But, despite the occurrence of acceleration atelectasis, S_{aO2} remains above the levels for breathing air during increased G exposures (13) (Table 9.11). Maximum levels of O_2 in the inhaled gas without inducing acceleration atelectasis is 50–70%.

The reduction in P_{aO2} during HSG exposure is also directly related to the duration of exposure. The G kinetics involving gas exchange in the lung at 8 G sustained for 60 seconds is determined in the following equation (6):

$$P_{aO_2} = 104 \, T^{-0.196} \qquad (8)$$

Where:

P_{aO_2} = same as Eq. 7

T = time at 8 G in seconds

A physiologic (blood gas) steady state does not occur during exposure to HSG, thus the level of P_{aO_2} reported for a G level can vary considerably between studies depending upon the duration of G. Even at lower G levels, a steady state does not occur as measured in several respiration parameters after several minutes at 3 G. Therefore, when evaluating most physiologic G effects, time at G is an important variable.

SYMPATHETIC RESPONSES AND GENERAL STRESS EFFECTS

Exposures to all levels of $+G_z$ on the centrifuge release increased amounts of epinephrine (E), norepinephrine (NE), and serum cortisol in the blood of subjects (14). The levels of these hormones that accompany physiologic stress and sympathetic responses are directly correlated with the G level (Fig. 9.13).

CENTRAL NERVOUS SYSTEM

The principal acute limiting factors to $+Gz$ exposure involving the central nervous system are the loss of vision and consciousness. These conditions are the result of decreased retinal and central nervous system (CNS) perfusion. Regulation of blood flow near the G-tolerance limit provides cerebellum and brain stem blood flow when blood flow to the higher CNS levels is diminished. CNS blood flow under normal conditions is controlled primarily by autoregulation; however, during G, flow is maintained by a combination of autoregulatory vasodilatation and the

Table 9.11.
Effect of Increasing Inspired Oxygen Concentration on Arterial Oxygen Saturation (S_{aO_2}) During a SACM (13)

Inspired O_2 (percent)	21%	50%	70%	82.5%	95%	100%
S_{aO_2}	87.5* ± 4.28	91.6 ± 4.42	95.0 ± 2.78	95.8 ± 2.43	96.6 ± 5.18	97.8 ± 2.60

*Mean ± S.D.

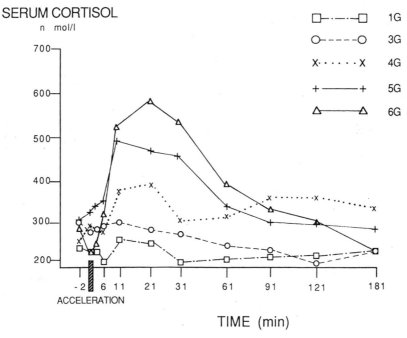

Figure 9.13. Physiologic stress responses to different 60s G levels. Subjects were not wearing anti-G suits. Reprinted with permission from Mills FJ. The endocrinology of stress. Aviat Space Environ Med 1985;56: 642–650.

siphon effect. The siphon effect occurs from a pressure gradient established between the afferent carotid arterial system and the efferent jugular venous system. This pressure gradient and consequent blood flow are maintained with low cerebral perfusion pressures.

Vision

Maintenance of adequate retinal blood flow is necessary for a full field of vision. Loss of peripheral vision followed by loss of central vision leading to a complete blackout results from decremental retinal blood flow. These visual symptoms begin to occur when P_a at eye level falls below 50 mmHg; blackout occurs when P_a equals the intraocular pressure of approximately 20 mmHg. In a series of retinal photographs taken at intervals during a rapid-onset centrifuge run at $+3.1$ G_z on a human subject whose head-level P_a was measured, blackout occurred at peak G plus 1.6 seconds and lasted to peak G

plus 8.0 seconds. This condition coincided with a collapse of both the central retinal artery and vein and with a concurrent fall in head-level P_a. At 8.0 seconds, a recovery of pressure was observed with the expected baroceptor carotid sinus vasoconstriction response coincident with a filling of the retinal artery (15) (Fig. 9.14). It is important to recognize that with any asymmetry in the location of the eyes in the $+G_z$ field, as might occur with an aviator looking over his or her shoulder to acquire a target, loss of vision will occur first in the eye highest in the G field. There are also some individual differences in the exact visual symptoms that are probably related to variations in vascular anatomy within the eye and CNS.

G-Induced Loss of Consciousness

The major acceleration threat that confronts every fighter pilot on every sortie—a threat that can abruptly result in pilot incapacitation,

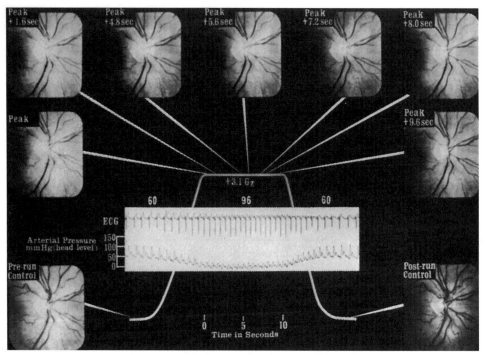

Figure 9.14. Retinal photographs taken at intervals during a centrifuge run to +3.1 G_z during the onset of blackout and return of vision. From Leverett SD Jr, Newsom WA. Photographic observations of the human fundus oculi during +G_z blackout on the USAF School of Aerospace Medicine centrifuge. In: Lunc M, ed. XIXth international astronautical congressbook 4: Bioastronautics. New York: Pergamon Press, 1971; 75–80.

mission compromise, loss of the aircraft, and loss of life—is G-induced loss of consciousness (G-LOC). A mismatch of the pilot's G tolerance with the G-envelope capability of the aircraft and the requirements of the mission is ever present. Everyone has a G-tolerance limit which, even with existing protective technology, can be exceeded and result in G-LOC. From the beginning of aeromedical acceleration research, the thrust toward solving the G-LOC problem had been aimed at the cardiovascular system and techniques to augment its ability to provide a continuous supply of blood to the central nervous system (CNS). Although generally successful, more recent research has focused on the nervous system (16–21).

The G-LOC Syndrome

G-induced loss of consciousness is the *transition* from normal consciousness to a state of unconsciousness that results when blood flow to the nervous system is reduced below the critical level necessary to support conscious function (1). In flight, with the attendant loss of motor control that occurs with a G-LOC episode, the

Figure 9.15. Schematic of the states of incapacitation and consciousness resulting from G-LOC. A visual master-caution light and auditory tone were used to determine the end of the relative incapacitation period shown in the upper figure. Reprinted with permission from Whinnery JE, Burton RR, Boll PA, et al. Characterization of the resulting incapacitation following unexpected +G_z-induced loss of consciousness. Aviat Space Environ Med 1987;58:631–636. The sequence of symptomatology of G-LOC is shown in the lower figure. Reprinted with permission from Whinnery JE. The G-LOC syndrome. Report No. NADC-91042-60, Naval Air Development Center, Warminster, PA, 1991.

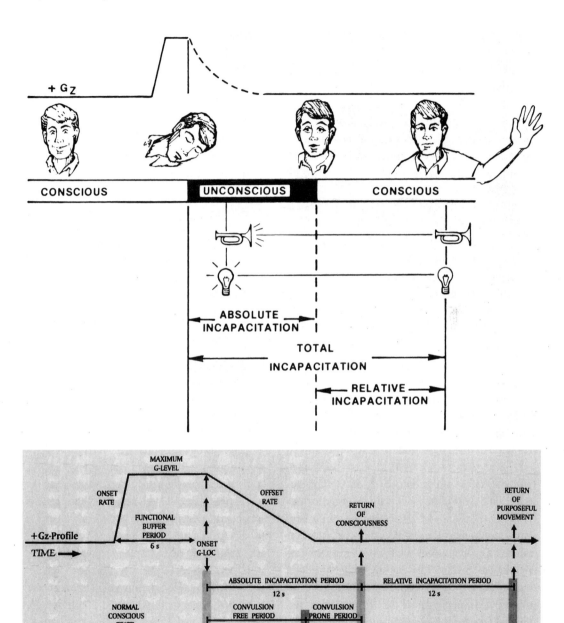

flight controls are released and the level of G is rapidly reduced allowing CNS blood flow and subsequent consciousness to return. A multitude of symptoms are produced during a G-LOC episode in a healthy human. The entire symptom complex, along with the physiologic alterations, is a normal response to transient G-induced CNS ischemia and is referred to as the G-LOC syndrome (17). The symptoms occur in a specific sequence, as shown in Figure 9.15, for the usual rapid-onset HSG exposure. The G-LOC syndrome includes both the loss of and recovery of consciousness.

For the flight surgeon, the importance of recognizing this discrete symptom complex as the G-LOC syndrome is important in understanding this normal response. Loss of consciousness and seizure activity are generally disqualifying if exhibited by an aviator, as is delta wave activity observed on an electroencephalogram (EEG). Conversely, G-LOC is a normal response when an individual exceeds his or her G tolerance. The myoclonic jerking in association with the G-LOC episode is not epileptic activity. The EEG response during the usual G-LOC episode has no spike or other activity in temporal association with the myoclonic activity. The delta wave activity is closely associated with the time of unconsciousness and is normal. By the same token, any symptoms observed that are not a part of the G-LOC syndrome, such as incontinence or tongue biting, should be reason for aeromedical concern and possible clinical evaluation. Aviators are no longer automatically restricted and disqualified from flying duties when they experience the G-LOC syndrome as they were up until the 1980s. Implicit in this position is that there is no permanent residual from the G-LOC syndrome. Recovery is complete and without pathologic consequences.

G-LOC Incapacitation

Pilot incapacitation associated with a G-LOC episode poses the main threat for an aircraft mishap. Centrifuge research has quantified and kinetically related the symptoms of the G-LOC

syndrome. The overall or total incapacitation associated with a G-LOC episode can be divided into two periods: (a) absolute incapacitation and (b) relative incapacitation. The average absolute incapacitation period lasts 12 seconds with a range of 2–38 seconds. During this period, the pilot is unconscious (Fig. 9.15). This is followed by a period of confusion/disorientation which lasts on the average of 15 seconds with a range of 2–97 seconds. A pilot is unable to maintain aircraft control during either of these periods, the sum of which is the total incapacitation period, averaging 28 seconds with a range of 9–110 seconds. Because of this potentially long incapacitation period, when flying high speed fighter-type aircraft, it is not surprising that G-LOC has been responsible for the loss of aircraft and aircrew.

Myoclonic Convulsive Activity

Observations in the centrifuge suggest that approximately 70% of the individuals who have G-LOC episodes also have associated uncoordinated myoclonic jerking of the upper and lower extremities and head. The usual pattern of myoclonic jerking resulting from rapid-onset HSG is such that the average 12-second absolute incapacitation period can be separated into an initial 8-second convulsion free period and a terminal 4- second convulsion prone period. The myoclonic jerking averages 4 seconds and ends coincident with the return of consciousness. There is no evidence (except for muscular artifact) of this activity on the standard EEG, which generally remains in a delta rhythm. Close inspection of the small muscle groups of the face and extremities reveals their inclusion in the myoclonic activity.

The importance of myoclonic jerking activity, from the flight surgeon's perspective is that: (a) it is a normal component of the G-LOC syndrome, (b) it may be a key in recognizing that a G-LOC episode has occurred, and (c) it may result in inadvertant flight control (and other cockpit switch) input during flight. The importance of myoclonic jerking activity for the acceleration scientist is that it provides insight into the extent of CNS ischemia that is induced by HSG. Evidence shows that when a G-LOC episode occurs, myoclonic convulsive activity is more often associated with longer incapacitation periods.

Dreamlets

The importance to flight surgeons and acceleration physiologists of the dreamlets associated with the G-LOC syndrome is similar to the myoclonic convulsions. They seem to have all the characteristics of sleep dreams, except for their recognizably short duration—hence dreamlets. The concurrent EEG throughout the dreamlets and myoclonic convulsion periods remains an unchanged delta wave pattern (3 to 6 per second of high amplitude 50 to 200 mv) that is characteristic of the entire absolute incapacitation period. Analysis of the dream content of a large number of G-LOC dreamlets reveals that the physiologic stimuli that exist during the dream period can become incorporated into the dreamlet. For example, an individual with myoclonic jerking that includes the upper extremities may report a dream of a near-drowning episode involving thrashing about in the water. This physiologic stimuli incorporation into the dream experiences is the logic behind trying to define exactly when the dreamlet occurs.

Memory

The G-LOC syndrome is associated with a transit interruption of the normal memory process. The interruption of memory is generally only for the duration of the absolute incapacitation period. Depending on the type of G profile and the resulting ischemic insult, memory may be compromised for several seconds before or after the loss of consciousness. The significance of the memory compromise for the flight surgeon is related to potential difficulty for the pilot to remember or recognize that a G-LOC episode has occurred. The reluctance of aircrew to report a G-LOC episode, because of the threat to continued flying duties, combined with the memory compromise that may prevent recognition of the

event makes it difficult to accurately assess the actual incidence of in-flight G-LOC. When G-LOC results in a fatal mishap, it frequently becomes a diagnosis by exclusion of all other possible causes. Surveys of pilots of high performance aircraft from several countries agree that approximately 25% have experienced a recognizable G-LOC episode at least once in their flying careers. This is likely a conservative estimate based on the compromise of memory associated with G-LOC.

Once again, the importance of defining the exact kinetics of the memory compromise associated with the G-LOC syndrome for the acceleration scientist is related to it providing insight into the physiologic mechanism. What is remembered provides the indication of exactly when memory is lost and regained.

Psychologic Impact

A G-LOC episode has a psychologic impact on the aviator. This impact is related to the characteristics of the ischemic insult and frequently lingers well beyond the immediate recovery of full consciousness. It is at least partially because of this transient but persisting psychologic change in the aviator that the recommendation for an efficient return to base and restriction from further flying for the remainder of that day be followed. A period of sleep is recommended before an aviator returns to flying after a G-LOC episode.

Theory of the Induction of G-LOC

The underlying theory of the G-LOC syndrome is related to G-induced ischemia affecting the cephalic areas of the nervous system (18). The symptoms and physiologic changes result from regional ischemic differences within the cephalic nervous system. The relationship between functional and nonfunctional areas produce symptoms characteristic of essentially different functional configurations of the nervous systems. The characteristics of the G stress that determines the ischemic pattern of the nervous system and resulting neuronal response (tolerance) must be considered in determining the extent of the G effect.

Current theory development was based on data from more than 500 G-LOC episodes in normal humans (19). The G-LOC syndrome is regarded as a protective mechanism that has evolved to prevent injury to the nervous system and the organism as a whole when exposed to a magnitude of G exposure above tolerance levels. The G-LOC syndrome is sequentially induced when the cardiovascular system is overwhelmed by HSG. Many of the G-LOC syndrome symptoms occur as adequate blood flow is returning to the nervous system. The protective sequence therefore involves not only protection of the nervous system directly, but in addition, protection of the organism as a whole in a hostile environment by enhancing rapid and complete recovery of consciousness.

Electroencephalogram (EEG) Changes

EEG results have been compared on subjects exposed to HSG with and without G-LOC. Without G-LOC, alpha waves were replaced by high-frequency, low-amplitude waves that were identified as stressful and probably caused by compensatory cardiovascular changes associated with the high G exposure. However, with G-LOC, the EEG response changed significantly progressively slower delta waves (3 to 6 per second) of high amplitude (50 to 200 volts) that occurred during most of the G-LOC episode. The delta wave pattern was not different in subjects with convulsions (22). More recent studies confirm the shift in power of the delta and theta frequencies with G-LOC, including a reduction in beta activity.

RENAL SYSTEM

Renal blood flow dictates the functional capacity of the kidneys. Because blood flow is reduced in the human with standing and exercise, a reduction in kidney function during exposure to

Table 9.12.
Effects of +G$_z$ on Renal Blood Flow in Miniature Swine (23)

	Cortex	J-M	Medulla
+3 G$_z$ exposure			
Control	428 ± 50	292 ± 63	57 ± 21
During +G$_z$	161 ± 61	91 ± 43	2 ± 1
10 MP	310 ± 39	196 ± 39	35 ± 13
+5 G$_z$ exposure			
Control	432 ± 43	303 ± 43	73 ± 21
During +G$_z$	3 ± 2	2 ± 1	0.1 ± 0.1
10 MP	247 ± 27	176 ± 22	50 ± 12
+7 G$_z$ exposure			
Control	578 ± 51	430 ± 38	61 ± 13
During +G$_z$	36 ± 28	40 ± 27	3 ± 2
10 MP	191 ± 35	155 ± 40	28 ± 10

Mean blood flows are means ± SE in ml • min^{-1} • 100 g^{-1}; cortex, outer cortex; J-M juxtamedullary cortex; and 10 MP measurements made 10 min after +G$_z$ exposure.

HSG is anticipated. Renal blood flow of the outer cortex, juxtamedullary cortex, and medulla were significantly reduced in miniature swine at +3, 5, and 7 G (Table 9.12). Particularly affected was the medulla. Ten minutes after G exposure, blood was still reduced to about 50% of control values (23). In support of this animal research, oliguria for 1 hour post-G exposure occurs in humans along with some sodium and potassium retention. Plasma renin (of the renin-angiotensin system) increases in the human with 30-minute exposures to 2.0–2.5 G.

ACCELERATION-ASSOCIATED PATHOLOGIC CHANGES

Flight surgeons and acceleration physiologists are particularly sensitive to the possibility that HSG exposure causes pathologic changes in the body. The clinical aeromedical research community must understand the possible pathologic changes associated with exposure to potentially hazardous flight environments as part of aviation occupational medicine.

Although pathologic changes associated with G stress have been sought, their absence is notable. Acute neck injuries are the most common

G-related malady in aircrew of high performance aircraft. Other spinal injuries have also been reported (24). The heart and lung would appear to be at risk in this environment, but the absence of symptoms and the results of centrifuge studies suggest otherwise. Yet, serious G-induced pathologies do occur in laboratory animals, usually at high G levels well above their physiologic tolerances.

Neurological Pathology

In the late 1950s, a young military flight student experienced 9 G during an emergency maneuver that caused symptoms suggesting cerebellar injury. All symptoms disappeared after 6 months and he returned to flying status. Axial sleeving of the brain stem has been suggested as the cause of that injury and others reported in an aerobatic pilot and several in high speed vehicular accidents in which the head is pitched forward with $+G_z$ exposure (24).

A single case of left hypoglossal neurapraxia occurring at levels of approximately 7 G during aircrew centrifuge training has been reported with subsequent restriction from flight duties in fighter-type aircraft. After aircrew centrifuge training, which involved a single G-LOC episode, a reported case of cerebral lacunar infarct with mild functional deficit was thought to potentially be related to the G exposure. The pilot was, however, eventually returned to flying duties. Left phrenic nerve injury causing hemidiaphragmatic paralysis occurred in a Spanish pilot with accidental excessive inflation of an anti-G suit during flight. This accident impaired respiratory dynamics with permanent disqualification from flying duties.

The vestibular system has adaptive properties that may render it symptom free even though some pathology exists. Symptoms of otoconial separation have been reported post-centrifugation. Benign paroxysmal positional vertigo resulting from otolithic disruption occurred in a research subject during exposure to a complex seat-tilting G profile which involved significant

levels of $+G_x$. The symptoms resolved over approximately 2 weeks and did not recur; however, the subject was disqualified from further experimental participation. High G animal studies reported a loss of otoconia in guinea pigs (24).

Cardiac Pathology

Because all HSG exposures cause significant changes in the cardiovascular system, the heart has received extensive investigation for possible G-related pathologic changes. Most of the early reports dealt with goats, dogs, rats, and swine exposed to G levels (both $+G_z$ and $-G_z$) well in excess of the animals' tolerances. Although miniature swine studies have reported myocardial injury from tolerable levels of HSG, no pathologic changes have been detected in human centrifuge subjects. In addition, no pathologic cardiac findings suggestive of G-induced lesions have been found during autopsies carried out at the Armed Forces Institute of Pathology on high-performance fighter pilots killed in aircraft accidents. Electrocardiographic changes do not provide any evidence of suspected myocardial damage. Therefore, it is unlikely that myocardial damage resulting from HSG exposures occurs within the cardiovascular tolerance limits of normal humans. Evidence suggests that coronary circulation is adequate in humans during HSG (9). It should be noted, however, that one case of an anterolateral myocardial infarction associated with aircrew centrifuge training has been reported. The 37-year-old aviator with significant risk factors was subsequently found to angiographically have a 95% obstructive lesion in the left anterior descending coronary artery. Similar results have been observed in a miniature swine exposed to HSG with coronary artery disease.

Musculoskeletal Pathology

Acute spinal injuries of sustained G are most commonly associated with extremely high, rapid-onset sustained acceleration forces such as during aerial combat, aerobatics, or centrifuge exposure. But relatively few instances of serious spinal injury have been reported. Two cases of a ruptured intervertebral disc from in-flight $+G_z$ have been described. The first case, which reportedly occurred at 9 G, involved the lumbar region between L-4 and L-5. The second case, occurring at 5 G, affected the lumbosacral region. Both cases occurred during increased G with the back in a flexed and rotated position. It was suggested that this awkward, flexed position under G loading could result in severe strain on the posterior longitudinal ligament and its adjacent annulus fibrosis. The probability of posterior herniation of the nucleus pulposus was also increased. Recent magnetic resonance imaging (MRI) studies of senior Finnish fighter pilots reported cervical disc bulges in 3 pilots after in-flight neck pain. Disc bulging at the C3–4 level was reported in an aviator with cervical dystonia (spasmodic torticallis) after in-flight aerial combat maneuvering in an F-14. Although the aviator recovered, intramuscular botulinum toxin was required for several months to relieve the pain.

Chronic-type degenerative diseases in these regions may occur but have not been confirmed by controlled studies. Always a complicating issue is deciding if certain skeletal abnormalities, lifestyles, or age predispose an individual to problems related to diseases of HSG. Studies of senior Finnish fighter pilots using MRI techniques found a significant increase in degenerative disc changes of the C3–4 vertebrae. However, the Naval Air Warfare Center conducted MRI studies of several experimental research subjects who had been exposed long-term to sustained levels of G as high as $+10\,G_z$, and they were not found to have any pathologic spinal abnormalities. An AGARD Conference (April 1989) on this subject resulted in the publication of an AGARD/AMP Aeromedical Review (AGARD-AR 317) entitled "The Musculoskeletal and Vestibular Effect of Long-Term Repeated Exposure to Sustained High G" (24).

However, regardless of the absence of controlled data on this subject, flight surgeons at fighter aircraft bases are well aware of the high frequency of neck-related problems. Several reports show acute neck injury in pilots of high performance aircraft to be as high as 70%. These problems are rarely of a long-lasting, severe nature, but they do result in a decrement in performance, some loss of flight time, and reduced G tolerance. Pilots of F-18, F-16, and F-15 aircraft are encouraged to regularly perform neck strengthening exercises, and immediately before aerial combat sorties, exercise the neck and shoulder muscles as a warm-up before pulling G. Undoubtedly, the use of heavy helmets with an undesirable center of gravity and the location of the headbox exacerbates the problem. In the future, helmet and seat designers must address this problem with high performance aircraft.

Preexisting abnormalities, such as excessive scoliosis, Scheuermann's disease, Schmorl's nodes, spondylolysis, spondylolisthesis, and degenerative disease of the vertebral column, are usually considered disqualifying for experimental centrifuge subjects. Indeed, these spinal abnormalities should also be closely scrutinized for high-performance fighter aircrew.

Cases of uncomplicated (lower) rib fractures have been found in experimental subjects (one male and one female) wearing extended coverage anti-G suits at levels of 8–10 G. Similar uncomplicated cases, although rare, have also occurred in aircrew wearing standard anti-G suits participating in centrifuge training. A single case of a complete fracture of the right femoral head occurred in a pilot during aircrew centrifuge training. No associated preexisting hip pathology was found. The pilot ultimately returned to flying duties in aircraft with low G capability.

In animals exposed to extremely high G, there is an increase in plasma levels of tissue isoenzymes CPK, LDH, and SGOT. The results varied among individual animals, but generally there was a maximum effect 3 days post-acceleration and a return to normal levels after 14 days. These increases in isoenzymes appear to result from skeletal muscle tissue damage. Increases in the mm fraction of CPK, total CPK, and LDH, denoting some muscle damage, commonly occurs in humans after exposure to HSG, but these are not considered medically or operationally important because much higher increases routinely occur in people after strenuous muscular effort at 1 G. A case in point was a Canadian pilot with massive myoglobinuria (CPK ranged from 2,000–3,000) after aircrew centrifuge training. Recovery was complete with ultimate return to unrestricted flying duties. These CPK levels that peaked 24 hours post-G are near pre-G levels after 72 hours of the G exposure.

Pulmonary Pathology

The lungs undoubtedly are stressed during HSG with respect to ventilation and perfusion abnormalities, mechanical distortion, and organ displacement. These anatomic/physiologic changes are quickly reversible with the termination of acceleration. No lung pathologies have been reported with in-flight or high G centrifuge exposures in healthy individuals. The possibility of a spontaneous pneumothorax could be expected since pneumothorax occurs during usual strenuous physical activities. However, experience up to 10 G has not produced any pulmonary pathologic changes of that nature.

Although HSG has not been associated with lung pathology, the HSG use of positive pressure breathing (PBG) continues to be examined in the laboratory and is the focus of operational surveys. Recent miniature swine studies have shown that medical concerns about elevated transmural and differential pressures in the heart and lung with PBG are without any physiologic basis.

Acceleration (or aero-) atelectasis syndrome is associated with HSG exposure in pilots breathing oxygen-enriched gas mixtures (>70% oxygen) and wearing an inflated anti-G suit. This condition has been documented in U.S. Naval fighter pilots who are operationally required to breathe 100% oxygen. Symptoms include retrosternal chest pain or discomfort, dys-

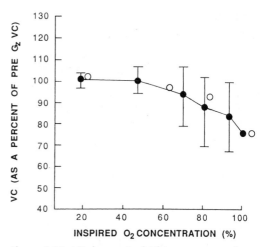

Figure 9.16. Vital capacity (VC) is a measure of lung function that is reduced atelectasis with increased inspired O_2. Reprinted with permission from Haswell MS, Tacher WA, Balldin UI, et al. Influence of inspired oxygen concentration on acceleration atelectasis. Aviat Space Environ Med 1986; 57:432–437.

pnea, and paroxysmal coughing episodes. No residual effects are known to result from this condition. This G-induced syndrome is caused by the downward movement of the lung contacting the upward shift of the diaphragm; the inflation of the abdominal bladder of the anti-G suit compresses the lungs and closes distal alveolae. Oxygen in these alveolae is rapidly absorbed into the blood. If high partial pressures of oxygen are in these alveolae, they will collapse, causing atelectasis. A significant presence of the more slowly absorbing nitrogen gas will prevent the occurrence of atelectasis. Therefore, the problem can be eliminated by breathing oxygen-rich mixtures that have sufficient levels of nitrogen. Studies have found that a maximum of 70% oxygen with 30% slowly-absorbable gas (nitrogen or argon) will prevent acceleration atelectasis (13) (Fig. 9.16). Dilutor-demand breathing gas regulators, such as those used by the U.S. Air Force, provide adequate nitrogen to prevent the routine occurrence of atelectasis in most aviators. There is a high degree of individual susceptibility to acceleration atelectasis; tobacco smoking increased its incidence in U.S. Naval aviators.

Vascular Pathology

Symptoms related to the peripheral vascular system are the most frequent problems experienced by individuals exposed to HSG. Small, pinpoint, cutaneous petechiae occur in the dependent and unsupported areas of the body during $+G_z$ exposure. Most common areas are the feet and ankles, followed in decreasing frequency in the legs and arms. The distribution of the petechiaesis is highly dependent on the seat configuration and the anti-G protective equipment worn. With an increasing $+G_x$ component (F-16 seat configuration), the buttocks and back become more frequently involved. Occasionally in severe cases, the petechiaes may coalesce into large purpuric areas. The probable cause of petechiaesis is either rupturing of capillaries or diapedesis in response to high intravascular pressure. The petechiae, referred to by fighter pilots as "high-G measles," resolve in several days without sequelae. Experience at the Armstrong Laboratory and Naval Air Warfare Center with G research subjects finds that frequent high G exposures result in a reduced occurrence of petechiae.

A less common but more painful problem results from the rupture of a larger blood vessel. One case of a G-induced scrotal hematoma occurred at the Armstrong Laboratory during SACM as the subject performed a vigorous AGSM. The hematoma resolved without sequelae, but initially, it was very painful. The subject returned after complete resolution and continued to participate in high G acceleration research without further problems. At least one case of an in-flight incapacitation has been documented in an aviator with a varicocele who lost consciousness because of extreme pain during aerobatic training in a T-37 aircraft.

Bilateral superficial phlebitis of the lower extremities after aircrew centrifuge training occurred in a Marine aviator. He was exposed to $+9\ G_z$ and then soon after performed strenuous physical activity. These together may have led to the phlebitis. The pilot completely recovered

and returned to flying high performance aircraft. A somewhat similar case occurred in a female exposed to $+5.6\ G_z$ with subsequent vigorous physical activity. Also, the individual was a smoker, taking contraceptives, and had developed stress myositis, although venous thrombosis in the left calf was considered a possibility. Full recovery was uneventful.

Prostatic edema and bleeding have been reported in centrifuge subjects after exposures up to $+9\ G_z$. The severity of the lesions was directly related to the level of G (25).

Pathology Summary

The majority of the pathology that has resulted from exposure to HSG, both in centrifuges and in fighter-type aircraft, generally does not fit a pattern and has probably occurred in uniquely susceptible individuals. The clear exception to this is with respect to the musculoskeletal injuries of the neck. The increased risk of neck problems in aircrew during actual flight, in comparison to the centrifuge environment, suggests that the combination of HSG in individuals wearing headgear while performing complex head and torso movements manifests neck injury. Substantial benefits are found with neck strengthening exercises in aircrew. The pathologic problems discussed in the preceding paragraphs are the result of acute exposure to G. Occupational health surveillance that spans entire careers of repeated exposures to HSG should be systematically conducted to determine the cumulative effects of the ACM environment (24).

SELECTION CRITERIA AND STANDARDS FOR HIGH $+G_z$ ENVIRONMENTS

Increased $+G_z$ tolerance demands will continue to be placed on aircrew flying high-performance aircraft. Indeed, future fighter aircraft promise even higher G environments. Consequently, future fighter pilot selection criteria may well include at least minimum G-tolerance standards. Also, it is important to determine if certain medical irregularities are associated with reduced G tolerance and if the condition is exacerbated with high G exposures. Medical standards should evaluate this information on G sensitivity that could compromise acceptable human performance and pilot safety.

Centrifuge Research Standards

Reasons for exposing humans to increased G on a centrifuge include orientation, training, medical evaluation, and research. Although safety concerns are fundamental, different standards exist for humans exposed to G for various reasons. Use of volunteer subjects for research usually requires long-term intermittent exposure to G. Frequently, G exposure levels are high and sustained until the individual has reached significant fatigue. Training, orientation, and medical evaluation, however, require fewer and lower G-level centrifuge exposures. Consequently, a thorough medical evaluation is required for individuals who volunteer as experimental subjects. The following is a list of the mandatory medical evaluation requirements for centrifuge volunteers, in the order of completion, as required by the Armstrong Laboratory at Brooks Air Force Base, Texas, and the Naval Air Warfare Center:

1. Air Force and Naval Flying class II physical examination
   a. History and physical examination
   b. 12-lead electrocardiogram
   c. Clinical laboratory tests (blood and urine)
   d. Chest radiographs (PA and lateral)
2. Centrifuge orientation
   a. Medical evaluation protocol
   b. Minimum G tolerance (ROR, 7 G × 15 s)[d]
3. Maximal treadmill exercise test
4. Echocardiogram
5. Complete spinal MRI

Incidentally, reasons for performing several of these tests frequently differ from those of a clinician who is looking for abnormalities. The

[d] See following methods for ROR description.

Table 9.13.
Type and Number of G_z Induced Symptoms Over a 3-Year Period on the Armstrong Laboratory Centrifuge (Brooks Air Force Base, Texas)

Number of Occurrence	Symptom Description
16	Abdominal pain
16	Arm pain
1	Clonic movements
5	Disorientation, vertigo
3	Hyperventilation
67	Loss of consciousness
2	Loss of consciousness with severe convulsion
15	Neck pain
16	Petechial hemorrhages
2	Scrotal hematoma/discomfort

above medical requirements have been successful in that no permanently disabling medical problems have been encountered. The symptomatology and its incidence resulting from hundreds of G exposures over 3 years at the Armstrong Laboratory are summarized in Table 9.13. In spite of this list of minor symptomatology, all volunteers who are to be exposed to G must be briefed on an extensive list of numerous potential hazards, as required by the Advisory Committee on Human Experimentation (Table 9.14).

With the approval for women to fly in fighter-type aircraft during combat in several countries, more tolerance information is now needed for women in the HSG environment to ensure that gender-related problems are explored. Also, the requirements that women cannot be excluded as research volunteers in the G environment based solely on gender, has significantly increased their opportunity to participate. However, care must be taken to ensure that the subjects are not pregnant. Certainly, absolute assurance of nonpregnancy in research subjects represents a significant challenge, however, methodologies to accomplish these goals are in place in centrifuge research facilities. Aeromedical standards that protect fetuses have been established that minimally affect the flying careers of female aviators.

Table 9.14.
Topics Required to be Briefed to Human Volunteers Before $+G_z$ Exposure

1. Symptoms
   a. Blackout
   b. Loss of consciousness
   c. Seizures, convulsions, amnesia, confusion
   d. Vertigo
   e. Motion sickness, vomiting
   f. Dyspnea
   g. Pain, fatigue
2. Trauma
   a. Pneumothorax
   b. Muscle soreness
   c. Vertebral body compression fractures
   d. Herniated nucleus pulposus
   e. Petechial hemorrhages
   f. Swelling of the lower extremities
   g. Scrotal hematoma
   h. Hernia
   i. Vestibular alterations
3. Cardiac stress
   a. Dysrhythmias (tachycardia and bradycardia)
   b. Heart blocks
   c. Stress cardiomyopathy

Clinical Aeromedical Centrifuge Evaluation

Certain aircrew members undergoing conventional aeromedical evaluation may be referred for centrifuge testing to determine whether their medical condition is sensitive to $+G_z$. A medical evaluation with G-tolerance testing provides information about the G sensitivity of aircrew for assignment to a high-performance aircraft for obvious safety reasons. Although it is argued that only aviators with "normal" clinical evaluations should be selected for flying high-performance fighter aircraft, the following two situations counter that philosophy: (a) accurately defining a "normal" clinical evaluation is difficult and (b) the expertise, personal, and financial losses associated with pilot disqualification.

Methods Used for Clinical G-Tolerance Determination

Clinical $+G_z$ tolerance measurement has been carried out using several techniques at different acceleration laboratories. Two separate types of runs generally are used as defined by the G onset rate: (a) rapid-onset rate (ROR) and (b) gradual-onset rate (GOR). These runs assess an individual's G-level tolerance and cardiovascular responses. Consequently, the rate of gradual-onset runs should be slow enough to allow cardiovascular compensation to occur with the acceleration increase during the exposure. This type of GOR has a rate slower than 0.25 G/sec. At the Armstrong Laboratory, the GOR is 0.067 G/sec. An ROR must have a rate greater than 0.33 G/sec. At the Armstrong Laboratory, an ROR is 6 G/sec. Seatback angles and footrest positions used are the same as the pilot has when flying; e.g., an F-16 pilot will have an elevated heel line and a 30° seatback angle.

The aeromedical G protocol usually consists of a series of runs that include an initial relaxed GOR(1), a series of RORs, a second relaxed GOR(2), and a final GOR with the pilot performing the protective straining maneuver, GOR(S). The test results include various G-tolerance measurements, the electrocardiographic response, and any symptoms that occurred during the test period. The use of GORs, both relaxed and using a protective straining maneuver, measures tolerance to acceleration, the integrity of cardiovascular reflexes, and the performance proficiency of the AGSM. This protocol may be modified according to specific problems as requested by the referring flight surgeon. Frequently, specific profiles similar to an in-flight profile that caused a problem for the aviator are used to supplement the clinical evaluation profiles.

The G tolerance and heart rate response standards for this aeromedical evaluation protocol are given in Table 9.15. These standards were established using 425 healthy individuals on the Armstrong Laboratory centrifuge.

PLUS G_Z TOLERANCES

Aircrew are always directly exposed to the G environment seated upright—a vulnerable

Table 9.15.
G_z Tolerance Criteria for Centrifuge Profiles

		Profile Standard Values
Profile 1-GOR (1)	High	-5.6 or greater
	Low	-less than 4.0
	Average	-4.0–5.5
Profile 2-ROR (pass)	High	-4.1 or greater
	Low	-less than 3.1
	Average	-3.1–4.0
Profile 3-GOR (2)	High	-5.3 or greater
	Low	-less than 3.7
	Average	-3.7–5.2
Profile 4-GOR (S)	High	-6.0 or greater
	Low	-less than 4.6
	Average	-4.6–5.9

GOR = gradual-onset run (0.067 G/s)
ROR = rapid-onset run (1.0 G/s)

position. Consequently, their ability to tolerate this exposure is of major concern to the USAF/ USN operational communities and a challenge to acceleration physiologists. Methods used to measure these tolerances are the same as those used in any environment: (a) level of the exposure (its intensity and application of that intensity; i.e., G onset/offset) and (b) duration of exposure; i.e., G level and G duration. A detailed description of what cumulatively composes acceleration tolerance is available (20).

G-Level Tolerance

The ability to tolerate G exposure is primarily a function of adequate blood flow to the brain—the most vulnerable and vital organ regarding aircrew performance. Consequently, symptoms that relate to reduced blood flow in the head are used primarily as the measure of G-level tolerance.

The traditional method used to determine G-level tolerance is loss of vision symptoms in a relaxed upright seated subject at a level of G exposure. The loss of vision symptoms (commonly called greyout), loss of peripheral or tunnel vision, blackout, or loss of central vision all refer to a reduction in blood flow in the retina of the eye in conjunction with the opposing intraocular pressure. Usually light-loss criteria are

100% peripheral light loss (PLL) with 50% CLL. However, even with 100% CLL, blood flow to the head continues, supporting the brain and auditory systems so that complete consciousness and hearing remain undisturbed even though this person cannot see (i.e., blackout). Recovery from this interesting condition of blackout is *immediate* upon restoration of a higher level of P_a or a decrease in G (Fig. 9.14). If P_a at head level continues to drop, blood flow to the brain is significantly reduced or may even stop, then G-LOC occurs—a condition discussed earlier in this chapter. G-LOC was once used as the main criterion of G tolerance.

The most common method for measuring the light loss phenomenon is with a straight light bar that is 71 cm in length placed 76 cm in front of the subject at eye level. This light bar has a small green light (2.5-cm diameter) at each end and a single 2.5-cm diameter red light at the center. The subject looks straight ahead at the light bar without moving his eyes or head. When the peripheral green lights can no longer be seen but the center red light remains clear, 100% PLL or greyout occurs. When there is complete loss of vision (the red light disappears), 100% CLL or blackout occurs.

The classic G-level tolerance measurement of loss of vision is determined on subjects who are "relaxed" (as much as possible) and seated in the centrifuge gondola in an aircraft-type seat. This tolerance is called the relaxed G-level tolerance, and because it is a function of the dynamic response of the cardiovascular system—particularly the arterial system—to a reduction in eye-level P_a, the rate of applying G is extremely important. A rapid application of G at 1 G per second and higher onset rates in a relaxed person preempts an expected vasoconstriction response of the cardiovascular system mediated by the baroreceptors at the level of the carotid sinus. Therefore, this measurement, known as the relaxed rapid onset run (ROR) G tolerance, is about 1 G lower than the gradual onset run (GOR) tolerance that is measured with slower G-onset rates of 0.067–0.1 G per second. These

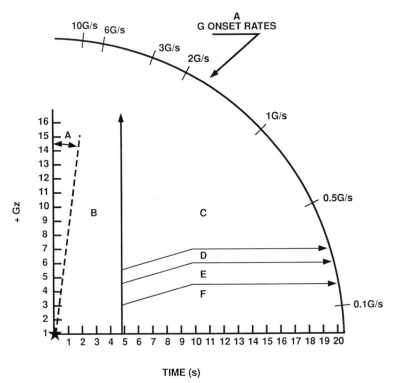

Figure 9.17. Nomogram of symptomatology expected at various G onset rates and G levels. With a straight-edge intersecting 1 G at 0 time and extending beyond the G onset rate curve, subject symptoms (G tolerance criteria) are predicted as a function of time as individual regions (e.g., B, C, D, E, or F) are transected. The G level of symptom occurrence is directly to the left of the vertical axis. See text for detailed explanation.

slower G-onset rates allow arterial vasoconstriction before light loss occurs, thereby increasing G-level tolerance.

Human studies using centrifuges with high G-onset capability (3 to 10 G/sec) have determined that a neurologic symptom-free period of 4 to 5 seconds occurs before the onset of G-LOC. This functional buffer period eliminates G-level "tolerances," but unfortunately it lasts only 4 to 5 seconds (20,26).

A G-level tolerance nomogram (provided in Fig. 9.17) allows the reader to identify "average" G-level tolerances with expected symptoms as a function of rate of onset of G and duration of G exposure.

This time-intense G-tolerance nomogram defines G limits regionally as they relate to *linear* G-onset rates (A) for *relaxed* subjects with average tolerances.

A = G/sec onset rate designates G tolerance, depending on symptomatology.

B Region = *Asymptomatic*—limited by the 4 to 5 second functional reserve of the eye-brain tissue.

Infinite tolerance (within structural limits) is theoretically possible with sufficient onset rate until LOC occurs when Region C is entered at 4–5 seconds.

C Region = *G-LOC*—obtained by either exceeding time exposure of B, or C level of D Region.

D Region = *Blackout*—100% CLL region that begins with about 20 mmHg of P_a at head level that amounts for 1 G of tolerance between the beginning of 100% CLL (top of Region E) and development of G-LOC (Region C).

E Region = *Light Loss*—defined by the first sign of PLL that occurs at 50 mmHg of P_a at the lower G level up to total loss of vision or 100% CLL of Region D.

F Region = *Asymptomatic*—limited not by time as is B Region, but by the G level. D, E, and F tolerances are increased during the 5–10 second time frame as a result of vasoconstriction mediated by the sympathetic nervous system via the baroreceptors that increase P_a at head level.

It is stressed here that this G intensity-duration tolerance nomogram is for a *relaxed* subject exposed to linearly increasing G because any significant muscular tensing increases G tolerance. It is not surprising, therefore, to learn that muscle tensing is used as the basis for the AGSM.

As demonstrated with this nomogram, the subject can "enter" these "symptom" regions at any time, depending upon the onset rate of G, and produce different levels of G tolerance, depending upon symptomatology. As an example, an onset rate of 6 G/sec to 7 G remaining for 2 seconds and returning to 1 G, also at 6 G/sec, would result in no symptoms of G intolerance. If however, the pilot was exposed to a G maneuver of 0.5 G/sec onset rate at 5 seconds, PLL would begin upon reaching 3 G at 10 seconds, blackout would start at 5.5 G, and 12 to 13 seconds into this maneuver, LOC would occur at 6.5 G. However, an onset of G at 0.1 G/sec or slower, as GOR tolerance is determined in the laboratory, PLL does not begin until after the baroceptors have responded, giving the subject an additional 1 G in tolerance during all stages of light loss. Another important characteristic of this nomogram is that a rapid onset rate of G within the functional reserve of the brain (B Region) to a high G level (more than 6 G) shows the absence of recognizable light loss (PLL or CLL) before G-LOC. Since PLL is used by pilots as a measure of their G tolerance, its unexpected absence can unsuspectingly lead to G-LOC.

Studies have measured relaxed ROR and GOR and straining GOR tolerances; each reports slightly different average values, but the most referenced study, conducted in the early 1950s, involved 1,000 relaxed male subjects with varying occupational backgrounds. Their mean ROR tolerances (1 G/sec onset rate) and wide ranges are shown in (27) Table 9.16. GOR tolerances for several hundred U.S. Air Force Air Combat Command (ACC), formerly Tactical Air Command (TAC), pilots using 100% PLL are shown in Figure 9.18. As expected, GOR relaxed tolerances of Figure 9.18 are about 1 G higher than the ROR tolerances of Table 9.16. The wide range of tolerances among individuals shown for both studies has implications for aircrew selection—perhaps aircrew of high performance aircraft could be selected with high G relaxed tolerances. However, a G-tolerance selection program to identify persons with high G-level tolerances has never been developed for several reasons, but persons with extremely low G tolerances (e.g., <3 G ROR) are advised to fly aircraft with low G capability. It is important to know, however, that people with relatively low relaxed G tolerances can increase their G tolerances by effectively using the AGSM and other G-protection methods to levels that are compatible with flying modern fighter aircraft (6). Yet, it is clear that pilots who cannot tolerate the maximum G-level capabilities of their aircraft after G training on the centrifuge are not able to utilize the maximum operational capabilities of their aircraft.

G-Level Tolerance Model

A simple mathematical model based on hydrostatic physical principles (see Eq. 4) is useful in understanding the important direct role that eye-level blood pressure, eye-heart vertical distance,

Table 9.16.
G-Level Tolerances of 1000 Relaxed Subjects Not Wearing Anti-G Suits at 1 g/sec Onset Rate (ROR) (27)

Criteria	Mean G	± S.D.	G Range
PLL	4.1	0.7	2.2–7.1
Blackout	4.8	0.8	2.7–7.8
Unconsciousness	5.4	0.9	3.0–8.4

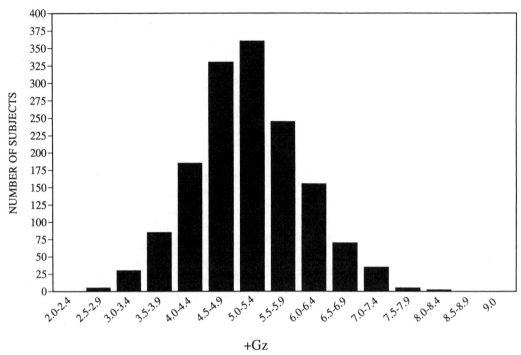

Figure 9.18. GOR relaxed tolerances of several hundred USAF fighter pilots seated in the F-16 seatback configuration not wearing an inflated anti-G suit.

and pulmonary (intrathoracic) pressure have on ROR G-level tolerances:

$$G_{LT} = [(P_a + P_I)/hd] + K \qquad (9)$$

Where:

G_{LT} = G-level tolerance (G)

P_a = arterial pressure of 100 mmHg at heart level

P_I = intrathoracic pressures in mmHg (dependent upon AGSM with a maximum of 100 mmHg)

h = eye-heart vertical distance (mm)

d = specific density of blood related to the specific density of Hg (1/13.6)

K = 1 G tolerance increase with the anti-G suit

This model with P_a set at 100 mmHg (i.e., 120 mmHg of systolic pressure at heart level—20 mmHg intraocular pressure), eye-heart vertical distance varied with body position, and P_I at a maximum of 100 mmHg has been validated with

centrifuge tolerance data (3). A "rule of thumb" to remember is that each G costs the arterial system approximately 25 mmHg because of the opposing hydrostatic pressure that develops with the eye-heart vertical distance of 330 mm in the human. A constant value of 1 G increase in tolerance is accurate with current operational anti-G suits. Advanced anti-G suit models that provide increased lower body coverage will provide more G tolerance. The derivation of this model is available to the interested reader (3).

This model accurately predicts the ROR relaxed G-level tolerance in a seated upright individual at 4 G, with the anti-G suit of 5 G, and with different AGSM efforts. Because high performance aircraft can rapidly reach 9 G, it is clear that an AGSM of 100 mmHg—about the maximum mean pressure that is humanly possible—is required to fly this aircraft to its maximum capability. Figure 9.19 shows G-level tolerances of pilots using various anti-G methods (see the section on protection against $+G_z$) (3).

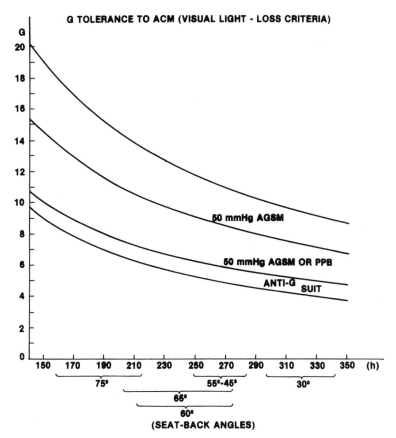

Figure 9.19. ROR G tolerances using PLL visual criteria of subjects using various anti-G methods related to the eye-heart vertical distance h. The h changes with different seatback angles. Reprinted with permission from Burton RR. A conceptual model for predicting pilot group G tolerance for tactical fighter aircraft. Aviat Space Environ Med 1986;57:733–744.

G-Duration Tolerance

Fighter aircraft are capable of sustaining high G maneuvers for several minutes (limited only by fuel capacity); thus, the ability of aircrew to tolerate these long-duration G exposures and frequently repeated short-duration exposures is an important operational consideration. Human performance limits have been the impetus for developing methods to measure G-duration tolerances.

The limiting physiologic factor of G-duration tolerance is the development of fatigue, which is used as a principal measurement endpoint. Simply, G-duration tolerance is the length of time in seconds that a subject can continue to maintain vision and perform a task while exposed to a repeating predetermined G profile that continues until the G exposure is stopped by the subject because of fatigue. This G profile is called a simulated aerial combat maneuver (SACM). A typical SACM profile used in a G-duration tolerance measurement is shown in Figure 9.20. Several modifications of this type of G profile are used in acceleration research but the cyclic nature of repeating low-high G epochs and the subjectively determined fatigue endpoint remain common to these profiles (28). A significant component of this tolerance is anaerobic; consequently, an increased level of blood lactate is frequently used to validate the subjective fatigue criterion. Of course, for this G-duration

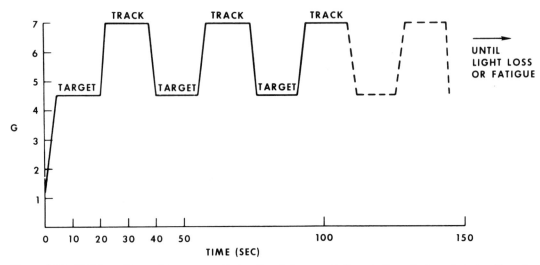

Figure 9.20. SACM profile used to measure G-duration tolerance. Fatigue is the criterion of choice. Target (shooting) and tracking are used occasionally to measure performance during the SACM. Reprinted with permission from Burton RR, Shaffstall RM. Human tolerance to aerial combat maneuvers. Aviat Space Environ Med 1980;51:641–648.

tolerance measurement to be reproducible, subjects must be well-trained in the use of the AGSM.

There is a direct correlation, to be sure, between G-level and G-duration tolerances, suggesting that if one (e.g., G level) is increased by the use of an "anti-G" system or method, then the other (G-duration tolerance) will also be increased; i.e., physiologically coupled (28).

G-duration tolerances have been measured for several sustained G levels up to 9 G (Fig. 9.21). Except for the 3 G exposure that was terminated because of an arbitrarily set limit of 1 hour (AL), the remaining tolerances were limited by subject fatigue (29).

G Tolerances in Women

Now that women are flying high performance aircraft in combat, considerable attention has been directed toward their G tolerances. Although laboratory studies are not yet complete on this topic, the G-level and G-duration tolerances that have been measured in women are not statistically different from those of men. The menstrual cycle does not affect G tolerances.

The important roles of muscular strength and anaerobic power in male SACM duration tolerances are well-known. This relationship translates to a highly significant correlation between SACM tolerance and lean body mass (38). Women have significantly less strength than men for the same body size. Yet, a qualitatively similar relationship between lean body mass and SACM tolerance exists for women, but with a much steeper slope; i.e., women have greater SACM tolerances with less lean body mass.

Factors Affecting G Tolerances

Physiologic/Anatomic

Physiologic/anatomic factors that increase relaxed G tolerance include age, reduced height (shorter h in Eq. 9), and high diastolic and systolic P_a. Using the Armstrong Laboratory aeromedical evaluation protocol, clinical parameters of aircrew were grouped according to relaxed high G tolerance (HTG) and low G tolerance (LTG) (Table 9.17). Clearly the HTG flyers are older and exhibit the physiologic changes that accompany the aging process; i.e., increased P_a and resting heart rate, increased body mass with

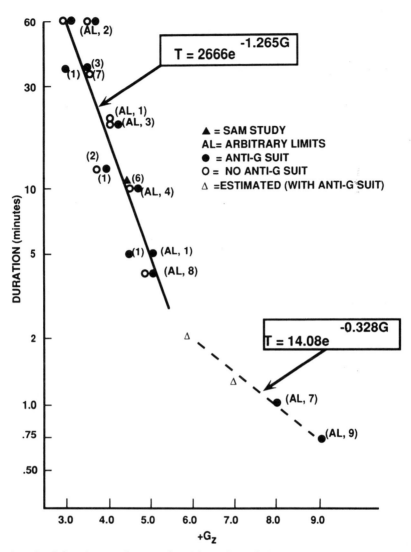

Figure 9.21. Sustained duration G tolerances for either subject fatigue or arbitrary limits (AL) criteria. Arbitrary limits were established by the study protocol. Number of subjects per data point is in parenthesis. Estimated values are based on data provided by the authors from past research studies. Reprinted with permission from AGARDograph No. 322. High G Physiological Protection Training, AMP Working Group 14, 1990; Hamilton R, Whinnery JE. The diagnosis of physiologically uncomplicated +G$_z$-induced loss of consciousness: a guide for the naval flight surgeon. Air Vehicle and Crew Systems Technology Department, Naval Air Development Center, Warminster, PA, 1990; Burton RR. Human responses to repeated high G simulated aerial combat maneuvers. Aviat Space Environ Med 1980;51:1185–1192.

increased triglycerides, cholesterol, and blood sugar. It should be remembered, however, that relaxed G tolerances represent less than half of the G level required to tolerate HSG.

Another attempt has been made to understand the physiologic bases of G tolerances by grouping subjects with high and low HSG tolerances with physiologic responses measured during G exposures (31) (Table 9.18). Clearly, those subjects that were most tolerant were least affected physiologically by the G exposure (i.e., their physiologic systems were most tolerant).

Analysis of the characteristics of fighter aircrew undergoing centrifuge training at the Naval

Table 9.17.
Clinical Parameters Associated With the High-G and Low-G Tolerance Subgroups*

Parameter	High-Tolerance Group (HTG)	Low-Tolerance Group (LTG)
Age (yr)	37 ± 5	32 ± 8
Height (in)	68.4 ± 1.6	71.3 ± 2.3
Weight (lb)	172 ± 23	157 ± 19
Flying hours	3196 (high-5000; low-650)	1798 (high-3860; low-0)
Treadmill test		
Maximum heart rate (beats/min)	176 ± 7	186 ± 6
Maximum time (min)	14.0 ± 3.1	14.1 ± 2.9
Maximum systolic blood pressure (mmHg)	184 ± 11	171 ± 8
Maximum distolic blood pressure (mmHg)	91 ± 13	72 ± 15
Rest		
Heart rate (beats/min)	75 ± 17	69 ± 13
Systolic blood pressure (mmHg)	135 ± 10	115 ± 13
Diastolic blood pressure (mmHg)	86 ± 19	68 ± 8
Lean body mass (lb)	132 ± 9	131 ± 19
Percent body fat	23 ± 8	18 ± 7
Hematocrit (%)	48.3 ± 0.8	45.2 ± 0.2
Hemoglobin (g%)	15.8 ± 0.6	15.1 ± 0.6
Cholesterol (mg%)	222 ± 35	165 ± 10
Triglyceride (mg%)	169 ± 77	92 ± 30
Blood sugar (mg%)	112 ± 14	106 ± 11
Urine specific gravity	1.026 ± 0.004	1.021 ± 0.007

* Mean ± S.D.

Table 9.18.
Comparison of Several Parameters Between Most-SACM Tolerant (Two Subjects) With Least-SACM Tolerant (Three Subjects) (31)

Parameter	Most Tolerant[a] (n = 10)[b]	Least Tolerant[a] (n = 15)	Difference[c] (%)
V_{O2}	0.62 ± 0.03	0.90 ± 0.05	+45
VC_{O2}	0.65 ± 0.04	0.99 ± 0.08	+52
R	1.05 ± 0.03	1.10 ± 0.04	
Lactate (SACM)	24.9 ± 2.5	49.9 ± 2.5	+100
Pyruvate (SACM)	0.49 ± 0.09	1.12 ± 0.12	+129
Glucose (SACM)	126 ± 7.4	134 ± 5.2	
Heart Rate			
Max (during SACM)	147 ± 1.7	196 ± 2.2	+15
30 s (recovery)	97.5 ± 4.2	135 ± 5.2	+38
Fatigue (1–10)[d]	1.5	6.7	
B.V. (% reduction)	11.8 ± 2.0	15.0 ± 0.9	
Sa_{O2}	86.4 ± 0.3	81.9 ± 0.6	−5
Pa_{O2}[e]	55	48	
Performance			
Error	120 ± 5.3	141 ± 8.2	−18

[a] X ± S.E.
[b] n = number of observations (five observations per subject)
[c] [(Least-most)/most] × 100 = % difference—determined if differences between groups are statistically different ($P < 0.05$)
[d] high number indicates more fatigue
[e] mmHg

Air Warfare Center has revealed specific correlations with respect to the occurrence of G-LOC episodes during the training profiles. From a group of 520 aviators, 98 individuals experienced a G-LOC episode during the training. In comparison to those that did not have a G-LOC episode, the G-LOC aircrew had a lower GOR relaxed tolerance, less tactical flying hours, were younger, and if a recent illness had occurred, they had fewer days since the illness resolved. The strongest predictor for having G-LOC during centrifuge training was the number of tactical aircraft flying hours—the least flying hours, the most likely to experience G-LOC.

Thermal

An increase in the ambient (cockpit) temperature that either increases the body core temperature or produces dehydration will significantly reduce both relaxed and SACM type G tolerances; e.g., 3% dehydration results in a 40% reduction in SACM tolerance times. Cold, if shivering is induced, will increase relaxed ROR tolerances by a net 0.4 G.

Inhaled Gas Mixtures

Inhaled gas mixtures that are hypo- or hyperoxic cause minor changes in relaxed G-level tolerances depending upon the direct effect on P_a. Hypoxia of 10% inhaled oxygen reduces P_a by 10 mmHg (about 0.5 G) and 100% oxygen increases P_a by 11 mmHg (about 0.5 G). However, with breathing 100% oxygen and exposure to increased G while wearing an anti-G suit, an undesirable pulmonary pathologic condition known as atelectasis may occur. Atelectasis exhibits symptoms of retrosternal chest pain and a dry cough.

Increased levels of CO_2 in the inhaled gas (7.6% CO_2) significantly increase P_a by 30 mmHg (an increase of more than 1 G) and cerebral blood flow by 75%. Because of these beneficial physiologic effects, CO_2 added to breathing gas has been considered an anti-G protection system. Hyperventilation will reduce P_{aCO_2} and temporarily increase P_a by 8 mmHg, a slight in-

crease in G-level tolerance. However, rapid breathing during G will probably not cause hypocapnia because right-to-left shunting in the lung venous admixtures keep the P_{aCO_2} relatively constant during increased ventilatory volumes that occur during the AGSM (Table 9.9).

G-Exposure Requirements

The ability to tolerate high-G ACM appears to decrease with reduced exposures. It is believed that at least one weekly exposure to high G is necessary to maintain maximum G tolerance. Certainly, aircrew who have not flown for several weeks should re-enter the high-G environment cautiously by first performing lower-level G maneuvers. If several months or years of not flying at high G have elapsed, flight surgeons should recommend AGSM refresher training on the centrifuge. Of particular concern should be illness, especially illness that includes bedrest (0 G simulation)—a condition that may exacerbate a decline in G tolerance.

Nutrition

The importance of nutrition to G tolerance is not completely understood. Relaxed G-level tolerance studies measured the effects of hypoglycemia induced with insulin injections. In one study, no changes in relaxed G tolerance were found with either hyperglycemia or hypoglycemia. However, in another study, a decrease of 0.6 G with hypoglycemia and an increase of 0.5 G above control levels occurred during the reactive portion of the hypoglycemia attack. These changes in G tolerance appear to follow hypoglycemia-related arterial blood pressure changes. A synergistic decrease in $+G_z$ tolerance was measured by slowed EEG activity with a combination of hyperventilation and hypoglycemia.

A stomach full of water appears to enhance G tolerance (< 1 G) although the variability is quite large. The mechanism for this action is controversial—the result of increased abdominal pressure or better support for the diaphragm. This latter effect would keep the diaphragm and heart from descending during acceleration, and consequently minimize the height of the heart-brain vascular column. Preventing a heart descent of 5 cm would provide increased tolerance by 0.3 G (Eq. 9)—about that observed for ingesting a liter of water.

Alcohol

Alcohol reduces G-tolerance, but much less than investigators had expected. Drinking 4 ounces of whiskey reduced the tolerance 0.2 G in a 2 to 4 hour period after ingestion. The effect is a result of peripheral vasodilation. The major detrimental effect of alcohol is not in reducing G tolerance, but in the synergistic effects with increased G that reduces performance. At a blood alcohol of 0.1% (i.e., legally drunk), 1 G performance was decreased about 40%, but when combined with acceleration, it was further reduced about 10% per G (at 5 G, it was decreased 90%).

Therefore, it is generally accepted, and for good reasons, that aircrew be prohibited from drinking alcohol a minimum of 12 hours before flight. The idea is, of course, that aircrew should not fly under the influence of alcohol. However, the 12-hour rule is not always enough, and recent experiments show that even if blood alcohol concentration is zero, aircrew performance can be impaired for 48 hours after intake of large amounts of alcohol because of the "hangover." Also dehydration, known to reduce G tolerance, is common the day after a night of excessive alcohol consumption.

Drugs

Acceleration studies have used drugs experimentally to either enhance or reduce G tolerance; clinical drugs have been tested for side effects that reduce G tolerance. Drugs used experimentally to increase G-level tolerance, such as epinephrine, ephedrine, and amphetamines, affect the sympathetic nervous system. They were not generally effective in raising G-level tolerances. Vasodilators or drugs used to abolish vasoconstriction that usually reduce G-level tolerance include tetraethyl ammonium salts and dibenzyline (phenoxybenzamine).

Clinical drugs, including aldactazide and propanolol, used for treating hypertension neither significantly reduce G-level tolerance nor affect P_a, although the increase in heart rate (HR) from the G exposure was significantly reduced in those individuals taking propanolol (IV 0.25 mg/kg body mass). This increase in HR was not required to maintain cardiac output (that was not altered) because there was an increase in peripheral resistance and stroke volume, probably resulting from the unmasked alpha activity (beta blockage from propanolol) that caused a compensating venoconstriction.

No information is available concerning the effects of illegal drugs on G tolerance. However, considering the synergistic effects of alcohol and increased G in reducing performance, their anticipated negative effects would be significant.

RECOVERY FROM HSG EXPOSURES

During the immediate post-G period, the physiologic recovery period is generally related to the physiologic basis of the activities that had occurred during the G exposure. These physiologic responses to HSG are generally characterized as sympathetic and stress responses with tachycardia, vasoconstriction, venous return that may be becoming inadequate, and accumulated lactic acid. In this physiologic recovery, there is a fast neurogenic component and slower hormonal components of epinephrine and cortisol acting long after the G exposure has ended. A sizable O_2 debt may have developed during the G exposure because of: (a) the increased metabolic requirement of the AGSM, (b) the reduced oxygen carrying capacity of the blood ($\dot{V}/\dot{Q}$ inequalities), (c) the reduced blood flow to the muscles, and (d) the anaerobic share of the AGSM. Elimination of the oxygen debt is an important consideration in the physiologic recovery of an individual to the high-G environment.

Cardiovascular

Cardiovascular recovery is unique in the HSG environment because, at its completion, a large volume of blood is rapidly shifted toward the heart. This blood volume shift distends the heart, causing increased stroke volume and cardiac output that raises P_a. Fortunately, during G exposure, circulating blood volume depletion has occurred so that less blood volume is circulating at the end of the G exposure. The cardiovascular system is limited with options to accommodate this shift in blood volume and control the P_a at the end of G: (a) systemic vasodilation, (b) slowed HR, (c) increased heart and lung blood volumes, and (d) increased blood flow in the muscles of the upper torso. Total blood volumes require about 20 minutes to return to control values after 5 repeated SACMs. Immediately after the last SACM, BV was reduced by 16.5%, 10.9% after 5 minutes, 6.3% at 10 minutes, and only 2.2% at 17.5 minutes post-G exposure (31).

Heart rhythm recovery has been discussed previously; there was an increased incidence in dysrhythmias most likely resulting from an excessive parasympathetic activity that followed an excessive sympathetic response. Development of marked sinus arrhythmia after an HSG exposure is typical. This dysrhythmia becomes particularly exaggerated approximately 1 minute after the G exposure ends. The heart rate can be reduced to lower than pre-G levels; thus, heart rate recovery and its physiologic basis are complex. Certainly, the baroceptors are attempting to *slow* the heart because of the increase in P_a (see the following section on P_a recovery). However, the volume receptors of the right heart, because of the immediate increase in venous return, are stimulating the cardiac center in the brain to *increase* the heart rate.

Heart rate recovery has been used as a measure of fatigue from G exposure. This measure of fatigue—developed by exercise physiologists and related to bicycle ergometry workload—is the sum of all of the heart beats after the G exposure until the pre-G (resting) HR returns (called

the "erholungspulssume" ESP). Although this determination is complicated by sinus arrhythmia that occurs post-G, it was useful in comparing the AGSM with unassisted PBG. An ESP of 108 ± 11.2 (mean $\pm$ S.E.) was found for an 8 G exposure using the AGSM and only 66.2 ± 12.8 with PBG. Smaller ESPs were found after lower G exposures (6). Complete recovery of HR after a high-G exposure may take several minutes. After 150 seconds of recovery, a mean HR of 104 was determined after a 10 G peak SACM with a pre-G (control) level of 72 bpm. Repeating this SACM five times with 4-minute rest periods between exposures prolonged this recovery period; i.e., mean HR was 111 bpm after 150 seconds of recovery.

The recovery of P_a after HSG includes a pressure "overshoot" that is directly related to the duration and level of the prior G. Carotid sinus denervation of cats prevents this P_a overshoot, suggesting that the vasoconstriction usually following the vasodilative inhibiting activity of the baroceptor is prevented.

Respiratory and Metabolic

Duration of the recovery of S_{aO_2} is a direct function of the previous level of G. After a 1-minute, 7 G exposure, recovery of S_{aO_2} took about 60 seconds, whereas it took 30 seconds to recover after a 3-G exposure. After a 95-second, 8-G peak SACM, S_{aO_2} recovery also took about 60 seconds. This recovery is hyperbolic; thus, the majority of recovery occurs within the first 30 seconds of 1 G. However, if the SACM begins before S_{aO_2} recovery is complete, cumulative reductions in S_{aO_2} will occur. Total expired gas flow, VO_2, and VCO_2 all appear to be recovered 5 to 10 minutes after the last of five repeated SACMs.

Pyruvate recovery to pre-G levels takes about 20 minutes after five SACM exposures. Glucose levels that increased during five repeated SACMs appear to recover to pre-G levels after resting for approximately 10 minutes at 1 G (24). Lactate recovery particularly signals metabolic recovery after HSG because a significant portion of the energy base for high G tolerance is anaerobic. Lactate blood levels increase significantly during G with an exponential recovery period of 15–20 minutes, although some elevation of blood lactate levels appear to persist after 20 minutes, indicating a continuing recovery of the energy capacity of the body. This response is similar to that of muscle fatigue after sustained isometric contractions at 1 G; i.e., generally, more than 90% recovery has occurred during a 20-minute rest period after fatiguing exercise, but recovery is still incomplete. The effect of this incomplete recovery upon the G-duration and G-level tolerances with successive SACMs is not known; it can be assumed after an SACM to fatigue that, without adequate rest, a repeated SACM would not be as well-tolerated—fatigue will become cumulative. Unfortunately we do not have specific data that verifies complete physiologic recovery from HSG exposures. During experiments, we do not usually expose subjects to an SACM to fatigue more often than once every other day because of fatigue-recovery concerns. Pilots of high performance aircraft should be aware that cumulative fatigue, such as that experienced flying repeated sorties (with ACMs) the same day, reduces G tolerances with an increased risk of G-LOC.

Subjective Fatigue

Subjective fatigue was not complete 20 minutes after five 10 G SACM exposures. The pre-G fatigue score was 12.4, which lowered to 7.8 immediately after the last SACM exposure (a lower score indicates more fatigue), and was 10.2 after 20 minutes of recovery (24). Fatigue recovery using the same subjective fatigue scoring was measured 20 minutes after a fatiguing 4.5–7 G SACM. Pre-SACM scores were 15–16 with immediate post-SACM scores of 6–8. After 20 minutes of recovery, fatigue scores had increased 11–12, but were still well below the pre-G exposure scores. Obviously, subjective recovery from the fatigue induced by HSG exposures is not complete after resting for 20 minutes.

PROTECTION AGAINST $+G_Z$

Several methods have been developed to increase G-level and/or G-duration tolerances. Although these are called methods of *protection*, it must be remembered that these aircrews are still experiencing G forces; i.e., in reality, these methods of increasing G tolerance increase the level of the hazard to which the aircrew are subjected.

Anti-G Suit and Its Inflation

The anti-G suit invented by David Clark in World War II remains operational today, with only minor changes. This anti-G suit is considered the basic component of anti-G protection systems. This suit, composed of five interconnected bladders, covers the legs and abdominal region (Fig. 9.22). It is pressurized during increases in G (controlled by the anti-G valve) with air from the jet engine compressor. Suit pressure is increased by 1.5 psi per G beginning at about 2 G to a maximum suit pressure of about 10 psi. For maximum anti-G suit protection, suit inflation must be completed within 1 second (maximum lag period of suit inflation) after

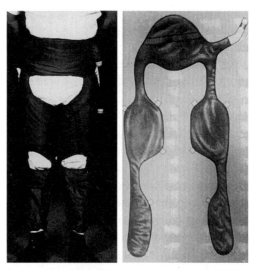

Figure 9.22. The USAF CSU-12/P anti-G suit with bladders.

obtaining the maximum G level. Too rapid anti-G suit inflation is uncomfortable and pre-G exposure inflation increases P_a above 120 mmHg, theoretically stimulating a baroceptor response with resulting vasodilation and an unwanted drop in P_a. The discomfort in the abdominal region that accompanies an extremely rapid abdominal bladder inflation is probably caused by diaphragm stretching.

The anti-G suit increases relaxed ROR and GOR G-level tolerance about 1–1.5 G. This suit protection includes 0.3–0.5 G that occurs with just putting on a properly fitted anti-G suit. About 80% of the remaining protection (1.0–1.2 G) is provided by the abdominal bladder. The abdominal bladder upwardly displaces the diaphragm and heart, reducing the eye-heart vertical distance (h of Eq. 9) and increasing vascular resistance in the splanchnic region; consequently, considerable venous blood is mobilized, rapidly enhancing venous return and cardiac output. The leg portion of the suit accounts for the remaining 20% of the (1.0-1.2 G) protection by increasing resistance of the leg vasculature.

The leg coverage of the anti-G suit has been recently increased with the development of the advanced technology anti-G suit (ATAGS). Flight-test results found improved comfort with an increase in G-level tolerance and a major increase in G-duration tolerance. The reduction in fatigue is probably a result of improved blood flow through the skeletal leg muscles used in the AGSM, removing lactic acid from the muscles. It increases the total vascular resistance below the heart, maintaining blood volume distribution within the body to that found in a 1-G environment. This more ''natural'' distribution of blood volume during high-G exposure provides a greater ''functional'' blood volume, eliminating the greatly increased right ventricular volume that occurs immediately after an increased G exposure. It possibly reduces cardiac dysrhythmias post-G as well.

The anti-G suit increases G-level tolerance by increasing eye-level P_a (Fig. 9.23) with greater vascular resistance, stroke volume (index), and cardiac output, and with less changes in heart rate (Table 9.2). G tolerance also increases somewhat because the eye-heart vertical distance is reduced by elevating the heart with the inflated abdominal bladder of the anti-G suit. The anti-G suit is also effective in reducing the physiologic stress response of the G exposure (Fig. 9.24) by reducing the amount of fluid shift below the heart (Fig. 9.25) and increasing blood flow to all organs of the body (Fig. 9.26).

Anti-G Straining Maneuver (AGSM)

The idea of a muscular straining maneuver to increase G tolerance was first proposed by Steinforth in England in 1933. It was further developed by Drs. Baldes and Wood at the Mayo Clinic (circa 1943); it became known as the M-1 maneuver when it was transitioned to fighter pilots. The M-1 used in conjunction with the anti-G suit proved effective in increasing G-level tolerance, which provided a substantial increase in aircraft capability in the European theater of operations in World War II. Developed nearly five decades ago, it still remains the principal means used to increase G tolerance *above* the 5 G of protection afforded by the operational anti-G suit (32).

The AGSM is a forced exhalation effort against a closed (L-1 maneuver) or partially closed (M-1 maneuver) glottis while tensing leg, arm, and abdominal muscles to maintain vision and consciousness. The higher G levels, to maintain higher intrathoracic pressure, require a greater straining effort. The major problem with the use of the AGSM is that it is fatiguing; it severely limits the duration of high-G that can be tolerated.

The respiratory aspect of the AGSM is an adaptation of the Valsalva maneuver that produces a high intrathoracic pressure (100 mmHg maximum). However, unlike the Valsalva maneuver test that challenges the circulatory system to cope with a reduced venous return, the AGSM interrupts the effort at 3 to 4 second intervals with a rapid expiration/inspiration effort (<1

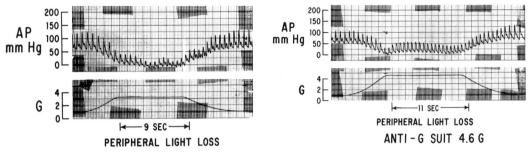

Figure 9.23. Light loss symptoms related to eye-level P_a with and without an inflated anti-G suit. G-level tolerance was increased 1.4 G with the anti-G suit.

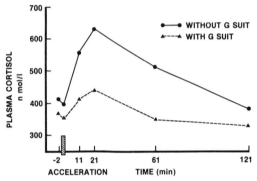

Figure 9.24. Plasma cortisol, an indicator of the physiologic stress response to 6 G for 1 min, is reduced with the anti-G suit. Reprinted with permission from Mills FJ. The endocrinology of stress. Aviat Space Environ Med 1985;56:642–650.

second) that for a brief period of time allows adequate venous return because of a low intrathoracic pressure. Although the head-level P_a falls to nearly zero in conjunction with a lowered thoracic pressure, the period of time is so brief (<1 second) that the brain and retinal tissue oxygen/energy reservoir maintains vision and consciousness. The relationship between the intrathoracic pressure (as measured with esophageal pressure) and eye-level P_a is shown in Figure 9.27. The P_a increase is immediate with an increase in intrathoracic (esophageal) pressure; i.e., an effective anti-G method.

In order to support venous return during the 3 to 4 second forced exhalation phase, anti-G suit inflation pressure must be four times greater than the intrathoracic pressure. This level of

anti-G suit pressure is always present because it increases sufficiently with increasing G. When the AGSM is required, adequate anti-G suit pressure is available; e.g., at 6 G when 0.5 psi (25 mmHg or 3.5 kPa) intrathoracic pressure (AGSM) is required, a minimum of 2 psi anti-G suit pressure is needed, but the anti-G suit is pressurized at 6 G to 6 psi (41.4 kPa). Nine G requires 2 psi (14 kPa) of intrathoracic pressure; the anti-G suit pressure is 10 psi or 70 kPa, yet only 8 psi is needed for a 4:1 pressure ratio.

The AGSM is a learned maneuver; therefore, it must be taught to aircrew. An effective and safe teaching platform is formal AGSM training on a human-use centrifuge. The Naval Air Warfare Center centrifuge training program particularly favors teaching the AGSM as the "hook" maneuver (33). Benefits of the hook maneuver include: (a) easy to teach, (b) easy to critique and correct during centrifuge training, (c) rapidly mastered, (d) easy to remember and rapidly recall (if it is needed, just say "hook"), (e) proven effectiveness, (f) proven to be highly acceptable by aircrew, (g) effective for evaluating AGSM performance from audio portion of inflight video recordings, and (h) facilitates inflight incident and mishap analysis of possible G-LOC when audio recordings are available. Aircrew nominated to fly high performance aircraft of most nations receive training in centrifuges dedicated to pilot training before they fly these aircraft. The USAF G-training centrifuge is located at Holloman AFB, New Mexico. The

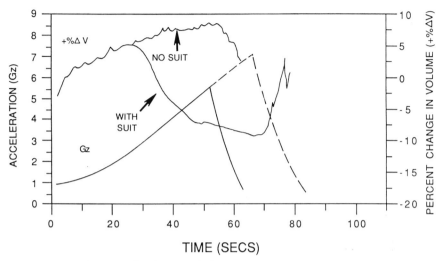

Figure 9.25. Percentage change in fluid volume below the heart is reduced during GOR with the anti-G suit. Reprinted with permission from Burton RR, Smith AH. Adaptation to acceleration environments. In: Fregly MJ, Blattis CM, eds. Handbook of physiology: environmental physiology. IV. the gravitational environment. New York: Oxford University Press, 1996; 943–970.

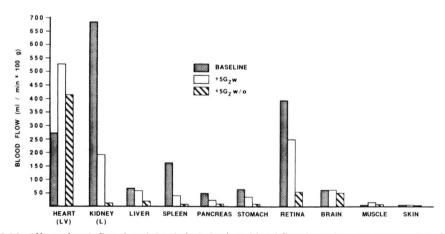

Figure 9.26. Effect of an inflated anti-G suit ($+5\,G_zw$) on blood flow in various organs at $+5\,G_z$ for 60 sec on unanesthetized baboons. Baseline is at $+1\,G_x$ (animal at rest on its back) immediately before the $+G_z$ exposure. Reprinted with permission from Whinnery JE. Observations on the neurophysiologic theory of acceleration ($+G_z$) induced loss of consciousness. Aviat Space Environ Med 1989;60:589–593.

USN centrifuge training is accomplished at Lemore NAS, California.

Physical Conditioning

The physiologic basis for the AGSM is primarily fueled anaerobically with muscular strength as a principal factor in its intensity that provides the G-level protection capability. Both anaerobic capacity and muscular strength can be increased with a weight-lifting, high-intensity, physical conditioning program. Research has shown that a 10 to 12 week weight-lifting program can increase G-duration tolerance approximately 50% compared with a nonexercising control group (34). Recent studies have shown a direct individ-

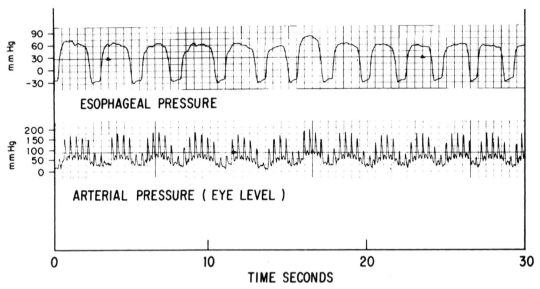

Figure 9.27. Mean eye-level arterial blood pressure and esophageal pressure changes during +G$_z$ in a subject performing an AGSM. Reprinted with permission from Burton RR, Smith AH. Adaptation to acceleration environments. In: Fregly MJ, Blattis CM, eds. Handbook of physiology: environmental physiology. IV. the gravitational environment. New York: Oxford University Press, 1996; 943–970.

ual correlation between muscular strength and G-duration tolerance (4). Aerobic conditioning, such as distance running, has no effect on G tolerance (Fig. 9.28). However, excessive aerobic conditioning in certain individuals may: (a) cause serious cardiac dysrhythmias associated with reduced G tolerance, (b) increase susceptibility to motion sickness on the centrifuge, and (c) increase the length of time of incapacitation with G-LOC. Some aerobically conditioned individuals had episodes of marked cardiac slowing; the longest sinus arrest we have observed was 12 seconds, and was associated with loss of consciousness lasting more than 30 seconds. Therefore, jogging excessively should be approached with caution.

Current recommendations suggest that jogging should not exceed 9 miles (14.5 km) per week. The 1988 publication "Physical Fitness Program to Enhance Aircrew Tolerance" (a joint USAF/USN report, USAFSAM-SR-88-1, NAMRL-1334) is recommended as a physical training guide for aircrew of high performance aircraft. The information in reference 4 is also relevant to this topic.

Positive Pressure Breathing

Assisted positive pressure breathing during G (PBG), as a method of reducing the fatigue associated with the AGSM, is the latest G protection method. The USAF version, named "combat edge," uses a chest-counterpressure garment (jerkin) that is worn and inflated at the same pressure as the mask that increases the intrapulmonary pressure. This jerkin counteracts high levels of positive pressures required for G protection (e.g., 60 mmHg or 7.5 kPa). In conjunction with the use of a standard type anti-G suit with a standard inflation rate, the mask and jerkin are pressurized at 15 mmHg (1.9 kPa) per G, beginning at 4 G to a maximum at 9 G of 60 mmHg (7.5 kPa). Higher PBG pressures do not appear to add to G protection. These pressures are controlled by a single anti-G valve with dual controlled simultaneous pressurization schedules for the anti-G suit and PBG system. For safety reasons, this valve is programmed so that if anti-G suit pressurization fails, PBG cannot occur. Centrifuge studies and early flight-test data suggest that the fatigue that develops during

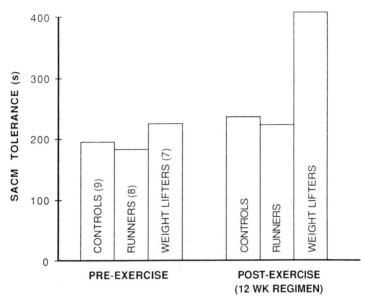

Figure 9.28. Effects of 12 weeks of aerobic training (runners) or strength training (weight lifters) compared with control subjects (no physical conditioning) on SACM tolerance (4,34).

high G maneuvers with the AGSM is reduced by about 50%; i.e., a 5 to 9 G SACM tolerance time is doubled with PBG. Basically, positive pressure within the lung at 60 mmHg accounts for about 2 G of protection that reduces the requirement for the AGSM by 50% at 9 G. With this system, the AGSM, essentially eliminated at 7 G, significantly reduces fatigue. The PBG/ATAGS combination ideally will offer high anti-G protection that will allow many pilots to tolerate 9 G sustained with minimal or no AGSM.

Water Immersion Protection

Anti-G suits filled with water instead of with air have been developed with less than satisfactory results. The concept of immersing an individual in water, providing external hydrostatic pressures for protection against intravascular hydrostatic pressures, theoretically holds great promise. Early in World War II, Dr. Franks from Canada developed a water-filled anti-G suit that was used sparingly in combat. As an extra benefit, it provided additional water for fighter pilots shot down in the desert. But with the develop-

ment of the air-filled anti-G suit system, Dr Franks' flying suit (FFS) was soon replaced in combat aircraft. The water-filled anti-G suit is heavy, must cover the body to the neck, must be leakproof, has mobility problems, and fails to provide the expected G protection. Recent attempts with modern materials and advanced water-filled suit designs provide less G protection than PBG with ATAGS.

Postural Modification

The most effective method for enhancing G tolerance and protecting the pilot is to reduce the vertical (effective) height of the eye-heart vascular column (h in Eq. 9). This reduction in h is made possible by either having the subject tilt forward (prone) or backward (supine) relative to the $+G_z$ vector. The idea of changing the position of the pilot relative to the G vector is not new. In the 1930s, German designers developed several reclining seats, some of which were flight tested, but none became operational. Their first seat was the DVL-1, or so-called ''flop back seat,'' that was developed and flight tested in 1938. It automatically reclined to a completely horizontal position at 3 G, resuming the conventional upright position upon a reduction of G forces. Other more sophisticated devices have been developed; some were flight tested, but the required major changes in cockpit design with new seat configurations and pilot positioning have prevented advanced development. The fixed 30° seat-back angle of the F-16 with a significant angle of attack (>10°) will position the pilot in the $+G_z$ vector so that some G protection is available. In one centrifuge study, duration was increased 38% and the GOR 15% (28). But pilots must sit back into the seat to gain this G advantage. It is generally agreed that F-16 pilots most frequently sit upright in the seat during the majority of ACM to increase their visual field of view. In the tilt-back seat, the most popular concept (over pronation) at the present time, the pilot can recline (become supine), decreasing the eye to heart distance (specifically the eye to aortic arch). The improvement in G tolerance, proportionally exponential to the decrease in vertical distance between the eye and heart, pervades all methods of G protection (Fig. 9.19). The beneficial effects of supination on reducing G stress is shown in Figure 9.29. Leg discomfort associated with HSG is reduced in tilt-back seats.

PHYSIOLOGIC EFFECTS OF OTHER ACCELERATIONS

The cardiovascular effects of the $+G_z$ environment (especially P_a effects) were found to be a function of the eye-heart vertical distance (h) that defined various G tolerances. This relationship was mathematically described in Equations 4 and 9. Therefore, as defined by these equations, subject orientation within G environment that significantly affects either the h distance (i.e., $\pm G_x$ or $\pm G_y$) or h direction (i.e, $\pm G_z$) profoundly affects P_a that, in turn, determines G tolerances and cardiovascular functions. Hence, as h is reduced, G tolerance increases and cardiovascular responses are diminished. If the subject becomes inverted (i.e., direction of h effect is

reversed, $-G_z$) then the cardiovascular system generally responds inversely from $+G_z$ exposure.

Negative ($-G_z$) Acceleration

Negative G_z is not usually an operational concern with fighter pilots because, during ACM, a simple roll maneuver will reverse the direction of the G on the pilot, thereby maintaining a $+G_z$ maneuver. However, some naval aviators use a push-over maneuver in combat that introduces a $-G_z$ component. Usually though, negative G_z is avoided during maneuver if possible because of discomfort and possible injury to the brain, although the latter has never been proved. In that regard, and as an example, an F-4 pilot during an in-flight accident was exposed to $-9\ G_z$ for approximately 30 seconds without serious pathologic sequelae. Some reversible soft tissue injury in the head region did occur; i.e., subcutaneous edema and hemorrhages. However, negative G_z is commonly flown during civilian aerobatics; exposures up to $-6\ G_z$ occur in outside loops (discussed later in this chapter, "Civilian Aerobatic Environment").

Cardiovascular Effects

The most profound cardiovascular effect of $-G_z$ is a decrease in heart rate that occurs in response to the baroreceptors located in the carotid sinus. Resting heart rates of about 100 bpm are reduced to 90 bpm at -1.5 G and 50 bpm at $-3\ G_z$. During civilian aerobatics, the mean maximum heart rate during the $+G_z$ maneuvers is about 165 bpm. Heart rate will quickly change during $-G_z$ maneuvers to 68 bpm (in one case, a low of 32 bpm was recorded at $-3.8\ G_z$). Individual heart rate changes, from 175 bpm to 50 bpm within 5 sec, are common during cycles of $\pm G_z$. Premature atrial and ventricular contractions are found, but are considered nonsignificant stress dysrhythmias. Repeated daily exposures to $-G_z$ over several weeks appear to reduce this cardiovascular response—a condition known as the "batman syndrome."

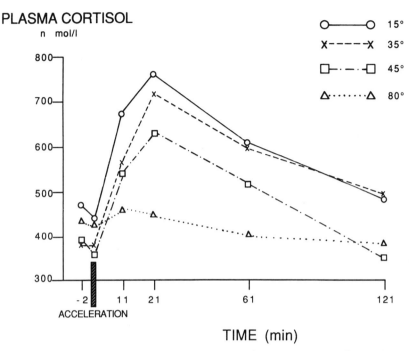

Figure 9.29. Reclining the seat back reduces physiologic stress from 6 G exposure for 1 min as measured with plasma cortisol levels. Reprinted with permission from Mills FJ. The endocrinology of stress. Aviat Space Environ Med 1985;56:642–650.

At one time, it was thought that a common symptom of $-G_z$ was a reddening of the visual field, called "red-out" or the "pink mist." However, "red-out" symptoms are not commonly reported by acrobatic pilots who are routinely exposed to $-G_z$ levels up to -5 G_z.

A concern with $-G_z$ relates to capillary fragility that could cause brain hemorrhage. Normally, pressure differences between brain tissue (cerebral spinal fluid—CSF) and blood vessels of 100 mmHg are considered sufficient to rupture small vessels, and because the pressure at the level of the brain will increase 25 mmHg per $-G_z$, physical limits could be reached at 3–3.5 $-G_z$. This pressure differential is the basis for the multiple petechial hemorrhages that appear under the unprotected skin in the lower body regions during $+G_z$ exposures and in the soft facial tissues (especially the eyes and conjunctival) in people subjected to higher levels of $-G_z$. However, studies with goats and cats found increases in cerebral venous and arteriolar pres-

sures in the brain that were similar to increases in the cerebral spinal fluid during G that afforded adequate protection for both types of vessels.

Pulmonary Effects

The knowledge of the effect of $-G_z$ on respiration in humans is quite limited because of concerns about the discomfort and safety of subjects and the lack of operational relevance of this environment. It is known, however, that inverting an individual—going from $+1$ G_z to -1 G_z—will provide more uniform lung perfusion. Subjects exposed to -3 G_z have reductions of: (a) 150 cc in total lung volume (TLV), (b) 400 cc in functional reduce capacity (FRC), and (c) 1 L in vital capacity (VC).

Prone/Supine $+G_x$ Acceleration

Supine exposure ($+G_x$) to acceleration has interested aviation physiologists for many decades; G-level tolerances can be significantly increased if subjects are reclined before the onset of G. German physiologists were aware of this G protection as early as 1935. However, the major problem with this method of increasing G tolerance is a limited visual field of view. Complex engineering problems are involved in a reclining cockpit position; neither supination nor pronation has been operationally used to increase G tolerance.

However, the National Aeronautics and Space Administration (NASA) did use $+G_x$ to protect astronauts in the Mercury and Apollo space programs from high G exposures during lift-off and reentry. In these situations, because takeoff and landing were essentially automated, the absence of specific visual fields of view were not an important consideration. Considerable research on the physiologic effects of $+G_x$ was conducted by NASA during the '50s and '60s. This physiologic information, especially on $+G_x$ exposure on the respiratory and cardiovascular systems, is available.

Cardiovascular Effects

Because h of Equation 9 is greatly reduced during prone or supine body positioning, the physical effects of $+G_x$ on the cardiovascular system of humans are considerably attenuated. A comparison of the effects between moderate levels of $+G_z$ and $+G_x$ on several cardiovascular parameters in six men is made in Table 9.19. Not surprisingly, the cardiovascular

effects of $+G_x$ are much less than with $+G_z$; i.e., cardiac output is decreased during $+G_z$ but increased during $+G_x$. Negative G_x (prone position) cardiovascular effects are generally similar to those of $+G_x$ (as are those of $\pm G_y$).

Atrial pressure is increased three- to fourfold at $+5$ G_x. If the head is elevated during $+G_x$ exposures, heart rate increases, indicating some baroceptor (carotid sinus) effect. At $+8$ G_x, heart rates (HR) are similar to HR for $+5$ G_x in pilots, but were increased 2 to 10% in nonpilot subjects. A reduction of 5 bpm with greater duration of exposure occurs with subjects breathing 100% oxygen with positive pressure breathing (PPB) of 3 mmHg per G.

As expected, heart arrhythmias are rare during $+G_x$. In one study involving nine men, premature atrial contraction (PAC) occurred at $+5$ G_x at 15 seconds in only one subject. At $+7$ G_x during 45-second exposures, three occurrences of PAC (one with aberrant conduction—AC) were found. Doubling the exposure to 90 seconds only doubled the occurrence of PAC with AC. At the onset of $+9$ G_x exposures and during the first 15 seconds, four occurrences of PAC (one with AC) were found. Certain subjects are more prone to G_x-induced arrhythmias.

No significant change was seen in QRS angle, but a statistically significant decrease in mean spatial vector was observed in a study of 15 men

Table 9.19.
Comparison of Relative Cardiovascular Effects of $+G_z$ and $+G_x$—Percentage Changes from Control (1 G_z) Values of Various Cardiovascular Parameters Found During Increased $+G_z$ or $+G_x$ Acceleration of 20–40 sec Duration in Subjects not Wearing Anti-G Suits (7)

G Field	Cardiac Output	Heart Rate	Stroke Volume	Mean Arterial Blood Pressure	Peripheral Resistance
± 2 G_z	-7%	$+14$	-24	$+9$	$+7$
± 3 G_z	-18	$+35$	-37	$+21$	$+41$
± 4 G_z	-22	$+56$	-49	$+27$	$+59$
± 2 G_x	-18	-4	-20	$+17$	$+36$
± 3.5 G_x	$+16$	$+19$	-1	$+19$	$+6$
± 5 G_x	$+11$	$+35$	-20	$+17$	$+10$

at 1 minute each at $+6$, $+8$, and $+10$ G_x. This change in the spatial vector is considered a G_x-cumulative effect.

Pulmonary/Respiration Effects

There is considerable difference between $+G_x$ and $-G_x$ regarding lung volumes and ventilation. These differences occur because during $-G_x$ the lung is not restricted by the spinal area as is the case during increased $+G_x$ with the subject in the supine position.

At $+6$ G_x, VC is reduced 50 to 75% over 1 G values, whereas at -6 G_x, there is only a reduction of 15%. At higher $+G_x$ levels, the inability of the subject to expand the chest wall upward (breathe) against the $+G_x$ force limits $+G_x$ human tolerance to about 15 G.

Distribution of ventilation in $+G_x$ is compartmentalized as for $+G_z$; closure occurs at about the same regional minimal volumes. Closure lung volumes, as a percent of total lung volume, increase with $+G_x$ exposure levels; there is a progressive reduction in FRC. Closure volumes at $+5$ G_x are doubled from 30% to 60% of total lung capacity (TLC) and FRC is reduced by half—40% to 20% of TLC. A reduction in FRC does not occur during $-G_x$; in fact, FRC may increase. Compliance of the lung during $+G_x$ is considerably reduced by as much as 40% at $+4$ G_x over a one liter tidal volume.

Breathing effort during increased $+G_x$ becomes greater and, with reduced functional lung volumes, a higher breathing frequency occurs; i.e., an increase in functional dead space. The increased breathing effort during $+G_x$ is caused by a major increase in the elastic component and total breathing effort (doubled at $+4$ G_x over 1 G). Respiratory frequency increases from 11 bpm at rest to 22 bpm at 5 G_x to 30 bpm at 8 G_x. Minute volumes increase from 8 L/min to 10.9 L/min at 5 G_x to 12.2 at 8 G_x. Oxygen consumption increases from 300 ml/min at 1 G to 350 ml/min at 5 G_x. Much of this increase in O_2 consumption is a function of the increase in breathing effort.

The increase in ventilation frequency from

10.7 at 1 G to 14.5 at 4 G, and with an increase in unperfused and underventilated alveolae, P_{ACO_2} decreases from 39 mmHg at 1 G to 32 mmHg at $+4$ G_x. However, because of the increase in underventilated alveolae, total alveolar ventilation (V_A) during $+G_x$ is reduced by 6% per increase in each G level; i.e., at $+8$ G_x, V_A is reduced by 50%. Conversely, at -8 G_x, with increasing lung volume, V_A is increased to 150% of 1 G values.

Lung perfusion during $+G_x$, much like $+G_z$, is unevenly distributed within the lung; there is increased blood volume (shunting from right to left) in the lung near the back "bottom" of the lung and no perfusion at the "top" of the lung at the sternum. Pulmonary right-to-left shunting at $+6$ G_x amounts to 42% of total lung blood volume. Alveolae that are ventilated near the "top" of the lung are not perfused, and richly perfused alveolae at the "bottom" of the lung are not ventilated. Consequently, this mismatch in $\dot{V}/\dot{Q}$ ratio significantly reduces S_{aO_2} while breathing air above $+2$ G_x. In breathing air at 4 G for 2 minutes, S_{aO_2} goes to 90% and to 80% after 2 minutes at 5.4 G. The time factor for a decreasing S_{aO_2} is a 3% reduction every 10 seconds at $+7$ Gx until an 80% S_{aO_2} is reached. Breathing air with PPB at 30 mmHg per G does not affect this reduction in S_{aO_2}. However, breathing 100% O_2 with or without PPB prevents any reduction in S_{aO_2} at $+7$ G_x for 90 seconds. Therefore, most of the right-to-left shunting is physiologic. $-G_x$, however, has little effect on S_{aO_2} while breathing air. One minute at -6 G_x results in no reduction in arterial saturation.

Acceleration atelectasis occurs at $+5.6–6.4$ G_x in a subject breathing 100% oxygen who is not wearing an anti-G suit. Remember, the anti-G suit is required to produce acceleration atelectasis during $+G_z$. It is not required during $+G_x$ exposure because lung volumes are limited by the spinal area. Lung volumes are not restricted during $-G_x$, thus acceleration atelectasis is not a problem.

TOLERANCES TO OTHER ACCELERATIONS

Negative Acceleration

Discomfort because of head/face soft tissue swelling limits a human's *voluntary* tolerance to $-G_z$. Although no maximum tolerance determinations have been made in humans, pilots tolerate -6 G_z routinely during aerobatics. Also, remember that the USAF pilot who was exposed to -9 G_z for approximately 30 seconds survived without permanent medical sequelae. It appears, therefore, that human tolerances to $-G_z$ are considerably greater than previously imagined because of the high cerebral spinal fluid pressures that protect the cerebral vascular system.

In a study of 305 episodes of negative 1–1.8 G_z with immediate re-exposure to increased $+G_z$, there was a reduction of about 40% in $+G_z$ tolerance. Pilots who develop $-G_z$ during push-over maneuvers that are followed by increased $+G_z$ should be aware of this $+G_z$ tolerance deficiency.

Prone/Supine Acceleration

The horizontal position of the body in the G field essentially reduces h of Equation 9 to a very small number. Therefore, $+G_x$ tolerance is totally independent of the physical effects of G on the cardiovascular physiology. Hence, a time intensity relaxed tolerance curve as determined for $+G_z$ based on cardiovascular responses (Fig. 9.17) is inappropriate. A limiting tolerance factor for some subjects during $+G_x$ appears to be increased effort during inspiration. Specific subject complaints include difficulty in breathing, discomfort in the throat region, and soft tissue edema (swelling) that lead to termination of the G exposure. If this pain can be tolerated for a long period, hypoxemia from reduced alveolar ventilation and V/Q inequalities will theoretically become limiting during $+G_x$ exposures. However, fatigue

from breathing effort primarily limits $+G_x$ tolerance, which in humans is about $+15$ G_x. In one study, $+12$ G_x was tolerated for 60 seconds, 10 G for 2 minutes, 8 G for 2.5 minutes, 6 G for 4.5 minutes, 4 G for 8 minutes, and 3 G for 15 minutes. Similar duration tolerances were found for $-G_x$ exposures.

THE IN-FLIGHT ENVIRONMENT

Military Environment

The military in-flight environment is uniquely multivariant. Its acceleration profiles are aircraft- and mission-dependent. The most stressful of military in-flight environments is probably that of ACM. A representative description of the in-flight acceleration environment includes (35):

1. Durations of the entire flight and of the G maneuvering
2. Rate of G onset/offset
3. Peak G
4. G-time integration

These parameters closely parallel the in-flight acceleration environment used in the aeromedical research laboratory. Physiologic stress responses using subjective and biochemical indicators of F-15 and F-106 pilots following ACM activities between these different aircraft showed that the ACM was fatiguing and elicited a moderate stress response—an increase in urinary epinephrine (54%), norepinephrine (19%), and 17-OHCS (20%) (35).

G-time recording of ACMs for the F-15 showed a maximum of $+7.5$ G_z. The maximum rate of onset was greater than $+6$ G_z/sec. The maneuvering time was approximately 300 seconds. The maximum $-G_z$ was -0.5 G_z. In-flight recordings of 1-hour aerial combat sorties (F-16 versus F-16) showed maximum $+9.0$ G_z levels. The maximum rate of onset

Table 9.20.
Mean and Maximum Values for Aerial Combat Maneuvers for Various Aircraft for Specific Numbers of Engagements (36)

Aircraft		Max G-onset Rate (G/s)	Peak G Load (G)	Time Spent at or Above:				Engage. Duration (s)	Fraction of Enge. Spent at or Above				# of Peaks at or Above			
				5G (s)	6G (s)	7G (s)	8G (s)		5G	6G	7G	8G	5G	6G	7G	8G
F-4E (7 engagements)	Mean	1.13	6.0	13.1	1.2	0	0	176	.07	0	0	0	2.9	0.7	0	0
	Max	1.8	6.8	29.9	3.5	0	0	332	.12	.01	0	0	5	2	0	0
F-5G (12 engagements)	Mean	1.13	5.9	9.5	1.4	0.4	0	66	.15	.02	0	0	2	0.8	0.2	0.1
	Max	3.0	8.2	25.0	10.5	4.4	0.5	158	.37	.20	.08	.01	10	6	1	1
F-15G (58 engagements)	Mean	2.06	6.83	21.8	8.4	1.3	0	143	.17	.07	.01	0	3.7	2.1	0.6	0.1
	Max	6.3	8.2	72.2	45.5	18.1	0.8	303	.60	.30	.10	0	14	9	6	1
F-16G (21 engagements)	Mean	1.73	7.11	20.3	7.8	2.0	0.2	160	.14	.06	.02	0	3.1	1.7	0.8	0.14
	Max	3.0	8.4	56.4	33.1	10.2	1.9	292	.51	.29	.16	.02	11	3	3	1

was greater than $+6$ G/sec. The maximum $-G_z$ was -0.2 G_z. The maximum angle of attack was directly related to the maximum $+G_z$ level.

Acceleration profiles of four models of high performance aircraft performing ACM have been developed and summarized in Table 9.20 (36). The "usual ACM" has peak loads of 9 G that can recur frequently with varying G levels for several minutes, several G onset per second, with an average integrated $\times$ G time of 1000 G/sec for a 3-minute ACM. This ACM can be repeated several times a day, several days per week, per month, per year. It is possible that over a "lifetime" career flying high performance for 20 years, a pilot will be exposed to 18,720,000 G $\times$ sec representing a total of 36 days exposed to an average of 6 G—a G level that requires the use of an AGSM.

Aircraft-Centrifuge G-Tolerance Comparisons

Generally, studies of acceleration tolerance are performed on centrifuges—where conditions

Table 9.21.
Relaxed Tolerances Compared in Aircraft or on the Centrifuge Without Anti-G Suits (37)

Criteria (Light Loss)	Centrifuge	Aircraft	
		Passenger	Pilot
Dim	3.3	4.0	4.6
PLL	3.6	4.3	5.0
CLL	3.9	4.7	5.3

are controlled, and acceleration field strength is the only variable. However, in aircraft, the environment is much less uniform: (a) fluctuations in cockpit temperature, (b) frequently changed body positions, (c) anticipation of the flight, and (d) various other human factor reasons that can introduce variables that alter tolerance limits in flight significantly from those determined on the centrifuge.

Tolerance comparisons have been made between the aircraft and centrifuge using experimental subjects and pilots (same individuals) exposed to both environments without anti-G suits (37). The results are shown in Table 9.21. The higher pilot relaxed G tolerance relative to that for the passenger is, to a large extent, the result of pulling on the stick during the maneuver; i.e., tensing only one arm will increase G tolerance by 0.6 G, which is an important contribution to the AGSM. The difference between the tolerances as a passenger in the airplane and as a subject on the centrifuge is primarily a result of the increased sympathetic activity attributed to the anticipation of the flight.

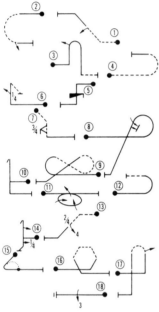

Figure 9.30. Typical Aresti Diagram for an advanced civilian aerobatic flight.

Civilian Aerobatic Environment

There are differences in the military and the civilian G environment, although the civilian environment is by no means less stressful. The Aresti diagram for a typical "advanced known" aerobatic flight in a Pitts S-1 is shown in Figure 9.30. The G_z profile for that aerobatic flight is shown in Figure 9.31. Civilian aerobatics frequently involve substantial negative G_z exposures. In that regard, an increased $+G_z$ exposure after increased $-G_z$ is known to increase G-LOC susceptibility. Simultaneous heart rate and G_z recordings made during aerobatics show significantly increased heart rate with $+G_z$ and decreased heart rate with $-G_z$ —a minimum heart rate of 32 beats/min at $-3.8\ G_z$. The heart rate before the onset of aerobatic maneuvering was 118 beats/min. The maximum heart rate was 188 beats/min at $+7.0\ G_z$. It decreased from 175 to 40 beats/min within five beats during $+G_z$ to $-G_z$ maneuvering. The maximum rate of onset of $+G_z$ was $+6$ G/sec; for $-G_z$ it was -6 G/sec. Excursions from $+5\ G_z$ to $-5\ G_z$ within 3 seconds have been observed (38).

It is important that the civilian aerobatic community realize the hazards inherent in such high $+G$ maneuvers. High-risk exposures should be documented and the information provided to competitors and safety supervisors to achieve safety without unnecessarily limiting vigorous aerobatic competition.

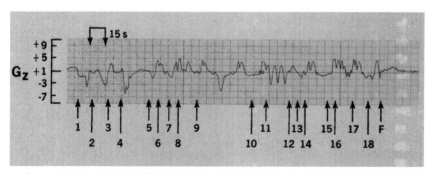

Figure 9.31. The continuous electrocardiographic G_z profile for the Aresti diagram flight shown in Figure 9.30. The numbers refer to the start of the specific maneuvers. Note the rather high degree of $-G_z$ exposure.

REFERENCES

1. Burton RR. G-induced loss of consciousness—definition, history, current status. Aviat Space Environ Med 1988;59:2–5.
2. Armstrong HG, Heim JW. The effect of acceleration on the living organism. J Aviat Med 1938;9:199–215.
3. Burton RR. A conceptual model for predicting pilot group G tolerance for tactical fighter aircraft. Aviat Space Environ Med 1986;57:733–744.
4. AGARDograph No. 322. High G Physiological Protection Training, AMP Working Group 14, 1990.
5. Parkhurst MS, Leverett SD Jr, Shubrooks S. Human tolerance to high, sustained $+G_z$ accelerations. Aerosp Med 1972;43:708–712.
6. Burton RR, Leverett SD Jr, Michaelson ED. Man at high sustained $+G_z$; a review. Aerospace Med 1974; 45:1115–1136.
7. Wood EH, Sutterer WF, Marshall HW, Lindberg EF, Headley RN. Effect of headward and forward accelerations on the cardiovascular system. WADD-TR-60–634, Wright-Patterson AFB, 1961.
8. Laughlin MH, Burns JW, Parnell MJ. Regional distribution of cardiac output in unanesthetized baboons during $+G_z$ stress with and without an anti-G suit. Aviat Space Environ Med 1982;53:133–141.
9. Laughlin MH. An analysis of the risk of human cardiac damage during $+G_z$ stress; a review. Aviat Space Environ Med 1982;53:423–431.
10. Lamb LE. Cardiopulmonary aspects of aerospace medicine. In: Randel HW, ed. Aerospace medicine. 2nd ed. Baltimore: Williams & Wilkins Co., 1971.
11. Glaister DH. The effects of gravity and acceleration on the lung. AGARDograph 133. England: Technivision Services, 1970.
12. Burton RR, Smith AH. Adaptation to acceleration environments. Fregly MJ, Blattis CM, eds. In: Handbook of physiology: environmental physiology. IV. the gravitational environment. New York: Oxford University Press, 1996; 943–970.
13. Haswell MS, Tacher WA, Balldin UI, Burton RR. Influence of inspired oxygen concentration on acceleration atelectasis. Aviat Space Environ Med 1986;57: 432–437.
14. Mills FJ. The endocrinology of stress. Aviat Space Environ Med 1985;56:642–650.
15. Leverett SD Jr, Newsom WA. Photographic observations of the human fundus oculi during $+G_z$ blackout on the USAF School of Aerospace Medicine centrifuge. In: Lunc M, ed. XIXth international astronautical congressbook 4: bioastronautics. New York: Pergamon Press, 1971; 75–80.
16. Whinnery JE, Burton RR, Boll PA, Eddy DR. Characterization of the resulting incapacitation following unexpected $+G_z$-induced loss of consciousness. Aviat Space Environ Med 1987;58:631–636.
17. Whinnery JE. The G-LOC syndrome. Report No. NADC-91042–60, Naval Air Development Center, Warminster, PA, 1991.

18. Whinnery JE. Observations on the neurophysiologic theory of acceleration ($+G_z$) induced loss of consciousness. Aviat Space Environ Med 1989;60:589–593.
19. Whinnery JE, Whinnery AM. Acceleration induced loss of consciousness. Arch Neurol 1990;47:764–776.
20. Whinnery JE. On the theory of acceleration tolerance. Report No. NADC-88088–60, Naval Air Development Center, Warminster, PA, 1988.
21. Hamilton R, Whinnery JE. The diagnosis of physiologically uncomplicated $+G_z$-induced loss of consciousness: a guide for the naval flight surgeon. Air Vehicle and Crew Systems Technology Department, Naval Air Development Center, Warminster, PA, 1990.
22. Franks WR, Kerr WK, Rose B. Some neurological signs and symptoms produced by centrifugal force in man. J Physiol 1945–46;104:108–118.
23. Laughlin MH, Witt MW, Whittaker RN Jr. Renal blood flow in miniature swine during $+G_z$ stress and anti-G suit inflation. J Appl Physiol 1980;49:471–475.
24. The musculoskeletal and vestibular effects of long-term repeated exposure to sustained high-G. Aeromedical Report 317, AGARD/Aerospace Medical Panel, 1994.
25. Barer AS, Okhobotov AA, Sorokina YI, Tardov VM. Some pathological signs in pelvis minor organs after exposure to long-term high-level $+G_z$ acceleration. Kosm Biol Avia Med 1986;20:81–82.
26. Beckman EL, Duane TD, Ziegler JE, Hunter HN. Some observations on human tolerance to accelerative stress: phase IV. Human tolerance to high positive G applied at a rate of 5 to 10 G per second. J Aviat Med 1954; 25:50–66.
27. Cochran LB, Gard PW, Norsworthy ME. Variations in human G tolerance to positive acceleration, USN SAM/NASA/NM 001–059.020.10, Pensacola, FL, 1954.
28. Burton RR, Shaffstall RM. Human tolerance to aerial combat maneuvers. Aviat Space Environ Med 1980;51: 641–648.
29. Burton RR. Human physiologic limitations to G in high-performance aircraft. In: Farhi LE, Paganelli CV, eds. Environmental physiology. New York: Springer-Verlag, 1989.
30. Wiegman JF, Burton RR, Forster EM. The role of anaerobic power in human tolerance to simulated aerial combat maneuvers. Aviat Space Environ Med 1995;66: 938–942.
31. Burton RR. Human responses to repeated high G simulated aerial combat maneuvers. Aviat Space Environ Med 1980;51:1185–1192.
32. Wood EH, Lambert EH, Baldes EJ, Code CF. Effects of acceleration in relation to aviation. Fed Proc 1946; 5:327–344.
33. Whinnery JE, Murray DC. Enhancing tolerance to acceleration ($+G_z$) stress: the "hook" maneuver. Report No. NADC-90088–60, Air Development Center, Warminster, PA, 1990.
34. Epperson WL, Burton RR, Bernauer EM. The influence of differential physical conditioning regimens on simulated aerial combat maneuvering tolerance. Aviat Space Environ Med 1982;53:1091–1097.

35. Burton RR, Storm WF, Johnson LW, Leverett SD Jr.
Stress responses of pilots flying high-performance aircraft during aerial combat maneuvers. Aviat Space Environ Med 1977;48:301–307.

36. Gillingham KK, Plentzas S, Lewis NL. G environments
of F-4, F-5, F-15, and F-16 aircraft during F-15 tactics
development and evaluation. USAFSAM-TR-85–51,
1985.

37. Lambert EH. Effects of positive acceleration on pilots
in flight, and a comparison of the responses of pilots
and passengers in an airplane and subjects on a human
centrifuge. Aviat Med 1950;21:195–220.

38. Bloodwell RD, Whinnery JE. Acceleration exposure
during competitive civilian aerobatics. Reprints of the
Annual Scientific Meeting of the Aerospace Medical
Association, Bal Harbour, FL, 1982.

39. Smith AH. Introduction to gravitational biology. In:
Principles of biodynamics. USAFSAM-TR-74-44,
1974;1:12.

GLOSSARY

a	acceleration
A	anterior
AC	aberrant conduction
ACC	Air Combat Command (formerly TAC)
ACM	aerial combat maneuver
AFB	Air Force Base
AGARD	Advisory Group for Aerospace Research and Development
AGSM	anti-G straining maneuver
AL	arbitrary limit
AMP	Aeromedical Panel in AGARD
AR	advisory report
ATAGS	advanced technology anti-G suit
AV	atrioventricular
BV	blood volume
C	cervical vertebra
CLL	central light loss
CNS	central nervous system
CO_2	carbon dioxide
CPK	creatine phosphokinase
CSF	cerebral spinal fluid
d	specific density of blood
DVL-1	reclining seat of World War II designed by the Institute of Aviation Medicine, German Research Institute of Aeronautics (DVL)
E	epinephrine
ECG	electrocardiogram or -graph
EEG	electroencephalogram or -graph
ESP	erholungspulssume (sum of heart beats)
F	force
FFS	Frank's flying anti-G suit
FRC	functional reserve capacity
g	gravity or centripetal force
G	Acceleration induced inertial force
G-LOC	G induced loss of consciousness
GOR	gradual onset rate
$+G_x$	positive transverse G (A to P)
$-G_x$	negative transverse G (P to A)
$\pm G_y$	positive/negative lateral G (side to side)
$+G_z$	positive vertical G
$-G_z$	negative vertical G
h	blood column height (mm)
H^+	hydrogen ion
HR	heart rate (beats per minute)
HSG	high sustained G
HTG	high-G tolerance group
I	inspired
IAM	Institute of Aviation Medicine
K	constant of 1 G tolerance increase (Eq. 9)
km	kilometer
kPa	kilopascal
L	lumbar vertebra
L-1	type of AGSM
LDH	lactate dehydrogenase
LOC	loss of consciousness
LTG	low-G tolerance group
m	mass or meter
mmHg	mm mercury
MRI	magnetic resonance imaging
M-1	Maneuver number 1; a type of AGSM
NAMRL	Naval Aeromedical Research Laboratory
NASA	National Aeronautics and Space Administration
NATO	North Atlantic Treaty Organization
NAWC	Naval Air Warfare Center
NE	norepinephrine
O_2	oxygen
P	posterior or pressure
P_a	arterial blood pressure (mmHg)
P_A	pulmonary alveolar pressure
PAC	premature atrial contraction
PBG	positive pressure breathing during G exposure
P_H	hydrostatic pressure (mmHg)
PLL	peripheral light loss
psi	pounds of pressure per square inch
PVC	premature ventricular contraction
Q	blood perfusion rate
r	centrifuge radius (m)
RAF	Royal Air Force of the UK
ROR	rapid onset rate
S_a	arterial oxygen saturation
SACM	simulated ACM
SGOT	serum glutamic-oxaloacetic transaminase
SR	special report
TAC	Tactical Air Command
TLC	total lung capacity
TLV	total lung volume
UK	United Kingdom
USAF	United States Air Force
USAFSAM	United States Air Force School of Aerospace Medicine
USN	United States Navy
V	pulmonary ventilation rate
VC	vital capacity
ω	radians per sec
w	weight
17-OHCS	17-hydroxy corticosteroid

Chapter 10

Vibration, Noise, and Communication

Henning E. von Gierke

and Charles W. Nixon

Whoever, in the pursuit of science, seeks after immediate practical utility may generally rest assured that he will seek in vain.

Herman L.F. Helmholtz, Academic Disclosure 1862

Aerospace systems produce perhaps the most severe noise and vibration environments experienced by man. These biomechanical force environments, singly and in combination, threaten the health, safety, and well-being of persons associated with or exposed to aerospace operations. Mechanical vibration transmitted to human operators can induce fatigue, degrade comfort, interfere with performance effectiveness, and, under severe conditions, influence operational safety and occupational health. Excessive exposure to airborne acoustic energy may interfere with routine living activities, induce annoyance, degrade voice communication, modify physiologic functions, reduce the effectiveness of performance, and cause noise-induced hearing loss. Both vibratory and acoustic effects may occur simultaneously with the onset of the stimulus or may be manifest only with the passage of time and repeated exposure; for example, noise-induced hearing loss and vibrational disease. The problems generated by the closely related phenomena of noise and vibration are addressed by the unifying field of biodynamics and are dealt with on an individual or group basis by the field of aerospace medicine.

Human exposure to moderate vibratory and acoustic energy can be controlled to acceptable levels that do not jeopardize either the persons involved or the operational aerospace mission. Severe whole-body vibration and intense noise exposures to aerospace air and ground crews, however, may affect performance and even contribute to accidents. The results of noise and vibration research on physiologic and psychologic effects and on performance and comfort have provided an extensive technology pool that serves as the basis of exposure guidelines, criteria, and standards. Scientifically developed prediction schemes allow the nature and magnitude of biodynamic environments to be reliably estimated. Appropriate action may be initiated to minimize the impact of most exposures by treating the source, the propagation of the energy, and the exposed, and by monitoring the influence of such exposures over time with hearing tests and medical observations. Certainly, research must continue to address the many gaps that exist in our knowledge of severe noise and vibration exposures, as well as of less intense exposures, to allow such environments to be controlled with even greater confidence. This chapter addresses the variety of effects on humans of the vibratory and acoustic energy experienced in aerospace activities, and the major operational control methods and procedures presently available and in use.

MEASUREMENTS AND ANALYSIS OF SOUND AND VIBRATION ENVIRONMENTS

Definitions and Measurement Units

Vibration Stimulus

Vibration is generally defined as the motion of objects relative to a reference position, which is usually the object at rest. Specifically, vibration is a series of oscillations of velocity, an action that necessarily involves displacement and acceleration. Acceleration is typically used as the fundamental measure of vibration environments and is expressed as multiples of gravitational acceleration of the earth, G (G = 9.8 m/sec^2). Vibration is described relative to its effects on man in terms of frequency, intensity (amplitude), direction (with regard to anatomic axes of the human body), and duration of exposure.

Frequency

The frequency of periodic motion (sound and vibration) is the number of complete cycles of motion taking place in a specific unit of time, usually 1 second. The international standard unit of frequency is the hertz (Hz), which is 1 cycle/sec. Vibration in aerospace systems and activities is usually nonperiodic or random in nature. Random vibratory motion is adequately described in terms of frequency spectra using appropriate spectral analysis techniques. Vibrations with the energy concentrated in narrow regions or at discrete frequencies may be analyzed by the measurement in frequency bands by Fourier analyzers or by observation of the oscilloscope.

Amplitude

The amplitude of vibration is defined as the maximum displacement about a position of rest. The displacement unit of choice in vibration

work is the meter (m). The term amplitude is often used with a descriptor such as velocity-amplitude or acceleration-amplitude to describe the value of a vibration. Velocity and acceleration may be determined by the following formulas for sinusoidal vibrations for which the frequency and amplitude are known. Given the frequency, f, and the (displacement) amplitude, A:

$$\text{Velocity amplitude} = 2\pi fA$$

$$\text{(1)}$$

$$\text{Acceleration amplitude} = 4\pi^2f^2A$$

The same formulas may be used with narrow-band random vibration.

The intensity of nonperiodic or complex vibrations is a computed, time-averaged, or root-mean-square (rms) value. In sinusoidal vibration, the rms value is $1/\sqrt{2}$ (0.707) times the maximum (peak) value. The relationships between sinusoidal vibration frequency, displacement, velocity, and acceleration may be determined from the nomograph in Figure 10.1.

Direction of Vibration

Vibration can have three linear and three rotational degrees of freedom. Man's response to linear vibration depends on the direction in which the force acts on the body. The directions of vibration entering the human body have been standardized relative to the anatomic axes illustrated in Figure 10.2. The description of the vibration should apply to the force or motion at the point of entry into the body when evaluating the vibration's effects on man. Care should be taken in the use of vibration data to ensure that its measurement relates to the coordinate system of anatomic axes and is not remote from the man. Rotational accelerations around a center of rotation are separated into pitch (rotation around the Y-axis), roll (rotation around the X-axis), and yaw (rotation around the Z-axis).

Duration Of Vibration Exposure

In general, human tolerance to continuous vibration declines with increasing duration of

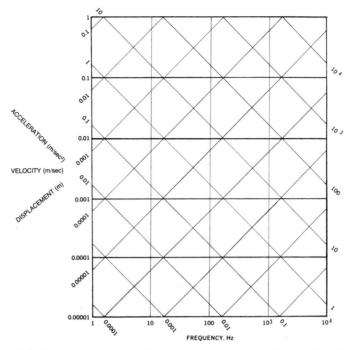

Figure 10.1. Nomograph relating the principal parameters of sinusoidal vibration.

exposure (1). Adaptation or habituation to vibration stress remains an open question because it has received little research attention. Long-term vibration sometimes denotes exposures exceeding one hour, whereas short-term (or short-duration) vibration usually identifies exposures lasting one minute to one hour. Vibration lasting only a few seconds or a few cycles of motion can usually be treated as transient vibration, shock motion, or sometimes as impact.

Sound Stimulus

Sound waves are variations in air pressure above and below the ambient pressure. Sound is described in terms of its intensity, spectrum, and time history (2).

Intensity

The intensity of a sound wave is the magnitude that the pressure varies above and below the ambient level. It is measured by a logarithmic scale that expresses the ratio of sound pressure to a reference pressure in decibels (dB). The decibel is a unit used to describe levels of acoustic pressure, power, and intensity.

Atmospheric or ambient pressure is measured in newtons/m^2 (N/m^2). The smallest ambient pressure change (sound wave), varying at a rate of about 1000 times per second, that can be detected by man is a pressure amplitude of about 0.00002 N/m^2. This just detectable pressure is the standard reference sound pressure for the decibel scale for sound measurement in gases in terms of sound pressure level (SPL). The intensity of a pressure (P), in terms of SPL, is defined as follows:

$$SPL = 20 \log_{10} \frac{P}{P_0} \qquad (2)$$

where $P_0 = 0.00002$ N/m^2 and the SPL value is quoted in decibels referenced to 0.00002 N/m^2. The relationship between sound pressure and SPL is shown in Table 10.1. Complex sounds are usually expressed in terms of time-averaged rms values.

Spectrum

The spectrum of sound represents the sound pressure present distributed across frequency

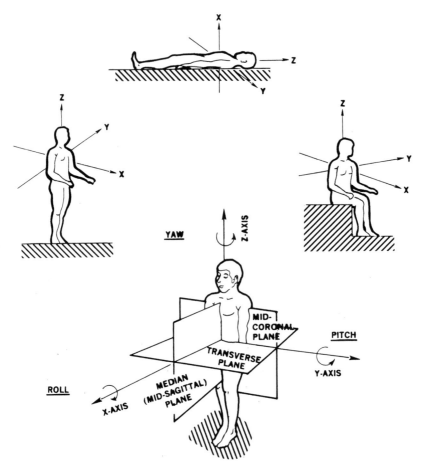

Figure 10.2. Directions of coordinate system used in biodynamics for mechanical vibrations influencing humans.

Table 10.1.
Common Scales Used to Describe the Magnitude of Acoustic Energy

Sound Pressure Level (dB)	Sound Pressure (μbar)	Sound Pressure (N/m^2)	Pressure (lb/in^2)
174	100,000	10,000	1.47
134	1000	100	14.7×10^{-3}
94	10	1	147.0×10^{-6}
74	1	0.1	14.7×10^{-6}
54	0.1	0.01	1.47×10^{-6}
14	0.001	0.0001	14.7×10^{-9}
0	0.0002	0.00002	2.94×10^{-9}

(defined under vibration stimulus). It is commonly described in terms of levels in successive passbands of octave, half-octave, and third-octave bandwidths but can be in a successive bandwidth of any size. Noises of concern to aerospace medicine are frequency-dependent in terms of their effects on man. The spectrum of acoustic energy important to man's perception ranges from less than 1 to over 20,000 Hz. The young, normal human ear is sensitive to acoustic energy of about 15 to 20,000 Hz, which is termed the audio frequency range. Infrasound, energy below about 15 Hz, can be perceived at high intensity levels. Ultrasound is classically defined as acoustic energy above 20,000 Hz;

however, the term is applied to energy as low as 8,000 to 10,000 Hz and above.

Time History

Pressure-time histories describe variations in the sound pressure of a signal as a function of time. The frequency content is not quantified in pressure-time histories of signals. Analytic techniques must be applied to the signal to obtain frequency or spectrum characteristics. Steady-state sounds are those with a time course or duration greater than one second. Impulse sounds, individual pressure pulses of sudden onset and brief duration, are those with a duration of less than one second and a peak-to-rms ratio greater than 10 dB. Impulse sounds are typically described by their rise time, peak level, duration, and number of events or repetitions. The frequency content of impulsive sounds is determined by spectral-energy-density analysis.

Propagation

Theoretically, sound waves in open air spread spherically in all directions from an idealized point source. As a result of the spherical dispersion, the sound pressure is reduced to half of its original value as the distance is doubled, which is a 6 dB reduction in SPL. Sound propagation is further affected by such factors as atmospheric attenuation, air temperature, and topography, which generally result in propagation loss and distortion. The speed of sound in air is temperature-dependent and is about 344 m/sec at a temperature of 21° C.

Aerospace noises do not radiate uniformly in all directions, but follow forms or patterns characteristic of the source. This directivity of sound radiation must be included in the evaluation of noise to ensure the appropriate placement of personnel and to avoid overexposure of communities in the vicinity of the noise sources.

Instrumentation

Vibration Measurement Instruments

The basic instrumentation components used for vibration measurement include a transducer, an amplifier, and a readout stage. The transducer is an acceleration (velocity or displacement) pickup that is available in models for measurement in one, two, or three (triaxial) mutually perpendicular directions, each with different frequency and sensitivity ranges. Except for the transducer, the instrumentation is similar to that used for acoustic measurement, providing information on the level of the vibration and the frequency components present in the signal. The measurement of rotational vibration is infrequently accomplished because it is more sophisticated, requiring special pickups (rate gyros) and more complicated calibration.

A variety of vibration meters are available for general-purpose measurements, for monitoring, and for evaluating human response to vibration. Most devices operate in acceleration, velocity, and displacement modes. The amount of energy present at the various frequencies is obtained using conventional frequency analysis techniques and instrumentation. The frequency analysis component of the instrumentation is important for vibration measurement because the reduced comfort, fatigue-decreased proficiency, and safety criteria are presented in frequency or third-octave bands as a function of acceleration and exposure duration (1). Care must be taken to ensure that all instrumentation components cover the whole frequency range of interest. Vibration measurement instrumentation incorporating the various weighting functions to evaluate human response to whole-body vibration, building vibration, and hand-arm vibration has been standardized and is commercially available.

Sound Measurement Instruments

The basic instrumentation components used for sound measurement consist of a microphone, an amplifier, and a readout device. The basic sound level meter contains these components and responds to sound pressure levels referenced to 0.00002 N/m^2. It provides a single-number overall reading of the sound pressure level in the audible frequency range. Most sound level meters contain three standardized electrical weighting or filter networks—A, B, and C—which enable the instrument to measure the approximate loudness response of the human ear at the respective sound levels of 40, 70, and 100 dB. The sound level meter is an important instrument because most noise exposure standards and criteria are based on sound measurements made with the A-weighting scale of the device.

The sound level meter is used for general-purpose and survey work such as continuous monitoring of noise at a work station or the identification of noise-hazardous areas. When noise conditions exceed exposure criteria and noise control measures are indicated, an analysis of sound pressure level as a function of frequency is usually required. Instruments that perform this function are frequency analyzers, which commonly assess levels in frequency bandwidths of one octave or one-third octave and may be used independently or with sound level meters. Frequency analyzers are important because effective noise control measures deal with the problem areas in the frequency spectrum identified by octave or one-third octave descriptions of the sound.

Noise Dosimeters

Personal noise dosimeters are small, lightweight devices worn by individuals to indicate their noise exposure over a specified time period, typically for hearing-conversation purposes. A dosimeter consists of a microphone, a unit that integrates acoustic energy over time, and a readout that displays the exposure or dose at the time the unit is read. A dosimeter is designed with a specific built-in noise exposure standard like the Occupational Safety and Health Act standard of 90 dB(A) for 8 hours. Ideally, a 90 dB(A) exposure for 8 hours would read a dose of 100%, with greater and lesser exposures reading doses higher and lower than 100%, respectively. Various commercially available noise dosimeters differ somewhat in operation and readout, with some providing continuous 24-hour monitoring; however, the general principle of operation is essentially the same, with the final output indicating the percentage of the allowable daily noise dose actually experienced by the individual wearing the unit.

Aerospace Noise and Vibration Sources

Aerospace noises and vibrations that may affect man generally have common sources that are further influenced by the type of system, kind of operation, and environmental factors. A primary source, and usually the most intense, is the propulsion system required to power the aerospace vehicle (3). This energy source not only affects crew and support personnel, but it is radiated into surrounding areas and communities. Auxiliary ground equipment required for the maintenance and preflight support of both aircraft and space vehicles, as well as static engine firing, also produce a variety of noise and vibration environments. Onboard life-support systems generate different types and levels of acoustic energy that may be accompanied by vibration. Aerodynamic sources, wind gusts, and air turbulence also cause numerous combinations of biodynamic environments that gradually increase as vehicles fly closer and closer to the ground and subside at increasing altitude as the density of the atmosphere decreases, eventually to disappear for vehicles in space.

Substantial vibration is often present in the operation of aviation and space vehicles (4). The primary sources during space operations are the propulsion systems, aerodynamic factors, and onboard powered systems and equipment. The intense combustion and powerful thrust required to propel a large space vehicle generate noise and movement that are transmitted throughout the structure and internally to the crew stations. Noise and vibration are worst during the maximum aerodynamic loads that occur immediately after launch as the vehicle is gathering speed and decrease it as it moves through the more rarefied atmosphere into space. A similar but briefer effect occurs and subsides as the speed of the spacecraft is greatly reduced during the initial moments of reentry prior to deployment of the parachutes or landing of vehicles such as the Space Shuttle. Vibration from onboard equipment and apparatus may be present and even observable in some circumstances but is generally not a problem. Exceptions might be a low-level vibration that persists throughout the flight and is judged to be objectionable for a very delicate manual task, the performance of which is affected by the vibration.

The maximum intensity of aerodynamically induced vibrations and noise occur when the aerospace vehicles are under the highest aerodynamic pressures. For space systems, this maximum intensity occurs during the first few minutes of acceleration after launch and during deceleration upon reentry into the atmosphere. Aerodynamically induced energy is maximum for aircraft during lift-off, climb-out, dives, supersonic dashes, and maneuvers. These categories of vibratory and acoustic energy are relatively high frequency and are more easily controlled than the low-frequency energy.

Crew and community noise exposure and the potential environmental impact from space operations are summarized in Table 10.2. Examples of aviation and space noise environments are compared with automobile and subway noises in Figure 10.3. Most aerospace noises shown are relatively intense; however, hearing protection and audio communications equipment provide adequate protection and information transfer in these hostile environments.

The crew is subjected to the highest maneuvering loads and vibration loads caused by air turbulence during the high-speed, low-altitude flight of military maneuvers. The transition in the force spectrum from low-frequency vibration to alternating G exposures to which the crew is exposed is continuous, and any dividing line between these areas is arbitrary and usually based on the difference in laboratory simulation equipment (centrifuge versus vibration table).

THE HUMAN BODY AS RECEIVER OF NOISE AND VIBRATION

Energy Absorption and Transmission

When the human body is exposed to airborne noise fields or comes into contact with vibrating structures such as aircraft floors or fuselage walls, there is a response to the physical force. Obviously, the alternating pressures or forces are transmitted to and propagated inside the body tissue. Basically, there is no longer any difference between sound and vibration once the energy is inside the tissue. There is a big difference, however, in the transmission of energy from air to body tissue compared with the transmission from a vibrating structure. Structures are solids and are similar to body tissue in their mechanical characteristics; consequently, vibrations are easily transmitted from the vibrating structure to tissue. At the body surface, the contact area of the tissue will be excited to the same vibration amplitude, acceleration, or velocity as the exciting structure. Most energy is transmitted from the structure to the body and propagates without much attenuation inside the tissue (5). The situation is different, however, with respect to airborne sound waves. When they impinge on a solid surface, the wave is almost stopped, and the particle velocity at the interface is reduced to a small fraction of its free-field value. The sound wave is reflected at the body surface due to what is called the "mismatch" of the media, and only a small percentage of the sound energy enters the tissue.

The sound in our environment can carry important information to us about events, as well as messages from our fellow man; consequently, the ear has evolved as a special receiver of sound energy. By its intricate, dynamic design the mammalian outer and middle ear matches the receiver organ, the cochlea, to the acoustic characteristics of air. The tympanic membrane is the only part of the human body surface that absorbs almost 100% of the acoustic energy arriving through air in the frequency range of interest

Table 10.2.
Summary of Space Operations, Noise Exposure, and Potential Environmental Impact

Operation	Exposure	Spacecrew	Groundcrews	Community
Industrial support of space systems	Noise	Not applicable	Industrial noise exposure; 8 hr/day compliance with U.S. Dept. of Labor, 90 dB(A) criteria	Potential problems where noises intrude into neighboring communities
Launch	Noise	Brief exposures of 125–130 dB SPL in crew area; less than 120 dB at ear; hearing protection and voice communication adequate with current systems; no adverse effects due to protection and brief exposures	Very intense levels as high as 150 dB SPL at 600 ft from pad; adverse effects without protection provided by structures and/or hearing protectors	Intense levels perceived at great distances; low frequencies of 115 db 3 miles from pad; 105 dB at 10 miles infrequent occurrence, brief duration contributes to acceptability
	Sonic boom	Not perceptible	Not perceptible	Not perceptible
Cruise	Noise	Onboard systems; ambient levels of 60–70 dB; noise levels higher during certain operations; levels tolerable for brief missions of several days; acceptable levels for missions of 6–18 mo not determined	Not applicable	Not applicable
Reentry	Noise	Noise similar to maximum aerodynamic noise at launch; greater duration; requires voice communication capability for space shuttle type reentry	Brief, low-level exposures at landing	Negligible; infrequent
	Sonic boom	Not perceptible	Not perceptible; boom occurs some distance from landing site	Space shuttle-type reentry may expose large areas of Earth's surface; impact depends on number of people exposed.
Static firing	Noise	Not applicable	Very intense levels of 150 dB at 600 ft; must use protection; durations and frequency of occurrence much greater than launch	Noise propagates a far distance into communities; duration of runs; frequency of occurrence, time of day, will contribute to acceptability; this may be worst community exposure situation

and transmits it to the cochlea to stimulate the receiver.

Mechanical Impedance

The amount of mechanical energy transmitted from one medium to another is best described by the match or mismatch of the mechanical impedance of the media. This mechanical impedance is the ratio of the force or pressure at the contact area to the velocity from this force. For a simple sinusoidal motion, force and velocity can be out of phase. If the phase angle between force and velocity is $+90°$, one speaks of a mass reactance, that is, the medium acts at the interface like a pure inertial loading. If the phase angle is $-90°$, one speaks of an elastic

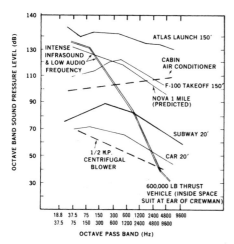

Figure 10.3. Representative sources of acoustic energy depicting a variety of sound spectra and levels.

reactance; that is, a pure spring. For phase angle 0°, one speaks of a frictional resistance, that is, the energy transmitted through the boundary is completely absorbed by the receiving medium.

Whole-Body Impedance

For an example of whole-body impedance, look at the mechanical impedance of a sitting human subject exposed to vibration (Fig. 10.4). At the low frequencies (below approximately 3 Hz), the body acts like a pure mass corresponding to the body weight (represented theoretically by the line $m\omega$). Depending on body dimensions, composition, muscle tension, and posture, there is a maximum of the impedance between 3 and 7 Hz, which is called a resonance. Above this frequency, the impedance decreases and more and more energy is absorbed by the elasticities of soft tissue and the damping inherent in the latter. Such impedance curves are important and useful for the following reasons:

1. The impedance indicates in which frequency range maximum energy is transmitted to the subject, namely, in the resonance range. Where the maximum energy is transmitted, the maximum physiologic and potentially maximum psychologic effects of the energy

must be expected. It certainly explains why some frequencies are potentially more traumatic than others.

2. The impedance explains quantitatively why all vibration effects depend critically on body posture, restraint, and support. It indicates how to modify the energy transmission to the body.

3. The impedance is the first clue as to the mechanical structure of the human body and indicates how to describe this structure in mechanical/engineering terms. For example, for the standardized nominal impedance shown in Figure 10.4, a standardized engineering representation is shown in the insert. The network of masses, springs, and dampers of this mechanical system simulates at the input interface the complex mechanical impedance of the human body. The engineer considering vibration-attenuating seats or reduction of aircraft or automobile vibration can calculate numerically the effectiveness of vibration control measures by means of mechanical equivalents of the human body like the one shown in Figure 10.4 (3,6). He can also design a physical analog of the human body; that is, a dynamic dummy that loads the seat or the vibration source dynamically the same way as a human subject. The impedance also indicates that anthropometric dummies, which simulate only dimensions and inertial properties of man without considering the elastic characteristics, cannot be expected to represent realistic loads above approximately 3 Hz and can lead to misleading results if used in tests containing higher frequencies.

The impedance of man is only linear as a first approximation; that is, the impedance value changes above certain displacements at constant frequency. For the same reason, the impedance changes with the static or inertial preload. For example, a person in an aircraft or space vehicle exposed to sustained acceleration maneuvers or to a zero-G environment reacts differently to vibration environments than in the normal environment on earth. These impedance changes are

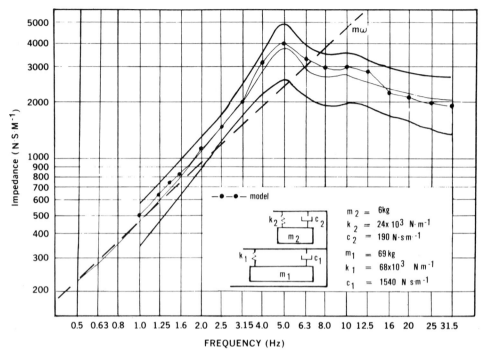

Figure 10.4. Mechanical impedance of a human subject in the sitting position (standardized values for the mean, 20th percentile, and 80th percentile experimental data) on a rigid, flat seat; the subject's feet on a footrest moving with the seat. Test accelerations are 1 to 2 m/sec^2. The subject's body weight is 51 to 94 kg. The impedance curve of a simple mechanical analog is also indicated. If the body would move as a rigid mass, the impedance would follow the $m\omega$ line.

illustrated in Figure 10.5 (3). The curves explain why vibration and buffeting are perceived as less severe under acceleration preloads.

Because human susceptibility to transient acceleration and impact can be calculated for the simplified linear response condition from the steady-state response, the vibration response discussed also is helpful in understanding human response to and protection against impact loads (see Chapter 8). The inertial preload effects illustrated in Figure 10.5 can alter and decrease human impact response. It is also the reason why vibration and impact response under zero G has been hypothesized to be more severe.

Acoustic Impedance

As another example of mechanical impedance, Figure 10.6 illustrates the acoustic impedance (mechanical impedance divided by the square of the area) of a small body area. The impedance of a 1 cm^2 surface area overlying soft tissue behaves at low frequencies like a mass reactance, whereas bony areas under the skin change the behavior to an elastic reactance. This figure also shows impedance values for the tympanic membrane and their proximity to the characteristic impedance of air. The transformer action of the middle ear is responsible for the high sensitivity of the ear to airborne sound compared with the rest of the body surface (curves a and b). Preloading of the tympanic membrane with static pressure—for example, as due to atmospheric pressure changes during ascent to or descent from altitude without pressure equalization through the eustachian tube—shifts the elasticity of the transmission chain into the nonlinear range. As a result of this pressure differential, a decrease in auditory acuity or a temporary hearing loss of as much as 8 to 10 dB for frequencies below 1500 and above 2300 Hz can occur.

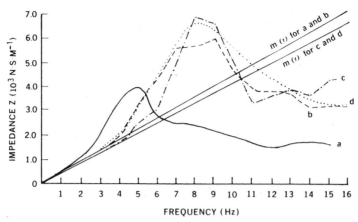

Figure 10.5. The mechanical impedance of the sitting human body: (a) under normal gravity; (b) under $+2\ G_z$; (c) under $+3\ G_z$; and compared with (d) the mechanical impedance of a simple mass-spring-damper system with $f_o = 8$ Hz, $m = 65{,}000$ dyne sec²/cm, and $\delta = 0.575$ (3).

Transmission of Mechanical Energy

Impedance measurements at the body surface tell us how much energy enters the body; however, these measurements do not indicate how the energy is propagated and distributed inside the body. With respect to the human ear, the energy transmission from the tympanic membrane to the hair cells of the inner ear is well understood, and even the mechanical filtering and electrical filtering of the frequency components in the cochlea and peripheral nervous system are known in principle. The ear and auditory system as energy receivers hide no big secrets; however, the auditory system as information processor, analyzer, and pattern recognizer is still a serious challenge to science. Solving this puzzle will not only aid the medical therapy of speech and hearing disorders but also lead to further progress in the technology of automatic speech recognition, synthetic speech, and speech understanding.

Transmission of vibration and impact through the body structure is of primary interest with respect to explaining undesirable effects and trauma. Except for the case of direct energy transmission to the head, the effects are usually confined to the frequency range below 100 Hz and to the displacement of larger body parts such as the abdominal viscera, the arm and hand, or the head and eye. The measurements of the transmission characteristics are available (Fig. 10.7); understandably, they vary greatly with the direction and the body support and restraint.

In explaining and describing energy transmission, mathematical models of the whole body and its subsystems have been of great assistance (8,9). Although lumped parameter models (Fig. 10.8) with discrete masses, elasticities, and dampers can explain the basic behavior and have the advantage of illustrative insight, finite element models exercised on digital computers provide a geometric fidelity and detail of mechanical stress definition far beyond verification by available measurements. For example, the head-spine model, which is indicated in the computer graphics in Figure 10.8, not only incorporates details of the skeleton structure and the mechanical properties of the skeletal system, but also the properties of the major tendons and muscles and of the internal organs. It allows calculation of relative displacement and deformation of major body parts, such as the head, spine, or abdominal viscera, and also compressive and bending stresses on vertebral bodies and disks. When excited at the buttocks with Z-axis vibrations, the head-spine model predicts the impedance of a sitting subject as measured. Today, the primary tool in predicting and assessing the mechanical

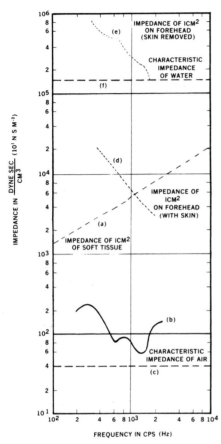

Figure 10.6. Acoustic impedance at various locations on the body surface: (a) impedance of a 1 cm² area overlying soft tissue; (b) impedance measured at the tympanic membrane; (c) characteristic impedance of air; (d) impedance on the forehead; (e) impedance on the forehead without skin; and (f) characteristic impedance of water (5).

response of human subjects to vibration, rotational oscillation, and impact are models such as the ones illustrated.

Sound and Vibration Reduction and Protection

Noise and vibration exposures exceeding established safety, health, or performance interference criteria must be reduced to desirable levels. Depending on the stimulus-response relationship considered, some criteria are defined by the effective exposure, that is, the product of stimu-

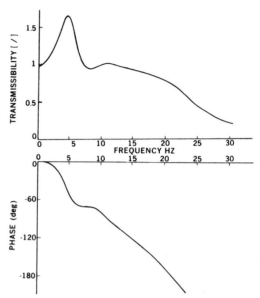

Figure 10.7. Transmissibility (feet or buttocks to head) for the standing or sitting human subject. The transmissibility is essentially the same for both positions (7).

lus intensity and exposure time, whereas other criteria give the desirable limits solely in terms of maximum or average sound pressure level or vibration.

To protect an operator from long-term health effects, exposure intensity and time are the factors requiring control. In the case of single events, such as impulse noise or shock, the intensity and number of events per day or week are the parameters to control. Therefore, in most cases, it is desirable and economical to consider the whole system from the noise or vibration source over the transmission path to the human receiver and to analyze the feasibility of control at the source, in the intervening medium, or at the receiver. Engineering control and operational control through changes of the exposure time and exposure pattern are possibilities.

Noise Reduction

Noise control from the source to the receiver is a well-established engineering discipline that is amenable to quantitative analysis and design. Noise reduction of stationary sources on the

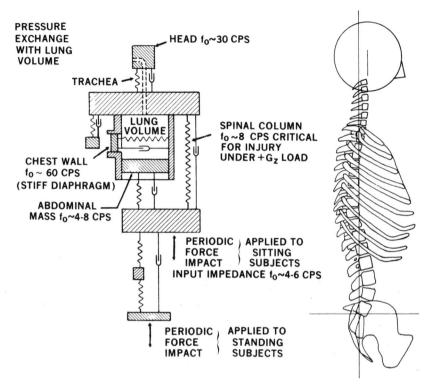

Figure 10.8. Models for describing and predicting vibration response. The left side of the figure shows the lumped parameter model. The right side of the figure shows the finite element upper torso model.

ground can be accomplished through conventional engineering approaches, such as isolation, shock mounting, damping, shielding, or enclosing the source to eliminate the radiation of airborne noise. Mufflers and hush houses for jet engines and aircraft are effective. Practical limits in noise control are dictated by operational and/or economical constraints. For example, the maintenance time of jet engines is increased because of the use of ground runup noise suppressors.

In closed facilities occupied by personnel, noise control is accomplished by sound treatment tailored to the specific noise situation. In aerospace vehicles, internal noise from air conditioners, blowers, and pneumatic pumps and external noise from the propulsion units and aerodynamic flow over the fuselage must be considered and controlled. Because weight and space are at a premium in flight vehicles, noise reduction is usually not designed to satisfy optimum

comfort criteria but to guarantee allowable safe exposure conditions and communication capability for crew members. Whenever possible and practical, increasing the distance between the noise source and the receiver is a very effective noise control measure. The amount of attenuation to be expected can be grossly estimated by the inverse square law, which predicts a 6 dB change of sound pressure level for each halving or doubling of the distance between source and receiver.

Personal Hearing Protection (10,11)

In most operational noise environments, the use of personal hearing protection devices (i.e., earplugs, earmuffs, helmets) is the only feasible means of reducing noise to an acceptable level at the ears of exposed personnel. The attenuation achieved by individuals under operational conditions varies considerably among the different devices depending on factors such as the

TYPE OF PROTECTION	THIRD-OCTAVE BAND CENTER FREQUENCIES (Hz)						
	125	250	500	1000	2000	4000	8000
EARPLUGS (Premolded, User formable)	10–30	10–30	15–35	20–35	20–40	30–45	25–45
FOAM EARPLUGS (Varies with depth of insertion)	20–35	20–35	25–40	25–40	30–40	40–45	35–45
EARPLUGS (Custom Molded)	5–20	5–20	10–25	10–25	20–30	25–40	25–40
SEMI-INSERT EARPLUGS	10–25	10–25	10–30	10–30	20–35	25–40	25–40
EARMUFFS (With or without communications)	5–20	10–25	15–30	25–40	30–40	30–40	25–40
EARPLUGS AND EARMUFFS (In combination)	20–40	25–45	25–50	30–50	35–45	40–50	40–50
ACTIVE NOISE REDUCTION HEADSETS	15–25	15–30	20–45	25–40 (IDENTICAL TO EARMUFFS ABOVE 1000 Hz)	30–40	30–40	25–40
HELMETS	0–15	5–15	15–25	15–30	25–40	30–50	20–50
SPACE HELMET (Total head enclosure)	8–12	10–15	15–25	15–30	25–40	30–50	30–60

Figure 10.9. The ranges of attenuation shown for good hearing protection devices represent the approximate minimum and maximum protection available.

selection, care, use, and effectiveness of the hearing protectors. All personnel should receive training on hearing protection devices and hearing conservation. Representative ranges of mean attenuation values of various types of hearing protection devices are summarized in Figure 10.9. The mean values are the ''real-ear attenuation'' determined in the laboratory by a standardized psychophysical method with human subjects wearing the devices. The average attenuation values are extended to cover 98% of the population by subtracting two standard deviations from the means. The attenuation obtained with hearing protectors in the operational situation is much less than that measured in the laboratory (after the standard deviation correction),

by about 10 dB to 20 dB for earplugs and 5 dB to 10 dB for earmuffs. These differences are due to the high attenuation measured under ideal conditions in the laboratory compared to the low attenuation resulting from factors in the work place such as lack of training, incorrect size and fit, poor motivation, deterioration of devices, and modifications to the devices by employees. The maximum attenuation of 40 dB to 50 dB achievable with the best hearing protection devices is not typically obtained because of air leaks, vibration of the protector, and sound passing through the materials. Even with maximum attenuation, intense levels of sound bypass the hearing protection device, enter the head and upper torso through areas not covered by the protectors, and reach the inner ear through tissue and bone conduction.

The performance of a hearing protection device can be conveniently described as a single number rating, such as the Noise Reduction Rating (NRR) required by the Environmental Protection Agency in its regulation on the noise labeling of hearing protectors (12). The NRR is calculated using the octave-band attenuation measured for the protector and it provides a single number attenuation value of the device. The A-weighted sound level under the device is estimated by subtracting the NRR from the C-weighted level of the noise. For example, a wearer of a device with an NRR of 25 dB is exposed to an effective level at the ear of 80 dB when the C-weighted level of the noise is 105 dB. Considerable accuracy is lost when the NRR is subtracted from the A-weighted level of the noise and a large safety factor must be included in the computation.

Active noise reduction (ANR) (13) hearing protection devices reduce the low frequency noise at the ear under the earcup by means of cancellation. An average ANR increase of 15 to 20 dB in attenuation over that provided by the passive earcup may be obtained in the frequency range below 2000 Hz, with as much as 25 dB at some frequencies. Active noise reduction headsets reduce the low-frequency sound at the ear, which provides better intelligibility, increased comfort, less hearing loss, and less fatigue than the same headset with only passive attenuation.

Speech and Other Acoustic Signals With Hearing Protectors

Speech communication is slightly easier for normal hearing persons when earplugs or earmuffs are worn than without them in broad band noises ranging from 85 dB to about 105 dB. This occurs because both the speech and noise are reduced and the aural distortion due to the high level sounds is minimized. Non-normal hearing persons with high frequency hearing losses may not experience this communication advantage

while wearing hearing protection in noise. Ordinarily, recognition of auditory warning signals is the same either with or without hearing protection devices, even though they may sound different, because the levels of both the noise and the auditory signal are equally attenuated. However, non-normal hearing wearers may have some recognition difficulty while wearing hearing protectors depending upon the nature of the hearing loss and of the auditory signal.

Earmuffs that electronically transmit the speech signal from the outside to the inside of the earmuff are used in noise environments which fluctuate frequently between noise and quiet. The transmission of speech occurs at ambient levels of noises of about 85 dB and below. The electronics do not operate in levels of noise above 85 dB where only the passive attenuation of the earmuff is provided to the wearer.

Sound Protection at Infrasonic and Ultrasonic Frequencies

Hearing protection provided by good insert earplugs at infrasonic frequencies (i.e., sounds at frequencies below 20 Hz) is about the same as that observed at the 125 Hz center frequency (cf) one-third octave band. Very little protection is provided by earmuffs and sound may even be amplified at some of these infrasonic frequencies. Very good protection is provided by conventional earplugs or earmuffs at the ultrasonic frequencies above about 20,000 Hz. Attenuation exceeding 30 dB is generally provided for frequencies from 10,000 to 30,000 Hz.

Vibration Reduction

Protection against undesirable vibration is accomplished by two means: (1) attenuation of the vibration delivered to the crew or isolation of the crew; and (2) restraining of the crewmember to the seatback and armrest to reduce relative displacement with respect to the seat, displays, and control handles and to minimize displacement of one body segment relative to another. Safety and performance criteria require vibration protection primarily in the frequency range below 12 Hz. Unfortunately, for many aerospace situations, the requirements for safety, comfort, and performance capability are not necessarily mutually compatible. In the low-frequency range, effective vibration isolation of a whole person requires large stroke distances, which are undesirable as long as displays and controls do not move with the person and are intolerable in space systems and military aircraft equipped with an ejection seat. Impact acceleration loads transmitted through an elastic seat or soft seat cushion usually lead to an amplification of the dynamic response of the human structure and an increased injury risk. The most common compromise is a seat cushion with a nonlinear stress-strain relationship. A soft elastic top layer provides comfort and isolation from annoying high-frequency vibration and the stiffer lower layers bottom out under high-amplitude impact accelerations.

Whole-body restraint in both commercial and military aircraft requires a compromise between acceleration, vibration, and impact protection and the mobility requirements for satisfying performance capability and comfort. Inertia reel-locking mechanisms employed for crash protection are actuated at higher forces and displacements than are usually involved in aircraft and spacecraft vibrations but can offer some protection against high-amplitude oscillations and displacement from the seat due to unexpected severe turbulence.

Another compromise to be considered in military aircraft and space systems is with respect to body positioning. Human tolerance to sustained G is maximum in the G_x (chest-to-back) direction, a fact which led to the use of the space couch for launch and reentry and the reclined seat proposals for high-performance military fighters. G_x vibrations transmitted to the crew through a couchlike body support expose the human head directly to the unattenuated input vibrations without the benefit of head isolation through the body structure in the seated position. Exposure criteria for this situation are available and must be considered.

Reducing direct vibration inputs to the hands, arms, or head usually presents no serious engineering problem once the necessity is predicted or recognized. Serious problems can exist with respect to occupational exposure to vibrations transmitted directly to the hand and arm from hand tools such as chipping hammers, pneumatic tools, and chain saws. Safety standards established for such exposures must be met for frequencies up to at least 1,000 Hz by appropriate tool design, the wearing of protective gloves, and operational exposure time control.

EFFECTS OF AEROSPACE NOISES

The effects of aerospace noises on man have been divided into physiologic and psychologic responses. Physiologic responses, both auditory and nonauditory, involve changes in physiologic mechanisms or functions attributed to the noise. Auditory effects are confined to direct influences on the peripheral auditory system and the hearing function. Acoustic energy exposures can also affect the vestibular system, the autonomic nervous system, sleep, and startle and induce fatigue; however, with few exceptions, these nonauditory effects also are mediated through the auditory system. Psychologic response behavior to noise is influenced by man's perceptions, judgments, attitudes, and opinions, which may be either related or unrelated to the noise itself. Most noise exposures stimulate elements of both types of responses, which clearly affect and interact with one another (14).

Human Hearing Function (15)

The human auditory system is an extremely sensitive and highly specialized mechanism that is also quite resistant to the adverse effects of acoustic energy unless abused (Fig. 10.10) (11). The audible frequency range in the normal, young human ear extends from about 16 to 20,000 Hz. The most sensitive region of hearing is from about 500 to 4,000 Hz; this band is most important for understanding speech and is

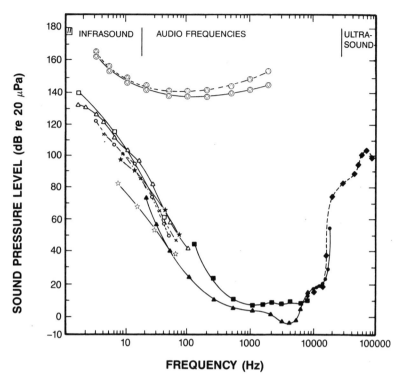

Figure 10.10. Human auditory sensitivity and pain threshold levels. □ = Von Bekesy (1960) Data-Minimum Audible Pressure (MAP); ○ = Yeowart, Bryan, and Tempest (1969) Data-MAP; △ = Whittle, Collins, and Robinson (1972) Data-MAP; X = Yeowart, Bryan, and Tempest (1969) Data-MAO for bands of noise; ■ = Standard reference threshold values-MAP (American National Standard on Specifications For Audiometers, 1969); ▲ = ISO R226-Minimum Audible Field (1961); ● = Northern, et al. (1972) Data; ◆ = Corso (1963) Data-Bone conduction minus 40 dB; ◎ = Von Bekesy (1960) Data = Tickle, pain; ◉ = Benox; ▩ = Static Pressure-Pain; ☆ = Yamada et. al. (1986) Average hearing threshold; ★ = Yamada et. al. (1986) Minimum hearing threshold. Adapted from Nixon CW. Excessive noise exposure. In: Singh S, ed. Measurement procedures in speech, hearing, and language. Baltimore: University Park Press, 1975.

expressed in decibels relative to the normal threshold of hearing or standard hearing reference zero. In the infrasound region, below 20 Hz, signal detection by the human ear requires high sound-pressure levels, and tonal quality is lost below about 16 Hz. Airborne ultrasound, energy above 20,000 Hz, is not ordinarily perceived by the human ear. The harmonics of infrasound and subharmonics of ultrasound may be perceived outside their respective frequency regions. Although well below the upper boundary of hearing, intense acoustic signals do produce tickle, discomfort, and even pain in the ear.

Hearing level is an individual's hearing sensitivity for standard test frequencies expressed in decibels relative to the normative hearing refer-

ence values. The range of normal hearing sensitivity is from −10 to 25 dB for a pure-tone air-conduction audiogram (Fig. 10.11). Hearing levels greater than 25 dB are considered below normal and constitute hearing loss. Conductive-type hearing losses, caused by impairment of outer and middle ear function, are relatively the same value for each test frequency and appear flat on the audiogram. Sensorineural or perceptive hearing loss, usually attributed to inner ear impairment, characteristically displays a growing loss of sensitivity with increasing frequency beginning around 1000 to 2000 Hz. Persons with hearing losses greater than 35 to 40 dB in the speech-frequency range (400 to 4000 Hz) are potential candidates for a hearing aid. Many conductive-

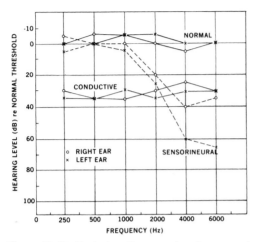

Figure 10.11. Typical audiograms showing normal hearing, a conductive-type hearing loss that is relatively flat, and a sensorineural or perceptive hearing loss with the characteristic loss of sensitivity with increasing frequency.

type problems are amenable to medical treatment, whereas sensorineural problems usually consist of permanent intractable losses.

Excessive noise exposure is one of the situations that may produce either or both of these hearing loss syndromes. Conductive hearing problems involving acoustic damage or mechanical stress to the tympanic membrane-middle ear system and sensorineural problems involve damage to the inner ear sensory system. The middle ear, mechanical-type acoustic trauma is the characteristic flat conductive hearing loss in which there is no sensorineural involvement. Noise-induced sensorineural hearing loss characteristically involves the higher audio frequencies and is a slow loss of sensitivity progressive with exposure time that is first observed between 2000 and 6000 Hz, with the greatest and most rapid decrease usually occurring at 4000 Hz. This loss increases in magnitude and spreads in frequency with continued exposure. The progression of noise-induced sensorineural loss with the number of years of exposure has been widely documented (15). Mixed hearing losses include both conductive and sensorineural components.

A number of protective actions operate in the

region of the middle ear to reduce the amount of acoustic energy transmitted to the inner ear. At high sound intensities, the motion of the stapes changes from a piston-like to a rocking action in the oval window due to temporary dislocation of the ossicular joints, thus reducing the efficiency of transmission. Also, the stapedic and tensor tympanic muscles contract, increasing the stiffness and the damping of the ossicular chain. The response latency of this muscle reflex varies from 25 to over 100 milliseconds; consequently, it operates too slowly to provide protection against brief, impulsive sounds shorter than about 20 milliseconds.

Temporary Threshold Shift (TTS) and Permanent Threshold Shift (PTS)

Noise-induced hearing loss may be either temporary or permanent. Temporary threshold shift is a loss of sensitivity that returns to normal or preexposure hearing levels within a reasonable time following cessation of the noise exposure. Permanent threshold shift is a loss of hearing that persists, with no recovery of sensitivity, regardless of the time away from the noise. Relationships have been established between recent noise exposure and TTS, and between PTS and noise exposure experienced in daily activities performed over many years. Noise-induced TTS is considered to be an integral part of an essential precursor to noise-induced PTS. It is further assumed that noise exposures that do not produce TTS will not produce PTS, that PTS develops similarly to TTS but on a slower time scale, and, finally, that different noise exposures which produce equal amounts of TTS also are considered equally noxious with regard to PTS. These assumptions, based on TTS data from the laboratory and TTS/PTS data from actual field noise exposures, have provided a basis for formulating noise exposure standards and hearing risk criteria that relate noise exposure with hearing loss (16,17).The development and statistical distribution of noise-induced hearing loss in a population as a function of daily noise exposure for exposure times from 10 years to 40 years can be estimated by standardized procedures (17).

Presbycusis

Noise-induced sensorineural hearing loss may be confounded by presbycusis (15), which is the gradual loss of high-frequency auditory sensitivity that accompanies advancing age. Loss of sensitivity attributed to accidents, disease, or ototoxic substances is called nosoacusis and that attributed to non-occupational noise exposure is called sociacusis. On the average, auditory sensitivity diminishes as a function of age at frequencies from 500 to 6000 Hz, beginning in the third decade of life. The higher the frequency, the greater the loss, with the maximum loss appearing at 4000 Hz. Aerospace medical evaluations of noise-induced hearing loss should estimate that portion of the loss, if any, which is contributed by presbycusis. This may be accomplished statistically by subtracting the average presbycusis value for a non-noise-exposed population from the hearing loss values at each frequency. Present data bases suggest less presbycusis loss for females than for males, whereas there appears to be no gender differences with respect to noise-induced hearing loss (17). The remaining loss of hearing may be attributed to the noise exposure history of the individual, other factors considered.

Auditory Pain

Auditory pain due to intense noise is associated with excessive mechanical displacement of the middle ear system and is believed to occur in the threshold region where damage begins. Noise-induced auditory pain occurs almost independent of frequency at levels of 130 to 140 dB SPL and above. No pain is associated with overexposure of the inner ear; however, ringing or similar sounds in the ear produced by the noise do suggest that acceptable exposure limits have been exceeded and that the responsible exposure should not be repeated.

Static Air Pressure

Differential pressures may occur across the tympanic membrane with variations in pressure associated with changing atmospheric (flight) conditions and a eustachian tube that remains closed. Although a high pressure differential may cause noticeable discomfort or pain, lower pressure differences could cause an undetected decrease in hearing sensitivity of 8 to 10 dB for frequencies below 1500 and above 2300 Hz. These effects are usually transitory and may be relieved by the Valsalva maneuver or other means of equalizing ambient and middle ear pressures.

Individual Susceptibility

Individual ears vary greatly in their susceptibility to the adverse effects of noise. Although the ability to determine the noise susceptibility of an ear would be most valuable prior to a work assignment in noise, no satisfactory method for quantifying susceptibility has been developed. Exposure standards and criteria do not include a susceptibility factor because of this wide variance and the inability to predict TTS for a specific ear.

Nonauditory Effects of Continuous Noise

Generally, humans adapt quite well to stimuli such as noise; however, adaptation has not been demonstrated by the responses of a variety of nonauditory systems. Changes in physiologic responses to noise have been measured under laboratory conditions and in real-life situations; however, the magnitudes of these changes are frequently no greater than those experienced under typical daily living conditions. Although some physiologic reactions to certain noises occur at levels as low as 70 dB, the state of understanding is still unclear as to relationships between potential adverse physiologic effects and general noise exposure, as well as to the significance to general health and well-being of the changes that do occur (14,15).

General Physiologic Responses

Because most nonauditory effects are mediated through the auditory system, they may be avoided with the use of adequate hearing protection, which, unfortunately, is impractical in many situations (Fig. 10.9). Even with maximum hearing protection, exposure to sound pressure levels in excess of 150 dB should be prohibited because of mechanical stimulation of receptors other than the ear. Noise spectra containing intense low-frequency and infrasonic energy may excite body parts such as the chest, abdomen, eyes, and sinus cavities, causing concern, annoyance, and fatigue. The response of the vestibular system to extremely high levels of noise apparently mediated through the auditory system manifests itself by disorientation, motion sickness, and interference with postural equilibrium.

A number of investigators have reported general and specific physiologic responses to sound. The reported responses include effects on the peripheral blood flow, respiration, galvanic skin response, skeletal muscle tension, gastrointestinal motility, cardiac response, pupillary dilation, and renal and glandular function. Recent emphasis has been directed toward hypertension, elevated blood pressure, and cardiovascular responses. Review of the European literature on the cardiovascular and related responses to noise primarily in industrial settings shows that the effects varied from study to study; however, the overall findings indicated adverse effects on the general health parameters investigated. Similar work in the United States has not demonstrated the same degree of adverse effects as shown in these European studies. A recent analysis of the potential association between noise-induced hearing loss and cardiovascular diseases in United States Air Force aircrew members was completely negative and raised the question how important a negative attitude towards the noise and the motivation might have been in the studies with positive results (16). Nevertheless, this area of concern is especially significant, and additional work is required to ensure that reasonable decisions that are safe for the exposed individuals are possible. In addition to these studies, subjective reports of fatigue, loss of appetite, irritability, nausea, disorientation, headache, and even loss of memory continue to be attributed to high and extended noise exposure. Caution should be exercised, however, in attributing such adverse effects solely to noise in various aerospace and industrial situations where numerous other factors may contribute to or create physiologic problems. The contribution of conditions such as temperature extremes, poor ventilation, threat of accidental injury or death, special task demands, and other non-noise elements that tend to grow as noise intensity grows cannot be ascertained without being controlled in test populations.

Subjective reports of disorientation, vertigo, nausea, and interference with postural equilibrium during high-intensity noise exposure suggest stimulation of the vestibular system. Empirical efforts to demonstrate the vestibular response to acoustic energy have been inconclusive; however, the evidence does suggest the vestibular system as the most probable site responding to the acoustic stimulation. Other than the vestibular system, mechanoreceptors and proprioreceptors may be the primary mediators of physiologic responses at SPLs above 140 dB.

Sleep Interference

Interference with sleep due to noise could be a serious effect because there is widespread agreement that adequate sleep is a physiologic necessity. Two general kinds of sleep interference are due to noise: Actual arousal or wakening, and changes within the sleeping individual who does not awaken. Sleep occurs in stages or levels, which are revealed by patterns of electrical activity in the brain. Individuals are more susceptible to awakening during some stages of sleep than during others. During sleep stage 2, subjects are more susceptible to behavioral wakening than during the other stages; they are more resistant to wakening during stage 4 and REM (rapid eye movements with dreaming) sleep. Sleeping individuals not awakened in response to noise stimuli still have shown changes in electroencephalographic recordings, as well as in peripheral vasoconstriction and heart rate. These responses confirm that measurable effects of noise on biologic responses occur in man during sleep, even though the sleeper is totally unaware of the acoustic exposure.

An interesting investigation of sleep was conducted by Myasnikov, who exposed subjects to broadband continuous noise at levels of 75 to 78 dB during simulated space flight. A dichotomy emerged: Subjects who fell asleep rapidly slept well and awakened feeling well, and subjects who fell asleep with difficulty did not sleep well and did not feel well on awakening. Other effects were generally bimodal, corresponding to the two types of sleepers. Myasnikov concluded that the selection of candidates for astronauts should include screening of sleep characteristics to eliminate poor sleepers, especially for lengthy missions.

Startle

Startle may be evoked by a wide variety of stimuli but is particularly susceptible to sudden, unexpected noises. This response is more consistent among individuals than almost any other behavioral pattern. The physiologic aspects of the startle response are reasonably independent of the stimulus and include increased pulse rate, increased blood pressure, and diversion of blood flow to the peripheral limbs and gross musculature. Startle responses do not occur frequently or with any regularity in aerospace environments; consequently, they have not been an operational problem. The universality and uniformity of this reaction from one person to another suggests that startle is an inborn reaction that is modified little by learning and experience.

Several studies have been cited to point out that nonauditory physiologic responses to acoustic energy have been observed and measured among selected populations. At the same time, it should be emphasized that these findings are not sufficiently clear or consistent to demonstrate relationships reliable enough to generalize about any typical populations. The aerospace physician must evaluate potential adverse effects of aerospace noise environments on an individual basis, especially when they fall outside the conditions specified in existing standards and criteria for allowable noise exposures.

Psychologic Responses

Numerous psychologic factors in the lives of individuals, such as their perceptions, beliefs, attitudes, and opinions, contribute to the manner in which they respond to noise from aerospace activities. These responses are generally treated in terms of annoyance, performance, and speech communication, which is a special task addressed in a separate section of this chapter.

Annoyance

Acoustic energy is undesirable when attention is called to it unnecessarily or when it interferes with routine activities in the home, office, shop, recreational area, or elsewhere. Individuals become annoyed when the amount of interference becomes significant. Numerous techniques based on measurement of the physical stimulus are used to assess noise exposure effects on people in work and living spaces and to estimate community reaction to noise. One concept maintains that the human reaction to a sound is determined by the annoyance or unwantedness of the sound instead of its loudness. This subjectively judged unwantedness of sounds is described as perceived noisiness (PN). Perceived noisiness may be adequately determined by using the physical measurements of the sound to calculate perceived noisiness in decibels, or PNdB.

Relationships between various PNdB levels and the nature of community reactions that correspond to them have been defined on the basis of data from airport noise experiences, as well as both laboratory and field research. These relationships are compiled for use in estimating reactions, and a step-by-step procedure is available for arriving at PNdB values from the measurement data of the noise. A comprehensive discussion of the concept of perceived noisiness is presented in detailed form in Kryter's discussion (15).

A different concept of estimating annoyance incorporates both the duration and magnitude of all the acoustic energy occurring during a given time period. The measurement unit is the average sound level and is called the equivalent continuous sound level (Leq). The noise energy content of the continuous A-weighted level is equivalent to that of the actual fluctuating noise existing over the total observation period. Leq, which is the energy mean noise level, is defined as the level of the steady-state continuous noise having the same energy as the actual time-varying noise. The problem of quantifying environmental noise is greatly simplified using the statistical measures of the Leq. The Leq is one of the most important measures of environmental noise for assessing effects on humans, because experimental evidence suggests that it accurately describes the development of noise-induced hearing loss and that it applies to human annoyance due to noise.

The equivalent continuous sound level (Leq) measured over a 24-hour period is the day-night average sound level (Ldn), which is weighted for night time exposures with a 10-dB penalty. Ldn is used to relate noise exposures in residential environments to interference with daily living activities and sleep, as well as to chronic annoyance. Most daily noise environments are repetitive in nature, with some variations occurring over weekends and with seasonal changes. It has been found useful to treat environmental noise as a long-term, yearly average of the daily levels to account for these variations.

Performance

The effects of noise on cognitive and sensorimotor performance remain unclear and very complex. The same general experimental conditions have produced performance enhancement on some occasions and performance degradation on others. However, performance degradation due to noise has been reported with reasonable consistency in a number of task situations. The efficiency of vigilance tasks (requiring alertness) over long periods of time was degraded in noise environments of about 100 dB. Mental counting tasks were influenced in a complex manner, and time judgments were found to be distorted. High-frequency noise of sufficient intensity produces more harmful effects on performance than low-frequency noises. Sudden and unexpected changes in noise level, either up or down, may produce momentary disturbances. Noise ordinarily increases the number of errors but does not reduce the speed at which work is performed. High-level and moderate-level noises may act as stress factors and contribute to general fatigue and irritability. The general level of performance may be influenced by these responses.

Sleep and Startle

Both startle and sleep interference have substantial psychological components in addition to the clear-cut physiologic components discussed earlier. In fact, the major adverse reaction of annoyance is usually caused by being startled or awakened and not because of the changes in physiologic response that also occur. The personal feelings of the exposed individual regarding factors such as the reason for the disturbance, concern over those who are causing the disturbance, attempts to minimize and eliminate the disturbance, and other factors usually determine the degree of acceptance or annoyance to the acoustic energy.

Impulse Noise and Blast (18)

Noise exposures generated by weapons fire, explosions, impact devices in industry, and sonic booms are impulsive or transient in nature and are not covered by most continuous noise exposure data. Guidelines for the exposure to various kinds of impulses generated by these sources are contained in established standards and criteria. Some typical values of peak SPL for impulse noise are presented in Table 10.3. The standard method for the estimation of noise-induced hearing impairment includes instantaneous sound pressures (impact or impulse noise) not exceed-

Table 10.3.
Some Typical Values of Peak Sound Pressure Levels (SPL) For Impulse Noise

SPL (in dB re 20 micropascals)	Example
190+	Within blast zone of exploding bomb
160–180	Within crew area of heavy artillery piece or naval gun when shooting
140–170	At shooter's ear when firing handgun
125–160	At child's ear when detonating toy cap or firecracker
120–140	Metal-to-metal impacts in many industrial processes (e.g., drop-forging, metal-beating)
110–130	On construction site during pile-driving

ing 140 dB at the ear (e.g., potentially under the hearing protection device) in the averaged A-weighted sound exposure used to calculate hearing impairment (17).

Noise exposures with rapid rise times and durations of less than 1 second have been described as impulse noises. When impulsive noises occur repeatedly or at high levels, their potential for producing adverse effects on the auditory system is relatively high. Temporary threshold shift is systematically treated in the various exposure criteria cited above. The higher the peak pressure level of the impulse, the greater the risk of TTS. Other things being equal, longer impulse durations, higher repetition rates, and greater high-frequency energy in the spectrum of the impulse also pose greater risks to hearing. Although various impulsive sound exposures differ a great deal, TTS usually occurs in the 4000- to 6000-Hz region of hearing. Impulses repeated at a constant rate produce TTS that is generally predictable; however, TTS from single impulses and recovery both from single impulses and from serial impulses are more erratic and less predictable than from steady-state exposures.

The acoustic shock wave or blast noise generated by explosions is treated similarly to impulse noise by the ear even though the levels are much higher and the durations longer. The relationships between impulsive noise and the auditory system and function are generally the same for blast noise.

The eardrum may be ruptured by intense levels of blast noise or impulse noise. The high amplitude causes the operation of the middle ear system to exceed its mechanical limits, causing eardrum rupture and, in severe cases, disarticulation and damage to the ossicular chain. Acoustic signals of sufficient severity to rupture the eardrum membrane also often cause some sensorineural involvement. Eardrum rupture, however, which causes a flat 20 to 40 dB hearing loss, is usually repairable if it does not heal itself, and the conductive hearing loss is restored. Eardrum rupture in response to these intense signals is considered to be a safety function that prevents the acoustic energy from reaching the inner ear. If the eardrum does not rupture, severe PTS at the high frequencies can be the result of the exposure. The threshold of eardrum rupture is about 5 psi, with 50% of eardrums failing at 15 psi. The threshold for lung damage also is estimated to be in the region of 15 psi.

Sonic Boom

Research on the effects of sonic booms on people was concentrated in the late 1960s and early 1970s relative to potential over flights of land by commercial supersonic aircraft (19). Decisions to stop the United States supersonic transport (SST) program and to prevent commercial flights over land at supersonic speeds resulted in sharply reduced research on sonic boom effects. Today's knowledge of sonic booms is, with few exceptions, based on research conducted in those years (Table 10.4).

The sonic boom is again becoming an important issue for aerospace operations. The increasing numbers of high-performance aircraft being acquired by the United States Department of

Table 10.4.
Sonic Boom and Blast Exposures: Measurements and Estimations

Peak Exposures			Predicted and/or Measured Effects
lb/ft^2	dynes/cm^2		
0–1	0–478		No damage to ground structures; no significant public reaction day or night
1.0–1.5	478–717	Sonic booms from normal operational altitudes	Very rare minor damage to ground structures; probable public reaction
1.5–2.0	717–957	typical community exposure (seldom above 2 lb/ft^2)	Rare minor damage to ground structures; significant public reaction, particularly at night
2.0–5.0	957–2393		Incipient damage to structures
20–144	9.57×10^3 6.8×10^4		Measured sonic booms from aircraft flying at supersonic speeds at minimum altitude; experienced by human without injury
720	3.44×10^5		Estimated threshold for eardrum rupture (maximum overpressure)
2160	1.033×10^6		Estimated threshold for lung damage (maximum overpressure)

From von Gierke HE and Nixon CW: Human Response to sonic boom in the laboratory and the community. J Acoust Soc Am Part 2, *31:*5, May 1966.

Defense have resulted in urgent requirements for new air space for supersonic training where some sonic booms will not be a problem. Present and future space programs will use vehicles that produce sonic booms during launch and reentry at more frequent intervals. Certain space-launch flight trajectories, as well as reentry from space at supersonic speeds, generate sonic booms that reach the ground. The impact on the population of these space vehicle-generated sonic booms, however, is expected to be small. These booms are generated at high altitudes with very long propagation distances and at infrequent intervals. The actual effects on communities of more frequent sonic booms anticipated for the future are yet to be determined.

Generally, sonic booms do not cause direct injury to humans, although both physiologic and psychologic changes may be stimulated by the sudden, unexpected loud sound. The potential effects of such acoustic exposures over many years, if any, have yet to be determined. The human auditory mechanism has shown no adverse effects of sonic booms in individuals exposed under special field and laboratory test conditions to numbers and intensities of booms greater than those that could occur under typical living conditions (20).

Although alleged health effects of sonic booms have been reported, the major problems continue to be annoyance with the reaction caused by startle, fear associated with startle, interruption of activities, shaking and rattling of structures and buildings, sleep and rest interference, and attitudes toward those causing the sonic booms.

COMMUNICATION IN AEROSPACE ENVIRONMENTS

Voice communications effectiveness is influenced by environmental, personal, message, and equipment factors in aerospace operations (21). Noise, both acoustic and electrical, is the most predominant environmental factor; however, acceleration, whole-body vibration, artificial atmospheres, combinations of stressors, special task requirements, and environmental threats to personal safety also can alter communications. Audio communications may be further affected by personal speech habits, dialects, word usage, hearing loss, the amount and type of communication experience, and even the emotional state of the individual. Communications are also affected by speech elements that include message set, type of material, vocabulary size, both familiar and unexpected terms, and infrequently used phrases. Communication equipment can be optimized for human speech using peak-clipping, spectrum-shaping, adequate passband, appropriate impedance, and other methods to result in very little equipment degradation of speech.

Definition and Assessment of Speech Intelligibility

Various standardized methodologies measure the performance of the total voice communication system, or of the various individual elements of the communication chain, with or without the man in the loop. These methodologies are based on the subjective measurement of intelligibility, which is the percentage of a given sample of speech presented to an observer that is correctly perceived, as well as the physical measurement of the communication system and environment. Everyday speech is difficult to quantify and measure, so that smaller collections of speech have been organized into groups of syllables, words, phrases, or sentences that can be more precisely specified relative to everyday communications. Most of these groups of materials, or tests of speech intelligibility, have been standardized with human operators in the loop to provide reliable measurements that can be generalized to other populations. Relating the physical measurements of the communications systems and environments to the speech intelligibility measurements allows the assessment of speech communications effectiveness.

The major operational threat to voice communications is noise that may mask or drown out the speech or produce a temporary hearing loss that interferes with the listener's ability to understand the message. Speech communication assessment techniques use physical measurements of the noise to assess the masking effect but do not account for temporary hearing loss that may be experienced by the communicators. Overall, the least sophisticated measurement method for estimating communications effectiveness is the sound level or the A-weighted sound level

(dB(A)). Speech interference levels (SIL) is the simplest method using octave-band descriptions of the noise. A more refined method developed for use in a wide range of applications is noise criteria (NC). The most comprehensive method for predicting speech communications in noise environments is the articulation index (AI). The most direct approach is to simulate the communication environmental and system variables and directly measure the intelligibility response of interest.

Communication versus Sound Level

The A-weighting approximates sensitivity of the normal human ear to moderate-level sound. The measured values in Figure 10.12 provide relationships between communication capability and noise (dB(A)). Speech communication effectiveness as a function of type of communication and A-weighted sound level is provided in Table 10.5. This procedure is ideal for predicting intelligibility for survey and monitoring purposes; however, it is unsuited for noise control and engineering purposes because detailed spectral information is lacking in the descriptor. Additional accuracy with sound level data may be obtained using the correction factor for noise spectrum described in *Handbook of Noise Control* (21).

Speech Interference Level

Speech interference level (SIL) procedures allow estimates of the maximum acceptable noise levels for satisfactory speech communication based on octave-band descriptions of the noise. The SIL is the arithmetic average of the sound pressure levels (dB) of the noise in the octave bands centered at 500, 1000, 2000, and 4000 Hz. SIL values for reliable communications at various distances and voice levels are shown in Figure 10.12.

Noise Criteria

Noise criteria (NC) are an expansion of SIL from a single number to sets of numbers representing octave-band values. The term NC is used

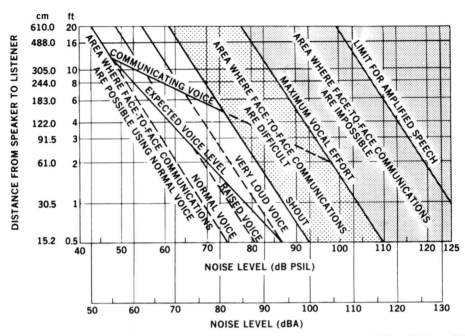

Figure 10.12. Measures of noise level and corresponding communications capabilities (PSIL an dB(A)).

Table 10.5.
Speech Communication Capabilities Versus A-Weighted Sound Level dB(A) of the Background Noise

Communication	Below 50 dBA	50 to 70 dBA	70 to 90 dBA	90 to 100 dBA	110 to 130 dBA
Face-to-face (unamplified speech)	Normal voice at distances up to 6 m	Raised voice at distances up to 2 m	Very loud or shouted voice level at distances up to 50 cm	Maximum voice level at distances up to 25 cm	Very difficult to impossible, even at a distance of 1 cm
Telephone	Good	Satisfactory to slightly difficult	Difficult to unsatisfactory	Use press-to-talk switch and an acoustically treated booth	Use special equipment
Intercom system	Good	Satisfactory to difficult	Unsatisfactory using loudspeaker	Impossible using loudspeaker	Impossible using loudspeaker
Type of earphone to supplement loudspeaker	None	Any	Using any earphone	Using any in earmuff or helmet except bone conduction-type	Use insert-type or over-ear earphones in helmet or in earmuffs; good to 120 dBA on short-term basis
Public-address system	Good	Satisfactory	Satisfactory to difficult	Difficult	Very difficult
Type of microphone required	Any	Any	Any	Any noise-cancelling microphone	Good noise-cancelling microphone

Table 10.6.
Octave-Band Sound Pressure Level (SPL) Values Associated With the Recommended 1971 Preferred Noise Criterion (PNC) Curves

Preferred Noise	31.5	63	125	250	500	1000	2000	4000	8000
Criterion Curves	Hz	Hz	Hz	Hz	Hz	Hz	Hz	Hz	Hz
PNC-15	58	432	35	28	21	15	10	8	8
PNC-20	59	46	39	32	26	20	15	13	13
PNC-25	60	49	43	37	31	25	20	18	18
PNC-30	61	52	46	41	35	30	25	23	23
PNC-35	62	55	50	45	40	35	30	28	28
PNC-40	64	59	54	50	45	40	35	33	33
PNC-45	67	63	58	54	50	45	41	38	38
PNC-50	70	66	62	58	54	50	46	43	43
PNC-55	73	70	66	62	59	55	51	48	48
PNC-60	76	73	69	66	63	59	56	53	53
PNC-65	79	76	73	70	67	64	61	58	58

interchangeably with preferred noise criterion (PNC). Noise criteria allow estimations of the quality of speech communication that may be expected with various indoor functional activities. Octave-band sound pressure levels for these functional activities are described in Table 10.6. To estimate the quality of communication for a given noise environment:

1. The noise in the octave bands must be described.
2. The octave-band spectrum must be compared with the appropriate PNC curve in Table 10.6.
3. The criterion value just above the highest octave-band level must be used to describe the noise environment.
4. The quality of communication to be expected for that environment must be determined (Table 10.7).

Articulation Index

The articulation index (AI) is calculated from physical measurements made on a communication system that describes the intelligibility that might be expected for that system under actual conditions. The speech spectrum and effective masking spectrum at the ear of the listener are required for the computation. The method is applicable for communication situations that involve male talkers.

Procedures for calculating the AI are based on the spectrum level of the noise and of speech present in 20 contiguous bands of frequencies, octave bands, or one-third octave bands of frequencies. The greatest precision is obtained with the 20-band procedure, the least precision is obtained with the octave-band method. An appropriate worksheet must be used to calculate the AI. A sample worksheet is shown in Figure 10.13, and Figure 10.14 is a sample calculation of an AI by the octave-band method for a relatively flat noise spectrum of moderate intensity. This calculation procedure may be followed in the example in Figure 10.14, which provides an AI of 0.54. The procedure is as follows:

1. The octave-band of the steady-state noise reaching the listener's ears must be plotted.
2. The idealized speech peaks curve must be adjusted to reflect the speech curve in the system under test.
3. The difference in decibels at the band center frequencies between the speech and the noise spectra must be determined. (Assign zero to differences less than one and 30 to differences greater than 30.)
4. The difference values in each band must be multiplied by the weighting factor for that band and the resulting numbers added to obtain the AI.

Table 10.7.
Recommended Noise Criteria Ranges For Steady Background Noise as Heard in Various Indoor Functional Areas

Type of Space (and Acoustic Requirements)	PNC Curve	Approximate Sound Level dB(A)
For sleeping, resting, relaxing, bedrooms, sleeping quarters, hospitals, residences, apartments	25–40	34–47
For fair-listening conditions; laboratory work spaces, drafting and engineering rooms, general secretarial areas	40–50	47–56
For moderately fair-listening conditions; light maintenance shops, office and computer equipment rooms	45–55	52–61
For just-acceptable speech and telephone communication; shops, garages, powerplant control rooms, Levels above PNC-60 are not recommended for any office or communication situation	50–60	56–66
For work spaces where speech or telephone communication is not required, but where there must be no risk of hearing damage	60–75	66–80

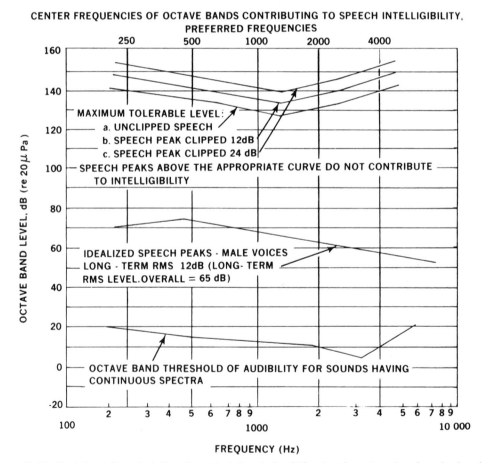

Figure 10.13. Worksheet for calculating the articulation index (AI) using the octave-band method and preferred frequencies.

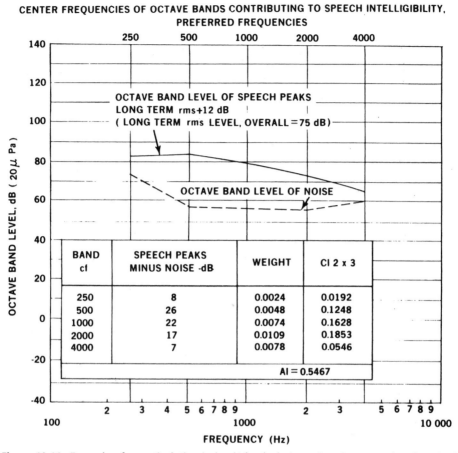

Figure 10.14. Example of an articulation index (AI) calculation using the octave-band method.

A number of factors that influence speech intelligibility scores, either individually or in combination, may be quantitatively evaluated using the AI. Some of the factors are: (1) masking by steady-state noise; (2) masking by nonsteady-state noise, including the interruption rate; (3) frequency distortion of the speech signal; (4) amplitude distortion of the speech signal; (5) reverberation time; (6) vocal effort; and (7) visual cues. The many factors not evaluated by AI include (1) the gender of the talker; (2) multiple transmission paths; (3) combinations of distortions; (4) monaural versus binaural presentation; and (5) asymmetric clipping, frequency shifting, and fading.

The relationship of AI to the various measures

of speech intelligibility is shown in Figure 10.15. The intelligibility score is dependent on the constraints placed on the message—that is, the greater the constraint, the higher the intelligibility score. No single-value AI can be established as a universally acceptable communications criterion because of variations in the proficiency of talkers and listeners and in the nature of the messages to be transmitted. The AI is a consistent, reliable procedure for predicting the relative performance of communications systems operating under given conditions. Modern communications systems usually have design goals of AIs in excess of 0.5. An AI of 0.7 appears appropriate as a goal for systems that will operate under a variety of stress conditions and with

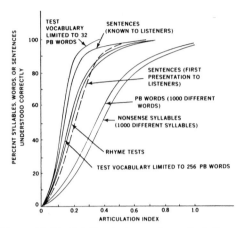

Figure 10.15. Relation between the articulation index and the various measures of speech intelligibility. These relationships are approximate.

many different talkers and listeners of varying degrees of skill.

The Room Acoustics Speech Transmission Index (RASTI) (22) is a procedure using specialized instrumentation which estimates the quality of speech intelligibility in rooms, lecture halls, churches, and auditoriums. An artificial talker generates a specific test signal at the talker's position, and a small device with a microphone receives the test signal at the listener's position in the room. An analysis of the received test signal yields an index value which indicates the speech intelligibility for that particular talker and listener position in the room. Although the RASTI provides accurate estimations of speech intelligibility in a wide variety of rooms, it has not been generally accepted yet for use with voice communications systems.

Measurements of Intelligibility

In some situations, the speech and/or noise characteristics may not satisfy the basic assumptions underlying the standard calculation procedures. Unusual noise environments, whole-body vibration in noise, audio communications jamming, and artificial atmospheres are examples. The communication efficiency with talkers and/ or listeners in the environment of interest must then be measured. Three procedures for measur-

ing speech intelligibility have been standardized and are described in ANSI-S3.2–1989. The most sensitive of these is the Phonetically Balanced (PB) Monosyllable Word Intelligibility Test (23). This test consists of trained talkers reading lists of phonetically balanced material to trained listeners using the communication system features being evaluated. A score of about 70% on the PB word lists corresponds to more than 90% intelligibility for sentences. The Modified Rhyme Test (MRT) is a test of choice for evaluating the performance of aerospace voice communications systems in the presence of environmental noise. Trained talkers read to trained listeners material that consists of lists of 50 one-syllable words that are equivalent in intelligibility. Test words are presented imbedded within a carrier phrase that is the same for each item. The MRT is easy to administer, score, and evaluate, and it does not require extensive training of the listeners. The MRT word intelligibility has been sufficiently standardized to allow the relative intelligibility of such materials as closed message sets and sentences to be estimated on the basis of corresponding measured MRT scores. Scores of 80% and above are acceptable for aerospace and military systems; scores of 70% to 80% are generally marginal, and scores below 70% represent unacceptable voice communications for such applications. The Diagnostic Rhyme Test (DRT) consists of lists of common, monosyllabic English words which are presented in pairs to the listeners who must select the correct response. A carrier phrase is not used. The DRT words differ only in their initial consonant and are based on distinctive features of speech, such as voicing, nasality, and sibilation instead of speech sounds. The test can be administered very quickly, scored in different ways, and is effective for diagnosing deficiencies of a communication system, which affect particular distinctive features of speech.

Effects of Noise on Speech Reception

The primary effect of noise on speech communication is interference with or masking of the speech signal. Intense noise levels at the ear also may cause aural overload and distortion that accompany the masking, producing additional interference with reception. The effectiveness of the acoustic masker varies with the frequency content of the noise and with the ratio of the signal level to the noise level (S/N ratio). The most effective noise masking speech contains the same energy that is present in the long-term average speech spectrum of the signal to be masked. Long-term average speech spectra vary slightly from talker to talker, and substantially for different levels of vocal effort (23). Although there is some upward spread of masking, intelligibility generally increases when the noise spectrum is the maximum above or below the speech spectrum.

Generally, the speech signal level must be greater than the noise level at the ear for good intelligibility. Intelligibility as a function of the S/N ratio, however, does vary with the type of speech material. The intelligibility of sentences is approximately 0% correct at -12 dB S/N and greater than 95% correct at 0 dB S/N (range of 12 dB), whereas nonsense syllables that are also 0% correct at -12 dB S/N ratio require about $+15$ dB S/N to exceed 95% correct (range of 27 dB). Both the spectra and level of aerospace noises must be considered to avoid masking of the speech signal and ensure successful communication.

Direct Communication

The relationships between background noise, in terms of A-weighted sound level and SIL, and the distances between talker and listener, where face-to-face communication is satisfactory, are summarized in Figure 10.12. These data show that satisfactory communication, about 90 to 95% correct perception of sentences, is expected with a normal voice at a distance of about 3 m in a noise at a level of 55 dB(A) (48 dB SIL). At the same distance apart, direct communications are difficult at a noise level of about 74 dB(A), where talkers must shout to be understood. As the background noise reaches a level

where the talker must increase his vocal output, the voice level is increased from 3 dB (lower noise levels) to 6 dB (higher noise levels) for every 10 dB increase in noise level.

The data in Figure 10.12 show the effect of noise on voice communication and demonstrate that conversation with a normal voice is not possible in most high-noise environments at distances greater than about 1 m. This means that aerospace work environment noises that require an above-normal voice effort place additional stress on both the talkers and listeners. The amount of stress on the communicator and strain on the vocal cords is dependent on the amount of vocal effort and frequency or amount of communication required. Infrequent or occasional raised voices and shouts may be tolerable; however, personnel should not be required to maintain frequent or continuous face-to-face communication under conditions requiring above-normal vocal effort. Electronically aided communications should be considered for these situations to protect the health and well-being of the personnel and to minimize errors due to inadequate communications.

Communication Equipment Effectiveness

State-of-the-art communications systems and accompanying terminal equipment are satisfactory for most modern speech communications tasks in noise. The equipment is designed to optimize the speech signal by techniques that include a passband similar to the long-term average speech spectrum, peak-clipping, low impedance, and automatic gain control. Microphones and earphones are housed in noise-excluding shields and earcups and designed with frequency responses idealized for human speech. Noise-cancelling microphones significantly reduce the sensitivity of the microphone to low-frequency noise without affecting their sensitivity to the speech signal. In some aerospace environments, such as helicopters, navy flight decks, jet engine test stands, and near field rocket firings, improved voice communications effectiveness is still needed. The use of insert earplugs under communications headsets and helmets can often provide the additional voice communications required in these very high level noises. The earplug provides equal attenuation of the noise and the speech signal. Increasing the gain of the system raises the level of the voice signal while the level of the noise remains unchanged, providing a significant improvement in the speech-to-noise ratio at the ear and in the speech intelligibility. In these situations, the noise-excluding features of the terminal equipment are not always adequate for the high levels of noise in which the equipment is used; however, in most other situations, the equipment does not contribute to degradation of voice communications.

Communication in In-Flight Environments

The noise exposure at an in-flight crew station is composed of some combination of propulsion system, auxiliary equipment, and aerodynamic noise. The noise exposure for a particular flight sequence or profile can be analyzed in terms of frequency content, levels, durations, and appropriate equipment selected to operate under the worst-case conditions. All aircraft and space vehicles must contend with these propulsion system, auxiliary equipment, and aerodynamic noises. The duration of intense propulsion system noise and aerodynamic noise during space launches is so brief that communications equipment can be selected to operate in the presence of the lower noise levels of the equipment operating during cruise. These auxiliary and life-support system noises ordinarily pose no threat to voice communications, so that small, lightweight headset-microphone systems are satisfactory. High-performance aircraft require voice communications equipment to be integrated with the flight helmet-oxygen mask system. Typically, this includes a high-performance, altitude-compensated earphone inside the helmet and a noise-cancelling microphone in the oxygen mask. Both the helmet and oxygen mask act as noise shields. Crewmembers of other types of military aircraft may use the flight helmet with a noise-cancelling microphone mounted on

a boom or simply a headset with a noise-cancelling boom microphone. These terminal equipment items typically have been designed specifically for the kinds of noise environments in which they are used, and their performance is usually reliable.

The flight crew compartments of most commercial passenger aircraft have been sufficiently sound-treated to minimize or eliminate noise as a voice communications problem. The situation is different with general aviation aircraft where cabin noise can pose a threat to voice communications. Communications terminal equipment—that is, the headset-microphone system—should be selected specifically for the cabin noise environment in which it will be used because the performance of such systems in noise may vary widely. It is interesting to note that the preferred ambient noise levels for commercial airline passengers is about 67 dB(A), a level that generally masks conversations at a distance of about 1 m from the talker. Ambient noise levels below this value do not provide acoustic privacy for conversations of passengers seated close to one another and result in speech interference and dissatisfied passengers.

In helicopters, present communications equipment may become marginal or inadequate for special phases of flight. This is particularly true for air crew members required to work in large open vehicles or to be outside the vehicle fuselage. For example, medical rescue personnel immediately outside the helicopter in the direct downwash of the rotating blades may find both the transmission and reception of voice communication to be marginal to unacceptable. Part of the problem can be attributed to the helicopter noise spectrum, which is particularly high in the low-frequency regions where the noise-attenuating properties of flight helmets are least effective. Although substantial progress has been made in the development of noise-excluding headwear, some helicopter situations need continued improvement in communications equipment. Active noise reduction headsets which provide low-frequency (below 2000 Hz) noise cancellation provide significant help to helicopter crew members. ANR headsets are effectively used in general aviation aircraft.

Communication in Ground Environments

Ground communication headset-microphones provide adequate to marginal communications in noise levels up to 130 to 135 dB SPL. Units consist of noise-cancelling microphones housed in noise shields and high-output earphones mounted in noise-excluding earcups. These units must be properly manufactured and in good working order to provide the maximum design performance. The Air Force standard ground communication headset-microphone (H-133) can be modified to provide satisfactory voice communications in some environments that exceed 140 dB. The modification involves the use of a custom-molded earplug (with long canal) equipped with a button microphone that is worn under the earcup. The standard earphone is removed and the lead reconnected to the button earphone. This modification has provided adequate voice communications in jet engine test cell noise, where communications were not satisfactory with the standard unit. Although demonstrated on the Air Force system, this modification concept should improve voice communications of most earcup-enclosed earphone terminal equipment.

Voice communications problems may occur in locations such as in-flight control centers, air traffic control facilities, C^3 (command, control, and communications), and surveillance operations due to noise generated by the equipment in use, as well as by external sources. Many of these problems can be alleviated by the identification and treatment of the noise source. Such treatment may range from the use of sound-absorbing materials and enclosures to rearrangement of the equipment to locate noise sources away from the crew positions. When the noise at crew positions is not adequately reduced by treatment of the source and propagation, it may be necessary to add noise-cancellation and noise-exclusion features to the headset-microphones in use.

Machine Speech Recognition and Production

Aerospace operations comprise a very fertile area for the successful application of developing new technologies of voice control and voice response. Voice control using automatic speech recognition has been, for several decades, a technologic goal with virtually unlimited applications. The ultimate functional objective is a totally reliable, talker-independent device that requires virtually no training and will operate with an unlimited vocabulary. Human speech has proven to be a much more complex and sophisticated acoustic signal for this application than initially estimated; consequently, these objectives have necessarily been revised to realistically correspond to the present limited voice control technology. Voice response devices, those generating synthetic speech, are seen in numerous applications such as educational toys, games, status report systems, novelties, and prompting. The voice response technology is growing much faster than voice control primarily because the problems associated with its generation and use are relatively less difficult and challenging than those associated with voice control technology.

Automatic Speech Recognition (Voice Control)

Automatic speech recognition systems are commercially available and in various stages of development for use in situations relatively free of interfering environmental factors. Although these systems operate using techniques such as template matching, linear predictive coding, or phoneme recognition, they are characterized in terms of vocabulary size, speaker dependency, word or phrase recognition, and reliability. Vocabulary size may vary from as few as 20 words to as many as a few hundred words. Speaker-dependent systems require training by each talker and retraining before use by another talker. Training consists of from one to numerous repetitions of the total vocabulary by the talker, depending on the system. Speaker-independent systems theoretically can be directly used by any talker without their participation in the training. Isolated word recognition systems ordinarily require a brief pause between words to allow each word to be recognized. Connected-word or connected-speech systems function more quickly and allow several words to be spoken as a phrase. The reliability of present systems is degraded by unfavorable operating conditions. Reliability or correct word recognition may vary from 95% to more than 99% under ideal conditions but may drop to essentially 0% under the most severe conditions such as high-level ambient noise environments.

Present automatic speech recognition systems are being evaluated and developed for adaptation to different applications, with varying degrees of success. Among these applications are human operator interfaces with data processing equipment; voice queries for information; the filing of information such as flight plans; voice instead of manual control of buttons, switches, and knobs; as well as of naval and aircraft avionics, flight controls, and weapons delivery. One of the areas of highest potential payoff is that of excessive human operator work load, which consists of too many visual and manual tasks, time-critical tasks, or highly specialized situations, such as high-speed, low-level flight, where looking down into the cockpit to perform a manual task is a threat to safety. Clearly, numerous situations exist that would profit from the use of a voice interactive system, having crewmembers speak appropriate key words, to control various aerospace vehicle operations typically activated with manual controls.

A major problem with current systems is their vulnerability to environmental stressors, which in aerospace operations means noise, vibration, and acceleration. Several programs are presently under way to produce robust versions of voice interactive systems that will operate in various aerospace vehicles, including helicopters, tactical aircraft, and space vehicles. The comparatively severe stressors present in helicopter and tactical aircraft environments require a much more robust system than demanded by the cruise portions of space flight. For example, voice control of cameras during most portions of a space mission is within the state of the art. Generic systems are being developed and adapted to tasks instead of being designed for specific applications that require robust systems; perhaps this approach, along with the limitations in speech technology, is contributing to the difficulties experienced in achieving satisfactory systems for stress environments.

Advances in neural net technology, computer processing time, increased memory, coding techniques, and microprocessor development hold high promise for expanded application and increased reliability of voice interactive systems in spite of the absence of recent significant breakthroughs in speech recognition technology. Numerous companies are actively working in the voice recognition technology area, and specific applications in nonstressed environments are being implemented. The full application of voice control in the hostile environments of various aerospace systems, however, is not expected in the immediate future.

Machine Voice Response

Voice response systems are appearing on the commercial market in increasing numbers and at decreasing costs, resulting in a ready supply for applications activities. Microprocessors provide a wide variety of preprogrammed words and phrases in reasonably typical male or female voices. Speech synthesis systems can be custom-developed for a particular user and application, including specific vocabulary and male or female voice. Speech synthesis already has been successfully demonstrated in numerous contemporary situations where radios, automobiles, computers, clocks, games, educational toys, and various other devices provide information by "talking." The technology is well developed and will continue to be refined with virtually unlimited applications opportunities.

Machine voice response does not experience the same vulnerability to environmental stressors as voice control. It is susceptible to noise-making, and favorable synthetic speech-to-noise ratios are required for effective operation. Different voice response systems produce speech that varies in quality or naturalness, and many systems sound cryptic, disconnected, poorly articulated, and are lacking in inflection. In some applications, such as voice warning, the unnaturalness may be desirable as an "attention-getter," whereas during long-term space missions, natural-sounding synthetic speech would be preferred. Although preliminary, there are some indications that human responses to synthetic speech may differ slightly from responses to human speech; for example, the reaction time to synthetic speech was observed to be slightly longer than to human speech.

Among the aerospace applications of machine voice responses are advisory, validation, and warning functions. Appropriate rules for information management via the auditory, visual, and other sensory channels must be developed; however, many of the status conditions of aerospace vehicles could be provided by synthetic speech. These audio advisories would greatly relieve many of the visual requirements for monitoring dials, gauges, and annunciator panels. Validation functions could operate as feedback loops, actually telling the operator by voice the action that was performed, such as confirming "wheels down," talking avionics, repeating the newly tuned radio frequency, and stating other changes in aircraft control as activated by the crewmember. In space, or missile control centers, and air traffic control-type environments, voice responses can accompany selected visual displays as a redundant means of increasing the effectiveness of audiovisual information transfer.

High interest has been shown in optimizing and integrating voice warning into the total warning networks of aerospace systems. The initial voice warning system in the United States Air Force B-58 Hustler aircraft consisted of tape recordings of words and phrases spoken by a female. Although novel at the time and of scientific interest, the technical approach eventually proved unacceptable. Present microprocessor-type systems are highly flexible and can be developed to be adaptive in terms of message management, including priorities. Additional investigative work is needed to develop a data base of the trade-offs and optimum usage of voice warnings. The application of this voice response data base involves the effective integration of voice warning with nonvoice-warning signals, visual displays, annunciator indicators, and the audio communications function.

Future Communication in Aerospace Environments

Aerospace requirements for secure, reliable communications have fostered the application of rapidly developing technologies to audio communications. The procedures involved in providing secure, jam-resistant communication use a variety of voice-processing techniques that may alter or even completely transform the signal. These techniques generally require a very wide bandpass, reduced sensitivity to noise, digitizing, and multiplexing, as well as other features that are not normally present in contemporary communications equipment. Future communications systems, including aerospace radios, must be designed to incorporate these new developments, as well as those of noise cancellation for communications systems, fiber optic technology, adaptive frequency response, and voice control. These highly advanced systems will display marked miniaturization of components, extremely high reliability, and robustness. They will be completely wireless, resulting in essentially personal communication units, which together will comprise a communications system or net.

EFFECTS OF VIBRATION ON AVIATION PERSONNEL

Operational Vibration Exposures

Operators and passengers of all types of transportation vehicles, be they in air, space, on the ground, or underwater, are exposed to some kind of vibration during some phases of the operation. The oscillations of the vehicle motions around a reference stationary state, at rest, or during constant velocity and/or acceleration are transmitted to the occupants through the supporting seat and floor, or through wall vibrations or vibrating handles. This transmission results in motions of the whole human body or body parts. In studying biochemical interaction, it is somewhat artificial to separate body motions into sustained, transient, rotational, or impact acceleration and linear oscillations, although this is driven in part by our analytic, experimental, and laboratory simulation tools. In taking this conventional approach, it is important to keep its limitations in mind and not to forget that vibra-

tions are only a small part of the total mechanical force or motion spectrum. The physical, physiologic, and performance effects to be discussed for the vibration spectrum of interest, from 0.5 Hz to a few hundred hertz, often occur simultaneous with and are modified by the effects of sustained and/or transient accelerations. Table 10.8 indicates the simultaneous occurrence of some of these mechanical environments during various phases of aerospace flight and denotes the degree of performance capability usually required or desired. Low-altitude, high-speed flight in military operations and storm and clear-air turbulence in commercial and general aviation cause the most severe vibration exposures of concern. Their severity depends on the input gust velocities and acceleration spectra, as well as on the aerodynamic properties and flexibility of the aircraft. In military aircraft with manual or automatic terrain-following control systems, maneuvering loads with maxima between 0.01 and 0.1 Hz are superimposed on the gust-response spectra of the aircraft and crew. Prediction of human effects and protective measures required for all phases indicated in Table 10.8

Table 10.8.
Vibration, Acceleration, and Other Environments Associated With Aerospace Flight

Environment	Military		General Aviation		Space		
	Escape	Low-Altitude, High-Speed Flight	Storm and Clear-Air Turbulence	Helicopter and V/STOL Operations	Boost Phase of Spaceflight	Reentry Phase of Spaceflight	Weightlessness
Simple sustained acceleration	M	C	—	—	C	C	—
Complex sustained acceleration	M	C	C	—	C	C	—
Angular and linear vibration	E	C	C	C	C	C	C
Rotation	E	—	—	—	—	—	C
Transient acceleration	E	C	C	C	—	E	—
Complex transient acceleration	E	C	C	C	—	E	C
Overpressure	E	—	—	—	—	—	—
Windblast	E	—	—	—	—	—	—
Infrasonic noise	—	—	—	—	C	—	—
Acoustic noise	E	R	R	R	C	C	—
Thermal extremes, fire	E	C	—	C	—	C	—
Reduced atmospheric pressure	E	—	—	—	—	R	R
Ballistic impact	E	—	—	—	—	—	—

The level of performance required is indicated by the letter code. The presence of a letter code indicates that the environment occurs during the indicated aerospace operation. Performance code: E = retain ability to escape and evade; M = retain monitor function; C = retain ability to control vehicle; and R = perform during repeated exposure.

requires the forecasting or measurement of the environments in all six degrees of freedom and for the total mechanical spectrum.

Pathophysiologic and Physiologic Effects of Vibration

As elaborated in the earlier section entitled "The Human Body as a Receiver of Noise and Vibration," which part of the human body is exposed to maximum vibration stress and responds most severely depends on the frequency range and the exposure conditions. Unlike sound exposure, in which most effects are mediated through the ear, there is no specific target area or organ for low-frequency, whole-body vibration, and the mechanical stresses imposed can potentially lead to interference with bodily functions and tissue damage in practically all parts of the body (24). Fortunately, operational stresses are almost never that high, and vibration exposures remain below injury and interference levels. Severe buffeting in one military aircraft led to a few oscillations best described as repetitive impacts that resulted in spinal fractures. Based on scanty human evidence and animal studies, damage to renal functions and pulmonary hemorrhages are suspected of being the first sign of injury from acute overexposure in the frequency range of maximum abdominal response (4 to 8 Hz). Whole-body vibration of intensities voluntarily tolerated by human subjects up to the limit of severe discomfort or pain has not resulted in demonstrable harm or injury (25). Minor kidney injuries in truck and tractor drivers have been suspected to be due to vibration exposure of long duration at levels that produce no apparent acute effects, but epidemiologic studies have yet to prove any clear correlation. Similarly higher incidents of back pain in helicopter pilots and tractor operators have been assumed to be related to the vibration produced by the vehicles; in spite of several studies and plausible arguments, clear dose-response relationships are lacking and difficult to obtain. Modern exposure limits for health and safety reasons are, therefore, primarily based on voluntary tolerance limits, pain

thresholds, and experiences with occupational exposures assumed to be safe. Most physiologic effects in the 2 to 12 Hz frequency range are associated with the resonance of the thoracoabdominal viscera. It has been shown to be responsible for pain occurring in the 1 to 2 g_z (peak) and 2 to 3 g_x ranges, suspected to be caused by the stretching of the perichondrium and periosteum at the chondrosternal and interchondral joint capsules and ligaments. Movement of abdominal viscera in and out of the thoracic cage, in both X- and Z-axis excitation, is responsible for the interference of vibration with respiration. It causes the involuntary oscillation of a significant volume of air in and out of the lungs, leading to an increase in minute volume, alveolar ventilation, and oxygen consumption. In some experimental exposures to g_z vibrations, Pco_2 decreased and clinical signs of hypocapnia were observed, suggesting hyperventilation. Dyspnea results from short exposures to high amplitudes.

Cardiovascular functions change similarly in response to X-axis, and Y-axis, and Z-axis excitation (16). The test results, indicating an increase in mean arterial blood pressure, cardiac index, and heart rate in humans, are illustrated in Figure 10.16. In general, the combined cardiopulmonary response to vibration in the 2 to 12 Hz range resembles the response to exercise. Although the increased muscular effort of bracing against the vibration and psychologic factors may account for some of the response, observance of the same general pattern in anesthetized animals speaks for the stimulation of various mechanoreceptors.

The resonance of the abdominal viscera, with its resulting distortions and stretching, is also responsible for the epigastric or periumbilical discomfort and testicular pain reported at high amplitudes. Headache is frequently associated with exposure to frequencies above 10 Hz. Particularly in $G_x \pm g_x$ and $G_x \pm g_y$ exposures (space couch positions), vibrations are transmitted to the head directly from the headrest, which can lead to extremely uncomfortable and disturbing impacts of the head against the headrest.

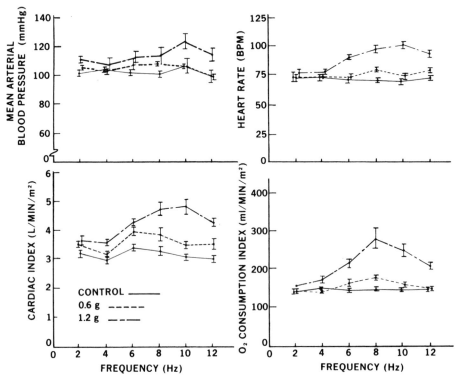

Figure 10.16. Effect of amplitude and frequency of $G_z \pm g_x$ sinusoidal whole-body vibration on mean arterial blood pressure, cardiac index, heart rate, and oxygen consumption.

Raising the head away from the headrest and attempts to counteract the forces leads to neck muscle strain, spasm, and soreness. Restraining the head to follow the motion can result in disorientation during the exposure.

Rubbing the body surfaces against the seat, backrest, or restraint straps (e.g., "back scrub" in some tractor or vehicle arrangements) can lead to discomfort and skin injuries.

The severe vibration responses and injuries observed in animal experiments have not been reported in humans due to appropriate safety criteria (27–29). In interpreting animal experiments, it is of utmost importance to consider appropriate scaling laws due to the changed body dimensions and resonances, and, therefore, maximum-effects frequencies are considerably higher in small animals.

The Vibration Syndrome

The only specific vibration-induced disease with well-supported etiologic data is the vibration disease, or "white finger syndrome," caused by habitual occupational exposure over months and years to the vibration of machinery and certain hand tools such as chain saws, chipping hammers, and other pneumatic tools (30,31). Although epidemiologic research over the last decade has documented various patterns and stages of the disease affecting the blood vessels, nerves, bones, joints, muscles, or connective tissues of the hand and forearm, the earliest and most clearly established manifestations are Raynaud's phenomenon, impairment of the blood circulation to the hands, or disorders of the peripheral nervous system. Individual susceptibility to the disease and the influence of other factors affecting peripheral circulation such as cold and smoking are not yet well understood. The physical impact of the handtool vibrations is clearly modified by working methods (tightness of handgrip, i.e., "let the tool do the work") and the intermittency of exposure. With respect to the effectiveness of various frequencies, constant input velocity appears to result in equal injury potential over most of the effective frequency range (8 to 1000 Hz). Consequently, curves of equal risk of developing disorders from exposure to hand-transmitted vibration are assumed to have the shape shown in Figure 10.17, and filters with the inverse function have been standardized for measuring and weighting hand-arm vibrations. The overall weighted level—obtained in approximately 40 studies in various countries on workers exposed to hand-transmitted vibrations in their job for periods of up to 25 years—has been related to the exposure time for the onset of vascular disorders in selected percentiles of the population (Fig. 10.18). This dose-effect relationship allows the estimation of the risk involved in various exposure conditions (32,33). The particular curves in Figure 10.17 predict for a weighted acceleration of 2.9

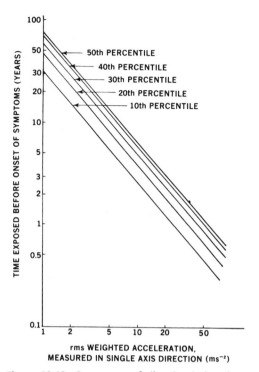

Figure 10.18. Occurrence of vibration-induced vascular symptoms in various percentiles of a population using hand tools on a daily basis as a function of the weighted hand acceleration.

m/sec² the onset of disorders in 50% of the population after 25 years. The lower curve A is for the broad-band spectrum that reaches the curve in each third-octave frequency band; the upper curve is for a weighted acceleration spectrum coinciding with the curve in a third-octave band only while all other bands are 20 dB lower. All other possible spectra with the same weighted acceleration value will fall between these two curves (34). Analysis of recent data questions the steep increase of the weighting curves of Figure 10.17 above 16 Hz and proposes flat weighting up to 1000 Hz and even 5000 Hz. However, this proposal has not yet been accepted as general guidance for all types of hand tools.

Effects on Task Performance (3,29)

The whole body vibration environment can interfere with the sensory and motor aspects of

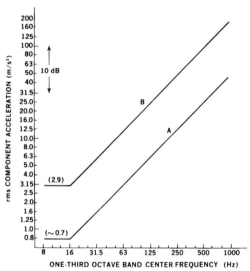

Figure 10.17. Weighting curves for hand-arm vibrations. Both curves correspond to a weighted overall acceleration level of 2.9 m/sec²: curve A applies to broad band spectra, of which all one-third octave band levels coincide with the curve; curve B applies to spectra that are composed of a single band, which coincides with the criteria curve. Both curves represent curves of equal risk of the onset of disorders in 50% of a population after 25 years of using hand tools for approximately 4 hours per day.

tasks. It has less effect on cognitive performance and central nervous system processing through its general stress component. The performance requirements under vibration conditions during various phases of aerospace flight are indicated in Table 10.8. They can vary from the gross monitoring of instrument panels and single gross motor tasks to detailed monitoring, reading of complex displays, and high work load motor functions required to control an aircraft in turbulent, low-level flight. In military missions, low-level navigation and weapon delivery and the maneuvering loads associated with pull-ups and push-overs for terrain following increase task demands as well as environmental stress. With manual control, pull-ups are in the range of $+2.0$ G_x, push-overs in the range of $+0.5$ G_x. Aircraft and spacecraft design specifications with respect to vibration acceptability for satisfactory performance are based primarily on flight test data and subjective pilot evaluations. Realistic simulations of the vibration environment on moving-base simulators adds to this body of knowledge and gives confidence to specific designs or task requirements. Controlled laboratory experiments are designed to explore in detail interference effects as a function of frequency, amplitude, task design, and exposure time. These studies are the keys to improved designs of vibration-resistant controls and displays.

Motor Performance

The involuntary motions of the body and the extremities introduced by vibrations are superimposed as disturbances on the active control motions of a human operator. The greater the vibration amplitude of hand or foot in comparison with the required control motion (through strong original excitation or through resonance reinforcement), the larger the undesirable interference. The complexity of the overall control situation and of the various interference paths is shown in Figure 10.19. In laboratory tracking experiments, errors increase in the 2 to 12 Hz frequency range at seat accelerations above ap-

proximately 0.05 g_z rms. The maximum decrement is usually in the range of 4 Hz, which is the main body resonance. For X-axis and Y-axis vibration, the largest decrements are at 1.5 to 2 Hz. In all cases, tracking errors tend to be largest in the direction of the disturbing vibration stimulus. The magnitudes of the decrements cannot be generalized because they depend too much on the specific details of the control task (e.g., position, velocity or force control, amplitude of required control motion) and the hand-arm or foot-leg support. Design guides for vibration-resistant controls are available, however. The ability to perform fine manipulative tasks such as writing or setting cursors should be verified by simulation before relying on them in operational situations.

The severity of the vibration interference can be influenced to some extent by the operator's control strategy. For example, under turbulent flight conditions, pilots often postpone motor activity during short bursts of high-amplitude vibrations and introduce corrective action as soon as the burst is over. Under sustained turbulence, very low frequencies can excite "pilot-induced oscillations," which are caused by inappropriate control inputs. The pilot apparently has time to correct for the disturbance inputs, but due to misinterpretations of kinesthetic cues or the response characteristics of the motor system, he does not do it in an appropriate way at some frequencies and adds through his inputs to aircraft instabilities.

Effects on Vision (35)

Difficulties in reading instruments and performing visual searches occur when vibrations introduce relative movement of the eye with respect to the target. Although persons and instruments might be excited by the same structural vibrations, their response is completely different, causing different displacements in different frequency ranges. A complex relationship exists between all of the relevant parameters, such as vibration frequency, amplitude and direction, viewing distance, illumination, contrast, and the

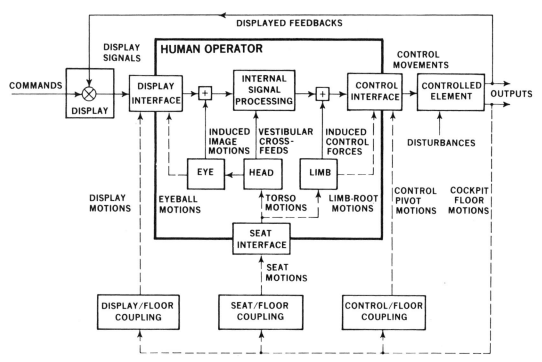

Figure 10.19. The human operator performing a manual task in a biodynamic environment.

shape of the viewed object. Large effects on the resolution of visual detail occur under Z-axis, whole-body vibration and for Y-axis and Z-axis vibration of viewed objects. The main difference between the object versus the subject vibration is the compensating ocular reflexes mediated by the vestibular system (vestibulo-ocular reflex) and by proprioceptors in the head (colliculo-ocular reflex), which enable the eye to compensate for body and head motions, thereby fixating the gaze on the target. Although effectiveness of the vestibulo-ocular reflex drops off above 1 Hz, the reflex has been shown to affect results up to 8 Hz. Analysis and prediction of visual capability are further complicated by the fact that translational body motion results not only in translational but also in rotational head movements. The latter influence passive eye movement, as well as vestibular feed-back. The same compensatory reflexes have been shown to degrade remarkably visibility on head-mounted or helmet-mounted displays under vibration when the display moves with the head.

Although mechanical eye resonances have been investigated in several studies up to 90 Hz, their influence on vision is apparently of secondary importance, and no sharp resonance phenomena as a function of frequency have been observed.

Unfortunately, the large number of test results cannot yet be presented in uniform curves allowing the prediction of visual decrement. The large number of variables prevent generalization of the results. These variables include, for example, small changes in subject posture and restraint, affecting translational and rotational head responses, and large intersubject intervariability among others. The examples of Figure 10.20, therefore, should be accepted as specific test results and not as generally valid design guidance. The levels of vibration below which no interference with visual acuity normally is expected are indicated.

For $G_z \pm g_x$, g_y, and g_z vibrations and for $G_x \pm g_z$ vibrations, the largest effects were found in the 11 to 15 Hz range. Decoupling the head

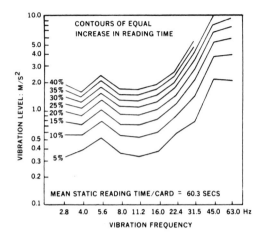

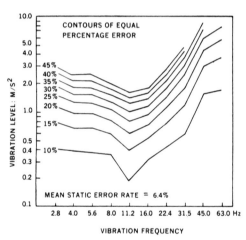

Figure 10.20. Mean vibration levels required to produce contours of equal percentage reading errors and equal percentage increases in reading time, ten subjects.

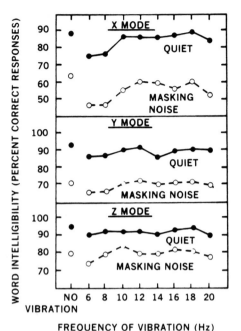

Figure 10.21. Mean word intelligibility of talkers exposed to $G_x \pm g_x, g_y$, or g_z whole-body sinusoidal vibration (0.35 g (rms)). Quiet condition was with 70 dB speech and no masking noise; noise condition was with 70 dB speech and 70 dB masking noise.

from the headrest improved capability in this frequency range, whereas head restraints generally reduced reading errors at 6 Hz and below. The type of helmet and restraint, however, is crucial for these experiments. All of these results underline the previously stated conclusion that because of the complexity and large number of variables, important vehicle performance requirements should be tested for each specific configuration in realistic simulations.

Effects on Speech Communication

Although hearing ability is practically not affected by vibration, the quality of speech can be impaired. Movements of the thoracoabdominal viscera induce modulations of the airflow in the respiratory system and, consequently, cause a tremolo-type modulation of the voice with the frequency of vibration. Vibrated speech is masked by noise to a greater extent than might be expected. Speech progressively deteriorates with increasing intensity of vibration. In addition, the pitch of the voice is increased, presumably due to the increased muscle tension. As a result of all these effects, speech intelligibility can be slightly impaired at some frequencies and amplitudes, as shown in Figure 10.21. In addition, the rate of talking can be slowed down.

Effects on Cognitive Functions

The central nervous system appears to be relatively unaffected by the vibration stress. Simple cognitive functions were unaffected in laboratory tests (pattern recognition and monitoring of dials and warning lights); more demanding tasks involving mental arithmetic and short-term memory during a 0.5 g_z (peak) vibration at frequencies below 15 Hz resulted in significantly slower performance. Other studies, however, indicate that vibration can increase the level of arousal similar to observations in noise, depending on the exposure intensity, exposure time pattern, and the activity of the subject. This effect was particularly demonstrated in several studies on the combined effects of vibration and noise. In one such test, 100 dB(A) noise and 0.36 rms g_z vibration (5 sinusoids from 2.6 to 16 Hz combined) were used as stressors individually and in combination while the subjects performed a complex counting task. The task was sensitive to both the noise and vibration. Vibration and noise combined, however, resulted in less performance decrement than either of these stimuli alone.

The possibility of nonspecific central nervous system alterations due to continuous long-term exposure to vibrations in industrial situations and its contribution to general fatigue has been addressed in several studies, primarily in eastern European countries. The results are not uniform and not convincing. Habituation to monotonous vibration environments in aircraft or on ships is probably a central nervous system phenomenon, although some adaptation on the receptor level has been proposed.

Exposure and Design Guidance

General Basis for Guidelines

Discussion of the various vibration-induced physiologic and psychologic effects in the previous sections should have made it clear that no simple exposure limits and assessment procedures are applicable to all environmental, human posture and restraint, and task performance conditions. Too many factors can influence these conditions. A detailed interference analysis and simulation is desirable whenever expensive or irreversible decisions are at stake, particularly for the design of aircraft cockpits and spacecraft command modules when new environments or

new visual or manipulatory tasks are involved. For the evaluation of existing situations and the assessment of complaints and guidance with respect to good preventive medicine and ergonomic practices, however, the following guidelines should be helpful. These guidelines are a summary of present national and international standards and military specifications on this subject.

EXPOSURE CRITERIA. The guidelines give exposure criteria, considered on the basis of laboratory and field experiences, as protective with respect to the potential consequences stated (27,29). They should not be exceeded without considered and compelling reasons. Criteria are proposed for the following conditions:

1. Preservation of health and safety exposure limits. These limits should not be exceeded without special justification and awareness of a potential health risk to a nonselected population. The limits are approximately doubled in amplitude in military specifications, where they are close to the pain threshold for healthy young subjects.
2. Preservation of working efficiency "fatigue or decreased proficiency boundary." As discussed, this limit cannot apply uniformly to all tasks and work loads. It is representative, however, of typical control situations in transportation vehicles and to a large extent based on aircraft pilot evaluations.
3. Preservation of comfort or reduced comfort boundary.

The fatigue-decreased proficiency boundaries for Z-axis, Y-axis vibration are shown in Figure 10.22. To obtain the exposure limits, the curves should be raised by a factor of 2 (6 dB). The reduced comfort boundaries are obtained by dividing the curves in Figure 10.22 by 3.15 (10 dB). The dependence of the criteria on the vibration frequency is assumed to be the same for all three types of criteria: the Z-axis curve has maximum sensitivity in the resonance range of the thoracoabdominal system (4 to 8 Hz),

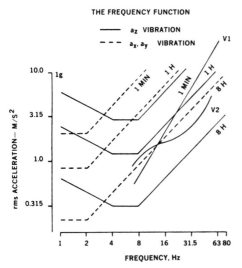

THE FREQUENCY FUNCTION

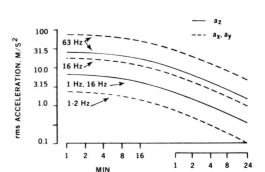

THE EXPOSURE TIME FUNCTION

Figure 10.22. Vibration exposure criteria for the g_x, g_z, g_y directions. The curves represent the "fatigue-decreased efficiency" boundary. For "exposure limit," curves should be raised by a factor of two. For "reduced comfort," curves should be divided by 3.15. Object vibrations above curve V_1 and whole-body vibration above curve V_2 will lead to reductions in visual acuity.

Figure 10.23. "Fatigue-decreased efficiency" exposure criteria as a function of daily exposure time.

whereas the X-axis and Y-axis curves have their maximum sensitivity below 2 Hz. The curves apply to the seated or standing subject without significant support by a backrest. A backrest will primarily affect the X-axis curve and make it increase less with frequency. In Figure 10.22, all criteria are a function of the average daily exposure time. This dependence, which might apply primarily to the exposure limits and the comfort boundary and is questionable with respect to task performance, is illustrated in Figure 10.23. The boundaries are defined in terms of rms value for single-frequency exposure or rms value in the third-octave band for broad-band vibration. The limits presented are valid at least for crest factors (maximum peak value to rms value over a 1-minute or longer period) of 3. Weighted accelerations with crest factors as great as 6 are still meaningfully interpreted by this approach.

Weighted Acceleration

Frequently, it is desirable to characterize a vibration environment by a single quantity. Recent research on comfort and performance has shown that filtering the acceleration signal between 1 and 80 Hz with an electronic network having an insertion loss equivalent to the response curves of Figure 10.22 results in a single weighted acceleration value that correlates well with comfort and performance. The method weights each frequency according to its relative effectiveness with respect to human response. This weighting method is coming into wider and wider use, and the filtering networks for evaluating X-axis, Y-axis, and Z-axis whole-body vibrations and for evaluating hand-arm vibrations are incorporated into commercial human-response vibration meters. The overall weighted acceleration values are to be compared with the boundary values in the most sensitive frequency bands (4 to 8 Hz for Z-axis and 1 to 2 Hz for X-axis and Y-axis vibration). Depending on the vibration spectrum, particularly if the spectrum rises outside the most sensitive frequency band, this weighting method can result in an over-conservative assessment of the environment compared with the one-third octave-band analysis method. In this case, when the weighted values are close to the limits of acceptability, the one-third octave-band method should be used for numeric comparison with the criteria.

Multidirectional and Rotational Vibrations

If vibrations are present in several directions simultaneously, the accelerations for each direction are to be assessed separately by the corresponding exposure criteria. When the g_x and g_y acceleration components multiplied by 1.4 have similar values to the g_z component, the combined motion can be more severe than the individual components would indicate. In this case, it is recommended that the weighted accelerations, g_w, be combined in the following way:

$$g_w = \sqrt{(1.4\ g_{xw})^2 + (1.4\ g_{yw})^2 + g_{zw}^2}\ (3)$$

This amount of the vector sum can be compared for comfort and performance evaluations with the weighted acceleration values for Z-axis vibration.

Data on the acceptability of rotational or angular vibrations have been collected only recently, and generalized or standardized criteria are not available. Pure roll was perceived as producing more discomfort than the same amplitude and frequency of pure pitch oscillations. Examples of such data are shown in Figure 10.24. Yaw

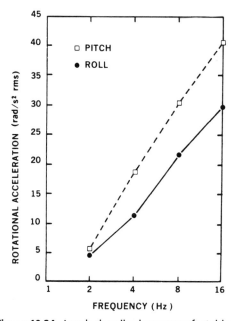

Figure 10.24. Levels described as uncomfortable for pure rotational vibration.

discomfort appears to vary considerably with a backrest support. If the operator is seated away from the axis of rotation, both the rotational vibration and the translational component must be considered. For many situations, prediction of response is adequate if only the most severe component is taken into consideration.

Vibrations Producing Motion Sickness

Although the symptoms and causes of and therapeutic measures for motion sickness are discussed in Chapters 11 and 18, the frequency and amplitude range of vibrations producing the discomfort or acute distress associated with motion sickness will be mentioned briefly in this chapter. The frequency range for vertical (Z-axis) vibration leading to this disability extends downwards from 1 Hz on, i.e., it starts right below the frequency range so far discussed. Motion sickness symptoms cause the curves shown in Figure 10.22 to drop sharply below 1 Hz. A continuous transition of the criteria curves shown in Figure 10.22 (e.g., of the reduced comfort boundary) is not desirable because the sensations, symptoms, and susceptibility of the population are quite different in the motion sickness range and are not comparable to those described for the higher vibrations. Because vibration-caused motion sickness can occur in most transportation systems, and controlling vibrations in one frequency range can easily magnify the amplitudes in another frequency range, design guidance with respect to motion sickness will be mentioned here briefly. Curves of equal sensitivity in the 0.1 to 1 Hz range have the shape shown in Figure 10.25 (29). The absolute levels for severe discomfort after 30-minute, 2-hour, and 8-hour exposures are very tentative and open to many variables. The boundaries as presented apply to infrequent, inexperienced travelers and are assumed to cover approximately 95% of such a population (5% probably never adapt to motion below 1 Hz). Civil and military vehicle operators and many travelers clearly have much higher discomfort and tolerance thresholds due to habituation and selection.

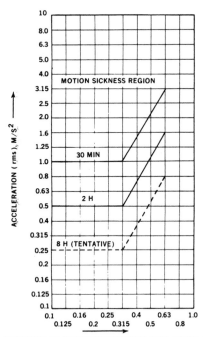

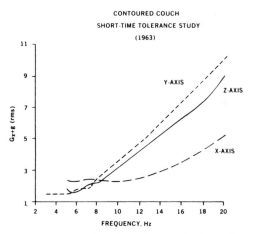

CONTOURED COUCH

SHORT-TIME TOLERANCE STUDY

(1963)

Figure 10.26. Acceleration tolerance in three directions of vibration in a contoured couch.

Figure 10.25. Motion sickness weighting function for g_z oscillations. These are approximate boundaries for severe discomfort for a general population not accustomed to motion.

The Supine Position

The criteria in Figure 10.22 apply to the normal standing or sitting position. Vibration transmission is changed in the supine or semisupine position, which is used in space operations and experimental military applications for its increased protection against sustained acceleration. In this position, X-axis vibrations are most unpleasant and disturbing because of the direct transmission of the vibrations to the head (Fig. 10.26). Helmet properties are most significant, influencing tolerance as well as visual and speech capabilities.

Sustained Acceleration Combined With Vibration

Limited experimental evidence suggests that accelerations and vibrations are not synergistic. On the contrary, it appears as if vibration tolerance at 11 Hz 3 g_x was increased by the simultaneous application of 3.8 G_x. This finding can

be theoretically explained by the inertial preload effect of the sustained acceleration, which at the same time has a static preload or restraining effect on the subject. On the other hand, it can be argued that the vibrations partially alleviate or counteract the circulatory and respiratory manifestations of sustained acceleration.

In this chapter, after reviewing the basic definitions and units of sound (decibel) and vibration (g [rms]) environments and their frequency ranges (in Hertz), examples of their occurrence and intensity inside aerospace vehicles and radiating from the vehicles were discussed. The human body as receiver of mechanical energy was explained, including the absorption and reflection of sound at the body surface and the transmission of sound and vibration through the body structure. The special transformer design of the middle ear enables the high sensitivity and broad-band-width of the human auditory system so essential for speech communication. The requirements and technical possibilities for noise reduction and vibration control were elaborated. The effects of aerospace noise were reviewed in detail: The sensitivity (temporary and permanent threshold shift), the physiologic effects, potential health effects, startle, and annoyance. The measure of speech intelligibility, the masking of speech communication by noise, and the communication quality and reliability required operationally were described. Communication equipment effectiveness and the rapidly advancing bareas of mechanical speech recognition and production were assessed.

Whole-body vibration exposure can result on various pathologic and physiologic effects located in different body regions, which are determined by the exposure frequency. For most operational exposures, however, effects on task performance and interference with activities were found to be of primary concern. The only well-documented vibration-induced disease is the "white finger syndrome" caused by habitual exposure to vibrating hand tools. The standards for safety, performance capability, and comfort for whole-body vibration (1 to 80 Hz) and for risk assessment of hand-tool vibration (8 to 1000 Hz) were recommended as practical guidelines for the assessment of operational vibration exposure. The guidance for the evaluation of vibration in air, spacecraft, and other transportation vehicles was supplemented by weighting curves (0.1 to 0.63 Hz) to estimate the incidence of motion sickness in vertical vibrating motions.

The information and references presented should be adequate for the evaluation of existing and future aerospace medical noise and vibration problems (36).

REFERENCES

1. von Gierke HE, and Goldman DE. Effects of shock and vibration on man. In: Harris CM, ed. Shock and Vibration Handbook. 2nd Ed. New York: McGraw-Hill Book Co., 1979.
2. Harris CM, ed. Handbook of Noise Control. 2nd Ed. New York: McGraw-Hill Book Co., 1979.
3. von Gierke HE, Nixon CW, and Guignard J: Noise and vibration. In: Foundations of Space Biology and Medicine. Vol. II Book 1. Joint USA/USSR Publication. Washington, D.C.: National Aeronautics and Space Administration, 1975.
4. von Gierke HE, ed.: Vibration and combined stress in advanced systems. Springfield, Virginia: NTIS, AGARD Conference Proceedings No. 145, 1975.
5. von Gierke HE: Transmission of vibratory energy through body tissue. In: O Glassner, ed. Medical Physics III. Chicago: Yearbook Medical Publishers, Inc., 1960; 651–80.
6. International Standards Organization (ISO). Vibration and shock—mechanical driving point impedance of the human body, ISO 5982, 1981.
7. International Standards Organization (ISO), Mechanical transmissibility of the human body in the Z direction, ISO 7962, 1987.
8. Symposium on biodynamic models and their application. Aviat Space Environ Med, 1978; 49:109–348.
9. von Gierke HE. To predict the body's strength. Aviat Space Environ Med, 1988; 59:A107–A115.
10. Nixon CW and Berger EH. Hearing protection devices. In: Harris CM, ed. Handbook of noise measurement and control. 3rd Ed. New York: McGraw-Hill Book Co., 1990.
11. Nixon CW. Excessive noise exposure. In: Singh S, ed. Measurement procedures in speech, hearing, and language. Baltimore: University Park Press, 1975.
12. Environmental Protection Agency. Noise labeling requirements for hearing protectors. Washington, DC: Federal Register, 42 (190), (40 CFP Part 211), 56120–56147, 20460, 1979.
13. Meeker WE. Active ear defender systems: Component considerations and theory, Part I, Development of a laboratory model, Part II. Dayton, OH: WADC TR 57–368, (ASTIA Document No. AD 130806), 45433, 1958.
14. Environmental Health Criteria 12: Noise. Geneva, Switzerland: World Health Organization, 1980.
15. Kryter KD. The effects of noise on man. New York: Academic Press, 1970.
16. Kent SJ, Tolen GD, and von Gierke HE. Analysis of the potential association between noise-induced hearing loss and cardiovascular disease in USAF air crew members. Aviat Space Environ Med; 57: 348–361, 1986.
17. Acoustics, determination of occupational noise exposure and estimation of noise-induced hearing impairment. ISO 1999–2nd Ed. 1990. International Standards Organization, 1990.
18. Hammernik RP, Henderson D, and Salvi R, eds. Noise-induced hearing loss. New York: Raven Press, 1980.
19. Proceedings of the sonic boom symposium. J Acoust Soc Am Part 2, 31:5, May, 1966.
20. von Gierke HE and Nixon CW. Human response to sonic boom in the laboratory and the community. J Acoust Soc Am; 51:766–782, 1972.
21. Webster J. Effects of noise on speech communication. In: Harris CM, ed. Handbook of noise control. 2nd. Ed. New York: McGraw-Hill Book Co., 1979.
22. Houtgast T and Steeneken HJM. A multi-language evaluation of the RASTI-method for estimating speech intelligibility in auditoria. Soesterberg, The Netherlands: Report IZF 1981–12, IZF-TNO, 1981.
23. American National Standards Institute (ANSI). Method for measuring the intelligibility of speech over communication systems. S3.2–1989, Acoustical Society of America, 1989.
24. Dupuis H and Zerlett G. The effects of whole-body vibration. New York and Tokyo: Springer—Verlag, Boston, Heidelberg, 1986.
25. Lippert S, ed. Vibration research. New York: Pergamon Press, 1963.

26. Hood CM, et. al. Cardiopulmonary effects of whole-body vibration in man. J Appl Physiol; 21:1725–1731, 1966.
27. Guide for the evaluation of human exposure to whole-body vibration. New York: ANSI S3. 18–1979, Standards Secretariat, Acoustical Society of America, 1979.
28. American National Standard guide to the evaluation of human exposure to vibration in buildings, ANSI S3.29–1983, Acoustical Society of America, 1983.
29. International Standards Organization. Evaluation of human exposure to whole-body vibration. Part 1: General requirements, ISO 2631/1. 1985. Part 2: Continuous and shock induced vibration in buildings (1–80 Hz), ISO 2631/2, 1989. Part 3: Evaluation of exposures to whole body vibration: z-axis vertical vibration in frequency range 0.1 to 0.63 Hz, 1985.
30. Taylor W, and Pelmear PL, ed. Vibration white finger in industry. New York: Academic Press, 1975.
31. U.S. Department of Health and Human Services, National Institute for Occupational Safety and Health. Occupational exposure to hand-arm vibration. DHHS (NIOSH), Publication No, 89–166, 1989.
32. American National Standards guide for the measurement and evaluation of human exposure to vibration transmitted to the hand, ANSI S3.34–1986, Acoustical Society of America, 1986.
33. Guide for the measurement and assessment of human exposure to vibration transmitted to the hand. ISO 5349–1985. International Standards Organization, 1985.
34. Taylor W and Wasserman DE, ed. Proceedings of the international occupational hand-arm vibration conference. Washington, DC: United States Department of Health, Education and Welfare, Publication No. 77–170. Government Printing Office, 1977.
35. Griffin MJ and Lewis CH. A review of the effects of vibration on visual acuity and continuous manual control. Part I: Visual acuity, Part II: Continuous manual control. J. Sound and Vibration, 56(3), 1978.
36. Guidelines for noise and vibration levels for the space station, Committee on Hearing, Bioacoustics and Biomechanics (CHABA). Washington, DC: National Research Council, NASA Contractor Report 178310, 1987.

Chapter 11

Spatial Orientation in Flight

Kent K. Gillingham

and Fred H. Previc

Appearances often are deceiving.

Aesop

MECHANICS

Operators of today's and tomorrow's air and space vehicles must understand clearly the terminology and physical principles relating to the motions of their aircraft so they can fly with precision and effectiveness. These crewmembers also must have a working knowledge of the structure and function of the various mechanical and electrical systems of which their craft is comprised to help them understand the performance limits of their machines and to facilitate trouble-shooting and promote safe recovery when the machines fail in flight. So, too, must practitioners of aerospace medicine understand certain basic definitions and laws of mechanics so that they can analyze and describe the motional environment to which the flyer is exposed. In addition, the aeromedical professional must be familiar with the physiologic bases and operational limitations of the flyer's orientational mechanisms. This understanding is necessary to enable the physician or physiologist to speak intelligently and credibly with aircrew about spatial disorientation and to enable him or her to contribute significantly to investigations of aircraft mishaps in which spatial disorientation may be implicated.

Motion

We shall discuss two types of physical motion: *linear motion* or *motion of translation,* and *angular motion* or *motion of rotation.* Linear motion can be further categorized as rectilinear, meaning motion in a straight line, or curvilinear, meaning motion in a curved path. Both linear motion and angular motion are composed of an infinite variety of subtypes, or motion parameters, based on successive derivatives of linear or angular position with respect to time. The most basic of these motion parameters, and the most useful, are displacement, velocity, acceleration, and jerk. Table 11.1 classifies linear and angular motion parameters and their symbols and units and serves as an outline for the following discussions of linear and angular motion.

Linear Motion

The basic parameter of linear motion is linear displacement. The other parameters— velocity, acceleration, jerk—are derived from the concept of displacement. Linear displacement, x, is the distance and direction of the object under consideration from some reference point; as such, it is a vector quantity, having both magnitude and direction. The position of an aircraft located at 25 nautical miles on the 150° radial of the San

Table 11.1.
Linear and Angular Motion—Symbols and Units

Motion Parameter	Linear		Angular	
	Symbols	Units	Symbols	Units
Displacement	x	meter (m); nautical mile (= 1852 m)	θ	degree; radian (rad) (= 360/2π degree)
Velocity	v, $\dot{x}$	meter/second (m/sec); knot ($\approx$0.514 m/sec)	ω, $\dot{\theta}$	degree/sec; rad/sec
Acceleration	$\bar{a}$, $\check{v}$, $\bar{x}$	m/sec^2; g ($\approx$9.81 m/sec^2)	α, $\dot{\omega}$, $\ddot{\theta}$	degree/sec^2; rad/sec^2
Jerk	j, $\dot{a}$, $\ddot{v}$, $\dddot{x}$	m/sec^3		degree/sec^3; rad/sec^3
		g/sec	γ, $\dot{\alpha}$, $\ddot{\omega}$, $\dddot{\theta}$	

Antonio vortac, for example, describes completely the linear displacement of the aircraft from the navigational facility serving as the reference point. The meter (m), however, is the unit of linear displacement in the International Systems of Units (SI) and will eventually replace other units of linear displacement such as feet, nautical miles, and statute miles.

When linear displacement is changed during a period of time, another vector quantity, linear velocity, occurs. The formula for calculating the mean linear velocity, v, during time interval, Δt, is as follows:

$$v = (x_2 - x_1)/\Delta t \qquad (1)$$

where x_1 is the initial linear displacement and x_2 is the final linear displacement. An aircraft that travels from San Antonio, Texas to New Orleans, Louisiana in 1 hour, for example, moves with a mean linear velocity of 434 knots (nautical miles per hour) on a true bearing of 086°. Statute miles per hour and feet per second are other commonly used units of linear speed, the magnitude of linear velocity; meters per second (m/sec), however, is the SI unit and is preferred. Frequently, it is important to describe linear velocity at a particular instant in time, that is, as Δt approaches zero. In this situation, one speaks of instantaneous linear velocity, $\dot{x}$ (pronounced "x dot"), which is the first derivative of displacement with respect to time, dx/dt.

When the linear velocity of an object changes over time, the difference in velocity, divided by the time required for the moving object to make the change, gives its mean linear acceleration, a. The following formula:

$$a = (v_2 - v_1)/\Delta t \qquad (2)$$

where v_1 is the initial velocity, v_2 is the final velocity, and Δt is the elapsed time, is used to calculate the mean linear acceleration, which like displacement and velocity, is a vector quantity with magnitude and direction. Acceleration is thus the rate of change of velocity, just as velocity is the rate of change of displacement. The SI unit for the magnitude of linear acceleration is meters per second squared (m/sec^2). Consider, for example, an aircraft that accelerates from a dead stop to a velocity of 100 m/sec in 5 seconds: the mean linear acceleration is 100 m/sec − 0 m/sec ÷ 5 seconds, or 20 m/sec^2. The instantaneous linear acceleration, $\ddot{x}$ ("x double dot") or $\dot{v}$, is the second derivative of displacement or the first derivative of velocity d^2x/dt^2 or dv/dt, respectively.

A very useful unit of acceleration is g, which for our purposes is equal to the constant g_o, the amount of acceleration exhibited by a free-falling body near the surface of the earth— 9.81 m/sec^2. To convert values of linear acceleration given in m/sec^2 into g units, simply divide by 9.81. In the above example in which an aircraft accelerates at a mean rate of 20 m/sec^2, one divides 20 m/sec^2 by 9.81 m/sec^2 per g to obtain 2.04 g.

A special type of linear acceleration, radial or centripetal acceleration, results in curvilinear, usually circular, motion. This acceleration acts along the line represented by the radius of the curve and is directed toward the center of the curvature. Its effect is a continuous redirection of the linear velocity, in this case called tangential velocity, of the object subjected to the acceleration. Examples of this type of linear acceleration are when an aircraft pulls out of a dive after firing on a ground target or flies a circular path during aerobatic maneuvering. The value of the centripetal acceleration, a_c, can be calculated if one knows the tangential velocity, v_t, and the radius, r, of the curved path followed:

$$a_c = v_t^2/r \qquad (3)$$

For example, the centripetal acceleration of an aircraft traveling at 300 m/sec (approximately 600 knots) and having a radius of turn of 1500 m can be calculated. Dividing $(300 \text{ m/sec})^2$ by 1500 m gives a value of 60 m/sec^2, which when divided by 9.81 m/sec^2 per g, comes out to 6.12 g.

One can go another step in the derivation of linear motion parameters by obtaining the rate of change of acceleration. This quantity, j, is known as linear jerk. Mean linear jerk is calculated as follows:

$$j = (a_2 - a_1)/\Delta t \qquad (4)$$

where a_1 is the acceleration, a_2 is the final acceleration, and Δt is the elapsed time. Instantaneous linear jerk, $\dot{x}$ or $\dot{a}$, is the third derivative of linear displacement or the first derivative of linear acceleration with respect to time, that is d^3x/dt^3 or da/dt, respectively. Although the SI unit for jerk is m/sec^3, it is generally more useful to speak in terms of g-onset rate, measured in g's per second (g/sec).

Angular Motion

The derivation of the parameters of angular motion follows in a parallel fashion the scheme used to derive the parameters of linear motion. The basic parameter of angular motion is angular displacement. For an object to be able to undergo angular displacement it must be polarized, that is, it must have a front and back, so that it can face or be pointed in a particular direction. A simple example of angular displacement is seen in a person facing east. In this case, the individual's angular displacement is 90° clockwise from the reference direction, which is north. Angular displacement, symbolized by θ, is generally measured in degrees, revolutions (1 revolution = 360°), or radians (1 radian = 1 revolution ÷ 2π, or approximately 57.3°). The radian is a particularly convenient unit to use when dealing with circular motion (e.g., motion of a centrifuge) because it is necessary only to multiply the angular displacement of the system, in radians, by the length of the radius to find the value of the linear displacement along the circular path. The radian is the angle subtended by a circular arc the same length as the radius of the circle.

Angular velocity, ω, is the rate of change of angular displacement. The mean angular velocity occurring in a time interval, Δt, is calculated as follows:

$$\omega = (\theta_2 - \theta_1)/\Delta t \qquad (5)$$

where θ_1, is the initial angular displacement and θ_2 is the final angular displacement.

Instantaneous angular velocity is $\dot{\theta}$, or $d\theta/dt$. As an example of angular velocity consider the standard-rate turn of instrument flying, in which a heading change of 180° is made in 1 minute. Then $\omega = (180° - 0°) \div 60$ seconds, or 3 degrees per second (degrees/sec). This angular velocity also can be described as 0.5 revolutions per minute (rpm) or as 0.052 radians per second (rad/sec) (3 degrees/sec divided by 57.3 degrees/rad). The fact that an object may be undergoing curvilinear motion during a turn in no way affects the calculation of its angular velocity: an aircraft being rotated on the ground on a turntable at a rate of half a turn per minute has the same angular velocity as one flying a standard rate instrument turn (3 degrees/ sec) in the air at 300 knots.

Because radial or centripetal linear acceleration results when rotation is associated with a radius from the axis of rotation, a formula for calculating the centripetal acceleration, a_c, from the angular velocity, ω, and the radius, r, is often useful:

$$a_c = \omega^2 \, r \qquad (6)$$

where ω is the angular velocity in radians per second. One can convert readily to the formula for centripetal acceleration in term of tangential velocity if one remembers the following:

$$v_t = \omega \, r \qquad (7)$$

To calculate the centrifuge having a 10-m arm and turning at 30 rpm, equation 6 is used after first converting 30 rpm to π radians per second. Squaring the angular velocity and multiplying by the 10-m radius, a centripetal acceleration of $10 \, \pi^2$ m/sec^2, or 10.1 g is obtained.

The rate of change in angular velocity is angular acceleration, α. The mean angular acceleration is calculated as follows:

$$\alpha = (\omega_2 - \omega_1)/\varDelta t \qquad (8)$$

where ω_1 is the initial angular velocity, ω_2 is the final angular velocity, and $\varDelta t$ is the time interval over which angular velocity changes. $\dot\theta$, $\ddot\omega$, $d^2\theta/dt^2$ and $d\omega/dt$ all can be used to symbolize instantaneous angular acceleration, the second derivative of angular displacement or the first derivative of angular velocity with respect to time. If a figure skater is spinning at 6 revolutions per second (2160 degrees/sec, or 37.7 rad/ sec) and then comes to a complete stop in 2 seconds, the rate of change of angular velocity, or angular acceleration, is (37.7 rad/sec) $\div$ 2 seconds, or -18.9 rad/ sec^2. One cannot express angular acceleration in g units, which measure magnitude of linear acceleration only.

Although not commonly used in aerospace medicine, another parameter derived from angular displacement is angular jerk, the rate of change of angular acceleration. Its description is completely analogous to that for linear jerk, but angular rather than linear symbols and units are used.

Force, Inertia, and Momentum

Generally speaking, it is not the linear and angular motions themselves, but the forces and torques which result in or appear to result from linear and angular velocity changes that stimulate or compromise the crewmember's physiologic mechanisms.

Force and Torque

Force is an influence that produces, or tends to produce, linear motion or changes in linear motion; it is a pushing or pulling action. Torque produces, or tends to produce, angular motion or changes in angular motion; it is a twisting or turning action. The SI unit of force is the newton (N). Torque has dimensions of force and length because torque is applied as a force at a certain distance from the center of rotation. The newton meter (N m) is the SI unit of torque.

Mass and Rotational Inertia

Newton's Law of Acceleration states the following:

$$F = m \, a \qquad (9)$$

where F is the unbalanced force applied to an object, m is the mass of the object, and a is linear acceleration.

To describe the analogous situation pertaining to angular motion, the following equation is used:

$$M = J \, \alpha \qquad (10)$$

where M is unbalanced torque (for moment) applied to the rotating object, J is rotational inertia (moment of inertia) of the object, and α is angular acceleration.

The mass of an object is thus the ratio of the force acting on the object to the acceleration resulting from the force. Mass, therefore, is a measure of the inertia of an object—its resistance to being accelerated. Similarly, rotational inertia is the ratio of the torque acting on an object to the angular acceleration resulting from that torque—again, a measure of resistance to acceleration. The kilogram (kg) is the SI unit of mass and is equivalent to 1 N/(m/sec²). The SI unit of rotational inertia is merely the N m/(radian/sec²).

Because $F = m\ a$, the centripetal force, F_c, needed to produce a centripetal acceleration, a_c, of a mass, m, can be calculated as follows:

$$F_c = m\ a_c \qquad (11)$$

Thus, from equation 3:

$$F_c = (m\ v_t^2)/r \qquad (12)$$

or from equation 6:

$$F_c = m\ \omega 2\ r \qquad (13)$$

where v_t, is tangential velocity and ω is angular velocity.

Newton's law of Action and Reaction, which states that for every force applied to an object there is an equal and opposite reactive force exerted by that object, provides the basis for the concept of inertial force. Inertial force is an apparent force opposite in direction to an accelerating force and equal to the mass of the object times the acceleration. An aircraft exerting an accelerating forward thrust on its pilot causes an inertial force, the product of the pilot's mass and the acceleration, to be exerted on the back of the seat by the pilot's body. Similarly, an aircraft undergoing positive centripetal acceleration as a result of lift generated in a turn causes the pilot's body to exert inertial force on the bottom of the seat. More important, however, are the

inertial forces exerted on the pilot's blood and organs of equilibrium because physiologic effects result directly from such forces.

At this point it is appropriate to introduce G, which is used to measure the strength of the gravitoinertial force environment. (Note: G should not be confused with G, the symbol for the universal gravitational constant, which is equal to 6.70×10^{-11} N m²/kg².) Strictly speaking, G is a measure of relative weight:

$$G = w/w_o \qquad (14)$$

where w is the weight observed in the environment under consideration and w_o is the normal weight on the surface of the earth. In the physical definition of weight,

$$w = m\ a \qquad (15)$$

and

$$w_o = m\ g_o \qquad (16)$$

where m is mass, a is the acceleratory field (vector sum of actual linear acceleration plus an imaginary acceleration opposite the force of gravity), and g_o is the standard value of the acceleration of gravity (9.81 m/sec²). Thus, a person having a mass of 100 kg would weigh 100 kg times 9.81 m/sec² or 981 N on earth (although conventional spring scales would read "100 kg"). At some other location or under some other acceleratory condition, the same person could weigh twice as much—1962 N—and cause a scale to read "200 kg." He or she would then be in a 2-G environment, or, if that person were in an aircraft, he or she would be "pulling" 2 G. Consider also that since

$$G = w/w_o = m\ a/\ m\ g_o$$

then

$$G = a/g_o \qquad (17)$$

Thus, the ratio between the ambient acceleratory field (a) and the standard acceleration (g_o) also can be represented in terms of G.

Therefore, g is used as a unit of acceleration (e.g., $a_c = 8$ g), and the dimensionless ratio of weights, G, is reserved for describing the resulting gravitoinertial force environment (e.g., a force of 8 G, or an 8-G load). When in the vicinity of the surface of the earth, one feels a G force equal to 1 G in magnitude directed toward the center of the earth. If one also sustains a G force resulting from linear acceleration, the magnitude and direction of the resultant gravitoinertial G force can be calculated by adding vectorially the 1-G gravitational force and the inertial G force. An aircraft pulling out of a dive with a centripetal acceleration of 3 g, for example, would exert 3 G of centrifugal force. At the bottom of the dive, the pilot would experience the 3-G centrifugal force in line with the 1-G gravitational force, for a total of 4 G directed toward the floor of the aircraft. If the pilot could continue his or her circular flight path at a constant airspeed, the G force experienced at the top of the loop would be 2 G because the 1-G gravitational force would subtract from the 3-G inertial force. Another common example of the addition of gravitational G force and inertial G force occurs during the application of power on takeoff or on a missed approach. If the forward acceleration is 1 g, the inertial force is 1 G directed toward the tail of the aircraft. The inertial force adds vectorially to the 1-G force of gravity, directed downward, to provide a resultant gravitoinertial force of 1.414 G pointing 45° down from the aft direction.

Just as inertial forces oppose acceleration forces, so do inertial torques oppose acceleratory torques. No convenient derived units exist, however, for measuring inertial torque; specifically, there is no such thing as angular G.

Momentum

To complete this discussion of linear and angular motion, the concepts of momentum and impulse must be introduced. Linear momentum is the product of mass and linear velocity— m and v. Angular momentum is the product of rotational inertia and angular velocity, J ω. Momentum is a quantity that a translating or rotating body conserves, that is, an object cannot gain or lose momentum unless it is acted on by a force or torque. A translational impulse is the product of force, F, and the time over which the force acts on an object, Δt, and is equal to the change in linear momentum imparted to the object. Thus:

$$F \ \Delta t = m \ v_2 - m \ v_1 \qquad (18)$$

where v_1 is the initial linear velocity and v_2 is the final linear velocity.

When dealing with angular motion, a rotational impulse is defined as the product of torque, M, and the time over which it acts, Δt. A rotational impulse is equal to the change in angular momentum. Thus:

$$M \ \Delta t = J \ \omega_2 - J \ \omega_1 \qquad (19)$$

where ω_1 is the initial angular velocity and ω_2 is the final angular velocity.

The above relations are derived from the Law of Acceleration, as follows:

$$F = m \ a$$

$$M = J \ \alpha$$

since $\alpha = (v_2 — v_1)/\Delta t$
and $\alpha = (\omega_2 — \omega_1)/\Delta t$

Directions of Action and Reaction

A number of conventions have been used in aerospace medicine to describe the directions of linear and angular displacement, velocity, and acceleration and of reactive forces and torques. The more commonly used of those conventions will be discussed in the following sections.

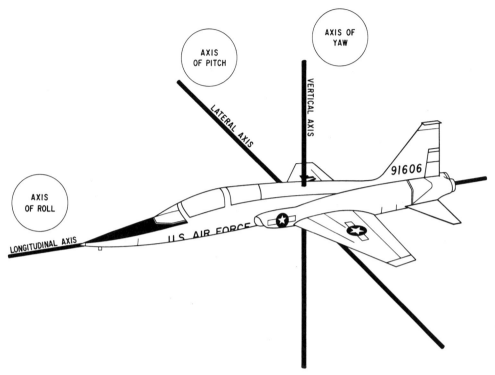

Figure 11.1. Axes of linear and angular aircraft motions. Linear motions are longitudinal, lateral, and vertical, and angular motions are roll, pitch and yaw.

Vehicular Motions

Because space is three-dimensional, linear motions in space are described by reference to three linear axes and angular motions by reference to three angular axes. In aviation, it is customary to speak of the longitudinal (fore-aft), lateral (right-left), and vertical (up-down) linear axes and the roll, pitch, and yaw angular axes, as shown in Figure 11.1.

Most linear accelerations in aircraft occur in the vertical plane defined by the longitudinal and vertical axes because thrust is usually developed along the former axis and lift is usually developed along the latter axis. Aircraft capable of vectored thrust are now operational, however, and vectored-lift aircraft are currently being flight-tested. Most angular accelerations in aircraft occur in the roll plane (perpendicular to the roll axis) and, to a lesser extent, in the pitch plane. Angular motion in the yaw plane is very limited in normal flying, although it does occur during spins and several other aerobatic maneuvers. Certainly, aircraft and space vehicles of the future can be expected to operate with considerably more freedom of both linear and angular motion than do those of the present.

Physiologic Acceleration and Reaction Nomenclature

Figure 11.2 depicts a practical system for describing linear and angular accelerations acting on man (1). This system is used extensively in aeromedical scientific writing. In this system, a linear acceleration of the type associated with a conventional takeoff roll is in the $+a_x$ direction, that is, it is a $+a_x$ acceleration. Braking to a stop during a landing roll results in $-a_x$ acceleration. Radial acceleration of the type usually developed during air combat maneuvering is $+a_z$ acceleration—foot-to-head. The right-hand rule for describing the relationships between three

PHYSIOLOGIC ACCELERATION NOMENCLATURE

PHYSIOLOGIC REACTION NOMENCLATURE

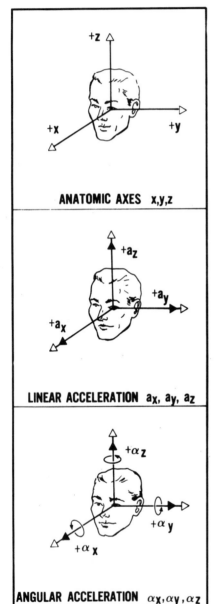

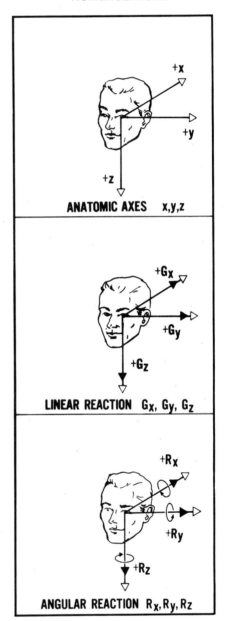

Figure 11.2. System for describing accelerations and inertial reactions in humans. (Adapted from Hixson WC, Niven JI, Correia MJ. Kinematics nomenclature for physiological accelerations, with special reference to vestibular applications. Monograph 14. Naval Aerospace Medical Institute, Pensecola, Florida, 1966.)

orthogonal axes aids recall of the positive directions of a_x, a_y, and a_z accelerations in this particular system: if one lets the forward-pointing index finger of the right hand represent the positive x-axis and the left-pointing middle finger of the right hand represent the positive y-axis, the positive z-axis is represented by the upward-pointing thumb of the right hand. A different right-hand rule, however, is used in another convention, one for describing vehicular coordinates. In that system, $+a_x$ is noseward acceleration, $+a_y$ is to the right, and $+a_z$ is floorward; an inverted right hand illustrates that set of axes.

The angular accelerations, a_x, a_y, and a_z, are roll, pitch and yaw accelerations, respectively, in the system shown in Figure 11.2. Note that the relations between the positive x-axis, y-axis, and z-axis are identical to those for linear accelerations. The direction of positive angular displacement, velocity, or acceleration is described by another right-hand rule, wherein the flexed fingers of the right hand indicate the direction of angular motion corresponding to the vector represented by the extended, abducted right thumb. Thus, in this system, a right roll results from $+a_x$ acceleration, a pitch down results from $+a_y$ acceleration, and a left yaw results from $+a_z$ acceleration. Again, it is important to be aware of the inverted right-hand coordinate system commonly used to describe angular motions of vehicles. In that convention, a positive roll acceleration is to the right, positive pitch is upward, and positive yaw is to the right.

The nomenclature for the direction of gravitoinertial (G) forces acting on humans is also illustrated in Figure 11.2. Note that the relation of these axes to each other follows a backward, inverted, right-hand rule. In the illustration convention, $+a_x$ acceleration results in $+G_x$ inertial force, and $+a_z$ acceleration results in $+G_z$ force. This correspondence of polarity is not achieved on the Y-axis, however, because $+a_y$ acceleration results in $-G_y$ force. If the $+G_y$ direction were reversed, full polarity correspondence could be achieved between all linear accelerations and all reactive forces, and that con-

vention has been used by some authors. An example of the usage of the symbolic reaction terminology would be: "An F-16 pilot must be able to sustain $+9.0$ G_z without losing vision or consciousness."

The "eyeballs" nomenclature is another useful set of terms for describing gravitoinertial forces. In this system, the direction of the inertia reaction of the eyeballs when the head is subjected to an acceleration is used to describe the direction of the inertial force. The equivalent expressions, "eyeballs-in acceleration" and "eyeballs-in G force," leave little room for confusion about either the direction of the applied acceleratory field or the resulting gravitoinertial force environment.

Inertial torques can be described conveniently by means of the system shown in Figure 11.2, in which the angular reaction axes are the same as the linear reaction axes. The inertial reactive torque resulting from $+a_x$ (right roll) angular acceleration is $+R_x$ and $+a_z$ (left yaw) results in $+R_z$; however $+a_y$ (downward pitch) results in $-R_y$. This incomplete correspondence between acceleration and reaction coordinate polarities again results from the mathematical tradition of using right-handed coordinate systems.

It should be apparent from all of this that the potential for confusing the audience when speaking or writing about acceleration and inertial reaction is great enough to make it a virtual necessity to describe the coordinate system being used. For most applications, the "eyeballs" convention is perfectly adequate.

VISUAL ORIENTATION

Vision is by far the most important sensory modality subserving spatial orientation, especially so in moving vehicles such as aircraft. Without it, flight as we know it would be impossible, whereas this would not be necessarily the case in the absence of the vestibular or other sensory systems that provide orientation information. For the most part, the function of vision in spatial orientation is obvious, so a discussion proportional in size to the importance of that function in orientation will not be presented here. Certain special features of visual orientation deserve mention, however. First, there are actually two separate visual systems, and they have two distinct functions: object recognition and spatial orientation. A knowledge of these systems is extremely important, both to help in understanding visual illusions in flight and to appreciate the difficulties inherent in using flight instruments for spatial orientation. Second, visual and vestibular orientation information are integrated at very basic neural levels. For that reason spatial disorientation frequently is not amenable to correction by higher-level neural processing.

Anatomy and the Visual System

General

The retina, an evaginated portion of the embryonic brain, consists of an outer layer of pigmented epithelium and an inner layer of neural tissue. Contained within the latter layer are the sensory rod and cone cells, the bipolar and horizontal cells that comprise the intraretinal afferent pathway from the rods and cones, and the multipolar ganglion cells, the axons of which are the fibers of the optic nerve. The cones, which number approximately 7 million in the human eye, have a relatively high threshold to light energy. They are responsible for sharp visual discrimination and color vision. The rods, of which there are over 100 million, are much more sensitive to light than the cones; they produce the ability to see in twilight and at night. In the retinal macula, near the posterior pole of the eye, the cone population achieves its greatest density; within the macula, the fovea centralis—a small pit totally comprised of tightly packed slender cones—provides the sharpest visual acuity and is the anatomic basis for foveal, or central, vision. The remainder of the eye is capable of far less visual acuity and subserves paracentral and peripheral vision.

Having dendritic connections with the rods and cones, the bipolar cells provide axons that synapse with the dendrites or cell bodies of the multipolar ganglion cells, whose axons in turn course parallel to the retinal surface and converge at the optic disk. Emerging from the eye as the optic nerve, they meet their counterparts from the opposite eye in the optic chiasm and then continue in one of the optic tracts, most likely to terminate in a lateral geniculate body, but possibly in a superior colliculus or the pretectal area. Second-order neurons from the lateral geniculate body comprise the geniculocalcarine tract, which becomes the optic radiation and terminates in the primary visual cortex, the striate area of the occipital cortex (Area 17). In the visual cortex, the retinal image is represented as a more or less point-to-point projection from the lateral geniculate body, which receives a similar topographically structured projection from both retinae. The lateral geniculate and the primary visual cortex are thus structurally and functionally suited for the recognition and analysis of visual images. The superior colliculi project to the visual association areas (Areas 18 and 19) of the cerebral cortex via the pulvinar, and also eventually to the motor nuclei of the extraocular muscles and muscles of the neck, and appear to provide a pathway for certain gross ocular reflexes of visual origin. Fibers entering the pretectal area are involved in pupillary reflexes. In addition, most anatomic and physiologic evidence indicates that information from the occipital visual association areas, parietal cerebral cortex, and frontal eye movement area (Area 8) is relayed through the paramedian pontine reticular formation to the nuclei of the cranial nerves innervating the exraocular muscles. Via this pathway and perhaps others involving the superior colliculi, saccadic (fast) and pursuit (slow) eye movements are initiated and controlled.

Visual-Vestibular Convergence

Vision in humans and other primates is highly dependent on cerebral cortical structure and function, whereas vestibular orientation primarily involves more primitive anatomic structures.

Yet visual and vestibular orientational processes are by no means independent. We know that visually perceived motion information and probably other visual orientational data reach the vestibular nuclei in the brain stem (2,3), but it appears that a major integration of visual and vestibular orientational information is first accomplished in the cerebral cortex.

The geniculostriate projection system is divided both anatomically and functionally into two parts: that incorporating the parvocellular layers of the lateral geniculate body (the "parvo" system) and that incorporating the magnocellular layers (the "magno" system). These systems remain partly segregated in the primary visual cortex, undergo further segregation in the visual association cortex, and ultimately terminate in the temporal and parietal lobes, respectively. The parvo system neurons have smaller, more centrally located receptive fields that exhibit high spatial resolution (acuity), and they respond well to color; they do not, however, respond well to rapid motion or high flicker rates. The magno cells, by comparison, have larger receptive fields and respond better to motion and flicker, but are relatively insensitive to color differences. Magno neurons generally exhibit poorer spatial resolution, although they seem to respond better than parvo neurons at low luminance contrasts. In general, the parvo system is better at detecting small, slowly moving, colored targets located near the center of the visual field, while the magno system is more capable of processing rapidly moving and optically degraded stimuli across larger regions of the visual field.

What is important about these two components of the geniculostriate system is that the parvo system projects ventrally to the inferior temporal areas, which are involved in visual search, pattern recognition, and visual object memory, while the magno system projects dorsally to the posterior parietal and superior temporal areas, which are specialized for motion information processing. The cerebral cortical areas to which the parvo system projects receive vir-

tually no vestibular afferents; the areas to which the magno system projects, on the other hand, receive significant vestibular and other sensory inputs, and are believed to be involved to a greater extent in maintaining spatial orientation.

The posterior parietal region projects heavily to cells of the pontine nuclei, which in turn provide the mossy-fiber visual input to the cerebellar cortex. Via the accessory optic and central tegmental tracts, visual information also reaches the inferior olives, which provide climbing fiber input to the cerebellar cortex. The cerebellar cortex, specifically the flocculonodular lobe and vermis, also receives direct mossy-fiber input from the vestibular system. Thus, cerebellar cortex is another area of very strong visual-vestibular convergence. Furthermore, the cerebellar Purkinje cells have inhibitory connections in the vestibular nuclei and possibly even in the vestibular end-organs; so visual-vestibular interactions mediated by the cerebellum also occur at the level of the brain stem, and maybe even peripherally.

Finally, there is a confluence of visual and vestibular pathways in the paramedian pontine reticular formation. Integration of visual and vestibular information in the cerebellum and brain stem appears to allow visual control of basic equilibratory reflexes of vestibular origin. As might be expected, there also are afferent vestibular influences on visual system nuclei; these influences have been demonstrated in the lateral geniculate body and superior colliculus.

Visual Information Processing

Primary control of the human ability to move and orient ourselves in three-dimensional space is mediated by the visual system, as exemplified by the fact that individuals without functioning vestibular systems ("labyrinthine defectives") have virtually no problems with spatial orientation unless they are deprived of vision. The underlying mechanisms of visual orientation-information processing are revealed by receptive-field studies, which have been accomplished for the peripheral retina, relay structures, and primary visual cortex. Basically, these studies show that there are several types of movement-detecting neurons and that these neurons respond differently to such features as the direction of movement, velocity of movement, size of the stimulus, its orientation in space, and the level of illumination.

As evidenced by the division of the primate geniculostriate system into two separate functional entities, however, vision must be considered as two separate processes. Some researchers emphasize the role of the ventral (parvo) system in object recognition (the ''what'' system) and that of the dorsal (magno) system in spatial orientation (the ''where'' system); others categorize the difference in terms of form (occipito-temporal) versus motion (occipito-parietal) processing. A recent theory suggests that the dorsal system is primarily involved in processing information in peripersonal (near) space during reaching and other visuomotor activity, whereas the ventral system is principally engaged in visual scanning in extrapersonal (far) visual space (4). In the present discussion, we shall refer to the systems as the ''focal'' and ambient'' visual systems, respectively, subserving the focal and ambient modes of visual processing. Certain aspects of yet another visual process, the one responsible for generating eye movements, will also be described.

Focal Vision

Liebowitz and Dichgans (5) have provided a very useful summary of the characteristics of focal vision:

[The focal visual mode] is concerned with object recognition and identification and in general answers the question of ''what.'' Focal vision involves relatively fine detail (high spatial frequencies) and is correspondingly best represented in the central visual fields. Information processed by focal vision is ordinarily well represented in consciousness and is critically re-

lated to physical parameters such as stimulus energy and refractive error.

Focal vision uses the central 30 degrees or so of the visual field. While it is not primarily involved with orienting the individual in the environment, it certainly contributes to conscious percepts of orientation, such as those derived from judgments of distance and depth and those obtained from reading flight instruments. Tredici (6) categorized the visual cues to distance and depth as monocular or binocular. The monocular cues are (1) size constancy, the size of the retinal image in relation to known and comparative sizes of objects; (2) shape constancy, the shape of the retinal image in relation to the known shape of the object (e.g., the foreshortening of the image of a known circle into an ellipsoid shape means one part of the circle is farther away than the other); (3) motion parallax (also called optical flow), the relative speed of movement of images across the retina such that when an individual is moving linearly in his or her environment, the retinal images of nearer objects move faster than those of objects farther away; (4) interposition, the partial obstruction from view of more distant objects by nearer ones; (5) gradient of texture, the apparent loss of detail with greater distance; (6) linear perspective, the convergence of parallel lines at a distance; (7) illumination perspective, which results from the tendency to perceive the light source to be above an object and from the association of more deeply shaded parts of an object with being farther from the light source; and (8) aerial perspective, the perception of objects to be more distant when the image is relatively bluish or hazy. The binocular cues to depth and distance are (1) stereopsis, the visual appreciation of three-dimensional space that results from the fusion of slightly dissimilar retinal images of an object; (2) vergence, the medial rotation of the eyes and the resulting direction of their gaze along more or less converging lines, depending on whether the viewed object is closer or farther, respectively; and (3) accommodation, or focusing of the image by changing the curvature of the lens of the eye. Of all the cues listed, size and shape constancy and motion parallax appear to be most important for deriving distance information in flying because they are available at and well beyond the distances at which binocular cues are useful. Stereopsis can provide orientation information at distances up to only about 200 m; it is, however, more important in orientation than vergence and accommodation, which are useless beyond about 6 m.

Ambient Vision

Liebowitz and Dichgans (5) have provided a summary of ambient vision:

The ambient visual mode subserves spatial localization and orientation and is in general concerned with the question of "where." Ambient vision is mediated by relatively large stimulus patterns so that it typically involves stimulation of the peripheral visual field and relatively coarse detail (low spatial frequencies). Unlike focal vision, ambient vision is not systematically related to either stimulus energy or optical image quality. Rather, provided the stimulus is visible, orientation responses appear to be elicited on an "all or none" basis . . . .The conscious concomitant of ambient stimulation is low or frequently completely absent.

Ambient vision, therefore, is primarily involved with orienting the individual in the environment. Furthermore, this function is largely independent of the function of focal vision. This becomes evident in view of the fact that one can fully occupy central vision with the task of reading while simultaneously obtaining sufficient orientation cues with peripheral vision to walk or ride a bicycle. It is also evidenced by the ability of certain patients with cerebral cortical lesions to maintain visual orientation responses even though their ability to discriminate objects is lost.

While we commonly think of ambient vision as dependent on stimulation of the peripheral

visual field, it is more accurate to consider ambient vision as involving large areas of the total visual field, which of course usually include the periphery. In other words, ambient vision is not so much location-dependent as it is area-dependent. Moreover, ambient vision is stimulated much more effectively by large images or groups of images perceived to be at a distance than by those appearing to be close.

The function of ambient vision in orientation can be thought of as two processes, one providing motion cues and the other providing position cues. Large, coherently moving contrasts detected over a large area of the visual field result in vection, i.e., a visually induced percept of self-motion. If the moving contrasts revolve relative to the subject, he or she perceives rotational self-motion, or angular vection (also called circular vection), which can be in the pitch, roll, yaw, or any intermediate plane. If the moving contrasts enlarge and diverge from a distant point, become smaller and converge in the distance, or otherwise indicate linear motion, the percept of self-motion that results is linear vection, which also can be in any direction. Vection can, of course, be veridical or illusory, depending on whether actual or merely apparent motion of the subject is occurring. One can appreciate the importance of ambient vision in orientation by recalling the powerful sensations of self-motion generated by certain scenes in widescreen motion pictures (e.g., flying through the Grand Canyon in an IMAX theater).

Position cues provided by ambient vision are readily evidenced in the stabilization of posture that vision affords patients with defective vestibular or spinal proprioceptive systems. The essential visual parameter contributing to postural stability appears to be the motion of the retinal image that results from minor deviations from desired postural position. Visual effects on posture also can be seen in the phenomenon of height vertigo. As the distance from (height above) a stable visual environment increases, the amount of body sway necessary for the retinal image movement to be above threshold increases. Above a certain height, the ability of this visual mechanism to contribute to postural stability is exceeded and vision indicates posture to be stable despite large body sways. The conflict between visual orientation information, indicating relative stability, and the vestibular and somatosensory data, indicating large body sways, results in the unsettling experience of vertigo.

One more distinction between focal and ambient visual function should be emphasized. In general, focal vision serves to orient the perceived object relative to the individual, whereas ambient vision serves to orient the individual relative to the perceived environment. When both focal and ambient vision are present, orienting a focally perceived object relative to the ambient visual environment is easy, whether the mechanism employed involves first orienting the object to oneself and then orienting oneself and the object to the environment or whether the object is oriented directly to the environment. When only focal vision is available, however, it can be difficult to orient oneself correctly to a focally perceived environmental orientation cue because the natural tendency is to perceive oneself as stable and upright and to perceive the focally viewed object as oriented with respect to the stable and upright egocentric reference frame. This phenomenon can cause a pilot to misjudge his or her approach to a night landing, for example, when only the runway lights and a few other focal visual cues are available for spatial orientation.

Eye Movements

We distinguish between two fundamental types of eye movement: smooth movements, including pursuit, vergence, and those driven by the vestibular system; and saccadic (jerky) movements. Smooth eye movements are controlled at least in part by the posterior parietal cerebral cortex and surrounding areas, as evidenced by functional deficits resulting from damage to these areas. Eye movements of vestibular origin are primarily generated by very

basic reflexes involving brain stem mechanisms; and because visual pursuit eye movements are impaired by vestibular and certain cerebellar lesions, the vestibular system appears to be involved in the control of smooth eye movements even of visual origin. Saccadic eye movements are controlled mainly by the frontal eye fields of the cerebral cortex, which work with the superior colliculus in generating the movements. The frontal eye fields receive their visual input from the cortical visual association areas.

The maintenance of visual orientation in a dynamic motional environment is greatly enhanced by the ability to move the eyes, primarily because the retinal image of the environment can be stabilized by appropriate eye movements. Very powerful and important mechanisms involved in reflexive vestibular stabilization of the retinal image will be discussed in the section dealing with vestibular function. Visual pursuit movements also serve to stabilize the retinal image, as long as the relative motion between the head and the visual environment (or object being observed in it) is less than about 60 degrees/sec: targets moving at higher relative velocities necessitate either saccadic eye movements or voluntary head movements for adequate tracking. Saccadic eye movements are used voluntarily or reflexively to acquire a target, i.e., to move it into focal vision, or to catch up to a target that cannot be maintained on the fovea by pursuit movements. Under some circumstances, pursuit and saccadic eye movements alternate in a pattern of reflexive slow tracking and fast back-tracking called optokinetic nystagmus. This type of eye-movement response is typically elicited in the laboratory by surrounding the subject with a rotating striped drum; however, one can exhibit and experience optokinetic nystagmus quite readily in a more natural setting by watching railroad cars go by while waiting at a railroad crossing. Movement of the visual environment sufficient to elicit optokinetic nystagmus provides a stimulus that can either enhance or compete with the vestibular elicitation of eye movements, depending on whether the visually perceived motion is compatible or incompatible, respectively, with the motion sensed by the vestibular system.

Vergence movements, which aid binocular distance and motion perception at very close range, are of relatively minor importance in spatial orientation when compared with the image-stabilizing pursuit and saccadic eye movements. Vergence assumes some degree of importance, however, under conditions where a large visual environment is being simulated in a confined space. Failure to account for vergence effects can result in loss of simulation fidelity: a subject who must converge his or her eyes to fuse an image representing a large, distant object will perceive that object as small and near. To overcome this problem, visual flight simulators display distant scenes at the outer limit of vergence effects (7–10 meters) or use lenses or mirrors to put the displayed scene at optical infinity.

Even though gross stabilization of the retinal image aids object recognition and spatial orientation by enhancing visual acuity, absolute stability of an image is associated with a marked decrease in visual acuity and form perception. This stability-induced decrement is avoided by continual voluntary and involuntary movements of the eyes, even during fixation of an object. We are unaware of these small eye movements, however, and the visual world appears stable.

Voluntary scanning and tracking movements of the eyes are associated with the appearance of a stable visual environment, but why this is so is not readily apparent. Early investigators postulated that proprioceptive information from extraocular muscles provides not only feedback signals for the control of eye movements but also the afferent information needed to correlate eye movements with retinal image movements and arrive at a subjective determination of a stable visual environment. An alternative mechanism for oculomotor control and the subjective appreciation of visual stability is the "corollary discharge" or feed-forward mechanism, first proposed by Sperry (7). Sperry concluded: "Thus, an excitation pattern that normally re-

sults in a movement that will cause a displacement of the visual image on the retina may have a corollary discharge into the visual centers to compensate for the retinal displacement. This implies an anticipatory adjustment in the visual centers specific for each movement with regard to its direction and speed." The theoretical aspects of visual perception of movement and stability have been expanded over the years into various models based on "inflow" (afference), "outflow" (efference), and even hybrid sensory mechanisms.

In developing the important points on visual orientation, we have emphasized the "focal-ambient" dichotomy. As visual science matures further, this simplistic construct will likely be replaced by more complex but valid models of visual processes. Presently we are enthusiastic about a theory in which the dichotomy emphasized is that between the peripersonal (near) and focal extrapersonal (far) visual realms (4). This theory argues that the dorsal cortical system and its magno projection pathways are more involved in processing visual information from peripersonal space, while the ventral system and its parvo projections attend to the focal extrapersonal visual environment. The theory also suggests that visual attention is organized to be employed more efficiently in some sectors of three-dimensional visual space than in others (e.g., far vision is biased toward the upper visual field and utilizes local form processing, while near vision is biased toward the lower visual field and is better at global form processing), and that ambient extrapersonal information is largely excluded from attentional mechanisms. Certainly, the current state of knowledge concerning visual orientation is fluid.

VESTIBULAR FUNCTION

The role of vestibular function in spatial orientation is not so overt as that of vision but is extremely important for three major reasons. First, the vestibular system provides the structural and functional substrate for reflexes that serve to stabilize vision when motion of the head and body would otherwise result in blurring of the retinal image. Second, the vestibular system provides orientational information with reference to which both skilled and reflexive motor activities are automatically executed. Third, the vestibular system provides, in the absence of vision, a reasonably accurate percept of motion and position, as long as the pattern of stimulation remains within certain naturally occurring bounds. Because the details of vestibular anatomy and physiology are not usually well-known by medical professionals and because a working knowledge of them is essential to the understanding of spatial disorientation in flight, these details will be presented in the following sections.

Vestibular Anatomy

End-Organs

The vestibular end-organs are smaller than most people realize, measuring just 1.5 cm across. They reside well-protected within some of the densest bone in the body, the petrous portion of the temporal bone. Each temporal bone contains a tortuous excavation known as the bony labyrinth, which is filled with perilymph, a fluid much like cerebrospinal fluid in composition. The bony labyrinth consists of three main parts: the cochlea, the vestibule, and the semicircular canals (Fig. 11.3). Within each part of the bony labyrinth is a part of the delicate, tubular, membranous labyrinth, which contains endolymph, a fluid characterized by its relatively high concentration of positive ions. In the cochlea, the membranous labyrinth is called the cochlea duct or scala media; this organ converts acoustic energy into neural information. In the vestibule lie the two otolith organs, the utricle and the saccule. They translate gravitational and inertial forces into spatial orientation information—specifically, information about the angular position (tilt) and linear motion of the head. The semicircular ducts, contained in the semicircular canals, convert inertial torques into information about angular motion of the head. The three semicircular canals and their included semicircular ducts are oriented in three mutually perpendicular planes, thus inspiring the names of the canals: anterior vertical (or superior), posterior vertical (or posterior), and horizontal (or lateral).

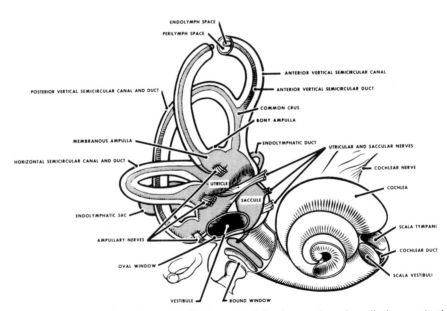

Figure 11.3. Gross anatomy of the inner ear. The bony semicircular canals and vestibule contain the membranous semicircular ducts and otolith organs, respectively.

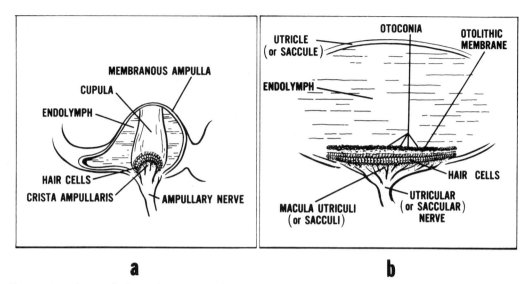

Figure 11.4. The vestibular end-organs. *a*. The ampulla of the semicircular duct, containing the crista ampullaris and cupula. *b*. A representative otolith organ, with its macula and otolithic membrane.

The semicircular ducts communicate at both ends with the utricle, and one end of each duct is dilated to form an ampulla. Inside each ampulla lies a crest of neuroepithelium, the crista ampullaris. Atop the crista, occluding the duct, is a gelatinous structure called the cupula (Fig. 11.4A). The hair cells of which the crista ampullaris is composed project their cilia into the base of the cupula, so that whenever inertial torques of the endolymph ring in the semicircular duct deviate the cupula, the cilia are bent.

Lining the bottom of the utricle in a more or less horizontal plane is another patch of neuroepithelium, the macula utriculi, and on the medial wall of the saccule in a vertical plane is still another, the macula sacculi (Fig. 11.4B). The cilia of the hair cells comprising these structures project into overlying otolithic membranes, one above each macula. The otolithic membranes are gelatinous structures containing many tiny calcium carbonate crystals, called otoconia, which are held together by a network of connective tissue. Having almost three times the density of the surrounding endolymph, the otolithic membranes displace endolymph and shift position relative to their respective maculae when subjected to changing gravitoinertial forces. This shifting of the otolithic membrane position results in bending of the cilia of the macular hair cells.

The hair cell is the functional unit of the vestibular sensory system. It converts spatial and temporal patterns of mechanical energy applied to the head into neural information. Each hair cell possesses one relatively large kinocilium on one side of the top of the cell and up to 100 smaller stereocilia on the same surface. Hair cells thus exhibit morphologic polarization, that is, they are oriented in a particular direction. The functional correlate of this polarization is that when the cilia of a hair cell are bent in the direction of its kinocilium, the cell undergoes an electrical depolarization, and the frequency of action potentials generated in the vestibular neuron attached to the hair cell increases above a certain resting frequency; the greater the deviation of the cilia, the higher the frequency. Similarly, when its cilia are bent away from the side with the kinocilium, the hair cell undergoes an electrical hyperpolarization, and the frequency of action potentials in the corresponding neuron in the vestibular nerve decreases (Fig. 11.5).

The same basic process described above occurs in all of the hair cells in the three cristae

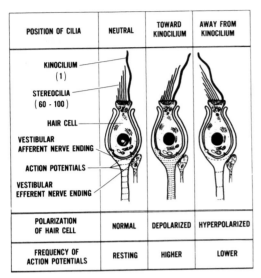

POSITION OF CILIA	NEUTRAL	TOWARD KINOCILIUM	AWAY FROM KINOCILIUM
KINOCILIUM (1) STEREOCILIA (60 - 100) HAIR CELL VESTIBULAR AFFERENT NERVE ENDING ACTION POTENTIALS VESTIBULAR EFFERENT NERVE ENDING			
POLARIZATION OF HAIR CELL	NORMAL	DEPOLARIZED	HYPERPOLARIZED
FREQUENCY OF ACTION POTENTIALS	RESTING	HIGHER	LOWER

Figure 11.5. Function of a vestibular hair cell. When mechanical forces deviate the cilia toward the side of the cell with the kinocilium, the hair cell depolarizes and the frequency of action potentials in the associated afferent vestibular neuron increases. When the cilia are deviated in the opposite direction, the hair cell hyperpolarizes and the frequency of action potentials decreases.

and both maculae; the important differences lie in the physical events that cause the deviation of cilia and in the directions in which the various groups of hair cells are oriented. The hair cells of a crista ampullaris respond to the inertial torque of the ring of endolymph contained in the attached semicircular duct as the reacting endolymph exerts pressure on the cupula and deviates it. The hair cells of a macula, on the other hand, respond to the gravitoinertial force acting to displace the overlying otolithic membrane. As indicated in Figure 11.6A, all of the hair cells in the crista of the horizontal semicircular duct are oriented so that their kinocilia are on the utricular side of the ampulla. Thus, utriculopetal endolymphatic pressure on the cupula deviates the cilia of these hair cells toward the kinocilia, and all the hair cells in the crista depolarize. The hair cells in the cristae of the vertical semicircular ducts are oriented in the opposite fashion, i.e., their kinocilia are all on the side away from the utricle. In the ampullae of the vertical semicircu-

lar ducts, therefore, utriculopetal endolymphatic pressure deviates the cilia away from the kinocilia, causing all of the hair cells in these cristae to hyperpolarize. In contrast, the hair cells of the maculae are not oriented unidirectionally across the neuroepithelium: the direction of their morphologic polarization depends on where they lie on the macula (Fig. 11.6B). In both maculae, there is a central line of reflection, on opposing sides of which the hair cells assume an opposite orientation. In the utricular macula, the kinocilia of the hair cells are all oriented toward the line of reflection, whereas in the saccular macula, they are oriented away from it. Because the line of reflection on each macula curves at least 90°, the hair cells, having morphologic polarization roughly perpendicular to this line, assume virtually all possible orientations on the plane of the macula. Thus, the orthogonality of the planes of the three semicircular ducts enables them efficiently to detect angular motion in any plane, and the perpendicularity of the planes of the maculae plus the omnidirectionality of the orientation of the hair cells in the maculae allow the efficient detection of gravitoinertial forces acting in any direction (8).

Neural Pathways

To help the reader better organize the potentially confusing vestibular neuroanatomy, a somewhat simplified overview of the major neural connections of the vestibular system is presented in Figure 11.7. The utricular nerve, two saccular nerves, and the three ampullary nerves converge to form the vestibular nerve, a portion of the VIIIth cranial or statoacoustic nerve. Within the vestibular nerve lies the vestibular (or Scarpa's) ganglion, which is comprised of cell bodies of the vestibular neurons. The dendrites of these bipolar neurons invest the hair cells of the cristae and maculae; most of their axons terminate in the four vestibular nuclei in the brain stem—the superior, medial, lateral, and inferior nuclei—but some axons enter the phylogenetically ancient parts of the cerebellum to terminate in the fastigial nuclei and in the

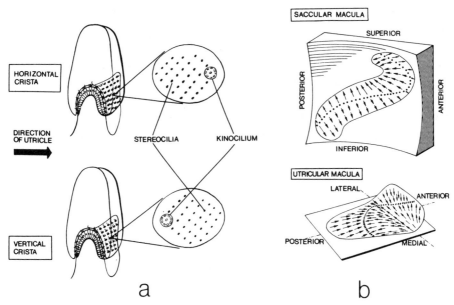

Figure 11.6. Morphologic polarization in vestibular neuroepithelia. *a.* All the hair cells in the cristae of the horizontal semicircular ducts are oriented so that their kinocilia are in the direction of the utricle; those hair cells in the cristae of the vertical ducts have their kinocilia directed away from the utricle. *b.* The maculae of the saccule (above) and utricle (below) also exhibit polarization—the arrows indicate the direction of the kinocilia of the hair cells in the various regions of the maculae. (Adapted from Spoendlin, HH. Ultrastructural studies of the labyrinth in squirrel monkeys. In: The role of the vestibular organs in the exploration of space. NASA-SP-77, Washington, D.C.: National Aeronautics and Space Administration, 1965.)

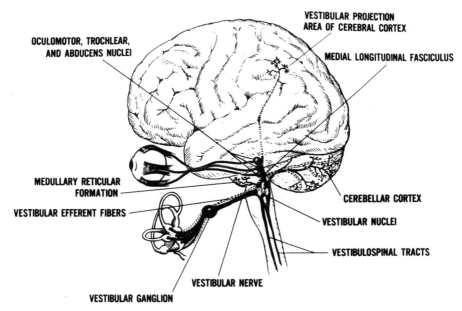

Figure 11.7. Major connections and projections of the vestibular system.

cortex of the flocculonodular lobe and other parts of the posterior vermis.

The vestibular nuclei project via secondary vestibular tracts to the motor nuclei of the cranial and spinal nerves and to the cerebellum. Because vestibulo-ocular reflexes are a major function of the vestibular system, it is not surprising to find ample projections from the vestibular nuclei to the nuclei of the oculomotor, trochlear, and abducens nerves (cranial nerves III, IV, and VI, respectively). The major pathway of these projections is the ascending medial longitudinal fasciculus (MLF). The basic vestibulo-ocular reflex is thus served by sensor and effector cells and an intercalated three-neuron reflex arc from the vestibular ganglion to the vestibular nuclei to the nuclei innervating the extraocular muscles. In addition, indirect multisynaptic pathways course from the vestibular nuclei through the paramedian pontine reticular formation to the oculomotor and other nuclei. The principle of ipsilateral facilitation and contralateral inhibition via an interneuron clearly operates in vestibulo-ocular reflexes, and numerous crossed internuclear connections provide evidence of this. The vestibulo-ocular reflexes that the various ascending and crossed pathways support serve to stabilize the retinal image by moving the eyes in the direction opposite to that of the motion of the head. Via the descending MLF and medial vestibulospinal tract, crossed and uncrossed projections from the vestibular nuclei reach the nuclei of the spinal accessory nerve (cranial nerve XI) and motor nuclei in the cervical cord. These projections form the anatomic substrate for vestibulocollic reflexes, which serve to stabilize the head by appropriate action of the sternocleidomastoid and other neck muscles. A third projection is that from primarily the lateral vestibular nucleus into the ventral gray matter throughout the length of the spinal cord. This important pathway is the uncrossed lateral vestibulospinal tract, which enables the vestibulospinal (postural) reflexes to help stabilize the body with respect to an inertial frame of reference by means of sustained and transient vestibular in-

fluences on basic spinal reflexes. Secondary vestibulo-cerebellar fibers course from the vestibular nuclei into the ipsilateral and contralateral fastigial nuclei and to the cerebellar cortex of the flocculonodular lobe and elsewhere. Returning from the fastigial and other cerebellar nuclei, crossed and uncrossed fibers of the cerebellobulbar tract terminate in the vestibular nuclei and in the associated reticular formation. There are also efferent fibers from the cerebellum, probably arising in the cerebellar cortex, which terminate not in nuclear structures but on dendritic endings of primary vestibular afferent neurons in the vestibular neuroepithelia. Such fibers are those of the vestibular efferent system, which appears to modulate or control the information arising from the vestibular end-organs. The primary and secondary vestibulocerebellar fibers and those returning from the cerebellum to the vestibular area of the brain stem comprise the juxtarestiform body of the inferior cerebellar peduncle. This structure, along with the vestibular end-organs, nuclei, and projection areas in the cerebellum, collectively constitute the so-called vestibulocerebellar axis, the neural complex responsible for processing primary spatial orientation information and initiating adaptive and protective behavior based on that information.

Several additional projections, more obvious functionally than anatomically, are those to certain autonomic nuclei of the brain stem and to the cerebral cortex. The dorsal motor nucleus of cranial nerve X (vagus) and other autonomic cell groups in the medulla and pons receive secondary vestibular fibers, largely from the medial vestibular nucleus; these fibers mediate vestibulovegetative reflexes, which are manifested as the pallor, perspiration, nausea, and vomiting—motion sickness—that can result from excessive or otherwise abnormal vestibular stimulation. Via vestibulothalamic and thalamocortical pathways, vestibular information eventually reaches the primary vestibular projection area of the cerebral cortex, located in the parietal and parietotemporal cortex. This projection area is provided with vestibular, visual, and somato-

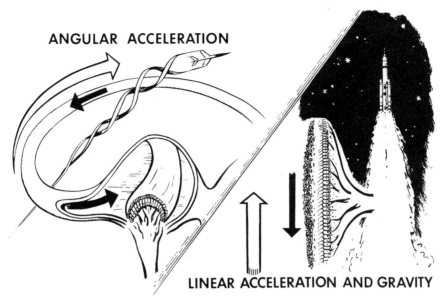

Figure 11.8. The cardinal principle of vestibular mechanics: angular accelerations stimulate the semicircular ducts; linear accelerations and gravity stimulate the otolith organ.

sensory proprioceptive representation and is evidently associated with conscious spatial orientation and with integration of sensory correlates of higher-order motor activity. In addition, vestibular information can be transmitted via long polysynaptic pathways through the brain stem reticular formation and medial thalamus to wide areas of the cerebral cortex; the nonspecific cortical responses to vestibular stimuli that are evoked via this pathway appear to be associated with an arousal or alerting mechanism.

Vestibular Information Processing

As the reader probably deduced while reading the discussion of the anatomy of the vestibular end-organs, angular accelerations are the adequate, that is, physiologic, stimuli for the semicircular ducts, and linear accelerations and gravity are the adequate stimuli for the otolith organs. This statement, illustrated in Figure 11.8, is the cardinal principle of vestibular mechanics. How the reactive torques and gravitoinertial forces stimulate the hair cells of the cristae and maculae, respectively, and produce changes in the fre-

quency of action potentials in the associated vestibular neurons, has already been discussed. The resulting frequency-coded messages are transmitted into the various central vestibular projection areas as raw orientational data to be further processed as necessary for the various functions served by such data. These functions are the vestibular reflexes, voluntary movement, and the perception of orientation.

Vestibular Reflexes

As stated so well by Melvill Jones (12), '' . . . for control of eye movement relative to space the motor outflow can operate on three fairly discrete anatomical platforms, namely: (1) the eye-in-skull platform, driven by the external eye muscles, rotating the eyeball relative to the skull; (2) the skull-on-body platform driven by the neck muscles; and (3) the body platform, operated by the complex neuromuscular mechanisms responsible for postural control.''

In humans, the retinal image is stabilized mainly by vestibulo-ocular reflexes, primarily those of semicircular-duct origin. A simple demonstration can help one appreciate the contribution of the vestibulo-ocular reflexes to retinal-image stabilization. Holding the extended fingers half a meter or so in front of the face, one can move the fingers slowly from side to side and still see them clearly because of visual (optokinetic) tracking reflexes. As the frequency of movement increases one eventually reaches a point where the fingers cannot be seen clearly—they are blurred by the movement. This point is about 60 degrees/sec or 1 or 2 Hz for most people. Now, if the fingers are held still and the head is rotated back and forth at the frequency at which the fingers became blurred when they were moved, the fingers remain perfectly clear. Even at considerably higher frequencies of head movement, the vestibulo-ocular reflexes initiated by the resulting stimulation of the semicircular ducts function to keep the image of the fingers clear. Thus, at lower frequencies of movement of the external world relative to the body or vice versa, the visual system stabilizes the retinal image by means of optokinetic reflexes. As the frequencies of such relative movement become greater, however, the vestibular system, by means of vestibulo-ocular reflexes, assumes progressively more of this function, and at the higher frequencies of relative motion characteristically generated only by motions of the head and body, the vestibular system is responsible for stabilizing the retinal image.

The mechanism by which stimulation of the semicircular ducts results in retinal image stabilization is simple, at least conceptually (Fig. 11.9). When the head is turned to the right in the horizontal (yaw) plane, the angular acceleration of the head creates a reactive torque in the ring of endolymph in (mainly) the horizontal semicircular duct. The reacting endolymph then exerts pressure on the cupula, deviating the cupula in the right ear in a utriculopetal direction, depolarizing the hair cells of the associated crista ampullaris and increasing the frequency of the action potentials in the corresponding ampullary nerve. In the left ear, the endolymph deviates

the cupula in a utriculofugal direction, thereby hyperpolarizing the hair cells and decreasing the frequency of the action potentials generated. As excitatory neural signals are relayed to the contralateral lateral rectus and ipsilateral medial rectus muscles, and inhibitory signals are simultaneously relayed to the antagonists, a conjugate deviation of the eyes results from the described changes in ampullary neural activity. The direction of the conjugate eye deviation is the same as that of the angular reaction of the endolymph, and the angular velocity of the deviation is proportional to the pressure exerted by the endolymph on the cupula. The resulting eye movement is, therefore, compensatory; that is, it adjusts the angular position of the eye to compensate for changes in angular position of the head and thereby prevents slippage of the retinal image over the retina. Because the amount of angular deviation of the eye is physically limited, rapid movements of the eye in the direction opposite to the compensatory motion are employed to return the eye to its initial position or to advance it to a position from which it can sustain a compensatory sweep for a suitable length of time. These rapid eye movements are anticompensatory, and because of their very high angular velocity, motion is not perceived during this phase of the vestibulo-ocular reflex.

With the usual rapid, high-frequency rotations of the head, the rotational inertia of the endolymph acts to deviate the cupula as the angular velocity of the head builds, and the angular momentum gained by the endolymph during the brief acceleration acts to drive the cupula back to its resting position when the head decelerates to a stop. The cupula-endolymph system thus functions as an integrating angular accelerometer, i.e., it converts angular acceleration data into a neural signal proportional to the angular velocity of the head. This is true for angular accelerations occurring at frequencies normally encountered in terrestrial activities; when angular accelerations outside the dynamic response range of the cupula-endolymph system are experienced, the system no longer provides accurate

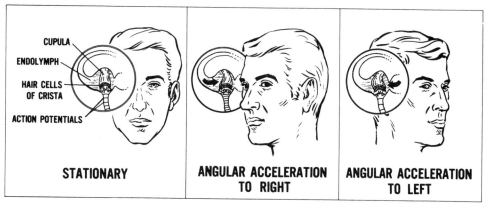

Figure 11.9. Mechanism of action of a horizontal semicircular duct and the resulting reflex eye movement. Angular acceleration to the right increases the frequency of action potentials originating in the right ampullary nerve and decreases in those of the left one. This pattern of neural signals causes extraocular muscles to rotate the eyes in the direction opposite to that of head rotation, thus stabilizing the retinal image with a compensatory eye movement. Angular acceleration to the left has the opposite effect.

angular velocity information. When angular accelerations are relatively sustained or when the cupula is kept in a deviated position by other means, such as caloric testing, the compensatory and anticompensatory phases of the vestibulo-ocular reflex are repeated, resulting in beats of ocular nystagmus (Fig. 11.10). The compensatory phase of the vestibulo-ocular reflex is then called the slow phase of nystagmus, and the anticompensatory phase is called the fast or quick phase. The direction of the quick phase is used

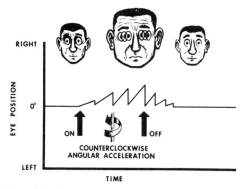

Figure 11.10. Ocular nystagmus—repeating compensatory and anticompensatory eye movements—resulting from vestibular stimulation. In this case, the stimulation is a yawing angular acceleration to the left, and the anticompensatory, or quick- phase, nystagmic response is also to the left.

to label the direction of the nystagmus because the direction of the rapid motion of the eye is easier to determine clinically. The vertical semicircular ducts operate in an analogous manner, with the vestibulo-ocular reflexes elicited by their stimulation being appropriate to the plane of the angular acceleration resulting in that stimulation. Thus, a vestibulo-ocular reflex with downward compensatory and upward anticompensatory phases results from the stimulation of the vertical semicircular ducts by pitch-up ($-\alpha_y$) angular acceleration; and with sufficient stimulation in this plane, up-beating vertical nystagmus results. Angular accelerations in the roll plane result in vestibulo-ocular reflexes with clockwise and counterclockwise compensatory and anticompensatory phases and in rotary nystagmus. Other planes of stimulation are associated with other directions of eye movement such as oblique or horizontorotary.

As should be expected, there also are vestibulo-ocular reflexes of the otolith-organ origin. Initiating these reflexes are the shearing actions that bend the cilia of macular hair cells as inertial forces or gravity cause the otolithic membranes to slide to various positions over their maculae (Fig. 11.11). Each position that can be assumed by an otolithic membrane relative to its macula evokes a particular spatial pattern of frequencies

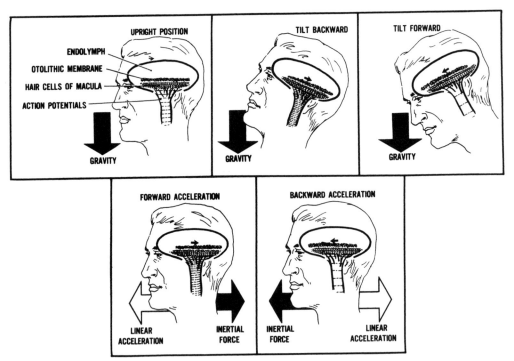

Figure 11.11. Mechanism of action of an otolith organ. A change in direction of the force of gravity (above) or a linear acceleration (below) causes the otolithic membrane to shift its position with respect to its macula, thereby generating a new pattern of action potentials in the utricular or saccular nerve. Shifting of the otolithic membranes can elicit compensatory vestibulo-ocular reflexes and nystagmus, as well as perceptual effects.

of action potentials in the corresponding utricular or saccular nerve, and that pattern is associated with a particular set of compatible stimulus conditions such as backward tilt of the head or forward linear acceleration. These patterns of action potentials from the various otolith organs are correlated and integrated in the vestibular nuclei and cerebellum with orientational information from the semicircular ducts and other sensory modalities; appropriate orientational percepts and motor activities eventually result. Lateral (a_y) linear accelerations can elicit horizontal reflexive eye movements, including nystagmus, presumably as a result of utricular stimulation. Similarly, vertical (a_z) linear accelerations can elicit vertical eye movements, most likely as a result of stimulation of the saccule; the term elevator reflex is sometimes used to describe this response because it is readily provoked by the vertical linear accelerations associated with riding in an elevator. The utility of these horizontal and vertical vestibulo-ocular reflexes of the otolith-organ origin is readily apparent: like the reflexes of semicircular-duct origin, they help stabilize the retinal image. Less obvious is the usefulness of the ocular countertorsion reflex (Fig. 11.12), which repositions the eyes about their visual (anteroposterior) axes in response to the otolith-organ stimulation resulting from tilting the head laterally in the opposite direction. Presumably, this reflex contributes to retinal image stabilization by providing a response to changing directions of the force of gravity.

Our understanding of the vestibulocollic reflexes has not developed to the same degree as our understanding of the vestibulo-ocular reflexes, although some clinical use has been made of measurements of rotation of the head on the neck in response to vestibular stimulation. Per-

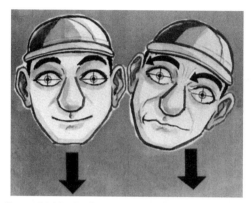

Figure 11.12. Ocular countertorsion, a vestibulo-ocular reflex of otolith-organ origin. When the head is tilted to the left, the eyes rotate to the right to assume a new angular position about the visual axes, as shown.

haps this situation reflects the fact that vestibulocollic reflexes are not as effective as the vestibulo-ocular reflexes in stabilizing the retinal image, at least not in humans. Such is not the case in other species, however; birds exhibit extremely effective reflex control of head position under conditions of bodily motion—even nystagmus head movements are quite easy to elicit. The high level of development of the vestibulocollic reflexes in birds is certainly either a case or a consequence of the relative immobility of birds' eyes in their heads. Nonetheless, the ability of a human (or any other vertebrate with a mobile head) to keep the head upright with respect to the direction of applied gravitoinertial force is maintained by means of tonic vestibular influences on the muscles of the neck.

Vestibulospinal reflexes operate to assure stability of the body. Transient linear and angular accelerations, such as those experienced in tripping and falling, provoke rapid activation of various groups of extensor and flexor muscles to return the body to the stable position or at least to minimize the ultimate effect of the instability. Everyone has experienced the reflex arm movements that serve to break a fall, and most have observed the more highly developed righting reflexes that cats exhibit when dropped from an upside-down position; these are examples of vestibulospinal reflexes. Less spectacular, but nevertheless extremely important, are the sustained vestibular influences on posture that are exerted through tonic activation of so-called ''antigravity'' muscles such as hip, knee, and calf extensors. These vestibular reflexes, of course, help keep the body upright with respect to the direction of the force of gravity.

Voluntary Movement

It has been shown how the various reflexes of vestibular origin serve to stabilize the body in general and the retinal image in particular. The vestibular system is also important in that it provides data for the proper execution of voluntary movement. To realize just how important such vestibular data are in this context, one must first recognize the fact that skilled voluntary movements are ballistic; that is, once initiated, they are executed according to a predetermined pattern and sequence, without the benefit of simultaneous sensory feedback to the higher neural levels from which they originate. The simple act of writing one's signature, for example, involves such rapid changes in speed and direction of movement that conscious sensory feedback and adjustment of motor activity are virtually precluded, at least until the act is nearly completed. Learning an element of a skill thus involves developing a computer-program-like schedule of neural activations that can be called up, so to speak, to effect a particular desired end product of motor activity. Of course, the raw program for a particular voluntary action is not sufficient to permit the execution of that action: information regarding such parameters as intended magnitude and direction of movement must be furnished from the conscious sphere, and data indicating the position and motion of the body platform relative to the surface of the earth must be furnished from the preconscious sphere. The necessity for the additional information can be seen in the signature-writing example cited above: one can write large or small, quickly or slowly, and on a horizontal or vertical surface. Obviously, different patterns or neuromuscular activation, even grossly different muscle groups, are needed to accomplish a basic act under varying spatial and temporal conditions; the necessary adjustments are made automatically, however, without conscious intervention. Vestibular and other sensory data providing spatial orientation information for use in either skilled voluntary or reflexive motor activities are processed into a preconscious orientational percept that provides the informational basis upon which such automatic adjustments are made. Thus one can decide what the outcome of his or her action is to be and initiate the command to do it, without consciously having to discern the direction of the force of gravity, analyze its potential effects on planned motor activity, select appropriate muscle groups and modes of activation to compensate for gravity, and then activate and deactivate each muscle in proper sequence and with proper timing to accomplish the desired motor activity. The body takes care of the details, using stored programs for elements of skilled motor activity, and the current preconscious orientational percept. This whole process is the major function and responsibility of the vestibulocerebellar axis.

Conscious Percepts

Usually as a result of the same information processing that provides the preconscious orientational percept, one also is provided a conscious orientational percept. This percept can be false, in which case the individual is said to experience an orientational illusion, or to have spatial disorientation. One can be aware, moreover, that what his or her body is signalling is not what he or she has concluded from the other orientational information, such as flight instrument data. Conscious orientational percepts thus can be either natural or derived, depending on the source of the orientation information and the perceptual process involved, and an individual can experience both natural and derived conscious orientational percepts at the same time. Because of this, pilots who have become disoriented in flight commonly exhibit vacillating control inputs, as they alternate indecisively between responding first to one percept and then to the other.

Thresholds of Vestibular Perception

Often, an orientational illusion occurs because the physical event resulting in or from a change in bodily orientation is below the threshold of perception. For that reason, the student of disorientation should be aware of the approximate perceptual thresholds associated with the various modes of vestibular stimulation.

The lowest reported threshold for perception of rotation is 0.035 degrees/sec^2, but this degree of sensitivity is obtained only with virtually continuous angular acceleration and long response latencies (20 to 40 seconds). Other observations put the perceptual threshold between roughly 0.1 and 2.0 degrees/sec^2; reasonable values are 0.14, 0.5 and 0.5 degrees/sec^2 for yaw, roll, and pitch motions, respectively. It is common practice, however, to describe the thresholds of the semicircular ducts in terms of the angular acceleration-time product, or angular velocity, which results in just perceptible rotation. This product, known as Mulder's constant, remains fairly constant for stimulus times of about 5 seconds or less. Using the reasonable value of 2 degrees/sec for Mulder's constant, an angular acceleration of 5 degrees/sec^2 applied for half a second would be perceived because the acceleration-time product is above the 2-degree/sec angular velocity threshold. But a 10-degree/sec^2 acceleration applied for a tenth of a second would not be perceived because it would be below the angular velocity threshold; nor would a 0.2-degree/sec^2 acceleration applied for 5 seconds be perceived. Inflight experiments have shown that blindfolded pilot subjects are unable to perceive consistent roll rates of 1.0 degree/sec or less, but can perceive a roll when the velocity is 2.0 degrees/sec or higher. Pitch rate thresholds in flight are also between 1.0 and 2.0 degrees/sec. But when aircraft pitch motions are coupled with compensatory power adjustments to keep the net G force always directed toward the aircraft floor, the pitch threshold is raised well above 2.0 degrees/sec (10).

The perceptual threshold related to otolith-organ function necessarily involves both an angle and a magnitude because the otolith organs respond to linear accelerations and gravitoinertial forces, both of which have direction and intensity. A 1.5° change in direction of applied G force is perceptible under ideal (experimental) conditions. The minimum perceptible intensity of linear acceleration has been reported by various authors to be between 0.001 and 0.03 g, depending on the direction of acceleration and the experimental method used. Values of 0.01 g for a_z and 0.006 g for a_x accelerations are appropriate representative thresholds, and a similar value for a_y acceleration is probably reasonable. Again, these absolute thresholds apply when the acceleration is either sustained or applied at relatively low frequencies. The threshold for linear accelerations applied for less than about 5 seconds is a more or less constant acceleration-time product, or linear velocity, of about 0.3 to 0.4 m/sec.

Unfortunately for those who would like to calculate exactly what orientational percepts results from a particular set of linear and angular accelerations, such as might have occurred prior to an aircraft mishap, the actual vestibular perceptual thresholds are, as expressed by one philosopher, "constant except when they vary." Probably the most common reason for an orientational perceptual threshold to be raised is inattention to orientational cues because attention is directed to something else. Other reasons might be a low state of mental arousal, fatigue, drug effects, or innate individual variation. Whatever the reason, it appears that a given individual can monitor his or her orientation with considerable sensitivity under some circumstances and with relative insensitivity under others, which inconsistency can itself lead to perceptual errors that result in orientational illusions.

Of paramount importance in the generation of orientational illusions, however, is not the fact that absolute vestibular thresholds exist or that vestibular thresholds are time-varying. Rather, it is the fact that the components of the vestibular system, like any complex mechanical or electrical system, have characteristic frequency responses, and stimulation by patterns of acceleration outside the optimal, or "design," frequency-response ranges of the semicircular ducts and otolith organs causes the vestibular system to make errors. In flight, much of the stimulation resulting from the acceleratory environment is indeed outside of the design frequency-response ranges of the vestibular end-organs; consequently, orientational illusions occur in flight. Elucidation of this important point is provided in the section entitled "Spatial Disorientation."

Vestibular Suppression and Enhancement

Like all sensory systems, the vestibular system exhibits a decreased response to stimuli that are persistent (adaptation) or repetitious (habituation). Even more important to the aviator is the fact that with time and practice, one can develop the ability to suppress natural vestibular responses, both perceptual and motor. This ability is termed vestibular suppression. Closely related to the concept of vestibular suppression is that of visual dominance, the ability to obtain and use spatial orientation cues from the visual environment despite the presence of potentially strong vestibular cues. Vestibular suppression seems to be exerted, in fact, through visual dominance because it disappears in the absence of vision. The opposite effect, that of an increase in perceptual and motor responsiveness to vestibular stimulation, is termed vestibular enhancement. Such enhancement can occur when the stimulation is novel, as in an amusement park ride, as in an aircraft spinning out of control, or whatever spatial orientation is perceived to be especially important. It is tempting to attribute to the efferent vestibular neurons the function of controlling the gain of the vestibular system so as to effect suppression and enhancement, and some evidence exists to support that notion. The actual mechanisms involved appear to be much more complex than would be necessary to merely provide gross changes in the gain of the vestibular end-organs. Precise control of vestibular responses to anticipated stimulation, based on sensory efferent copies of voluntary commands for movement, is probably exercised by the cerebellum via a feed-forward loop involving the vestibular efferent system. Thus, when discrepancies between anticipated and actual stimulation generate a neural error signal, a response is evoked, and vestibular reflexes and heightened perception occur. Vestibular suppression, then, involves the development of accurate estimates of vestibular responses to orientational stimuli repeatedly experienced and the active countering of anticipated responses by spatially and temporally patterned sensory efferent activity. Vestibular enhancement, on the other hand, results from the lack of available estimates of vestibular responses because of the novelty of the stimulation, or perhaps from a revision in neural processing strategy obligated by the failure of normal negative feed-forward mechanisms to provide adequate orientation information. Such marvelous complexity of vestibular function assures adaptability to a wide variety of motional environments and thereby promotes survival in them.

Other Senses of Motion and Position

Although the visual and vestibular systems play a dominant role in spatial orientation, the contributions of other sensory systems to orientation cannot be overlooked. Especially important are the nonvestibular proprioceptors—the muscle, tendon, and joint receptors—and the cutaneous exteroceptors, because the orientational percepts derived from their functioning in flight generally support those derived from vestibular information processing, whether accurate or inaccurate. The utility of these other sensory modalities can be appreciated in view of the fact that, in the absence of vision, our vestibular, muscle, tendon, joint, and skin receptors allow us to maintain spatial orientation and postural equilibrium to a great extent, at least on the

earth's surface. Similarly, in the absence of vestibular function, vision and the remaining proprioceptors and cutaneous mechanoreceptors are sufficient for good orientation and balance. When two components of this triad of orientational senses are absent or substantially compromised, however, it becomes impossible to maintain sufficient spatial orientation to permit postural stability and effective locomotion.

Nonvestibular Proprioceptors

Sherrington's "proprioceptive" or "self-sensing" sensory category includes the vestibular (or labyrinthine), muscle, tendon, and joint senses. Proprioception generally is spoken of as though it means only the nonvestibular components, however.

Muscle and Tendon Senses

All skeletal muscle contains within it complex sensory end-organs, called muscle spindles (Fig. 11.13A). These end-organs are comprised mainly of small intrafusal muscle fibers that lie parallel to the larger, ordinary, extrafusal muscle fibers and are enclosed over part of their length by a fluid-filled bag. The sensory innervation of these structures consists mainly of large, rapidly conducting afferent neurons that originate as primary (annulospiral) or secondary (flower-spray) endings on the intrafusal fibers and terminate in the spinal cord on anterior horn cells and interneurons. Stretching of the associated extrafusal muscle results in an increase in the frequency of action potentials in the afferent nerve from the intrafusal fibers; contraction of the muscle results in a decrease or absence of action potentials. The more interesting aspect of muscle spindle function, however, is that the intrafusal muscle fibers are innervated by motoneurons (gamma efferents and others) and can be stimulated to contract, thereby altering the afferent information arising from the spindle. Thus, the sensory input from the muscle spindles can be biased by descending influences from higher

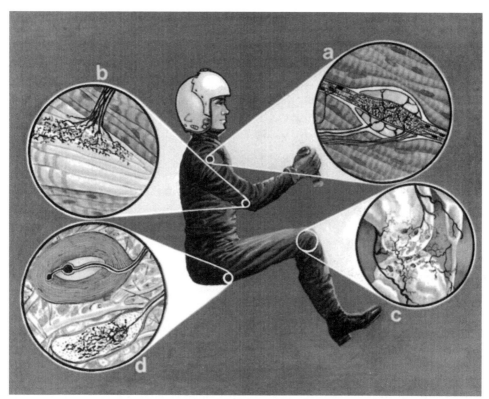

Figure 11.13. Some of the nonvestibular proprioceptive and cutaneous exteroceptive receptors subserving spatial orientation. *a.* Muscle spindle, with central afferent (sensory) and more peripheral efferent (fusimotor) innervations. *b.* Golgi tendon organ. *c.* Lamellated, spray-type, and free-nerve-ending joint receptors. *d.* Two of the many types of mechanoreceptors found in the skin: lamellated Pacinian corpuscles and spray-type Ruffini corpuscles.

neural centers such as the vestibulocerebellar axis.

Although the muscle spindles are structurally and functionally in parallel with associated muscle groups and respond to changes in their length, the Golgi tendon organs (Fig. 11.13B) are functionally in series with the muscles and respond to changes in tension. A tendon organ consists of a fusiform bundle of small tendon fascicles with intertwining neural elements, and is located at the musculotendinous junction or wholly within the tendon. Unlike that of the muscle spindle, its innervation is entirely afferent.

The major function of both the muscle spindles and the tendon organs is to provide the sensory basis for myotatic (or muscle stretch) reflexes. These elementary spinal reflexes operate to stabilize a joint by providing, in response to an increase in length of a muscle and concomitant stimulation of its included spindles, monosynaptic excitation and contraction of the stretched agonist (e.g., extensor) muscle and disynaptic inhibition and relaxation of its antagonist (e.g., flexor) muscle through the action of an inhibitory interneuron. In addition, tension developed on associated tendon organs results in disynaptic inhibition of the agonist muscle, thus regulating the amount of contraction generated. The myotatic reflex mechanism is, in fact, the foundation of posture and locomotion. Modification of these and other basic spinal reflexes by organized facilitatory or inhibitory intervention originating at higher neural levels, either through direct action on skeletomotor (alpha) neurons or through stimulation of fusimotor (primarily gamma) neurons to muscle spindles, results in sustained postural equilibrium and other purposive motor behavior. Some researchers have speculated, moreover, that in certain types of spatial disorientation in flight, this organized modification of spinal reflexes is interrupted as cerebral cortical control of motor activity is replaced by lower brain-stem and spinal control. Perhaps the ''frozen-on-the-controls'' type of disorientation-induced deterioration of flying ability is a reflection of primitive reflexes made manifest by disorganization of higher neural functions.

Despite the obvious importance of the muscle spindles and tendon organs in the control of motor activity, there is little evidence to indicate that their response to orientational stimuli (such as occur when one stands vertically in a 1-G environment) results in any corresponding conscious proprioceptive percept. Nevertheless, it is known that the dorsal columns and other ascending spinal tracts carry muscle afferent information to medullary and thalamic relay nuclei and thence to the cerebral sensory cortex. Furthermore, extensive projections into the cerebellum, via dorsal and ventral spinocerebellar tracts, ensure that proprioceptive information from the afferent terminations of the muscle spindles and tendon organs is integrated with other orientational information and is relayed to the vestibular nuclei, cerebral cortex, and elsewhere as needed.

Joint Sensation

In contrast to the stimulation with the so-called ''muscle sense of position'' just discussed, it has been well established that sensory information from the joints does reach consciousness. In fact, the threshold for perception of joint motion and position can be quite low: as low as 0.5 degree for the knee joint when moved greater than 1.0 degree/sec. The receptors in the joints are of three types, as shown in Figure 11.13C: (1) lamellated or encapsulated Pacinian corpuscle-like end-organs; (2) spray-type structures, known as Ruffini-like endings

when found in joint capsules and Golgi tendon organs when found in ligaments; and (3) free nerve endings. The Pacinian corpuscle-like terminals are rapidly adapting and are sensitive to quick movement of the joint, whereas both of the spray-type endings are slowly adapting and serve to signal slow joint movement and joint position. There is evidence that polysynaptic spinal reflexes can be elicited by stimulation of joint receptors, but their nature and extent are not well understood. Proprioceptive information from the joint receptors projects via the dorsal funiculi eventually to the cerebral sensory cortex and via the spinocerebellar tracts to the anterior lobe of the cerebellum.

One must not infer from this discussion that only muscles, tendons, and joints have proprioceptive sensory receptors. Both lamellated and spray-type receptors, as well as free nerve endings, are found in fascia, aponeuroses, and other connective tissues of the musculoskeletal system, and they presumably provide proprioceptive information to the central nervous system.

Cutaneous Exteroceptors

The exteroceptors of the skin include: the mechanoreceptors, which respond to touch and pressure; the thermoreceptors, which respond to heat and cold; and the nociceptors, which respond to noxious mechanical and/or thermal events and give rise to sensations of pain. Of the cutaneous exteroceptors, only the mechanoreceptors contribute significantly to orientation.

A variety of receptors are involved in cutaneous mechanoreception: spray-type Ruffini corpuscles, lamellated Pacinian and Meissner corpuscles, branched and straight lanceolate terminals, Merkel Cells, and free nerve endings (Fig. 11.13D). The response patterns of mechanoreceptors also are numerous: eleven different types of response, varying from high-frequency transient detection through several modes of velocity detection to more or less static displacement detection, have been recognized. Pacinian corpuscles and certain receptors associated with hair follicles are very rapidly adapting and have the highest mechanical frequency responses, responding to sinusoidal skin displacements in the range of 50 to 400 Hz. They are thus well suited to monitor vibration and transient touch stimuli. Ruffini corpuscles are slowly adapting and, therefore, respond primarily to sustained touch and pressure stimuli. Merkel cells appear to have a moderately slowly adapting response, making them suitable for monitoring static skin displacement and velocity. Meissner corpuscles seem to detect primarily velocity of skin deformation. Other receptors provide other types of response, so as to complete the spectrum of mechanical stimuli that can be sensed through the skin. The mechanical threshold for the touch receptors is quite low—less than 0.03 dyne/cm^2 on the thumb. (In comparison to the labyrinthine receptors subserving audition, however, this threshold is not so impressive: a 0-dB sound pressure level represents 0.0002 dyne/cm^2, more than 100 times lower.) Afferent information from the described mechanoreceptors is conveyed to the cerebral cortex mainly by way of the dorsal funiculi and medullary relay nuclei into the medial lemnisci and thalamocortical projections. The dorsal spinocerebellar tract and other tracts to the cerebellum provide the pathways by which cutaneous exteroceptive information reaches the cerebellum and is integrated with proprioceptive information from muscles, tendon, joints, and vestibular end-organs.

Auditory Orientation

On the surface of the earth, the ability to determine the location of a sound source can play a role in spatial orientation, as evidenced by the fact that a revolving sound source can create a sense of self-rotation and even elicit reflex compensatory and anticompensatory eye movements called audiokinetic nystagmus. Differential filtering of incident sound energy by the external ear, head, and shoulders at different relative locations of the sound source provides the ability to discriminate sound location. Part of this discrimination process involves analysis of interaural differences in arrival time of congruent sounds; but direction-dependent changes in spectral characteristics of incident sound energies allow the listener to localize sounds in elevation, azimuth, and to some extent range, even when the interaural arrival times are not different. In aircraft, binaural sound localization is of little use in spatial orientation because of high ambient noise levels and the absence of audible external sound sources. Pilots do extract some orientational information, however, from the auditory cues provided by the rush of air past the airframe: the sound frequencies and intensities, characteristic of various airspeeds and angles of attack are recognized by the experienced pilot, and he or she uses them in conjunction with other orientation information to create a percept of velocity and pitch attitude of the aircraft. As aircraft have become more capable, however, and the pilot has become more insulated from such acoustic stimuli, the importance of auditory orientation cues in flying has diminished.

SPATIAL DISORIENTATION

The evolution of humans saw us develop over millions of years as an aquatic, terrestrial, and even arboreal creature, but never an aerial one. In this development, we subjected ourselves to and were subjected to many different varieties of transient motions, but not to the relatively sustained linear and angular accelerations commonly experienced in aviation. As a result, humans acquired sensory systems well suited for maneuvering under our own power on the surface of the earth but poorly suited for flying. Even the birds, whose primary mode of locomotion is flying, are unable to maintain spatial orientation and fly safely when deprived of vision by fog or clouds. Only bats seem to have developed the ability to fly without vision, and then only by replacing vision with auditory echolocation. Considering our phylogenetic heritage, it should come as no surprise that our sudden entry into the aerial environment resulted in a mismatch between the orientational demands of the new environment and our innate ability to orient. The manifestation of this mismatch is spatial disorientation.

Illusions in Flight

An illusion is a false percept. An orientational illusion is a false percept of one's position or motion—either linear or angular—relative to the plane of the earth's surface. A great number of orientational illusions occur during flight: some named, others unnamed; some understood, others not understood. Those that are sufficiently impressive to cause pilots to report them, whether because of their responsibility or because of their emotional impact, have been described in the aeromedical literature and will be discussed here. The illusions in flight are categorized into those resulting primarily from visual misperceptions and those involving primarily vestibular errors.

Visual Illusions

We shall organize the visual illusions in flight according to whether they involve primarily the focal mode of visual processing or primarily the ambient mode. Although this categorization is somewhat arbitrary and may seem too coarse in some cases, it serves to emphasize the dichotomous nature of visual orientation information processing. We shall begin with illusions involving primarily focal vision.

Shape Constancy

To appreciate how false shape constancy cueing can create orientational illusions in flight, consider the example provided by a runway that is constructed on other than level terrain. Figure 11.14A shows the pilots view of the runway during an approach to landing and demonstrates the linear perspective and foreshortening of the runway that the pilot associates with a 3° approach slope. If the runway slopes upward 1° (a rise of

only 35 m for a 2-km runway), the foreshortening of the runway for a pilot on a 3° approach slope is substantially less (i.e., the height of the retinal image of the runway is greater) than it would be if the runway were level. This can give the pilot the illusion that he or she is too high on the approach. The pilot's natural response to such an illusion is to reshape the image of the runway by seeking a shallower approach slope (Fig. 11.14B). This response, of course, could be hazardous. The opposite situation results when the runway slopes downward. To perceive the accustomed runway shape under this condition, the pilot must fly a steeper approach slope than usual (Fig. 11.14C).

Size Constancy

Size constancy is very important in judging distance, and false cues are frequently responsible for aircraft mishaps due to illusions of focal visual origin. The runway width illusions are particularly instructive in this context. A runway that is narrower than that to which a pilot is accustomed can create a hazardous illusion on the approach to landing. Size constancy causes the pilot to perceive the narrow runway to be farther away (i.e., that he or she is higher) than is actually the case, and the pilot may flare too late and touch down sooner than he or she expects (Fig. 11.15B). Likewise, a runway that is wider than what a pilot is used to can lead to the illusion of being closer to the runway (i.e., lower) than he or she really is, and the pilot may flare too soon and drop in from too high above the runway (Fig. 11.15C). Both of these runway-width illusions are especially troublesome at night when peripheral visual orientation cues are largely absent. The common tendency for pilots to flare too high at night results at least partly from the fact that the runway lights, being displaced laterally from the actual edge of the runway, make the runway seem wider, and therefore closer, than it actually is. A much more serious problem at night, however, is the tendency for pilots to land short of the runway when arriving at an

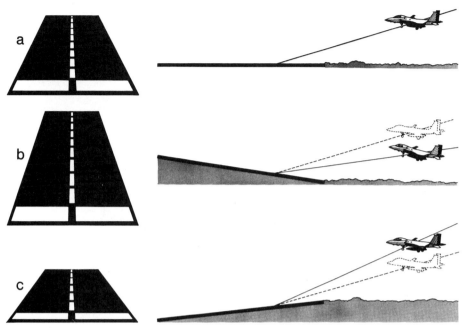

Figure 11.14. Effect of runway slope on the pilot's image of runway during final approach (left) and the potential effect on the approach slope angle flown (right). *a.* Flat runway—normal approach. *b.* An up-sloping runway creates the illusion of being high on approach—pilot flies the approach too low. *c.* A downsloping runway has the opposite effect.

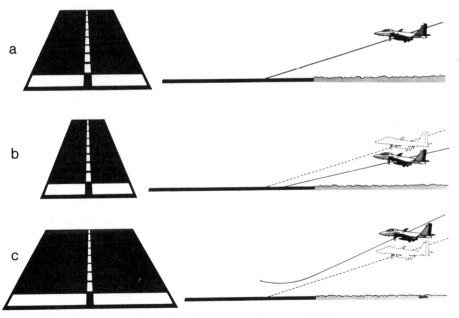

Figure 11.15. Effect of runway width on the pilot's image of runway (left) and the potential effect on approach flown (right). *a.* Accustomed width—normal approach. *b.* A narrow runway makes the pilot feel he is higher than he actually is, so he flies the approach too low and flares too late. *c.* A wide runway gives the illusion of being closer than it actually is—the pilot tends to approach too high and flares too soon.

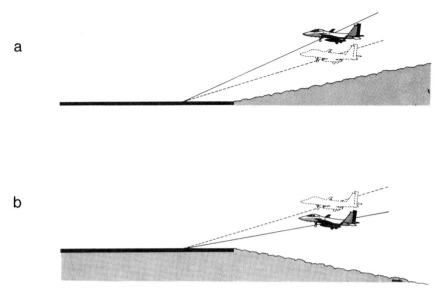

Figure 11.16. Potential effect of the slope of the terrain under the approach on the approach slope flown. *a.* The terrain slopes down to the runway; the pilot thinks he is too shallow on the approach and steepens it. *b.* Upsloping terrain makes the pilot think he is too high, so he corrects by making the approach too shallow.

unfamiliar airport having a runway that is narrower than the one to which they are accustomed.

The slope and composition of the terrain under the approach path also can influence the pilot's judgment of his or her height above the touchdown point. If the terrain descends to the approach end of the runway, the pilot tends to fly a steeper approach than he or she would if the approach terrain were level (Fig. 11.16A). If the approach terrain slopes up to the runway, on the other hand, the pilot tends to fly a less steep approach than he or she would otherwise (Fig. 11.16B). Although the estimation of height above the approach terrain depends on both focal and ambient vision, the contribution of focal vision is particularly clear: consider the pilot who looks at a building below the aircraft and, seeing it to be closer than such buildings usually are, seeks a higher approach slope. By the same token, focal vision and size constancy are responsible for the poor height and distance judgments pilots sometimes make when flying over terrain having an unfamiliar composition (Fig. 11.17). A reported example of this is the ten-

dency to misjudge height when landing in the Aleutians, where the evergreen trees are much smaller than those to which most pilots are accustomed. Such height-estimation difficulties are by no means restricted to the approach and landing phases of flight. One fatal mishap occurred during air combat training over the Southwest desert when the pilot of a high-performance fighter presumably misjudged his height over the desert floor because of the small, sparse vegetation and was unable to arrest his deliberate descent to a ground-hugging altitude.

Aerial Perspective

Aerial perspective also can play a role in deceiving the pilot, and the approach-to-landing regime again provides examples. In daytime, fog or haze can make a runway appear farther away as a result of the loss of visual discrimination. At night, runway and approach lights in fog or rain appear less bright than they do in clear weather and can create the illusion that they are farther away. It has even been reported that a pilot can have an illusion of banking to the right, for example, if the runway lights are brighter on

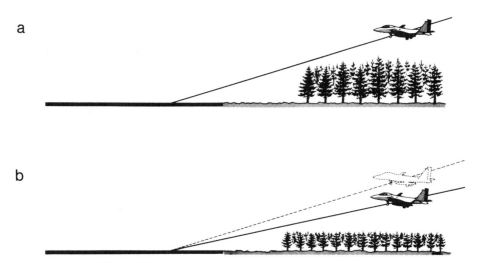

Figure 11.17. Potential effect of unfamiliar composition of approach terrain on the approach slope flown. *a.* Normal approach over trees of familiar size. *b.* Unusually small trees under the approach path make the pilot think he is too high, so he makes his approach lower than usual.

the right side of the runway than they are on the left. Another hazardous illusion of this type can occur during approach to landing in a shallow fog or haze, especially during a night approach. The vertical visibility under such conditions is much better than the horizontal visibility, so that descent into the fog causes the more distant approach or runway lights to diminish in intensity at the same time that the peripheral visual cues are suddenly occluded by the fog. The result is an illusion that the aircraft has pitched up, with the concomitant danger of a nose-down corrective action by the pilot.

Absent Focal Cues

A well-known pair of approach-to-landing situations that create illusions because of the absence of adequate focal visual orientation cues are the smooth-water (glassy-water) and snow-covered approaches. A seaplane pilot's perception of height is degraded substantially when the water below is still: for that reason, he or she routinely just sets up a safe descent rate and waits for the seaplane to touch down, rather than attempting to flare to a landing when the water is smooth. A blanket of fresh snow on the ground and run-

way also deprives the pilot of visual cues with which to estimate his or her height, thus making his or.her approach extremely difficult. Again, approaches are not the only regime in which smooth water and fresh snow cause problems. A number of aircraft have crashed as a result of pilots maneuvering over smooth water or snow-covered ground and misjudging their height above the surface.

Absent Ambient Cues

Two runway approach conditions that create considerable difficulty for the pilot, requiring focal vision to accomplish by itself what is normally accomplished with both focal and ambient vision, are the black-hole and whiteout approaches. A black-hole approach is one that is made on a dark night over water or unlighted terrain to a runway beyond which the horizon is indiscernible, the worst case being when only the runway lights are visible (Fig. 11.18). Without peripheral visual cues to help him or her orient relative to the earth, the pilot tends to feel that the aircraft is stable and situated appropriately but that the runway itself moves about or remains malpositioned (is downsloping, for example). Such illusions make the black-hole

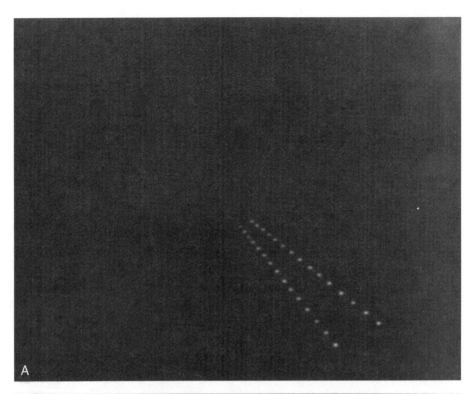

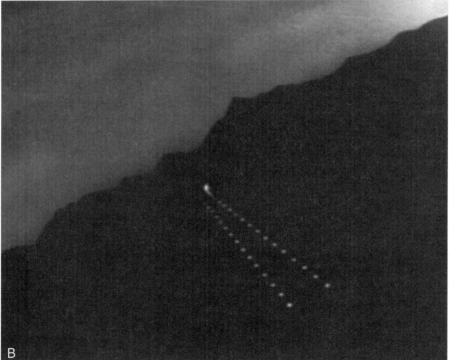

Figure 11.18. Effect of loss of ambient visual orientation cues on the perception of runway orientation during a black-hole approach. *A.* When ambient visual orientation cues are absent, the pilot feels horizontal and (in this example) perceives the runway to be tilted left and upsloping. *B.* With the horizon visible, the pilot orients himself correctly with peripheral vision and the runway appears horizontal in central vision.

approach difficult and dangerous and often result in a landing far short of the runway. A particularly hazardous type of black-hole approach is one made under conditions wherein the earth is totally dark except for the runway and the lights of a city on rising terrain beyond the runway. Under these conditions, the pilot may try to maintain a constant vertical visual angle for the distant city lights, thus causing his or her aircraft to arc far below the intended approach as he or she gets closer to the runway (Fig. 11.19). An alternative explanation is that the pilot falsely perceives through ambient vision that the rising terrain is flat and he or she lowers the approach slope accordingly.

An approach made under whiteout conditions can be as difficult as a black-hole approach, and for essentially the same reason—lack of sufficient ambient visual orientation cues. There are actually two types of whiteout, the atmospheric whiteout and the blowing-snow whiteout. In the atmospheric whiteout, a snow-covered ground merges with a white overcast, creating a condition in which ground textural cues are absent and the horizon is indistinguishable. Although visibility may be unrestricted in the atmospheric whiteout, there is essentially nothing to see except the runway markers; an approach made in

this condition must therefore be accomplished with a close eye on the altitude and attitude instruments to prevent spatial disorientation and inadvertent ground contact. In the blowing-snow whiteout, visibility is restricted drastically by snowflakes, and often those snowflakes have been driven into the air by the propeller or rotor wash of the affected aircraft. Helicopter landings on snow-covered ground are particularly likely to create blowing-snow whiteouts. Typically, the helicopter pilot tries to maintain visual contact with the ground during the sudden rotor-induced whiteout, gets into an unrecognized drift to one side, and shortly thereafter contacts the ground with sufficient lateral motion to cause the craft to roll over. Pilots flying where whiteouts can occur must be made aware of the hazards of whiteout approaches, as the disorientation induced usually occurs unexpectedly under visual rather than instrument meteorological conditions.

Another condition in which a pilot is apt to make a serious misjudgment is in closing on another aircraft at high speed. When the pilot has numerous peripheral visual cues by which to establish both his or her own position and velocity relative to the earth and the target's position and the velocity relative to the earth, the pilot's

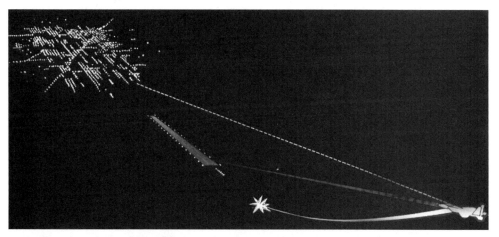

Figure 11.19. A common and particularly dangerous type of black-hole approach, in which the pilot perceives the distant city to be flat and arcs below the desired approach slope.

tracking and closing problem is not much different from what it would be on the ground if he or she were giving chase to a moving quarry. When relative position and closure rate cues must come from foveal vision alone, however, as is generally the case at altitude, at night, or under other conditions of reduced visibility, the tracking and closing problem is much more difficult. An overshoot, or worse, a midair collision, can easily result from the perceptual difficulties inherent in such circumstances, especially when the pilot lacks experience in an environment devoid of peripheral visual cues.

A related phenomenon that pilots need especially to be aware of is the dip illusion. It occurs during formation flying at night, when one aircraft is in trail behind another. To avoid wake turbulence and maintain sight of the lead aircraft, the pilot in trail needs to keep his or her aircraft at a small but constant angle below the lead aircraft. The pilot does this by placing the image of the lead aircraft in a particular position on his or her windscreen and keeping it there. Now suppose the pilot is told to "take spacing" (separate) to 10 km (5 nautical miles). For every 1° below lead the pilot in trail flies, he or she is lower than lead by 1.7 percent (sin 1°) of the distance behind lead. Thus, if the pilot is 2° below lead and keeps the image of the lead aircraft at the same spot on the windscreen all the way back to 10 km, his or her aircraft will descend to 350 m (1100 ft) below the lead aircraft. To make matters worse, when the aircraft in trail slows down to establish separation, its pitch attitude increases by several degrees; and if the pilot does not compensate for this additional angle and tries to maintain the lead aircraft image in the same relative position, he or she can double or even triple the altitude difference between the two aircraft. In the absence of ambient visual orientation cues, the pilot can not detect the large loss of altitude unless he or she monitors the flight instruments and may inadvertently "dip" far below the intended flight path. Clearly this situation would be extremely hazardous if it were to occur at low altitude or during maneu-

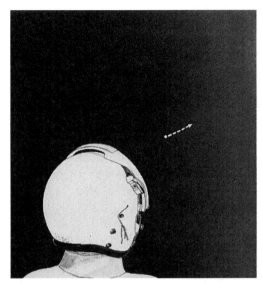

Figure 11.20. Visual autokinesis. A small, solitary light or small group of lights seen in the dark can appear to move, when in fact they are stationary.

vers in which altitude separation from other aircraft is critical.

Autokinesis

One puzzling illusion that occurs when ambient visual orientation cues are minimal is visual autokinesis (Fig. 11.20). A small, dim light seen against a dark background is an ideal stimulus for producing autokinesis. After 6 to 12 seconds of visually fixating the light, one can observe it to move at up to 20 degrees/sec in a particular direction or in several directions in succession, but there is little apparent displacement of the object fixated. In general, the larger and brighter the object, the less the autokinetic effect. The physiologic mechanism of visual autokinesis is not understood. One suggested explanation for the autokinesis phenomenon is that the eyes tend to drift involuntarily, perhaps because of inadequate or inappropriate vestibular stabilization, and that checking the drift requires unrecognized oculomotor efferent activity having sensory correlates that create the illusion.

Whatever the mechanism, the effect of visual autokinesis on pilots is of some importance. Anecdotes abound of pilots who fixate a star or a stationary ground light at night, and seeing it move because of autokinesis, mistake it for another aircraft and try to intercept or join up with it. Another untoward effect of the illusion occurs when a pilot flying at night perceives a relatively stable aircraft, one that he or she must intercept or follow, to be moving erratically when in fact it is not; the unnecessary and undesirable control inputs that the pilot makes to compensate for the illusory movement of the target aircraft represent increased work and wasted motion at best and an operational hazard at worst.

To help avoid or reduce the autokinetic illusion, the pilot should try to maintain a well-structured visual environment in which spatial orientation is unambiguous. Because this is rarely possible in night flying, it has been suggested that (1) the pilot's gaze should be shifted frequently to avoid prolonged fixation of a target light; (2) the target should be viewed beside or through and in reference to a relatively stationary structure such as a canopy bow; (3) the pilot should make eye, head, and body movements to try to destroy the illusion; and (4) as always, the pilot should monitor the flight instruments to help prevent or resolve any perceptual conflict. Equipping aircraft with more than one light or with luminescent strips to enhance recognition at night probably has helped reduce problems with autokinesis.

Vection Illusions

So far, this chapter has dealt with visual illusions created by excessive orientation-processing demands being placed on focal vision when adequate orientation cues are not available through ambient vision or when strong but false orientation cues are received through focal vision. Ambient vision can itself be responsible for creating orientational illusions, however, whenever orientation cues received in the visual periphery are misleading or misinterpreted. Probably the most compelling of such illusions are the vection illusions. Vection is the visually induced perception of self-motion in the spatial environment and can be a sensation of linear motion (linear vection) or angular motion (angular vection).

Nearly everyone who drives an automobile has experienced one very common linear vection illusion: when a driver is waiting in his or her car at a stoplight and a presumably stationary vehicle in the adjacent lane creeps forward, a compelling illusion that his or her own car is creeping backward can result (prompting a swift but surprisingly ineffectual stomp on the brakes). Similarly, if a passenger is sitting in a stationary train and the train on the adjacent track begins to move, he or she can experience the strong sensation of self-motion in the opposite direction (Fig. 11.21A). Linear vection is one of the factors that make close formation flying so difficult because the pilot can never be sure whether his or her own aircraft or that of the pilot's lead or wing-man is responsible for the percieved relative motion of the aircraft.

Angular vection occurs when peripheral visual cues convey the information that one is rotating; the perceived rotation can be in pitch, roll, yaw, or any other plane of movement. Although angular vection illusions are not common in everyday life, they can be generated readily in a laboratory by enclosing a stationary subject in a rotating striped drum. Usually within 10 seconds after the visual motion begins, the subject perceives that he or she rather than the striped drum is rotating. A pilot can experience angular vection if the rotating anticollision light on his or her aircraft is left on during flight through clouds or fog: the revolving reflection provides a strong ambient visual stimulus signaling rotation in the yaw plane.

Another example of vection illusions is the so-called ''Star Wars'' effect, named after the popular motion picture by that name because of its vection-creating visual effects. This phenomenon involves linearly and angularly moving reflections of ground lights off of the curved inside surface of a fighter aircraft canopy, which create in the pilot disconcerting sensations of motion

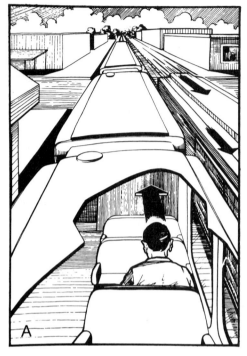 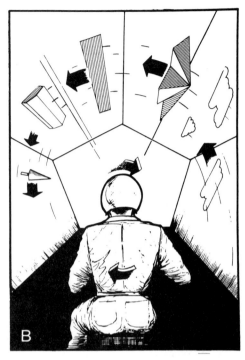

Figure 11.21. Vection illusions. *A.* Linear vection. In this example, the adjacent vehicle seen moving aft in his peripheral vision causes the subject to feel as though he is moving forward. *B.* Angular vection. Objects seen revolving around the subject in the flight simulator leads to a sense of self-rotation in the opposite direction—in this case, a rolling motion to the right.

that conflict with the actual motion of the aircraft.

Fortunately, vection illusions are not all bad. The most advanced flight simulators depend on linear and angular vection to create the illusion of flight (Fig. 11.21B). When the visual flight environment is dynamically portrayed in wide-field-of-view, infinity-optics flight simulators, the illusion of actual flight is so compelling that additional mechanical motion is not even needed (although mechanically generated motion-onset cues do seem to improve the fidelity of the simulation).

False Horizons and Surface Planes

Often the horizon perceived through ambient vision is not really horizontal. Quite naturally, this misperception of the horizontal creates hazards in flight. A sloping cloud deck, for example, is very difficult to perceive as anything but horizontal if it extends for any great distance into the

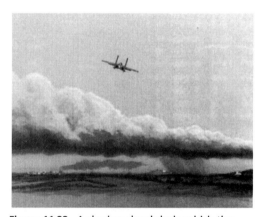

Figure 11.22. A sloping cloud deck, which the pilot misperceives as a horizontal surface.

pilot's peripheral vision (Fig. 11.22). Uniformly sloping terrain, particularly upsloping terrain, can create an illusion of horizontality with disastrous consequences for the pilot thus deceived. Many aircraft have crashed as a result of the pilot's entering a canyon with an apparently level floor, only to find that the floor actually rose faster than his or her airplane could climb. At night, the lights of a city built on sloping terrain can create the false impression that the extended plane of the city lights is the horizontal plane of the earth's surface, as already noted (Fig. 11.19). A distant rain shower can obscure the real horizon and create the impression of a horizon at the proximal edge (base) of the rainfall. If the shower is seen just beyond the runway during an approach to landing, the pilot can misjudge the pitch attitude of his or her aircraft and make inappropriate pitch corrections on the approach.

Pilots are especially susceptible to misperception of the horizontal while flying at night (Fig. 11.23A and B). Isolated ground lights can appear to the pilots as stars, and this can lead to the illusion that they are in a nose-high or one-wing-low attitude. Flying under such a false impression can, of course, be fatal. Frequently, no stars are visible because of overcast conditions. Unlighted areas of terrain can then blend with the dark overcast to create the illusion that the unlighted terrain is part of the sky. One extremely hazardous situation is that in which a takeoff is made over an ocean or other large body of water that cannot be distinguished visually from the night sky. Many pilots in this situation have perceived the shoreline receding beneath them to be the horizon, and some have responded to this false ''pitch-up'' percept with disastrous consequences.

Pilots flying at high altitudes can sometimes experience difficulties with control of aircraft attitude, because at high altitudes the horizon is lower with respect to the plane of level flight than it is at the lower altitudes where most pilots are accustomed to flying. As a reasonable approximation, the angle of depression of the horizon in degrees equals the square root of the altitude in kilometers. A pilot flying at an altitude of 15 km (49,000 ft) thus sees the horizon almost 4° below the extension of his or her horizontal plane. If the pilot visually orients to the view from the left cockpit window, he or she might be inclined to fly with the left wing 4° down to

level it with the horizon. If the pilot does this and then looks out through the right window, the right wing would be seen 8° above the horizon, with half of that elevation due to his or her own erroneous control input. The pilot also might experience problems with pitch control because the depressed horizon could cause him or her to perceive falsely a 4° nose-high pitch attitude.

Another result of false ambient visual orientational cueing is the lean-on-the-sun illusion. On the ground, we are accustomed to seeing the brighter visual surround above and the darker one below, regardless of the position of the sun. The direction of this gradient in light intensity thus helps us orient with respect to the surface of the earth. In clouds, however, such a gradient usually does not exist, and when it does, the lighter direction is generally toward the sun and the darker direction is away from it. But the sun is almost never directly overhead; as a consequence, a pilot flying in a thin cloud layer tends to perceive falsely the direction of the sun as directly overhead. This misperception causes him or her to bank in the direction of the sun, hence the name of the illusion.

Other False Ambient Cues

One very important aspect of ambient visual orientational cueing in flight is the stabilizing effect of the surrounding instrument panel, glare shield, and canopy bow or windshield frame, especially the reflection of panel lights and other cockpit structures off of the windshield or canopy at night. When the aircraft rolls or pitches while the pilot is inattentive, the stable visual surround provided by these objects tends to cause the motion not to be perceived, even though it may be at a rate well above the usual threshold for vestibular motion perception. While flying at night or in instrument weather, a pilot may thus have a false sense of security because of the lack of perceived motion, as his or her dominant orientational sense locks onto an apparently stable ambient visual environment. Of course, this falsely stabilizing effect

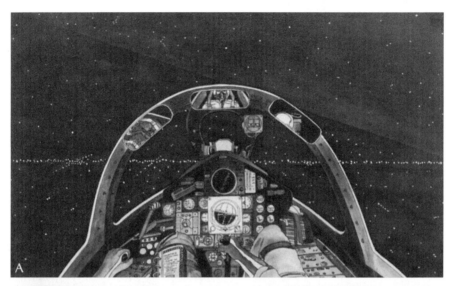

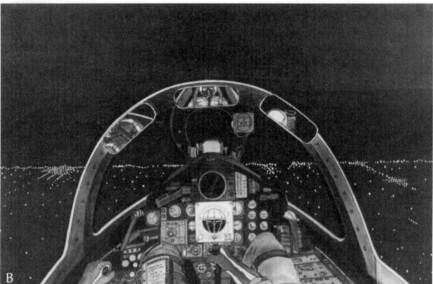

Figure 11.23. Misperception of the horizontal at night. *A.* Ground lights appearing to be stars cause the earth and sky to blend and a false horizon to be perceived. *B.* Blending of overcast sky with unlighted terrain or water causes the horizon to appear lower than is actually the case.

does not occur when the visual environment contains the usual, valid, spatially orienting ambient visual references (natural horizon, earth's surface, etc.).

Finally, the disorienting effects of the northern lights and of aerial flares should be mentioned. Aerial refueling at night in high northern latitudes often is made quite difficult by the northern lights, which provide false cues of ver-

ticality to the pilot's peripheral vision. Similarly, when aerial flares are dropped, they may drift with the wind, creating false cues of verticality. Their motion also may create vection illusions. Another phenomenon associated with use of aerial flares at night is the ''moth'' effect. The size of the area on the ground illuminated by a dropped flare slowly decreases as the flare descends. Because of the size constancy mechanism of visual orientation discussed earlier, a pilot circling the illuminated area may tend to fly in a descending spiral with gradually decreasing radius. Another important factor is that the aerial flares can be so bright as to reduce the apparent intensity of the aircraft instrument displays and thereby minimize their orientational cueing strength.

Vestibular Illusions

The vestibulocerebellar axis processes orientation information from the vestibular, visual, and other sensory systems. In the absence of adequate ambient visual orientation cues, the inadequacies of the vestibular and other orienting senses can result in orientational illusions. It is convenient and conventional to discuss the vestibular illusions in relation to the two functional components of the labyrinth that generate them—the semicircular ducts and the otolith organs.

Somatogyral Illusion

A somatogyral illusion is a false sensation of rotation (or absence of rotation) that results from misperceiving the magnitude or direction of an actual rotation. In essence, somatogyral illusions result from the inability of the semicircular ducts to register accurately a prolonged rotation, i.e., sustained angular velocity. When a person is subjected to an angular acceleration about the yaw axis, for example, the angular motion is at first perceived accurately because the dynamics of the cupula-endolymph system cause it to respond as an integrating angular accelerometer (i.e., as a rotation-rate sensor) at stimulus frequencies in the physiologic range (11) (Fig. 11.24). If the acceleration is followed immediately by a deceleration, as usually happens in the terrestrial environment, the total sensation of turning one way and then stopping the turn is quite accurate (Fig. 11.25). If, however, the angular acceleration is not followed by a deceleration and a constant angular velocity results instead, the sensation of rotation becomes less and

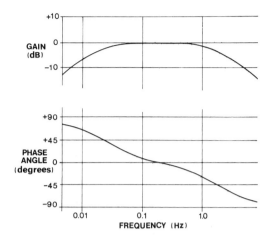

Figure 11.24. Transfer characteristics of the semicircular duct system as a function of sinusoidal stimulus frequency. Gain is the ratio of the magnitude of the peak perceived angular velocity to the peak delivered angular velocity; phase angle is a measure of the amount of advance or delay between the peak perceived and peak delivered angular velocities. Note that in the physiologic frequency range (roughly 0.05 to 1 Hz), perception is accurate; that is, gain is close to unity (0 dB) and phase shift is minimal. At lower stimulus frequencies, however, the gain drops off rapidly and the phase shift approaches 90°, which means that angular velocity becomes difficult to detect and that angular acceleration is perceived as velocity. (Adapted from Peters RA. Dynamics of the vestibular system and their relation to motion perception, spatial disorientation, and illusions. NASA-CR-1309. Washington, D.C.: National Aeronautics and Space Administration, 1969.)

less and eventually disappears as the cupula gradually returns to its resting position in the absence of an angular acceleratory stimulus (Fig. 11.26). If the rotating subject is subsequently subjected to an angular deceleration after a period of prolonged constant angular velocity, say after 10 seconds or so of constant-rate turning, his or her cupula-endolymph system signals a turn in the direction opposite that of the prolonged constant angular velocity, even though the person is really only turning less rapidly in the same direction. This is because the angular momentum of the rotating endolymph causes it to press against the cupula, forcing the cupula to deviate in the direction of endolymph flow, which is the same direction the cupula

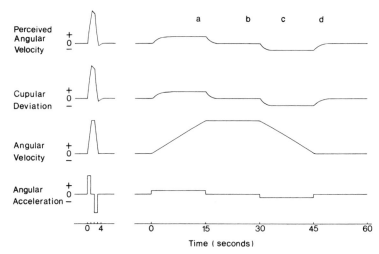

Figure 11.25. Effect of the stimulus pattern on the perception of angular velocity. On the left, the high-frequency character of the applied angular acceleration results in a cupular deviation that is nearly proportional to, and perceived angular velocity that is nearly identical to, the angular velocity developed. On the right, the peak angular velocity developed is the same as that on the left, but the low-frequency character of the applied acceleration results in cupular deviation and perceived angular velocity that appear more like the applied acceleration than the resulting velocity. This causes one to perceive: (a) less than the full amount of the angular velocity; (b) absence of rotation while turning persists; (c) a turn in the opposite direction from that of the actual turn; and (d) that turning persists after it has actually stopped. These false percepts are somatogyral illusions.

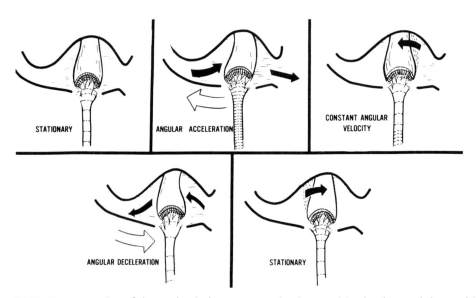

Figure 11.26. Representation of the mechanical events occurring in a semicircular duct and the resulting action potentials in the associated ampullary nerve during somatogyral illusions. The angular acceleration pattern applied is that shown in the right side of Figure 11.25.

would deviate if the subject were to accelerate in the direction opposite to his or her initial acceleration. Even after rotation actually ceases, the sensation of rotation in the direction opposite to that of the sustained angular velocity persists for several seconds—half a minute or longer with a large decelerating rotational impulse. Another more mechanistic definition of somatogyral illusion is "any discrepancy between actual and perceived rate of self-rotation that results from an abnormal angular acceleratory stimulus pattern." The term "abnormal" in this case implies the application of low-frequency stimuli outside the useful portion of the transfer characteristics of the semicircular duct system.

In flight under conditions of reduced visibility, somatogyral illusions can be deadly. The graveyard spin is the classic example of how somatogyral illusions can disorient a pilot with fatal results. This situation begins with the pilot intentionally or unintentionally entering a spin, let's say to the left (Fig. 11.27). At first, the pilot perceives the spin correctly because the angular acceleration associated with entering the spin deviates the cupulae the appropriate amount in the appropriate direction. The longer the spin persists, however, the more the sensation of spinning to the left diminishes as the cupulae return to their resting positions. If the pilot tries to stop the spin to the left by applying the right rudder, the angular deceleration causes him or her to perceive a spin to the right, even though the only real result of the pilot's action is termination of the spin to the left. A pilot who is ignorant of the possibility of such an illusion is then likely to make counterproductive left-rudder inputs to negate the unwanted erroneous sensation of spinning to the right. These control inputs keep the airplane spinning to the left, which gives the pilot the desired sensation of not spinning but does not bring the airplane under control. To extricate himself or herself from this very hazardous situation, the pilot must read the aircraft flight instruments and apply control inputs to make the instruments give the desired readings (push right rudder to center the turn

needle, in this example). Unfortunately, this may not be so easy to do. The angular accelerations created by both the multiple-turn spin and the pilot's spin-recovery attempts can elicit strong but inappropriate vestibulo-ocular reflexes, including nystagmus. In the usual terrestrial environment, these reflexes help stabilize the retinal image of the visual surround; in this situation, however, they only destabilize the retinal image because the visual surround (cockpit) is already fixed with respect to the pilot. Reading the flight instruments thus becomes difficult or impossible, and the pilot is left with only his or her false sensations of rotation to rely on for spatial orientation and aircraft control (12).

Although the lore of early aviation provided the graveyard spin as an illusion of the hazardous nature of somatogyral illusions, a much more common example occurring all too often in modern aviation is the graveyard spiral (Fig. 11.28). In this situation, the pilot has intentionally or unintentionally gotten himself or herself into a prolonged turn with a moderate amount of bank. After a number of seconds in the turn, the pilot loses the sensation of turning because the cupula-endolymph system cannot respond to the constant angular velocity. The percept of being in a bank as a result of the initial roll into the banked attitude also decays with time because the net gravitoinertial force vector points toward the floor of the aircraft during coordinated flight (whether the aircraft is in a banked turn or flying straight and level), and the otolith organs and other graviceptors normally signal that down is in the direction of the net sustained gravitoinertial force. As a result, when the pilot tries to stop the turn by rolling back to a wings-level attitude, he or she not only feels a turn in the direction opposite that of the original turn, but also feels a bank in the direction opposite to the original bank. Unwilling to accept this sensation of making the wrong control input, the hapless pilot rolls back into the original banked turn. Now the pilot's sensation is compatible with his or her desired mode of flight, but the instruments indicate that the aircraft is losing altitude (because the banked turn is

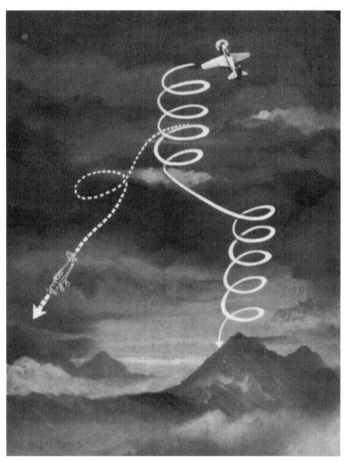

Figure 11.27. The graveyard spin. After several turns of a spin the pilot begins to lose the sensation of spinning. Then, when he or she tries to stop the spin, the resulting somatogyral illusion of spinning in the opposite direction makes the pilot reenter the original spin. (The solid line indicates actual motion; the dotted line indicates perceived motion.)

wasting lift) and still turning. So the pilot pulls back on the stick and perhaps adds power to arrest the unwanted descent and regain the lost altitude. This action would be successful if the aircraft were flying wings-level, but with the aircraft in a banked attitude it tightens the turn, serving only to make matters worse. Unless the pilot eventually recognizes his or her error and rolls out of the unperceived banked turn, he or she will continue to descend in an ever-tightening spiral toward the ground, hence the name graveyard spiral.

Oculogyral Illusion

Whereas a somatogyral illusion is a false sensation or lack of sensation of self-rotation in a subject undergoing unusual angular motion, an oculogyral illusion is a false sensation of motion of an object viewed by such a subject. For example, if a vehicle with a subject inside is rotating about a vertical axis at a constant velocity and suddenly stops rotating, the subject experiences not only a somatogyral illusion of rotation in the opposite direction, but also an oculogyral illusion of an object in front of him or her moving in the opposite direction. Thus, a somewhat oversimplified definition of the oculogyral illusion is that it is the visual correlate of the somatogyral illusion; however, its low threshold and lack of total correspondence with presumed cupular deviation suggest a more complex

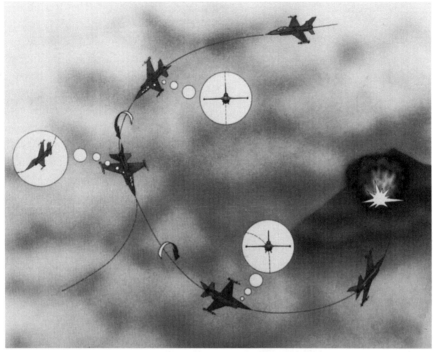

Figure 11.28. The graveyard spiral. The pilot in a banked turn loses the sensation of being banked and turning. Upon trying to reestablish a wings-level attitude and stop the turn, the pilot perceives a banked turn in the opposite direction from the original one. Unable to tolerate the sensation of making an inappropriate control input, the pilot banks back into the original turn.

mechanism. The attempt to maintain visual fixation during a vestibulo-ocular reflex elicited by angular acceleration is probably at least partially responsible for the oculogyral illusion. In an aircraft during flight at night or in weather, an oculogyral illusion generally confirms a somatogyral illusion: the pilot who falsely perceives that he or she is turning in a particular direction also observes the aircraft's instrument panel to be moving in the same direction.

Coriolis Illusion

The vestibular Coriolis effect, also called the Coriolis cross-coupling effect, vestibular cross-coupling effect, or simply the Coriolis illusion, is another false percept that can result from unusual stimulation of the semicircular duct system. To illustrate the phenomenon, let us consider a subject who has been rotating in the plane of his or her horizontal semicircular ducts (roughly the yaw plane) long enough for the endolymph in

those ducts to attain the same angular velocity as the head: the cupulae in the ampullae of the horizontal ducts have returned to their resting positions, and the sensation of rotation has ceased (Fig. 11.29A). If the subject then nods his or her head forward in the pitch plane, let's say a full 90° for the sake of simplicity, he or she is completely removing the horizontal semicircular ducts from the plane of rotation and inserting the two sets of vertical semicircular ducts into the plane of rotation (Fig. 11.29B). Although the angular momentum of the subject's rotating head is forcibly transferred at once out of the old plane of rotation, the angular momentum of the endolymph in the horizontal duct is dissipated more gradually. The torque resulting from the continuing rotation of the endolymph causes the cupulae in the horizontal ducts to be deviated, and a sensation of angular motion occurs in a new plane of the horizontal ducts— now the roll plane relative to the subject's body.

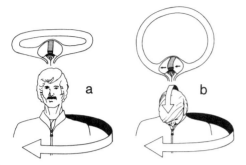

Figure 11.29. Mechanism of the Coriolis illusion. A subject rotating in the yaw plane long enough for the endolymph to stabilize in the horizontal semicircular duct (*a*) pitches his head forward (*b*) Angular motion of the endolymph deviates the cupula, causing the subject to perceive rotation in the new plane of the semicircular duct, even though no actual rotation occurred in that plane.

Simultaneously, the endolymph in the two sets of vertical semicircular ducts must acquire angular momentum because these ducts have been brought into the plane of constant rotation. The torque required to impart this change in momentum causes deflection of the cupulae in the ampullae of these ducts, and a sensation of angular motion in this plane—the yaw plane relative to the subject's body—results. The combined effect of the cupular deflection in all three sets of the semicircular ducts is that of a suddenly imposed angular velocity in a plane in which no actual angular acceleration relative to the subject has occurred. In the example given, if the original constant-velocity yaw is to the right and the subject pitches his or her head forward, the resulting Coriolis illusion experienced is a sudden rolling to the left.

A particular perceptual phenomenon experienced occasionally by pilots of relatively high-performance aircraft during instrument flight has been attributed to the Coriolis illusion because it occurs in conjunction with large movements of the head under conditions of prolonged constant angular velocity. It consists of a sensation of rolling and/or pitching that appears suddenly after the pilot diverts his or her attention from the front instruments and moves his or her head to view some switches or displays else-

where in the cockpit. The illusion is especially deadly because it is most likely to occur during an instrument approach, a phase of flight in which altitude is being lost rapidly and cockpit chores (e.g., radio frequency channels) repeatedly require the pilot to break up the instrument cross-check. The sustained angular velocities associated with instrument flying are insufficient to create Coriolis illusions of any great magnitude. However, another mechanism (the G-excess effect) has been proposed to explain the illusory rotations experienced with head movements in flight. Even if not responsible for spatial disorientation in flight, the Coriolis illusion is useful as a tool to demonstrate the fallibility of our nonvisual orientation senses. Nearly every military pilot living today has experienced the Coriolis illusion in the Barany chair or some other rotating device as part of his or her physiological training, and for most of these pilots it was then that they first realized their own orientation senses really cannot be trusted—the most important lesson of all for instrument flying.

Somatogravic Illusion

The otolith organs are responsible for a set of illusions known as somatogravic illusions. The mechanism of illusions of this type involves the displacement of otolithic membranes on their maculae by inertial forces so as to signal a false orientation when the resultant gravitoinertial force is perceived as gravity (and therefore vertical). Thus, a somatogravic illusion can be defined as a false sensation of body tilt that results from perceiving as vertical the direction of a nonvertical gravitoinertial force. The most common example of somatogravic illusions, the illusion of pitching up after taking off into conditions of reduced visibility, is perhaps the best illustration of this mechanism. Consider the pilot of a high-performance aircraft holding his or her position at the end of the runway waiting to take off. Here, the only force acting on the otolithic membranes is the force of gravity, and the positions of those membranes on their maculae signal accurately that down is towards the floor of the aircraft. Suppose the aircraft now accelerates down the runway, rotates, takes off, cleans up gear and flaps, and maintains a forward acceleration of 1 g until reaching the desired climb speed. The 1 G of inertial force resulting from the acceleration displaces the otolithic membrane towards the back of the pilot's head. In fact, the new positions of the otolithic membranes are nearly the same as they would be if the aircraft and pilot had pitched up 45°, because the new direction of the resultant gravitoinertial force vector, if one neglects the angle of attack and climb angle, is 45° aft relative to the gravitational vertical (Fig. 11.30). Naturally, the pilot's percept of pitch attitude based on the information from his or her otolith organs is one of having pitched up 45°; and the information from the pilot's nonvestibular proprioceptive and cutaneous mechanoreceptors senses supports this

false percept, because the sense organs subserving those modalities also respond to the direction and intensity of the resultant gravitoinertial force. Given the very strong sensation of a nose-high pitch attitude, one that is not challenged effectively by the focal visual orientation cues provided by the attitude indicator, the pilot is tempted to push the nose of the aircraft down to cancel the unwanted sensation of flying nose-high. Pilots succumbing to this temptation characteristically crash in a nose-low attitude a few miles beyond the end of the runway. Sometimes, however, they are seen to descend out of the overcast nose-low and try belatedly to pull up, as though they suddenly regained the correct orientation upon seeing the ground again. Pilots of carrier-launched aircraft need to be especially wary of the somatogravic illusion. These pilots experience pulse accelerations lasting 2 to 4

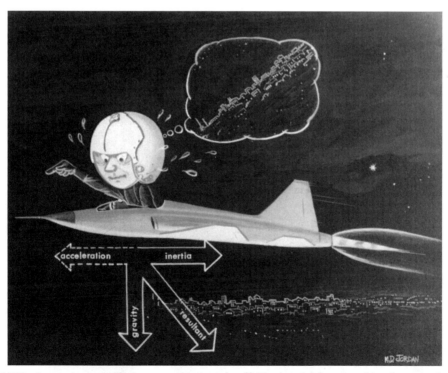

Figure 11.30. A somatogravic illusion occurring on takeoff. The inertial force resulting from the forward acceleration combines with the force of gravity to create a resultant gravitoinertial force directed down and aft. The pilot, perceiving down to be in the direction of the resultant gravitoinertial force, feels in an excessively nose-high attitude and is tempted to push the stick forward to correct the illusory nose-high attitude.

seconds and generating peak inertial forces of $+3$ to $+5$ G_x. Although the major acceleration is over quickly, the resulting illusion of nose-high pitch can persist for half a minute or more afterward, resulting in a particularly hazardous situation for the pilot who is unaware of this phenomenon (13).

Do not be misled by the above example into believing that only pilots of high-performance aircraft suffer the somatogravic illusion of pitching up after takeoff. More than a dozen air transport aircraft are believed to have crashed as a result of the somatogravic illusion occurring on takeoff (14). A relatively slow aircraft, accelerating from 100 to 130 knots over a 10-second period just after takeoff, generates $+0.16$ G_x on the pilot. Although the resultant gravitoinertial force is only 1.01 G, barely perceptibly more than the force of gravity, it is directed 9° aft, signifying to the unwary pilot a 9° nose-up pitch attitude. Because many slower aircraft climb out at 6° or less, a 9° downward pitch correction would put such an aircraft into a descent of 3° or more—the same as a normal final-approach slope. In the absence of a distinct external visual horizon or, even worse, in the presence of a false visual horizon (e.g., a shoreline) receding under the aircraft and reinforcing the pitch-up vestibular illusion, the pilot's temptation to push the nose down can be overwhelming. This type of mishap has happened at one particular civil airport so often that a notice has been placed on navigational charts cautioning pilots flying from this airport to be aware of the potential for loss of attitude reference.

Although the classic graveyard spiral was indicated earlier to be a consequence of the pilot's suffering a somatogyral illusion, it also can be said to result from a somatogravic illusion. A pilot who is flying ''by the seat of the pants'' applies the necessary control inputs to create a resultant G-force vector having the same magnitude and direction as that which his or her desired flight path would create. Unfortunately, any particular G vector is not unique to one particular condition of aircraft attitude and motion,

and the likelihood that the G vector created by a pilot flying in this mode corresponds for more than a few seconds to the flight condition desired is remote indeed. Specifically, once an aircraft has departed a desired wings-level attitude because of an unperceived roll, and the pilot does not correct the resulting bank, the only way he or she can create a G vector that matches the G vector of the straight and level conditions is with a descending spiral. In this condition, as is always the case in a coordinated turn, the centrifugal force resulting from the turn provides a G_y force that cancels the G_y component of the force of gravity that exists when the aircraft is banked. In addition, the tangential linear acceleration associated with the increasing airspeed resulting from the dive provides a $+G_x$ force that cancels the $-G_x$ component of the gravity vector that exists when the nose of the aircraft is pointed downward. Although the vector analysis of the forces involved in the graveyard spiral is somewhat complicated, a skillful pilot can easily manipulate the stick and rudder pedals to cancel all vestibular and other nonvisual sensory indications that the aircraft is turning and diving. In one mishap involving a dark-night takeoff of a commercial airliner, the recorded flight data indicate that the resultant G force which the pilot created by his control inputs allowed him to perceive his desired 10 to 12° climb angle and a net G force between 0.9 and 1.1 G for virtually the whole flight, even though he actually leveled off and then descended in an accelerating spiral until the aircraft crashed nearly inverted.

Inversion Illusion

The inversion illusion is a type of somatogravic illusion in which the resultant gravitoinertial force vector actually rotates backward so far as to be pointing away from rather than toward the earth's surface, thus giving the pilot false sensation that he or she is upside down. Figure 11.31 shows how this can happen (15). Typically, a steep climbing high-performance aircraft levels off more or less abruptly at the desired altitude. This maneuver subjects the aircraft and

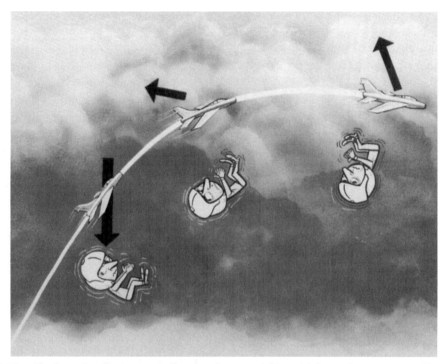

Figure 11.31. The inversion illusion. Centrifugal and tangential inertial forces during a level-off combine with the force of gravity to produce a resultant gravitoinertial force that rotates backward and upward with respect to the pilot, causing a perception of suddenly being upside down. Turbulent weather can produce additional inertial forces that contribute to the illusion. (Adapted from Martin JF, Jones GM. Theoretical man-machine interaction which might lead to loss of aircraft control. Aerospace Med, 1965; 36:713–716.)

pilot to a $-G_z$ centrifugal force resulting from the arc flown just prior to level-off. Simultaneously, as the aircraft changes to a more level attitude, airspeed picks up rapidly, adding a $+G_x$ tangential inertial force to the overall force environment. Adding the $-G_z$ centrifugal force and the $+G_x$ tangential force to the 1- G gravitational force results in a net gravitoinertial force vector that rotates backward and upward relative to the pilot. This stimulates the pilot's otolith organs in a manner similar to the way a pitch upward into an inverted position would. Even though the semicircular ducts should respond to the actual pitch downward, for some reason this conflict is resolved in favor of the otolith-organ information, perhaps because the semicircular-duct response is transient while the otolith-organ responses persists, or perhaps because the information from the other mechanoreceptors rein-

force the information from the otolith organs. The pilot who responds to the inversion illusion by pushing forward on the stick to counter the perceived pitching up and over backwards only prolongs the illusion by creating more $-G_z$ and $+G_x$ forces, thus aggravating the situation. Turbulent weather usually contributes to the development of the illusion; certainly, downdrafts are a source of $-G_z$ forces that can add to the net gravitoinertial forces producing the inversion illusion. Again, do not assume one must be flying a jet fighter to experience this illusion. Several reports of the inversion illusion involve crew of large airliners who lost control of their aircraft because the pilot lowered the nose inappropriately after experiencing the illusion. Jet upset is the name for the sequence of events that includes instrument weather, turbulence, the inability of the pilot to read his or her instruments, the inversion illusion, a pitch-down control input, and difficulty recovering the aircraft because of resulting aerodynamic or mechanical forces (16).

G-Excess Effect

Whereas the somatogravic illusion results from a change in the direction of the net G force, the G-excess effect results from a change in G magnitude. The G-excess effect is a false or exaggerated sensation of body tilt that can occur when the G environment is sustained at greater than 1 G. For a simplistic illustration of this phenomenon, let us imagine a subject is sitting upright in a $+1G_z$ environment and tips the head forward 30° (Fig. 11.32). As a result of this change in head position, the subject's otolithic membranes slide forward the appropriate amount for a 30° tilt relative to vertical, say a distance of $\times$ μm. Now suppose that the same subject is sitting upright in a $+2G_z$ environment and again tips the head 30° forward. This time, the subject's otolithic membranes slide forward

more than $\times$ μm because of the doubled gravitoinertial force acting on them. The displacement of the otolithic membranes, however, now corresponds not to a 30° forward tilt in the normal 1-G environment but to a much greater tilt, theoretically as much as 90° (2 sin 30° = sin 90°). The subject has initiated only a 30° head tilt, however, and expects to perceive no more than that. The unexpected additional perceived tilt is thus referred to the immediate environment; i.e., the subject perceives his or her vehicle to have tilted by the amount equal to the difference between the actual and expected percepts of tilt. The actual perceptual mechanism underlying the G-excess effect is more complicated than the illustration suggests: first, the plane of the utricular maculae is not really horizontal but slopes upward 20–30° from back to front; second, the saccular maculae contribute in an undetermined manner to the net percept of tilt; and third, as is usually the case with vestibular illusions, good visual orientational cues tend to attenuate the illusory percept. But experimental evidence clearly demonstrates the existence of the G-excess effect. Perceptual errors of 10° to 20° are generated at 2 G, and at 1.5 G the errors are about half that amount (17,18).

In fast-moving aircraft, the G-excess illusion can occur as a result of the moderate amount of G force pulled in a turn—a penetration turn or procedure turn, for example. If the pilot has to look down and to the side to select a new radio frequency or to pick up a dropped pencil while in a turn, he or she should experience an uncommanded tilt in both pitch and roll planes due to the G-excess illusion. As noted previously, the G-excess illusion may be responsible for the false sensation of pitch and/or roll generally attributed to the Coriolis illusion under such circumstances. The G-excess has recently become a suspect in a number of mishaps involving fighter/attack aircraft making 2- to 5.5-G turns at low altitudes in conditions of essentially good visibility. For some reason, the aircraft were overbanked while the pilots were looking out of the cockpit for an adversary, wingman, or some other object of visual attention, and as a result

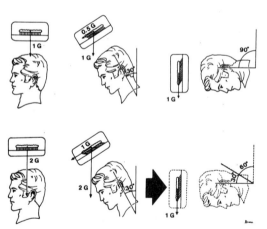

Figure 11.32. Mechanism of the G-excess illusion. The subject in a 1-G environment (upper half of figure) experiences the result of a 0.05-G pull on his utricular otolithic membranes when the head is tilted 30° off the vertical, and the result of a 1-G pull when the head is tilted a full 90°. The subject in a 2-G environment (lower half of figure) experiences the result of a 1-G pull when upon tilting the head only 30°. The illusory tilt perceived by the subject is attributed to external forces (lower right).

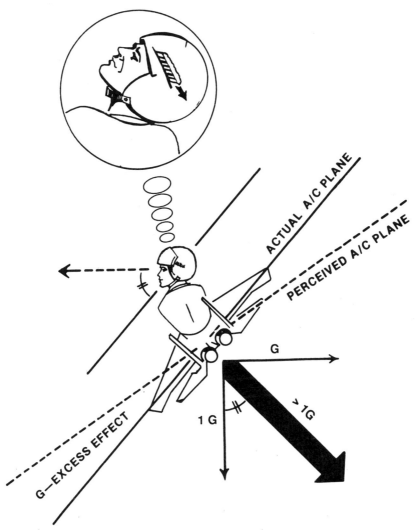

Figure 11.33. The G-excess illusion during a turn in flight. G-induced excessive movement of the pilot's otolithic membranes causes him or her to feel an extra amount of head and body tilt, which is interpreted as an underbank of the aircraft when the pilot looks up to the inside of the turn. Correcting for the illusion, the pilot overbanks the aircraft and it descends.

they descended into the terrain. The theory is that the G-excess effect causes the pilot to have an illusion of underbank if his or her head is either facing the inside of the turn and elevated (Fig. 11.33) or facing the outside of the turn and depressed. If facing forward, the pilot would have an illusion of pitching up (i.e., climbing) during the turn. Thus, in any of these common circumstances, if the pilot were to fail to maintain a continuous visual reference to the earth's surface, he or she would likely cause the aircraft

to descend in response to the illusory change of attitude caused by the G-excess effect. Perhaps in some of the mishaps mentioned, the pilot's view of the spatial environment was inadequate because he or she was looking at sky rather than ground, or perhaps G-induced tunnel vision was responsible for loss of ambient visual cues. In any case, it is apparent that the pilots failed to perceive correctly their attitude, vertical velocity, and height above the ground, i.e., they were spatially disoriented.

The elevator illusion is a special kind of G-excess effect. Because of the way the urticular membranes are variably displaced with respect to their maculae by increases and decreases in $+G_z$ force, false sensations of pitch and vertical velocity can result even when the head remains in the normal upright position. When an upward acceleration (as occurs in an elevator) causes the net G_z force to increase, a sensation of climbing and tilting backward can occur. In flight, such an upward acceleration occurs when an aircraft levels off from a sustained descent. This temporary increase in $+G_z$ loading can make the pilot feel a pitch up and climb if his or her view of the outside world is restricted by night, weather, or head-down cockpit chores. Compensating for the illusory pitch up sensation, the pilot would likely put the aircraft back into a descent, all the while feeling that the aircraft is maintaining a constant altitude. In one inflight study of the elevator illusion, blindfolded pilots were told to maintain perceived level flight after a relatively brisk level-off from a sustained 10m/sec (2000-ft/min) descent: the mean response of the six pilots was a 6.6 m/sec (1300-ft/min) descent (10). Clearly this tendency to re-establish a descent is especially dangerous during the final stage of a non-precision instrument approach at night or in weather. Upon leveling off at the published minimum descent altitude, the pilot typically starts a visual search for the runway. If the pilot fails to monitor the flight instruments during this critical time, the elevator illusion can cause him or her unwittingly to put the aircraft into a descent and thus squander the altitude buffer protecting the aircraft from ground impact.

Oculogravic Illusion

The oculogravic illusion can be thought of as a visual correlate of the somatogravic illusion and occurs under the same stimulus conditions. A pilot who is subjected to the deceleration resulting from the application of speed brakes, for example, experiences a nose-down pitch because of the somatogravic illusion. Simultane-ously, he or she observes the front instrument panel to move downward, confirming the sensation of tilting forward. The oculogravic illusion is thus the visually apparent movement of an object that is actually in a fixed position relative to the subject during changing of the direction of the net gravitoinertial force. Like the oculogyral illusion, the oculogravic illusion probably results from the attempt to maintain visual fixation during a vestibulo-ocular reflex, elicited in this case by the change in direction of the applied G vector rather than by angular acceleration.

The elevator illusion was originally thought of as a visual phenomenon like the oculogravic illusion, except that the false percept was believed to result from a vestibulo-ocular reflex generated by a change in magnitude of the $+G_z$ force instead of by a change in its direction. When an individual is accelerated upward, as in an elevator, the increase in $+G_z$ force elicits a vestibulo-ocular reflex of otolith organ origin (the elevator reflex) that drives the eyes downward. Attempting to stabilize visually the objects in a fixed position relative to the observer causes those objects to appear to shift upward when the G force is increased. The opposite effect occurs when the individual is accelerated downward; the reduction in the magnitude of the net gravitoinertial force to less than $+1\ G_z$ causes a reflex upward shift of the direction of gaze, and the immediate surroundings appear to shift downward. (The latter effect also has been called the oculoagravic illusion because of its occurrence during transient weightlessness.) Although the described visual effect undoubtedly contributes to the expression of the elevator illusion, it is not essential for its generation, since the illusion can occur even in the absence of vision, as noted above.

The Leans

By far the most common vestibular illusion in flight is the leans. Virtually every instrument-rated pilot has had or will get the leans in one form or another at some time during his or her flying career. The leans consists of a false percept of angular displacement about the roll axis, i.e., is an illusion of bank, and it is frequently associated with a vestibulospinal reflex, appropriate to the false percept, that results in the pilot's actually leaning in the direction of the falsely perceived vertical (Fig. 11.34). The usual explanations of the leans invoke the known deficiencies of both otolith-organ and semicircular-duct sensory mechanisms. As indicated previously, the otolith-organs are not reliable sources of information about the exact direction of the true vertical because they respond to the resultant gravitoinertial force, not to gravity alone. Furthermore, other sensory inputs can sometimes override otolith-organ cues and result in a false perception of the vertical, even when the gravitoinertial force experienced is truly ver-

tical. The semicircular ducts can provide such false inputs in flight by responding accurately to some roll stimuli but not responding at all to others because they are below threshold. If, for example, a pilot is subjected to an angular acceleration in roll so that the product of the acceleration and its time of application does not reach some threshold value, say 2 degrees/sec, he or she will not perceive the roll. Suppose the pilot, who is trying to fly straight and level, is subjected to an unrecognized and uncorrected 2-degree/sec roll for 10 seconds: a 20° bank results. If the pilot suddenly notices the unwanted bank and corrects it by rolling the aircraft back upright with a suprathreshold roll rate, say 15 degrees/sec, only half of the actual roll motion that took place (the half resulting from the correcting roll)

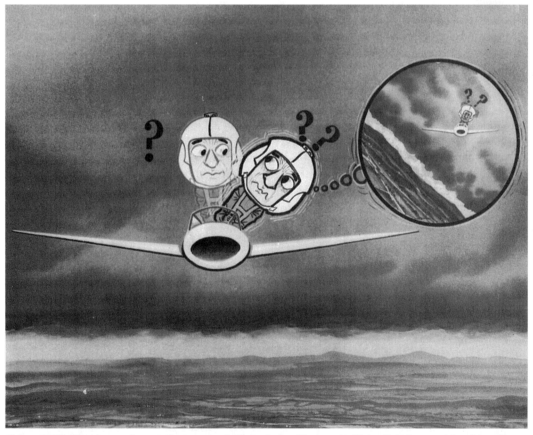

Figure 11.34. The leans, the most common of all vestibular illusions in flight. Falsely perceiving himself to be in a right bank, but flying the aircraft straight and level by means of the flight instruments, this pilot leans to the left in an attempt to assume an upright posture compatible with his illusion of bank.

is experienced. As the pilot started from a wings-level position, he or she is left with the illusion of having rolled into a 20° bank in the direction of the correcting roll, even though the aircraft is again wings-level. At this point, the pilot has the leans; and even though he or she may be able to fly the aircraft properly by the deliberate and difficult process of forcing the attitude indicator to read correctly, this illusion can last for many minutes, seriously degrading the pilot's flying efficiency during that time.

Interestingly, pilots frequently get the leans after prolonged turning maneuvers and not because of alternating subthreshold and suprathreshold angular motion stimuli. In a holding pattern, for example, the pilot rolls into a 3-degree/sec standard-rate turn, holds the turn for 1 minute, rolls out and flies straight and level for 1 minute, turns again for 1 minute, and so on until traffic conditions permit him or her to proceed towards the destination. During the turning segments, the pilot initially feels the roll into the turn and accurately perceives the banked attitude. But as the turn continues, his or her percept of being in a banked turn dissipates and is replaced by a feeling of flying straight and level, both because the sensation of turning is lost when the endolymph comes up to speed in the semicircular ducts (somatogyral illusion) and because the net G force being directed toward the floor of the aircraft provides a false cue of verticality (somatogravic illusion). Then when the pilot rolls out of the turn, he or she feels a roll into a banked turn in the opposite direction. With experience, a pilot learns to suppress this false sensation quickly by paying strict attention to the attitude indicator. Sometimes, however, the pilot cannot dispel the illusion of banking—usually when he or she is particularly busy, unfortunately. The leans also can be caused by misleading peripheral visual orientation cues, as mentioned in the section entitled "Visual Illusions." Roll angular vection is particularly effective in this regard, at least in the laboratory. One thing about the leans is apparent: there is no single explanation of this illusion.

The deficiencies of several orientation-sensing systems in some cases reinforce each other to create an illusion; in other cases, the inaccurate information from one sensory modality for some reason is selected over the accurate information from others to create the illusion. Stories have surfaced of pilots suddenly experiencing the leans for no apparent reason at all or even of experiencing it voluntarily by imagining the earth to be in a different direction from the aircraft. The point is that one must not think that the leans, or any other illusion for that matter, occurs as a totally predictable response to a physical stimulus: there is much more to perception than stimulation of the end-organs.

Disorientation

Definitions

An orientational percept is a sense of one's position and motion relative to the plane of the earth's surface. It can be primary (i.e., natural), meaning that it is based on ambient visual, vestibular, or other sensations that normally contribute to our orientation in our natural environment; or it can be secondary (i.e., synthetic), meaning that it is intellectually constructed from focal visual, verbal, or other symbolic data, such as that presented by flight instruments. While the former type of orientational percept is essentially irrational (not subject to analysis and interpretation) and involves largely preconscious mental processing, the latter type is rational and entirely conscious. A locational percept, to be distinguished from an orientational percept, is a sense of one's motion and position in (as opposed to relative to) the plane of the earth's surface. An accurate locational percept is achieved by reading a map or knowing the latitude and longitude of one's location.

Spatial disorientation is a state characterized by an erroneous orientational percept, i.e., an erroneous sense of one's position and motion relative to the plane of the earth's surface. Geographic disorientation, or "being lost," is a state characterized by an erroneous locational percept. These definitions together encompass all the possible positions and velocities, both translational and rotational, along and about three orthogonal earth-referenced axes. Spatial orientation information includes those parameters that an individual on or near the earth's surface with eyes open can reasonably be expected to process accurately on a sunny day. Lateral tilt, forward-backward tilt, angular position about a vertical axis, and their corresponding first derivatives with respect to time are the angular positions and motions included; height above ground, forward-backward velocity, sideways velocity, and up-down velocity are the linear positions and motions included. Absent from this collection of spatial orientation information parameters are the location coordinates, the linear position dimensions in the horizontal plane. In flight, orientation information is described in terms of flight instrument-based parameters (Fig. 11.35). Angular position is bank, pitch, and heading; and the corresponding angular velocities are roll rate, pitch rate and turn rate (or yaw rate). The linear position

parameter is altitude; and the linear velocity parameters are airspeed (or groundspeed), slip/skid rate, and vertical velocity. Inflight navigation information is comprised of linear position dimensions in the horizontal plane, such as latitude and longitude or bearing and distance form a navigation reference point.

United States Air Force Manual 51–37, *Instrument Flying* (19), categorizes flight instruments into three functional groups: control, performance, and navigation. In the control category are the parameters of aircraft attitude (i.e., pitch and bank) and engine power or thrust. In the performance category are airspeed, altitude, vertical velocity, heading, turn rate, slip/skid rate, angle of attack, acceleration (G loading), and flight path (velocity vector). The navigation category includes course, bearing, range, latitude/longitude, time, and similar parameters useful for determining location on the earth's surface. This categorization of flight instrument parameters allows us to construct a useful operational definition of spatial disorientation: it is an

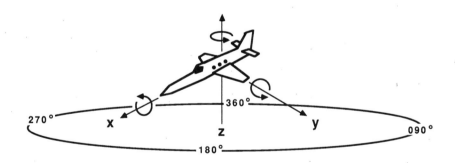

AXIS	ANGULAR		LINEAR	
	POSITION	VELOCITY	POSITION	VELOCITY
x	Bank	Roll rate	*	Airspeed
y	Pitch	Pitch rate	*	Slip/skid rate
z	Heading	Turn rate	Altitude	Vertical velocity

* Navigation information

Figure 11.35. Flight instrument-based parameters of spatial orientation. Spatial disorientation is a state characterized by an erroneous sense of any of these parameters.

erroneous sense of any of the flight parameters displayed by aircraft control and performance instruments. Geographic disorientation, in contrast, is thus: an erroneous sense of any of the flight parameters displayed by aircraft navigation instruments. The practical utility of these operational definitions is that they can establish a common understanding of what is meant by spatial disorientation among all parties investigating an aircraft mishap, whether they be pilots, flight surgeons, aerospace physiologists or experts in some other discipline. If the answer to the question, "Did the pilot not realize his or her actual pitch attitude and vertical velocity (and/or other control or performance parameters)?" is "Yes," then it is obvious that the pilot was spatially disoriented, and the contribution of the disorientation to the sequence of events leading to the mishap is clarified.

Sometimes aircrew tend to be imprecise when they discuss spatial disorientation, preferring to say that they "lost situational awareness" rather than "became disoriented," as though having experienced spatial disorientation stigmatizes them. Situational awareness involves a correct appreciation of a host of conditions, including the tactical environment, location, weather, weapons capability, own capabilities, administrative constraints, etc., as well as spatial orientation. Thus, if the situation about which a pilot lacks awareness is his or her position and motion relative to the plane of the earth's surface, then that pilot has spatial disorientation, specifically, as well as loss of situational awareness, generally.

Types of Spatial Disorientation

We distinguish three types of spatial disorientation in flight: Type I (unrecognized), Type II (recognized), and Type III (incapacitating). In Type I disorientation, the pilot does not consciously perceive any of the manifestations of disorientation: i.e., he or she experiences no disparity between natural and synthetic orientational percepts, has no suspicion that a flight instrument (e.g., attitude indicator) has malfunc-

tioned, and does not feel that the aircraft is responding incorrectly to his or her control inputs. In unrecognized spatial disorientation the pilot is oblivious to the fact that he or she is disoriented, and controls the aircraft completely in accord with and in response to a false orientational percept. To distinguish Type I disorientation from the others, and to emphasize its insidiousness, some pilots and aerospace physiologists call Type I spatial disorientation "misorientation."

In Type II disorientation, the pilot consciously perceives some manifestation of disorientation. The pilot may experience a conflict between what he or she feels the aircraft is doing and what the flight instruments indicate that it is doing. Or the pilot may not experience a genuine conflict, but merely conclude that the flight instruments are faulty. The pilot also may feel that the aircraft is attempting to assume a pitch or bank attitude other than the one he or she is trying to establish. Type II disorientation is the kind to which pilots are referring when they use the term "vertigo," as in "I had a bad case of vertigo on final approach." Although Type II spatial disorientation is labeled "recognized," this does not mean that the pilot must necessarily realize he or she is disoriented: the pilot may only realize he or she has a problem controlling the aircraft, not knowing that the source of the problem is spatial disorientation.

With Type III spatial disorientation the pilot experiences an overwhelming—i.e., incapacitating—physiologic response to physical or emotional stimuli associated with the disorientation event. Pilots may have vestibular nystagmus to such a degree that they can neither read the flight instruments nor obtain a stable view of the outside world (vestibulo-ocular disorganization). Or they may have such strong vestibulo-spinal reflexes that they cannot control the aircraft. Pilots may even be so incapacitated by fear that they are unable to make a rational decision—they may freeze on the controls. The important feature of Type III spatial disorientation is that the pilot is disoriented and most likely knows it, but can't do anything about it.

Examples of Disorientation

The last of four F-15 Eagle fighter aircraft took off on a daytime sortie in bad weather, intending to follow the other three in a radar in-trail departure. Because of a navigational error committed by the pilot shortly after takeoff, he was unable to find the other aircraft on his radar. Frustrated, the pilot elected to intercept the other aircraft where he knew they would be in the arc of the standard instrument departure, so he made a beeline for that point, presumably scanning his radar diligently for the blips he knew should be appearing at any time. Meanwhile, after ascending to 1200 m (4000 ft) above ground level, he entered a descent of approximately 750 m/min (2500 ft/min) or 13 m/sec as a result of an unrecognized 3° nose-low attitude. After receiving requested position information from another member of the flight, the pilot either suddenly realized he was in danger of colliding with another aircraft or he suddenly found the other aircraft on the radar because he then made a steeply banked turn, either to avoid a perceived threat of collision or to join up with the rest of the flight. Unfortunately, he had by this time descended far below the other aircraft and was going too fast to avoid the ground, which became visible under the overcast just before the aircraft crashed. This mishap resulted from an episode of unrecognized, or Type I, disorientation. The specific illusion responsible appears to have been the somatogravic illusion, which was created by the forward acceleration of this high-performance aircraft during takeoff and climb-out. The pilot's preoccupation with the radar task compromised his instrument scan to the point where the false vestibular cues were able to penetrate his orientational information processing. Having unknowingly accepted an inaccurate orientational percept, he controlled the aircraft accordingly until it was too late to recover.

Examples of recognized, or Type II, spatial disorientation are easier to obtain than are examples of Type I because most experienced pilots have anecdotes to tell about how they "got vertigo" and fought it off. Some pilots were not so fortunate, however. One F-15 Eagle pilot, after climbing his aircraft in formation with another F-15 at night, began to experience difficulty in maintaining spatial orientation and aircraft control upon leveling off in the clouds at 8,200 m (27,000 ft). "Talk about practice bleeding," he commented to the lead pilot. Having decided to go to another area because of the weather, the two pilots began a descending right turn. At this point, the pilot on the wing told the lead pilot, "I'm flying upside down." Shortly afterward, the wingman considered separating from the formation, saying, "I'm going lost wingman." Then he said, "No, I've got you," and finally, "No, I'm going lost wingman." The hapless wingman then caused his aircraft to descend in a wide spiral and crashed into the desert less than one minute later, even though the lead pilot advised the wingman several times during the descent to level out. In this mishap, the pilot probably suffered an inversion illusion upon leveling off in the weather, and entered a graveyard spiral after leaving the formation. Although he knew he was disoriented, or at least recognized the possibility, he still was unable to control the aircraft effectively. That a pilot can realize he is disoriented, see accurate orientation information displayed on the attitude indicator, and still fly into the ground always strains the credulity of nonaviators. Pilots who have had spatial disorientation, who have experienced fighting oneself for control of an aircraft, are less skeptical.

The pilot of an F-15 Eagle, engaged in vigorous air combat tactics training with two other F-15s on a clear day, initiated a hard left turn at 5200 m (17,000 ft) above ground level. For reasons that have not been established with certainty, his aircraft began to roll to the left at a rate estimated at 150 to 180 degrees/sec. He transmitted, "out-of-control autoroll," as he descended through 4600 m (15,000 ft). The pilot made at least one successful attempt to stop the roll, as evidenced by the momentary cessation of the roll at 2400 m (8000 ft); then the aircraft began to roll again to the left. Forty seconds elapsed between the time that the rolling began and the time that the pilot ejected—but too late. Regardless of whether the rolling was caused by a mechanical malfunction or was an autoroll induced by the pilot, the likely result of his extreme motion was vestibulo-ocular disorganization, which not only prevented the pilot from reading his instruments but also kept him from orienting with the natural horizon. Thus, Type III disorientation probably prevented him from taking appropriate corrective action to stop the roll and keep it stopped; if not that, it certainly compromised his ability to assess accurately the level to which his situation had deteriorated.

Statistics

Because the fraction of aircraft mishaps caused by or contributed to by spatial disorientation has doubled over the four decades between 1950 and 1990, one might conclude that continuing efforts to educate pilots about spatial disorientation and the hazard it represents have been to no avail. Fortunately, the total number of major mishaps and the number of major mishaps per million flying hours have dropped considerably over the same period (at least in the United States), so it appears that such flying safety educational efforts actually have been effective. A number of statistical studies of spatial disorientation mishaps in the United States Air Force will provide an appreciation of the magnitude of the problem in military aviation.

In 1956, Nuttall and Sanford (20) reported that, in one major air command during the period of 1954 to 1956, spatial disorientation was responsible for 4% of all major aircraft mishaps and 14% of all fatal aircraft mishaps. In 1969, Moser (21) reported a study of aircraft mishaps in another major air command during the 4-year period from 1964 to 1967: he found that spatial disorientation was a significant factor in 9% of major mishaps and 26% of fatal mishaps. In 1971, Barnum and Bonner (22) reviewed the Air

Force mishap data from 1958 through 1968 and found that in 281 (6% of the 4679 major mishaps) spatial disorientation was a causative factor; fatalities occurred in 211 of those 281 accidents, accounting for 15% of the 1462 fatal mishaps. A comment by Barnum and Bonner summarizes some interesting data about the "average pilot" involved in a spatial disorientation mishap: "He will be around 30 years of age, have 10 years in the cockpit, and have 1500 hours of first pilot/instructor-pilot time. He will be a fighter pilot and will have flown approximately 25 times in the three months prior to his accident." In an independent 1973 study, Kellogg (23) found the relative incidence of spatial disorientation mishaps in the years 1968 through 1972 to range from 4.8% to 6.2% and confirmed the high proportion of fatalities in mishaps resulting from spatial disorientation.

The major (Class A) Air Force mishaps over the ten-year period from 1980 through 1989 were reviewed by Freeman (personal communication, 1990). He found that 81 (13%) of the 633 major mishaps during that period, and 115 (14%) of the 795 fatalities, were due to spatial disorientation. If we consider only the mishaps caused by operator error, disorientation accounted for approximately one-fourth of these (81 out of 356). If we only consider the Air Force's front-line fighter/attack aircraft, the F-15 and F-16, nearly one-third (26 of 86) of the losses of these aircraft resulted from spatial disorientation. The cost of the Air Force aircraft destroyed each year in disorientation mishaps until the decade of the 1980s was on the order of $20 million per year. From 1980 through 1989, over half a billion dollars worth of Air Force resources were lost as a result of spatial disorientation. Currently the average dollar cost of spatial disorientation to the Air Force is on the order of $100 million; but occasional losses of particularly expensive aircraft result in much higher figures in some years.

Regarding the fractions of disorientation-related mishaps for which the various types of spatial disorientation are responsible, the conventional wisdom is that more than half of the mishaps involve Type I disorientation, most of the remainder involve Type II, and very few involve Type III. The same wisdom suggests that the source of the disorientation is visual illusions in about half of the mishaps, and vestibular/somatosensory illusions in the other half, with combined visual and vestibular illusions accounting for at least some of the mishaps. An analysis of Air Force aircraft mishaps in 1988 in which spatial disorientation was suspected by the investigating flight surgeon revealed that all eight involved Type I disorientation; two apparently resulted from visual illusions, three from vestibular illusions, and three from mixed visual and vestibular illusions (24).

The recent experience of the United States Navy with spatial disorientation is also instructive (25). During the years 1980 through 1989, 112 Class A flight mishaps involved spatial disorientation as a definite, probable, or possible causal factor. Of the 40 mishaps in the "definite" category, 20 occurred in daytime and 20 happened at night; 17 occurred during flight over land, and 23 resulted during flight over water. Thirty-two aircraft, including 15 fighter/attack aircraft, six training aircraft, and 11 helicopters, were destroyed; and 38 lives were lost in the 13 fatal mishaps out of 40 Class A mishaps. The mean experience level for the Navy pilots involved in spatial disorientation mishaps was 1488 hours (median: 1152 hours), nearly the same as that for Air Force pilots. Surprisingly, the incidence of spatial disorientation-related mishaps for the Air Force, Navy, and Army have been remarkably similar over the years, even though the flying missions of the several military services are somewhat different.

One problem with the mishap statistics presented above is that they are conservative, representing only those mishaps in which disorientation was stated to be a possible or probable factor by the Safety Investigation Board. In actuality, many mishaps resulting from spatial disorientation were not identified as such because other factors—such as distractions, task saturation,

and poor crew coordination—initiated the chain of events resulting in the mishap; these factors were considered more relevant or more amenable to correction than the disorientation that followed and ultimately caused the pilot to fly the aircraft into the ground or water. In the Air Force from 1980 through 1989, 263 mishaps and 425 fatalities, at a cost of over two billion dollars, resulted from "loss of situational awareness" (Freeman, J.E.; personal communication, 1990). It is apparent that the great majority of those mishaps would not have happened if the pilots had at all times correctly assessed their pitch/bank attitude, vertical velocity, and altitude—i.e., if they had not been spatially disoriented. Thus we can infer that spatial disorientation causes considerably more aircraft mishaps than the disorientation-specific statistics would lead us to believe, probably two or three times as many.

Although statistics indicating the relative frequency of spatial disorientation mishaps in air-carrier operations are not readily available, it would be a serious mistake to conclude that there have been no air-carrier mishaps caused by spatial disorientation. Fourteen such mishaps occurring between 1950 and 1969 were reportedly due to somatogravic and visual illusions that resulted in the so-called "dark-night takeoff accident." (14) In addition, 26 commercial airliners were involved in jet-upset incidents or accidents during the same period (16). Spatial disorientation also is a problem in general (non-military, non-air-carrier) aviation. Kirkham and colleagues (26) reported in 1978 that although spatial disorientation was a cause or factor in only 2.5% of all general aviation aircraft accidents in the United States, it was the third most common cause of fatal general aviation accidents. Of the 4012 fatal general aviation mishaps occurring in the years 1970 through 1975, 627 (15.6%) involved spatial disorientation as a cause or factor. Notably, 90% of general aviation mishaps in which disorientation was a cause or factor were fatal.

Dynamics of Spatial Orientation and Disorientation

Visual Dominance

It is naive to assume that a certain pattern of physical stimuli always elicits a particular veridical or illusory perceptual response. Certainly, when a pilot has a wide, clear view of the horizon, ambient vision adequately supplies virtually all orientation information, and potentially misleading linear or angular acceleratory motion cues do not result in spatial disorientation (unless, of course, they are so violent as to cause vestibulo-ocular disorganization). When a pilot's vision is compromised by night or bad weather conditions, the same acceleratory motion cues can cause him or her to develop spatial disorientation; but, the pilot usually avoids it by referring to the aircraft instruments for orientation information. If the pilot is unskilled at interpreting the instruments, if the instruments fail or, as frequently happens, if the pilot neglects to look at the instruments, those misleading motion cues inevitably cause disorientation. Such is the character of visual dominance, the phenomenon in which one incorporates visual orientation information into his or her percept of spatial orientation to the exclusion of vestibular and nonvestibular proprioceptive, tactile, and other sensory cues. Visual dominance falls into two categories: the congenital type, in which ambient vision provides dominant orientation cues through natural neural connections and functions, and the acquired type, in which orientation cues are gleaned through focal vision and are integrated as a result of training and experience into an orientational percept. The functioning of the proficient instrument pilot illustrates acquired visual dominance: he or she has learned to decode with foveal vision the information on the attitude indicator and other flight instruments and to reconstruct that information into a concept of what the aircraft is doing and where it is going, which concept is referred to when controlling the aircraft. This complex skill must be developed through training and maintained through practice, and its fragility is one of the factors that make spatial disorientation such a hazard.

Vestibular Suppression

The term vestibular suppression often is used to denote the active process of visually overriding undesirable vestibular sensations or reflexes of vestibular origin. An example of this aspect of visual dominance is seen in well-trained figure skaters who, with much practice, learn to abolish the postrotatory dizziness, nystagmus, and postural instability that normally result from the high angular decelerations associated with suddenly stopping rapid spins on the ice. But even these individuals, when deprived of vision by eye closure or darkness, have the very dizziness, nystagmus, and falling that we would expect to result from the acceleratory stimuli produced. In flight, the ability to suppress unwanted vestibular sensations and reflexes is developed with repeated exposure to the linear and angular accelerations of flight. As is the case with the figure skaters, however, the pilot's ability to prevent vestibular sensations and reflexes is compromised when he or she is deprived of visual orientation cues by night, weather, and inadequate flight instrument displays.

Opportunism

Opportunism on the part of the primary (ambient visual and vestibular) orientation-information processing systems refers to the propensity of those systems to fill an orientation-information void swiftly and surely with natural orientation information. When a pilot flying in instrument weather looks away from the artificial horizon for only a few seconds, this is usually long enough for erroneous ambient or visual or vestibular information to break through the pilot's defenses and become incorporated into his or her orientational percept. In fact, conflicts between focal visual and ambient visual or vestibular sources of orientation information often tend to resolve themselves very quickly in favor of the latter, without providing the pilot an opportunity to evaluate the information. It is logical that any orientation information reaching the vestibular nuclei—whether vestibular, other proprioceptive, or ambient visual—should have an advantage in competing with focal visual cues for expression as the pilot's sole orientational percept because the vestibular nuclei are primary terminals in the pathways for reflex orientational responses and are the initial level of integration for any eventual conscious concomitant of perception of spatial orientation. In other words, although acquired visual dominance can be maintained by diligent attention to synthetic orientation cues, the challenge to this dominance presented by the processing of natural orientation cues through primitive neural channels is very potent and ever present.

The lack of adequate orientation cues and conflicts between competing sensory modalities are only a part of the whole picture of a disorientation mishap. Why so many disoriented pilots, even those who know they are disoriented, are unable to recover their aircraft has mystified aircraft accident investigators for decades. There are two possible explanations for this phenomenon. The first suggests that the psychologic stress of disorientation results in a disintegration of higher-order learned behavior, including flying skills. The second describes a complex psychomotor effect of disorientation that causes the pilot to feel the aircraft itself is misbehaving.

Disintegration of Flying Skill

The disintegration of flying skill perhaps begins with the pilot's realization that his or her spatial orientation and control over the motion of the aircraft have been compromised. Under such circumstances, the pilot pays more heed to whatever orientation information is naturally available, monitoring it more and more vigorously. Whether the brain stem reticular activating system or the vestibular efferent system or both are responsible for the resulting heightened arousal and enhanced vestibular information flow can only be surmised; the net effect, however, is that more erroneous vestibular information is processed and incorporated into the pi-

lot's orientational percept. This, of course, only makes matters worse. A positive-feedback situation is thus encountered, and the vicious circle can now be broken only with a precisely directed and very determined effort by the pilot. Unfortunately, complex cognitive and motor skills tend to be degraded under the conditions of psychologic stress that occur during Type II or Type III spatial disorientation. First, there is a coning of attention. Pilots who have survived severe disorientation have reported that they were concentrating on one particular flight instrument instead of scanning and interpreting the whole group of them in the usual manner. Pilots also have reported that they were unaware of radio transmissions to them while they were trying to recover from disorientation. Second, there is the tendency to revert to more primitive behavior, even reflex action, under conditions of severe psychologic stress. The highly developed, relatively newly acquired skill of instrument flying can give way to primal protective responses during disorientation stress, making appropriate recovery action unlikely. Third, it is often suggested that disoriented pilots become totally immobilized—frozen to the aircraft controls by fear or panic—as the disintegration process reaches its final state.

Giant Hand

The giant hand phenomenon described by Malcolm and Money (16) undoubtedly explains why many pilots have been rendered hopelessly confused and ineffectual by spatial disorientation, even though they knew they were disoriented and should have been able to avoid losing control of their aircraft. The pilot suffering from this effect of disorientation perceives falsely that the aircraft does not respond properly to his or her control inputs because every time the pilot tries to bring the aircraft to the desired attitude, it seems actively to resist his or her effort and fly back to another, more stable attitude. A pilot experiencing disorientation about the roll axis (e.g., the leans or graveyard spiral) may feel a force—like a giant hand—trying to push one

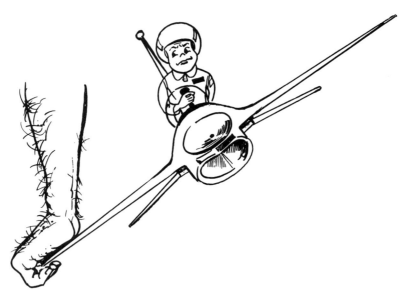

Figure 11.36. The giant hand phenomenon. This pilot, who is disoriented with respect to roll attitude (bank angle), feels the aircraft is resisting his conscious attempt to bring it to the desired attitude according to the flight instruments, as though a giant hand is holding it in the attitude compatible with his erroneous natural sense of roll attitude.

wing down and hold it there   (Fig. 11.36), whereas the pilot with pitch-axis disorientation (e.g., the classic somatogravic illusion) may feel the airplane subjected to a similar force trying to hold the nose down. The giant hand phenomenon is not rare: one report states that 15% of pilots responding to a questionnaire on spatial disorientation had experienced the giant hand (27). Pilots who are unaware of the existence of this phenomenon and experience it for the first time can be very surprised and confused by it and may not be able to discern the exact nature of their problem. A pilot's radio transmission that the aircraft controls are malfunctioning should not, therefore, be taken as conclusive evidence that a control malfunction caused a mishap: spatial disorientation could have been the real cause.

What mechanism could possibly explain the giant hand? To try to understand this phenomenon, we must first recognize that an individual's perception of orientation results not only in the conscious awareness of his or her position and motion but also in a preconscious percept needed for the proper performance of voluntary motor

activity and reflex actions. A conscious orientational percept can be considered rational in that one can subject it to intellectual scrutiny, weigh the evidence for its veracity, conclude that it is inaccurate, and to some extent modify the percept to fit facts obtained from other than the primary orientation senses. In contrast, a preconscious orientational percept must be considered irrational, in that it consists only of an integration of data relayed to the brain stem and cerebellum by the primary orientation senses and is not amenable to modification by reason. So what happens when a pilot knows he or she has become disorientated and tries to control the aircraft by reference to a conscious rational percept of orientation that is at variance with a preconscious, irrational one? Because only the data comprising one's preconscious orientational percept are available for the performance of orientational reflexes (e.g., postural reflexes) and a large part of skilled voluntary motor activity (e.g., walking, bicycling, flying), it is to be expected that the actual outcome of these types of actions will often deviate from the rationally intended outcome whenever the orientational data on which they depend are different from the rationally perceived orientation. The disoriented pilot who consciously commands a roll to recover aircraft control may experience a great deal of difficulty in executing the command, because the informational substrate in reference to which his or her body functions indicates that such a move is counterproductive or even dangerous. Or the pilot may discover that the roll, once accomplished, must be reaccomplished repeatedly, because preconsciously influenced arm motions automatically keeps returning the aircraft to its original flight attitude despite his or her conscious efforts and actions to regain control. Thus, the preconscious orientational percept influences Sherrington's "final common pathway" for both reflex and voluntary motor activity, and the manifestation of this influence on the act of flying during an episode of spatial disorientation is the giant hand phenomenon. To prevail in this conflict between will and skill, the pilot must decouple his or her voluntary acts from automatic flying behavior. It has been suggested that using the thumb and forefinger to move the control stick, rather than using the whole hand, can effect the necessary decoupling and thereby facilitate recovery from the giant hand.

Conditions Conducive to Disorientation

From a knowledge of the physiologic basis of the various illusions of flight, the reader can readily infer many of the specific environmental factors conducive to spatial disorientation. Certain visual phenomena produce characteristic visual illusions such as false horizons and vection. Prolonged turning at a constant rate, as in a holding pattern or procedure turn, can precipitate somatogyral illusions or the leans. Relatively sustained linear accelerations, such as occur on takeoff, can produce somatogravic illusions, and head movements during high-G turns can elicit G-excess illusions.

But what are the regimes of flight and activities of the pilot that seem most likely to allow these potential illusions to manifest themselves?

Certainly, instrument weather and night flying are primary factors. Especially likely to produce disorientation, however, is the practice of switching back and forth between the instrument flying mode and the visual, or contact, flying mode; a pilot is far less likely to become disoriented if he or she gets on the instruments as soon as out-of-cockpit vision is compromised and stays on the instruments until continuous contact flying is again assured. In fact, any event or practice requiring the pilot to break his or her instrument cross-check is conducive to disorientation. In this regard, avionics control switches and displays in some aircraft are located where the pilot must interrupt the instrument cross-check for more than just a few seconds to interact with them and are thus known as "vertigo traps." Some of these vertigo traps require substantial movements of the pilot's head during the time his or her cross-check is interrupted, thereby providing both a reason and an opportunity for spatial disorientation to strike.

Formation flying in adverse weather conditions is probably the most likely of all situations to produce disorientation; indeed, some experienced pilots get disoriented every time they fly wing or trail in weather. The fact that a pilot has little if any opportunity to scan the flight instruments while flying on the lead aircraft in weather means that he or she is essentially isolated from any source of accurate orientation information, and misleading vestibular and ambient cues arrive unchallenged into the orientational sensorium.

Of utmost importance to the pilot in preventing spatial disorientation is competency and currency in instrument flying. A noninstrument-rated pilot who penetrates instrument weather is virtually assured of developing spatial disorientation within a matter of seconds, just as competent instrument pilots would develop it if they found themselves flying in weather without functioning flight instruments. Regarding instrument flying skill, one must "use it or lose it," as they say. For that reason, it is inadvisable and usually illegal for one to act as a pilot in command of an aircraft in instrument weather if he or she has not had a certain amount of recent instrument flying experience.

Even highly capable instrument pilots are susceptible to spatial disorientation when their attention is diverted away from the flight instruments and they neglect the primary task of flying the airplane. This can happen when other duties, such as navigation, communication, operating weapons, responding to malfunctions and managing inflight emergencies, place excessive demands on the pilot's attention and he or she becomes "task saturated." In fact, virtually all aircraft mishaps involving Type I spatial disorientation occur as a result of the pilot's failure to prioritize properly his or her several tasks. "First, fly the airplane; then do other things as time allows," is always good advice for pilots, especially for those faced with a high mental workload. Not to prioritize in this manner can result in disorientation and disaster.

Finally, conditions affecting the pilot's physical or mental health must be considered capable of rendering the pilot more susceptible to spatial disorientation. The unhealthy effect of alcohol ingestion on neural information processing is one obvious example; however, the less well-known ability of alcohol to produce vestibular nystagmus (positional alcohol nystagmus) for many hours after its more overt effects have disappeared is probably of equal significance. Use of other drugs, such as barbiturates, amphetamines, and especially the illegal "recreational" drugs (marijuana, cocaine, etc.), certainly could contribute to the development of disorientation and precipitate aircraft mishaps. Likewise, physical and mental fatigue, as well as acute or chronic emotional stress, can rob the pilot of the ability to concentrate on the instrument cross-check and can, therefore, have deleterious effects on his or her resistance to spatial disorientation.

Prevention of Disorientation Mishaps

Spatial disorientation can be attacked in several ways. Theoretically, each link in the physiologic chain of events leading to a disorientation mishap can be broken by a specific countermeasure (Fig. 11.37). Many times, spatial disorientation can be prevented by modifying flying procedures to avoid those visual or vestibular motion and position stimuli that tend to create illusions in flight. Improving the capacity of flight instruments to translate aircraft position and motion information into readily assimilable orientation cues will help the pilot to avoid disorientation. Through repeated exposure to the environment of instrument flight, the pilot becomes proficient

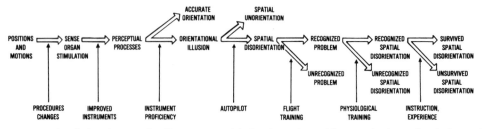

Figure 11.37. The chain of events leading to a spatial disorientation mishap, and where the chain can be attacked and broken. From the left: Flight procedures can be altered to generate less confusing sensory inputs. Improved instrument presentations can aid in the assimilation of orientation cues. Proficiency in instrument flying helps to assure accurate orientational percepts. In the event the pilot suffers an orientational illusion, having the aircraft under autopilot control avoids disorientation by substituting unorientation. Flight training helps the pilot prioritize his various tasks properly so he or she can recognize quickly that the aircraft is not flying the desired flight path. Once the pilot knows that a problem exists, the pilot's physiological training helps him or her realize that the problem is spatial disorientation. With appropriate instruction and/or firsthand experience, the pilot with recognized spatial disorientation can apply the correct control forces to recover the aircraft and survive the disorientation incident.

in instrument flying; this involves developing perceptual processes that result in accurate orientational percepts rather than orientational illusions. If a pilot who experiences an illusion is relegating primary control of flight parameters to an autopilot rather than directly controlling the aircraft, the fact that he or she has an orientational illusion is essentially irrelevant (i.e., the pilot has spatial unorientation rather than disorientation).

Use of an autopilot cannot only help prevent disorientation, but it can also help the pilot recover from it: i.e., the disoriented pilot can engage the autopilot and ride as a passenger until safely able to reclaim primary control of the aircraft. (Indeed, some fighter aircraft have a special "panic switch" which the disoriented pilot can activate to bring the aircraft back to a wings-level attitude.) If a pilot who has developed spatial disorientation can be made to recognize that he or she is disoriented, that pilot is well along the road to recovery. Recognizing disorientation is not necessarily easy, however. First, the pilot must be aware that he or she is having a problem holding altitude or heading; this the pilot cannot do if he or she is concentrating on something other than the flight instruments—the radar scope, for instance. Only through proper flight training can the appreciation of the need for appropriate task prioritization and the discipline of continuously performing the instrument cross-check be instilled. Second, the pilot must recognize that his or her difficulty in controlling the aircraft is a result of spatial disorientation. This ability is promoted through physiological training. Finally, a pilot's ability to cope with the effects of disorientation on his or her control inputs to the aircraft comes through effective flight instruction, proper physiological training, and experience in controlling a vehicle in an environment of conflicting orientation cues—the pilot's simply being aware that he or she is disoriented by no means ensures survival.

Education and Training

Physiological training is the main weapon against spatial disorientation at the disposal of the flight surgeon and aerospace physiologist. The training ideally should consist of both didactic material and demonstrations. There is no paucity of didactic material on the subject of disorientation: numerous films, videocassette tapes, slide sets, handbooks, and chapters in books and manuals have been prepared for the purpose of informing the pilot about the mechanisms and hazards of spatial disorientation. Although the efforts to generate information on spatial disorientation are commendable, there is a tendency for such didactic material to dwell too much on the mechanisms and effects of disorientation without giving much practical advice on how to deal with it.

We now emphasize to pilots a two-stage approach to preventing disorientation mishaps. First, minimize the likelihood of spatial disorientation by monitoring frequently and systematically the critical flight parameters (bank, pitch, vertical velocity, altitude) displayed by the flight instruments or a valid natural reference; conversely, expect to become disoriented if attention to these flight parameters is allowed to lapse as a result of misprioritizing the tasks at hand. Second, when disorientation does occur, recognize it as such and act. In the past, the standard advice was "Believe the instruments." Now we feel this message by itself is inadequate, because the pilot in a stressful, time-critical situation needs to know what to do to extricate himself or herself from the predicament, not merely how to analyze it. If a pilot is told "Make the instruments read right, regardless of your sensation," he or she has simple, definite instructions on how to bring the aircraft under control when disorientation strikes. We strongly advise that every presentation to pilots on the subject of spatial disorientation emphasize (1) the need to avoid disorientation by making frequent instrument cross-checks, and (2) the need to recover from disorientation by making the instruments read right.

The traditional demonstration accompanying lectures to the pilots on spatial disorientation is a ride on a Barany chair or some other smoothly rotating device. Sitting in the device with eyes closed, pilot traineees are accelerated to a constant angular velocity and asked to signal their perceived direction of turning. After a number of seconds (usually from 10 to 20) at constant angular velocity, the trainee loses the sensation of rotation and signals this fact to the observers. The instructor then suddenly stops the rotation, whereupon the trainee immediately indicates that he or she feels turning in the direction opposite to the original direction of rotation. Pilot trainees usually are asked to open their eyes during this part of the demonstration and are amazed to see that they are actually not turning, despite the strong vestibular sensation of rotation. After the described demonstration of somatogyral illusions, the trainee is again rotated at a constant velocity with eyes closed, this time with his or her head down (facing the floor). When the pilot trainee indicates his or her sensation of turning has ceased, the trainee is asked to raise his or her head abruptly so as to face the wall. The Coriolis illusion resulting from this maneuver is one of a very definite roll to one side: the startled trainee may exhibit a protective postural reflex and may open his or her eyes to help visually orient during this falsely perceived upset. The message delivered with these demonstrations is not that such illusions will be experienced in flight in the same manner, but that the vestibular sense can be fooled (i.e., is unreliable) and that only the flight instruments provide accurate orientation information.

Over the years, at least a dozen different training devices have been developed to augment or supplant the Barany chair for demonstrating various vestibular and visual illusions and the effects of disorientation in flight. These devices fall into two basic categories: orientational illusion demonstrators and spatial disorientation demonstrators. The majority are illusion demonstrators, in which the trainee rides passively and experiences one or more of the following: somatogyral, oculogyral, somatogravic, oculogravic, Coriolis, G-excess, vection, false horizon, and autokinetic illusions. In an illusion demonstra-

tor, the trainee typically is asked to record or remember the magnitude and direction of the orientational illusion and then is told or otherwise allowed to experience his or her true orientation. A few devices actually put the trainee in the motion control loop and allow him or her to experience the difficulty in controlling the attitude and motion of the device while being subjected to various vestibular and visual illusions. Figure 11.38 shows two such spatial disorientation demonstrators presently in use.

Although the maximal use of ground-based spatial disorientation training devices in the physiological training of pilots is to be encouraged, it is important to recognize the great potential for misuse of such devices by personnel not thoroughly trained in their theory and function. Several devices have aircraft-instrument tracking tasks for the trainee to perform while he or she is experiencing orientational illusions but is not actually controlling the motion of the trainer. The temptation is very strong for unsophisticated operating personnel to tell the trainee he or she is ''fighting disorientation'' if he or she performs well on the tracking task while being subjected to the illusion-generating motions. Because the trainee's real orientation is irrelevant to the tracking task, any orientational illusion is also irrelevant and he or she experiences no conflict between visual and vestibular information in acquiring cues on which to base the control responses. This situation, of course, does not capture the essence of disorientation in flight, and the trainees who are led to believe they are fighting disorientation in such a ground-based demonstration may develop a false sense of security about their ability to combat disorientation in flight. The increasing use of spatial disorientation demonstrators in which the subject must control the actual motion of the trainer by referring to true-reading instruments while under the influence of orientational illusions will reduce the potential for misuse and improve the effectiveness of presentations to pilots on the subject of spatial disorientation.

Flight training provides a good opportunity to

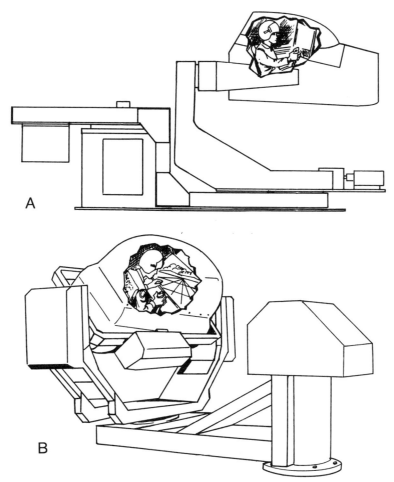

Figure 11.38. Two spatial disorientation demonstrators currently available for physiological training—the Model 2400 Vertifuge (*A*) and the Gyrolab 3000 (*B*). Both devices use somatogyral, somatogravic, and other vestibular illusions, as well as focal and ambient visual illusions, to create disorientation in the trainee, who "flies" the cockpit by reference to flight instruments.

instruct pilots about the hazards of spatial disorientation. In-flight demonstrations of vestibular illusions are included in most formalized pilot training curricula, although the efficacy of such demonstrations is highly dependent on the motivation and skill of the individual flight instructor. Somatogyral and somatogravic illusions and illusions of roll attitude usually can be induced in a student pilot by a flight instructor who either understands how the vestibular system works or knows from experience which maneuvers consistently produce illusions. The vestibular illusion demonstrations should not be confused with the unusual-attitude-recovery demonstrations in the typical pilot training syllabus: the objective of the former is for the student to experience orientational illusions and recognize them as such, whereas the objective of the latter is for the student to learn to regain control of an aircraft in a safe and expeditious manner. In both types of demonstration, however, control of the aircraft should be handed over to the student pilot with the instruction, "Make the instruments read right."

Part of flight training is continuing practice to maintain flying proficiency, and the importance of such practice in reducing the likelihood of having a disorientation mishap cannot be overemphasized. Whether flying instruments in formation or in aerobatic maneuvering, familiarity with the environment (based on recent exposure to it) and proficiency at the flying task (based on recent practice at it) result not only in a greater ability to avoid or dispel orientational illusions but also in a greater ability to cope with disorientation when it does occur.

Inflight Procedures

If a particular in-flight procedure frequently results in spatial disorientation, it stands to reason that modifying or eliminating that procedure should help to reduce aircraft mishaps due to disorientation. Night formation takeoffs and rejoins are examples of in-flight procedures that are very frequently associated with spatial disorientation, and the United States Air Force wisely has officially discouraged these practices in most of its major commands.

Another area of concern is the ''lost wingman'' procedure, which is used when a pilot has lost sight of the aircraft on which he or she has been flying wing. Usually the loss of visual contact is due to poor visibility and occurs after a period of vacillation between formation flying and instrument flying; this, of course, invites disorientation. The lost wingman procedure must, therefore, be made as uncomplicated as possible while still allowing safe separation from the other elements of the flight. Maintaining a specified altitude and heading away from the flight until further notice is an ideal lost wingman procedure in that it avoids frequent or prolonged disorientation-inducing turns and minimizes cognitive workload. Often, a pilot flying wing in bad weather does not lose sight of the lead aircraft but suffers so much disorientation stress as to make the option of going lost wingman seem safer than that of continuing in the formation. A common practice in this situation is for the wingman to take the lead position in the formation, at least until the disorientation disappears. This avoids the necessity of having the disoriented pilot make a turn away from the flight to go lost wingman, a turn that could be

especially difficult and dangerous because of his or her disorientation. One should question the wisdom of having a disoriented pilot leading a flight, however, and some experts in the field of spatial disorientation are adamantly opposed to this practice, with good reason.

Verbal communication can help keep a pilot from becoming disoriented during formation flying in weather, when workload is high and the pilot's visual access to the flight instruments is by necessity infrequent. The leader of the flight should report periodically to the wingman what the flight is doing; i.e., lead should announce his or her pitch and bank attitude, altitude, vertical velocity, heading, and airspeed as necessary to allow the wingman to construct a mental image of his or her own spatial orientation. If the wingman has already become disoriented, the lead pilot still needs to tell the wingman the correct orientation information, but also needs to provide some potentially life-saving advice about what to do. Unfortunately, no clear-cut procedure exists for ensuring appropriate communications. Should disoriented pilots be hounded mercilessly with verbal orders to get on the instruments or should they be left relatively undistracted to solve their orientation problem? The extremes of harassment and neglect are definitely not appropriate; a few forceful, specific, action-oriented commands probably represent the best approach. ''Level the artificial horizon!'' and ''Roll right 90°!'' are examples of such commands. One must remember that the pilot suffering from spatial disorientation may be either so busy or so functionally compromised that complex instructions may fall on deaf ears. Simple, emphatic directions may be the only means of penetrating the disoriented pilot's consciousness.

To illustrate how official recommendations regarding inflight procedures are disseminated to pilots in an effort to prevent spatial disorientation mishaps, a message from a major United States Air Force command headquarters to field units is excerpted here:

. . .Review SD procedures in [various Air Force manuals] . . . Discuss the potential for SD during flight briefings prior to flight involving night, weather, or conditions where visibility is significantly reduced . . . Recognize the [SD] problem early and initiate corrective actions before aircraft control is compromised.

A. Single ship:

(1) Keep the head in the cockpit. Concentrate on flying basic instruments with frequent reference to the attitude indicator. Defer nonessential cockpit chores.

(2) If symptoms persist, bring aircraft to straight and level flight using the attitude indicator. Maintain straight and level flight until symptoms abate—usually 30 to 60 seconds. Use autopilot if necessary.

(3) If necessary, declare an emergency and advise air traffic control. Note: It is possible for SD to proceed to the point where the pilot is unable to see, interpret, or process information from the flight instruments. Aircraft control in such a situation is impossible. A pilot must recognize when physiological/psychological limits have been exceeded and be prepared to abandon the aircraft.

B. Formation flights:

(1) Separate aircraft from the formation under controlled conditions if the weather encountered is either too dense or turbulent to insure safe flight.

(2) A flight lead with SD will advise his wingmen that he has SD and he will comply with procedures in Paragraph A. If possible, wingmen should confirm straight and level attitude and provide verbal feedback to lead. If symptoms do not abate in a reasonable time, terminate the mission and recover the flight by the simplest and safest means possible.

(3) Two-ship information. Wingman will advise lead when he experiences significant SD symptoms.

(a) Lead will advise wingman of aircraft attitude heading, and airspeed.

(b) The wingman will advise lead if problems persist. If so, lead will establish straight and level flight for at least 30 to 60 seconds.

(c) If the above procedures are not effective, lead should transfer the flight lead position to the wingman *while in straight and level flight.* Once assuming lead, maintain straight and level flight for 60 seconds. If necessary, terminate the mission and recover by the simplest and safest means possible.

(4) More than two-ship formation. Lead should separate the flight into elements to more effectively handle a wingman with persistent SD symptoms. Establish straight and level flight. The element with the SD pilot will remain straight and level while other element separates from the flight.

Cockpit Layout and Flight Instruments

One of the most notorious vertigo traps is the communications-transceiver frequency selector or transponder code selector located in an obscure part of the cockpit. To manipulate this selector requires the pilot not only to look away from the flight instruments, which interrupts the instrument scan, but also to tilt his or her head to view the readout, which potentially subjects the pilot to G-excess and Coriolis illusions. Aircraft designers are now aware that easy accessibility and viewing of such frequently used devices minimize the potential for spatial disorientation; accordingly, most modern aircraft have communications frequency and transponder code selectors and readouts located in front of the pilot near the flight instruments.

The location of the flight instruments themselves is also very important. They should be clustered directly in front of the pilot and the attitude indicator, the primary provider of orientation cueing and the primary instrument by

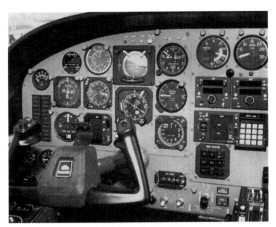

Figure 11.39. A well-designed instrument panel, with the attitude indicator located directly in front of the pilot and the other flight instruments clustered around it. Radios and other equipment requiring frequent manipulation and viewing are placed close to the flight instruments to minimize interruption of the pilot's instrument scan and to obviate his or her having to make head movements that could precipitate spatial disorientation. (Photo courtesy of Gen-Aero Inc. of San Antonio, Texas.)

which the aircraft is controlled, should be in the center of the cluster (Fig. 11.39). When this principle is not respected, the potential for spatial disorientation is increased. One modern fighter aircraft, for example, was designed to have the pilot sitting high in the cockpit to enhance the field-of-view during air-to-air combat in conditions of good visibility. This design relegates the attitude indicator to a position more or less between the pilot's knees. As a result, at night and during instrument weather, the pilot is subjected to potentially disorienting peripheral visual motion and position cueing by virtue of his or her being surrounded by a vast expanse of canopy, while he or she tries to glean with central vision the correct orientation information from a relatively small, distant attitude indicator. The net effect is an unusually difficult orientation problem for the pilot and a greater risk of developing spatial disorientation in this aircraft than in others with a more advantageously located attitude indicator.

The verisimilitude of the flight instruments is

a major factor in their ability to convey readily assimilable orientation information. The old "needle, ball, and airspeed" indicators (a needle pointer showing the direction and rate of turn, a ball showing whether the turn is being properly coordinated with the rudders, and an airspeed indicator showing whether the airplane is climbing or diving) required a lot of interpretation for the pilot to perceive his or her spatial orientation through them; nevertheless, this combination sufficed for nearly a generation of pilots. When the attitude indicator (also known as the gyro horizon, artificial horizon, or attitude gyro) was introduced, it greatly reduced the amount of work required to spatially orient during instrument flying because the pilot could readily imagine the artificial horizon line to be the real horizon. In addition to becoming more reliable and more versatile over the years, it became even easier to interpret: the face was divided into a gray or blue "sky" half and a black or brown "ground" half, with some models even having lines of perspective converging to a vanishing point in the lower half. Such a high degree of similarity to the real world has made the attitude indicator the mainstay of instrument flying today.

A relatively new concept in flight instrumentation, the head-up display (HUD), projects numeric and other symbolic information to the pilot from a combining glass near the windscreen, so that he or she can be looking forward out of the cockpit and simultaneously monitoring flight and weapons data. When the pilot selects the appropriate display mode, the pitch and roll attitude of the aircraft are observed on the "pitch ladder" (Fig. 11.40) and heading, altitude, airspeed, and other parameters are numerically displayed elsewhere on the HUD. Its upfront location and its close-together arrangement of most of the required aircraft control and performance data make the HUD a possible improvement over the conventional cluster of instruments with regard to minimizing the likelihood of spatial disorientation. Pilot's acceptance and use of the HUD for flying in

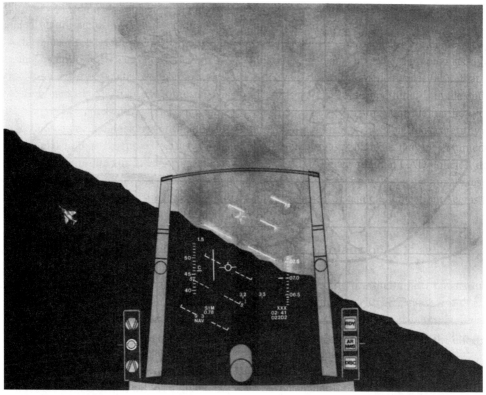

Figure 11.40. A typical head-up display (HUD). The pitch ladder in the center of the display provides pitch and roll attitude information.

instrument weather has not been universal, however. Many pilots prefer to use the HUD under conditions of good outside visibility and use the conventional instruments for flying at night and in weather.

This is understandable, because in some ways the HUD is inferior to the conventional flight instruments in being able to provide spatial orientation information that can readily be assimilated. One reason is that the HUD presents a relatively narrow view of the outside world—a "vernier" view with high resolution—while the conventional attitude indicator gives an expansive, "global" view of the spatial environment. Another reason is that the relative instability of the HUD pitch ladder and the frequency with which the zero-pitch line (horizon) disappears from view make the HUD difficult to use during moderately active maneuvering, as would be necessary during an unusual-attitude recovery

attempt. A third reason may be that the horizon on the conventional attitude instrument looks more like the natural horizon than does the zero-pitch line on the HUD pitch ladder. Nevertheless, at the time of this writing, the HUD is the sole source of primary (aircraft control and performance) flight information in at least one aircraft (the US Navy F/A-18 Hornet), and the United States Air Force is planning to approve the use of the HUD as the primary flight reference in its HUD-equipped aircraft. Attempts to eliminate the potpourri of HUD symbologies and arrive at a maximally efficient, standardized display are also being made.

As good as they are, both the attitude indicator and the HUD leave much to be desired as flight instruments for assuring spatial orientation. Both suffer from the basic design deficiency of presenting visual spatial orientation information to the wrong sensory system—the focal visual system. Two untoward effects result. First, the pilot's focal vision not only must serve to discriminate numeric data from a number of instruments but also must take on the task of spatially orienting the pilot. Thus, the pilot has to employ focal vision system in a somewhat inefficient manner during instrument flight, with most of his or her time spent viewing the attitude indicator or pitch ladder, while ambient vision remains unutilized (or worse, is being bombarded with misleading orientational stimuli). Second, the fact that focal vision is not naturally equipped to provide primary spatial orientation cues causes difficulty for pilots in interpreting the artificial horizon directly. There is a tendency, especially among novice pilots, to interpret the displayed deviations in roll and pitch backward and to make initial roll and pitch corrections in the wrong direction. Several approaches have been taken to try to improve the efficiency of the pilot's acquisition of orientation information from the attitude indicator and associated flight instruments. One has been to make the artificial horizon stationary but to roll and pitch the small aircraft on the instrument display to indicate the motion of the real aircraft (the so-called ''outside-in'' presentation, as opposed to the ''inside-out'' presentation of conventional attitude displays). Theoretically, this configuration relieves the pilot of having to orient himself or herself spatially before trying to fly the aircraft: rather, the pilot merely flies the small aircraft on the attitude instrument and the real aircraft follows. Another approach involves letting the artificial horizon provide pitch information but having the small aircraft on the attitude instrument provide roll information (e.g., the Crane Flitegage). Neither of these approaches, however, frees foveal vision from the unnatural task of processing spatial orientation information. Another concept, the peripheral vision display (PVD), also known as the Malcolm horizon, attempts to give pitch and roll cues to the pilot through his or her peripheral vision, thus sparing foveal vision for tasks requiring a high degree of visual discrimination. The PVD projects across the instrument panel a long, thin line of light representing the true horizon; this line of light moves directly in accordance with the relative movement of the true horizon (Fig. 11.41). The PVD has been incorporated into at least one military aircraft, but its limited pitch display range and certain other characteristics have prevented an enthusiastic acceptance of this display concept.

The eventual solution to the spatial disorientation problems lies, we believe, in head-mounted display (HMD) technology. The revolution in computer image-generation capability and advances in optical and acoustic techniques will ultimately allow the display of a synthesized representation of the natural spatial environment over the full visual field at optical infinity and in three dimensions of auditory space (Fig. 11.42). HMDs are already being used in military aircraft to provide targeting and basic flight control and performance information. Further development is needed, however, to reach the point where an electronically enhanced visual and auditory spatial environment is displayed superimposed on the real world, so that the pilot can spatially orient in a completely natural fashion, using a synthetic device.

Other Sensory Phenomena

Flicker vertigo, fascination, and target hypnosis are traditionally described in conjunction with spatial disorientation, although, strictly speaking, these entities involve alterations of attention rather than aberrations of perception. Neither is the break-off phenomenon related directly to spatial disorientation, but the unusual sensory manifestations of this condition make a discussion of it here seem appropriate.

Flicker Vertigo

As most people are aware from personal experience, viewing a flickering light or scene can be distracting, annoying, or both. In aviation, flicker is sometimes created by helicopter rotors or idling airplane propellers interrupting direct sunlight or, less frequently, by such things as several

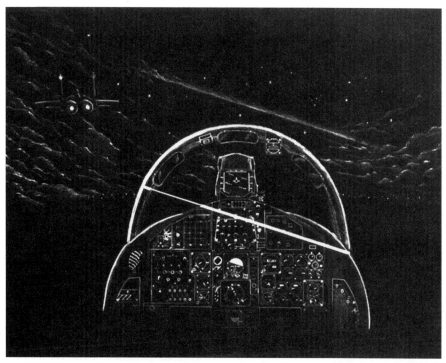

Figure 11.41. The peripheral vision display (PVD), or Malcolm horizon. An artificial horizon projected across the instrument panel moves in accordance with the real horizon, and the pilot observes the projected horizon and its movement with ambient vision.

anticollision lights flashing in nonunison. Pilots report that such conditions are indeed a source of irritation and distraction, but there is little evidence that flicker induces either spatial disorientation or clinical vertigo in normal aircrew. In fact, one authority insists there is no such thing as flicker vertigo and that the original reference to it was merely speculation (28). Certainly, helicopter rotors or rotating beacons on aircraft can produce angular vection illusions because they create revolving shadows or revolving areas of illumination; However, vection does not result from flicker. Symptoms of motion sickness also conceivably result from the sensory conflict associated with angular vection but, again, these symptoms would be produced by revolving lights and shadows and not by flicker.

Nevertheless, one should be aware that photic stimuli at frequencies in the 8- to 14-Hz range, that of the electroencephalographic alpha rhythm, can produce seizures in those rare individuals who are susceptible to flicker-induced epilepsy. Although the prevalence of this condition is very low (less than 1 in 20,000), and the number of pilots affected are very few, some helicopter crashes are thought to have been caused by pilots suffering from flicker-induced epilepsy.

Fascination

Coning of attention is something everyone experiences every day, but it is especially likely to occur when one is stressed by the learning of new skills or by the relearning of old ones. Pilots are apt to concentrate on one particular aspect of the flying task to the relative exclusion of others when that aspect is novel or unusually demanding. If this concentration is of sufficient degree to cause the pilot to disregard important information to which he or she should respond, it is termed fascination. An extreme example of fascination is when the pilot becomes so intent

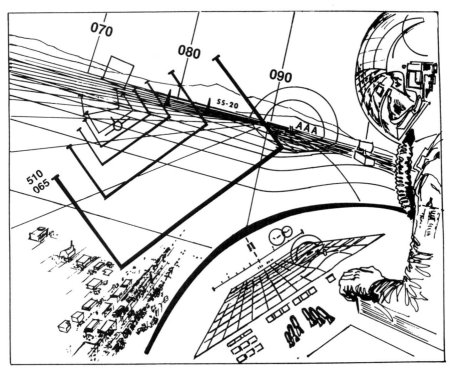

Figure 11.42. Artist's concept of an advanced helmet-mounted display. A computer-generated image of the plane of the earth's surface and other critical flight information are displayed on the helmet visor at optical infinity, superimposed on the real world.

on delivering weapons to the target that he or she ignores the obvious cues of ground proximity and flies into the ground. Mishaps of this sort are said to result from target hypnosis; no actual hypnotic process is suspected or should be inferred, however. Other examples of fascination in aviation are: 1) the monitoring of one flight instrument rather than cross-checking many of them during particularly stressful instrument flight; 2) paying so much attention to flying precise formation that other duties are neglected; and 3) the aviator's most ignominious act of negligence, landing an airplane with the landing gear up, despite the clearly perceived warning from the gear-up warning horn. These examples help us to appreciate the meaning of the original definition of fascination by Clark and colleagues: "a condition in which the pilot fails to respond adequately to a clearly defined stimulus situation in spite of the fact that all the necessary cues are present for a proper response and the

correct procedure is well known to him'' (29). From the definition and the examples given, it is clear that fascination can involve either a sensory deficiency or an inability to act, or perhaps both. It also is known that fascination, at least the type involving sensory deficiency, occurs not only under conditions of relatively high work load but also can occur when work load is greatly reduced and tedium prevails. Finally, the reader should understand that coning of attention, such as occurs with fascination, is not the same thing as tunneling of vision, which occurs with G stress: even if all pertinent sensory cues could be made accessible to foveal vision, the attentional lapses associated with fascination still could prevent those cues from being perceived or eliciting a response.

Break-off

In 1957, Clark and Graybiel (30) reported a condition that is perhaps best described by the title of their paper: "The break-off phenomenon—a feeling of separation from the earth experienced by pilots at high altitude." They found that 35% of 137 United States Navy and Marine Corps jet pilots interviewed by them had had feelings of being detached, isolated, or physically separated from the earth when flying at high altitudes. The three conditions most frequently associated with the experience were: 1) high altitude (approximately 5000 to 15,000 with a median of 10,000 m or 15,000, 45,000 and 33,000 ft, respectively); 2) being alone in the aircraft; and 3) not being particularly busy with operating the aircraft. The majority of the pilots interviewed found the break-off experience exhilarating, peaceful, or otherwise pleasant; over a third, however, felt anxious, lonely, or insecure. No operational importance could be ascribed to the break-off phenomenon; specifically, it was not considered to have any significant effect on a pilot's ability to operate the aircraft. The authors nevertheless suggested that the break-off experience might have significant effects on a pilot's performance when coupled with preexisting anxiety or fear, and for that reason, the phenomenon should be described to pilots before they go alone to high altitudes for the first time. Break-off may, on the other hand, have a profound, positive effect on the motivation to fly. Who could deny the importance of this experience to John Gillespie Magee, Jr., who gave us "High Flight," the most memorable poem in aviation?

"Oh, I have slipped the surly bonds of the earth . . . Put out my hand, and touched the face of God."

MOTION SICKNESS

Motion sickness is a perennial aeromedical problem. The important syndrome is discussed in this chapter to emphasize the critical importance of the spatial orientation senses in its pathogenesis; so closely entwined, in fact, are the mechanisms of spatial orientation and those of

motion sickness that orientation is sometimes (and legitimately) used as the general term for the category of related conditions that are commonly referred to as motion sickness.

Definition, Description, and Significance of Motion Sickness

Motion sickness is a state of diminished health characterized by specific symptoms that occur in conjunction with and in response to unaccustomed conditions existing in one's motional environment. These symptoms usually progress from lethargy, apathy, and stomach awareness to nausea, pallor, and cold eccrine perspiration, then to retching and vomiting, and finally to total prostration if measures are not taken to arrest the progression. The sequence of these major symptoms is generally predictable; and vestibular scientists have devised a commonly used scale, consisting of five steps from mild malaise to frank sickness, to quantify the severity of motion sickness according to the level of symptoms manifested (31). Under some conditions, however, emesis can occur precipitously, i.e., without premonitory symptoms. Other symptoms sometimes seen with motion sickness are headache, increased salivation and swallowing, decreased appetite, eructation, flatulence, and feeling warm. Although vomiting provides temporary relief from the symptoms of motion sickness, the symptoms usually will return if the offending motion or other condition continues, and the vomiting will be replaced by nonproductive retching, or "dry heaves." A wide variety of motions and orientational conditions qualify as offensive, so there are many species of the generic term motion sickness. Among them are seasickness, airsickness, car sickness, train sickness, amusement-park-ride sickness, camel sickness, motion-picture sickness, flight-simulator sickness, and the most recent addition to the list, space motion sickness.

Military Experience

Armstrong (32) has provided us with some interesting statistics on airsickness associated with the World War II military effort:

. . . it was learned that 10 to 11 percent of all flying students became air sick during their first 10 flights, and that 1 to 2 percent of them were eliminated from flying training for that reason. Other aircrew members in training had even greater difficulty and the airsickness rate among them ran as high as 50 percent in some cases. It was also found that fully trained combat crews, other than pilots, sometimes became air sick which affected their combat efficiency. An even more serious situation was found to exist among air-borne troops. Under very unfavorable conditions as high as 70 percent of these individuals became air sick and upon landing were more or less temporarily disabled at a time when their services were most urgently needed.

More recent studies of the incidence of airsickness in United States and British military flight training reveal that approximately 40% of aircrew trainees become airsick at some time during their training. In student pilots, there is a 15% to 18% incidence of motion sickness that is severe enough to interfere with control of the aircraft. Airsickness in student aviators occurs almost exclusively during the first several training flights, during spin training, and during the first dual aerobatic flights. The adaptation of which most people are capable is evidenced by the fact that only about 1% of military pilot trainees are eliminated from flight training because of intractable airsickness. The percentage of other aircrew trainees eliminated because of airsickness is considerably higher, however.

Although trained pilots almost never become airsick while flying the aircraft themselves, they surely can become sick while riding as a copilot or as a passenger. Other trained aircrew, such as navigators and weapon systems operators, are likewise susceptible to airsickness. Particularly provocative for these aircrew are flights in turbulent weather, low-level "terrain-following" flights, and flights in which high G forces are repeatedly experienced, as in air combat training and bombing practice. Both the lack of foreknowledge of aircraft motion, which results

from not having primary control of the aircraft, and the lack of a constant view of the external world, which results from having duties involving the monitoring of in-cockpit displays, are significant factors in the development of airsickness in these aircrew.

Simulator Sickness

Flight simulator sickness is getting increased attention now as aircrew spend more and more time in flight simulators capable of ever greater realism. Currently used high-quality military flight simulators are reported to elicit symptoms in 40% to 70% of trainees. Generally these symptoms are the usual drowsiness, perspiration, and nausea that occur in other forms of motion sickness; vomiting rarely occurs because simulated flights can readily be terminated prior to reaching the point of emesis. Symptoms associated with eyestrain (headache, blurring of vision) are also quite common. But of particular aeromedical interest is the fact that simulator exposure also frequently results in post-flight disturbances of posture and locomotion, transient disorientation, involuntary visual flashbacks, and other manifestations of acute sensory rearrangement. Simulator sickness is more likely to occur in simulators that employ wide-field-of-view, optical-infinity, computer-generated visual displays, both with and without motion bases, than in those providing less realistic ambient visual stimulation. Helicopter simulators are especially likely to generate symptoms, probably because of the greater freedom of movement available to these aircraft at low altitudes. Interestingly, simulator sickness is more likely to occur in pilots having considerable experience in the specific aircraft that is being simulated than in pilots without such experience. Symptoms usually disappear within several hours after termination of the simulated flight, but a small percentage of subjects have symptoms of disequilibrium persisting as long as one day after exposure. Because of the possibility of transient sensory and motor disturbances following intensive training in a flight simulator, it is recommended that aircrew not resume normal flying duties in real aircraft until the day after training in simulators known to be capable of inducing simulator sickness. As is the case with other motion environments, repeated exposure to the simulated motion environment usually renders aircrew less susceptible to its effects.

Civil Experience

The incidence of airsickness in the flight training of civilians can only be estimated, but is probably somewhat less than that for their military counterparts because the training of civil pilots usually does not include spins and other aerobatics. Very few passengers in today's commercial air-transport aircraft become airsick, largely because the altitudes at which these aircraft generally fly are usually free of turbulence. This cannot be said, however, for passengers of most lighter, less capable, general aviation aircraft, who often must spend considerable portions of their flights at the lower, "bumpier" altitudes.

Space Motion Sickness

The challenge of space flight includes coping with space motion sickness, a form of motion sickness experienced first by cosmonaut Titov and subsequently by approximately 50% of spacecrew. The incidence of space motion sickness has been significantly greater in the larger space vehicles (e.g., Skylab, Shuttle), in which crew members make frequent head and body movements, than in the smaller vehicles (e.g., Apollo), in which such movements were more difficult. Although space motion sickness resembles other forms of motion sickness, the emesis occurring in space vehicles often is not associated with the customary prodromal nausea and cold sweat, but rather occurs precipitously. This same phenomenon can occur, however, in other novel orientational environments when the level of stimulation is very low and prolonged or very intense and sudden. Because of the similarity between the sudden vomiting associated with space flight and the "projectile" vomiting

frequently seen in patients with increased intracranial pressure, a theory was proposed that the sickness precipitated by space flight was due to a cephalad fluid shift resulting from the zero-G environment. This fluid shift theory is no longer popular, having been replaced by the more conservative consensus that the symptoms generated by space flight have the same origin as those of ordinary motion sickness—hence the commonly accepted terminology, "space motion sickness."

The time course of space motion sickness symptom development and resolution is presented graphically in Figure 11.43. Symptoms usually appear within a few minutes to several hours after exposure, plateau for hours to several days, and rapidly resolve by 36 hours on average. One feature of space motion sickness that bears special mention is a characteristic adynamic ileus, evidenced by the profound lack of bowel sounds. Because of this absence of normal gastrointestinal activity, nutrition is compromised until adaptation occurs. As a consequence of their adaptation to the zero-G environment, some spacecrew again experience motion sickness upon their return to Earth, although the severity and duration of symptoms tend to be less than they were during their initial exposure to space. Spacecrew are also reported to be especially resistant to other forms of motion sickness (e.g., airsickness, seasickness) for up to several weeks after returning from space.

Space motion sickness has a definite negative effect on the efficiency of manned space operations, with on the order of 10% of crewmembers being affected to the point that their performance is significantly impaired. Thus, the potential impact of space motion sickness on manned space operations must be minimized by appropriate mission planning. If possible, duties involving less locomotion should be scheduled early in the flight. Because of the possibility of space motion sickness-induced emesis into a space suit and the consequent risk of life and mission success, extravehicular activity (EVA) should not be undertaken before the third day of a space mission.

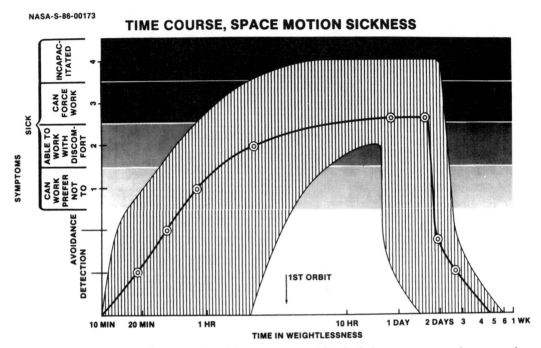

Figure 11.43. Time course of space motion sickness symptoms. The shaded area represents the range of symptoms recorded from Space Shuttle crewmembers. (From Thornton WE, et al. Clinical characterization and etiology of space motion sickness. Aviat Space Environ Med 1987;58:A1–A8.)

By that time adaptation to the novel environment is largely complete, and the head and body movements concomitant with EVA are much less likely to provoke symptoms than they would have been prior to adaptation. (Of interest is the fact that pitching motions of the head are the most provocative, followed by rolling and yawing motions, and that such motions are more provocative with eyes open than with eyes closed. Those observations suggest that otolith-organ-mediated changes in vestibulo-ocular reflex gain during altered gravitational states constitute at least part of the underlying mechanism of space motion sickness (33).)

Another type of space sickness will be encountered in the event that larger space stations are rotated to generate G-loading for the purpose of alleviating the fluid shift, cardiovascular deconditioning, and skeletal demineralization that occur in the zero-G environment. Vestibular Coriolis effects created in occupants of such rotating systems are very potent procedures of mo-

tion sickness and would be expected to plague the occupants for several days after arrival. Of course, after the space station personnel have become adapted to the rotating environment, they would be disadapted to the nonrotating one and would suffer from motion sickness upon returning to Earth.

Etiology of Motion Sickness

We have speculated about the causes of and reasons for motion sickness for thousands of years. Largely because of the scientific interest in motion sickness that has been generated by naval and aerospace activities of the present century, we may now have a satisfactory explanation for this puzzling malady.

Correlating Factors

As already mentioned, motion sickness occurs in response to conditions to which one is not accustomed in the normal motional environment. Motional environment means all of the linear and angular positions, velocities, and accelerations that are directly sensed or secondarily perceived as determining one's spatial orientation. The primary quantities of relevance here are mechanically (as opposed to visually) perceived linear and angular acceleration—i.e., those stimuli that act on the vestibular end-organs. Certainly, the pitching, rolling, heaving, and surging motions of ships in bad weather are clearly correlated with motion sickness, as are the pitching, rolling, yawing, and positive and negative G-pulling of aircraft during maneuvering. Abnormal stimulation of the semicircular ducts alone, as with a rotating chair, can result in motion sickness. So also can abnormal stimulation of the otolith organs alone, as occurs in an elevator or a four-pole swing. Whether the stimulation provided is complex, as is usually the case on ships and in aircraft, or simple, such as that generated in the laboratory, the important point is that abnormal labyrinthine stimulation is associated with the production of motion sickness. Not only is a modicum of abnormal vestibular stimulation sufficient to cause motion sickness, but some amount of vestibular stimulation is also necessary for motion sickness to occur. Labyrinthectomized experimental animals and humans without functioning vestibular end-organs (so-called "labyrinthine defectives") are completely immune to motion sickness.

The visual system can play two very important roles in the production of motion sickness. First, self-motion sensed solely through vision (i. e., vection) can make some people sick. Examples of this phenomenon are: motion-picture sickness, in which wide-screen movies of rides on airplanes, roller-coasters, and ships in rough seas are provocative; microscope sickness, in which susceptible individuals cannot tolerate viewing moving microscopic slides; and flight-simulator sickness, in which wide-field-of-view visual motion systems create motion sickness in the absence of any mechanical motion. Abnormal stimulation of ambient vision rather than of focal vision appears to be the essential feature

of visually induced motion sickness. The fact that orientation information processed through the ambient visual system converges on the vestibular nuclei helps to reconcile the phenomenon of visually induced motion sickness with the necessity for functioning vestibular end-organs. The second role of vision in the etiology of motion sickness is illustrated by the well-known fact that the absence of an outside visual reference makes persons undergoing abnormal motion more likely to become sick than they would be if an outside visual reference were available. Good examples of this are the sailor who becomes sick below deck but prevents the progression of motion sickness by coming topside to view the horizon, and the aircrewman who becomes sick while attending to duties inside the aircraft (e.g., radarscope monitoring) but alleviates the symptoms by looking outside.

Other sensory systems capable of providing primary spatial orientational information also are capable of providing avenues for motion-sickness-producing stimuli. The auditory system, when stimulated by a revolving sound source, is responsible for audiogenic vertigo, audiokinetic nystagmus, and concomitant symptoms of motion sickness. Nonvestibular proprioceptors may contribute to the development of motion sickness when the pattern of stimulation of these senses by linear and angular accelerations is unfamiliar. Perhaps more important than the actual sensory channel employed or the actual pattern of stimulation delivered, however, is the degree to which the spatial orientational information received deviates from that anticipated. The experience with motion sickness in various flight simulators bears witness to the importance of unexpected patterns of motion and unfulfilled expectations of motion. Instructor pilots in the 2-FH-2 helicopter hover trainer, for example, were much more likely to become sick in the device than were student pilots. It is postulated that imperfections in flight simulation are perceived by pilots who, as a result of their experience in the real aircraft, expect certain orientational stimuli to occur in response to certain control inputs. Pilots without time in the real aircraft, on the other hand, have no such expectations, and therefore notice no deviations from them in the simulator. Another example of the role played by the expectation of motion in the generation of motion sickness is seen in the pilot who does not become sick as long as he or she has control of the airplane but does become sick when another pilot is flying the same maneuvers in the same airplane. In this case, the pilot's expectation of motion is always fulfilled whenever he or she is controlling the airplane but is not fulfilled when someone else is flying.

Several other variables not primarily related to spatial orientation seem to correlate well with motion sickness susceptibility. Age is one such variable: susceptibility increases with age until puberty and then decreases thereafter. Sex is another: women are more susceptible to motion sickness than men (two-thirds more women than men become seasick on ocean-going ferry boats, for example). In concordance with popular opinion, there is some scientific evidence that having eaten just prior to motion exposure tends to increase motion sickness susceptibility. There is also evidence suggesting that a high level of aerobic conditioning increases one's susceptibility to motion sickness, possibly as a result of increased parasympathetic tone. The personality characteristics of emotional lability and excessive rigidity are also positively correlated with motion sickness susceptibility. Whether one is mentally occupied with a significant task during exposure to motion or is free to dwell on orientation cues and the state of one's stomach seems to affect susceptibility—the latter, more introverted state is more conducive to motion sickness. Likewise, anxiety, fear, and insecurity, either about one's orientation relative to the ground or about one's likelihood of becoming motion sick, seem to enhance susceptibility. We must be careful, however, to distinguish between sickness caused by fear and sickness caused by motion: a paratrooper who vomits in an aircraft while waiting to jump into battle may be suffering from fear or from motion sickness, or both.

Finally, it must be recognized that many things, such as mechanical stimulation of the viscera and malodorous aircraft compartments, do not in themselves cause motion sickness, even though they are commonly associated with conditions that result in motion sickness.

A mildly interesting but potentially devastating phenomenon is conditioned motion sickness. Just as Pavlov's canine subjects learned to salivate at the sound of a bell, student pilots and other aircrew, with repeated exposure to the conditioning stimulus of sickness-producing aircraft motion, can eventually develop the autonomic response to motion sickness to the conditioned stimulus of being in or even just seeing an aircraft (Fig. 11.44). For this reason, it is advisable to initiate aircrew gradually to the abnormal motions of flight and to provide pharmacologic prophylaxis against motion sickness, if necessary, in the early instructional phases in flight.

Unifying Theory

Current thinking regarding the underlying mechanisms of motion sickness has focused on the "sensory conflict," or "neural mismatch," hypothesis proposed originally by Claremont in 1931. In simple terms, the sensory conflict hypothesis states that motion sickness results when incongruous orientation information is generated by various sensory modalities, one of which must be the vestibular system. In virtually all examples of motion sickness, one can, with sufficient scrutiny, identify a sensory conflict. Usually the conflict is between the vestibular and visual senses or between the different components of the vestibular system, but conflicts between vestibular and auditory or vestibular and nonvestibular proprioceptive systems are also possible. A clear example of sickness resulting from vestibular-visual conflict is that which occurs when an experimental subject wears reversing prisms over the eyes so that his or her visual perception of self-motion is exactly opposite in direction to his or her vestibular perception of

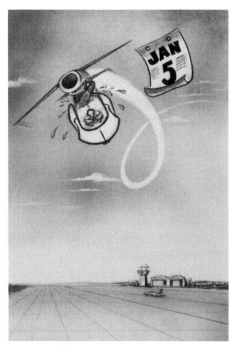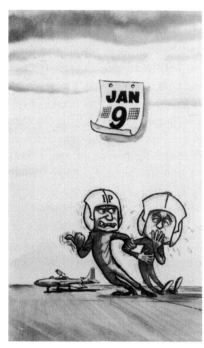

Figure 11.44. Conditioned motion sickness. A student aviator who repeatedly gets airsick during flight can become conditioned to develop symptoms in response to the sight or smell of an aircraft even before flight. Use of antimotion-sickness medicine until the student adapts to the novel motion can prevent conditioned motion sickness.

it. Another example is motion-picture sickness, where conflict arises between visually perceived motion and a vestibularly perceived stationary state. Airsickness and seasickness are most often a result of vestibular-visual conflict: the vestibular signals of linear and angular motion are not in agreement with the visual percept of being stationary inside the vehicle. Vestibular-visual conflict need not even be in relation to motion but can be in relation to static orientation: some people become sick in "antigravity" houses, which are built in such a way that the visually apparent vertical is quite different from the true gravitational vertical. Intravestibular conflict is an especially potent means of producing motion sickness. When vestibular Coriolis effects cause the semicircular ducts to signal falsely that angular velocity about a nonvertical axis is occurring, and the otolith organs do not confirm a resulting change in angular position, the likelihood of developing motion sickness is great. In a zero-gravity environment, when an individual makes head movements, the semicircular ducts sense rotation but the otolith organs cannot sense any resulting change of angular position relative to a gravity vector: many scientists believe the generation of the intravestibular conflict to be the underlying mechanism of space motion sickness. Conceptually similar is the "otolith-organ tilt-translation reinterpretation" hypothesis, which states that space motion sickness results from a visual-vestibular conflict that occurs until one learns to interpret otolith-organ stimulation in the zero-G condition correctly (i.e., as resulting from linear acceleration rather than from the force of gravity). This model is the basis of a promising scheme to preadapt astronauts to the conflictual sensory effects of the weightless environment (34). Another hypothesis is that the altered gain of vestibular-ocular reflexes in microgravity creates conflicts between visually perceived orientation and that perceived through the vestibular sense, or even the anticipated and the actually experienced visual orientations. A more subtle hypothesis is that morphological asymmetry and/or asymmetric functioning of the left and right otolith organs, for which compensation has occurred in the one-G environment, results in conflicting vestibular orientation information in other than the one-G environment. Whatever explanation of space motion sickness eventually prevails, sensory conflict will likely remain a central theme.

What determines whether orientation information is conflicting or not? It is one's prior experience in the motional environment and the degree to which orientation information expected on the basis of that experience agrees with the actual orientation information received. The important sensory conflict is thus not so much an absolute discrepancy between information from the several sensory modalities as it is between anticipated and actual orientation information. Evidence of this can be seen in the gradual adaptation to sustained abnormal motional environments, such as the sea, space, slow rotation room, and prism-reversing environments, and in the readaptation to the normal environment that must take place upon returning to it. It can also be seen that being able to anticipate orientation cues confers immunity to motion sickness, as evidenced by the fact that pilots and automobile drivers almost never make themselves sick and by the fact that we actively subject ourselves to many motions (jumping, dancing, acrobatics) that would surely make us sick if we were subjected to them passively. It appears, then, that the body refers to an internal model of orientational dynamics, both sensory and motor, to effect voluntary and involuntary control over orientation. When transient discrepancies between predicted and actual orientation data occur, corrective reflex activity is initiated or the internal model is updated or both. But when sustained discrepancies occur, motion sickness is the result.

Neurophysiology

The neurophysiology of motion sickness remains an enigma, although some progress in this area has been made recently. We now know that the chemoreceptive emetic trigger zone (CTZ) in the lower brain stem is not essential for motion-induced vomiting in experimental animals, as was once believed: thus, there is more than one pathway to the medullary vomiting center. A popular hypothesis has been that motion sickness results mainly from a stimulated imbalance of lower brainstem neuronal activity, which is normally in a state of dynamic balance between muscarinic cholinergic (parasympathetic) and noradrenergic (sympathetic) activity. The focus of attention thus has been on the vestibular nuclei, reticular formation, and automatic control centers of the lower brain stem. Appearing to support this hypothesis have been the observations that scopolamine, a muscarinic cholinergic receptor blocker, and dextroamphetamine, an adrenergically active compound that stimulates norepinephrine release, are highly effective pharmacologic agents for controlling motion sickness, especially in combination. But neuropharmacologic studies have not demonstrated significant lower brainstem sites of activity of these drugs; accordingly, there has been productive speculation that other anatomic structures, in particular the limbic system and basal ganglia, are of critical importance in the development and treatment of motion sickness. Kohl (35) points out that limbic structures are very important in the selection of sensory systems in the mechanisms of attention: he argues that the sensory conflict that is an essential feature of motion sickness pathogenesis, as well as the profound dependence on vision which develops with adaptation to a conflict-generating motional environment, both strongly suggest that limbic attentional mechanisms are heavily involved in the production and resolution of motion sickness. Kohl also argues that the known effects of scopolamine on limbic structures (particularly the septohippocampal tract) and the ability of dextroamphetamine to enhance dopamine transmission (particularly in the nigrostriatal and mesolimbic systems) constitute evidence that limbic structures and the basal ganglia are involved in motion sickness pathogenesis. Kohl and Lewis (36) believe that those structures subserve ''a higher sensory integrative process that acts upon sensory discordance and suppresses or activates reflexes which produce autonomic symptomatology.'' Although the neurophysiology and neuropharmacology of motion sickness and its treatment have not been determined definitively, current evidence removes the important sites of action from the vestibular end-organs and lower brain stem and places them in the higher subcortical regions.

Teleology

Even if the mechanism of motion sickness could be described completely in terms of cellular and subcellular functions, the question would remain: ''What purpose, if any, does motion sickness serve?'' The idea that a chance mutation rendered countless generations of vertebrates potential victims of motion sickness, and that the relatively recent arrival of transportation systems gave expression to that otherwise innocuous genetic flaw, strains credulity. A satisfactory answer, in our opinion, is that of Treisman (37), who proposed that the orientation senses, in particular the vestibular system, serve an important function in the emetic response to poisons. When the animal ingests a toxic substance and experiences its effects on the central nervous system, namely, deterioration of the finely tuned spatial orientation senses and consequent degraded predictability of sensory responses to motor activity, reflex vomiting occurs and the animal is relieved of the poison. The positive survival value of such a mechanism to eliminate ingested poisons is obvious. The essentiality of the vestibular end-organs and certain parts of the cerebellum, and the role of sensory conflict as manifested through the functioning of those structures, are provided a rational basis in Treisman's theory. Finally, experimental support for

Treisman's theory recently has been provided: labyrinthectomized animals, in addition to being immune to motion sickness, exhibit marked impairment of the emetic response to certain naturally occurring poisons.

Prevention and Treatment of Motion Sickness

The variety of methods at our disposal for preventing and treating motion sickness is less an indication of how easy motion sickness is to control than it is of how incompletely effective each method can be. Nevertheless, logical medical principles are generally applicable; several specific treatments have survived the test of time and become traditionalized, and some newer approaches appear to have great potential. Additional information on the treatment of airsickness is contained in Chapter 18, ''Neuropsychiatry in Aerospace Medicine.''

Physiologic Prevention

An obvious way to prevent motion sickness is to avoid the environments that produce it. For most individuals in today's world, however, this is neither possible nor desirable. The most common and ultimately most successful way is to adapt to the novel motional environment through constant or repeated exposure to it. The rapidity with which adaptation occurs is highly variable, depending mainly on the strength of the challenge and on the adaptability of the individual involved. Usually, several days of sustained exposure to mild orientational challenges (like sea and space travel) or several sessions of repeated exposure to vigorous challenges (like aerobatics or centrifuge riding) will confer immunity. The use of antimotion-sickness medications to prevent symptoms during the period of adaptation does not appear to compromise the process of adaptation and is recommended where practicable.

An important concept that must be considered when attempting to preadapt passengers or crew to a novel orientational environment is that adaptation to motion appears to have both a general and a specific component (38). Thus, the greater the similarity of the stimuli used in the preadaptation regimen to the stimuli expected in the novel environment, the greater the probability of successful adaptation. As a case in point, exposure to high-G aerobatics prior to zero-G space flight might help increase resistance to space motion sickness because of a general effect, but it could have the opposite outcome as a result of a specific effect. A possibly more efficacious procedure would involve head movements and locomotion during zero-G parabolic flights in aircraft or training in a device specifically designed to promote otolith-organ tilt-translation reinterpretation, as the stimuli would be more like those encountered in space flight.

The selection of individuals resistant to motion sickness, or screening out those unusually susceptible to it, has been considered as a method for reducing the likelihood of motion sickness in certain operations, such as military aviation training. The fact that susceptibility to motion sickness is so complex a characteristic makes selection less efficacious a means of prevention than might be supposed. At least three separate factors are involved in motion sickness susceptibility: (1) receptivity, the degree to which a given orientational information conflict is perceived and the intensity with which it is experienced and responded to; (2) adaptability, the rate at which one adjusts to a given abnormal orientational environment as evidenced by his or her becoming less and less symptomatic; and (3) retentivity, the ability to remain adapted to the novel environment after leaving it. These factors appear to be independent. This means that a particular prospective aviator with high receptivity also might very rapidly adapt and remain adapted for a long time, so that it would be unwise to eliminate him or her from flying training on the basis of a history of motion sickness or even a test of susceptibility. Nevertheless, although the great majority of aircrew trainees do adapt to the aerial environment, use of

vestibular stimulation tests and motion sickness questionnaires reveals that sensitivity to motion sickness tends to be inversely related to success in flight training. Furthermore, sound judgment dictates that an attempt to select against crewmembers with a high probability of becoming motion sick is appropriate for some of the more critical and expensive aerospace operations.

Some promising results have been obtained with biofeedback-mediated behavior modification and other methods for desensitizing fliers with chronic airsickness. These techniques are discussed in Chapter 18.

Physiologic Treatment

Once symptoms of motion sickness have developed, the first step to take to bring about recovery is to escape from the environment that is producing the symptoms. If this is possible, relief usually follows rapidly; symptoms can still progress to vomiting, however, and nausea and drowsiness can sometimes persist for many hours, even after termination of the offending motion. If escape is not possible, assuming a supine position or just stabilizing the head seems to offer some relief. As mentioned previously, passengers subjected to motion in enclosed vehicles can help alleviate symptoms by obtaining a view of the natural horizon. One of the most effective physiologic remedies is turning over control of the vehicle to the symptomatic crewmember. Generations of flight instructors have used this technique to avert motion sickness in their students, even though they were probably unable to explain how it works in terms of reducing conflict between anticipated and actual orientation cues. Another procedure that has proven useful in practice is to cool the affected individual with a blast of air from the cabin air vent; such thoughtfulness on the part of their instructors has saved many student pilots from having to clean up the cockpit.

Pharmacologic Prevention

The most effective single medication for prophylaxis against motion sickness is scopolamine

(0.3 to 0.6 mg) taken orally 30 minutes to 2 hours before exposure to motion. Unfortunately, the side effects of scopolamine when taken in orally effective doses (i.e., drowsiness, dry mouth, pupillary dilation, and paralyzed visual accommodation) make the routine oral administration of this drug to aircrew highly inadvisable. When prophylaxis is needed for prolonged exposure to abnormal motion (e.g., an ocean voyage), oral scopolamine can be administered every 4 to 6 hours; again, the side effects are troublesome and may preclude repeated oral administration. One approach to the problem of prolonged prophylactic administration of scopolamine is the transdermal therapeutic system (TTS), in which 0.5 mg of scopolamine is delivered transcutaneously over a 3-day period from a small patch worn on the skin behind the ear. For maximum effectiveness, the patch should be applied at least 8 hours prior to exposure to the environment that causes sickness. The cognitive, emotional, and visual side effects associated with this route of administration are considerably less than with oral scopolamine.

The antimotion-sickness preparation most useful for aircrew is the "scop-dex" combination, which is 0.6 mg of scopolamine and 5 or 10 mg of dextroamphetamine taken orally 2 hours prior to exposure to motion. A second dose of scopolamine, 0.6 mg, and dextroamphetamine, 5 mg, can be given after several hours if needed. Not only is this combination of drugs more effective than scopolamine alone, but the stimulant effect of the dextroamphetamine counteracts the drowsiness provided by the scopolamine. Another useful oral combination is 25 mg of promethazine and 50 mg of ephedrine, taken approximately 1 hour before exposure. Because the individual response to the several effective antimotion-sickness preparations is variable, it may be worthwhile to perform individual assessments of different drug combinations and dosages to obtain the maximum benefit.

Pharmacologic Treatment

If motion sickness progresses to the point of nausea, and certainly if vomiting occurs, oral medication is useless. If the prospect of returning soon to the accustomed motional environment is remote, it is important to treat the condition to prevent the dehydration and electrolyte loss that result from protracted vomiting. The intramuscular injection of scopolamine, 0.5 mg, or promethazine, 50 mg, is recommended: intramuscular promethazine has, in fact, been used with a high degree of success in treating space motion sickness on Space Shuttle flights. Scopolamine administered intravenously or even by nasal spray or drops is also effective. Promethazine rectal suppositories are used to control vomiting in many clinical situations, and their use in treatment of motion sickness also should be successful. If the parenteral administration of scopolamine or promethazine does not provide relief from vomiting, sedation with intravenous phenobarbital may be necessary to prevent progressive deterioration of the patient's condition. Of course, fluid and electrolyte losses must be replaced in patients who have been vomiting for prolonged periods.

Aeromedical Use of Antimotion-Sickness Preparations

As mentioned previously, the routine use of antimotion-sickness drugs in aircrew is not appropriate because of the undesirable side effects of these drugs. Prophylactic medication can be very useful, however, in helping the student aviator cope with the novel motions that can cause sickness during flight training—thus promoting better conditions for learning and preventing the development of conditioned motion sickness. Prophylaxis also can help reduce a student's anxiety over becoming motion sick, which could otherwise develop into a self-fulfilling vicious circle. After using medication, if necessary, for two to three dual training sorties (usually at the beginning of flight training and again during the introduction of aerobatics), student pilots should no longer need antimotion- sickness drugs. The use of drugs for solo flight should absolutely be forbidden. A more liberal approach can perhaps be taken with other aircrew trainees, such as navigators, because of their greater propensity to become motion sick and their less critical influence on flight safety. Trained aircrew, as a rule, should not use antimotion-sickness drugs. An exception to this rule is made for spacecrew, whose exposure to the zero-gravity condition of space flight is usually very infrequent and whose premission adaptation by other means cannot be assured. Spacecrew also should be expected to need prophylaxis for reentry into the normal gravitational environment of Earth after a prolonged stay at zero gravity. Airborne troops, who must arrive at the battle zone fully effective, are also candidates for antimotion-sickness prophylaxis under certain circumstances, such as prolonged low-level flight in choppy weather. In all such cases, the flight surgeon must weigh the risks associated with the developing motion sickness against the risks associated with the side effects of the antimotion-sickness drugs and arrive at a judgment of whether to medicate. Decisions of this sort are the very essence of his or her profession.

CONCLUSION

Thus we see how the recent transition of humans into the aerospace motional environment has introduced us not only to new sensations but also to new sensory demands. If they fail to appreciate the fallibility of our natural orientation senses in the novel environment, pilots can succumb to spatial disorientation. By recognizing our innate limitations, however, pilots can meet the demands of the environment and function effectively in it. We see also how our phylogenetic heritage, by means of orientational mechanisms, renders us susceptible to motion sickness. That same heritage, however, enables us to adapt to new motional environments. The profound and pervasive influence of our orientation senses in aerospace operations cannot be denied or ignored; through knowledge and understanding, however, it can be controlled.

ACKNOWLEDGEMENT

Shortly after completion of this chapter, Dr. Kent K. Gillingham was killed in an aircraft accident. This contribution, together with his many others, is a memorial to the life of the USAF's leading expert in the area of spatial disorientation.

REFERENCES

1. Hixson WC, Niven JI, Correia MJ. Kinematics nomenclature for physiological accelerations, with special reference to vestibular applications. Monograph 14. Pensacola, Florida: Naval Aerospace Medical Institute, 1966.
2. Henn V, Young LR, Finley C: Vestibular nucleus units in alert monkeys are also influenced by moving visual fields. Brain Res 1974;71:144–149.
3. Dichgans J, Brandt T. Visual-vestibular interaction: Effects on self-motion perception and postural control. In: Held R, Liebowitz H, Teuber HL, eds. Handbook of sensory physiology. Volume VIII. Perception. Berlin: Springer-Verlag, 1978.
4. Previc, FH. Functional specialization in the lower and upper visual fields in humans: Its ecological origins and neurophysiological implications. Behav Brain Sci, 1990;13:471–527.
5. Liebowitz HW, Dichgans J. The ambient visual system and spatial orientation. In: Spatial disorientation in flight: Current problems. AGARD-CP-287. Neuilly-sur-Seine, France: North Atlantic Treaty Organization, 1980.
6. Tredici TJ. Visual illusions as a probable cause of aircraft accidents. In: Spatial disorientation in flight: Current problems, AGARD-CP-287. Neuilly-sur-Seine, France: North Atlantic Treaty Organization, 1980.
7. Sperry RW. Neural basis of the spontaneous optokinetic response preceded by visual inversion. J Comp Physiol Psych 1950;43:482–489.
8. Spoendlin HH. Ultrastructural studies of the labyrinth in squirrel monkeys. In: The role of the vestibular organs in the exploration of space. NASA-SP-77. Washington, DC: National Aeronautics and Space Administration, 1965.
9. Jones GM: Disturbance of oculomotor control in flight. Aerospace Med 1965;36:461–465.
10. Fulgham D, Gillingham K. Inflight assessment of motion sensation thresholds and disorienting maneuvers. Presented at the Annual Scientific Meeting of the Aerospace Association, Washington, DC, May, 1989.
11. Peters RA. Dynamics of the vestibular system and their relation to motion perception, spatial disorientation, and illusions. NASA-CR-1309. Washington, DC: National Aeronautics and Space Administration, 1969.
12. Jones GM. Vestibulo-ocular disorganization in the aerodynamic spin. Aerospace Med 1965;36:976–983.

13. Cohen MM, Crosbie RJ, Blackburn LH. Disorienting effects of aircraft catapult launchings. Aerospace Med 1973;44:37–39.

14. Buley LE, Spelina J. Physiological and psychological factors in ''the dark-night takeoff accident.'' Aerospace Med 1970;41:553–556.

15. Martin JF, Jones GM: Theoretical man-machine interaction which might lead to loss of aircraft control. Aerospace Med 1965;*36*:713–716.

16. Malcolm R, Money KE. Two specific kinds of disorientation incidents: Jet upset and giant hand. In: The disorientation incident. AGARD-CP-95. Part 1. Benson J, ed. Neuilly-sur-Seine, France: North Atlantic Treaty Organization, 1972.

17. Schone H. On the role of gravity in human spatial orientation. Aerospace Med 1964;35:764–722.

18. Correia MJ, Hixson WC, Niven JI. On predictive equations for subjective judgments of vertical and horizon in a force field. Acta Otolaryng Suppl. 230, 1968;1–20.

19. AFM 51–37, Instrument flying. Washington, DC: Department of the Air Force, Headquarters US Air Force, 1986.

20. Nuttall JB, Sanford WG. Spatial disorientation in operational flying. Publication M-27–56. United States Air Force Directorate of Flight Safety Research, Norton Air Force Base, California, Sept. 12, 1956.

21. Moser R. Spatial disorientation as a factor in accidents in an operational command. Aerospace Med 1969;40:174–176.

22. Barnum F, Bonner RH. Epidemiology of USAF spatial disorientation aircraft accidents, 1 Jan. 1958–31 Dec 1968. Aerospace Med 1971;42:896–898.

23. Kellogg RS. Letter report on spatial disorientation incidence statistics. From The Aerospace Medical Research Laboratory, Wright-Patterson Air Force Base. Ohio to AMD/RDL; Mar 30, 1973.

24. Lyons TJ, Freeman JE. Spatial disorientation (SD) mishaps in the US Air Force—1988. Avait Space Eviron Med 1990;61: 459 (abstract).

25. The Naval Safety Center Aeromedical Newsletter. Number 90–3. Norfolk, Virginia: Naval Safety Center, 1990.

26. Kirkham WR, Collins WE, Grape PM, et al. Spatial disorientation in general aviation accidents. Aviat Space Environ Med 1978;49:1080–1086.

27. Lyons TJ, Simpson CG: The giant hand phenomenon. Aviat Space Environ Med 1990;60:64–66.

28. Wick RL. No flicker vertigo. Letter to the editor. Business/Commercial Aviat 1982;51:16.

29. Clark B, Nicholson M, Graybiel A.: Fascination: A cause of pilot error. J Aviat Med 1953;24:429–440.

30. Clark B, Graybiel A. The break-off phenomenon—a feeling of separation from the earth experience by pilots at high altitude. J Aviat Med 1957;28:121–126.

31. Miller EF II, Graybiel A. Comparison of five levels of motion sickness severity as the basis for grading susceptibility. Aerospace Med 1974;45:602–609.

32. Armstrong HG. Air sickness. In: Armstrong, HG, ed. Aerospace Medicine. Baltimore: Williams & Wilkins, 1961.

33. Lackner JR, Graybiel A. Head movements in low and high gravitoinertial force environments elicit motion sickness: Implications for space motion sickness. Aviat Space Environ Med 1987;58:A212–A217.

34. Parker DE, Reschke MF, von Gierke HE, et al. Effects of proposed preflight adaptation training on eye movements, self-motion perception, and motion sickness: A progress report. Aviat Space Environ Med 1987;58:A42–A49.

35. Kohl RL. Mechanisms of selective attention and space motion sickness. Aviat Space Environ Med 1987;58:1130–1132.

36. Kohl RL, Lewis MR. Mechanisms underlying the antimotion sickness effects of psychostimulants. Aviat Space Environ Med 1987;58:1215–1218.

37. Treisman M. Motion sickness: An evolutionary hypothesis. Science 1977;197:493–495.

38. Dobie TG, May JG. Generalization of tolerance to motion environments. Aviat Space Environ Med 1990;61:707–711.

Chapter 12

Thermal Stress

Sarah A. Nunneley

Cold hands, warm heart.

Folk Saying

Human flight has always involved thermal stress in some form. Pioneering aeronauts encountered increasing cold as their balloons ascended, and open-cockpit powered aircraft added wind to the problem. As late as WW II, aircrew members wore sheepskin clothing to combat the chill of long-duration flights at high altitude. Although pressurized, heated cabins now eliminate the chill from most flying, aerospace personnel may still encounter cold through exposure to high altitude, winter ground operations, post-accident survival in cold weather, or ditching into water.

Heat stress became a problem as aviation spread to hot climates, where closed cockpits produced oven-like conditions on the ground and during low-level flight. Heat casualties were a serious problem at airfields in North Africa in World War II. Even with the advent of air-conditioned aircraft, heat stress remains a factor because onboard cooling capacity is usually limited; problems often arise during startup procedures, ground standby and low-level flight. Supersonic aircraft and re-entering spacecraft produce aerodynamic heating which can cause serious problems if thermal control systems fail. In addition, both aircrew members and support personnel must often wear protective clothing which tends to trap metabolic heat and thus creates heat stress in otherwise comfortable environments. Post-crash survival may expose fliers to hot desert or tropical conditions.

The level of thermal stress which is acceptable for aerospace personnel varies with the task and the required safety margin. Maintenance tasks must often be performed outdoors or in shop areas with little or no thermal control, resulting in exposure of workers to extremes of heat and cold. While aircrew members are generally protected from outdoor temperatures, the critical nature of flight tasks means that performance may be impaired by seemingly mild levels of thermal stress. Aeromedical personnel therefore need to understand the factors which contribute to thermal stress, the range of human responses to heat and cold, methods for analyzing thermal problems, and options for ameliorating unacceptable stress. They may also be expected to provide advice on matters of thermal comfort and emergency criteria for the design of artificial environments such as orbiting spacecraft, space suits, and underwater habitats.

HUMAN THERMOREGULATION

In humans and other homeotherms, deep body or core temperature (T_{co}) must be maintained at a high level and within a narrow range to support normal functioning of the brain and other vital organs. Temperature is vitally important because it affects the rates of the multitude of biochemical reactions which underlie all physiological processes.

Internal Control System

Normal T_{co} in humans is generally given as 37° C (98.6° F), although the actual value varies with site of measurement, activity level and time of day. The latter is a strong influence: A person at rest under neutral thermal conditions shows a 24-hour temperature cycle with an amplitude of approximately 1° C. This circadian rhythm forms a shifting baseline for temperature changes due to fever, exercise, or climatic extremes, and its desynchronization is an important component of "jet lag." The small basal temperature shift which occurs in women upon ovulation has no practical effect on tolerance for thermal stress.

Maintenance of a stable T_{co} requires the continuous elimination of metabolic heat as well as compensation for any environmental heat gain or loss. Body temperature is regulated by a complex system as diagrammed in Figure 12.1. A control center in the hypothalamus integrates temperature inputs from both central and peripheral (shell) sites and adjusts various heat transfer mechanisms to hold T_{co} at the required level. Under natural conditions, heat produced in the core moves outward to the skin by tissue conduction and circulatory convection, and then dissipates to the environment. Thermal comfort is largely determined by mean

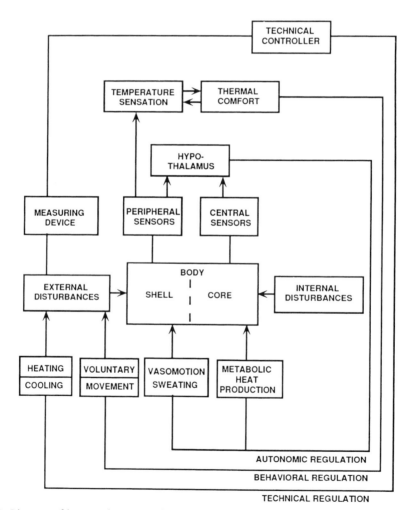

Figure 12.1. Diagram of human thermoregulation including autonomic, behavioral and technical components. After Hensel H. Thermoreception and temperature regulation. Monographs of the Physiological Society No. 38. London: Academic Press, 1981.

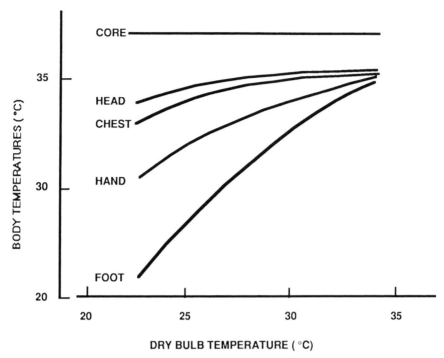

Figure 12.2. Temperatures at various locations on the body during steady-state exposures to a range of dry bulb temperatures. Core temperature was measured rectally. After Hardy JD, DuBois EF. Basal metabolism, radiation, convection and vaporization at temperatures of 22 to 35° C. J Nutr 1938;15:477–497.

skin temperature (T_{sk}) and perhaps heart rate, as core temperature per se produces no conscious sensation. The T_{sk} which is associated with comfort is 33° C in resting individuals, but this number covers a temperature distribution which varies from the head to the hands and feet, the gradient increasing in colder environments (Figure 12.2). Furthermore, the T_{sk} which is consistent with comfort declines as metabolic rate rises, reflecting the need for a greater core-skin gradient to externalize additional metabolic heat.

In physiological terms, humans cope better with heat stress than with cold, a fact which probably reflects our tropical origins. The body's first line of defense against thermal imbalance is control of cutaneous blood flow, which determines the rate of convective heat transport between the central blood pool and the subcutaneous circulation (1). The skin is unique among organs because its circulation is controlled centrally instead of responding only to local metabolic requirements. Cutaneous perfusion rises dramatically as T_{sk} traverses the range from 30° C to 40° C; Figure 12.3 shows the accompanying changes in cardiac output and its distribution. Cold-induced vasoconstriction creates a superficial "shell" of cool tissue which includes the skin itself, subcutaneous fat, and inactive muscle. Heat is further conserved in the extremities through countercurrent exchange: Venous return shifts from superficial vessels to the *venae commitantes* surrounding the axial arteries, so that warm arterial blood as it travels outward transfers heat to the adjacent veins, while the returning venous blood is rewarmed before it reaches the core.

Thermal stress is defined here as any set of conditions where vasomotor control alone cannot maintain thermal balance. When this occurs, the hypothalamic control center initiates

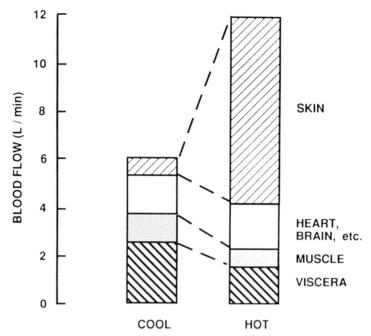

Figure 12.3. Blood flow distribution for a human at rest under cool and hot conditions. After Rowell LB. Cardiovascular adjustments to thermal stress. Chapter 27 in Handbook of Physiology, Section 2 The Cardiovascular System, Volume 3 Peripheral Circulation Part 2. Bethesda, MD: American Physiological Society, 1983.

Table 12.1.
Metabolic Heat Production for Various Activities

Task (Watts)	Heat Production (kcal · min^{-1})	
Sleep	84	1.2
Desk work	140	2.0
Piloting transport	175	2.5
Vehicle repair	245	3.5
Brisk walk	280	4.0
Heavy digging	628	9.0
Running	1395	20.0

sweating (evaporative cooling) or shivering (increased heat production), as well as behavioral changes to reduce discomfort (Figure 12.1). Thermal defense mechanisms are discussed further in the sections on heat and cold stress.

Physical Work

Table 12.1 lists the oxygen uptake (V_{O2}) associated with selected tasks. The heat production for a given task is primarily a function of the external work load. The resulting physiological strain depends upon the worker's body size (work load per unit muscle mass) and fitness level (work load as a fraction of capacity). Small and unfit individuals are therefore at a considerable disadvantage for working at a forced pace. Overweight individuals must work harder if the task involves moving around, as in walking or climbing.

When a person begins a bout of work, T_{co} rises over a period of 30–40 min to a plateau which depends on the steady state work load as a proportion of the individual's aerobic capacity. Given the option of self-pacing, most people will settle on a work rate which uses about 40% of their capacity and produces a T_{co} of about 38° C; the extreme sustained effort of a trained marathon runner produces stable temperatures of up to 41° C. Once the plateau is reached, all metabolic heat must be transferred to the environment to prevent continued, unphysiological increase in body temperature. Recovery from exercise heat loading again takes 30–40 min under cool conditions and cannot ordinarily be accelerated: a cold shower improves comfort by lowering T_{sk}, but once the water is turned off, the need to externalize stored heat will quickly assert itself in the form of renewed sweating.

Metabolism is relatively low for pilots in flight, since mental effort does not measurably alter metabolism, and work performed on aircraft controls or in anti-g maneuvers is intermittent and isometric in character. Even the most stressful flying produces a time-averaged metabolic rate of only 200–300 W (170–250 kcal/h), although heat production may be higher for crew members who must handle cargo. Groundcrew members and others working around aircraft may be required to maintain high physical work loads for prolonged periods.

Environmental Heat Exchange

Heat moves between the human body and its surroundings through conduction, convection, radiation and evaporation. Detailed analyses of the physical aspects of environmental heat exchange are available elsewhere (2–4). Body heat balance under natural conditions can be summarized by the following equation:

$$S = (M - W) - (C + R + E) \quad (12.1)$$

where S = body heat storage, M = metabolic energy transformation, W = external work (force $\times$ displacement), C = convective heat transfer with air and/or water, R = radiant heat exchange, E = evaporative heat transfer, and all quantities are correctly expressed in Watts. Resting human subjects will voluntarily tolerate environment-driven changes in T_{co} of about $\pm 2°$ C.

The term M is always positive and lies within the range shown in Table 12.1. Since the human body is only 15–20% efficient, positive external work (W) is accompanied by a relatively large increase in M, although individual variation in efficiency may slightly modify M for tasks requiring skill. Radiant heat transfer involves electromagnetic waves and is related to the temperature gradient between opposing surfaces independent of air temperature. The term E includes passive water loss from the respiratory tract and skin, as well as evaporation of secreted sweat. Storage remains zero and temperature is therefore stable only when there is equality between heat production ($M - W$) and heat loss to the environment ($C + R + E$).

With the exception of M, all variables in the equation can have either positive or negative signs, i.e. may act as heat sources or sinks. For instance, very high air temperatures produce convective heating and may raise T_{sk} above T_{co}, thus reversing the body's internal temperature gradient so that heat flows from skin to core. Similarly, although it is usual to have positive external work and evaporation of sweat from the skin, special conditions may reverse these processes: Negative external work such as walking downhill imposes mechanical heat input to the muscles, and condensation of water on the skin (as in a steam bath) adds heat to the body.

Although the term for conductive exchange with solids (K) is usually a negligible factor in terms of overall heat balance, contact of unprotected skin (usually hands and feet) with solids can cause discomfort or thermal injury. The limits for ability to grasp hot materials with bare hands are a function of both the temperature and the physical properties of the surfaces involved (5).

Thermal Effects of Altered Barometric Pressure

At high altitude, the scarcity of gas molecules reduces convective thermal exchange. At the same time, low barometric pressure permits ready evaporation of water and sublimation of ice. The latter is used for dissipation of heat from the cooling system carried by astronauts during extra-vehicular activity.

Diving involves not only increased pressure but also substitution of various inert gases for nitrogen, greatly increasing convective heat exchange (6). Saturation diving chambers require precise temperature control because the close thermal linkage between the body and hyperbaric gas severely narrows the comfort range. In addition, respiratory heat loss becomes a potential problem at depth if inspired gas is not warmed above the local water temperature.

Clothing—Protection and Burden

Protection from extreme heat loads may be provided by clothing made of special materials such as the flameproof garments worn by military aircrews and the aluminized suits which allow firefighters to face enormous radiant heat loads. At the other end of the spectrum are winter clothing assemblies and the more specialized anti-exposure (immersion) suits.

Clothing can also be a thermal liability as it impedes all forms of heat exchange between body and environment. Aerospace personnel must often use special ensembles to protect themselves from nonthermal hazards such as altitude, acceleration and toxic substances. Unfortunately, such clothing may trap body heat and increase the metabolic cost of physical work, creating a hot, humid microclimate next to the skin.

Figure 12.4 provides an example of clothing-induced heat stress for work in a mild environment. The conflict between clothing burden and benefit provides grounds for the longstanding debate over the amount of chronic discomfort which can be justified in the name of protection from extremely rare events.

Clothing is generally characterized in terms of its thermal insulation value and its permeability to water vapor. Thermal insulation is often expressed in clo units, where one clo equals $0.155 \text{ m}^2 \cdot {}^\circ\text{C} \cdot \text{W}^{-1}$ ($0.18 {}^\circ\text{C} \cdot \text{kcal}^{-1} \cdot (\text{m}^2)^{-1} \cdot \text{h}^{-1}$), equivalent to the insulation worn by an office worker in a comfortable environment. For comparison, physiological tissue insulation for

a lean individual ranges from 0.2 clo in heat to about 0.8 clo with maximal vasoconstriction. Insulation values for a variety of clothing appear in Table 12.2. Other clothing characteristics of interest include vapor permeability, wind resistance, waterproofness, and ability to reflect radiant heat. Simple physical measurements are performed using fabric swatches, while more complex determinations require entire outfits placed on heated metal manikins which may simulate simple human motion.

For conventional clothing, both insulation and vapor permeability are related to the thickness of the material, i.e., the depth of the still air layer trapped within the clothing. Figure 12.5 depicts this relationship and shows how it shifts by the use of an impermeable membrane or down-filled materials. Although in vitro methods of clothing assessment are accurate and repeatable, other important variables are much harder to measure, e.g., the effect of fit and body motion on air exchange through the clothing (pumping). It is difficult to simulate a sweating skin, and it is unclear to what extent the evaporation of sweat from various clothing layers actually cools the skin.

"High-Tech" Materials

In recent years a number of manufacturers have produced textiles for which they claim special thermal advantages. An example is material which incorporates a waterproof membrane which is supposed to allow passage of water vapor and thus decrease the thermal burden associated with rainwear, immersion suits, and the like. While such materials are measurably more permeable than traditional coated fabrics, the membrane still limits the evaporation of sweat under realistic conditions of use. Similarly, although synthetic materials may offer light and durable insulation, the concept of "thin" insulation is a contradiction in terms. These "high-tech" materials are usually quite expensive, and should be evaluated with care not only for their thermal advantages under realistic conditions,

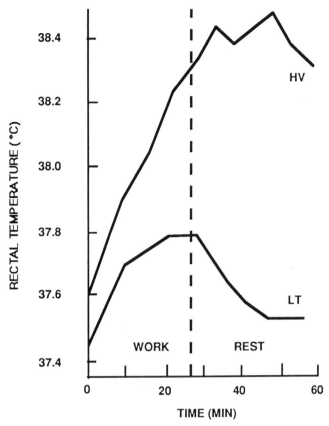

Figure 12.4. Mean core (rectal) temperature for groups of men performing moderate work in a warm climate wearing either light (LT) or heavy (HV) clothing.

but also for their durability in the face of repeated soaking with sweat, laundering, and physical abuse.

Active Microclimate Control

Aerospace operations sometimes involve unacceptable thermal stress when the severity of the exposure cannot be modified. In these cases, the only remedy may be installation of an active thermal control system which heats or cools the microclimate within the clothing. For example, electrically heated socks and gloves are sometimes used for high-altitude sailplane flights. However, most aerospace applications involve use of an external heat sink to provide chilled air or cool water for control of heat stress. Both media have been used in flight-qualified systems.

Table 12.2.
Examples of Clothing Insulation Values

Item	Insulation (clo)[a]
Cotton coveralls	0.8
Business suit	1.0
Military fatigues	1.5
Summer flight suit	1.8
Chem. defense flight suit	2.5
Arctic outfit (maximum)	4.0
Sleeping bag (maximum)	8.0

[a] 1 clo = $0.18°C \cdot m^2 \cdot h \cdot kcal^{-1}$

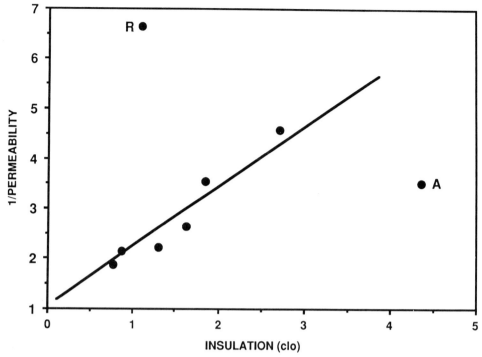

Figure 12.5. Clothing permeability vs. insulation measured in vitro. For conventional materials, permeability to water vapor is inversely related to thermal insulation. Two special cases are included: R (rainsuit) incorporates a waterproof membrane; A (arctic) represents an expedition-quality down outfit.

A ventilated suit distributes air over the skin through a system of ducts or a spacer-garment. Cooling occurs by convection and/or evaporation of sweat, but since the specific heat of air is low, evaporation usually does most of the cooling. Ventilated garments tend to be quite comfortable and remain fairly dry; potential problems include kinked ducting, suit inflation and noise from the air source. A typical suit requires a flow of 425 L · min^{-1} (15 ft^3 · min^{-1}).

Liquid cooled garments consist of underwear through which small-bore plastic tubing is woven. Cool water circulates in the tubing to pick up body heat, then passes through a heat-removing device before recirculating in the garment. The external heat sink may consist of an ice pack or a refrigeration system. Liquid circulation rates are typically about 1 L · min^{-1}. The high specific heat of water means that liquid is better than air for high work loads, but liquid systems also require closer control of inlet temperature for comfort.

HEAT STRESS AND HEAT DISORDERS

Heat stress originates from one or more factors among a triad which includes environmental conditions, work load and clothing. The undesirable consequences of heat stress range from discomfort to impaired performance, illness, collapse and even death (7).

Physiological Responses to Heat Stress

The primary physiological defense against heat stress is secretion of sweat to produce evaporative cooling. Sweating is normally associated with discomfort which stimulates behavioral changes such as stopping work, removing clothes and/or seeking a cooler location, but aerospace operations often preclude some or all of these behaviors.

Sweat Production and Evaporation

As air temperature rises toward core temperature, evaporation becomes the dominant means

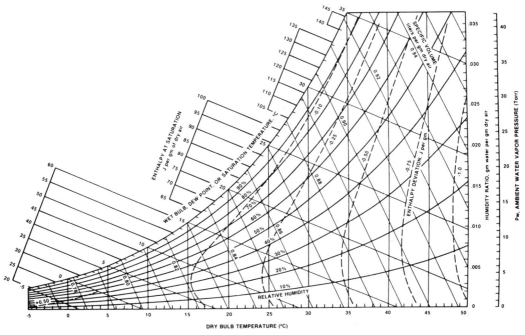

Figure 12.6. Psychrometric chart showing relationships among dry bulb temperature (T_{db}), water vapor pressure, and other measurements of humidity. Adapted from Chambers AB. Psychrometric chart for physiological research. J Appl Physiol 1970;29:406–412.

of dissipating body heat. Each liter of evaporated water carries away 2.43×10^6 J (580 kcal) of heat. Human sweat rate (SR) often reaches 1 L/h and may exceed 2 L/h for persons working hard in hot environments. Sweating is centrally controlled, commencing at some threshold core temperature and increasing linearly as T_{co} rises until reaching the maximal SR for the individual (8). The threshold varies with mean skin temperature, so that a hot environment causes onset of sweating at a lower T_{co}.

Evaporation of sweat is driven by the difference in water vapor pressure between warm, moist skin and the ambient air; relative humidity is not an adequate measure of this relationship. A psychrometric chart (Figure12.6) depicts the complex relationships among dry bulb (air) temperature (T_{db}) and several indices of humidity including wet bulb temperature (T_{wb}), relative humidity (RH), and dewpoint temperature (T_{dp}). Measurement of any two of these variables permits estimation of the others from the chart (2).

High ambient humidity and clothing impede

evaporation of sweat from the skin. Unevaporated sweat causes both discomfort and gradual dehydration without the benefit of cooling. Some physiological adjustment occurs, as hours of continuous exposure to hot-wet conditions cause a gradual decline in SR known as "sweat suppression."

Dehydration and Fluid Replacement

Dehydration (or hypohydration) is the term applied to depletion of body water below the level seen in normal, unstressed individuals. Dehydration by 1% of body weight (BW) has minimal physiological effects. As dehydration progresses there is little change in plasma volume, and most water for sweating is taken from interstitial and intracellular spaces rather than from the circulation. Loss of 2–3% BW causes increased core temperature, elevated heart rate, diminished saliva production and awareness of thirst. Further dehydration is associated with increasing discomfort, inability to continue work, and signs of central nervous system disturbance.

Acute dehydration can be delayed by preloading, i.e., consuming up to a liter of fluid immediately before the onset of heat stress. The antidiuretic effects of heat and exercise limit the diuresis which would otherwise occur upon water loading. For exposures exceeding an hour, the only means of preventing dehydration is to replace lost fluid at frequent intervals, at least every hour. Thirst is often an inadequate guide for rehydration, as most people fail to drink sufficient water to replace losses, producing a phenomenon known as "voluntary dehydration." This tendency can be largely counteracted by training combined with ready access to cool, palatable water. In some cases it is necessary to have workers drink known amounts of water under supervision, a procedure known as "drink-to-command." Work under severe heat stress can produce sweat rates which exceed the body's ability to absorb water through the gut. Under these conditions, progressive dehydration is inevitable unless work is scheduled around longer breaks designed for rehydration.

Figure 12.7 presents the daily water requirements of individuals working in the desert, which shows why the water supply for desert expeditions constitutes a major logistic problem. Unlike some animals, humans cannot adapt to

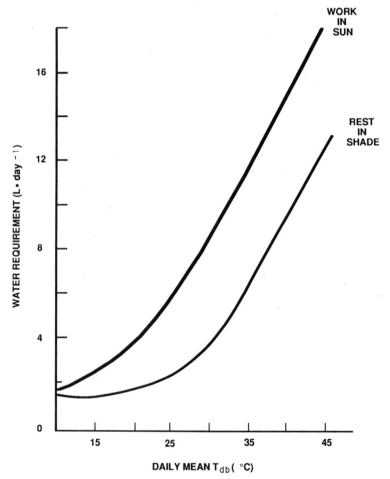

Figure 12.7. Water intake per 24 h required to maintain normal hydration for men living in the desert. After Adolph EF and Associates. Physiology of Man in the Desert. New York: Hafner Publishing Co. (facsimile of 1947 edition), 1969.

water deprivation; sweat secretion and urine production are obligatory processes. Water requirements can be lowered only by reducing environmental and/or metabolic heat loads on the body.

Dehydration can be prevented or remedied only by volume water intake. Water must be conveniently available in canteens or large cups, as fountains and little cups tend to limit consumption. Drinks should be cool but not ice-cold; chilling and carbonation tend to inhibit further drinking and may interfere with absorption of water from the gut. Flavors improve palatability, but may present hygiene problems (7).

Much discussion in recent years has centered on the possible value of adding electrolytes to drinks used for oral rehydration. Electrolyte deficit is not ordinarily a problem, as sweat is hypotonic and the modern diet contains an excess of salt; it is estimated that each gram of excess salt adds 1 L to the daily water requirement. In fact, heat stress is associated with hemoconcentration and elevated serum levels of sodium and potassium, especially if muscle damage has occurred. Thus, the primary need is water replacement, and the addition of electrolytes and nutrients to drinks should be considered only for prolonged exposure to heat stress when meals are missed (7).

Physiological Tolerance Limits

Tolerance for environmental heat stress is a function of both the severity and the duration of exposure. Studies of resting, unclothed subjects yield a two-part tolerance curve (Figure 12.8). Ordinarily, tolerance time is determined by heat storage and the accompanying rise in T_{co} to 39.0–39.5° C when the subject feels generally ill or faint. However, exposures to extreme conditions are pain-limited because T_{sk} rises past the pain threshold at 45° C.

As mentioned earlier, exercise raises T_{co} in a predictable manner; combining work with a hot

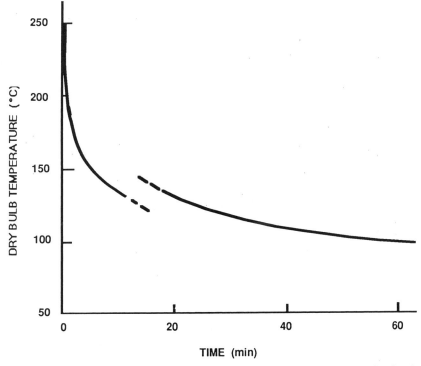

Figure 12.8. Time-tolerance limits for passive exposure to various environmental heat loads. The dashes show an indeterminate area where either factor may be limiting. After Iampietro PF. Tolerances to thermal extremes in aerospace activities. Aerospace Med 1970;41:1278–1281.

environment or heavy clothing elevates T_{co} beyond the physiological rise, producing either a higher plateau value or progressive heat storage to the point of physical collapse. Even when apparent thermal equilibrium is reached, tolerance for work in heat may be time-limited due to fluid depletion and/or circulatory decompensation.

Tolerance for work in heat improves significantly with repeated exposures, a process termed acclimatization. The minimum effective exposure appears to be 2 hours per day of stressful

work in heat. Adaptive changes include increased sweating, decreased heart rate, lower skin and core temperatures, and diminished electrolyte concentration in sweat (4,8). Complete acclimatization requires ten days, but a major portion of the adaptation occurs in the first 2–3 days (Figure 12.9). People who undergo daily aerobic exercise are partly heat acclimatized through the sustained temperature rise which accompanies training; such fit individuals adapt to heat stress more quickly and easily than do

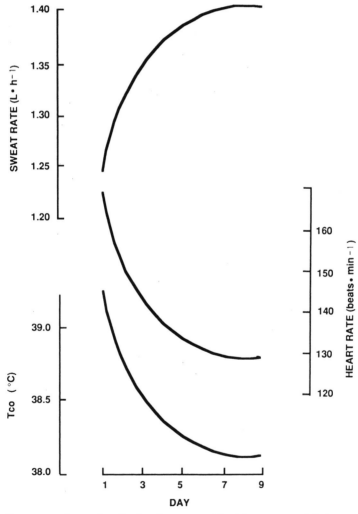

Figure 12.9. The time course for acclimatization in a group of subjects exposed daily to two hours of treadmill walking in a hot chamber. The curves indicate the mean final values for each day's exposure. On Day 1 none of the subjects was able to complete the 2-h session. Core temperature was measured rectally. After Lind AR, Bass DE. Optimal exposure time for development of acclimatization to heat. Fed Proc 1963; 22:704–708.

sedentary persons. Acclimatization begins to recede after a few days away from heat stress, so that return to hot work requires readaptation.

Human tolerance for heat stress shows wide individual variation and may be reduced by a variety of factors, including low aerobic capacity, lack of acclimatization, dehydration, subclinical illness, drugs, or toxins. A small percentage of individuals appear inherently incapable of adapting to heat stress and remain highly vulnerable to heat illness. Overweight per se does not increase vulnerability to heat illness, since the cutaneous circulation is superficial to the fat layer, but obese individuals carry a greater load of body weight and are often unaccustomed to physical stress.

Performance Effects of Heat Stress

Flying duties typically involve only limited amounts of physical work, usually in spaces with some type of thermal control. The occurrence of incapacitating heat illness is therefore rare among aircrew members. On the other hand, relatively mild heat stress may prove significant in the flight environment, which often requires peak mental performance during exposure to a combination of physiological and psychological stresses. Mild hyperthermia and dehydration may be associated with performance changes, exacerbated fatigue, and increased susceptibility to physical stressors. Considering the possibly disastrous consequences of pilot error, the acceptable level of heat stress may be very low, especially in high-performance military aircraft and agricultural aircraft. Pilots of such aircraft should not experience a rise in T_{co} of more than $1°$ C and/or dehydration of greater than 1% BW (9).

Strongly motivated individuals can maintain peak performance on a single task until physical collapse occurs, but this fact has limited relevance for the aerospace environment. More to the point is the extensive literature concerning heat effects on performance of complex tasks. The results often appear confusing or even contradictory; a wide variety of tests have been used, and earlier authors tended to report either the environmental conditions or the physiological (thermal) status of the subjects, but not both. Performance changes which have appeared in multiple studies include: shortened simple reaction time; increased error rate; narrowed attention with neglect of secondary tasks ("tunneling"); diminished capacity for learning and/or response to unusual events.

Arguments continue regarding the possible mechanisms underlying the performance effects of heat stress. One possibility is that central hyperthermia affects neurochemical processes and hence simple reaction time, while peripheral heat and discomfort tend to raise error rate. Like hypoxia, hyperthermia is insidious, the subject usually remaining unaware of performance degradation. Efforts to produce generalized time-tolerance curves for the onset of performance decrement have proven only partly successful, and none of the curves has received independent experimental validation. An alternative approach is a proposed open-ended scoring system for aircrew heat stress effects (10).

Heat Aboard Aircraft

The interior temperature of an aircraft rises rapidly when it is left on the ramp in hot weather. Sunlight heats the metal skin and penetrates transparencies, where it heats interior surfaces and raises air temperature (the "greenhouse effect"). Cockpit temperatures in bubble-canopy aircraft commonly exceed $50°$ C ($122°$ F). Heat aboard parked aircraft is a serious problem for maintenance personnel trying to work on board, as well as when aircrew members first enter the aircraft. Relief can be provided by shading the aircraft, covering transparencies, or using ground carts to cool occupied spaces. Reflective canopy materials would diminish the greenhouse effect, but they are rarely used due to their adverse impact on the pilot's outside vision.

Heat sources in flight may include sunlight, high external air temperatures, and/or aerodynamic heating of external surfaces, microwave

COCKPIT HEAT SOURCES

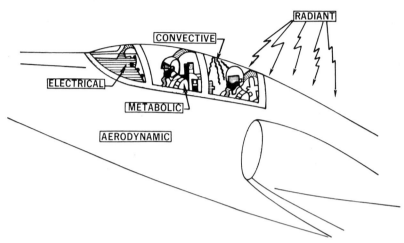

Figure 12.10. Heat sources in the cockpit.

radiation, and waste heat from onboard systems (avionics) (Figure 12.10). In light aircraft and helicopters, cockpit thermal control may be limited to simple ventilation (open doors or windows) or ram air. More powerful aircraft carry active cooling systems, but they often perform poorly on the ground and during pattern flying, when engines are throttled back; cockpit T_{db} in fighters during low-level flight over desert is often in the range 25–30° C (77–86° F). Helicopters and utility aircraft flying at low levels are generally hotter than the ambient air.

Aircrew heat stress increases with the need to wear protective clothing such as pressure suits or jerkins, anti-g suits, or chemical defense clothing. Measurements on pilots show that hot-weather flying produces high skin temperatures, with T_{co} reaching 38° C and dehydration by 1–3% BW by the end of one mission. Unfortunately, cockpit cooling may not provide a practical solution; in order to provide thermal comfort for a pilot wearing chemical defense clothing in summer weather, cockpit temperature would have to be at or below freezing.

Heat stress effects on high-performance flight include lower acceleration tolerance, increased fatigue, and possibly potentiation of the effects of hypoxia and susceptibility to motion sickness.

The newer fighter aircraft can sustain $+G_z$ acceleration which exceeds the best human tolerance limits, so that any heat-related limit on human performance will diminish the effective safe operating envelope of the aircraft. Military aircrew members are often aware that heat lowers their grayout threshold, and centrifuge studies indicate that a hot environment lowers $+G_z$ acceleration tolerance 0.5 to 1.0 G, primarily because vasodilation promotes pooling of blood in the legs. In addition, dehydration by 2–3% BW seriously reduces the tolerance of subjects for high-G exposure (Figure 12.11).

Thermal Problems in Space Flight

Space habitats and suits for extravehicular activity are thermally isolated to protect them from the extreme radiant heating and cooling of space. At the same time, they must have a means of dissipating the heat generated on board by electrical and chemical systems as well as by living occupants. Without provision for cooling, a suited astronaut would become hyperthermic within minutes of beginning work. Cooling by ventilation is impractical due to the volume of gas which would be required. Instead, the astronaut is fitted with an undergarment which is

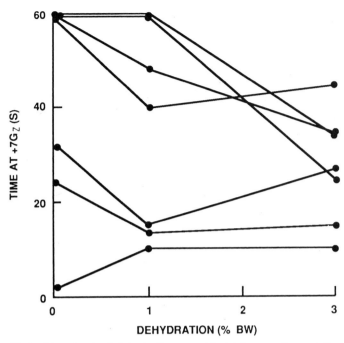

Figure 12.11. The effect of two levels of dehydration on subject tolerance for centrifuge exposure to +7 G$_z$ with anti-g suit and straining. After Nunneley SA Stribley RF. Heat and acute dehydration effects on acceleration response in man. J Appl Physiol Respirat Environ Exercise Physiol 1979;47:197–200.

laced with small-bore plastic tubing through which cool water circulates. The water then passes through the life-support pack, where heat is removed through sublimation of ice to space. The wearer adjusts cooling by means of a valve which varies the proportion of the water flow which bypasses the heat sink before recirculating to the undergarment.

The absence of gravity directly affects human thermoregulation in the "shirt sleeve" environment of a space station. Natural convection does not exist in zero-g, and unevaporated sweat does not drip off the body but instead forms a thick layer on the skin. Onboard systems must therefore provide for good air circulation and removal of water vapor sufficient to maintain comfort for people engaged in activities ranging from sleep to hard work; the task of system design is made more challenging due to the need to minimize the weight of components and expendable supplies.

Return from orbit involves potential heat stress due to reentry heating and landing at desert sites. Persons who have been in orbit long enough to suffer cardiovascular deconditioning may respond poorly to the combination of renewed exposure to 1 g together with even mild heat stress. Possible countermeasures for these problems include artificial expansion of plasma volume and use of anti-g suits.

Physical Work as Heat Stress

Flightline workers are often exposed to severe climatic heat while working outdoors or in thermally uncontrolled spaces such as hangars or powered-down aircraft. Metabolic heat production may be a factor, as groundcrew members perform work which may include sustained heavy exertion. In addition, they must sometimes wear protective clothing such as fuel-handler suits and respirators. The combination of environmental heat, work load and clothing may lead to progressive heat storage. As with industrial conditions, it is recommended that T_{co} remain at or below 38° C, although brief peaks to higher levels may be acceptable during periods of heavy exertion. Dehydration should be kept to <2% BW. Exposure limits for industry generally apply on the flight line and are described elsewhere in detail (11).

Heat-Related Illness

Heat illness occurs when stress either wears down or overwhelms the physiological defense mechanisms. Problems are more likely to develop among individuals who are unaccustomed to work in heat or who are otherwise stressed, e.g., through sleep loss, gastroenteritis, fever, recent immunization or ingestion of drugs (7).

Work in heat can lead to heat exhaustion through dehydration and/or electrolyte disorders without remarkable elevation in core temperature. Victims often suffer painful, wandering cramps in major muscle groups. The patient should be removed from the heat and given replacement fluid and electrolytes orally if possible, otherwise by intravenous infusion. Appropriate treatment should produce prompt recovery and return to duty in a matter of hours.

Severe central hyperthermia produces the life-threatening syndrome known as heat stroke (12). Diagnostic features include confusion or unconsciousness and hyperpyrexia (T_{co} usually exceeding 42° C). Cessation of sweating may occur but is not required for diagnosis. Mortality is directly related to the duration and severity of hyperthermia, and immediate treatment therefore consists of aggressive cooling by any available means. If there is some delay before the patient is examined, T_{co} may be reduced, and diagnosis then depends on the history with later confirmation through elevated enzyme levels indicating multisystem damage. Victims of heat stroke require hospitalization; in addition to cooling and rehydration, they may need seizure control and life support, and should be monitored for damage to the central nervous system, heart and kidneys. Coagulopathy may also

occur. Recovered heat-stroke victims exhibit an increased susceptibility to later heat injury and should be tested for heat intolerance before returning to activities involving heat stress (12).

Heat Stress Indices

The literature contains a variety of equations and nomograms which express net heat stress as a single number. The best known indices are compared and discussed elsewhere in review articles (3,8,13). Unfortunately, no one index is suitable for all purposes, as each involves certain limiting assumptions. Two which are commonly used in aerospace applications:

1. Effective Temperature (ET). This index is based on short-term experiments in which lightly clothed subjects were asked to compare paired environments representing different combinations of heat and humidity. The ET is suitable for use with moderate environments only, since a single value can represent more than one level of physiological stress. Effective Temperature is determined from a nomogram using as inputs T_{db} (or T_{bg}), T_{wb} and V (3).

2. Wet Bulb Globe Temperature (WBGT). The WBGT was developed to prevent heat casualties among troops training in hot weather. The WBGT is simple to calculate, but requires measurement of three variables to fulfill the equation,

$$WBGT = .7\ T_{wb} + .2\ T_{bg} + .1\ T_{db}$$

The heavy weight given to T_{wb} reflects the importance of evaporation in normal human thermal control. While WBGT does not perfectly predict human response to the environment, it is widely used as an industrial safety guideline (11), and there is a wide base of experience with this index. More recently, a simple instrument termed Wet globe Thermometer or Botsball has been used to estimate the WBGT;

it works well in humid heat, but introduces systematic errors under hot, dry (desert) conditions.

COLD STRESS AND COLD INJURY

Cold stress as used here denotes any combination of conditions which produces discomfort, loss of manual dexterity, or shivering. Undesirable consequences include impaired performance of tasks, local tissue damage, systemic hypothermia and possible death.

Shivering

When persistent heat loss occurs despite maximal vasoconstriction, the sole physiological defense is increased heat production through muscle tension, shivering, or exercise. Shivering is centrally controlled and depends upon both T_{co} and the rate of change in T_{sk}. The latter explains why sudden exposure to cold produces an immediate burst of shivering which subsides when T_{sk} stabilizes, only to reappear when T_{co} falls (Figure 12.12). Shivering offers only limited protection because peak heat production is only 3–4 times resting metabolism. Highly motivated subjects who are exposed to cold will generally tolerate a decrease in T_{co} to 35° C; temperatures below that level constitute clinically significant hypothermia, characterized by slow mentation, depressed reflexes, amnesia, and coma.

Repeated exposure to cold produces habituation and thereby improves ability to carry out useful work, but physiological acclimatization is difficult to prove, in part because humans generally avoid repetitive hypothermia. The search for signs of acclimatization has included both air and water exposure in natural and laboratory settings; various authors have reported suppression of shivering, increased resting metabolism and greater functional tissue insulation (14,15). It appears that cold acclimatization is difficult to produce and relatively weak compared to normal human adaptation to repeated heat stress.

Performance Effects of Cold Stress

The vasoconstriction which conserves body heat also promotes cooling of the extremities as they become part of the insulating shell. Manual dexterity decreases as hand temperature falls below 15° C and numbness ensues at temperatures below 8° C, even when the rest of the body remains warm (16). Stiffened, numb hands and shivering severely impair performance, as well as producing discomfort or pain. This creates serious problems for maintenance personnel working outside as well as for aircrew members working in cold cockpits. Since peripheral vasoconstriction is slow to reverse, prevention is easier than remedial warming. Aircrews operating on the ground in cold aircraft should be monitored for thermal status until takeoff unless auxiliary heat is used to warm occupied compartments (17).

Water Immersion

Water is a potent heat sink: Its high specific heat and capacity for convective exchange give it cooling power far greater than that of air at the same temperature (6,14). When an unprotected person enters cold water, skin temperature falls rapidly to match that of the water (T_w). Core temperature may show a brief, paradoxical rise as vasoconstriction takes hold, then declines linearly as shown in Figure 12.12. The rate of heat loss is a function of T_w, water motion, metabolic rate, and body build. The maximum insulation for any individual is a direct function of subcutaneous fat thickness, which varies about three-fold (e.g., triceps skinfold 7–20 mm) among military aircrew members but can be much higher in the general population.

Even relatively warm water can steal body heat over a period of time; lean subjects sitting in a bath begin shivering within two hours unless water temperature is at or above 33° C. Shivering offers little advantage in water because it increases perfusion to the limbs and stirs the surrounding medium, both of which

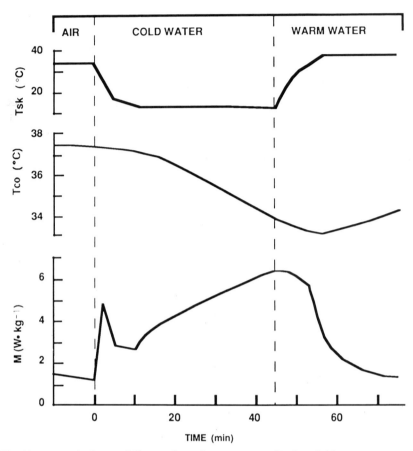

Figure 12.12. Mean metabolic rate (M), core (rectal) temperature (Tco) and skin temperature (Tsk) for a group of lean subjects immersed without clothing in water at 10° C. They were then placed in a warm bath to help them regain body heat. After Pozos RS, Wittmers LE, Jr., eds. Nature and treatment of hypothermia. Minneapolis: University of Minnesota, 1983.

increase convective heat loss. Similarly, swimming may speed the fall of T_{co} when T_w is less than 20° C (18). Successful channel swimmers combine a high level of aerobic fitness with a generous layer of subcutaneous fat which helps them to conserve the heat generated by their exertion (3).

When a person is rescued from cold water, T_{co} continues to decline for several minutes (Figure 12.12). This "afterdrop" probably represents a combination of two phenomena, one physical and the other physiological: a "wave of cold" continues to move inward by means of tissue conduction, and increased venous return brings to the core blood from chilled peripheral tissues.

Hypothermic Injury

Injury due to cold falls into two major categories: Localized damage and systemic hypothermia. Combined injuries often occur.

Localized Damage

Non-freezing injury develops with prolonged exposure to cold with restricted circulation. It is usually seen in the form of trench foot or immersion foot (4,14). Pathology consists of neuromuscular damage and venous thrombosis with redness, swelling and pain; wet gangrene and septicemia often follow. Treatment involves prolonged hospitalization, and residual effects include local neurological deficits, circulatory changes, and increased susceptibility to recurrent cold injury. Prevention consists primarily of good foot hygiene in the field.

Frostbite is the commonest injury under arctic conditions. The hands, feet, facial prominences and ears are especially susceptible to freezing because they have high surface-to-volume ratios, vasoconstrict readily upon cooling, and are difficult to insulate without compromising function. Superficial frostbite (frost nip) produces numbness and whitened skin, but has no permanent effect. More serious frostbite involves a greater thickness of frozen tissue which is white, firm, and numb. In cases of rescue from remote sites, thawing should be delayed if there is any danger of refreezing. The depth of injury cannot be assessed visually, and extremely conservative management is required to salvage all viable tissue. Prevention of frostbite depends upon appropriate use of clothing, conservative operational procedures, and training of both workers and supervisory personnel with regard to risks and preventive measures.

Systemic Hypothermia

Dry cold rarely produces systemic hypothermia in healthy adults, but may do so in persons immobilized by injury or impaired by disease or by drugs which interfere with physiological responses (15). Infants and the elderly are also vulnerable due to their diminished capacity for behavioral defense against cold.

On the other hand, even active, healthy adults become hypothermic quickly upon immersion or prolonged soaking with cold rain or spray. A plunge into icy water may occasionally precipitate death by cardiac arrest or uncontrollable hyperventilation. The victim who survives this "entry shock" undergoes rapid peripheral cooling, and chilled hands quickly lose their ability to manipulate objects such as rescue equipment and tools.

As T_{co} drops below 34° C, it produces progressive depression of the central nervous system with increased likelihood of drowning. In severe hypothermia ($T_{co} < 31°$ C) there is slowing of all physiological functions, and rescuers may have difficulty measuring vital signs. Core temperatures below 28° C are associated with fatal cardiac arrhythmias.

Severely hypothermic patients should be handled gently and rewarmed gradually in the field; aggressive rewarming should be reserved for hospital settings because the patient may require treatment for hypovolemic shock, electrolyte abnormalities, and cardiac dysrhythmias. Injection of drugs should be avoided in the presence of a hypodynamic circulation, and defibrillation is ineffective at temperatures below about 30° C. Hypothermia victims should not be given up until rewarming fails to produce signs of life.

Protective Measures

Protection from cold exposure generally involves providing appropriate clothing as well as training of personnel in preventive measures and response to emergency conditions.

Cold Air and Winter Survival

Protection from cold air implies control of convective cooling by means of thermal insulation and windproofing. Cold-weather clothing is worn in layers because insulation requirements vary widely over time with both weather conditions and metabolic rate (Figure 12.13). The greatest protection is needed during rest and sleep, while work generates the need to open or remove layers to preserve comfort. Overheating must be scrupulously avoided because sweat-dampened insulation loses its effectiveness and may prove dangerously deficient when work stops.

The feet are highly susceptible to cold injury but can be protected by bulky boots featuring thick insulation. Protection of the hands is much more difficult, as the high surface-to-volume ratio makes it difficult to provide adequate insulation in the form of gloves, and mittens seriously limit dexterity. Layering is again used, as workers can wear thin gloves for brief periods

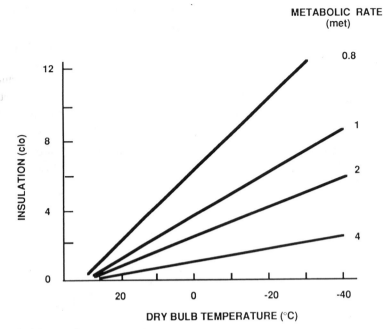

METABOLIC RATE
(met)

Figure 12.13. Clothing insulation required to maintain thermal comfort over a range of dry bulb temperatures for different metabolic rates. One met = resting metabolism; 0.8 met represents sleep. After Burton AC Edholm OG. Man in a cold environment. New York: Hafner Publishing Co. (facsimile of 1955 edition), 1969.

of hand work, then add thick gloves or mittens for long-term protection.

Although the face and ears vasoconstrict in cold, the scalp retains a high cutaneous perfusion rate and thereby becomes an important site for heat loss. A person sitting bareheaded in cold air may lose up to 40% of resting metabolic heat production through the surface of the head without incurring discomfort. Although heat loss from the head becomes less important during exercise, a warm hood can significantly improve systemic heat conservation for people at rest or asleep under arctic conditions.

Immersion Suits

Flying operations often entail the possibility that an aircraft may ditch into water. Most large bodies of water are below body temperature for at least part of the year, and thus pose a hypothermic hazard. Ordinary clothing allows free circulation of water and therefore offers negligible protection (0.03 clo immersed). On the other hand, special immersion suits can provide nearly infinite protection but they create unwanted warmth and bulk when worn during normal activities. Selection of appropriate clothing for over-water flights therefore represents a compromise between everyday comfort and the need for adequate emergency protection. In some circumstances "quick-don" suits may be provided for passengers or cabin crew, but in most cases only constant-wear suits meet the need for protection in emergencies. Immersion suits come in two basic types:

1. *Wet suits* allow water entry but limit convective cooling by trapping a layer of warmed water next to the skin. Such suits have a fixed insulation value and present serious heat stress potential under normal flying conditions because the material prevents evaporation of sweat. A major advantage of these suits is that they retain their protective characteristics even when damaged.

2. *Dry suits* exclude water and are worn with variable layers of insulation underneath. They must have seals at all openings (e.g. zippers, neck, wrists and ankles) and they become virtually worthless if the seals are loose or the material is torn. Entry of even limited amounts of water seriously degrades the insulating value of the undergarments.

Any immersion suit should include protection for the head and hands, possibly in the form of an inflatable hood and mittens stowed in the suit's pockets. Flotation devices can provide added thermal protection by decreasing the contact between the subject and the surrounding water. In the case of a life jacket or "personal flotation device" this may consist of a design which elevates the head and provides an inflatable hood or other device to prevent waves from washing over the scalp. A well designed life raft not only gets the victim out of the water but provides an inflated floor, a spray shield, and a bailing system to minimize convective cooling.

The effectiveness of immersion clothing is traditionally evaluated using human volunteers, but ethical and practical considerations limit the number and scope of such experiments. Furthermore, recent studies indicate that tests conducted in calm water do not accurately reflect suit performance under real-world conditions (19). A combination of manikin tests and computer modeling now provides a rational approach to limiting the need for hazardous human testing. Figure 12.14 summarizes time-tolerance predictions for various conditions. The Texas Model of human thermoregulation was used to predict how long it would take for T_{co} to reach 34° C, a level at which the victim becomes lethargic, loses the ability to co-operate in rescue measures, and is likely to drown even in calm water. The immersed clo values represent the following outfits: 0.06 clo = little or no protection (cotton shirt and trousers); 0.33 clo = waterproof suit without insulation; 0.50 clo = waterproof suit over a single layer of heavy underwear; 0.70 clo = waterproof suit over two layers of very

heavy underwear. Even without protection in the coldest water, humans may survive for an hour due to the thermal inertia of the body.

The curves in Figure 12.14 are based on the tenth percentile (thin) flying population and are specifically intended for use in determining the appropriate clothing to be worn on an over-water flight where approximate water temperature and maximum time to rescue are known. If estimates of survival time are being used to decide the duration of search-and-rescue efforts, it should be assumed that the individual exceeds the 90th percentile in fatness and therefore will survive much longer than is indicated in Figure 12.14 (20).

Windchill (Equivalent Chill Temperature)

The severity of cold air environments depends upon both the dry bulb temperature and the wind speed. Siple measured combined wind/temperature cooling power using a cylinder of water exposed to a range of extreme winter conditions in Antarctica (Figure 12.15). In addition, he observed time to frost nip for exposed facial skin, concluding that freezing of human flesh begins when cooling exceeds about 1400 $W \cdot m^{-2}$ (1200 $kcal \cdot m^{-2} \cdot h^{-1}$). The popular expression for "windchill" is the Equivalent Chill Temperature (ECT), the calm-air temperature which produces the same rate of cooling as the observed wind-temperature combination. Windchill cannot be used rigorously, and its application requires a generous dose of common sense. For instance, windspeed readings from a weather station often differ from local conditions due to location (shelter, siphon effects) or artificial air movement (prop wash, transport in open vehicles). Limitations of the windchill concept include: 1) It makes no allowance for clothing, activity, or body orientation to the wind. 2) It was not developed or validated as an index of discomfort. 3) No matter how miserable the conditions, frostbite cannot occur when air temperature is above freezing.

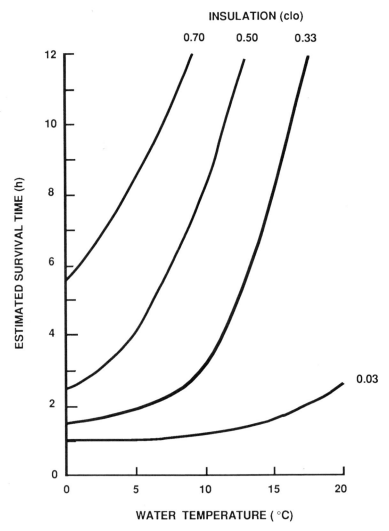

Figure 12.14. Predicted survival time plotted against water temperature for lean aircrew members. Curves indicate four levels of immersed clothing insulation. Air Standardization Coordinating Committee: Technical Basis for Specifying the Insulation of Immersion Protection Clothing. ASCC Air Standard 61/40A, 1984.

DEALING WITH THERMAL PROBLEMS

Analysis of a thermal problem involves evaluation of the environment, task, clothing, and the characteristics of the worker in order to identify both the sources of the difficulty and potential areas for improvement. Relevant areas of expertise include clinical medicine, physiology, engineering and human factors. The following techniques can be used to quantify the problem: 1) Preliminary information may be gained from a structured debriefing or survey of involved personnel; 2) Environmental contributions may be estimated from meteorological data, measurements at the work site, and observations hand- or voice-logged from simple instruments carried in flight; 3) Net physiological heat stress can be gauged from pre- and post-exposure measurement of body weight corrected for intake and output, where nude weight loss indicates sweat secreted, and clothed loss shows sweat evaporated; 4) More sophisticated instrumentation can

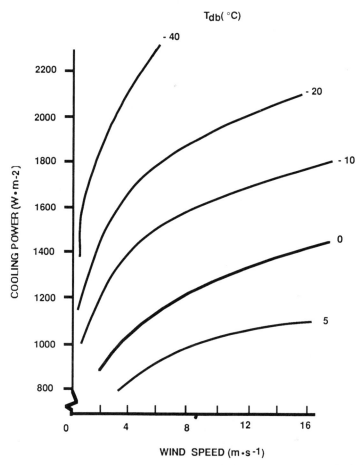

Figure 12.15. Cooling power of the atmosphere for a range of air temperatures and wind speeds. After Siple PA Passel CF. Measurements of dry atmospheric cooling in subfreezing temperatures. Proc Amer Philos Soc 1945;89:177–179.

be used for continuous records of environmental conditions and physiological variables such as core and skin temperatures and heart rate.

Core temperature can be estimated from timely rectal temperature readings. Oral temperatures are meaningless under stress conditions, and other sites such as the auditory canal and esophagus present major disadvantages. Although heart rate rises linearly with temperature, this effect is commonly obscured by changes in workload, emotional stress, and other sources of variability. It is well to remember that individuals vary widely in their response to a given thermal stress.

Possible solutions to thermal stress may in-

clude controlling the thermal environment, altering the physical work load or the duration of exposure, using different clothing, or raising tolerance through selection and training of workers. Any potential improvement(s) should be examined for the following factors:

1. Effectiveness—Does the proposed change reliably produce the required result?
2. Safety—Does the solution solve the thermal problem without introducing any other unacceptable hazards?
3. Practicality—Will the procedure or hardware item work in the real world, in terms of compliance, logistics and reliability?

4. Efficiency—Is this the best possible answer in terms of both initial investment and upkeep?

This chapter provides but a brief summary of the range of thermal stress problems which may be encountered in aerospace medicine. It is intended to help the reader appreciate the complexity of this subject and develop an approach for solving problems. The references should serve as an entry-point for anyone wishing to delve further into this field.

REFERENCES

1. Rowell LB. Human circulation: regulation during physical stress. New York: Oxford University Press, 1986.
2. American Society of Heating, Refrigeration and Air-Conditioning Engineers: Physical principals for comfort and health. ASHRAE Handbook of Fundamentals, 8.1–8.32. Atlanta: 1985.
3. Clark RP, Edholm OG. Man and his thermal environment. London: Edward Arnold Publishers, 1985.
4. Pandolf KB, Sawka MN, Gonzalez RR, eds. Human performance physiology and environmental medicine at terrestrial extremes. Indianapolis: Benchmark, 1988.
5. Stoll AM, Chianta MA, Piergallini JR. Thermal conduction effects in human skin. Aviat Space Environ Med 1979;50:778–787.
6. Webb P. Body heat loss in undersea gaseous environments. Aerospace Med 1970;41:1282–1288.
7. Air Standardization Coordinating Committee. Prevention of heat casualties during air operations in hot weather. ASCC Advisory Pub. 61/114L. Washington, D.C., 1991.
8. Leithead CS, Lind AR. Heat stress and heat disorders. Philadelphia: F.A. Davis Co., 1964.
9. Nunneley SA, Stribley RF. Fighter Index of Thermal Stress (FITS): Guidance for hot-weather aircraft operations. Aviat Space Environ Med 1979;50:639–642.
10. Air Standardization Coordinating Committee. Guidelines for the assessment of thermal stress in aircraft operations. ASCC Advisory Pub. 61/114G. Washington, D.C., 1991.
11. National Institute for Occupational Safety and Health: Occupational Exposure to Hot Environments, Criteria for a Recommended Standard. NIOSH Publication No. 86–13. Washington, D.C., U.S. Government Printing Office, 1986.
12. Hubbard RW, Armstrong LE. Symposium on exertional heat stroke: An international perspective. Med Sci Sports Exerc 1990;22:2–58.
13. Berenson PJ, Robertson WG. Temperature. In: Parker JF Jr., West VR, Bioastronautics data book. NASA SP-3006, 65–148, 1973.
14. Boutelier, C. Survival and protection of aircrew in the event of accidental immersion in cold water, AGARD-AG-211, 1979.
15. MacLean D, Emslie-Smith D. Accidental hyothermia. Oxford: Blackwell, 1977.
16. Fox, WF. Human performance in the cold. Hu Factors, 1967;9:203–220.
17. Air Standardization Coordinating Committee. Procedures for protecting aircrew during routine operations in cold climates. ASCC Advisory Publication 61/44. Washington, D.C., 1986.
18. Keatinge WR. Survival in cold water. Oxford: Blackwell, 1969.
19. Steinman AM, Hayward JS, Nemiroff MJ, et al. Immersion hypothermia: Comparative protection of anti-exposure garments in calm versus rough seas. Aviat Space Environ Med 1987;58:550–558.
20. Nunneley SA, Wissler EH, Allan JR. Immersion cooling: Effect of clothing and skinfold thickness. Aviat Space Environ Med 1985;56:1177–1182.

Chapter 13

Beyond the Biosphere

Arnauld E. Nicogossian and

Karen K. Gaiser

That's one small step for a man, one giant leap for mankind.

Neil Armstrong

The historical view of space has been that of an empty and alien realm sharing none of the characteristics we associate with our comfortable terrestrial biosphere. Although from the standpoint of the unprotected human, space is indeed inhospitable, in a physical sense the distinction between the two environments is not as clear-cut as was once believed. We now know that the earth's atmosphere and space are in equilibrium. Rather than being two completely distinct zones, they form a continuum whose shape and constitution are acted on by forces that are both terrestrial and extraterrestrial in origin. Within our solar system other bodies, notably the sun and planets, are likewise in physical equilibrium with space and impact our own local environment and equilibrium with space in various ways.

THE ORBITAL ENVIRONMENT

The Transition to Space

The gaseous envelope that forms our atmosphere is acted on principally by two forces: the terrestrial gravitational force that binds it to earth and solar thermal radiation, which causes its gases to expand into the surrounding space. Because these two forces are in relatively constant balance, the atmosphere exhibits a fairly distinct vertical profile of density and pressure. As the

distance from earth increases, the density of the gaseous medium decreases (Fig. 13.1). What we define as the border of the atmosphere occurs at the point where collisions between air molecules become immeasurably infrequent. This "collision limit" occurs at about 700 km above the earth's surface. Above this level is the exosphere, a zone of free-moving air particles that gradually thins out into true space. Even in space, however, the density of gas particles is about one to ten gas particles per cubic centimeter.

What concerns us as humans—as organisms adapted to life at the planet's surface—is the capacity of the atmosphere at various altitudes to support life. Predominant among these considerations are the atmosphere's breathability, its barometric pressure, and its protective effect as a shield against harmful radiation emanating from space. Each of these life-support capabilities of the atmosphere is diminished with increasing altitude, and at a certain point, each ceases to function. These functional limits of atmospheric effects determine, for man, the true border between the terrestrial biosphere and space. Although the physical border of the atmosphere is considered to be at 700 km, its functional limits are reached at considerably lower altitudes.

Manned flight in near-earth orbit, at altitudes in the order of 240 km, requires a space vehicle

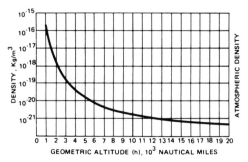

Figure 13.1. Atmospheric density as a function of altitude. The rapid decrease in density is correlated with a decrease in both the pressure and partial pressure of oxygen. (Adapted from Air Force Surveys in Geophysics, No. 115, August, 1959.)

well beyond functional limits of earth's biosphere. Designers of manned space vehicles must account for the new operating environment (weightlessness), the lack of life-supporting atmosphere, radiation, and the danger of collision with small objects in space (micrometeoroids).

Zero Gravity

The various forces that act, or cease to act, on an astronaut in space are an important feature of his environment because these forces can affect his work efficiency, his health, and even his survival. The most significant aspect of the force environment in orbital flight is the loss of the normal gravitational force that acts on us at all times on earth. The loss of gravity, or "weightlessness," occurs when the gravitational force vector is exactly counterbalanced by the centrifugal force imparted to the spacecraft as it travels tangentially to the earth's surface (Fig. 13.2).

To live and work in a world in which there is no gravity is a totally new experience for first-time space travelers. It is an experience characterized mostly by its novelty, but one having a broad range of important medical and behavioral consequences as well.

The dynamics of human existence are continuously shaped by the all-pervading force of gravity within the earth's biosphere. Every conscious movement is made in a manner that accounts for gravity. Such a simple motor act as

leaning forward brings into play a number of muscle systems that control the movement of the body as its center of gravity shifts. These are highly skilled acts, and yet they require no conscious thought. On initial entry into a gravity-free environment, however, each movement and act must be done differently, and a period of relearning is required. Fortunately, the problems of relearning have not proved to be as difficult as was predicted by some. Dr. Joseph Kerwin, in recounting his experience as a crewmember in Skylab 2, noted that, "The primary theme was one of pleasant surprise at all the things that didn't change, at all the things that were pleasant and easy to do" (1). Berry, summarizing the early Apollo experiences, noted that the absence of gravity could represent a bonus for locomotion because locomotion in zero gravity requires much less work than on earth (2). In addition, in-flight activities are frequently aided by the ease with which minimal velocities can be imparted to large objects that must be moved.

The zero-gravity environment also affects the physiologic functioning of major body systems; changes here are less obvious than the changes in locomotion but are greater medical consequences. On entry into weightlessness, the body fluids are redistributed. The function of the vestibular system, which is uniquely sensitive to gravity, is disturbed. Other systems begin a slow process of adaptation to the altered environment. For example, the cardiovascular system adjusts to a new situation in which the demands placed on it are greatly decreased. The result is a "deconditioned" system that functions appropriately for life in zero gravity but may have real difficulty when called on to readjust suddenly to a 1-g or greater environment.

Atmosphere

A major requirement for a manned spacecraft is the provision of a life-supporting atmosphere. The two key parameters of such an atmosphere are oxygen and pressure. Important additional requirements involve the control of carbon

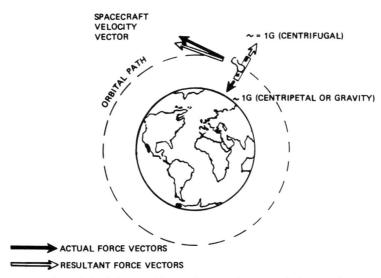

SPACECRAFT
VELOCITY
VECTOR

~ = 1G (CENTRIFUGAL)

ORBITAL PATH

~ 1G (CENTRIPETAL OR GRAVITY)

ACTUAL FORCE VECTORS
RESULTANT FORCE VECTORS

Figure 13.2. Representation of the balance of forces that produces weightlessness (0 G) in earth orbit.

dioxide and maintaining comfortable temperature and humidity levels.

Humans function well when oxygen is supplied at a pressure between 160 mm Hg (3.1 psi—equivalent to sea level) and 110 mm Hg (2.1 psi—equivalent to an altitude of 3048 m). Provided that an appropriate pressure level is maintained, the atmosphere can be 100% oxygen, with no nitrogen or other diluent gas present. Early spacecraft, such as that used in project Gemini provided a 100% oxygen atmosphere at a pressure of 5 psi. The obvious fire hazard found with a pure oxygen atmosphere was controlled to some extent in project Apollo through the use of a 60% oxygen and 40% nitrogen mixture at the time of launch. Through time, gas leakage was made up through the provision of oxygen only until the spacecraft achieved a 100% oxygen level, again at 5 psi. The suits used for extravehicular activity during project Apollo were pressurized with 100% oxygen at 3.8 psi. No problems with hypoxia, dysbarism, or oxygen toxicity were experienced during any of the Apollo missions.

Another key parameter of the atmosphere is that of pressure. When the body is exposed to reduced pressure, nitrogen in the tissues tends to form bubbles that then enter the vascular sys-

tem and can result in severe neurologic problems, which are termed "decompression sickness." Instances of this affliction occurring after exposure for an hour or longer at altitudes as low as 5486 m have been recorded. The pressure at 5486 m is 380 mm Hg (7.3 psi). Humans can function at lower pressures, such as the 5-psi pressure of the Apollo spacecraft, provided the tissue nitrogen is removed by breathing 100% oxygen for a period of several hours prior to exposure to the lower pressure.

The atmosphere in the space shuttle is essentially identical to that found at sea level on earth, with the oxygen supply, pressure, and humidity carefully controlled. The atmosphere consists of 22% oxygen and 78% nitrogen at a pressure of 760 mm Hg (14.7 psi) and provides complete comfort during normal shuttle activities. The only issue arises when astronauts must transfer into a pressurized suit for extravehicular work, generally conducted in the unpressurized cargo bay, the cabin is decompressed from 14.7 to 10.2 psi at 24 hours prior to the work to allow some nitrogen removal from tissues. During this lowering to 10.2 psi the EVA crew will pre-breathe for one hour. Then, based on the length of time, the crew will do a second pre-breathe. For an unscheduled EVA, the shuttle cabin will remain at 14.7 psi and the EVA crew pre-breathes for four hours. These procedures remain under review and may change when new equipment becomes available or as mission requirements dictate.

Radiation

The vacuum of space, although a more perfect vacuum than can be achieved in any facility on earth, nevertheless contains a great deal of matter that interests the planners of space missions. Radiation, particularly the submicroscopic particles of ionizing radiation, is a topic of major concern for biomedical scientists.

The radiation encountered during orbital flight can be classed as primary cosmic radiations, geomagnetically trapped radiations (Van Allen belts), and radiation due to solar flares. The latter two classes determine the unique quality of radiation found in near-earth space. Indeed, these two classes of radiation are important factors in determining the scheduling and trajectories of orbital flights. Anticipated radiation levels always are taken into account prior to a given mission.

The atmosphere of earth serves as a protective blanket to shield organisms on the surface from virtually all potentially damaging radiation. Particle radiation is slowed by collision with air atoms, whereas the ionosphere reflects most portions of the electromagnetic spectrum back into space. Only two "windows" in the ionosphere allow radiation from the sun and from deep space to pass through to the earth. One window covers the visible light frequencies and part of the ultraviolet and infrared frequencies. Another window covers radio frequencies of approximately 10^9 Hz. The protection afforded earth's inhabitants also has insulated us from knowledge of the radiation's physical characteristics. Thus, most of what has been learned concerning space radiation has come from space missions and probes flown during the past 30 years.

Cosmic Radiation

Galactic cosmic radiation consists of particles that originate outside the solar system, probably

resulting from cataclysmic events such as the supernova explosion witnessed by Chinese astronomers in the year 1054 A.D. Data from space probes show that these particles consist of 87% protons (hydrogen nuclei), 12% alpha particles (helium nuclei), and 1% heavier nuclei, ranging from lithium to iron. The individual particle energies are extremely high—in some instances up to 10^{20} eV. It has been estimated that this amount of energy per particle, if converted to mechanical work, could lift a normal-sized book about 1 m off the ground (3). The extreme particle energies mean that galactic cosmic particles, which fortunately are of very low flux density, are virtually unshieldable. At present, principal interest is in determining the extent to which periodic or continuous exposure to this radiation will affect career limits for space crewmen.

Trapped Radiation

In 1958, a project team led by Dr. James Van Allen conducted experiments in the United States Explorer satellite series, in which they discovered the existence of bands of geomagnetically trapped particles encircling the earth. These radiation belts consist of electrons and protons of the solar wind, which encounter the earth's magnetic field and become entrapped and begin to oscillate back and forth along the lines of magnetic force. The trapped particles follow the magnetic field completely around the earth (Fig. 13.3).

The Van Allen belts have two main portions, with effects being evident at altitudes as high as 55,000 km. The inner Van Allen belt begins at an altitude of roughly 300 to 1200 km, depending on latitude. The outer belt begins at about 10,000 km, with its upper boundary dependent on the activity of the sun.

In the low earth orbit to be followed in space shuttle missions, radiation from the Van Allen belts will be negligible. A discontinuity in the earth's geomagnetic field in the southern hemisphere, known as the South Atlantic anomaly, must be avoided to the extent possible in planning mission flight paths, however. At this location, which extends from about zero to 60°

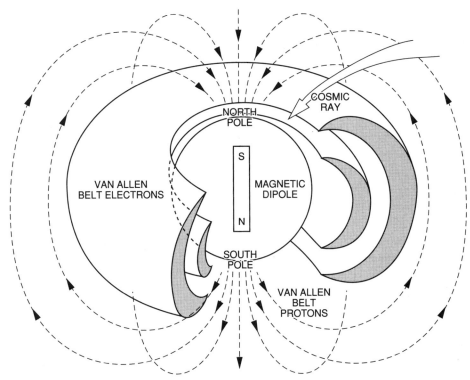

Figure 13.3. Solar wind electrons and protons are trapped by the Earth's magnetic field, forming the Van Allen belts.

west longitude and 20 to 50° south latitude, the intensity of trapped protons having energies more than 30 MeV is, at 161 to 322 km altitude, equivalent to that found at 1287 km altitude elsewhere.

Solar Flares

Solar flares are a major source of radiation concern, possibly the most potent of the radiation hazards (Fig. 13.4). The sun follows approximately an 11-year cycle of activity. When activity peaks, spectacular disturbances can occur on the surface of the sun. A solar flare is in fact a solar magnetic storm. These storms build up over several hours and last for several days. Although their occurrence cannot be forecast the onset of buildup can be detected. As the flare builds, an increase in visible light first takes place, accompanied by disturbances in the earth's ionosphere, which are probably due to solar x-rays. The principal problem, though, is

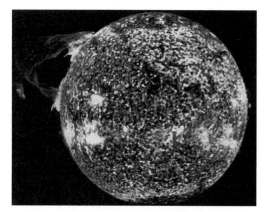

Figure 13.4. This photograph of the Sun shows one of the most spectacular solar flares (upper left) ever recorded, spanning more than 588,000 kilometers (367,000 miles) across the solar surface.

with the high-energy protons solar energetic particles that are produced during the storm. The energy of these protons ranges from about 10 million to about 500 million eV. The flux may be quite high. As a result, the radiation hazard for space crewmen could be quite serious, with a possibility of receiving a lethal dose (4).

The most important biological hazards associated with particles of high energy and high atomic number (HZE) are the so-called ''late effects'' occurring during the remaining life span of the individual after exposure. Life threatening and life shortening effects, in particular cancer, are of the greatest concern. Mutagenesis and other tissue damage, including cataract formation, are also significant health effects.

Other Radiation Effects

The Skylab missions provided an opportunity to evaluate yet another radiation hazard in space, the energetic neutron. Neutrons were recognized as one component of space radiation before Skylab, but the magnitude and, in particular, the source of this radiation were not well understood. Neutrons are of biomedical importance because, upon colliding with a hydrogen nucleus (a proton), there is a high probability of an energy exchange. Because humans contain an abundance of hydrogen-rich compounds, such as proteins, fat, and especially water, neutron exposure could cause considerable damage. Ambient neutron flux within a space vehicle, therefore, must be understood.

Free neutrons are not stable. With a half-life of 11 minutes, neutrons decay into a proton and an electron. Thus, neutrons detected in a space vehicle must be generated either within the spacecraft or within the earth's atmosphere and must represent products of the nuclear reactions caused by strikes of primary radiation. Skylab measurements showed that neutron flux within a spacecraft is higher than had been predicted — too high, in fact, to be attributed to solar neutrons, earth albedo neutrons, or even neutrons induced by cosmic rays in space-station materials. It was concluded that the neutrons were pro-

duced through bombardment of spacecraft material by trapped protons in the Van Allen belt. Fortunately, the flux level was not high enough to be considered a biologic hazard for crewmembers.

An interesting visual phenomenon that obviously was related to space radiation was first noted in the Apollo program. During the time of trans-earth coast, crewmembers of Apollo 11 reported seeing faint spots or flashes of light when the cabin was dark and they had become dark-adapted. From these reports and more systematic studies on later Apollo flights, it was concluded that the light flashes resulted from high-energy, heavy cosmic rays penetrating the spacecraft structure and the crewmembers' eyes. The fact that prior dark adaptation is necessary indicates that the phenomenon is connected with the retina rather than with a direct stimulation of the optic nerve.

Measures made during the Skylab program corroborated the light-flash finding of Apollo. Light-flash observations were made in two particular orbits to provide data on the effects of both latitude and the South Atlantic anomaly. During each session, the astronaut donned a blindfold, allowed 10 minutes for adaptation to darkness, and then recorded his observations of each flash. The results are shown in Figure 13.5. Two conclusions were drawn (3). First, the occurrence of light flashes correlates with the flux of cosmic particles. Second, the greatly increased number of flashes in the South Atlantic anomaly probably results either from trapped protons in this region or from trapped heavier nuclei.

Biomedical Significance

The biomedical significance of the radiation encountered in space flight can be assessed through a review of the radiation doses received by crewmen with varying times of exposure. Table 13.1 presents the measured radiation doses for astronauts in the Apollo program (5). These values are compared with the estimated total dose of radiation these individuals had

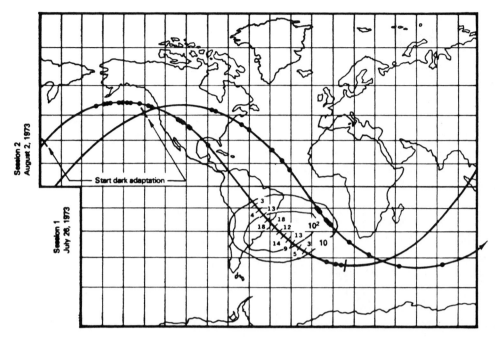

Figure 13.5. Light flashes observed during two particular orbits selected to provide data on the effects of latitude and the South Atlantic anomaly.

Table 13.1.
Average Mission Radiation Doses for Various U.S. Space Programs[a]

Program	Radiation Encountered	Missions Flown	Average Duration (d)	Average Mission Dose (mGy)
Mercury	Protons	6	0.37	0.07
Gemini	Protons	10	4.04	1.24
Apollo	GCR, Protons, Electrons	11	9.47	4.05
Skylab	Protons, GCR	3	57.17	43.20
Apollo-Soyuz	Protons	1	9.00	1.06
Shuttle[b]	Protons	43	6.28	1.31

[a] Correlation coefficient between average duration and average mission dose is 0.9966.
[b] Average Shuttle doses based on STS-1 through STS-48.
From *Mortality Among Astronauts Exposed to Space and Medical Radiation: General Patterns.* A presentation to the 1991 Annual meeting of NASA's Occupational Health Program. Kelsey-Seybold Clinic, Houston, Texas, and the Epidemiology Research Center, School of Public Health, University of Texas, Houston, Texas.

received, based on their age, from diagnostic radiographs and other sources of radiation on earth. When the space radiation dose is compared with the National Aeronautics and Space Administration (NASA) career limits, expressed in rem units for blood-forming organs, skin, and lens of the eye, these exposures are of negligible consequence. The Skylab 4 crewmen, who showed the highest exposures, could fly a mission comparable to one 84-day Skylab 4 mission per year for 50 years before exceeding the career limits for radiation exposure (6).

Micrometeoroids

A number of solid objects regularly pass through the orbital environment of the earth. The largest of these are the meteors, or "shooting stars," that appear on occasion as long streaks in the sky. Composed of solid material heated to incandescence by friction with the atmosphere, meteors are primarily of two types, with about 61% being stone, 35% iron, and 4% a mixture of the two. Remnants of meteors that reach the earth's surface are called meteorites.

The terms meteoroid and micrometeoroid describe the small object found in interplanetary and orbital space. Micrometeoroids often are referred to as interplanetary dust. Most of the extraterrestrial matter reaching the earth's surface, estimated at 10,000 metric tons per day, is in the form of micrometeorites.

The presence of micrometeoroids in space has long been recognized. The extent to which such objects might represent hazard for manned spaceflight, however, has not been known. Therefore, all missions have included some means of protection for crewmembers. In some instances, protection has been provided through the shielding afforded by the spacecraft itself. By contrast, during the Apollo program, astronauts who were scheduled for periods on the lunar surface were provided with an integrated thermal micrometeoroid garment.

The Skylab program presented an opportunity to obtain measures over an extended period of the incidence of micrometeoroids in orbital space. Because a number of these objects were expected to strike Skylab, an experiment was developed in which thin foils and polished metal plates were exposed on the exterior of the Skylab vehicle to record penetrations by micrometeoroids. On return to earth, the exposed materials were studied with optical microscopes and scanning electron microscopes at magnifications of 200X and 500X. Table 13.2 shows the results of these analyses. Because the exposed plates were located at different positions on Skylab and at different orientations, these figures represent an approximation of the micrometeoroid flux in orbit.

The size of the craters measured in the Skylab experiment showed all the impacting particles

Table 13.2.
Micrometeoroid Impacts Recorded During Skylab Experiments (Exposed Area = 1200 cm^2)

Sample Period (days)	Number of Impacts
1–34	23
2–46	17
3–34	21

Adapted from Lundquist CA ed. Skylab's Astronomy and Space Science. NASA SP-404. Washington, D.C.: Government Printing Office, 1979.

to be quite small, with only one believed to have been as large as 0.1 to 0.2 mm in diameter. The particles did have considerable power, as witnessed by their ability to produce craters in a stainless steel surface. Even though Skylab's micrometeoroid protective shield was lost during launch, however, the Orbital Workshop's wall, 3.8-mm thick, was not penetrated. There appears to be little, if any, micrometeoroid hazard to spacecraft in orbit with an exterior of such thickness.

The Long Deviation Exposure Facility (LDEF) was launched by the United States in 1984, The LDEF contained 57 onboard experiments designed to assist scientists and engineers better understand the environments of space and the effects of prolonged exposure to these environments. After almost six years in space, the LDEF was retrieved and numerous impacts by micrometeoroids and orbital debris were noted on the exterior of the facility. Analysis of the size, distribution, and composition of the impact material is currently underway.

Spacecraft Cabin Environment

In the absence of atmospheric protection, the space traveler is protected from these space factors by a pressurized space capsule containing various life-support systems. The hull itself provides the first line of protection against the near-vacuum of space, as well as against solar thermal radiation, particle radiation of various kinds, and micrometeoroids. Internal systems provide air and water regeneration while maintaining the necessary pressure, temperature, and humidity

Table 13.3.
Spacecraft Maximum Allowable Concentrations (ppm)

Chemical	Potential Exposure Period				
	1 hr	24 hr	7 d	30 d	180 d
2-Ethoxyethanol	10	10	0.8	0.5	0.7
Acetaldehyde	10	6	2	2	2
Acrolein	0.075	0.035	0.015	0.015	0.015
Ammonia	30	20	10	10	10
Carbon monoxide	55	20	10	10	10
Formaldehyde	0.4	0.1	0.04	0.04	0.04
Freon 113	50	50	50	50	50
Hydrogen	4100	4100	4100	4100	4100
Indole	1.0	0.3	0.1	0.05	0.05
Methane	5300	5300	5300	5300	5300
Methanol	70	20	10	10	10
Methyl Ethyl Ketone	100	50	10	10	10
Methyl hydrazine	0.002	0.002	0.002	0.002	0.002
Methylene chloride	200	50	10	3	3
Octamethyltrisiloxane	400	200	100	20	4
Trimethylsilanol	150	20	10	10	10
Vinyl chloride	130	30	1	1	1
Xylene	100	100	50	50	50

levels. The modern space vehicle is thus insulated against space and, in fact, constitutes a "shirt-sleeves environment" in which crewmembers can move, breathe, converse, and otherwise live in as normal a fashion as possible while they go about their daily routines.

The internal environment of the spacecraft, however, also includes factors that are significant in the overall health and well-being of the inhabitants. Although these environmental factors are generated by man and are thus not a "natural" aspect of the space environment, such as radiation and zero gravity, for instance, they are nonetheless space environmental issues in the context of manned missions.

The principal concern here is with contaminants present in the cabin atmosphere. Although materials used in the construction of manned spacecraft and onboard equipment are selected with great care, a certain amount of gassing of organic and inorganic products inevitably occurs. Many of these gases have toxicologic significance. In addition, contaminants are produced by the crew as metabolic by-products. Some of these contaminants are listed in Table 13.3, along with acceptable concentration levels in the onboard atmosphere.

PLANETARY ENVIRONMENTS

The spectacular successes of the American Pioneer, Viking, and Voyager unmanned missions and the Soviet Venera missions have provided a wealth of scientific information concerning the nature of our nearest planetary neighbors. In recent years, the rate of acquisition of data concerning the solar system has been such that it continues to be analyzed. Yet, even as we develop detailed descriptions of the solar planets, new questions are raised. For example, changes seen in the Martian polar regions have still not been explained; nor did the Viking missions provide insight as to the evolutionary processes that produced the puzzling differences between the martian surface and soil and those of Earth. Voyager spacecraft sent back photographs of the moons of Jupiter and the rings of Saturn that are striking beyond belief. The nature of the processes occurring in some of Jupiter's moons remains unclear, as do the physics involved in the configuration of some of Saturn's rings. An understanding of our solar system and, indeed, of our universe requires that questions such as these be answered.

Because the essence of the human spirit is that partial descriptions and unresolved scientific issues provoke action, man will inevitably venture past the moon and on into interplanetary space. Interplanetary missions will require a new era of research and planning if we are to be sustained during these long ventures and if we are to carry out all assigned activities. The information we now have concerning interplanetary space, as well as the orbital and surface environments of the planets, suggests that such missions will not be simple. The following brief descriptions of the four planets that have been probed most extensively to date indicate the kinds of issues to be confronted by biomedical scientists participating in the planning of interplanetary missions.

Venus

Venus, together with Earth, Mercury, and Mars, is known as a terrestrial planet, being composed of rocky materials and iron having a density quite similar to that of the earth. Passing 24 million miles from the earth at its point of closest approach, Venus is the earth's nearest planetary neighbor. It is a logical candidate for exploration missions within the solar system.

The first successful mission to Venus took place in 1962, when a United States Mariner 2 spacecraft flew to within 35,000 km of the planet and radioed back information concerning the near-environment of Venus. One of the most interesting of these discoveries was that Venus, for all practical purposes, has no surrounding magnetic field. From 1962 to 1982, the Soviet Union, with its Venera series, and the United States, with its Mariner and Pioneer programs, sent 17 spacecrafts to Venus.

Most of the information obtained in the American exploration of Venus has been through the Pioneer program. In December, 1978, the Pi-

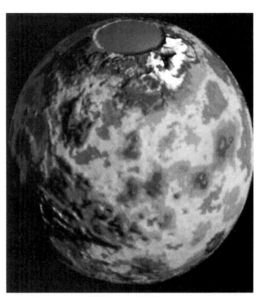

Figure 13.6. This global view of Venus was taken by the radar altimeter of the Pioneer spacecraft, so that the planet's cloud cover is eliminated. The large feature at the top of the picture is Venus' northern "continent," Ishtar. (Photo courtesy of the National Aeronautics and Space Administration.)

oneer-Venus spacecraft arrived in orbital flight around Venus. While the bus spacecraft remained in orbit, four entry probes were launched toward the Venusian surface. The gross topology of Venus was defined by a radar mapping system in the orbiting craft (Fig. 13.6). The probes provided much information on the structure of the atmosphere and more detailed surface effects. One probe transmitted for 67 minutes from the surface of Venus before heat rendered it ineffective.

The Soviet Venera spacecraft were the first to accomplish a landing on the planet's surface. The Venera-9 vehicle transmitted black-and-white photographs to earth on October 22, 1975, showing a Venusian landscape with considerably more light than had been expected under the heavy cloud cover and with sharply sided rocks indicating little of the expected erosion effects. More recently, in March, 1982, Venera 13 and 14 landed and transmitted photographs taken by imaging systems that permitted color reconstruction. Both landers also succeeded in analyzing samples of soil scooped up from their landing sites. In 1989, the United States launched the Magellan spacecraft which arrived at Venus 15 months later. During the first eight-month mapping cycle, the radar instrument obtained images of 84 percent of the planet's surface with resolution ten times greater than that achieved by the Soviets' earlier Venera 15 and 16 missions.

Although Venus has a number of features similar to earth, such as its size and density, there are some striking differences. The Venusian atmosphere is nearly 90 times more massive than that of the earth, and its predominate gaseous component is carbon dioxide. Sulfuric acid clouds encompass the entire planet, whereas the water clouds on earth only partially cover the planet. Water vapor and sulfur dioxide also have been detected in the lower atmosphere. Nitrogen is present, on the order of 3% by mass. The large volume and density of the atmosphere, however, mean that the amount of atmospheric nitrogen on Venus is about three times greater than on earth. The planet's surface temperature is extremely high — more than 450° C. Material analyzed by Venera 13 and 14 was shown to be basalt, an igneous rock similar to material found on volcanically active midocean ridges on earth. This finding suggests recent or ongoing volcanic activity on Venus.

Three fourths of the solar energy that impinges on Venus is reflected back into space by the planet's atmosphere and clouds, with 60% of the remainder absorbed in the heavy cloud layer. This layer consists chiefly of 1 to 3 mm particles that are believed to be sulfuric acid.

One of the more interesting findings during the earlier probes of Venus was evidence of lightning activity in the lower atmosphere. Both the American and Soviet data indicate that lightning discharges may occur as often as 25 times per second in relatively small areas above the Venusian surface. Terrestrial lightning, on the other hand, occurs only on the order of 100 times per second over the entire earth. The electrical

characteristics of Venusian storms, therefore, may be both different and more severe than those to which we are accustomed.

It was also learned that Venus has no planetary magnetic field to shield it from the solar wind. As a result, the Venusian ionosphere reacts strongly with the stream of particles from the sun. Both ion density and the height of the top of the ionosphere are affected by solar wind speed and pressure.

The picture of Venus pieced together from the various probes demonstrates that, although orbital observations certainly would be possible, the surface characteristics are not conducive to manned exploration of this planet. The great heat and barometric pressure at the surface and the composition and turbulence of the atmosphere make the planet quite inhospitable to human life. In addition to these physicochemical barriers, the rotation of Venus is much different from that to which we are accustomed, resulting in a day of 243 earth-days and a year of 224 earth-days. Thus, a day on Venus is longer than a Venusian year. Venus is not a planet that beckons visitors.

Mars

Mars is the closest neighbor of earth as one proceeds away from the sun. It also is a planet about which we have an unparalleled fund of scientific information, due mainly to data provided through Project Viking. By the beginning of the 1980s, the United States and the Soviet Union had sent 16 probes to Mars. The three most successful as planetary exploration missions were Mariner 9 and Viking 1 and 2.

The Viking program was a masterful blend of science and technology, for the first time carrying an automated scientific laboratory to a soft landing on the surface of another planet. The Viking 1 spacecraft landed on Mars on July 20, 1976 and was followed by Viking 2 on September 3. These spacecraft were each comprised of an orbiter-lander combination, which traveled through space as a single unit, separating only after orbit had been achieved around Mars and the appropriate landing site selected. The orbiter served as a relay station to transmit to earth information received from the lander. In addition, each orbiter took many thousands of high-resolution photographs of Mars as its orbit carried it over different areas of the planet. In combination, these four spacecraft have provided information concerning the Martian surface and its atmospheric environment that may be analyzed and studied fruitfully for many years.

The Martian atmosphere is totally unlike that found on Venus. For one thing, it is extremely thin. Pressures measured at various times by the Viking spacecraft were in the range from 6.5 to 7.7 mb, a value less than 1% of the earth's atmospheric pressure at sea level. Nevertheless, it is an active atmosphere. The Mariner 9 spacecraft, which orbited Mars in late 1971, photographed huge dust storms that obscured the surface for a 2-month period until they quieted enough for photographs to be made of the surface. The primary constituent of the Martian atmosphere is carbon dioxide, just as on Venus, with normal amounts of neon, argon, and oxygen.

Thanks to the remarkable photographs transmitted by Viking, the surface features of Mars are now familiar (Fig. 13.7). Mars has a very

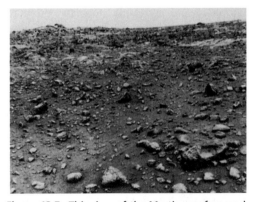

Figure 13.7. This view of the Martian surface and sky was taken by Viking 1. Color reconstruction showed that orange-red surface materials (possibly limonite) overlie darker bedrock and that the sky is pinkish-red. (Photo courtesy of the National Aeronautics and Space Administration.)

heterogeneous surface, with extensive cratering and evidence of volcanos over vast areas of the planet. Much of the northern hemisphere is covered by volcanic fields. Widespread evidence of catastrophic flooding is apparent, but no collection basins such as lakes or oceans have been found, and the source and sink of the water are still conjectural. The only water found on Mars to date occurs in the polar ice caps. These caps contain substantial amounts of water ice, are covered seasonally by carbon dioxide frost, and vary in size seasonally.

A major objective of the Viking project was to search for any indication of life on Mars. A number of photographs taken, some at close range, to determine if any organism — large or small — could be seen. The results were entirely negative. Beautiful pictures of the soil and rocks were obtained, but nothing lifelike was noted.

A more scientific approach to the detection of life was made through the use of the automated laboratory carried in the Viking landers. Samples of Martian soil were used for three experiments in the Biology Instrument Package, as follows:

1. *Gas exchange experiment.* This experiment was conducted in two parts. The first part tested whether the presence of moisture and appropriate environmental conditions would produce metabolic activity in simple, prebiologic organic complexes that might be present in the soil in a dormant state. Although gas chromatographic analysis indicated a chemical generation of oxygen, as well as physical desorption of some gases, nothing suggested the presence of metabolic activity. The second part of the experiment tested for the presence of heterotrophic organisms using organic compounds to satisfy their metabolic requirements. Extended incubation in the presence of organic nutrients and moisture resulted in a steady production of carbon dioxide, although no gases attributed to living systems were found.

2. *Pyrolytic release experiment.* It was assumed

that both carbon dioxide and carbon monoxide are found in the atmosphere of Mars; thus, organisms might have developed the capacity to assimilate one or both of these gases and convert them to organic matter. This experiment was conducted under conditions that approximate the Martian environment to the extent feasible. Incubations were carried out either in light or in dark for 5-day periods. Although weak responses were noted, the results appear to rule out any biologic explanation.

3. *Labeled-release experiment.* This experiment tested the assumption that Martian organisms would be capable of decomposing the simple organic compounds reported to be produced in the so-called "primitive reducing atmospheres" in laboratory simulations. The soil was moistened with nutrients tagged with carbon-14. Upon incubation, the sample immediately started to emit labeled gas. The radioactive gas release leveled off over the next several days until additional nutrients were added. Samples that had been heat-sterilized did not show this release of the gas. Young notes that, although the release of tagged carbon dioxide in a nominally terrestrial soil would have been indicative of an extremely active biota, under Martian conditions this might only suggest the presence of highly reactive soil-oxidizing agents (8). In short, the fact that the sterilized control samples did not show the reaction may mean either that the active run was biologic in nature or that the earlier heating of the sterilized samples had exhausted the reaction.

Since Viking, the only spacecraft to approach Mars has been the Soviet Phobos 2, which entered Mars orbit in early 1989, carrying instruments from 14 countries. Before losing contact with Earth two months later (as it was preparing to send landers to the surface of Mars' moon), the spacecraft transmitted high-quality television images of Mars and Phobos, along with the first data showing water vapor in Mars' atmosphere. Earlier, Phobos 1 had been disabled en route to Mars.

The U.S. Mars Observer, planned for launch from the Space Shuttle, will arrive at the red planet nearly one year later. Mapping the surface from orbit, Mars Observer will study the planet's geology and climate, investigate the composition and chemistry of the surface and the structure of the atmosphere, determine the inventory and distribution of volatiles. The spacecraft will gather data systematically over the course of two martian years, allowing us to observe and interpret seasonal changes in the atmosphere. Data from this mission will expand our understanding of the planet's topography, the dynamics of the interior, and Mars' gravitational field. The Mars Observer will add to the crucial database for a future sample return mission.

Preparation for human missions to Mars will require a series of robotic missions after Mars Observer to support and verify landing site selection, identify hazards to human explorers, and prepare for science experiments conducted by the crew. The Mars Environmental Survey (MESUR) mission, a series of landers planned for first launch early in the new millenium, will obtain high-resolution surface data and make seismological and meteorological measurements. MESUR's objectives include a better determination of the seismicity and internal structure of Mars. Other scientific objectives include an investigation of the characteristics and processes of the atmosphere (e.g., structure, temperature, pressure, circulation, dust and water transport), and further determination of the chemical composition of near-surface material.

The Mars Rover/Sample Return, projected for launch in 2005, will probably settle the question of indigenous martian life, extant or extinct, or organic matter. After a sample is obtained and transferred to the return vehicle, the rover will continue to traverse the surface and send back data. The goals of the mission include a better understanding of the evolution of Mars, its climate, geologic processes, physical and chemical properties of the surface regolith, and the composition of the crust and mantle. Other areas of inquiry include surface/atmosphere interactions and the fate of the liquid water that was very likely present on the surfaces ages ago. The return of the surface sample first to Space Station Freedom, then to laboratories on Earth, will enable a much greater range of iterative, in-depth experiments using state-of-the-art technology than would be possible on the Mars surface.

After the sample return mission, a Mars site reconnaissance orbiter will provide detailed imaging to characterize potential landing sites, assess landing site hazards, and provide a data base for subsequent rover traverses and pilot surface operations. Finally, several rover missions could certify sites with the greatest potential for piloted vehicle landing and outpost establishment.

The general conclusion is that the Martian surface is very different from Earth in terms of its chemistry and that this difference seriously affects the interpretation of the biology experiments. The bulk of the evidence, however, favors a nonbiologic explanation of the observed phenomena.

Mars remains an attractive candidate for further exploration. It has a thin atmosphere mostly compromised of carbon dioxide and a surface that could be traversed readily by exploration vehicles. The soil resembles that on earth but apparently has an intriguing increase in oxidative qualities. Of particular importance is the water supply contained in the large polar ice caps. This resource would be invaluable to an exploration team.

Jupiter

As one travels somewhat more than 240 million miles past Mars and on toward the outer solar system, the next planet to be encountered is Jupiter, the first of the giant planets. Jupiter is the largest planet, with a mass 318 times larger than the mass of earth. Its density (1.33 g/cm^3), however, is only one-fourth that of earth and just slightly greater than the density of water.

The United States has launched four success-

ful fly-by missions to Jupiter. The first of these, Pioneer 11, reached its closest point to the planet (130,000 km) on December 3, 1973. The most recent, Voyager 2, passed within 650,000 km of the planet on July 9, 1979. The two Pioneer and the two Voyager spacecraft returned a wealth of scientific information plus thousands of photographs of Jupiter. Although much of the interior of the planet remains a mystery, the outer surface of Jupiter, its satellites, and the conditions in the space surrounding it are now well documented. This information is contributing much to an understanding of the processes whereby the solar system was formed.

Jupiter is a gas planet, more massive than all of the other planets combined. It has no surface, in the usual sense, and many scientists believe that Jupiter is an entirely fluid planet with no solid core. Recent studies, however, postulate that the planet may have a small core of rocks and ice that constitutes about 4% of its mass.

In many respects Jupiter resembles a star; in fact, had it been 70 times more massive, it would have contracted during the time of its early formation into a star. Had this occurred, the sun would have been a double star and the solar system would be much different. Since 1969, it has been known that Jupiter radiates more than it receives from the sun. Thus, Jupiter must have an internal heat source. The internal heat is believed to represent the conversion of gravitational potential energy from the contraction of a giant cloud of gas beginning some 4.6 billion years ago. The surface heat, about 10^{17} W of power, flows from the dynamic processes within its luminous interior, which is believed to be about 30,000°K. Jupiter is composed of the same elements as the sun and stars, primarily hydrogen and helium. Most of its interior is metallic hydrogen held under enormous pressure, with normal molecular hydrogen appearing nearer the surface. In the upper regions, the hydrogen is gas.

The great mass of Jupiter and its powerful gravity mean that all gases and solids available during the early stages of condensation should

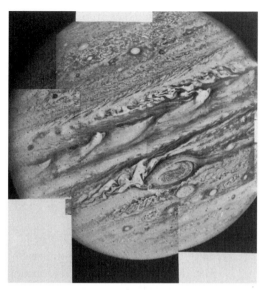

Figure 13.8. This mosaic of Jupiter was assembled from nine individual photographs taken by Voyager 1 when it was 7.8 million km from the planet. Shown are the Great Red Spot, the banded cloud features, and several white ovals. (Photo courtesy of the National Aeronautics and Space Administration.)

remain today. Jupiter, therefore, has the same basic composition as the sun, with hydrogen and helium being the two principal constituents. There is an abundance of additional elements and compounds, however.

The atmosphere of Jupiter is a mass of complex motion. Some of the atmospheric changes are quite fleeting; others, such as the Great Red Spot, remain relatively unchanged for centuries. The dominant features in the atmosphere of Jupiter are banded belts and zones, the Great Red Spot, and three white ovals (Fig. 13.8). The Great Red Spot is larger than the earth, and the ovals are about the size of our moon. All show anticlonic, counterclockwise motion. Materials within the Great Red Spot can be seen to rotate about once every 6 days.

Within the Jovian atmosphere, clusters of lightning bolts have been seen on the night side of the planet. One Voyager photograph showed the electrical discharges of 19 "superbolts" of lightning. This evidence of extensive electrical

activity confirms the disturbed condition of the atmosphere of Jupiter.

The similarities between the weather systems of Jupiter and Earth are matched by likenesses in the surrounding magnetic fields. The interior pressures of Jupiter are so great that hydrogen becomes an electrical conductor. The rotation of the planet thus causes a current to flow through the metallic core to produce a surrounding magnetic field. The strength of the Jupiter field, however, is about 4000 times that found around earth. A key effect of this field is to trap atomic particles arriving as part of the solar wind. The boundaries of the magnetosphere, in the direction toward the sun, lie between 4 and 8 million km from the planet. Within the magnetosphere, charged particles can be accelerated to high energies, with some subsequent escaping and being encountered far from Jupiter. On Voyager 1, one stream of hot plasma was encountered almost 50 million km from the planet. Certain "hot spots" are inside the magnetosphere. Voyager 1 also detected such a plasma about 5 million km from Jupiter and measured its temperature at 300 to 400 million degrees. This is the highest temperature encountered anywhere within the solar system. (It should be noted that the low particle densities found in such a stream make the concept of temperature almost meaningless from a physiologic standpoint.)

One of the most spectacular features of the Voyager missions was the photographs taken of the principal satellites of Jupiter. Jupiter now is known to have at least 14 satellites, with the four largest being termed the Galilean moons, in consideration of their discovery by Galileo in 1610. These moons (Io, Europa, Ganymede, and Callisto) are considered "terrestrial" space bodies. They are similar to the planets of the inner solar system, including earth, in both size and composition. Io, the innermost Galilean satellite, gained a measure of fame when it was found, by chance observation, to have an active volcano. A more careful search then revealed that there were no fewer than eight active volcanos on Io throwing up plumes from 70 to 300 km high. The next satellite, Europa, was found to be crisscrossed by stripes and bands that may represent filled fractures in the satellite's icy crust. It is believed that water, in solid and liquid form, constitutes about 20% of Europa's mass. The next satellite, Ganymede, is the largest of Jupiter's moons. A most noticeable feature of this moon is an immense dark area, the remnant of an ancient crust showing the impact of many meteorites. Finally, there is Callisto, at a mean orbital distance of 1.8 million km from Jupiter. Callisto is about the size of the planet Mercury and shows the effects of billions of years of cratering. It also shows a number of concentric rings that encircle the satellite. These rings are believed to have been formed dynamically by the impact of a large body early in the developmental cycle of the satellite.

During the month of July 1994, the comet Levy 9 broke up into at least 21 fragments, the largest 2 km in diameter, and collided with Jupiter. This was the first collision of two Solar System objects ever to be observed.

In 1989, the United States launched the Galileo project that will provide the first direct sampling of the atmosphere of Jupiter and the first extended observations of the planet, its satellites, and intense magnetospheric environment. The Galileo arrived at Jupiter on December 7, 1995. On the same day, Galileo's atmospheric probe plunged into the planet. Due to damage to the communication system the return of data will be delayed. The orbiter's primary mission is planned to last 22 months at Jupiter and complete the planned 10 orbits of the planet.

The planet itself is most interesting because it retains many features from the early developmental period of the solar system. It also possesses a system of satellites that are quite different from one another and should offer unique insights into the dynamics of early planetary development. The region itself, however, is not hospitable. An immense band of trapped radiation surrounds Jupiter. The planet itself is extremely hot toward the interior and offers no reasonable landing site. Any conceivable manned mission would have to be to one of the satellites.

Saturn

The rings of Saturn are without doubt one of the most spectacular features in the solar system. These rings, which were first observed by Galileo in July, 1610, are the distinguishing characteristics of Saturn. Observations from earth could easily distinguish three of the rings but provided little insight of these rings until close observations were made by American spacecraft.

The Pioneer 11 spacecraft accomplished a successful fly-by mission to Saturn on September 1, 1979. Considerable scientific information was returned, including a number of images from a photopolarimeter, which achieved up to 20 times the resolution provided in earth-based photographs. A major accomplishment of Pioneer was its demonstration that a spacecraft can safely cross the ring plane of Saturn. Although Pioneer was struck at least five times during the encounter by particles at least 10 mm in diameter, there was no real threat to its survival. Pioneer paved the way for the much more ambitious Voyager flights that followed immediately.

The missions of the Voyager 1 and 2 spacecraft provided thousands of startling photographs of the features of Saturn (Fig. 13.9).

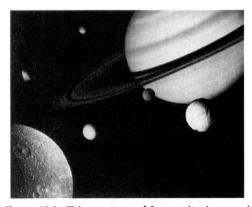

Figure 13.9. This montage of Saturn, its rings, and six of its moons was taken by Voyager 1. Shown clockwise from the right are Tethys, Mimas (with large crater), Enceladus, Dione (at lower left), Rhea, and Titan.

Voyager 1 made its closest approach to the cloud tops of Saturn on November 12, 1980. Thirty-eight months after launch and nearly 1.6 billion km from Earth, Voyager 1 passed the giant planet at a distance of 200,000 km. The Voyager 2 encounter with Saturn occurred on August 25, 1981 at a distance of less than 100,000 km. Each spacecraft photographed the planet, its rings, and its satellites. The passage of each spacecraft carried it through an area of the ring structure.

The surface of Saturn is covered by dense clouds, preventing any direct observation. Much is known of the structure of the planet, however. Saturn is a gas planet, like Jupiter. Its mass is 95 times that of earth. Recent estimates indicate that Saturn may have at the bottom of its gaseous and molten levels a solid core which could constitute about 25% of its mass. The outermost layer of the planet has a liquid mixture of hydrogen and helium, with the hydrogen in molecular form. Beneath this is a metallic liquid layer of hydrogen. The core is presumed to be made of rock and ice. It also is known that Saturn has a source of internal heat, presumably from conversion of gravitational potential energy.

The atmosphere of Saturn is similar to that of Jupiter, although muted by a thick haze layer. It contains dark belts, white-banded zones, and circulating storm regions. Maximum wind speeds are at the equator and can reach speeds of about 1600 km/hr. Temperatures near the cloud tops range from $-125°C$ to $-146°C$. Although auroral emissions have been seen near the poles, lightning has not yet been observed. Saturn also has been found to have a red spot, approximately 11,263 km in length, which resembles Jupiter's red spot. This relatively stable spot is believed to be the upper surface of a convective cell.

The rings of Saturn are most fascinating. The particles that make up these rings are believed to be primarily rock and ice. They have been described as having the size and appearance of "dirty snowballs." Voyager measurements indicate that the particle size in the ring structure ranges from micrometers to meters, with all sizes in between. The well-known A, B, and C rings were found to consist of hundreds of rings or ringlets, a few of which are elliptic in shape. The F ring is more complex and may consist of three interwoven rings that seem to be bounded by two "shepherding" satellites. It is believed that the "spokes" observed in the B rings may be due to fine, electrically charged particles above the ring, perhaps resulting from lightning occurring within the ring.

The flight of Voyager 1 resulted in the discovery of three new satellites of Saturn, bringing the total of known satellites to 15 at that time. Analyses of data from the Voyager 2 encounter, combined with new information from the Voyager 1 flight, now brings the number of known Saturnian satellites to between 21 and 23. The two "possible" satellites were seen in only one observation each, so their orbits could not be confirmed. Scientists at the Jet Propulsion Laboratory in California are continuing their extensive review of Voyager 2 data, and it is possible that additional satellites may yet be confirmed.

With the exception of one—the satellite Titan—all of the moons of Saturn are covered with water ice, and, in some instances, are composed mainly of water ice. For the most part, these satellites show evidence of heavy cratering through the years.

The most interesting of the moons is Titan. Voyager 1 passed within 7000 km of Titan, the closest encounter between cither of the Voyager spacecraft and any planet or moon. This was done to obtain as much information as possible. Titan is the second largest moon observed in the solar system, with a radius of 2575 km. It is the only moon in the solar system with a measurable atmosphere, found to be largely nitrogen with lesser amounts of methane, ethane, acetylene, ethylene, and hydrogen cyanide. The atmosphere of Titan is three times as dense and ten times as deep as that on earth. It also is quite cold, with a temperature near the surface of $-146°C$. The surface pressure is 1.6 bars, or 60% more than that found at the earth's surface. Titan's surface, which is not visible through the atmosphere, may be liquid methane or liquid nitrogen.

The real value of observations of Titan is that this moon, which in many ways resembles a primitive earth maintained in deep-freeze condition, might provide considerable information concerning the manner in which earth has developed. Titan might serve as a natural laboratory within which to realistically study the interaction of environmental forces and chemical factors.

The Voyager missions have shown Saturn and its environment to be a most complex and dynamic scene. There may be as many as 1000 identifiable bands within its complicated ring structure. The known moons of Saturn now number at least 21. The planet has a strong magnetic field and an extensive magnetosphere containing energetic charged particles. It also has the only satellite in the solar system, Titan, known to have a measurable atmosphere.

In all, future missions to Saturn would be a highly recommended step as we attempt to understand better the nature and origin of our solar system. Indeed, planning is being done now for possible insertion of an instrumented probe into the atmosphere of Titan. It is entirely feasible for such a probe to be launched from a manned laboratory orbiting within the near-space of Saturn. A manned mission, allowing direct control over the data collection plan and the operation of onboard instrumentation, would provide a wealth of scientific information and would represent a tremendous stride in the exploration of the solar system.

INTERSTELLAR SPACE

Today, manned spaceflight beyond the solar system remains a topic for science fiction. Probably within the next 100 years, however, serious planning will begin for manned missions beyond the most remote planets. Definitive data showing that the nearest stars have planetary systems similar to that of our sun certainly serves to spur such planning.

Missions into interstellar space will require new technologies. The challenges in engine development will be tremendous. Lightweight engines capable of imparting a continuous accelerative force over a period of days or months will be necessary. For the life sciences, a completely regenerative life-support system will be needed. Obviously, no opportunity will be available for resupply of any kind.

The interstellar environment within which a manned spacecraft will operate is sparse but by no means empty. Considerable gaseous matter is in the interstellar medium, although at densities substantially lower than the best vacuum achievable on earth. Approximately 90% of this gas is neutral hydrogen, radiating at a characteristic wavelength of 21 cm and thus readily detectable. Nearly all of the remaining 10% of gas is made up of atoms of helium. Most of the hydrogen is believed to have been formed during the explosive events that occurred in the creation of the universe approximately 13 to 15 billion years ago. Some of the helium perhaps was formed from primordial hydrogen at the same time, with the rest being manufactured in stars and distributed through supernova explosions. The remaining 1% or less of interstellar gases consists principally of carbon, nitrogen, oxygen, aluminum, and iron. All of these, including still scarcer elements such as aluminum, were formed in nuclear reactions within stars.

In recent years, complex molecules such as cyanogen and formaldehyde have been detected in interstellar space. These molecules are of considerable interest as possible precursors of living matter. They also demonstrate that, although much is being learned about the interstellar environment, a number of mysteries remain. For example, certain small, dense clouds of gas within the Milky Way appear to have substantial concentrations of formaldehyde molecules. Radio observations of these clouds show that the formaldehyde absorbs energy from its microwave background, rather than radiating energy. The formaldehyde appears to be 1.7°K colder than the background. Because one would expect that over time the formaldehyde normally would be warmed to match the temperature of the microwave background radiation, some unspecified action is working within the gas clouds to keep the formaldehyde chilled. Whether this interstellar refrigerator, as well as other features yet to be observed, is of any consequence for manned missions remains to be determined. The finding of such effects does underscore the work remaining before such missions can be attempted. When humanity looks up toward the heavens, it is looking toward its future.

REFERENCES

1. Kerwin JP. Skylab 2 crew observations and summary. In: Biomedical results from Skylab. Johnston RS Lietlein LF, eds. NASA SP-377. Washington, D.C.: Government Printing Office, 1977.
2. Berry CA. Biomedical findings on American astronauts participating in space missions: Man's adaptation to weightlessness. Paper presented at The Fourth International Symposium on Basic Environmental Problems of Man in Space. Yerevan, Armenia, U.S.S.R., October 1–5, 1971.
3. Lundquist CA, ed.: Skylab's Astronomy and Space Sciences. NASA SP-404. Washington, D.C.: Government Printing Office, 1979.
4. Radiation issues. Extracted from Extravehicular Crewman Work System (ECWS) Study Program (SP 04J77). Prepared by Hamilton Standard under Contract NAS 9–15290. Presented at the National Aeronautics and Space Administration, and the Lyndon B. Johnson Space Center, Houston, Texas, October, 1977.
5. Peterson LE. Mortality among astronauts exposed to space and medical radiation: General patterns. A presentation to the 1991 Annual Meeting of the NASA's Occupational Health Program. Kelsey—Seybold Clinic, Houston, Texas, and the Epidemiology Research Center, School of Public Health, University of Texas, Houston, Texas.
6. Bailey J V Hoffman RA English RA. Radiological protection and medical dosimetry for the Skylab crewmen. In: Biomedical results from Skylab. Edited by R.S. Johnston and L.F. Dietlein. NASA SP-377. Washington, D.C.: Government Printing Office, 1977.
7. LDEF—69 Months in Space. First Post-Retrieval Symposium, NASA CP-3134, 1992.
8. Young RS. Viking on Mars: A preliminary survey. Am Sci 1976;64(6):620–627.

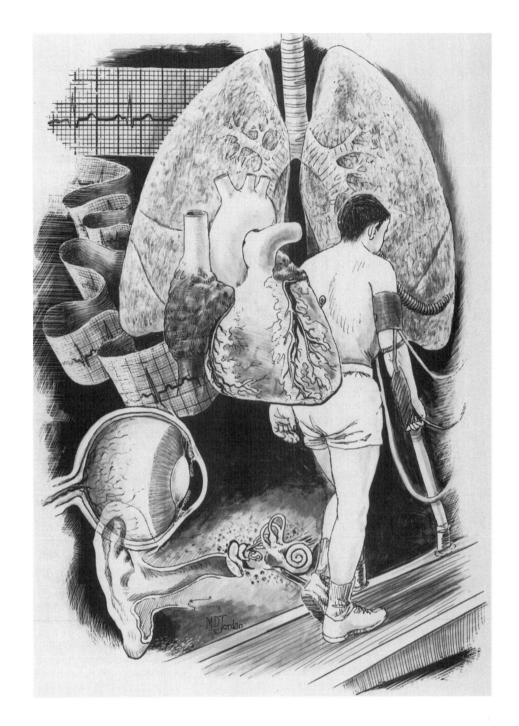

SECTION III
Clinical Practice of Aerospace Medicine

Because the aerospace environment can be demanding on an aviator or astronaut, it is recognized that those controlling flight need to meet a standard of medical fitness. Thus, it is usual for the candidate aircrew person to undergo a medical examination. The standards for the examination are dependent on the nature of the crew duty anticipated. Each body system may be examined, and standards have been developed over time that are appropriate to the sophistication of the examination techniques available and the dynamics of the flight experience.

Once performing aircrew duties, the crewman receives periodic health assessments. Again, the frequency and level of examination are dependent on the nature of the crew duties performed. The flight surgeon or aviation medical examiner can have a major impact on perspective health outcome during this periodic examination by taking advantage of the opportunity to advise on wellness and to institute a program of preventive health measures. Should the examination reveal the early signs of preclinical disease, active steps can be initiated to ameliorate the process.

In assessing the balance between the public safety and the desire of the crew member when disease becomes evident, it is frequently necessary to turn to the appropriate clinical specialist. A broad body of knowledge exists regarding the diseases of various body systems and their impact on continued activities in flying. This data is reviewed in the chapters that follow.

The medical status of the passenger or patient must be compatible with the anticipated stressors of flight. In this section, we are reminded that although aircraft are commonly used to move patients, the aeromedical evacuation aircraft is not a hospital.

Recommended Readings

Aircraft instrument and cockpit lighting by red or white light. Conference Proceedings No 26, Advisory Group for Aerospace Research and Development (AGARD)/ North Atlantic Treaty Organization (NATO), Washington, DC: October, 1967.

American College of Cardiology. Cardiovascular problems associated with aviation safety. Am J Cardiol, 1975:36;573–628.

American Medical Association. Neurological and neurosurgical conditions associated with aviation safety. Arch Neurol, 1979:36;729–812.

Armstrong HG, Heim JW. The effect of flight on the middle ear. JAMA, 1937:109;416.

Brown FM. Vertigo due to increased middle ear pressure. Six-year experience of the Aeromedical Consultation Service. Aerospace Med, 1971:42;999.

Genell L, National Flight Nurse Association. Flight nursing. St. Louis,MO: Mosby-Year Book, 1990.

Jensen RS, ed. Aviation psychology. Brookfield, VT: Gower, 1989.

Johnston N, McDonald N, Fuller R, eds. Aviation psychology in practice. Brookfield, VT: Ashgate, 1994.

Jones DR. Suicide by aircraft. Aviat Space Environ Med, 1977:48;454–455.

Pitts DG. Visual illusions and aircraft accidents. SAM-TR-67–28, United States Air Force School of Aerospace Medicine, Brooks Air Force Base, Texas, April, 1967.

Rayman RB. Clinical Aviation Medicine, 2nd ed. Philadelphia: Lea and Febiger, 1990.

Santy PA. Choosing the right stuff: the psychological selection of astronauts and cosmonauts. Westport, CT: Praeger Publishers, 1993.

Sarnoff CA. Medical aspects of flying motivation. United States Air Force School of Aviation Medicine, Brooks Air Force Base, Texas, 1957.

Sours JE, Ehrlich RE, Phillips PB. The fear of flying syndrome. A reappraisal. Aerospace Med, 1964:35; 156–166.

Chapter 14

Aircrew Health Care Maintenance

Russell B. Rayman

And it is well to superintend the sick to make them well, to care for the healthy to keep them well, also to care for one's own self, so as to observe what is seemly.

Hippocrates

What Hippocrates said centuries ago has as much relevance to today's practitioners of aerospace medicine as it did to the healers of ancient days. The aeromedical specialist is charged not only with the care of the aviator, but also with the prevention of illness and injury. To fulfill this obligation, the flight surgeon must fully understand the aviation environment and the physiologic stresses it imposes on aircrew members. Forearmed with this knowledge, that which was prescribed by Hippocrates can be fulfilled: to care for aviators when they are not well and to keep them healthy when they are well.

SELECTION OF AIRCREW

Historical Background

In the skies over Flanders Fields, Verdun, and other World War I battlegrounds, most Allied losses were due not to enemy fire, but rather to poor techniques in the selection of airmen and practically nonexistent physical standards. This stark realization prompted the founding of aeromedical laboratories such as the one at Mineola, Long Island, New York in 1917 to investigate losses and to establish physical standards for aviators. These early flight surgeons working in primitive laboratories revolutionized aircrew physical standards. Almost immediately, the number of losses over the battlefields of France, Germany, and the Low Countries was significantly reduced.

These early physical standards were only the beginning. Through the years, with the astounding worldwide proliferation of the airlines, general aviation, and military aviation and with the increasing experience of practitioners of aviation medicine, selection techniques and physical standards have continued to evolve.

One of the original selection tests that has survived to this day, introduced by Major Raymond F. Longacre in 1930, is the Adaptability Rating for Military Aeronautics (ARMA). The ARMA is a psychologic/personality inventory interview required of all United States Air Force aircrew candidates and is conducted by a flight surgeon. During this interview, the flight surgeon tries to determine the candidate's suitability for aviation by evaluating background, mental status, emotional stability, and motivation. Although the validity of this technique has not been proved, it is still an integral part of all Air Force aircrew candidate physical examinations and has been for over a half a century.

As World War II approached and it became

clear to many that airpower would play a decisive role in the conflict, there was renewed interest in aircrew selection in overseas countries, as well as in the United States. By this time, a large number of test batteries had been designed and adopted by flying organizations according to their own needs and their faith in the validity of these tests. In general, aircrew selection was governed not only by physical examination, but also by composite scores of psychologic and personality testing, general intelligence, emotional stability, and mechanical aptitude. In the United States Army, composite scores of the test battery were calculated and graded 1 through 9; the higher the score, the better. This system was known as the Standard 9, or Stanine. There appeared to be a direct correlation between Stanine score and the successful completion of pilot training.

Curiously, although new selection techniques are being studied, no giant steps have been taken since World War II in the area of aircrew selection. For example, the United States Air Force still depends very much on a paper/pencil general intelligence test, the Air Force Officer Qualification Test (AFOQT), which was adopted in 1955. Certainly, most flying organizations now have minimum educational requirements and have adopted newer aptitude testing techniques and test batteries. These tests, however, have basic similarities to their predecessors and, like their predecessors, purport to select those candidates with the greatest potential for success in flight training. The problem is further confounded in that success in flight training certainly does not guarantee success in flying operations later on in one's career. It is well known that some military student pilots who just got by were extremely effective in combat. From the military perspective, that far overrides grades and evaluations in school. Unfortunately, we continue to be frustrated in our quest for an aircrew selection test battery that consistently and convincingly selects the very best.

Conversely, aviation medicine has taken great strides in the development of the aircrew physi-

cal examination. Our diagnostic armamentarium is now much more sophisticated, and we have a much clearer understanding of what causes inflight pilot incapacitation, the adverse effects of illness and medication on pilot performance and flying safety, and the stresses of flight on the human organism. Consequently, we are now better able to detect and eliminate those individuals who, for medical reasons, are unsuitable for a career in aviation.

Cogent reasons clearly exist for an effective aircrew selection process: to preserve flying safety, to select those whose promise of a successful career is highest, to eliminate those unsuitable for aviation, and to minimize economic loss because of student pilot wastage. It has been estimated that of every 1000 applicants for flight training, 750 will be rejected for medical or psychologic reasons and 100 will be rejected due to flying deficiencies, leaving 150 candidates who will be able to complete the course successfully (1).

Aircrew Selection by Job Analysis and Testing

Although aircrew selection has long been of concern to flight surgeons and has been the subject of countless professional inquiries through the years, one needs only to consult Dr. Ross McFarland's classic textbook, *Human Factors in Air Transportation*, written 45 years ago, to understand the basic tenets as well as the inherent complexities of this subject. It was this pioneer of aviation medicine who recognized that the first step in the selection process of pilots is job or task analysis. That is, aircrew duties must be subjected to close scrutiny to identify their requirements in respect to reactions and responses, stresses, and component task skills. Next, those aptitudes must be identified that would be desirable in accomplishing each task in question. The final step is to devise tests that could then be used to identify training applicants who are best endowed with these aptitudes because they presumably would be the most likely to succeed.

Although this sequitur, at first glance, appears to be ingenuously logical, it is fraught with pitfalls that, to this day, remain unsolved. For example, one can never be certain that the job analysis is entirely accurate because the analysis itself is based on subjectivity, which, in turn, invites differences. For example, if two pilots, current in the same aircraft, were asked to analyze their cockpit responsibilities, there undoubtedly would be differences of opinion in substance as well as degree. Likewise, there would probably be inconsistencies if the pilots also were asked what they considered to be desirable traits or aptitudes to accomplish successfully their tasks. Finally, even if pilots unanimously agreed on job analysis and desirable aptitudes, how does one validate those tests or procedures used to select aircrew applicants? The validation of selection tests is very difficult regardless of whether the criterion is the successful completion of flight training or the ''success'' of a flying career, perhaps over a 5- to 10-year period. Thus, the complexities of aircrew selection become painfully clear.

Over the past 65 years, various types of selection tests have been designed, adopted, and administered by flying organizations. These have included general intelligence, mechanical, psychologic, and personality tests.

Mechanical/apparatus testing was given a great deal of attention in previous decades. Pilot candidates were evaluated with a multitude of contraptions — some ingenious, others primitive — for reaction time, stick and rudder control, instrument interpretation, and two-hand coordination tests, to mention only a few. A lot of time and effort was devoted to this science in the belief that there was a positive correlation of apparatus scores and training outcome. Until recent years, however, there appeared to have been a decline in interest in these tests, due, in part, to the cost of purchasing large numbers of expensive devices, as well as the administrative costs of bringing student applicants to their locations.

With advanced cockpit technology, the demands upon today's pilots have shifted, to some extent, from pure mechanical to information processing prowess. Hence, with the availability of computers, there has been renewed interest in testing methodology for the selection of student pilot applicants. One such new system being studied by the USAF is the PORTA-BAT (Portable Basic Attributes), now simply called the BAT, which features a sophisticated computerized battery of 15 psychometer and cognitive tests that promises to reduce attrition for pilot training and predict flying performance (2). Validation of BAT scores thus far has been very encouraging.

Another computer-administered test of cognitive function, which the USAF is currently evaluating, is CogScreen. Pending completion of studies, this test also holds great promise as a selection method.

Flight surgeons generally agree that certain personality types are better adapted than others for cockpit duties. For this reason, aircraft selection usually includes some type of personality inventory or evaluation. Those personality traits that are desirable for pilots were first described by McFarland four decades ago and are probably still relevant today. Among those desirable traits McFarland identified were mental ability, mechanical comprehension, judgment, alertness, observational ability, motor skill, emotional control, character, and leadership. Other investigators have found high correlations with intelligence, emotional stability, conscientiousness, and self-control.

Another method utilized by some flying organizations, the RAF in particular, is the group interaction technique, in which aircrew candidates are placed into groups and given problems to solve that require joint cooperation and coordination. By monitoring the group, skilled observers can identify those with leadership qualities, those who can function under stress, and those who effectively participate in problem solving. It is believed that these individuals would be eminently qualified for flight training, although not all flying organizations subscribe to this selection approach.

As an aside, a large American aircraft company published a comprehensive and detailed report outlining a program for the selection of fighter pilots who would be most effective in air-to-air combat (3). The report identifies 45 attributes that are essential to the most combat-effective air-to-air fighter pilot. The report further describes what testing is available to identify those applicants with these attributes. This study, although innovative, really is based on the original principles of job analysis that McFarland described many years ago.

Although much controversy remains regarding the efficacy and validity of the various test batteries, most of them, to some degree, have predictive value in the identification of pilot candidates who will be successful. Clearly, more research needs to be done in this area. In the meantime, flying organizations must incorporate those testing procedures into their aircrew selection process that are cost-effective and would most efficiently identify aircrewmen who will best accomplish the mission requirements of that flying organization.

PERIODIC MEDICAL ASSESSMENT

Purpose

Although flying organizations may employ different aircrew selection techniques and physical standards, individuals must be in a good state of health to pass any aviation medical department physical examination. With time, however, even healthy aviators will develop illnesses, whether acute or chronic, serious or benign, as would be expected in any adult population regardless of age or occupation. Because of the requirements of cockpit duties, as well as the obligation of aviation for safety in the air, airmen, to ensure continued good health, are required to have periodic medical assessment. The purpose of the periodic physical examination is really threefold: flying safety, health of the airman, and mission completion.

Scope

Aviation medical departments worldwide have, to some extent, different aeromedical programs and policies: what constitutes medical grounds for temporary or permanent removal from flying status, how often a periodic examination is required, and what physicians are qualified to administer the examination. This becomes apparent when one studies the policies of the International Civil Aviation Organization (ICAO), the Federal Aviation Administration (FAA), and the military services in the United States and abroad. To explore in detail these differences would not be particularly instructive because what may be policy one day may not be the next as flying organizations must readapt their standards to ever-changing conditions and requirements. Let it suffice to say that medical departments are obligated to establish physical standards tailored to their flying mission, with flying safety an uppermost consideration.

The periodic flight physical examination can be divided into five parts: history and physical examination, dental examination, laboratory procedures, subprofessional consultations, and specialty consultations. The history and physical examination is accomplished by the practitioner and because of its universality, little need be said other than to repeat that old adage — the physician should do a complete history and physical examination.

Although dental disease is an unlikely cause of in-flight incapacitation (the rare occurrence of aerodontalgia is perhaps the one exception), it is advisable that airmen maintain a healthy dental status. A toothache can cause both considerable discomfort and performance decrement should it occur in flight or in an isolated location where immediate dental care might not be available. There are also military implications in that many aviators who were prisoners of war during the Vietnam War suffered because of preexisting dental disease and practically nonexistent treatment during captivity. Long-term captivity for an airman with dental disease means not only pain, but possibly poor nutrition because of an inability to chew.

Laboratory tests may include a variety of determinations such as a complete blood count and urinalysis, with some medical departments adding to these a fasting blood glucose, serologic evaluation, and lipid profile among others. Procedures that are often part of the periodic flight physical include chest radiographs, spirometry, electrocardiogram, and electroencephalogram. As is true for so many screening laboratory tests and procedures, there is considerable debate regarding their cost-effectiveness and necessity. The chest radiograph is an example. Although the vast majority of chest radiographs taken in conjunction with the flight physical are normal, silent lesions occasionally are found such as a benign or malignant tumor, small pneumothorax, or sarcoid. The expense of the procedure and exposure to radiation weighed against the number of pathologic conditions detected brings into question its necessity. Because of this, many flying organizations have dropped the requirement, although in some countries, particularly those with a high prevalence of pulmonary disease, such as tuberculosis, a screening chest x-ray remains a part of the medical evaluation.

Spirometry is felt to be worthwhile in some quarters to detect obstructive pulmonary disease, particularly that caused by excessive cigarette smoking. Besides the known pulmonary association of cigarettes with lung cancer and emphysema, there is the aeromedical consideration of increased carbon monoxide levels reducing the oxygen-transport capability of hemoglobin. Hence, an explanation of this factor to the airman should reinforce the usual admonitions against smoking.

Because of the increased awareness of coronary artery disease during the past 20 years and its possible role in causing sudden in-flight incapacitation, aviation medical departments almost always require resting and/or stress electrocardiograms. Differences occur only in the frequency of testing, the method of stressing, and the interpretation of results. Clearly, the main reason for

a periodic electrocardiogram is to detect latent coronary artery disease.

Some medical departments require an electroencephalogram only on entry into flight training to identify those applicants with epileptogenic activity. Another reason is to have on record a baseline tracing that can be used for comparison should that individual sustain head trauma at some time in the future.

The paraprofessional portion of the examination is that which can be done by a technician. The physician's time need be spent only in the interpretation of abnormal findings. Measurements may include blood pressure and pulse determinations, audiometry, and several tests of vision. Because of the singular importance of vision in flight, the eye examination should include testing near and far visual acuity, phoria-tropia-diplopia, accommodation, depth perception, visual fields, and color and night vision. Tonometry to rule out glaucoma is also advisable for older airmen.

Specialty consultations must be available in the event that illness is suspected, the diagnosis and treatment of which is beyond the expertise of the flight surgeon. Such consultation is particularly useful if the specialists have had some training in the principles of aerospace medicine.

Effectiveness

The periodic flight physical examination can be considered a form of secondary preventive medicine, as defined by Lilienfeld:

Secondary preventive measures are designed to detect the disease at a sufficiently early stage to permit intervention in order to decelerate the rate of progression of the disease, and to prevent complications, sequelae, disability, and premature mortality (4).

To this definition the flight surgeon might add, "to remove from flying status, either temporarily or permanently, those aviators with illnesses that pose an added risk to flying safety."

Because the periodic physical examination really consists of a test battery (i.e., professional and paraprofessional examination and a number of laboratory procedures), it can be considered a form of multiphasic screening. Multiphasic screening has been a favorite, although controversial, subject of preventive medicine specialists in recent years. All of the arguments, pro and con, basically center on cost-effectiveness, that is, one questions whether, with limited health care delivery funds and finite physician time available, sufficient pathologic conditions are detected and effectively treated to make screening programs worthwhile.

For example, a study was done some years ago in the United States Air Force's Strategic Air Command to study efficacy of the periodic flight physical examination. It was found that in a 1-year period, 28,000 physical examinations were administered, with each examination consuming 30 minutes of a physician's time and a total of 200 minutes of time if laboratory procedures, dental examinations, and administration were included. The authors found that very little disease was detected by the physician; rather, the majority of the pathologic disorders were discovered by those measurable portions of the examination, such as blood pressure, radiography, electrocardiography, blood and urine tests, and visual and auditory testing, which can be done by a technician. Hence, it was concluded that too much time and money are given to the flight physical examination as we know it and that it would be far more economical to include only those measurable screening tests that can be performed by technicians.

Even if one accepts this, however, the flight surgeon reaps other benefits from the physical examination, which are unqualifiable in terms of cost-effectiveness yet clearly important. First, it affords the physician the opportunity to spend a little time with the flyer in the quiet and privacy of the office. This time can be well spent reviewing the aviator's medical history, particularly the interval history since the last examination and just talking with the aviator. During these min-

utes, the flight surgeon can get to know the airman a little better and possibly gain better insight into his or her personal situation. If given the opportunity, airmen will often confide in the flight surgeon various problems, either relating to health, family, or some other difficulties affecting job performance. The flight surgeon has a chance not only to intercede if it is appropriate, but also to enhance rapport with the airman, something that is very important to any aviation medicine program. Furthermore, in this day of emphasis on healthy life-styles and health education, the flight surgeon has the opportunity to help the aviator identify poor health habits and suggest ways of correcting such habits. For these reasons, the periodic flight physical examination is important and should continue to be an integral part of any aerospace medicine program.

THE FEMALE CREWMEMBER

Historical Background

The exigencies of World War II led to the creation of the famous Women's Army Service Pilots (WASPs) as a part of United States Army Aviation. Because every male crewmember was needed for combat assignments, this first group of female pilots was tasked with ferrying military aircraft within the United States and to overseas theaters. The saga of the WASPs and their success is now history. By ferrying hundreds of aircraft and logging thousands of hours, they clearly demonstrated that women could accomplish cockpit responsibilities. In spite of their illustrious record, however, women only in recent years have been admitted to commercial and military cockpits albeit with some degree of reluctance and skepticism. The controversial issues of women in the cockpit include anthropometric conformity to standard cockpit design, ability to withstand the stresses of flight, and pregnancy and menses.

In recent years, the aerospace medicine literature has devoted many pages to these subjects. It is to be expected, however, that more investigation will be accomplished as more experience is accrued in the coming years and as the military and commercial airlines gain confidence in their selection procedures of women crewmembers. However, women have clearly demonstrated thus far that their performance in the cockpit is on par with men.

Man-Machine Interface

The science of aviation anthropometrics was born in the early aeromedical research laboratories just prior to World War II. It was apparent that as cockpits were becoming more complicated and in-flight tasks more demanding, aeronautic engineers would have to take into consideration man's physical limitations. Consequently, cockpits, as well as flight clothing and life-support equipment, were designed to accommodate the physical size and strength characteristics of men between the 5th and 95th percentiles. All of these activities came under the rubric of "man-machine interface," which gives a subtle clue that those physical characteristics of women, size and strength in particular, were probably given little or no attention.

The average man is taller, heavier, and stronger than the average woman. A number of studies have clearly demonstrated that women have about 60% of the physical strength of men (5). Another study indicated that the maximum force of a significant percentage of women would fall below the design criteria of certain aircraft controls (Table 14.1). Although this disparity may not be true for all types of airplanes, the implication is that under extreme conditions, some women would not have sufficient strength to control the aircraft.

Over the years, cockpits have been designed to accommodate men anthropometrically, that is, sitting height, reach, and buttocks-to-knee distance, in the 5th to 95th percentiles. Surveys of anthropometrics of women reveal that a significant proportion of them fall below the 5th percentile of men in all measured parameters. For example, 77% of women fall below the 5th

Table 14.1.
Percent of Subjects Whose Maximum Force Was Below MIL-F-8782B Design Criteria

Control	Criteria		Percent Below Criteria	
	kg	lb	Males	Females
Stick forward	34	75	0	28
Stick back	23	50	0	40
Stick left	16	35	5	95
Stick right	16	35	50	100
Left rudder	82	180	7	11
Right rudder	82	180	0	5

From McDaniel JW. Male and female strength capabilities for operating aircraft controls. Preprints of the Scientific Program of the Aerospace Medical Association Meeting, May 4–7, 1981;12.

percentile for men in sitting height and 27% fall below the 5th percentile in buttocks-to-knee length (6). Hence, a significant percentage of women cannot be accommodated in today's cockpits. This is not due to any feminine deficiency, however, as much as to the engineering design and configuration of aircraft cockpits, which heretofore took into account only male physical characteristics. The solution, therefore, can be found in aeronautic engineering textbooks. Simply stated, if the military services and the airline companies see that it is in their interests to employ larger numbers of female crewmembers, engineers will consider the physical attributes of women and design cockpits accordingly.

The Stresses of Flight

The physiologic stresses of flight have been well defined through several decades of intense research. For the most part, however, the effects of these stresses and the limitations of human beings have focused on male crewmembers. We have now been examining how well women can tolerate these stresses and how the two sexes compare. Studies continue to be published on the female crewmember's tolerance of acceleration, hypoxia, decompression sickness, circadian rhythm, and noise and vibration, as well as a host of other physiologic stresses associated with aviation.

As an example of such research, the United States Air Force Armstrong Laboratory (formerly the United States Air Force School of Aerospace Medicine) has conducted studies on women and their tolerance to acceleration. These studies have revealed that women tolerate G forces as well as men (7).

These studies and others like it are now in progress in various research facilities around the world. More information will be forthcoming as an increasing number of female pilots are admitted to the cockpit and as their performance is observed. Thus far, no physiological factors of operational significance have been identified which would place women at a disadvantage to men.

Menses and Pregnancy

Menses and pregnancy are the two physiologic processes that clearly separate women and men. Because of their usual indispositions, women's fitness for cockpit duties has been questioned. There are those who argue that dysmenorrhea is very common and causes excessive absenteeism. Furthermore, there is the possibility that pain relief can be obtained only by medication, which might be disqualifying for flying duties. In support of this position, a study of 200 stewardesses indicated that 48% of them reported a change in menses—increased or decreased flow and/or pelvic pain and congestion—which was attributed to stress and internal desynchronization due to disruption of circadian rhythm (8). At this time, however, there is no solid evidence that menses causes performance decrement or increased absenteeism among female pilots.

Dysmenorrhea may be primary or secondary. The former occurs in the absence of an underlying disease while the latter may be associated with pelvic pathology such as endometriosis, congenital malformation, and pelvic inflammatory disease among others. Primary dysmenorrhea can be effectively treated with birth control pills and prostaglandin inhibitors, e.g., ibuprofen, thereby permitting aviatrices to perform in the cockpit as long as they get good relief and can tolerate the medication. For secondary dysmenorrhea, the underlying cause must be successfully treated.

Many questions regarding the pregnant pilot remain unanswered. What undesirable effects will the stresses of flight cause for the pregnant woman and the fetus and when should a pregnant crewmember stop flying? Most authorities agree that the physiologic stresses of flight in normal airline operations are so slight that they cannot really threaten a fetus. Even the mild hypoxia caused by cabin altitudes of 1524 to 2134 m will cause no adverse effects. Hence, physiologically, a pregnant woman with a normal pregnancy should be able to fly safely from the time of conception to the eve of delivery. In aviation, however, there are other considerations, especially performance decrement, which demand disqualification from the cockpit at some time during the course of the pregnancy. For example, most pregnant women will normally experience nausea and vomiting, increased fatigue, and emotional lability, not to mention an increase in size and weight. Although the time for removal is somewhat arbitrary and at the discretion of the many airline companies, flight attendants are usually disqualified between 20 and 27 weeks of gestation; primary crewmembers are often removed at the time of conception or shortly thereafter, depending upon airline policy.

Regarding military aircraft that subject crews to special physiologic stresses such as low barometric pressures, in-flight decompressions, and accelerative forces, it would be prudent to disqualify the pregnant crewmember at the time of conception because we have no knowledge at this time of the ill effects these would have on the conceptus.

MEDICAL DISABILITY

Temporary and Permanent Disability

Regardless of the stringent selection procedures for flight training and of the number of applicants that are disqualified because of preexisting disease, it can be expected that most aviators over the years will develop illness necessitating either temporary or permanent disqualification from flying duty or a medical waiver. Because aviators cannot be expected to maintain perfect health throughout their careers, flying organizations must employ some system that permits these deviations while compromising neither flying safety nor the health of the aviator. Financial factors also cannot be ignored in that permanent disqualification and pilot wastage will create enormous dollar losses in both commercial and military aviation. Disqualification and waiver policies necessarily differ among flying organizations because of both the differences of the aircraft flown and air operations. Although every flying organization has evolved its own rules and regulations governing these matters, in general, all of them have stringent entry physical examination requirements, with some degree of relaxation once the student crewmember or new employee is trained and operational.

In most cases, temporary disqualifications are for minor, self-limiting illness, illness requiring the temporary use of medication considered hazardous to the aviation environment (e.g., antihistamines, sedatives or analgesics), and treatable illness wherein cure is expected. In any event, once the condition is in remission and there are no sequelae that pose a threat to flying safety, it would be in order for the aeromedical specialist to recommend a return to flying status.

On the other hand, if the disease is of a more serious nature, permanent disqualification must be considered. Examples might include coronary artery disease, uncorrectable loss of visual acuity, or untreatable carcinoma. Again, all flying organizations determine those policies that govern permanent disqualification based on the type of aircraft flown and the flying mission.

Medical Waiver System

In some cases, crewmembers may develop illnesses that can be effectively treated, albeit with

a potential for progression. Glaucoma, glomerulonephritis, and hypertension are classic examples. Clearly, airmen with illnesses such as these can be granted medical waivers for flying duty as long as the defect is static and the disease itself or the treatment pose no threat to flying safety and there is assurance of periodic follow-up. On the other hand, if the disease process progresses, permanent disqualification from the cockpit would have to be considered. A sensible waiver policy and administrative mechanism tailored to the needs of every flying organization is necessary, without which there is the risk of eliminating airmen unnecessarily and unfairly.

The military services and the FAA have their own medical and administrative procedures, policies, and regulations for processing temporary and permanent disqualification and medical waiver requests. Let it suffice to say that in the military services, no formal appeal process exists should the airman not agree with the recommendation of the flight surgeon; that is, the aeromedical services makes its recommendation to operational commanders regarding disqualification, and in practically all cases, these recommendations are followed. In the case of the FAA, however, a system of appeals exists whereby individuals denied medical certification can petition the FAA, the National Transportation Safety Board, and even courts of law for an exemption. These procedures are described in greater detail in Chapter 26.

Waiver or exemption policy over the years has clearly become more liberal as aerospace medicine specialists have matured by acquiring more experience. This trend has been cautious, deliberative, and in most cases, sensible. Aviators today are actively flying—and flying safely—with waivers which would have been unthinkable in recent decades for various diseases and treatment regimens. There is no evidence that flying safety or personal safety have been compromised. One would expect a continued, steady course toward more liberal ground in the coming decade.

Consultation Services

Occasionally, airmen develop complex or obscure medical conditions for which continued flying status is questionable. To make a diagnosis and/or recommend aeromedical disposition, the United States Army, Navy, and Air Force have established their respective aeromedical consultation services. These consultation services are staffed by physicians with specialty training, as well as considerable training and experience in aerospace medicine. Crewmembers who are disqualified from flying duties because of complex or obscure medical conditions are referred from bases worldwide to these centers for diagnostic evaluation and recommendations for flying status. Over the years, the staffs of these consultation services have examined thousands of airmen with a legion of diseases involving all body systems. They have, because of their expertise in aviation medicine, saved the government a considerable sum of money by recommending a return to flying status for many airmen who otherwise would have been permanently disqualified.

OPERATIONAL STRESS

Since the infancy of aviation medicine, the physiologic stresses of flight have been the subject of intensive research in laboratories around the world. This great interest has been prompted by the realization that acceleration, hypoxia, vibration, and decreased barometric pressure, alone or in combination, pose a threat to flying safety of airmen. Through years of diligent research efforts, aerospace medicine scientists have developed excellent life-support equipment and systems to minimize this threat. Yet, even with these countermeasures, accidents and incidents continue to occur because of man's inability to fully accommodate to the extraterrestrial environment. It is for this reason that aviation organizations seek healthy, fit aircrew members whose constitutions are most resistant to the physiologic stresses of flight.

Acceleration

Although any type of aircraft can subject its crew to accelerative forces, we think more of aerobatics, aerial spraying, or high-performance military operations when discussing significant $+G_z$ or $-G_z$ stress. $+G_z$ affects primarily the cardiovascular system and can cause blackout or loss of consciousness—both clearly undesirable in flight—by decreasing blood flow to the eye and brain. Countermeasures include the use of an anti-G suit and the proper performance of the M-1 maneuver, the latter giving an additional 1 to 2 G_z of protection. With $-G_z$, blood is accelerated headward, causing stimulation of the carotid sinus and possible incapacitation by inducing various degrees of heartblock. Unfortunately, there are no effective countermeasures for this type of acceleration other than the avoidance of $-G_z$ maneuvers such as outside loops.

Accelerative forces are potentially incapacitating, although countermeasures are protective to some degree. This is of particular significance today because modern jet fighter aircraft are capable of sudden onset, sustained high-G loads—over $9+ G_z$. As a result, G-loss of consciousness (GLOC) has caused a number of aircraft accidents as well as near losses (9). Because $+G_z$ and $-G_z$ acceleration primarily affect the cardiovascular system, it is extremely important that individuals who fly G-inducing aircraft be free of cardiovascular disease. This is one reason why the cardiovascular system is given such intense scrutiny during initial and periodic physical examinations.

Hypoxia

Because most aircraft cockpits do not pressurize to sea level pressures during normal operations, crewmembers are frequently hypoxic to some degree. Healthy individuals, however, should still be able to perform their cockpit tasks without difficulty as long as they are not exposed to altitudes above 3048 m. At higher altitudes, everyone will develop hypoxic symptoms that can cause some degree of performance decrement. Crewmembers are well protected from hypoxia by sophisticated life-support systems, the foremost being the pressurized cabin. Furthermore, oxygen masks with continuous-flow or pressure-demand systems are commonplace in commercial and military aviation.

There is little question that a normal, healthy crewmember can tolerate mildly hypoxic environments without experiencing a significant performance decrement and without jeopardizing health. The same cannot be said, however, for individuals with cardiopulmonary disease. For example, in an hypoxic state, the coronary vessels must dilate to allow more blood to reach the oxygen-starved myocardium. The coronary vessels of individuals with coronary artery disease, however, do not dilate well, and this imposes an added burden on the heart muscle, which can have serious implications. Likewise, individuals with diseased lungs, such as those with emphysema, cannot absorb a normal complement of oxygen even under sea level conditions, and at altitude, oxygen absorption would be even more compromised.

Noise and Vibration

The noise emanating from any aircraft engine, jet or propeller, will eventually cause acoustic trauma if an unprotected individual is exposed for a sufficiently long time. This places not only aircrews at risk, but also the large work force normally employed in the various shops and activities in the vicinity of the flight line. Because of the potential for developing partial or complete deafness due to acoustic trauma, aviation medical departments conduct hearing conservation programs, the objective of which is to prevent hearing loss. Although these programs may vary somewhat in design, they are basically alike, with protocols that require the identification of flight-line and in-flight hazardous noise areas, the issuing of earplugs and/or muffs to those individuals at risk, and the administration of baseline and follow-up audiograms. Gener-

ally, audiologists agree that some form of ear protection is advisable if noise intensity levels exceed 85 dB.

It has been well established that vibrations between 1 and 12 Hz will cause performance decrement in the cockpit. For example, low-frequency vibration can induce motion sickness, fatigue, shortness of breath, and abdominal and chest pain. Furthermore, considerable blurring of the instrument panel can make accurate reading of the dials extremely difficult. For these reasons, aeronautic engineers have gone to great lengths in designing aircraft to eliminate or at least minimize potentially hazardous vibration.

Decreased Barometric Pressure

As one gains altitude from the Earth's surface, the barometric pressure decreases accordingly from a sea level value of 760 mm Hg to the vacuum of space. Because of this natural phenomenon, man is at risk, if without adequate protection, of becoming hypoxic or of developing decompression sickness and barotrauma. Decompression sickness manifests itself in various forms, causing symptoms by nitrogen bubble formation in the body fluids. Because significant bubble formation is unusual below altitudes of 5486 m (18,000 ft), decompression sickness is rarely encountered in those aircraft normally pressurized to 1524 to 2438 m (5000 to 8000 ft). The risk is far greater in some military aircraft, which fly with higher cabin altitudes. The symptoms of evolved gas decompression sickness are many and include joint pain (bends), chokes, central nervous system disturbances, and neurocirculatory collapse. Hence, this syndrome is of great aeromedical significance not only because it can cause in-flight incapacitation, but because it can be lethal.

Besides the ill effects of evolved gas, crewmembers can suffer serious discomfort if a pressure differential exists between the bony cavities, for example, the sinuses or middle ear, and the ambience. These forms of barotrauma can occur with any change in altitude, although they are most commonly associated with descent. The inability to freely exchange gas can incapacitate the crewmember by causing excruciating pain.

Circadian Rhythm

With the advent of long-range aircraft capable of crossing oceans and continents without refueling, the term circadian rhythm has become part of the aerospace medicine vocabulary. Today, it is not at all unusual for international flights to cross as many as five to ten time zones. Hence, an aircrew may depart on a flight en route to a destination with an 8-hour time difference. As a result, the sleep/wake/meal time cycle at the destination will not be synchronized with that of the crew. This desynchrony can result in some degree of personal discomfort and inefficiency at the destination because of fatigue during the day and wakefulness at night, commonly referred to as jet lag. As a rule of thumb, it takes approximately 1 day per time zone crossed to fully recover from jet lag.

Various diets and medications have been touted in minimizing the effects of jet lag, although none has passed the test of scientific scrutiny. Currently, melatonin has been advocated, although there is no solid evidence as to its efficacy in alleviating the symptoms of jet lag (10). A promising technique under investigation is bright light exposure preflight which, purportedly, entrains the internal clock very rapidly to the destination time.

It is well known that the above phenomenon is not just a psychologic idiosyncrasy but rather is due to diurnal biochemical reactions that occur at set times during the day and night. Therefore, when suddenly going to another part of the world with a significant time difference, the diurnal reactions are not in harmony with the time of day or night at the destination.

The physical and psychologic problems of circadian desynchrony are matters of special concern for those crossing numerous time zones for purposes other than recreation. Politicians, statesmen, athletes, business persons, and military personnel can all be affected by desynchronization, resulting in lower efficiency, poor decision making, and compromised negotiation ability. For most people, studies have established that fewer problems occur with movement across time zones in a westerly direction rather than easterly.

Temperature and Humidity

With the development of modern environmental systems, cockpit temperature and humidity are reasonably well controlled in commercial aircraft, although dryness is sometimes a problem. Regarding some military aircraft, cockpits have marginal environmental control and, consequently, are frequently hot and dry, causing some degree of dehydration, which can result in subjective discomfort and performance decrement. The stresses of cockpit heat are particularly threatening to military crews operating in tropical or desert climates. It is not at all unusual for pilots to spend 15 to 20 minutes in preflight readiness of their aircraft in a hot revetment area and then to sit in the cockpit wearing cumbersome flying equipment and without the benefit of effective air conditioning for another 30 minutes while completing checklists, taxiing, and arming prior to takeoff. Pilots frequently report that they are wringing wet from perspiration under such circumstances. Then, temperature control in flight is suboptimal in some fighter aircraft, causing further heat buildup during low-level or gunnery-range operations. The solution to the problem is improved engineering of environmental systems, which must come with future technologic advances.

Life-Support Equipment

Great technologic advances have occurred in life-support equipment over the years, without which flying operations as we know it would not be possible. Nevertheless, the benefits reaped are partially offset by the penalties, which, in the present state of the art, cannot be obviated. Some of the equipment is bulky and cumbersome, causing restriction of movement as well as heat retention and excessive perspiration—a significant imposition, particularly in hot, humid weather. These are special burdens in military aviation because a shirt-sleeves environment is the rule in commercial aircraft.

The fighter pilot's basic life-support equipment includes a helmet, visor, oxygen mask, anti-G suit, and survival vest, which are worn over the standard Nomex flight suit. It is easy to understand, therefore, how a buildup of body heat can occur, particularly when it takes as long as 30 minutes to do the preflight tasks, start the engines, taxi, arm, and take off. Another penalty pilots pay is restriction of visibility and limitation of movement of the head and neck due to the helmet/mask combination. This can be most critical in aerial combat maneuvers because scanning the skies and recognizing enemy aircraft early is a sine qua non of success in such operations. Furthermore, because the neck muscles must bear the entire weight of the helmet/oxygen mask combination, they tend to fatigue with repetitive G maneuvers. As night vision goggles become standard equipment, strain upon the head and neck will become even greater.

For high-flying aircraft that normally operate at altitudes above 15,240 m (50,000 ft), full- or partial-pressure suits must be worn. Although these suits can be lifesaving in the event of rapid decompression or ejection at high altitudes, they can cause considerable difficulties for pilots who must wear them—heat buildup, restriction of vision, and impaired movement of the head and limbs, to cite only a few problems.

An important addition to life-support systems is the chemical defense ensemble, the purpose of which is to protect airmen on the ground, as well as in flight should an enemy utilize chemical weapons. These suits provide excellent protection, but, like the pressure suit, they restrict vision and movement, although their greatest liability is heat retention. Today, scientists are avidly continuing the quest for an improved suit

that will protect the wearer while imposing minimum penalties.

Fatigue

The many operational stresses of flight induce fatigue to some degree. It can be said, perhaps, that fatigue is an inherent stress of aviation duties. Erratic schedules, hypoxic environments, noise and vibration, and imperfect environmental systems will eventually take their toll. Although fatigue can be neatly defined as acute, chronic, or cumulative and correlated to some extent with biochemical aberrations, we are not yet able to determine objectively at what point an airman is fatigued enough to cause performance decrement. Therefore, until we can do so, the risk of fatigue must be reduced by preventive measures such as ensuring that reasonable flying schedules and hours logged are maintained and that good food, quarters, and accommodations are provided.

SELF-IMPOSED STRESS

The physiologic stresses of flight, which have been briefly described, in themselves are potentially threatening to flying safety. Even under the most benign conditions, aviation will impose some degree of stress on airmen. Clearly, a healthy individual with a strong constitution will be more resistant to these physiologic stresses and, therefore, will function more efficiently and more safely. Unfortunately, many airmen degrade this resistance by self-imposed, unhealthy behavior patterns and life-styles.

Self-Medication

The side effects of commonly prescribed medications are well known to practicing aeromedical specialists. Because of the potential threat to flying safety, physicians in aerospace medicine are particularly sensitive to the actions of any medication prescribed for airmen. Consider, for example, the many medicines that, in addition to their primary pharmacologic effects, also cause degradation of visual acuity, impaired coordination, increased reaction time, drowsiness, or hypotension. Those that come immediately to mind are the antihistamines, anticholinergics, tranquilizers, sedatives, antihypertensives, and analgesics. It is likely that the vast majority of prescribed drugs would fall into one of these categories.

To discuss the hundreds of various routinely prescibed drugs and their side effects is beyond the scope of this chapter. Suffice it to say that practically every drug in the physician's pharmacopoeia has the potential for some untoward effects that could be detrimental in the cockpit. Because of this potential, it is advisable to temporarily remove airmen from flying duties for the duration of treatment. Although this is a universal principle in aerospace medicine, exceptions can and have been made for those medications that have been judged to be of minimal risk. Medical waivers for these exceptions can be safely granted with the proviso that there is a reasonably close following by the flight surgeon. Examples might include certain antibiotics, thiazides, and thyroid medication.

Organizational policies concerning medication and the aviator are somewhat difficult to enforce for several reasons. First, aviators may seek medical care from physicians who are unauthorized by the flying organization or who are not versed in aerospace medicine. Consequently, a physician may prescribe what is ordinarily considered a benign medication, not fully appreciating the in-flight implications. Perhaps a far greater problem is the availability of over-the-counter medicines that have enjoyed a remarkable proliferation over the past two decades. Many of these medicines, which purport to cure colds, headaches, myalgias, as well as a host of other ailments suffered by mankind, are no different than prescription drugs in that they may cause side effects that are undesirable in the cockpit. Crewmembers often purchase over-the-counter drugs for a minor illness without realizing the potential danger of this practice. For this

reason, self-medication can be considered one form of self-imposed stress.

It is the physician's obligation to discourage aircrew members from this practice and to encourage them to report illnesses to the appropriate authority. Only in this way can the proper medication be prescribed and proper follow-up be ensured. The flight surgeon can do this only by aircrew education in the form of talks and bulletins, as well as by establishing good rapport with the aviators of the organization.

Alcohol and Illicit Drug Abuse

The use of illicit drugs has become a global social phenomenon in recent decades, reaching all socioeconomic strata. Their availability, therefore, extends not only to the underprivileged, but also to the middle and affluent classes, to which most members of the aviation community belong. Hence, with the ubiquity of illicit drugs, as well as their social acceptability, airmen may be tempted to become experimenters or abusers. Today's newspapers and periodicals devote many pages to the subject of drugs and to the ''expert'' opinions of those who advocate their free and legal usage. Although controversy does exist concerning the short-term and long-term effects of many drugs, as well as the social implications of their use, they are clearly unacceptable in any cockpit. Most illicit drugs cause side effects (drowsiness, euphoria, impaired mentation, hallucinations, and flashbacks) that categorically threaten flying safety. For this reason, legal and moral considerations aside, these substances must be condemned. The aviation medicine practitioner is obligated to have some knowledge of illicit drugs and hallucinogens and to discourage their use among aviators.

Of the various types of self-imposed stress, the misuse of alcohol is unquestionably the leader as the cause of aircraft accidents and loss of life. Numerous investigations over the years revealed that 10 to 30% of general aviation pilots involved in fatal aircraft accidents due to pilot error had alcohol in their blood and tissues (11).

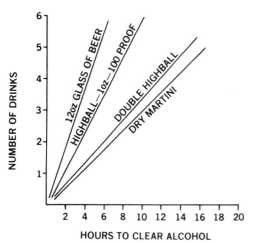

Figure 14.1. Time required for the body to eliminate alcohol.

Fortunately, aircraft accidents attributable to alcohol in United States airlines and military aviation are extremely rare. It has been well established that even small amounts of alcohol, 20 to 77 mg/dL, can cause significant performance decrement (12). This study is representative of many others, leading one to the inescapable conclusion that alcohol, even in modest amounts, has no place in the cockpit if flying safety is to be preserved.

Because alcohol is metabolized at an approximate rate of one-third ounce per hour it may take considerable time for its elimination from the body, particularly if larger amounts are ingested. This is well illustrated in Figure 14.1. Hence, flying organizations have instituted minimum bottle-to-throttle times. Besides the undesirable effects of a high blood alcohol level, there is also the problem of hangover to consider. Even if an individual's blood alcohol level approaches zero, the symptoms of hangover (e.g., headache, impaired mentation, and fatigue) can compromise flying safety.

Smoking

Today's practitioners of medicine are unanimous in their condemnation of cigarette smoking as a leading health hazard. Coronary artery disease, cancer, and chronic lung disease have been convincingly linked to this habit, which has been a part of our culture for many years. This should be reason enough for flight surgeons, as practitioners of preventive medicine, to discourage patients from smoking cigarettes. Even if public health considerations can be momentarily set aside, can we as aviation medicine specialists answer the question: Is cigarette smoking a threat to flying safety?

Theoretically, it would seem reasonable to assume that under certain circumstances of flight, smoking is indeed a threat to safety. Carbon monoxide, a byproduct of cigarette smoke, has an affinity for hemoglobin approximately 210 times that of oxygen. Hence, carbon monoxide will displace available oxygen from the hemoglobin molecule, reducing the oxygen-carrying capacity of the blood. Even at sea level, therefore, an individual who smokes will have a degree of hypoxia, albeit not necessarily to the point where symptoms will occur. Therefore, aviators who are slightly hypoxic at sea level because of cigarette smoke will be that much less resistant to the hypoxic environment of altitude, and this could be considered a threat to flying safety.

Investigators of the Civil Aeromedical Institute reviewed the literature on the subject of the hazards of smoking in aviation, reviewing 2660 fatal general aviation aircraft accidents occurring between 1973 and 1976 to see if they could find any evidence linking cigarette carbon monoxide to accidents (13). In this study, smoking was not identified as a causal factor but may have contributed to five of the accidents. These investigators, however, concluded that smoking cessation programs should still be pursued to improve health and maintain levels of performance and safety. Therefore, in spite of the negative findings of the above study, the positive recommendations of the authors should be endorsed by all flight surgeons, and aggressive campaigns against cigarette smoking should be pursued.

Improper Nutrition

Only in recent years have the medical community and the public at large become so aware of nutrition and weight control. As a result, the subject receives an unprecedented amount of space in lay periodicals and in the medical literature.

There is no question that it is unhealthy to be overweight and even worse, obese, in that there is an association with diabetes, heart disease, hypertension, and some cancers. Therefore, flight surgeons should advise overweight airmen accordingly and consult with a dietician if necessary. Patients should be discouraged from gimmick diets but rather encouraged to adhere to prescribed diets that are sensible and proven.

Likewise, as pointed out by the National Cholesterol Education Program, there is now ample evidence that cholesterol, LDL cholesterol in particular, is causally related to coronary heart disease (14). Hence, flight surgeons should monitor lipid levels and advise flying squadrons on lipid lowering diets.

Unfortunately, common sense and the basic principles of proper nutrition are too often forgotten by the public. Many people are frequently attracted to self-acclaimed nutritionists who advocate various crash programs, weight-reducing diets, and food fads that are often unphysiologic. Aeromedical specialists, in their role as preventive medicine specialists, should be strong advocates of acceptable nutritional principles and weight-reduction programs and educate airmen accordingly.

Regarding proper eating habits and cockpit duties, common sense again is the best guide to flying safety. Flight-line eating facilities and in-flight kitchens should be available to airmen day and night, depending on the flying operation. These facilities should be periodically inspected by aeromedical personnel to ensure not only the adequacy of the food selection but also sanitation in order to reduce the risk of food-borne illness. Airmen should be encouraged to utilize these facilities and to take their usual nourishment before flying, as well as in flight. The practice of having aircrew eat different meals at different times, which is required by some flying organizations, is to be commended in order to reduce the risk of an entire crew becoming ill. In spite of these precautions, there continues to be the occasional incident of in-flight "food poisoning" among aircrew.

For those airmen flying aircraft with cabin altitudes well in excess of 1524 to 2438 m (5000 to 8000 ft), special admonition is warranted. It is advisable for these crews to avoid pre-flight foods that are highly seasoned, greasy, or gas-forming (for example, cabbage, beans, and soft drinks). These foods can be extremely irritating to the gastrointestinal tract at altitude—recall that a given volume of gas in the gastrointestinal tract will be doubled at 5486 m (18000 ft). These dietary principles are well known to flight surgeons but need to be reviewed occasionally with aircrews.

Health Maintenance

The aviation environment, although not necessarily a hostile one, can be unfriendly to the aviator who is ill-prepared to accomplish his or her required duties. For this reason, a great amount of time and scientific effort have been directed toward studying the stresses of flight and developing appropriate life-support equipment to offer the airman maximum protection, and in this endeavor we have been eminently successful. The pressurized cabin is undoubtedly the single greatest development in life-support systems achieved during this century. Oxygen systems, flying clothing, temperature and humidity control, anti-G suits, and pressure suits are other contributions to aviation safety. For these advances, the aerospace medicine scientific community must be applauded not only for making flying safer, but also for having extended man's operational capabilities to the outer limits of physiologic tolerances.

Perhaps we have reached a point wherein self-imposed stress is now more threatening than operational stress. Smoking, alcohol, drugs, obesity, and unhealthy life-styles are commonplace in our culture. It is to these undesirable habits that physicians must direct their attention to ensure health maintenance of the aviation population. Today, the lay literature abounds with a multitude of recipes for a healthful life. Sometimes the advice is sensible, but too frequently it is not. After one has digested all of this material, a prescription for a healthy lifestyle can probably be best summarized in these words: moderation and common sense.

If these rules, long ago given to us by the Greek philosophers, were applied to our daily lives, many of our health-related problems could probably be avoided. Moderation and common sense dictate proper rest prior to flight, proper nutrition, the discreet use of alcohol, regular exercise, and avoidance of tobacco. As a preventive medicine specialist, the health maintenance of aviators should be an area of high interest for practitioners of aerospace medicine. Besides accomplishing periodic physical examinations as a preventive medicine function, the practitioner must actively participate in health education programs aimed at the flying population. Speaking at flying squadron meetings and consulting and advising commanders or organizational executives are excellent forums. Some flying organizations have embarked on even more ambitious programs that not only educate, but also intervene in life-style, the most popular example being the coronary artery disease risk factor intervention programs.

It is far too early to measure what success these programs will enjoy. In any event, they appear to be well founded and commensurate with the basic principles of preventive medicine. It is very much hoped that such intervention programs will reduce the incidence of coronary artery disease, which in turn would not only lessen the risk of an in-flight incapacitating event, but would also allow a longer and more productive career for the aviator.

REFERENCES

1. Hartman BO. Psychologic aspects of aerospace medicine. In: Aerospace Medicine. 2nd Ed. Randel RW, ed. Baltimore: Williams & Wilkins, 1971, p. 566.
2. Kantor JE Carretta TR. Aircrew selection systems. Aviat Space Environ Med 1988;59 (11, suppl.): A32–8.
3. Youngling EW Levine SH Mocharnuk JB Weston LM. Feasibility study to predict combat effectiveness for selected military roles: Fighter-Pilot effectiveness. St. Louis, Missouri: McDonnell-Douglas Corp., 1977.
4. Lilienfeld A. Chronic diseases. In: Preventive medicine and public health. 10th ed. Sartwell PE, ed. New York: Appleton-Century-Crofts, 1973, p. 498.
5. Baetjer AM. Industrial health. In: Preventive medicine and public health. 10th ed. Sartwell PE, ed. New York: Appleton-Century-Crofts, 1973, p. 964.
6. McDaniel JW. Male and female strength capabilities for operating aircraft controls. Preprints of the Scientific Program of the Aerospace Medical Association Meeting, AsMA, Washington, DC, May 4–7, 1981, p. 12.
7. Lyons T. Women in the fast jet cockpit—aeromedical considerations. Aviat Space Environ Med 1992;63: 809–818.
8. Iglesias R Teres A. Disorders of the menstrual cycle in airline stewardesses. Aviat Space Environ Med 1980; 51:518–520.
9. Burton RR. G-induced loss of consciousness: definition, history, current status. Aviat Space Environ Med 1988; 59(1):2–5.
10. Melatonin. Medical Letter. 1995;37(962):111–112.
11. Modell JG, Mountz JM. Drinking and flying—the problem of alcohol use by pilots. NEJM 1990;323(7): 455–461.
12. Aksnes EG. Effects of small dosages of alcohol upon performance in Link trainer. J Aviat Med 1954;25: 680–683.
13. Dille JR Linden MK. Effects of tobacco on aviation safety. Aviat Environ Med 1981;52:112–115.
14. Report of the National Cholesterol Education Program Expert Panel on Detection, Evaluation, and Treatment of High Blood Cholesterol in Adults. No author cited. Arch Int Med 1988;148:36–69.

Chapter 15

Clinical Aerospace Cardiovascular and Pulmonary Medicine

James R. Hickman, Jr.,

Gil D. Tolan, Gary W. Gray,

David H. Hull

Consequently, we must select a man who has a responsive, elastic system, capable of compensating for the strain which it will encounter.

Louis H. Bauer, MD

The cardiovascular system represents a frequent crossing point for aerospace medicine, physiology, and clinical medicine. Military aviation medicine has been especially challenged by the new generation of high-performance fighter aircraft. A number of subclinical conditions may be unmasked or exacerbated by high $+G_z$ loading, especially asymptomatic coronary artery disease (CAD). The decision rules for cardiovascular abnormalities in aircrew members discussed in this chapter are derived largely from experience and data from United States Air Force (USAF) aircrew. It is more difficult to apply discrete decision rules in civil aviation cases where exemptions for cardiovascular disease are oriented more toward functional testing.

One of the unique aspects of aviation cardiology is its close relationship to epidemiology. In many instances, abnormal cardiovascular findings, such as asymptomatic left bundle branch block, represent abnormal tests rather than a discrete disease entity. Alternatively, these abnormal findings do not always represent a disease

entity that can be defined in the subclinical state by available technology. Only through the elucidation of the natural history of these incidental findings in asymptomatic subjects will their significance become clear. In this regard, aeromedical policy is heavily dependent upon epidemiologic studies of disease subsets.

Aeromedical policy in the area of cardiovascular abnormalities has, of necessity, been quite conservative. This past conservatism has been due largely to the following three factors:

1. The diagnostic criteria for virtually all cardiovascular entities have been derived from "sick patient" populations. Decision rules which are derived from an understanding of an overt clinical state do not translate easily to the asymptomatic patient who has only had an abnormal test.

2. The natural history of most asymptomatic cardiovascular findings is unknown, and prognosis can only be estimated from clinical

populations. The bulk of the cofactor and endpoint research in aviation medicine remains to be accomplished.

3. The common use of invasive tools, such as coronary angiography, digital subtraction angiography, intracoronary angioscopy, intracoronary ultrasonography, and electrophysiologic studies, are relatively recent innovations in aerospace medicine.

Other noninvasive tools, such as two-dimensional Doppler echocardiography, transesophageal echocardiography, single-photon emission thallium tomography, ultrafast computed tomography of the coronary arteries, and full disclosure Holter monitoring, are all being used in clinical aviation medicine. The anatomic definition of the cardiovascular system has provided a previously unavailable baseline for natural history studies of asymptomatic disease.

Aeromedical standards are necessarily arbitrary when they are initially derived. Certification standards should be liberalized when the retrospective data for a given subset of aircrew with a discrete cardiovascular abnormality reveal a favorable trend. These groups of patients should then be conditionally waivered and prospectively followed closely over time. Subsequent standards should be relaxed or made more stringent based on these long-term observations.

The first section of this chapter describes the current recommendations for specific cardiovascular findings in apparently healthy male aircrew, especially in the areas of treadmill and Thallium testing, scalar electrocardiography, and rhythm disturbances. The final section addresses respiratory disease in aircrew.

CORONARY ARTERY DISEASE

The goal of early detection of CAD in aircrew is generally accepted worldwide, and sudden cardiac death has been documented in the loss of aircraft in both civilian and military aviation. However, accurate assessment of the role of CAD in aviation mishaps is difficult, if not impossible, due to a multitude of factors:

1. Pathologic specimens are often not recovered from the aircrew.
2. Even when the heart is recovered, evidence of fresh necrosis is virtually always absent because the appearance of the first visible histologic evidence of myocardial necrosis requires a survival of over five hours (1, 2).
3. Even when obstructive coronary disease is found in a recovered heart, it is still virtually impossible to determine whether the individual died with or of CAD. Asymptomatic CAD is so prevalent in older men of developed countries (3) that such a finding is insufficient to prove aircraft accident causality (4). A scar from an old "silent" myocardial infarction may exist for years without causing incapacitation. Discovery of an old infarction increases the probability of sudden incapacitation, but it is far from proof.
4. The laminar appearance of an antemortem blood clot may distinguish it from a postmortem thrombi, but the antemortem clot may lyse before necropsy (5). Pathologists at the National Heart, Lung, and Blood Institute studied the coronary arteries of 12 men, ages 50–68 (mean age: 57), who died within six hours of the onset of their presenting cardiac symptoms. None of the 12 had prior angina pectoris, congestive heart failure, left ventricular fibrosis, or left ventricular necrosis. None had thrombolytic therapy, angioplasty, or bypass surgery. Only one of the 12 had a clot found at necropsy (3).
5. Spasm is a common accompaniment of unstable angina; it often contributes to and occasionally causes coronary occlusion, but death releases the spasm (5).

How Common is CAD as a Cause of Sudden Incapacitation?

In one consecutive series where, by law, all unexpected deaths in the general population were

Table 15.1.
**Prevalence of Coronary Artery Stenosis in Men
Necropsied for Accidental Death (3)**

	White		Black	
Age	N	Prevalence	N	Prevalence
35–44	79	6%	78	1%
45–54	87	15%	62	5%
55–64	63	30%	39	15%
65–69	18	44%	7	14%

necropsied, 288 previously asymptomatic cau-
casian men, ages 31–55, had deaths that were
witnessed within one hour of the onset of symptoms. In most cases, the witness said the death
was instantaneous. Of these 288 unexpected sudden deaths, 92% were due to CAD (6). In New
Orleans between 1960 and 1963, coronary arteries were extensively examined in all necropsies
of accidental death. In men without myocardial
infarction who died from an accident, the prevalence of coronary artery stenosis increased with
age (3) (Table 15.1). Fortunately, since the peak
incidence around 1964, CAD mortality rates in
men have declined from 31% to 25% of all
deaths (7,8). Since 1979, age-adjusted CAD
mortality has decreased 3% per year (8, 9). Even
at this rate of decline, coronary heart disease will
remain the leading natural cause of death by a
wide margin (7). For example, in 1989, the mortality rate per 100,000 persons in the United
States was 200.6 deaths from coronary heart disease compared to stroke (59 deaths) and lung
cancer (57 deaths) (10). Although they generally
have less diabetes mellitus, uncontrolled hypertension, gross obesity, or tobacco use, aircrew
members are still susceptible to the number one
killer of the general population. In the 1980s, at
least 180 USAF-rated aviators were permanently grounded for proved CAD; over 200 more
were grounded for suspected CAD. Because of
the symptom denial, under reporting, and false-
negative screening, these cases represent only a
lower bound. In civilian airline pilots, cardiovascular disease accounts for more denials of medical certificates than all other causes combined
(11).

Although definitive proof of CAD as the
causal factor in aircraft accidents is often lacking, CAD continues to be a focal point for early
disease detection and prevention in aircrew because of its widespread prevalence, occurrence
in relatively young aircrew, and penchant for
presenting as a medical catastrophe without antecedent symptoms. CAD is the leading cause
of nontraumatic death in USAF aircrew, accounting for more than 70% of all medical
deaths. The rather striking occurrence of CAD
in young men was initially discovered during
battle casualty autopsies. During the Korean
War, in 300 autopsies (mean age: 22.1 years in
200 cases) some degree of atherosclerosis was
discovered on gross inspection in 77% of cases.
At least one 50% narrowing was noted in 15%
of cases, and one or more total occlusions noted
in 5% (12). In 105 autopsies from the Viet Nam
War battle causalties (mean age: 22 years), postmortem angiography and dissection demonstrated evidence of atherosclerosis in 45%. Five
percent had gross evidence of severe atherosclerosis, although postmortem angiography, with
its inherent limitations, was unable to confirm
significant narrowing (13). Nevertheless, the
amount of atherosclerotic substrate in this young
population was striking. In many respects, CAD
is a pediatric illness, often appearing clinically
during the active flying career of an aircrew
member.

Regarding the capricious presentation of
CAD, it should be noted that preinfarction angina often is absent before myocardial infarctions. Of those who died suddenly from CAD
in the Framingham or Albany studies, over half
had no warning symptoms (14). In 1949, the
Framingham study enrolled 2,282 men and
2,845 women, ages 30–62, without evidence of
coronary heart disease. These patients were then
followed with serial cardiovascular testing. Hospital admissions, death certificates, and medical
examiners' reports were also monitored. During
the first 14 years of this study, 334 initial myocardial infarctions occurred. Twenty-seven percent of these 334 patients suffered sudden, unex-

pected death before they could reach a hospital (15). In the first 30 years, 708 patients had new Q-waves (duration $\geq$ 40 msec) or lost initial QRS forces on the routine follow-up 12-lead ECG when compared to the tracing two years earlier. Eighty-four percent of these 708 patients had no angina pectoris before acute myocardial infarction (16). Ten percent of the men who manifested coronary artery symptoms in the first 26 years of the Framingham study died suddenly within one hour of initial symptoms (17). The alarming regularity of sudden cardiac death without premonitory symptoms has caused aviation medicine practitioners to place a great premium upon early detection of CAD.

The frequency with which myocardial infarctions often go clinically unrecognized is also a major factor in the decision to pursue CAD detection in aircrew. For example, 213 (30%) of the 708 unequivocal initial myocardial infarctions in the Framingham study were unrecognized in the acute phase. It is also important to note that age-adjusted prognoses were just as bad for unrecognized myocardial infarctions as for those who survived hospitalization for recognized infarctions. The 10-year, age-adjusted mortality rate of men with unrecognized infarcts equaled that of men with recognized infarctions, despite the earlier medical care given for recognized infarctions. In 1960, the Western Collaborative Group screened 3,524 men, ages 39–59, who were employed by 10 corporations. Previously unrecognized myocardial infarctions were discovered on the initial ECG in 42 men. The 3,182 men who were considered well on the initial screen were followed with annual examinations for an average of 4.5 years. During the follow-up period, 104 of these 3,182 men had myocardial infarctions. Twenty-three (22%) of the 104 initial myocardial infarctions were fatal within 10 days; half of these 23 died suddenly (18). Thirty-one of the 104 first myocardial infarctions were unrecognized during the acute phase.

Northwestern University screened 756 male utility employees, ages 50–59; 607 men had no evidence of coronary heart disease on initial screening and were studied prospectively for four years. Twenty patients developed new significant Q-waves on follow-up ECG; four of these 20 had myocardial infarctions that were unrecognized during the acute phase and three of those four were completely asymptomatic during the acute phase (19).

At the USAF School of Aerospace Medicine (USAFSAM), silent myocardial infarction was found on the routine ECG in 72 of 48,633 aircrew screened over a 10-year period. Of those aircrew who were interviewed, most recalled no symptoms and the remainder had atypical symptoms. The data from the above studies have great bearing on the necessity for cardiovascular surveillance in actively flying aircrew.

Other CAD Pathophysiologic Considerations Relevant in Aerospace Medicine

It is important to understand that neither critical obstruction nor reversible ischemia need always be present to precipitate a cardiac catastrophe. Recent advances in our knowledge of myocardial infarction, especially the dominant role of thrombosis in infarction, have underscored the concern in aviation medicine about thrombotic occlusions of moderate or even mild lesions. Sudden occlusion of noncritical lesions is often a malignant event because such lesions may not be collateralized, unlike more slowly growing high-grade lesions which may be well collateralized. Without protective collaterals, a sudden thrombotic occlusion can cause a catastrophic myocardial infarction (20).

In a series from Hammersmith Hospital, 10 patients free of unstable angina before their acute myocardial infarctions underwent coronary angiography one to six months after the acute event. In six of these 10 patients, the artery perfusing the infarction had diameter narrowings of less than 50% (21). By design, this series excluded patients with angioplasty or coronary bypass before follow-up catheterization. Excluded patients may well have represented more serious stenosis than the 10 reported; thus, the small series is biased toward having milder stenoses. Nevertheless, coronary diameter narrowings < 50% do cause infarctions without warning.

In another series, 386 patients were hospitalized within six hours of the onset of ischemic chest pain lasting at least 30 minutes with ST segment elevation ≥ 0.1 mV in at least two ECG leads. Ninety minutes after treatment with intravenous tissue plasminogen activator, coronary angiography revealed that 6% of the 386 had < 50% diameter narrowing of the coronary artery perfusing the acutely infarcted myocardial segment. Because lysis may not have been complete, 6% is a lower bound on the proportion of myocardial infarctions from atherosclerotic diameter narrowings < 50%. Another 38% of the 386 patients had flow into and out of the infarcted myocardium occur as promptly as flow in an uninvolved segment (22).

A 10-year follow-up study conducted after cardiac catheterization between January, 1964 and July, 1965 at the Cleveland Clinic in 521 medically treated patients found coronary death rates of 0.6% in the 357 patients with clean coronary arteries, 2% in the 101 patients with a maximum diameter narrowing < 30%, and 16% in the 63 patients with a maximum diameter narrowing of 30–50% (23). Seven-year follow-up of patients who underwent cardiac catheterization in the CASS Study between August, 1976 and June, 1979 found that after adjusting for age, smoking history, and BP, the survival of 3,136 subjects with clean coronary arteries was statistically better (p < 0.005) than for the 915 patients with the maximum coronary diameter narrowings of < 50% (24). The above clinical studies bear heavily upon the decision of aeromedical organizations to pursue subcritical CAD.

Epidemiologic Factors

Recent investigations evaluated not only the relationship of total cholesterol to the risk of CAD,

but also to the various forms in which cholesterol appears in the blood. High-density lipoprotein (HDL) cholesterol normally accounts for 20–25% of the total plasma cholesterol. The HDL level has shown a strong inverse relationship to CAD. The relationship between total serum cholesterol and HDL cholesterol is frequently expressed as a ratio of the two, and this ratio seems to be more sensitive in predicting coronary disease risk than either absolute value alone.

A retrospective analysis of this ratio in aircrew members with abnormal treadmill tests undergoing cardiac catheterization at the USAF-SAM revealed that a total cholesterol-to-HDL-cholesterol ratio of > six occurred in 88% of individuals with CAD, whereas a ratio of over six was seen in only 4% of those with no disease. Conversely, patients with a ratio of < 4.3 had a low prevalence of CAD (Figure 15.1). It should be noted that these results were in aircrew with abnormal exercise tests *and* a defined ratio. None was selected for testing because of lipids. Multiple preliminary studies regarding HDL subfractions and apolipoproteins are underway but no definitive correlative data in aircrew regarding anatomic CAD are available at present.

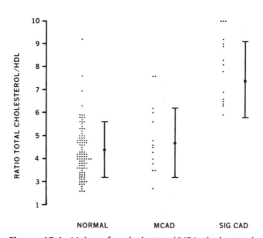

Figure 15.1. Values for cholesterol/HDL cholesterol ratio plotted according to angiographic classification (normal, minimal coronary artery disease [MCAD], and significant coronary artery disease [Sig CAD]). A ratio > 6.0 predicted Sig CAD. (From: Am J Cardiol 1981;48:903-910, published by permission.)

In the Framingham study, an HDL cholesterol level of $\leq$ 35 mg% was an independent risk factor. Klag et al. completed a 30-year prospective follow-up of 1,017 young men (mean age: 22 years at enrollment). In these patients, 125 cardiovascular events were recorded, 97 of which were CAD. The mean cholesterol was 192 at entry into the study. Serum cholesterol at baseline strongly correlated with coronary heart disease, cardiovascular mortality, and total mortality. Between the 25th and 75th percentile entry cholesterol levels, a 36 mg% difference, relative risks were calculated for the development of cardiovascular disease (1.72), coronary heart disease (2.01), mortality due to cardiovascular disease (2.02), and death before age 50 (1.64) (25).

The West Point study by Clark et al. was a longitudinal epidemiologic surveillance program of the entering class of 1952 at the United State Military Academy. These patients were followed with biennial serum lipids and lipoprotein levels as well as periodic physical examinations. Two rounds of hands on cardiovascular evaluations were performed when the patients were at mean ages of 42 and 57 years. Forty years of follow-up in 387 patients were completed. Using risk factors available before age 28, a multivariate regression formula was derived to predict the group with the highest likelihood of subsequent CAD. In the tertile with the highest risk related score, 17% manifested CAD by age 55, with the first event occurring at age 39. In the lowest risk tertile, 2% manifested CAD by age 51, with the first event occurring at age 51. (26). These data suggest that it is possible to select a lower risk population for aviation training.

Screening for CAD in Aircrew

The detection of asymptomatic CAD in aircrew members is a primary goal of aviation cardiology, superseded only by the goal of CAD prevention. Although angiographic disease in asymptomatic aircrew is usually single-vessel or low-grade multivessel disease, severe disease is still found with regularity. Even mild degrees of CAD may lead to sudden incapacitation during $+ G_z$ stress. Currently available screening methods include history, physical examination, resting ECG, exercise ECG, exercise scintigraphy, coronary fluoroscopy, ultrafast computed tomography, and risk estimation.

Scalar ECG

Although the routine resting 12-lead ECG continues to play a role in the screening of aircrew for CAD, it now seems clear that the application of the resting ECG as a standalone detection test is difficult to defend. After myocardial infarction, the scar often contracts, with the surviving myocardium undergoing hypertrophy. Consequently, even when ECG changes were obvious during the acute phase, the subsequent annual ECG may resolve to within the broad range of normal (15).

In the first seven years of the Framingham study, 49 patients suffered myocardial infarction recognized during the acute phase. These 49 patients had typical symptoms plus unequivocal ECG acute changes. In nine (18%) of these 49 patients, ECG had returned to normal by the time of the follow-up examination (27). In another series, 160 patients suffered their first recognized acute myocardial infarctions, documented by cardiac isoenzymes; 80 of these 160 patients were alive four years later without conduction abnormality, history of reinfarction, angioplasty, or bypass surgery. ECG changes reverted to normal in 20% of the 48 patients with inferior infarction, and 8% of 32 patients with anterior infarctions (28). This insensitivity for the grossest of cardiovascular abnormalities, myocardial infarction, is due to a combination of insufficient leads, obfuscating format, ambiguous measurements, within and between reader disagreement, and often unscientific and unverified criteria (29,30). Most criteria for old infarctions focus exclusively on the first 40 msec of ventricular depolarization. An occlusion of a nondominant circumflex coronary artery infarcts basal segments which only begin depolarization 40 msec *after* depolarization starts near the base of the papillary muscles (31). Classic criteria also miss 25% of myocardial infarctions in segments perfused by the dominant right coronary artery (30). In one study, readers applied three sets of criteria for myocardial infarctions to ECGs with posterior descending coronary artery infarctions mixed with tracings from healthy persons. The readers then applied three sets of criteria for inferior myocardial infarctions. The least sensitive criteria correctly diagnosed only 4% of these old infarctions. The best criteria diagnosed only 34% of these 83 patients, these criteria requiring Q-waves in lead AVF and lead III with duration $\geq$ 30 msec and amplitudes $\geq$ than 25% of the R-wave (32).

It should also be recognized that ECGs taken on aircrew members who subsequently have fatal accidents are also unlikely to show changes predictive of myocardial infarction. The Framingham study found that in the general population only one-third of the routine resting 12-lead ECGs taken < two years before an acute myocardial infarction gave any warning, even with 20/20 hindsight (15). It has long been a standard practice in aviation medicine to perform additional testing, such as treadmill testing, on pilots with ECG warnings, such as ST abnormalities. As will be discussed later in this chapter, this approach often unnecessarily penalizes the innocent. However, the other pitfall is that these ECG warnings are often waivered when follow-up testing, such as treadmill testing, is normal. Abnormal tests generally lead to angiography but many follow-up tests are often falsely negative. Exercise ECGs and thallium scans are meant to detect ischemia, but narrowings insufficient to cause ischemia may cause thromboembolic occlusion. The prospective Seattle Heart Watch Study followed asymptomatic patients after an exercise stress test. ECG response to the stress test was normal in the large majority of those who died suddenly during follow-up (4).

In another prospective study, 916 asymptomatic Indiana state policemen, ages 27–55, were followed for an average of 12.7 years with repeated medical evaluations including symptom-limited treadmill exercise tests. Initially, all 916 patients had no evidence of cardiac disease on clinical examination or resting ECG. Of the nine patients who suffered a witnessed sudden death within two hours of the onset of symptoms, seven had normal repolarization responses to exercise. Of the 27 who suffered myocardial infarctions, 25 had normal repolarization responses to exercise (33). Insensitivity of the scalar ECG (as well as treadmill testing) in asymptomatic men is a major reason for additional and focused CAD detection in aircrew.

Nonspecific ST- and T-wave changes, especially T-wave flattening or inversion and ST depression, may be indications of CAD. These changes are most useful when they occur in serial ECGs. However, they are markedly nonspecific, and only occasionally indicate the presence of CAD. During a one-year period at the USAF-SAM, 32,000 referral ECGs were reviewed. Treadmill tests were performed for various nondiagnostic serial ECG changes resulting in 923 exercise ECGs, of which 779 were normal. Of the 144 patients with abnormal exercise ECGs, 90 were evaluated by cardiac catheterization yielding 19 patients with any degree of CAD. Although the predictive value of an abnormal treadmill test in this population was low (21%), it was actually doubled from 10% to 21% by screening for serial nonspecific resting ECG changes.

Limitations to exercise testing exist, however, as shown by USAF aircrew who were exercised without regard to scalar ECG changes or risk factors. The absence of some pretest stratification that enhances predictive value was shown to severely limit the usefulness of the exercise test as a first order screening test in apparently healthy men. Although the scalar ECG is markedly limited as a first order standalone test in the detection of silent anatomic CAD, and resting ST-T changes only mildly enhance treadmill positive predictive value, ECG remains a valuable tool to detect silent myocardial damage in

Table 15.2.
Performance of a Test with 75% Sensitivity and 60% Specificity in a Population with 50% Prevalence of Disease

Patients	Number of Abnormal Tests	Number of Normal Tests
5000 with disease	3750 (TP)	1250 (TN)
5000 without disease	2000 (FP)	3000 (TN)
Total	5750	4250

Predicted value of abnormal test: 65.2%. Abbreviations: TP = true-positives; FN = false-negatives; FP = false-positives; and TN = true-negatives

Table 15.3.
Performance of a Test with 75% Sensitivity and 60% Specificity in a Population with 5% Prevalence of Disease

Patients	Number of Abnormal Tests	Number of Normal Tests
500 with disease	375 (TP)	125 (FN)
9000 without disease	3800 (FP)	5700 (TN)
Total	4175	5825

Predictive value of abnormal test: 8.9%. Abbreviations: TP = true-positives; FN = false-negatives; FP = false-positives; and TN = true-negatives

the 80% or more of infarctions in which the follow-up ECG remains abnormal.

Treadmill Testing in Asymptomatic Aircrew

A major limitation of treadmill testing in asymptomatic populations has been the occurrence of false-positive results. A rational approach to stress testing involves the application of Bayes' theorem. This theorem applies conditional probability analysis to any diagnostic test that is not perfect. The reliability of any less than perfect test is strongly influenced by the prevalence of the disease being sought in the study population. Understanding a few common epidemiologic terms is required. Positive predictive value is defined as the proportion of positive results that are truly positive and is dependent on the prevalence of the disease in the study population. Similarly, negative predictive value is the proportion of negative results that are truly negative. Sensitivity is the percentage of positive results in patients with disease. Specificity is the percentage of negative results among those patients without disease. For purposes of illustration, one should assume that a treadmill test with 75% sensitivity and 60% specificity is applied to a population of 10,000 patients with a disease prevalence of 50%. Table 15.2 illustrates the predictive value of an abnormal test under these conditions. Therefore, this treadmill test applied to a population with a disease prevalence of 50% would correctly identify 3750 of

5000 diseased patients and correctly classify 3000 of 5000 nondiseased individuals. A population with a disease prevalence of 5%, similar to the prevalence in healthy male aviators, would reveal a marked decrease in the predictive power of the identical test (Table 15.3).

A number of variables may be evaluated during exercise ECGs. Exercise ECG is abnormal when ST depression of a degree greater than a predetermined normal level develops with exercise or during recovery. All investigators accept horizontal or downsloping ST segment depressions of > 0.1 mV, when compared with baseline, as abnormal. Most investigators also accept upsloping ST segment depression as abnormal when the ST segment remains > 0.1 mV depressed 80 milliseconds after the termination of the QRS complex (the J point). We (JH and GT) consider ST segment depression 0.05–0.09 mV as "borderline," a category not universally recognized but one we feel requires further testing for CAD. Additional variables evaluated during exercise ECG include the occurrence of stress arrhythmias, maximum heart rate reached, maximum systolic BP, and total QRS and R-wave amplitude. Decreased peak heart rate or decreasing systolic BP with progressive exercise are possible indicators of CAD. Additional information, such as the inadequate rise of systemic BP, early appearance of ST segment depression, and prolonged duration of ST segment depression after exercise, also have diagnostic importance.

A combination of ECG, hemodynamic, and risk factor data may also be of diagnostic value in asymptomatic patients as shown in an exhaustive minute-by-minute analysis of 255 exercise tests of asymptomatic USAF aviators prior to angiography (34). The predictive value of > 0.1 mV of ST segment depression was 24%. ST segment depression alone did not increase predictive value until > 0.3 mV depression was reached, increasing the predictive value to 60%. The onset of > 0.1 mV depression in early exercise proved to be a poor predictor of angiographic disease in asymptomatic men. Exercise-induced R-wave amplitude increases (or no change in amplitude) enhanced the predictive value to 40% but were markedly insensitive (18%). Further, a decreased percentage of maximal predicted heart rate achieved and exercise double product failed to enhance significantly the predictive value of the exercise test in asymptomatic men. The exercise test variables that performed best were a total treadmill time of < 10 minutes on the USAFSAM protocol (35) (predictive value: 67%) and > 0.1 mV of ST segment depression persisting for at least six minutes after exercise (predictive value: 43%). Univariate analysis of cardinal risk factors did not increase the predictive value of the exercise test in asymptomatic men, but the value of the ST segment response was enhanced modestly by the presence of three risk factors. The combination of one or more risk factors with the three most predictive exercise variables (> 0.3 mV depression early in exercise, > 0.1 mV depression persisting six minutes after exercise, or < 10 minutes total performance) yielded a predictive value of > 80% for the detection of multivessel disease. Unfortunately, sensitivity was too poor to rely on this combination to rule out significant disease. Limitations exist in exercise testing of apparently healthy men, as well as diagnostic trade-offs between sensitivity and specificity as various criteria are examined. Of special concern in aerospace medicine is the usual loss in sensitivity when criteria of higher specificity are applied.

Exercise electrocardiography remains the most widely used screening procedure for asymptomatic CAD. A USAF study by Froelicher et al. analyzed the epidemiologic value of screening asymptomatic males with exercise electrocardiography (36). An abnormal ST segment response proved to be a potent predictor of subsequent symptomatic CAD. At USAFSAM, 640 aircrew members who underwent exercise ECG over a four-year period were reevaluated after a mean interval of 6.6 years. Marked differences were noted between those who originally had abnormal ST segment responses and those with normal responses. A 14-fold increase in the risk for subsequent coronary events was found in those with an abnormal result, as compared with the group who had normal tests. Although the treadmill test is an imperfect predictor of anatomic CAD, the potent epidemiologic risk of an abnormal result cannot be ignored.

Exercise Scintigraphy

Thallium scintigraphy was correlated with angiography in 845 asymptomatic USAF aircrew undergoing catheterization for noninvasive testing suggestive of myocardial ischemia. The positive predictive value for any degree of disease was 32%, and 17% for disease ≥ 50% luminal narrowing. However, the greatest value of this series was in the demarcation of the Bayesian aspects of scintigraphic results, especially declining negative predictive values with increasing disease prevalence. Table 15.4 displays the increasing positive predictive value with increasing age and increasingly unfavorable cholesterol-to-HDL ratios, calculated from the data.

Table 15.4.
Relationship of Positive Predictive Values of Thallium Scintigraphy in USAF Aircrew to Age and Lipids

Age in Years	Cholesterol to HDL Ratios		
	<4.5	4.5–6.0	>6.0
<45	8%	20%	41%
45	18%	43%	41%

Table 15.5.
Relationship of Negative Predictive Values of Thallium Scintigraphy in USAF Aircrew to Age and Lipids

Age in Years	Cholesterol to HDL Ratios		
	<4.5	4.5–6.0	>6.0
<45	96%	90%	87%
>45	93%	79%	72%

Positive predictive value increases, as expected, with increasing pretest likelihood of disease. Table 15.5 displays negative predictive values of thallium scintigraphy for the same conditions. Nondiagnostic tests were viewed as negative tests for this textbook chapter because most aviation services do not perform angiography on borderline tests. Note the 24% decrease in negative predictive values between an aviator under 45 with a good ratio compared to over 45 with unfavorable ratio. The declining negative predictive value of scintigraphy (or any other diagnostic test) as the disease becomes more dense must always be considered when aircrew members are stratified to test only those with the highest risks. Stratified testing, which utilizes multiple serial tests, is a safeguard against this aspect of the Bayesian problem.

Coronary Calcification Detection

Not only do treadmill tests and scintigrams function poorly in unstratified asymptomatic populations, there is little hope of detecting nonischemic stenoses which may produce malignant infarctions due to thrombosis. Nonischemic stenoses do not make an exercise test or a thallium scintigram abnormal, but in aviation medicine a great premium is placed upon early detection of mild-to-moderate disease. Such early detection of nonischemic thresholds is important from both a flying safety and a preventive medicine standpoint. Today, many of these nonischemic narrowings are detected by luck. For example, when the criteria for an exercise test are set to yield a specificity of 90%, then, by definition, 10% of the healthy patients will have a falsely

abnormal test for ischemia. Likewise, 10% of those with nonischemic CAD within the test population will also have a falsely abnormal test for ischemia. When we require angiography for abnormal tests suggestive of ischemia, we discover nonischemic narrowings by luck and mistakenly believe them to be ischemic. To increase sensitivity, we could lower the threshold for labeling an exercise test as abnormal, thereby increasing the yield of nonischemic stenoses, but in the process would place greater diagnostic burdens on more of the healthy aviators. Fortunately, better ways to screen for nonischemic coronary atherosclerosis exist.

In the decade beginning October, 1982, Loecker et al. at the USAF Aeromedical Consultation Service evaluated 712 asymptomatic male military aviators with selective coronary angiography and left ventriculography who had been screened with conventional cardiac fluoroscopy (37). These patients had also received symptom-limited treadmill exercise tests and thallium myocardial scintigraphy. An abnormal result on any one of these tests (fluoroscopy, treadmill, or scintigraphy) was a sufficient indication for left heart catheterization. Other catheterization indications, independent of other screening tests, were acquired left bundle branch block, some patients with supraventricular tachycardia, ventricular tachycardia, or some selected valvular lesions. Of these 712 asymptomatic flyers who elected to have coronary angiography, 36% had coronary diameter narrowing ≥ 10%, of whom 66% had definite calcium on fluoroscopy. Of the flyers without coronary stenosis on angiography, 81% were true negatives. Thirty-eight flyers had calcification on cardiac fluoroscopy as the *only* indication for left heart catheterization; 76% of those 38 flyers had coronary artery stenoses on angiography; eight of these 38 flyers had coronary artery diameter narrowing ≥ 50%.

Digital Subtraction Fluoroscopy for Calcification

Digital subtraction fluoroscopy has better sensitivity than conventional fluoroscopy but lower

Table 15.6.
Comparison of Conventional Fluoroscopy and Digital Subtraction Fluoroscopy for Calcification and Angiographic Correlations

		Coronary Diameter Narrowing			
		>50%	50%	0%	
Conventional	+	60	12	6	78
Fluoroscopy	−	36	22	55	113
Digital	+	88	20	13	121
Subtraction	−	8	14	48	70
Fluoroscopy					
		96	34	61	191

specificity. At the Cleveland Clinic, 191 consecutive patients without prior myocardial infarction had coronary angiography (38). Forty-eight percent had typical angina pectoris, 38% had atypical chest pain, and 14% were asymptomatic. Ages of patients ranged 34–78 years (mean age: 56 years), 63% of whom were men. Before cardiac catheterization, they underwent fluoroscopy both with and without digital subtraction. Readers were blinded to the results of the other two studies. Of the 68% with any coronary stenosis on angiography, 83% were true positives with digital subtraction fluoroscopy compared to 55% by conventional fluoroscopy. Of the patients with completely normal coronary angiography, 79% were true negatives with digital subtraction compared to 90% by conventional fluoroscopy. Table 15.6 compares these conventional fluoroscopy and digital subtraction fluoroscopy results.

Ultrafast Computed Tomography

Ultrafast computed tomography (CT) has better sensitivity than digital subtraction fluoroscopy but lower specificity. In one series of 313 patients scanned with ultrafast CT specifically searching for calcified coronary arteries, 73% of patients had coronary calcification, defined as a contiguous area ≥ 1.0 mm^2 with CT peak density > 130 Hounsfield units. Ninety-six of the 189 patients with coronary diameter narrowing $\geq 50\%$ on angiography had coronary calcium on ultrafast CT compared with 38% of the 124

with normal coronary angiography. The amount of calcium found on ultrafast CT increased with the severity of the coronary stenoses found on angiography (39,40). Similarly, 100 patients, ages 23–59 (mean age: 47 years) were scanned by the same technique except that coronary calcification was defined as a contiguous area ≥ 0.51 mm^2 (2 pixels) with peak density > 130 Hounsfield units. All patients underwent elective coronary angiography within one week, usually to evaluate symptoms suggestive of coronary ischemia. Ninety-four percent of the 71 patients with any coronary stenosis on angiography had coronary calcium on ultrafast CT compared with 28% of the 29 with completely normal angiograms (41).

A series of adequate sample size does not exist to compare ultrafast CT with conventional fluoroscopy. Further, ultrafast CT is more expensive and of limited availability to aerospace medicine practitioners.

General Philosophy of CAD Detection in Aircrew

As of this writing, treadmill testing, thallium scintigraphy, and conventional coronary fluoroscopy are generally available for aircrew evaluations. Further developments in ultrafast CT and digital subtraction techniques, as well as developments in cost and availability, may mean a wider use of these newer tools in the aviation environment. Due to the poor performance of conventional diagnostic techniques in a low prevalence environment, it seems clear that any strategy for the detection of silent CAD in aircrew must begin with some numerical or quantitative assignment of coronary risk to each aircrew member. Such stratification identifies a population of aircrew in whom second-order cardiovascular testing can be applied with greater diagnostic accuracy, while sparing those with little pretest likelihood of coronary disease from emotional duress, radiation, and diagnostic risks. Further, identification of those aircrew with the highest quantifiable coronary risks allows preventive strategies to be focused on those at highest risk.

The USAFSAM has derived a mathematical expression of coronary risk known as the USAF-SAM risk index. This risk index was derived retrospectively from angiographic data correlated with risk factors in almost 1000 aircrew members who had undergone angiography while asymptomatic. The index was derived specifically to allow the USAF to identify aircrew members requiring second-order cardiovascular testing. This index was based upon the fact that 90% of all predictive information in this highly selected group of aircrew who underwent coronary angiography was found in age, total cholesterol, and HDL. All prior reported angiographic results in aircrew have been exclusively based upon some second-order test, usually for reversible ischemia, without prior stratification. For the first time, the USAF undertook a small pilot series in a fighter command, performing tests based solely upon a coronary risk index. In a small, prospective series of 75 high-performance pilots, the coronary disease yield was essentially tripled (from 10% to 33%) when compared to the usual screening schema for the previous 47 months. The usual screening schema was based upon treadmill tests performed following serial ST and T changes on the resting scalar ECG. This increase in yield was gained at the expense of no additional angiographic studies when compared to the old method. Further field testing of such indices is underway in the US Army and Canadian armed forces.

Because stratified screening is heavily dependent upon accurate lipid determinations, stringent control of bias and total analytical error in supporting laboratories is essential. As various stratification tools are derived, arbitrary cut points should be avoided when using continuous risk factors like age. Such continuous risk factors should be multiplied by weighting factors, and then combined in a multivariate formula to calculate a composite risk that predicts CAD. Aircrew members should be ranked by this number. Those in the highest decile should be screened first, and fliers in the next lower decile should be screened only after the yield from screening the higher decile is known. Unanimity of opinion does not exist regarding the order of testing but many feel that the ECG response to a symptom-limited exercise test should be determined first because when such repolarization is abnormal, radiation from radiography and/or isotopes can be avoided.

An abnormal repolarization response in an aircrew member identified by stratification should be followed by angiography. If repolarization were normal in an aircrew member at high coronary risk, additional testing should follow. It is less obvious as to whether the search for calcium with radiography should precede a radioisotope scan. However, some reasons to search initially for coronary calcium with radiography do exist. With conventional fluoroscopy, the radiation burden to sensitive organs is less and the sensitivity for CAD is better. When stratifying candidates for second-order testing, it must be constantly kept in mind that positive predictive value increases steadily with increasing pretest probability of disease, but negative predictive value declines in a similar fashion. In an aircrew member at high coronary risk, one should not be tempted to offset an abnormal treadmill test by performing a thallium, and avoiding angiography based upon a negative scintigram. Negative predictive values of thallium decline markedly in the older aircrew with the highest cholesterol-to-HDL ratios. An abnormal treadmill in a high-decile-risk aircrew member, when the abnormal treadmill is at its most believable, should not be set aside for a negative thallium, when the negative thallium is at its least believable.

In the future, intravascular ultrasound measurements may precede usual coronary angiography. Ultrasound measurements of coronary stenoses correlate well with angiography for lumen narrowing (R = 0.96) and for lumen cross-sectional area (R = 0.95). Further, compared to angiography, intravascular ultrasound has far less radiation, actually detects more plaques, displays the internal elastic lamina for objectively measuring prestenosis lumen size, detects more plaque calcium and more intimal dissection, distinguishes thromboembolic from arteriosclerotic stenoses, and quantifies coronary artery distensibility. The role of intravascular ultrasound in aeromedical decision-making has yet to be defined. From a purely Bayesian standpoint, even with maximal stratification, many aircrew members with normal coronary vessels undergo invasive procedures. Intravascular ultrasound may be sufficient for the majority of aircrew members who undergo such procedures, thereby markedly reducing the average radiation dose of catheterizations to determine fitness to fly.

Aeromedical Disposition of CAD

Although in general, CAD is incompatible with flying safety, a long-term prospective study by the United States Air Force defined conditions under which aircrew members with minimal CAD (MCAD) may return to the cockpit in non-high-performance aircraft (42,43). This study defined minimal CAD as no single coronary lesion > 30% luminal narrowing, and no aggregate (sum) of lesions > 50%. These preliminary results suggested that such aircrew could be returned safely to the non-high-performance cockpit, provided repeated angiography was performed at no longer than three-year intervals, depending on the risk factor profile and the results of annual noninvasive testing, including myocardial scintigraphy. Ninety-six aircrew members who met the entry criteria were followed up at a mean of 6.1 years after angiography. Twenty-two had repeat angiography with five studies revealing progression. The single clinical endpoint (a case of angina) occurred nine years after angiography. This aircrew member retired one year after the initial angiography and did not receive any aircrew surveillance for eight years prior to the onset of angina pectoris. A second group of aircrew members (n = 24) had a retrospective followup of 14.5 years, yielding five endpoints (four myocardial infarctions and one case of angina pectoris). In this retrospective study, all patients with endpoints would have been disqualified for aeromedical cause long before the clinical endpoint occurred. The earliest clinical endpoint occurred 5.6 years after the initial angiography and the mean time from initial angiography to clinical event was 8.6 years. No events occurred in aircrew members while under active surveillance in the protocol. Based upon these retrospective data, the USAF increased the allowable aggregate to 100% (sum of lesions) in 1990.

The USAF also followed up retrospectively a second group of aircrew members with moderate CAD (maximum lesion: 31–50%). Ninety-two males, mean age 45.6 years, were followed up for a mean of 8.5 years. The study analyzed patients with maximal lesions equal to 50% stenosis (n = 54), as well as an additional group with lesions > 30% but < 50% (n = 38). The average annual incidence of events was 0.6% at five years and 0.4% at 10 years for lesions > 30% and < 50%. For lesions of 50%, the average annual incidence was 2.9% at five years and 2.3% at 10 years. Cardiac mortality was 0% at the 10-year mark for lesions > 30% and < 50%. For lesions of 50%, the cardiac mortality was 2.1% at five years and 3.3% at 10 years. The angina/myocardial infarction incidence in the > 30% but < 50% lesion group compared favorably with unscreened populations, such as Framingham, Massachusetts, and Rochester, Minnesota. At a threshold of 120% aggregate (sum of lesions), no events occurred in the group with lesions $\leq$ 40%. Based upon these data, the USAF is returning aircrew members with lesions $\leq$ 30%, and aggregates $\leq$ 100% to non-high-performance flying. The data do suggest that lesions of 40% with an aggregate of < 120% could also be waivered. Intensive, annual, noninvasive follow-up, and repeated angiography at no less than three years continues to be required. The current void in basic sciences data regarding coronary hemodynamics under high $+G_z$ precludes any current recommendation to return such aircrew to high-performance flying. The available data do not support returning to flying with asymptomatic lesions of 50% or more luminal narrowing. In an earlier natural study of USAF aircrew members with coronary lesions ≥ 50%, the annual event rate was 6% per annum (angina, infarction, or sudden death) with 75% of initial events occurring as angina. The rather marked increase in risk of lesions ≥ 50%, when compared to lesions < 30%, or even < 40%, makes a strong case for truncating CAD waivers to a maximum lesion within the 30-40% range.

Coronary Artery Bypass Surgery in Aircrew

Coronary artery bypass grafting precludes a return to flying in the military environment. The acknowledged differences in civil aviation and military aviation revolve around different missions, different aircraft demands, and combat considerations. Bypass grafting has been considered for return to civil aviation duties, including airline pilot duties, by the FAA and other civil aviation authorities. Such waivers usually require repeat angiography after bypass (usually at six months) to document graft patency and no reversible ischemia on noninvasive testing.

Many specialists in aerospace medicine consider bypass surgery to be a palliative procedure that does not diminish the potential for progression of the underlying disease. The disease substrate remains unchanged, and the disease may progress to involve vessels distal to the graft insertion, or the graft itself. Annual graft occlusion rates of approximately 3% per annum per graft pose an unacceptable risk in military aviation in the view of many aviation medicine specialists. Chaitman et al. reviewed the Coronary Artery Surgery Study data in an attempt to identify a group of bypass patients who would represent the most favorable five-year prognosis for consideration of return to flying (44). Of the 10,312 bypass patients, only 122 (1.1% of the registry) were identified as the most desirable patients. In this small group, the five-year event

rate was 2%, approximately four-fold the event rate of the general flying population. The entire basis of the USAF minimal CAD waiver policy was to select an angiographic group whose risks approached the unstudied group—the group from whom an actual replacement comes when a USAF flyer is permanently grounded. In the original USAF MCAD study group, the five-year event rate was 0%. For those with lesions from 31% to less than 50%, the annual event rate was 0.6% at the end of five years, and 0.4% at the end of 10 years. If that same standard of outcome were applied to bypassed aviators, no tenable waiver policy could currently be constructed for military aircrew. The unpredictable and capricious nature of atherosclerotic lesions does not currently allow for the formulation of a rational policy for the regular surveillance and return to the cockpit of military aviators who have had bypass surgery. It is conceivable that rare, acceptable candidates may be identified, and this issue needs to be periodically reviewed.

Coronary Angioplasty

No series of published angiographic results for aviators with angioplasty exists for review. In civil aviation, aircrew members with prior successful percutaneous coronary transluminal angioplasty (PCTA) have been waivered for all classes of flying following documented patency of the dilatation by angiography at six months and the absence of ischemia on noninvasive testing.

Is it possible to "turn back the clock" in aircrew by dilating a significant lesion down to a residual minimal stenosis and subsequently waivering the aircrew member for the military environment? If coronary artery decisions were based upon angiographic grading, would it be unreasonable to waiver such patients under minimal CAD decision rules? The first major issue is—how comparable are these dilated "minimal" lesions to native undilated minimal lesions? How comparable are the natural histories? The National Heart, Lung and Blood

Institute established an angioplasty registry, and impaneled angiographic experts to address the long-term issues in angioplasty. Of note, restenosis rates of up to 30% were noted within six months. These restenosis rates were largely clinically established, and the total rate of restenosis is unknown, 30% representing a lower bound. Thus, the dilated minimal lesion is not analogous to the minimal lesions discussed earlier in this chapter. Although restenosis after six months is much less common than during the first six months, most symptomatic patients receiving angioplasty do not have completely unifocal disease processes, and disease progression in the native vessels is quite common. Celio of the USAF has given an excellent analysis of the USAF's aircrew policies regarding angioplasty, as of 1993 (45). As with bypass surgery, this author noted that there are almost certainly acceptable angioplasty candidates for aircrew waiver, and the six-month restenosis problem can be overcome by a later repeated angiography. However, the USAF found virtually no acceptable candidates from multiple potential patients, but the policy is under continual review. The USAF is not, as of this writing, returning aircrew with PCTA to any category of flying. Progression in the undilated vessels in one angioplasty follow-up study revealed 36% progression at 34 months. Further, no concordance existed between the dilated vessel and the progressive disease.

It may be tempting to send aircrew to have dilatations of asymptomatic disease, whereas the morbidity of bypass surgery seems less attractive. Asymptomatic patients who do not have ominous anatomy are not usually candidates for any intervention on clinical grounds. It may be more appealing to dilate such symptomatic patients, but the angioplasty mortality exceeds or is similar to that of bypass surgery in many surgical centers, while emergency bypass surgery will be required in 3.4% of dilatations, and an additional 4.3% will suffer an infarction. Further, the types and kinds of asymptomatic lesions found in aircrew are quite likely to be of

mild or moderate degree. The restenosis of a mild-to-moderate lesion is not guaranteed to occur only to the level of the original lesion; for this reason, many invasive cardiologists avoid electively dilating a moderate lesion(s) that appears as a "target of opportunity" in the course of dilating the lesions responsible for the symptoms. Although it is possible that carefully selected angioplasty patients may be returned to flying status under minimal CAD policies, dilatation of lesions for purely occupational reasons in the absence of clinical indications seems unwise.

Myocardial Infarction

A documented myocardial infarction is viewed as disqualifying by virtually every aviation authority. A few such patients have been returned to flying status in civil aviation, virtually always following single-vessel, completed infarctions with favorable angiographic anatomy, normal left ventricular function, no resting or reversible ischemia, and no arrhythmias. The USAF's non-waiverability of myocardial necrosis was recently reviewed by comparing follow-up events, bypass surgery, and mortality in several groups of patients with asymptomatic infarctions (45). Event rates, including infarctions found in those with only minimal CAD, were far in excess of what was believed to be prudent for a military flying population, and certainly well above the benchmark levels of coronary events established in the USAF's minimal CAD study group.

Other Factors in the Disposition of CAD in Aircrew

Most asymptomatic lesions in aircrew members are discovered at angiography performed because of noninvasive tests suggestive of reversible ischemia. It is quite likely that many of the minimal lesions in the 30–40% range may actually not be producing reversible ischemia. However, pure angiographic topography is often a poor predictor of the metabolic consequences of a given stenosis. If one were to return aircrew with minimal disease to the cockpit, one must accept that some of these lesions would be producing reversible ischemia. However, the rate pressure products obtained in conventional testing for reversible ischemia are rarely reached in non-high-performance flying. For this reason, waivers for minimal coronary disease are restricted to non-high-performance systems. Further, coronary hemodynamics under $+G_z$ acceleration have not been sufficiently defined to waiver minimal CAD. A waiver policy in this regard may well change when this information void is filled.

Coronary Artery Risk in Selection for Flying Training

Stricter medical selection and retention standards for CAD risk factors could reasonably be expected to improve flying safety. The West Point (26) study by Clark et al. revealed that risk factor partitions can be discerned in a population of training age, and the long-term follow-up study by Klag et al. indicated that serum cholesterol alone is of some value (25). Screening applicants for flying training with total cholesterol alone would almost surely detect those with hereditary hyperlipidemia, but would be insufficient to eliminate the majority of those who will later jeopardize flying safety with CAD. Long-term prediction from risk factors remains inaccurate. For example, 20% of the cases of coronary heart disease in the Framingham study occurred in patients with total cholesterols of < 200 mg%. Prevalence data from the USAF Aeromedical Consultation Service agrees with Framingham incidence data: in the decade beginning July, 1978, 101 asymptomatic aviators had coronary artery narrowing ≥ 70% at angiography. Of these, 19% had preangiography serum total cholesterol levels ≤ 200 mg%, including six patients with narrowing ≥ 90%. None had diabetes, uncontrolled hypertension, or obesity. Coronary heart disease mortality in the United States population in 1989 was about 200.6 per

100,000 adults (10). Forty-four percent of adults in the United States have total serum cholesterol levels < 200 mg%. Thus, 40 (20% of the 200) coronary deaths per 100,000 occur in the 44% of the adults with total cholesterol levels < 200 mg%. Without adjusting for age and year of death, the coronary mortality rate is 40 per 44,000 or 92 per 100,000 in adults with total cholesterols < 200 mg%. It is interesting to note that these mortality figures exceed the rates for the second and third highest causes of death: stroke at 59 and lung cancer at 57 per 100,000. Because of the significant coronary mortality in those with cholesterols < 200 mg%, long-term prediction for flying training remains imprecise. Screening can be improved when based on the ratio of LDL to HDL cholesterol, on LP (a), and on the ratio of apolipoprotein B to apolipoprotein A1. After the elimination of those with obvious lipid dyscrasias, perhaps the best strategy should be to use risk factors as ancillary decision-making data in the competition between equally qualified candidates, rather than the setting of some arbitrary standard for these risk variables.

In a disease that is capricious, unpredictable, often presents as a catastrophe, and occurs early in life, the optimal approach is prevention rather than anatomic detection. The Bogalusa Heart Study necropsies of 88 deaths (98% by accident) in ages 7–24, found fatty streaks in the coronary arteries in all but six cases (46).

Lowering the ratio of serum LDL to HDL cholesterol by lifestyle changes is the first step. In conjunction with diet, a regular exercise program, consisting of low-impact, large-muscle rhythmic exercise for 20 minutes three to four times per week is the second major component of a risk reduction program. Exercise has salutary effects on both BP and stress management. A complete review of the diet-heart controversy and the exercise hypothesis are beyond the scope of this chapter. The reader is directed to reviews specifically addressing risk factors in aerospace medicine (47,48).

DISPOSITION OF ELECTROCARDIOGRAPHIC ABNORMALITIES IN AVIATORS

In this section, electrocardiographic abnormalities are discussed in the context of aeromedical significance. The prognostic implication of specific findings in electrocardiography traditionally have been based on clinical populations. The present criteria for the disposition of ECG abnormalities in aviators are based on findings within a flying population and on observation of the natural history of specific ECG characteristics. These recommendations are derived from the experience gained from the USAF Central ECG Library, which was established in 1957. Over 1 million ECGs are on file in this facility.

Electrocardiography is not an exact science. It must be correlated with the history and physical examination. Extensive cardiac evaluation may be required to clarify a given finding. The significance of a specific finding and its aeromedical implication depend heavily on the presence or absence of underlying cardiovascular disease.

This section is devoted primarily to a discussion of serial ST segment and T-wave changes, common arrhythmias, the Wolff-Parkinson-White ECG pattern, and conduction disturbances. The current aeromedical dispositions for these abnormalities are discussed. The disposition of individuals with certain of these ECG findings will remain flexible. Aeromedical recommendations continue to evolve as more experience is accumulated with the natural history of these asymptomatic cardiovascular findings.

ECG diagnostic criteria are not addressed in depth and the reader is referred to any one of the currently available textbooks on ECG.

The following is a list of ECG findings that are considered normal variants:

1. Sinus pause: < 2 seconds in duration.
2. Atrial premature beats: rare.
3. Junctional premature beats: rare.
4. Ventricular premature beats, uniform: rare.
5. Supraventricular rhythm, if slow (refers to a nonsinus supraventribular rhythm, such as atrial or junctional rhythm).
6. Supraventricular escape beats, occurring after a pause of < 2 seconds.
7. Wandering atrial pacemaker.
8. Terminal conduction delay in the QRS complex.
9. Right-axis deviation on an initial tracing in an individual younger than 35 years (QRS axis greater than $+120°$).
10. Left-axis deviation in an initial tracing (QRS axis more negative than $30°$).
11. $S_1S_2S_3$ pattern.
12. Short PR interval without tachyarrhythmias (PR of 0.10 seconds duration or less).
13. Indeterminate QRS axis.
14. Early repolarization pattern.
15. Incomplete right-bundle branch block pattern.

These variants, however, may require further evaluation to ensure that the aircrew member is free of cardiac disease. The rhythm disturbances listed above will, in many patients, require treadmill exercise testing and ambulatory electrocardiography for further evaluation. A normal variant ECG finding, by definition, must occur in an individual who is free of underlying heart disease. The recommended evaluation procedures listed in Table 15.7 should exclude the more commonly associated abnormalities. A repeated, fasting 12-lead ECG, with meticulous attention to lead placement, medication review, and history, should precede an evaluation for suspected normal variants.

Prevalence of ECG Abnormalities

In the USAF, all aviators receive an initial ECG on entry into flying duties and biennially after age 34. An analysis of all initial ECGs performed in the USAF flying population reveals that 82.5% are normal and 17.4% abnormal. Of the normal ECGs, 10% are labeled as normal variants. A normal variant is a finding that is common in normal individuals but not usually

Table 15.7.
Cardiovascular Evaluation of Electrocardiographic Findings That May Represent Normal Variant Patterns

Pattern	Evaluation Indicated
Sinus tachycardia (sinus rate >100 beats/min	Metabolic determinations to exclude hyperadrenergic state and hyperthyroidism
Voltage criteria for left ventricular hypertrophy (SV_1 plus RV_5 or SV_2 plus RV_6 of >55 mm in individuals below age 35 and >45 mm in individuals age 35 and older)	Echocardiographic study: if echo reveals LVH with hypertension or cardiomyopathy, patient permanently disqualify. If mild LVH, and exercise history is consistent with "athletic heart," repeat echo after three months of abstinence of exercise. If LVH regresses, return to flying indicated.
First-degree AV block (PR interval of >0.21 seconds)	Treadmill test: if PR fails to shorten, cardiac evaluation should be conducted for underlying conduction system disease.
Possible right ventricular hypertrophy (tall R in V_1 with or without secondary ST-T changes)	Echocardiographic study.
Evidence of left or right atrial abnormality	Echocardiographic study.
Left-axis deviation (serial change)	Treadmill and echocardiogram
Q-waves suggestive of myocardial abnormality	Inspiratory and expiratory ECGs with inferior Q's; vectorcardiography, echocardiographic study, and when indicated, nuclear cardiologic studies.

associated with underlying organic heart disease, incapacitating events, or a shortened lifespan. A normal variant ECG, however, may require an extensive evaluation to exclude organic heart disease.

A normal variant may be defined in two ways. The first definition is based on the prevalence of the finding in the population. The second definition is based on the presence or absence of

organic heart disease. The prevalence definition of an abnormal ECG means that the ECG is unlike the usually observed patterns. To judge an ECG as normal or abnormal from the state of health of an individual requires more information than is usually available to the ECG technician.

Diagnostic criteria based on prevalence are preferable to those based on the state of health in an asymptomatic population. In an asymptomatic population, especially a population of healthy aviators, an abnormal tracing must be considered the tracing of an individual at an increased risk of a cardiovascular event. Many ECG abnormalities when viewed alone are nonspecific, but when compared with previous ECGs may represent a significant serial change. The serial follow-up of resting ECGs has been a key feature of the USAF Central ECG Library. The detection of a serial change of the ECG represents a valuable indicator of possible underlying disease, particularly in those at high coronary risk. The scalar ECG remains a fundamental tool in the early detection of CAD, cardiomyopathy, and arrhythmias. Aeromedical ECG libraries are also rapidly becoming risk-factor repositories, from which stratified CAD screening programs can be operated. Figures 15.2 through 15.8are constructed from the USAF Central ECG Library data of Lancaster and Ord (49).

Specific ECG Findings by Age

Approximately 30% of aviators, ages 50 years or older, in the USAF have abnormal initial ECGs (Fig. 15.2). The most common abnormality is that of repolarization changes, especially ST segment and T-wave abnormalities (Fig. 15.3). The prevalence of repolarization changes on the initial ECG is lowest in the 20- to 34-year-old age group, an age range in which CAD, hypertension, and cardiomyopathy are infrequent. Further, most conduction disturbances and congenital heart diseases have been detected prior to this age. After an initial normal ECG, the

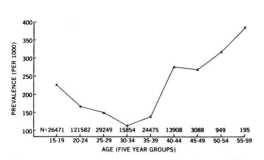

Figure 15.2. Prevalence of total ECG abnormalities on initial ECGs in five-year age groups of USAF aviators.

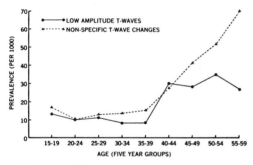

Figure 15.3. Prevalence of repolarization abnormalities on initial ECG in five-year age groups of USAF aviators.

prevalence of low-amplitude T-waves remains essentially unchanged, whereas the prevalence of nonspecific T-wave changes continues to increase to a maximum of 320 cases per 1000 aviators (Fig. 15.4). By ages 50–54 years, other repolarization abnormalities, consisting of ST-segment changes, have a strong correlation with age and are present in 28% of aviators by age 40.

Serial repolarization changes on a resting ECG increase the predictive value of the treadmill exercise test two-fold. Serial repolarization changes require a repeat fasting 12-lead ECG, risk factor analysis, and exercise ECG. The current policy among most aeromedical services is to evaluate asymptomatic serial repolarization changes with a repeat fasting 12-lead ECG, risk

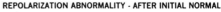
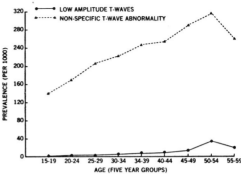

Figure 15.4. Prevalence of serial repolarization abnormalities after normal initial ECGs in five-year age groups of USAF aviators.

factor analysis, and maximal symptom-limited exercise test. Currently, no combined epidemiologic and angiographic series exists of aircrew who were chosen for second-order testing based solely on coronary risk. When such approaches are validated, it seems clear that many low-to-moderate coronary risk patients with nonspecific ST and T changes will be spared additional coronary disease testing. ST-T changes due to pericardial disease, metabolic disease, chamber enlargement, hypertension, and cardiomyopathy must, of course, be considered and evaluated. Aeromedical services that utilize a risk factor stratification program to determine the pursuit of nonspecific ST and T changes in aircrew usually perform treadmill tests first. Abnormal treadmills usually proceed to angiography. Myocardial scintigraphy's greatest value in such stratification programs lies in preventing a negative treadmill test from being accepted at face value in a subject at high coronary risk. Discarding an abnormal treadmill result in circumstances of high pretest probability of disease (high risk factor composite) is unwise. Because the negative predictive value of thallium scintigraphy is significantly degraded in circumstances of high pretest probability of disease, discarding an abnormal treadmill in such patients in favor of a negative scintigraphic result, is equally unwise. Negative thalliums in those with abnormal treadmills *and* high coronary risk must be suspect.

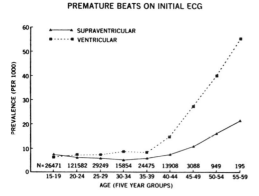

Figure 15.5. Prevalence of premature beats on initial ECGs in five-year age groups of USAF aviators.

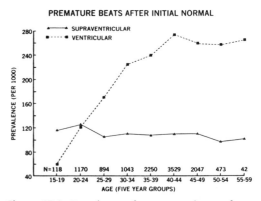

Figure 15.6. Prevalence of premature beats after normal initial ECGs in 5-year age groups of USAF aviators.

Coronary fluoroscopy of patients with high coronary risk and negative treadmill tests is preferred by some over scintigraphy because of the lower radiation exposure. For aeromedical services that do not use stratified screening, second-order studies should be ordered and interpreted with pretest coronary composite risk in mind.

Premature Beats

A study of premature beats on initial ECG reveals that ventricular premature beats are more common in the older age group (Fig. 15.5). Although the majority of individuals with premature atrial or ventricular beats have no clinical heart disease, the steady increase in the prevalence of ventricular ectopic beats with age parallels the increased prevalence of hypertension, CAD, and cardiomyopathy. After an initial normal ECG, the prevalence of supraventricular premature beats remains constant, whereas the prevalence of ventricular premature beats continues to increase, reaching a maximum prevalence of 260 aviators per 1000 at age 40 (Fig. 15.6).

Atrial Premature Beats

Atrial premature beats (APBs) or junctional premature beats (JPBs) are a common finding in ECGs. In one series, 56% of healthy patients had APBs on ambulatory ECG monitoring.

APBs have special significance as precursors of supraventricular arrhythmias, including atrial tachycardia, atrial fibrillation, and atrial flutter. APBs may, in some patients, be related to excess caffeine ingestion or other stimulants. Careful attention to symptoms of tachyarrhythmias is important. The presence of APBs warrants clinical evaluation including history, physical examination, and ambulatory ECG study. Exercise ECG, echocardiography, and thyroid function studies also may be needed.

Ventricular Premature Beats

Ventricular premature beats (VPBs) are a common finding in individuals with and without underlying heart disease. VPBs may be associated with organic heart disease, such as cardiomyopathy, hypertension, or CAD. Evaluation of an aviator with VPBs should include a careful history, physical examination, risk-factor analysis, and ambulatory ECG recording. The ambulatory ECG study is particularly important in detecting complex VPBs. If VPBs were < 1% of beats on Holter monitor, no further evaluation would be required. If VPBs > 1% were found, treadmill and echocardiogram should be performed. The pursuit of anatomic coronary disease by evaluating Holter ventricular ectopy in aviators has not been revealing on a population basis, according to Batchelor et al. (50). However, complex ventricular ectopy, including frequency >10% of beats must be evaluated for underlying organic heart disease. Ventricular arrhythmias are particularly dangerous in individuals with prolonged QT syndromes. Individuals with QT intervals that are prolonged for heart rate should be investigated carefully for underlying heart disease or associated arrhythmias.

Ventricular Ectopy During Stress

VPBs and complex ventricular arrhythmias that are absent in the resting state may be produced by increasing sympathetic tone in the normal individual during exercise. An unfavorable oxygen supply-demand imbalance may produce similar arrhythmias in individuals with subclinical ischemic heart disease. In addition, both mechanisms may be operating simultaneously. Further, the increasing parasympathetic tone seen in individuals immediately post $+G_z$ acceleration may lead to "breakthrough" ectopy as the heart slows.

VPBs are commonly seen during exercise stress. Their presence alone is poorly predictive of the existence of underlying CAD. In a USAFSAM study population, the prevalence, complexity, configuration, or time of VPB occurrence were not strong indicators of the presence of CAD among asymptomatic individuals. The absence of a statistical relationship between exercise-induced VPBs and angiographic coronary disease is reassuring but the true aeromedical significance of exercise ventricular ectopy must await long-term follow-up studies of aircrew with asymptomatic ectopy.

Exercise-induced Ventricular Tachycardia

Exercise-induced ventricular tachycardia (EIVT), defined as three or more consecutive ventricular beats at a rate of 100 beats/min or greater, is seen in some apparently healthy aviators during exercise testing. At USAFSAM, EIVT has been noted in 0.5% of treadmill tests. In a six-year retrospective follow-up study of 43 aviators with EIVT, nine individuals (21.2%) had cardiac events (angina, myocardial infarc-

tion, or sudden death). Among these nine individuals with cardiac events, three deaths occurred. The deaths occurred in patients with amyloidosis, myocardial infarction, and mitral valve prolapse at nine months, three years, and six years, respectively. Six nonfatal events occurred, with four individuals developing angina pectoris and two sustaining nonfatal myocardial infarctions.

In aviators with EIVT, none of the following discriminated between those with cardiac events and those without:

- length of the ventricular tachycardia,
- number of ventricular tachycardia episodes,
- rate of ventricular tachycardia,
- ventricular tachycardia configuration,
- heart rate at onset of ventricular tachycardia,
- ST segment response to exercise,
- ambulatory ECG data, or
- echocardiographic data.

Further, the presence of warning arrhythmias (> 10 VPBs per minute, pairing of VPBs, multiformity, or ventricular bigeminy) also did not separate those with and without events. All subjects were asymptomatic during EIVT. EIVT was usually unsustained, usually occurred in late exercise or early recovery at heart rates < 150 beats per minute, and was usually an isolated event. Antecedent complex arrhythmias were usually absent. Almost one-third of the EIVT patients were initially referred for noncardiac reasons.

Seventeen of the EIVT patients underwent cardiac catheterization with coronary angiography. Of these 17 individuals, 13 had normal coronary arteriograms and 4 had CAD. Although men with EIVT as a group were at increased risk for cardiac events, none of the aviators with normal arteriograms in this group had subsequent cardiac events during follow-up.

Disposition of Ventricular Tachycardia in Aircrew

Aviators with either Holter- or exercise-induced VT should be evaluated with a thorough clinical examination as well as echocardiography and treadmill testing. Holter monitoring should be performed monthly for three months to assess the pattern and frequency of any underlying ectopic substrate as well as to rule out any recurrence of VT. Aviators with significant substrate for ventricular arrhythmias or recurrence of VT should be disqualified and managed clinically. Those with no recurrence and no evidence of organic heart disease should undergo left heart catheterization. Although not all patients in the USAF EIVT retrospective study group underwent catheterization, available angiographic and epidemiologic data in this group support a policy of return to flying in those with normal left heart catheterizations. The required three Holter monitors also preclude angiography which would later become moot if recurrence were not established before such invasive studies were undertaken. Because no clinical indication for angiography exists in such cases, but only occupational indications, every effort must be made to assure that aircrew undergoing invasive studies are waiverable for flying on all other grounds, both for the body system in question and all other systems as well. Policy for invasive studies must assure that the entire and final waiver decision revolves around the angiography. This general principle applies to all aeromedical catheterizations because they are almost always performed in the absence of the usual clinical indications. Aviators with Holter- or exercise-induced ventricular tachycardia may be returned to non-high-performance flying with nonrecurrent, brief, isolated, monomorphic asymptomatic VT, without significant ventricular ectopic substrate, and with normal coronary arteriograms. Flying waivers for ventricular tachycardia, under carefully defined circumstances, is an acknowledgment that complex ventricular ectopy may certainly occur in those with normal hearts. Extension of VT waivers to the high-performance arena must await basic sciences information regarding the hemodynamic effects of ventricular tachycardia under $+G_z$.

Celio closely analyzed the work of others re-garding the implications of complex ectopy in asymptomatic persons (51). Based upon clinical outcomes, he concludes that VT in aircrew requires indepth evaluation with continued conservative policies.

Supraventricular Tachycardia

Supraventricular tachycardia (SVT) may cause sudden incapacitation. Even in the healthy individual, rapid, sustained tachycardias with short diastolic filling periods may lead to inadequate cardiac output with near or frank syncope. Further, individuals with subclinical CAD may develop symptoms of angina pectoris, heart failure, or cardiovascular collapse due to sustained tachyarrhythmia. Prior to 1974, all episodes of SVT were considered disqualifying for flying duties in the USAF. Subsequently, aviators with isolated asymptomatic episodes of SVT have been returned to flying status following stringent evaluations. The most favorable cases of SVT for return to flying status were those associated with classic precipitating factors for SVT in younger persons. The episodes of SVT often were related to a combination of fatigue, anxiety, hunger, alcohol, and stimulants, such as caffeine. SVT occurring in such circumstances is frequently referred to as the "holiday heart syndrome" and accounts for most cases of SVT seen in healthy aviators. Such episodes of SVT are usually self-limited events that seldom recur when precipitating factors are avoided.

The aeromedical disposition of SVT begins with a precise arrhythmia diagnosis. Whereas reentrant SVT and atrial fibrillation are potentially waiverable arrhythmias, atrial flutter is not generally waiverable because of the possibility of excessive ventricular rates. SVT with aberrancy must be distinguished from ventricular tachycardia.

Aeromedical Disposition Of Supraventricular Tachycardia

A landmark study in aircrew members with supraventricular tachycardia has resulted from the USAF SVT study group (52). Four hundred and thirty aircrew members with supraventricular tachycardia, as a referral or incidental diagnosis, occurring between 1955 and 1991, were followed up by the USAFSAM for a mean of 11.4 years. This study addressed the greatest clinical and aeromedical concern in tachyarrhythmias—hemodynamic compromise. Syncopal or presyncopal symptoms were carefully documented during this study. Ten percent (n = 42) of the SVT patients had hemodynamic compromise; hemodynamic compromise was actually the initial presenting symptom in 38 of these patients. The other four cases occurred during follow-up, three of which were recurrent, sustained supraventricular tachycardia, defined as two or more episodes $\geq$ 10 minutes duration. The fourth case had initially presented as a single, sustained episode of SVT. Five percent (n = 21) of the entire cohort had recurrent, sustained supraventricular tachycardia with hemodynamic compromise. Remarkably, 20 of these 21 (95%) had recurrent SVT as the initial presenting finding. Predictive information in this study revealed a relative risk of 15.6 for hemodynamic compromise in recurrent, sustained supraventricular tachycardia, and 3.8 for hemodynamic compromise in ventricular preexcitation. The risk ratio for recurrent, sustained SVT in preexcitation patients was 5.2.

Thus, recurrent, sustained supraventricular tachycardia was strongly predictive of hemodynamically unstable SVT, as was preexcitation. Preexcitation was also strongly predictive of the development of asymptomatic, recurrent SVT.

The study also provided invaluable data on the issue of predicting sustained events from the initial presentation. Only one of 214 (0.5%) of the initial, single, nonsustained SVTs developed subsequent sustained SVT. Further, only 2% of initial, recurrent, nonsustained SVTs developed sustained SVT during follow-up. However, 11% (three of 28) of initial, sustained cases developed sustained SVT during follow-up, and 22% (five of 23) of initial, recurrent, sustained SVTs developed sustained SVT during follow-up.

Based upon these studies, the USAF has concluded that aircrew with single, asymptomatic episodes of nonsustained supraventricular tachycardia of 3–10 beats can be evaluated locally with a history and physical to rule out precipitating causes, including thyroid function tests. One Holter test each month for three months is recommended to categorize the aircrew member's SVT. For episodes $\geq$ 11 beats, a more in depth examination with echocardiography and thallium scintigraphy is needed. No invasive studies are warranted except for tests consistent with reversible ischemia. An uneventful evaluation in either of the above cases usually means no further follow-up is required. Patients with recurrent, nonsustained SVT, or one or more episodes of sustained SVT require indepth evaluations at three-year intervals with Holter and exercise tests (for rhythm analysis). Underlying CAD should be sought in those older than age 35. Unrestricted flying waivers should be offered for single or recurrent, nonsustained SVT (< 10 minutes' duration) or a single, sustained SVT ($\geq$ 10 minutes' duration). The long-term follow-up data indicated that either of these diagnoses in association with mitral valve prolapse, sarcoidosis, bundle branch block, or valvular heart disease (excluding aortic insufficiency) is waiverable. Restrictive waivers for non-high-performance flying are recommended for recurrent, sustained SVT when the interval between episodes is $\geq$ three years. Such restricted waivers are also recommended for single or recurrent, nonsustained SVT with minimal CAD, asymptomatic ventricular tachycardia, or aortic insufficiency. Single, sustained supraventricular tachycardia is waiverable in conjunction with ventricular tachycardia and/or aortic insufficiency provided that the latter diagnoses are waiverable on their own.

Permanent disqualification is recommended for any hemodynamically unstable supraventricular tachycardia, recurrent, sustained supraventricular tachycardia less than three years apart, any SVT with preexcitation, or a single, sustained episode of SVT with gradable CAD.

In summary, hemodynamically unstable SVT occurred in 10% of all aircrew members with SVT. Asymptomatic, recurrent, sustained SVT occurred in 5% of all aircrew members with SVT. Recurrent, sustained SVT and SVT associated with preexcitation have an increased relative risk for developing hemodynamically unstable SVT. Aircrew members with nonsustained SVT in the absence of preexcitation have a benign prognosis, and aircrew members with a single sustained episode of SVT represent a small and aeromedically acceptable risk for continued flying duties. Aircrew members with recurrent, sustained SVT when the episodes are greater than three years apart also represent a small and aeromedically acceptable risk for continued flying duties. Maintenance medication to control SVT is not compatible with flying. This study did not address multifocal atrial tachycardia or atrial fibrillation.

In general, the other supraventricular arrhythmias should be evaluated for recurrence with multiple Holters. In the absence of underlying organic heart disease, nonrecurrent, hemodynamically stable supraventricular arrhythmias, such as atrial fibrillation and multifocal atrial tachycardia, are waiverable for all classes of flying. Particular attention must be paid to detecting atrial enlargement, pericardial disease, ischemic heart disease, and valvular disease, especially mitral valve disease. Euthyroid status should be documented in all waivered patients with supraventricular tachycardia.

Wolff-Parkinson-White ECG Finding

The Wolff-Parkinson-White (WPW) ECG finding consists of a short PR interval (< 0.10 seconds), a delta wave at the onset of the QRS complex, and a widened QRS complex. By definition, individuals with the WPW ECG finding who also have tachyarrhythmias have the WPW syndrome. The ECG finding of the WPW pattern indicates the presence of a bypass tract. The WPW ECG finding is disqualifying for entry into flight training in the USAF. This ECG finding may be waiverable for continued flying

duties when discovered in trained aviators in the absence of a history of tachyarrhythmia. Because the ECG finding of preexcitation may be intermittent, some cases of WPW are not discovered on entry into aircrew training and only appear on a subsequent ECG. Electrophysiologic studies for aeromedical assessment are not indicated in individuals with either the WPW ECG finding or in those with the WPW syndrome. An electrophysiologic study would not change the aeromedical disposition because the basic WPW pattern indicates the presence of a bypass tract, and the occurrence of tachyarrhythmias is a priori disqualifying in the WPW syndrome. The presence of the WPW pattern on the ECG requires thorough cardiovascular evaluation, including ambulatory ECG monitoring, treadmill exercise testing, and baseline thallium scintigraphy. As reported in the USAF SVT study group, significantly elevated relative risks for both hemodynamic compromise and recurrent, sustained SVT were noted in patients with preexcitation. SVT rates in WPW syndrome may be quite rapid, with short diastolic filling periods and reduced cardiac output. The SVT in the WPW syndrome may also occur as atrial fibrillation or, uncommonly, as atrial flutter. Rapid ventricular response rates may cause degeneration into ventricular fibrillation. For this reason, WPW ECG finding is disqualifying for entry into flying training in the USAF.

In the experience of USAFSAM, the WPW ECG pattern is not a marker for CAD. The occurrence of CAD in aviators with the WPW syndrome, however, is of special concern because coronary artery stenosis is the condition that individuals with rapid tachyarrhythmias are least able to tolerate. Although a young aviator without coronary disease may remain asymptomatic during paroxysmal tachycardia, the ability to tolerate the arrhythmia later in life may be compromised by the development of coronary disease. Coronary disease is the most frequently acquired heart disease in aviators. This fact, in our opinion, is another reason to prohibit the training of individuals with the anatomic substrate for paroxysmal tachyarrhythmias. Further, the ST segment becomes uninterpretable during exercise in the majority of individuals with the WPW pattern. The loss of the exercise test as a noninvasive cardiovascular surveillance tool is most unfortunate. The flight surgeon is thus deprived of a means to screen serially for the one condition that individuals with the WPW syndrome can least tolerate in the face of tachyarrhythmias: CAD. The presence of a large number of aviators with the WPW pattern and an uninterpretable ECG ST segment response to exercise would present a formidable medical follow-up problem and would seriously complicate surveillance for CAD in this group. The increased risk of sustained tachycardia and the logistic difficulty of cardiovascular surveillance in these patients continue to make this disorder disqualifying for entry into flight training in the USAF. Trained aviators without tachyarrhythmias may remain on flying status with periodic surveillance. Even brief, nonsustained runs of SVT in aviators with WPW is nonwaiverable. The sectioning or ablation of asymptomatic bypass tracts is to be discouraged. Some aviators with significant WPW syndrome may undergo bypass tract ablation on solid clinical grounds. Radio frequency ablation could conceivably result in a return to flying for those who have been managed with ablation, but insufficient experience during follow-up at this point does not allow such waivers. Early experience is encouraging. Currently, WPW syndrome, treated or untreated, remains disqualifying for all classes of flying.

Individuals with short PR intervals (< 0.10 seconds) who have histories of SVT without other features of the WPW syndrome are said to have the Lown-Ganong-Levine syndrome. Individuals with this syndrome are disqualified from flying duties in the USAF. Those individuals with a shortened PR interval and no history of tachyarrhythmia may be entered into or continued on flying status.

Right and Left Bundle Branch Block

Both right and left bundle branch block are rare conduction disturbances in the United States avi-

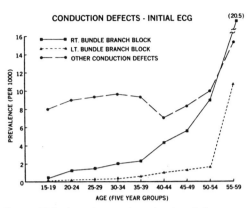

Figure 15.7. Prevalence of conduction defects on initial ECGs in five-year age groups of USAF aviators.

ation population (Fig. 15.7). Left bundle branch block (LBBB) occurs on the initial ECG in fewer than two of 1000 aviators under the age of 50. Right bundle branch block (RBBB) occurs on the initial ECG in fewer than six of 1000 aviators below age 50. Bifascicular and trifascicular blocks account for 90% of cases that ultimately develop complete heart block, whereas monofascicular blocks account for only 10% of cases that develop complete heart block.

Right Bundle Branch Block

Studies at USAFSAM have located the site of conduction delay in asymptomatic aviators with acquired RBBB. Using endocardial mapping techniques, investigators found that aviators with acquired RBBB had normal His bundle to RBB conduction times and prolonged His bundle to right ventricular outflow times. Normal control data were obtained from patients undergoing electrophysiologic studies for reasons other than acquired RBBB. The location of the block was in the distal arborization of the right bundle beyond the moderator band. Complete heart block developed in only one of 372 aviators with RBBB followed for an average of 10 years. Among the 164 aviators with RBBB previously evaluated at USAFSAM, 83% have been returned to flying duties. CAD was found in 13% of these aviators and an abnormal His bundle in 1%. Most cases of asymptomatic acquired right bundles were not due to CAD, as shown earlier by Lancaster et al. (53). Based on electrophysiologic and epidemiologic information, aviators with RBBB may be retained on flying status when a full, noninvasive evaluation, including exercise ECG and thallium scintigraphy, is normal. Electrophysiologic studies are still needed for aviators with RBBB if left axis deviation, marked right axis deviation, first-degree atrioventricular (AV) block, or second-degree AV block were present.

Canaveris and Halpern studied 261 aviators with incomplete RBBB; 136 patients were identified on the initial ECG (54). Prevalence was highest in patients 20–29 years of age; 4.6% of patients went on to develop complete RBBB. They recommended additional studies only in those with incomplete RBBB and additional conduction disturbances (54).

Left Bundle Branch Block

Coronary arteriography and electrophysiologic study are required by the USAF for all aviators with acquired LBBB. Wehrly's historical review of LBBB is an excellent summary of aeromedical policy evolution in this disorder (55). Aviators with LBBB have tended to be slightly older in the USAFSAM series and the prevalence of CAD and hypertension were slightly greater than that in a control population (53). Although the ST segment response to exercise is interpretable with RBBB, the ST segment response during exercise is uninterpretable with LBBB. R-wave amplitude changes with exercise in LBBB patients, however, may have diagnostic value. The USAFSAM experience indicates that some aviators with LBBB and normal coronary arteriograms have abnormal exercise thallium myocardial scintigrams. The presence of abnormal thallium scintigrams in individuals with LBBB and normal coronary arteriograms suggests that the basic defect in asymptomatic LBBB may be due to a process that is not confined to the conduction system but may stem from a common process affecting both myocardium and specialized conduction tissue. Aviators with acquired, asymptomatic LBBB will continue to be the focus of a natural history study.

In a group of 63 aviators with LBBB evaluated at USAFSAM, all of whom underwent left heart catheterization and electrophysiologic study, 46 (73%) were returned to flying status, 14 (22%) had CAD and were medically disqualified, and three (5%) were disqualified due to other causes, including one aviator with a prolonged H-Q interval.

Aviators with LBBB should have a complete cardiovascular evaluation with exercise ECG, thallium myocardial scintigraphy, coronary angiography, and electrophysiologic studies. A waiver may be considered for those aviators in whom no underlying cardiovascular disease is demonstrated.

Atrioventricular Block

Atrioventricular (AV) block is classified as first-degree, second-degree, and third-degree block. Second-degree AV block is further divided into Mobitz type I (Wenckebach) and Mobitz type II blocks. For USAF aviators, first-degree AV Block is defined as a PR interval on the resting ECG > 0.21 seconds in duration, irrespective of age and heart rate. The definition of first-degree AV block requires that, without exception, every sinus P-wave must be followed by a ventricular complex. First-degree AV block may occur anywhere in the AV conduction system proximal to Purkinje fibers. The site of the conduction delay in first-degree AV block is nearly always in the AV node. First-degree AV block is usually a normal variant secondary to increased vagal tone in healthy aviators. Associated sinus bradycardia is common. Aviators with first-degree AV block should undergo some vagal withdrawal maneuver, such as step climbing, running in place, or even a treadmill, to document electrocardiographically shortening of the PR interval and increasing heart rate. In an asymptomatic aviator with a normal physical examination and a normal

PR interval response to exercise, continuation of flying status is recommended. Follow-up examinations should include annual ECGs and repeat treadmill testing, when indicated.

In typical Mobitz type I block, the PR interval of successive beats lengthens progressively until a P-wave appears without a following QRS complex as expected. The next beat after the pause that follows the nonconducted P-wave has a shorter PR interval than any subsequent PR interval in the Wenckebach cycle. Electrophysiologic studies have revealed that block occurs within the AV node in most patients with Mobitz Type I block. Rarely is Mobitz Type I block caused by a conduction delay below the level of the AV node. Mobitz I AV block is a common finding in healthy, young athletic aircrew with high degrees of resting vagal tone. In the absence of a prolonged resting PR interval, usually no further studies are needed.

In Mobitz type II AV block, some of the P-waves are not followed by QRS complexes. No progressive increase occurs in the PR interval prior to the nonconducted P-wave, and no shortening of the PR interval follows the nonconducted P-wave. Mobitz type II block and third-degree AV block (complete heart block) will not be further discussed here because both of these conduction disorders are incompatible with flying safety.

Axis Deviation

Right axis deviation (RAD) is defined as a mean QRS axis of +120 degrees or more in the frontal plane. Left axis deviation (LAD) is defined as a mean QRS axis equal to or more negative than −30 degrees in the frontal plane. RAD in young aviators is usually due to a persistent juvenile pattern, but may rarely be due to undetected congenital heart disease. RAD detected before age 35 is usually a normal variant, requiring no further evaluation. When no serial tracings are available, or concern about underlying disease exists, an echocardiogram should be performed. Beyond age 35, acquired RAD should be care-

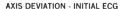

AXIS DEVIATION - INITIAL ECG

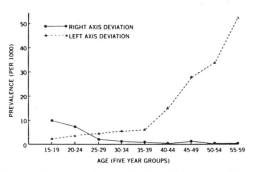

Figure 15.8. Prevalence of axis deviation on initial ECGs in 5-year age groups of United States Air Force aviators.

fully evaluated, including an echocardiographic study.

The prevalence of LAD on the initial ECG increases with age in USAF aircrew, occurring in 5 per 1000 below age 30, and 50 per 1000 by age 60 (Fig. 15.8). LAD may be related to conduction system disease, myocardial disease, or coronary disease. Long-standing LAD, in the absence of any other findings to suggest organic heart disease, is a normal variant. Canaveris et al. studied 247 patients with left-axis deviation, documenting the usual benign nature of the finding (56). Slowly developing LAD was the most common type, while LAD usually appeared first in patients who had associated RBBB. Tamura et al. studied 30 airline pilots at 48.5 years of age with a mean ECG follow-up of 22 years, confirming the lack of progression to complete LBBB, AV block, or cardiac events (57). Acquired LAD should be evaluated with an echocardiogram and an exercise test.

LAD may be a part of the left anterior fascicular block pattern (LAFB). LAFB also includes a small q-wave in leads I and aV1, small r-waves in leads II, III, and aVf, and s-waves in leads V_5 and V_6. Similarly, RAD may be a part of left posterior fascicular block (LPFB). LPFB is associated with small q-waves in leads II, III, and a Vf and with small r-waves in leads I and V1.

A 52-month follow-up of 15 pilots, ages 22

± 5 years revealed a benign course for LAFB in young aircrew. Echo parameters were identical to those of matched controls (58). The evaluation of the fascicular block patterns is determined by an assessment of the chronicity of the pattern. If the block were longstanding, an echocardiogram would suffice. When the block occurs as a serial change, echocardiography and a treadmill test should be performed.

Sinus Bradycardia

As a functional definition, the USAF chooses 50 beats/min or less rather than 60 beats/min to define sinus bradycardia. Sinus bradycardia often is seen in healthy, athletic individuals and frequently is found in military aviators. Sinus bradycardia, however, cannot always be presumed to be due to physical conditioning. In particular, sinus bradycardia, as a serial change in an unconditioned individual, may be a pathologic finding. In one study conducted at USAF-SAM, sinus bradycardia (≤ 50 beats/min over age 30, ≤ 43 beats/min age 30 and under) was searched for as a serial ECG change. Twenty percent of patients with newly diagnosed sinus bradycardia rarely engaged in exercise. Sinus bradycardia as a serial change should suggest the possibility of sinus node disease. Sinus node dysfunction also must be suspected in patients with sinus arrest, sinus node exit block, unexplained syncope, and in episodes of SVT in which a bradycardia-tachycardia syndrome may be the underlying disorder. In the USAF, evaluation for sinus bradycardia usually is triggered by heart rates under 40 beats/min. Evaluation of the aviator with sinus bradycardia should begin with a precise exercise history. A "Hoppogram" or running in place with an ECG lead attached should result in a doubling of the heart rate or an increase to 100 beats/min. In the absence of such a response, a treadmill and Holter should be performed. The Holter monitor may be helpful in detecting associated arrhythmias, advanced degrees of AV block, and correlating symptoms with rhythm. Failure of appropriate

Table 15.8.
Evaluation of Sinus Bradycardia in Aircrew

Clinical Finding	Recommended Evaluation
Sinus bradycardia <40 beats/min	Correlation with exercise history. Moderate exercise with rhythm strip.
Inadequate heart rate response to moderate exercise.	Maximal symptom-limited treadmill test.
Inadequate heart rate response to treadmill.	Electrophysiologic (pacing) study.

heart rate increase with exercise raises concern about sinus node disease. An electrophysiologic study should be performed in such patients. Sinus node disease is disqualifying for all classes of flying. Table 15.8 outlines the aeromedical evaluation of sinus bradycardia.

Sinus arrest must always be considered in the differential diagnosis of syncope or presyncope. Sinus pauses of > 2 seconds should be considered abnormal until normal sinus node function is demonstrated by further testing. The most common causes of sinus arrest are increased vagal tone, as seen in well-trained athletes, digitalis use, and sinus node disease.

Follow-up of Aviators with ECG Abnormalities

Aviators with ECG abnormalities who are returned to flying duties should receive adequate follow-up to ensure that the abnormal finding does not represent disease. Repetitive evaluations are mandatory because the natural history of many asymptomatic ECG abnormalities remains undefined. Only through detailed natural history follow-up studies will it be possible to determine the significance of certain ECG findings. Surveillance of aviators after an initial ECG should resume with biennial ECGs at age 35. ECGs in asymptomatic aviators are most useful when viewed in a serial fashion. The collection of natural history data on ECG abnormalities and normal variant patterns remains an important challenge in aviation cardiology.

VALVULAR HEART DISEASE

Valvular heart disease, both congenital and acquired, is found often enough in an apparently
healthy population to warrant a discussion of the
aeromedical disposition of these abnormalities.
Valvular lesions, when discovered incidentally
in asymptomatic aviators, usually represent subtle subclinical disease compatible with continued aviation duties. The aeromedical disposition
of each valvular lesion should include a consideration of all factors that could predispose the
patient to sudden incapacitation or aggravation
of coincidental disease processes, such as unsuspected CAD. These aeromedical considerations
include the following:

1. Risk of tachyarrhythmias
2. Risk of thromboembolic phenomena
3. Adverse effect of some valvular lesions on
   coronary perfusion
4. Risk of abrupt heart failure
5. Abnormal hemodynamics under $+G_z$ acceleration
6. Risk of bacterial endocarditis

Problem of Innocent Murmur

Aviation examiners should be intimately familiar with the innocent murmur because it will be
the most commonly encountered murmur in a
healthy, young population. It must be emphasized that an innocent murmur is produced by a
normal cardiovascular system. An innocent murmur does not mean a slight murmur produced
by a bicuspid aortic valve or a mitral regurgitant
murmur produced by a mildly deformed myxomatous or rheumatic valve. Such lesions frequently progress and the risk of endocarditis is
always present. Although the prevalence of innocent murmurs decreases steadily by the fourth
decade of life, they are by no means rare. Failure
to recognize an innocent murmur has serious
personal consequences for the person in whom
it is mistaken for an organic lesion. Such individuals are often needlessly restricted in lifestyle

and occupational pursuits, rated for insurance
purposes, or saddled with neurotic concerns
about their hearts. Conversely, failure to diagnose minimal organic valvular disease leaves the
risks of sudden incapacitation and endocarditis
unaddressed.

Evaluation of Valvular Lesions

The examination of all patients with suspected
valvular disease begins with a thorough history
and physical examination. Occasionally, the history may direct the physician toward the central
nervous system, as in mitral valve prolapse, or
the musculoskeletal system, as in ankylosing
spondylitis with aortic valvulitis. The physical
examination should include prolonged auscultation with the patient's chest completely bare.
Auscultation should be performed in a quiet
room that is free of air conditioner noise or other
distractions. Applicable postural, mechanical,
and pharmacologic interventions should be applied to differentiate the origin of the murmur.
For aeromedical purposes, valvular lesions generally should be evaluated with a full, noninvasive battery, as follows:

1. Resting ECG
2. Chest radiography
3. Exercise ECG
4. M-mode and two-dimensional Doppler echocardiography
5. Ambulatory ECG
6. Isotope ventriculography (in some cases)
7. Thallium scintigraphy (in some cases)

Thallium scintigraphy should be employed in
those patients with remarkable risk factors for
concomitant coronary disease or other noninvasive evidence of ischemia. Abnormal scintigrams may, of course, be due to noncoronary
factors, as in mitral prolapse, or due to oxygen
supply-demand imbalance in aortic valve disease. Gated blood pool studies with progressive
exercise are invaluable in the assessment of the
hemodynamic significance of regurgitant le-

sions. Cardiac catheterization should be performed for aeromedical indications if any uncertainty regarding the presence or degree of associated CAD were to remain. A high index of suspicion for coronary disease must be maintained because of the confounding effects of valvular and coronary disease. When a decision has been made to waiver the aviator with mild valvular disease for flying duties, serial, noninvasive surveillance must then be instituted, preferably on an annual basis. Echo/Doppler studies for assessment of left and right ventricular performance, gradients, regurgitation, and chamber size are invaluable in serial follow-up. Exercise echo, or sometimes radionuclide ventriculograms, offers excellent surveillance of valvular lesions. Repeat cardiac catheterization is occasionally necessary to assess any deterioration in noninvasive test results that suggest ischemia.

Aortic Valve Stenosis

The most common cause of isolated aortic valve stenosis is a congenitally bicuspid aortic valve, with 20–30% of isolated bicuspid valves eventually developing stenosis. Degenerative changes produce aortic valve stenosis, but this is uncommon in a young flying population. It is extremely unusual to find isolated aortic valve disease as a single valvular lesion in rheumatic heart disease. Calcific aortic stenosis in young adults is often rheumatic, although some congenital aortic defects may calcify early in life.

Pathophysiologic Factors

The aortic valve area is usually 2.5 to 3.5 cm^2. A valve area of 1.0 cm^2 or less leads to increased left ventricular work, whereas a valve area of < 0.75 cm^2 usually produces symptoms. The left ventricle responds to such stenosis with concentric hypertrophy, thereby maintaining normal wall stress despite elevated tension. This compensatory mechanism in the absence of other cardiac abnormalities maintains a normal cardiac output, even with significant aortic valve stenosis. The systolic gradient across the aortic valve is dependent on the rate of blood flow and the valve area. The hypertrophied ventricle has decreased diastolic compliance, thus producing an elevated left ventricular end-diastolic pressure. Left atrial contraction then becomes necessary for adequate filling of the stiff ventricle. Any cardiac rhythm disturbance that abolishes the atrial contribution to left ventricular filling can lead to pulmonary edema. In time, progressive stenosis results in congestive heart failure. Cerebral complaints, such as syncope, are common. Syncope usually occurs during or immediately following exercise. The failure of cardiac output to increase normally with exertion coupled with systemic vasodilatation related to effort results in decreased cerebral perfusion and loss of consciousness. Syncope may be dysrhythmic in origin. Coronary blood flow is decreased in aortic valve stenosis due to left ventricular hypertrophy, shortened diastolic filling time, systolic compression of the coronary blood vessels, a reduced gradient across the coronary vascular bed due to elevation of left ventricular end-diastolic pressure, and in some individuals, by associated aortic insufficiency. Increased myocardial oxygen demand and decreased coronary artery blood flow may produce angina pectoris, with or without associated coronary atherosclerosis.

Physical Examination

The carotid pulse is normal with minimal aortic valve stenosis, but with increased severity a slowly rising carotid pulse is characteristic. Palpation of the cardiac apex in the left lateral decubitus position reveals the sustained, forceful lift of left ventricular hypertrophy. The apical impulse may be bifid, the initial impulse corresponding to the S_4 gallop heard on auscultation. The systolic ejection murmur, which is usually loudest over the primary aortic area, transmits well to the carotid arteries and to the cardiac apex. In a young population, an aortic ejection click is frequently audible. The ejection click frequently disappears when the valve becomes relatively fibrotic, calcified, and immobile. The first heart sound is usually normal in aortic valve stenosis, and inspiratory splitting of the second heart sound usually is maintained until a delay in left ventricular ejection causes the second heart sound to be either single in inspiration or paradoxically split in expiration. Commonly, an associated diastolic murmur or aortic insufficiency occurs. An S_4 gallop is frequently audible due to the decrease in left ventricular diastolic compliance. The presence of an audible S_4 gallop usually correlates with at least moderate aortic valve stenosis in individuals under age 40. The recognition of an S_3 gallop in the younger population is not very meaningful. In individuals over age 40, however, the presence of an S_3 gallop may be one of the earliest signs of left ventricular decompensation.

Aeromedical Evaluation and Disposition

A complete cardiac noninvasive evaluation must be accomplished (see the list in the earlier section entitled ''Evaluation of Valvular Lesions''). ECG may reveal changes consistent with left ventricular hypertrophy. Chest radiography or cardiac fluoroscopy may reveal calcification in the aortic valve. Echocardiographic studies may reveal findings consistent with a bicuspid aortic valve, thickened aortic leaflets, and left ventricular hypertrophy. Doppler studies give an accurate estimate of transvalvular gradient and cardiac output. Left heart catheterization may be needed if the echo/Doppler study were inadequate or equivocal, or if concern were to exist about concomitant coronary disease. Aortic valve stenosis is potentially waiverable for flying duties when hemodynamically insignificant and asymptomatic. Isolated, asymptomatic aortic valvular stenosis is waiverable for continued flying in the USAF if the peak systolic gradient were 20 mm Hg or less, and exercise capacity exercise ejection fraction response, and other noninvasive studies were normal. No left ventricular hypertrophy should be found by any diagnostic mode. Any degree of coronary atherosclerosis, other than intimal roughening, should also be disqualifying for flying duties.

Although a report from the Eight Bethesda Conference of the American College of Cardiology would certify only those patients with a mean gradient ≤ 20 mm Hg and a normal left ventricular end-diastolic pressure (12 mm Hg) (59), we believe that the latter criterion is perhaps too restrictive because many normal patients with no valvular, coronary, or myocardial disease exceed this 12 mm Hg limit. Mandatory annual noninvasive examinations are necessary for aviators who are returned to active flying with aortic valve stenosis because the rate of progression of this lesion is unknown but is clearly capricious. SBE prophylaxis should be given. Entry into flight training for individuals with valvular heart disease is prohibited by the USAF, and exceptions made for mild lesions are reserved for those already trained to fly.

Aortic Valve Insufficiency

The most common cause of isolated aortic valve insufficiency is a congenitally bicuspid valve. It is extremely unusual to find isolated aortic insufficiency secondary to rheumatic heart disease. Other causes of aortic insufficiency are infections, trauma, and diseases that cause aortic root dilatation, such as Marfan syndrome.

Pathophysiologic Factors

Aortic valve insufficiency results in an increased volume load on the left ventricle. The resultant left ventricular dilatation produces increased myocardial wall stress, which stimulates an increase in left ventricular muscle mass. This increase in diastolic compliance accommodates a large volume of blood without an increase in the diastolic filling pressure. Aortic insufficiency is associated with wide pulse pressure. Ventricular ejection is quite rapid, decreasing wall tension during systole while maintaining a normal ejection fraction. The left ventricular stroke volume increases so as to maintain a normal net forward cardiac output, which is required to compensate for the regurgitant flow in aortic valve insufficiency. The amount of aortic regurgitation is dependent on the pressures in the aorta and left ventricle, peripheral resistance, and the duration of diastole. As compensatory mechanisms fail, ventricular failure results from elevation of left ventricular end-diastolic pressure and an increase in the time spent in systole by the left ventricle. Because the major portion of the coronary arterial blood flow occurs during diastole, the reduced time in diastole results in a discrepancy between left ventricular mass and myocardial oxygen demand. Angina pectoris is infrequent in pure aortic valve insufficiency, in contrast to patients with attendant aortic valve stenosis.

Physical Examination

With more than minimal aortic valve regurgitation, peripheral pulses are hyperdynamic and the carotid artery pulsation may have a bisferious quality. On palpation, the apical impulse is hyperdynamic, consistent with diastolic overload of the left ventricle. The typical diastolic murmur is best heard in the third left intercostal space at the left sternal border, with the patient learning forward during forced expiration. The murmur also may be heard in the primary aortic area, and it is not unusual for the murmur to transmit to the cardiac apex. Because the majority of cases of isolated aortic valve insufficiency are congenital in origin, an aortic valve ejection click is frequently audible. Because of the large stroke volume, an aortic ejection murmur most often is present, raising the possibility of associated aortic valve stenosis. The first heart sound may be decreased in intensity because of partial, premature closure of the mitral valve by the regurgitant flow into the left ventricle. The second heart sound maintains physiologic splitting until left ventricular failure ensues; paradoxic splitting may then occur. Aortic insufficiency commonly produces S_3 and S_4 gallops. An apical diastolic rumble in apparently pure aortic regurgitation is far more apt to represent an Austin Flint murmur (relative mitral valve stenosis) than anatomic mitral valve stenosis. Inhalation of amyl nitrite usually distinguishes the cause

of this diastolic rumble. Following amyl nitrite inhalation, increases in cardiac output, tachycardia, and a decrease in total peripheral resistance will increase the murmur of mitral valve stenosis, whereas the rumble associated with aortic valve insufficiency will decrease or disappear. Great care must be observed to avoid the administration of amyl nitrite to any patient with aortic valve stenosis.

Aeromedical Evaluation and Disposition

Complete, noninvasive cardiac evaluation must be accomplished. Chest radiography may demonstrate enlargement of the left ventricle and left atrium. The pulmonary vascular pattern is usually normal. ECG often demonstrates prominent QRS voltage due to the increased volume load placed on the left ventricle. Echocardiography is the noninvasive procedure of choice to detect chamber enlargement. Pulsed Doppler echocardiography with color flow mapping establishes the presence of aortic insufficiency and gives a reasonable quantification of the severity of the regurgitation. As ventricular muscle mass increases to handle the regurgitant load, coronary blood flow may be inadequate to prevent subclinical ischemia, even in the absence of obstructive coronary lesions Thus, abnormal thallium scintigrams in aortic regurgitation may not necessarily imply CAD.

Aortic insufficiency is acceptable for flying duties in hemodynamically insignificant and asymptomatic patients. Aortic insufficiency is well tolerated in a mild form for many years. In fact, the subclinical phase of this lesion extends throughout the active flying career of most military aviators. For flying recertification, no left ventricular hypertrophy should exist, and the angiographic grading of aortic valve insufficiency should be 2 + or less, with regurgitant fraction of 25% or less. The insufficiency should be due to a primary valvular abnormality. Aortic valve insufficiency secondary to aortic root disease is not waiverable for flying duties. Exercise capacity should be normal, with no significant exercise-induced arrhythmias. The lesion of aortic insufficiency is not usually a source of sudden incapacitation, and decrements in function are generally gradual and detectable. The USAF follows aviators with aortic insufficiency at one- to two-year intervals. Echocardiography and ejection fraction response to exercise with gated blood pool studies are the primary noninvasive procedures used for surveillance of this population. Progressive left ventricular dilatation and/ or a failure of the ejection fraction to increase appropriately with exercise (6% or greater increase) is grounds for disqualification, even if the aviator were asymptomatic. Flying waivers for aortic insufficiency have been limited to non-high-performance systems, based largely on theoretical considerations. A change in this restricted category waiver awaits more detailed hemodynamic data from primates in the $+G_z$ environment. Certainly, aviators with aortic valve insufficiency should not be retrained into high-performance aircraft. We do not recommend the selection of individuals with aortic insufficiency for initial aviation training.

Mitral Valve Insufficiency

Pathophysiologic Factors

Mitral regurgitation increases the volume load and dilates both the left atrium and left ventricle. Contractility is maintained by early, rapid decompression of the left ventricle. Forward cardiac output depends on the degree of mitral valve insufficiency and the total peripheral resistance. Effective forward cardiac output eventually decreases due to an increasing portion of the regurgitant stroke volume entering the left atrium. As the left atrium enlarges, mitral regurgitation begets more mitral regurgitation. Eventually, left ventricular failure occurs, further decreasing forward cardiac output.

It must be remembered that mitral insufficiency is a multifaceted disorder, which is best understood by considering all structures comprising the mitral valve apparatus. The mitral valve apparatus is a complex mechanism consisting of valve leaflets, chordae tendinae, papil-

lary muscles, mitral annulus, contiguous left ventricular wall, left atrial tissues, and the left ventricular outflow tract. Disease processes involving any of these structures may produce mitral valve insufficiency. Thus, one must make a decision as to whether the lesion is a primary leaflet abnormality or a more complex abnormality of the mitral valve apparatus.

Physical Examination

The left ventricular apical impulse is diffuse and hyperdynamic, consistent with a volume overload of the left ventricle. The typical murmur of chronic mitral valve insufficiency is a pansystolic, blowing murmur heard best at the cardiac apex in the left lateral decubitus position, transmitting well to the left axilla. The first heart sound may be decreased in intensity, whereas the second heart sound usually reveals exaggerated physiologic splitting due to rapid left ventricular decompression. The degree of mitral valve insufficiency may be assessed by listening carefully to early diastole in the left lateral decubitus position. The presence of an S_3 gallop in individuals over age 40 usually denotes moderate mitral regurgitation, whereas an S_3 gallop followed by a rumble usually indicates significant regurgitation. This should not be confused with an opening snap and rumble of true anatomic mitral valve stenosis. When diastole is quiet, the degree of regurgitation is usually mild.

Aeromedical Evaluation and Disposition

A complete, noninvasive evaluation is required. Echocardiography documents the presence and degree of regurgitation with Doppler color flow studies. Left heart catheterization, done for ischemic indications, may also document regurgitation. Exercise ejection fraction response to exercise should be documented serially with echocardiography or radionuclide ventriculogram. As in aortic regurgitation, certain practical and theoretical objections are raised to the exposure of aviators with mitral regurgitation to high $+G_z$ loads. The effect of repeated, marked increases in afterload during straining maneuvers could reasonably be expected to acutely and transiently increase mild preexisting mitral regurgitation. The effect of high-performance flying on the natural history of mild mitral regurgitation is unknown, but we believe that trained aviators with mitral regurgitation should not be placed into high-performance aircraft in our current state of knowledge. An aviator considered for return to a high-performance system should be evaluated with centrifuge stress to assess arrhythmic potentials. Cardiac catheterization should be performed to exclude coronary disease when suspected by noninvasive testing.

Aviators with mild valvular mitral regurgitation may be acceptable for flying duties when they are asymptomatic and regurgitation is not due to ruptured chordae tendinae, papillary muscle dysfunction, or left ventricular wall dysfunction. Further, no associated mitral valve stenosis, other valvular disease, left ventricular or left atrial enlargement, or arrhythmia can be present. Exercise capacity must be normal. Left ventricular end-diastolic pressure should be within the range of normal. Waivered aviators with mitral regurgitation must be evaluated annually. SBE prophylaxis is essential. Individuals with mitral regurgitation should not be enrolled in initial aviation training.

Mitral Valve Stenosis

Mitral valve stenosis is the most capricious of the valvular lesions and seldom occurs as an isolated finding. Because of the risk of sudden incapacitation from atrial tachyarrhythmias, thromboembolic events, and abrupt pulmonary venous hypertension, no degree of mitral valve stenosis is waiverable for aviation duties. For the same reasons, tricuspid stenosis is a nonwaiverable disorder.

Pulmonary Valve Stenosis

Pathophysiologic Factors

Congenital obstruction to right ventricular outflow can be valvular, subvalvular, or supra-valvular. Valvular pulmonary stenosis produces poststenotic dilatation of the main pulmonary artery and is often accompanied by dilatation of the left, but not the right, pulmonary artery. Valvular pulmonary stenosis commonly occurs as an isolated congenital anomaly. Rarely is the pulmonic valve bicuspid. Congenital valve stenosis is usually from the ring. Subvalvular and supravalvular pulmonary stenosis are uncommon as isolated anomalies and will not be discussed here. In pulmonary stenosis, the systolic gradient across the pulmonary valve produces increased right ventricular pressure. Pulmonary artery pressure may be normal or decreased, and concentric right ventricular hypertrophy may develop.

Physical Examination

The jugular venous pulse is normal in mild pulmonary stenosis, but with moderate-to-severe obstruction, a prominent a-wave is noted when the atrial septum is intact. A prominent v-wave and rapid descending y-wave occurs when associated tricuspid insufficiency is manifest. Precordial palpation may reveal a sustained and forceful left parasternal lift consistent with pressure overload of the right ventricle. Auscultation reveals a normal first heart sound. With mild pulmonary stenosis, the second heart sound reveals physiologic splitting and well-preserved pulmonic closure. A high-pitched, sharp ejection click is usually present and is heard best at the second through fourth left parasternal interspaces, loudest during expiration and decreasing during inspiration. This click is the only right-sided event that increases in intensity during expiration. A systolic ejection murmur, usually grade II to III/VI, is best heard at the second left intercostal space. The murmur usually increases in intensity during inspiration, is well transmitted to the left infraclavicular area, and may be heard in the left scapular region. A right ventricular S_4 gallop is not unusual. An S_3 gallop and murmur of tricuspid regurgitation may be present when right ventricular failure develops.

Aeromedical Evaluation and Disposition

Chest radiography may demonstrate an enlarged right ventricle, prominent pulmonary artery trunk, or dilated left pulmonary artery. The pulmonary vascular pattern is usually normal. ECG may demonstrate a pattern consistent with right ventricular hypertrophy. Echocardiography with color Doppler is usually sufficient when the valve can be well interrogated. Catheterization may be necessary in rare cases. Unlike aortic valve stenosis, pulmonic valve stenosis is usually not progressive, remains asymptomatic, and is well tolerated in moderate cases. Kruyer has suggested pulmonic valve stenosis waivers for asymptomatic patients with gradients under 20 mm Hg, no conduction abnormalities, no significant arrhythmias, and normal cardiac functions (60). Cardiovascular reevaluation at one-to two-year intervals is mandatory. Any evidence of increasing pulmonic stenosis, right ventricular dilatation and failure, or deterioration in any other noninvasive cardiac tests would render the aviator unfit for flying duties.

Other Congenital Lesions

In military aviation, congenital heart disease, even when corrected by surgery, is grounds for rejection upon application for flight training. Certain congenital lesions, however, when discovered in a trained aviator, may be waiverable for continued flying. Decisions regarding waiverability of specific lesions depend on the individual anatomy, method of repair, residual hemodynamic findings after repair, and the history of the postsurgical results (when available for a significant cohort of individuals followed closely for sequelae). In a trained aviator, successful closure of a secundum atrial septal defect without hemodynamic abnormalities or rhythm disturbances is sufficient for a return to flying status following a waiting period of six months. Completely normal cardiac function and successful repair should be documented by cardiac catheterization before a return to the cockpit is contemplated. Primum and sinus venosus defects are not waiverable after repair because of the high association of coexisting abnormalities. Ventricular septal defects which have been repaired are waiverable in trained aircrew, but not for flying training candidates in military aviation. Waiver criteria are essentially the same as for repaired atrial septal defect.

Although individuals with congenital heart disease, even when corrected by surgery, are unacceptable for military aviation training, increasing numbers of surgically treated adults with congenital heart disease are achieving such lifespans that their cases are no longer oddities in civilian aviation medicine practice. The Eighth Bethesda Conference (59) recommended that surgically treated atrial septal defect (secundum or sinus venosus), aortic coarctation, patent ductus arteriosus, tetralogy of Fallot, transposition of the great vessels, and ventricular septal defect are all potentially certifiable abnormalities following a minimum of one year's postoperative observation of the patient's clinical and hemodynamic state.

Bacterial Endocarditis Prophylaxis

All acquired and congenital lesions require bacterial endocarditis prophylaxis, irrespective of hemodynamic significance. The majority of the waiverable lesions discussed in the previous sections are mild and compatible with extended subclinical courses, during which the greatest risk is endocarditis. The risks begin to alter later in the course of the lesions as hemodynamic consequences occur, but the flight surgeon must ensure that the aviator is aware of the small, but definite, risk of endocarditis in asymptomatic valvular lesions. A program of prevention should include wallet cards and specific earmarking of dental and medical records, with special attention to allergic and idiosyncratic drug histories. Guidelines published by the American Heart Association or similar organizations should be followed with regard to prophylaxis.

Mitral Valve Prolapse

Mitral valve prolapse (MVP) is the most common valvular abnormality seen in the general population, occurring in approximately 5% of males and up to 10–12% of females. Prevalence figures for females vary widely, depending on selection factors. MVP may occur in a familial autosomal-dominant pattern with variable penetrance. MVP also occurs secondary to abnormalities, such as rheumatic heart disease, CAD, cardiomyopathy, and congenital heart disease.

Pathophysiologic Factors

In the common form of MVP, the spongiosa component of the valve proliferates, with acid mucopolysaccharide found in abnormal quantities. The pathologic changes in MVP are similar to those seen in Marfan syndrome and related connective-tissue disorders. Although increased spongiosa in the mitral leaflet occurs in apparently normal individuals of all ages, the changes are minor when compared with those of MVP. The term, myxomatous degeneration has been applied to this process, but little evidence supports a degenerative process. Secondary epithelial changes may initiate platelet-fibrin complexes, which may lead to embolization. Qualitative platelet abnormalities also have been found in MVP. It is unclear whether these coagulation phenomena are related to the abnormal valve or whether both are related to a common cause.

The leaflets in MVP are known to be thinned and voluminous. One or both leaflets bulge back into the left atrium during ventricular systole. It is believed that this prolapse places abnormal stress on the attached chordae tendinae and papillary muscles. Presumably, abnormal tension also is placed on the myocardium surrounding the papillary muscle. This ''ischemic theory'' of MVP may partially explain the ECG abnormalities, chest pain, thallium scintigraphic abnormalities, and arrhythmias.

Clinical Presentation

The majority of individuals with MVP are asymptomatic and never come under any medical surveillance. Chest pain, palpitations, fatigue, dyspnea, syncope, near-syncope, or symptoms of transient cerebral ischemia, however, may occur as an initial manifestation. Unfortunately, albeit rarely, MVP patients may experience catastrophic complications, including myocardial infarction, rupture of chordae tendinae, infective endocarditis, incapacitating chest pain, significant arrhythmias, or stroke. MVP is now recognized as a leading cause of strokes in patients younger than age 40. Although the risk of sudden death is still unsettled, patients with sudden death are reported to have MVP as the plausible cause. Disconcertingly, the subsets of patients with MVP at risk for catastrophic events have not been precisely identified. Data suggesting significant mitral regurgitation as a sudden death risk have been reported, and leaflet thickening was reported to be correlated with MVP complications. However, other studies found thickening to be a significant risk for endocarditis, surgical mitral valve disease, or severe regurgitation, but not for stroke or sudden death.

Physical Examination

The auscultatory hallmark of MVP is a midsystolic click, which may be associated with a late systolic murmur. The auscultatory findings vary with positional changes and pharmacologic interventions. A helpful way to view the dynamics in MVP is to observe that the mitral apparatus is functionally too large for the left ventricular cavity, and any maneuver or intervention that decreases cavity size will cause the valve to prolapse earlier in systole. Thus, the click and murmur will move toward the first heart sound. Any positional change or challenge that increases left ventricular cavity size will move the click and murmur later in systole, shortening the murmur. The intensity of the click and murmur depend on alterations in peripheral resistance. Figure 15.9 describes the effects of these interventions in MVP.

Other Findings

The resting ECG may reveal nonspecific ST-T-wave changes in the inferior and lateral leads.

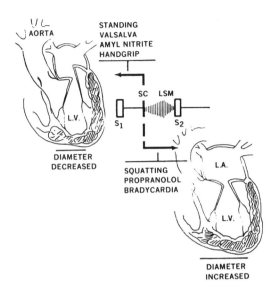

Figure 15.9. Effects of intervention on the click and murmur of mitral valve prolapse. (Reproduced with permission of Dr. Robert O'Rourke and the American Heart Association.)

Special attention must be paid to the QT interval because the prolonged QT syndrome is a recognized risk for sudden death in MVP, due to paroxysmal ventricular arrhythmias. Routine chest radiography usually demonstrates normal cardiac silhouette and pulmonary vascularity in the absence of significant mitral insufficiency. Thoracic skeletal anomalies, such as scoliosis, kyphosis, pectus abnormalities, and the straight back syndrome, also may be seen. A narrow anterioposterior chest diameter may compress the heart and increase the size of the cardiac silhouette in the posteroanterior view, mimicking cardiomegaly. MVP is a recognized cause of abnormal exercise tests in the absence of CAD. In one study, 25% of asymptomatic aviators with MVP had abnormal exercise ECGs (61). The suspicion of an ischemic mechanism in MVP has been strengthened by the observation of perfusion defects with thallium scintigraphy and normal coronary arteriograms. Abnormal responses to cardiovascular stress are especially remarkable, consistent with the observed autonomic lability found in this condition. Noncardiac presentations, such as neurop-

sychiatric symptoms, may be the initial manifestation in some patients with MVP.

Echocardiography

Two-dimensional echocardiography and M-mode echocardiography usually confirm the clinical diagnosis of MVP. An apparently normal echocardiogram, however, should not deter one from the diagnosis when the auscultatory findings are typical. In one series of MVP patients, using the midsystolic click as the "gold standard," echo sensitivity ranged from as low as 50% with M-mode alone, to 77% with M-mode combined with two-dimensional echo, to 93% with M-mode, 2D, and Doppler.

Inconstancy of Clinical Findings in MVP

It must be thoroughly appreciated that the auscultatory findings in MVP may be evanescent, often changing from examination to examination, largely due to volume status, but probably also due to the complex interplay of volume, autonomic tone, resistance, and contractility. Disputes over the presence or absence of MVP are often fueled by a lack of appreciation of the changeability of the findings. When competent observers recorded a click and/or a late systolic murmur, subsequent examiners may not hear the findings of MVP, and quite accurately record the absence of the auscultatory findings. However, this in no way negates the finding of previous examiners. The basic underlying physiology of prolapse accommodates such nonconcordance. On one day, one may hear the click and the murmur: on the next day, either one; and on a subsequent day neither. Such inconstancy also extends to the echocardiogram. Because of this phenomenon of evanescence, one who records a finding of MVP in an aircrew member should ask a colleague for confirmatory auscultation as immediately as possible.

Diagnosis of MVP

MVP may be diagnosed by the following:

1. Typical findings of a nonejection click with or without a late systolic murmur, which moves appropriately with maneuvers, or

2. 2 mm of late posterior motion or buckling behind the C-D line of the M-mode echocardiogram, or

3. 3 mm of holosystolic hammocking behind the C-D line on the M-mode echocardiogram, or

4. Systolic protrusion of either mitral leaflet into the left atrium beyond the mitral annulus on the 2-D parasternal long axis view only (the four-chambered view should not be used in MVP diagnosis).

The above criteria are currently in use in the USAF. In circumstances where the diagnosis is made from left ventricular cineangiography, leaflet protrusion posteriorly into the left atrium > 10 mm had a 100% specificity and a 75% sensitivity. When suspected mitral valve prolapse in the aircrew member is uncomplicated and no arrhythmias occur, it is not critical to separate possible or probable MVP from definite MVP in ''gray zone'' cases. However, when a disqualifying defect is present, such as ventricular tachycardia, the distinction becomes critical, because both diagnoses may be separately waiverable, but not both waiverable in the same aviator.

Aeromedical Considerations of Mitral Valve Prolapse

Most aviators with MVP are diagnosed incidentally during physical examinations. We believe that the healthy male aviator in whom MVP is discovered in the absence of chest pain, arrhythmias, or other symptoms represents the most benign end of the clinical spectrum of this disorder. Undoubtedly, some aviators with MVP are true normal variants with an excellent prognosis. Unfortunately, clinically identical subsets may experience sudden cardiac events. The current practitioner of aerospace medicine must recognize that the asymptomatic MVP subsets at risk for sudden events are not currently identifiable. The USAF is currently following over 400 aircrew MVP patients with serial clinical and noninvasive examinations in a long-term natural

history study. Waiver criteria currently utilized by the USAF include:

1. No ventricular tachycardia. Prospective results from the MVP study group revealed a 5.5% prevalence of ventricular tachycardia. A separate group of 193 ventricular tachycardia aircrew revealed 31 patients with MVP (16%). Of these 31, one died suddenly with no findings except MVP. A second MVP patient had recurrent presyncope attacks with recurrent polymorphic VT.

2. No SVT. In the MVP group, 8.5% had SVT. The USAF is currently considering waivers for nonsustained SVT and some cases of sustained SVT in the presence of MVP, but SVT and MVP in concert remain grounding as of this writing.

3. No significant chest pain.

4. No significant mitral regurgitation.

5. No evidence of a generalized myxomatous disorder, no aortic root disease, and no aortic valve disease.

6. No history of embolic events.

7. No history of syncope, except well-documented vasovagal syncope.

8. No history of endocarditis.

Aircrew members with MVP who fly high-performance systems should undergo centrifuge testing to screen for significant arrhythmias under $+ G_z$ acceleration.

Because of the small, but definite, excess risk for cerebrovascular events and arrhythmias, MVP should be disqualifying for entry into flying training. Not only are there usually well-qualified, alternative candidates, it seems unlikely that an MVP patient accepted for flying training will be maintained with no special surveillance. The USAF MVP study group revealed a 20% disqualification rate on the first MVP evaluation of trained aircrew, but an additional 15% cumulative grounding risk in follow-up examinations was also incurred. Thus, a normal initial evaluation for disqualifying cofactors in known MVP patients is no guarantee of future waiverability. The flying risks and the attendant cost of recurrent medical surveillance of MVP represent substantial barriers to the enrollment of candidates with MVP into costly aviation training.

While the risk of endocarditis is greater in those with murmurs than with clicks alone, it is difficult to adopt an endocarditis rule for aircrew in the face of the inconstancy of the murmur. Hence, we also recommend bacterial endocarditis prophylaxis for MVP patients with a click only.

ARTERIAL HYPERTENSION

Asymptomatic arterial hypertension increases tolerance to $+G_z$ acceleration, but this benefit is more than offset by the increased risk from stroke and CAD. Hypertension confers no benefit to the aviator flying nonaerobatic aircraft. Elevated BP, from any cause, raises the risk of aggravating preexistent cerebrovascular aneurysms and malformations. Acute elevations, such as practicing straining maneuvers without an opposing "G" field is unwise.

High BP should also be avoided to slow atherosclerosis. The lipid concentrations in veins and pulmonary arteries is the same as in systemic arteries, yet atherosclerosis is confined to the high-pressure vessels. This is not due to any difference in the intima. For example, when a vein becomes an arterial conduit, the vein develops atherosclerosis.

Although the concentrations of lipids are the same in all arteries, atherosclerosis is not uniform, developing at sites of turbulent flow. Just as with airflow over an airplane wing, turbulent flow increases the pressure on the intima compared to laminar flow. The atherosclerotic plaques themselves cause more turbulence, which accelerates atherosclerosis at that site. By lowering systemic BP, atherosclerosis should be slowed.

The definition of hypertension is both arbitrary and controversial. As people age, their BPs increase because they exercise less, gain weight, and their arteries become less compliant. This may be common, but it is not healthy. Arbitrary thresholds send the wrong message to those just below the cut point. A diastolic pressure below 90 torr may be defined as normal, but the risk of cardiovascular disease for someone with a diastolic pressure of 89 torr is about the same as someone at 91 torr. The risk of a diastolic pressure of 89 torr, however, is significantly more than for 60 torr (62). Waiting until a patient's BP exceeds some arbitrary threshold, such as the 95th percentile, before instituting lifestyle changes is to miss the opportunity to prevent atherosclerosis. Regular aerobic exercise, less sodium intake, and avoidance of android obesity should be prescribed for everyone to prevent hypertension and the vicious cycle of atherosclerosis from starting.

When is the risk from high BP too high to perform critical flying duties? Whatever rule is arbitrarily selected, it should allow for the marked day-to-day variation in BP. The following is a reasonable rule: If the average of ten measurements taken over five visits exceeds 140 torr systolic or 90 torr diastolic, then the flyer should be grounded until the five-day average is below this threshold and is at least 5 torr less than the pretreatment average. Some aeromedical services allow continued flying during a trial of nonpharmacologic therapy. A 5 torr reduction in diastolic BP lowers the risk of stroke by 42% and of coronary heart disease by 14% (62).

Methodology

Too often BP is measured improperly. The patient should be seated, awake, with less than five minutes rest. Conversation should be limited and bland. Pressure should be measured in both arms at each visit. The cuff bladder should completely encircle the arm. The cuff width should exceed the arm diameter. The examiner should have good hearing documented, preferably by an annual audiogram. The stethoscope ear pieces should fit inside the ear canal to make a seal. The examining room should be quiet. To increase agreement between observers, the disappearance of Karotkoff sounds should be used for diastolic pressure because muffling of Karotkoff sounds is more subjective. The cuff should be inflated to 20 torr above the expected systolic pressure, then deflated at a rate such that three beats are heard for each 10 torr drop in pressure. The first observation should be ignored if the original starting pressure were too low or the rate too fast. Before a measurement is repeated, the cuff should be fully deflated and the arm raised above the patient's heart to drain the venous pool. The pressure should be measured in the leg at least once if the average of arm pressures were elevated.

Some patients claim that their BPs are elevated only in the doctor's office. The actuarial and epidemiologic evidence for risk comes from measurements in doctors' offices. Even when the patient documents lower pressures at work or at home, the diagnosis of hypertension should be based on pressures measured in the doctor's office.

A search for secondary causes of hypertension should be limited to a careful history and inexpensive laboratory tests, such as urine analysis, fasting blood glucose, and serum potassium. Only when the pressures cannot be easily controlled should expensive or intrusive tests be pursued.

Treatment

Too often both the physician and patient fail to emphasize lifestyle changes because they control the BP by medication. For most mild hypertensive flyers, lifestyle changes should be the primary strategy. Prospective, controlled trials have shown that medication reduces the risk of stroke, but the effect on CAD has been less than expected by lifestyle changes. Aerobic exercise and weight control do more than lower BP: serum lipids improve and insulin is more effective. Even when they only partially control BP, lifestyle changes allow for pharmacologic treatment at a lower dose, which is less expensive and less prone to side effects.

Which medications are safe for flying? The following are criteria for selecting an antihypertensive medication for use in flyers:

1. Obtains control of five-day BP average;
2. Has no decrease in cognitive and motor performance with acceleration, heat, altitude, task saturation, and time-zone changes;
3. Has side effects that are:
   a. not sudden incapacitation,
   b. rare,
   c. predictable,
   d. treatable,
   e. found before the flyer is waivered.
4. Does not mask symptoms or signs of other diseases, such as β-blockers that hide cardiac ischemia;
5. Is long acting;
6. Does not require expensive or dangerous tests to detect side effects or performance decrements;
7. Has years of experience in other flyers;
8. Is low cost.

Thiazide diuretics meet all of these criteria, but remain controversial. We have over 25 years of favorable experience in thousands of flyers. The cost is two orders of magnitude less than agents still under patent like angiotensin converting (ACE) inhibitors. Diuretics decrease the incidence of stroke and CAD, but the reduction in CAD is less than expected from the decrease in BP (62). Factors, other than diuretics, account for much of this shortfall. Nevertheless, in some patients, thiazides increase insulin resistance, LDL and VLDL cholesterol, serum triglycerides, and uric acid. Many of these changes resolve after one year. Thiazides also decrease serum potassium in a few patients who then experience more ventricular ectopy.

Should thiazides be given to aviators? No drug is without side effects in all patients. Should aviators who can be controlled without side effects be denied a drug because others get side effects? If all side effects could be detected before returning to flying duty, then a drug would be potentially safe for flying in those without side effects. Use of a drug in an aviator necessitates a safe and effective response in the individual. Initially, aviators can be given a 30-day trial of a thiazide diuretic, starting at the lowest dose. Most patients do not require triamterene. If hypokalemia were found after a month of thiazide, then one should add triamterene only if the BP were controlled. One should switch to another drug, perhaps an indoline diuretic, or an ACE inhibitor if BP could not be controlled on a dose that causes hypokalemia. Even with triamterine added, a few patients on thiazides still lose potassium. Their thiazide and triamterene should be replaced with another drug. Only after exhausting all other drugs should potassium supplements be added to thiazide with triamterene. For all patients on diuretics, one should check serum potassium at least every six months.

To evaluate the effect of thiazides on risk factors requires a year of follow-up. This can be done while the aviator is on flying status if BP and serum potassium were normal. In all measurements of risk factors, considerable day-to-day variation occurs. Before committing aviators to lifetime regimens, they deserve at least a three-day pretreatment baseline of risk factors and a three-day follow-up started one year after the last increase in thiazide dose. When the all-risk factors for the median follow-up test are no worse than would be expected from day-to-day variation around the baseline median, then the drug should be safe for that individual.

β-Blockers hide CAD, the greatest medical risk for sudden incapacitation. Furthermore, β-blockers worsen risk factors for CAD.

In 1977, 32 USAF flyers were evaluated at the USAF Aeromedical Consultation Service before and after treatment with spironolactone and hydrochlorothiazide. Subsequent analysis found that this combination significantly increased cardiac irritability during exercise compared to hypertensive flyers treated with hydrochlorothiazide alone.

Indapamide is an indoline diuretic. It differs from thiazide diuretics in that it lacks a thiazide ring and has only one sulfonamide group; therefore, it should not be routinely waivered for use in flyers as an analogue of thiazides. Because it differs from thiazides, indapamide may be effective where thiazides have failed. Indapamide reportedly decreases peripheral resistance more than thiazides. The half-life of indapamide in blood is 14 hours. Unlike ACE inhibitors, the initial dose of 2.5 mg indapamide each morning is also the maximum dose; therefore, a trial at only one dose is sufficient to determine efficacy and side effects. Furthermore, indapamide has less hypercholesterolemia, less hypokalemia, less calcuria, more hyperuricemia, and similar hyperglycemia compared to thiazides. Hypokalemia occurs in 3% of patients; therefore, serum potassium should be checked as with thiazides. Indapamide is ten times more expensive than hydrochlorothiazide, but four times less expensive than the average dose to treat hypertension with an ACE inhibitor. A trial of indapamide should precede a trial of an ACE inhibitor because even if only 10% were controlled by indapamide, the cost saving over a lifetime would be substantial.

ACE inhibitors may meet the first six criteria for use in flyers. They have either no effect or favorable effect on risk factors for CAD. Their ability to prevent strokes and CAD awaits proof. Furthermore, ACE inhibitors are relatively new. Additional side effects may yet be discovered, especially in the flying environment. Because dizziness is the most common side effect, the one-month follow-up examination should test for decrements in equilibrium. Pregnant women and those trying to become pregnant should not take ACE inhibitors.

OTHER CARDIAC DISORDERS

Pericardial Disease

Resolved pericarditis is a waiverable abnormality for flying, and consideration for flying should not be made until six months after resolution of the acute attack. During this six-month observation, the etiology of pericarditis can be established with respect to serious underlying disease, such as autoimmune disorders, neoplastic disease, or chronic infections. Recurrence of acute viral pericarditis can also be detected during the observation. At the end of six months, the aviator should undergo echocardiography, treadmill exercise testing, and Holter monitoring. Unlimited flying status is recommended when myocardial function is normal, no residual effusion exists, and no significant arrhythmias occur. Evidence of constriction is disqualifying and usually nonwaiverable. Rare candidates with no arrhythmias, residual myocardial dysfunction, or myocardial scarring could conceivably be returned to flying after stripping of the pericardium for constriction. Lengthy postsurgical observation, at least one year in duration, is needed. All candidates considered for return to flying after any pericardial disease must be carefully investigated for the most common aeromedically-significant complication—atrial arrhythmias. High-performance pilots should be evaluated with monitored centrifuge stress before being returned to fighter aircraft. Waivered patients with pericarditis should be regularly reexamined.

Pericardial tumors, cysts, and involvement of the pericardium by neoplastic disease are all nonwaiverable.

Myocardial Disease

The list of primary cardiomyopathies is extensive and growing, with multiple etiologic, genetic, and functional categories. Cardiomyopathies carry risks of arrhythmias, sudden death, ischemia, thromboembolism, and global left ventricular dysfunction. Cardiomyopathies are nonwaiverable for any class of flying.

Viral myocarditis is potentially waiverable following six months of observation beyond the clinical resolution of acute illness. Recrudescence of myocarditis, low-grade smoldering

myocarditis, or clinically overt recurrences may all be detected during follow-up. ECG abnormalities, especially with concomitant pericarditis, are frequent. The acute phase of the illness should include acute serologic studies and nonexercise, noninvasive tests. Resting the myocardium is a significant therapeutic factor in myocarditis. Every effort should be made to avoid any exercise testing of the inflamed myocardium. At the six-month mark, waiver may be considered when all inflammatory indices are normal, regional and global left ventricular function is normal (both at rest and with exercise), and no arrhythmias are detected. Fliers waivered with past myocarditis must be periodically evaluated for several years, in order to detect recurrences or chronic inflammation.

On rare occasion, an aviator may be admitted to the hospital with chest pain and ECG changes suggestive of ischemia. A small CPK-MB increase may lead to the diagnosis of myocardial necrosis and grounding for presumed ischemic disease. Myo/pericarditis may also be accompanied by small enzyme elevations. Such cases are difficult to unravel later, even with normal coronaries because infarction is not ruled out by normal coronaries. A meticulous clinical history, a high index of suspicion for pericarditis in relatively young aircrew, and full, early noninvasive tests are critical.

Athletic Heart

The aircrew population usually includes aerobically fit individuals, and a small number who are extraordinarily fit. Voluminous studies have been compiled on such patients. Athletic heart is a normal variant, usually detected because of some combination of marked bradycardia, ventricular gallops, high ECG voltage with or without ST changes, enlarged cardiac silhouette, LVH, chamber enlargement, ejection murmurs, and Wenckebach phenomena. Significant arrhythmias are uncommon, but a wide variety of vagally-related arrhythmias are often investigated. Diastolic gallops, associated with the long diastolic filling period, are common. Noninvasive examination usually reveals increased left and right heart internal dimensions, and not uncommonly, mild-to-moderate LVH. Ventricular function is normal or above normal. Aircrew with left ventricular hypertrophy in a setting that suggests athletic heart, should be withdrawn from exercise and the echocardiogram repeated after two to three months of abstinence from exercise. Athletic heart is a normal variant. Abnormal noninvasives, ventricular gallops, and cardiomegaly in a nonexerciser should be viewed as pathologic and thoroughly investigated for organic causes.

Myocardial Sarcoidosis

Sarcoidosis is generally considered a benign and self-limiting disorder of young adults, although it requires special attention in aviators. A small percentage of patients (5–10%) will progress to serious pulmonary disability.

A more insidious clinical complication of sarcoidosis results from myocardial involvement. Autopsy studies revealed a prevalence of myocardial sarcoidosis that is 8–27% of all patients with sarcoidosis. The diagnosis of myocardial sarcoidosis is difficult and rarely made during life, even in cases of extreme involvement. A major difficulty in the diagnosis of myocardial sarcoidosis is the poor correlation of cardiac lesions with overt pulmonary involvement. In fact, some patients with symptomatic involvement of other organs may be less likely to have significant myocardial involvement. It is clear that patients with myocardial sarcoidosis generally have little or no clinical evidence of the disease in organs other than the heart. Because such patients are usually diagnosed only at autopsy, the time course between the initial onset and resolution of pulmonary findings and the appearance of myocardial granulomas is impossible to determine. Although some patients have died with massive myocardial involvement within months of the appearance of hilar adenopathy, this complication may develop years after the initial onset of disease.

A serious hazard to flying safety is caused by the sudden, catastrophic presentation of patients with myocardial sarcoidosis. A review of 113 necropsy patients with myocardial sarcoidosis revealed that 89 patients (79%) had cardiac dysfunction secondary to sarcoid involvement (63). Of these 89 patients, 60 (67%) died suddenly, presumably from arrhythmias. Of these 60 patients, sudden death was the initial manifestation of sarcoidosis in 10 individuals (17%). Several other reports confirmed the malignant nature of myocardial involvement. Cardiac abnormalities may be caused by active or healed granulomas. Such lesions may produce ventricular aneurysms, pericardial disease, conduction disturbances, and significant atrial and ventricular arrhythmias.

As concern about myocardial sarcoid surfaced, the USAF instituted a centralized evaluation of all aviator cases of myocardial sarcoid, beginning in 1978 (64). All cases of sarcoid were serially evaluated with clinical examinations and full, cardiac, noninvasive examinations, including thallium scintigraphy. A thorough eye examination, serum angiotensin-converting enzyme, and skin tests for PPD, mumps, and monilia were obtained. Initially, all aviators with sarcoid were grounded for two years and reevaluated at that time. By 1984, favorable follow-up led to a one-year grounding. By 1991, 82 aviators were followed up with a mean of three evaluations per patient. The mean clinical follow-up of six years was obtained in 75% of patients and a 100% 8.9 year mean follow-up was completed by telephone. Sixty-five percent of the aircrew were discovered on routine chest radiography; 35% were discovered due to symptoms. No sarcoid-related deaths occurred. Eleven of the initial 82 were grounded: one for syncope with VT and SVT, one for a fixed thallium defect, three for arrhythmias alone, one for neurosarcoid, one with active pulmonary sarcoid, and four with CAD. Of the 71 who were waivered to fly, 12 were grounded in follow-up for active sarcoid (four), arrhythmias (two), fixed thallium defect (one), and CAD or findings of CAD (five). The study group then had findings that would have been suggestive of myocardial involvement (four with arrhythmias and two with fixed thallium defects). Another 7.3% (six patients) had noncardiac sarcoid complications (one neurosarcoid, five pulmonary). Thus, the natural history of sarcoid, in terms of the development of myocardial sarcoid, was more favorable than expected. Those waivered experienced no incapacitating events. Although available technology may be inadequate to detect myocardial granuloma, clinical follow-up was encouraging enough for the USAF to revise the sarcoid waiver rules:

1. Aircrew may be evaluated locally with chest radiography, ACE level, chemistries, pulmonary function tests, and Holter monitors.
2. Waiver when local evaluation is normal, patient is asymptomatic, chest radiography is normal (or stable), and no evidence of other organ involvement exists.

Long-term follow-up of this cohort continues, but the first 12 years of the study were encouraging.

SUMMARY

Present aeromedical certification standards regarding cardiovascular disease, both military and civilian, reflect changes that are largely the result of natural history observations and rapid advancements in cardiovascular diagnosis. Nevertheless, the poor specificity of most diagnostic tests in a healthy population continue to be a difficult problem. Efforts to correct poor specificity usually have resulted in a loss of sensitivity. Poor specificity imposes additional expense, inconvenience, and occasional diagnostic risk on those who are screened for subclinical disease. Poor sensitivity, however, poses an even greater potential threat in aerospace medicine because aviators with significant disease

entities may be returned to the cockpit. Future aircrew screening for CAD must begin with some risk stratification before expensive and burdensome second-order tests are applied. The major challenge in aerospace cardiology is to accurately define the natural history of a host of abnormal tests and cardiovascular findings in the apparently healthy aviator. Such long-term studies should allow one to structure certification standards tailored to a variety of aviation categories. Epidemiologic studies should reveal disease subsets at the greatest risk of incapacitation, the poorest candidates for expensive aviation training, and define the serial cardiovascular tests that would be most useful. Careful natural history studies should benefit all certifying agencies because each agency can then clearly address selection and recertification criteria based on the demands of particular aerospace systems. Some asymptomatic cardiovascular findings may prove to be as unacceptable for high-performance jet flying as they are for recreational light-aircraft flying. If the aerospace medicine community is to serve the aviator best, we must pursue a data base that allows the widest latitude in aeromedical decision-making.

RESPIRATORY DISEASE IN AIRCREW

Respiratory diseases are of concern in the aviation environment for a number reasons. Some diseases (e.g., asthma or pneumothorax) may cause incapacitation and impact directly on flight safety. Diseases that adversely affect gas exchange by increasing ventilation-perfusion mismatch may aggravate mild hypoxia, causing more serious hypoxic symptoms with performance degradation. Minor effects of hypoxia on performance can be demonstrated, even at cabin altitudes of commercial aircraft; by impairing gas exchange on the cusp of the oxyhemoglobin dissociation curve, respiratory disease may produce more profound hypoxia. Smoking produces significant levels of carbon monoxide and may further aggravate hypoxia.

Intercurrent respiratory symptoms caused by atopy or infections are a major cause of temporary loss of flying status in aircrew. Candidates for flying training or aircrew employment should be carefully screened to identify individuals with a predilection for respiratory disease.

Screening Aircrew for Respiratory Disease

History/Examination

Chronic respiratory disease in adults often follows recurrent symptoms in childhood. Aircrew applicants should be screened for a history of childhood respiratory symptoms, including frequent coughs or infections requiring antibiotics, use of inhaled or oral bronchodilators, symptoms of hay fever, allergic rhinitis and eczema, recurrent sinusitis, and time off from school for respiratory problems. A family history of atopy and respiratory disease should be sought, as well as parental smoking history, which predisposes to childhood and adult respiratory disease. A personal smoking history should be obtained at selection and on each periodic medical examination.

Trained aircrew should be screened regularly for symptoms of respiratory disease, including frequent or persistent cough, wheeziness, or variable dyspnea on exertion.

Physical findings are generally minimal, but signs of atopic disease may be present with rhinitis (pale, boggy nasal mucosa), atopic faces, or eczema. Any wheezing detected on clinical examination should prompt further evaluation of airway reactivity.

Pulmonary Function Testing

Pulmonary function screening tests for small airway dysfunction include standard indices derived from maximum expiratory volume-time curves and flow-volume curves (65). Volume-time indices include forced vital capacity (FVC), forced expiratory volume in the first second (FEV1), and FEV1/FVC ratio; flow-volume analyses provide the FVC, maximum flow at 50% and 75% vital capacity (MEF50 and MEF75).

A modification of the flow-volume method to increase sensitivity for small airway dysfunction is the heliox test, which compares the MEF50 on air and after breathing a mixture of 80% helium with 20% oxygen for two minutes. In normal individuals, the majority of resistance to airflow is in large central airways where flow is turbulent and density-dependent; MEF50 increases by at least 20% in normal individuals after breathing the heliox mixture for three minutes. Flow in small airways is laminar and not density-dependent. Individuals with early, small airway disease fail to show a 20% increase in MEF50 with heliox.

The single-breath nitrogen washout test provides another assessment of small airway dysfunction through the closing volume, closing capacity, and slope of phase III (alveolar plateau). The closing volume represents the volume of gas expired after airway closure has occurred in dependent lung zones and is increased in small airway disease. The slope of the alveolar plateau is indicative of the homogeneity of gas mixing in the lungs; an increased slope indicates inhomogeneity due to small airway disease.

Individuals with a history of wheezing or asthma should be screened for bronchial hyperreactivity. The finding of an increase in MEF50 or MEF75 of 20% or greater after bronchodilator indicates increased bronchomotor tone consistent with asthma. Bronchial provocation tests (BPT) with methacholine or histamine have been standardized and provide an objective assessment of airway reactivity (66). Aircrew applicants with a history suggesting asthma even in childhood or who have significant atopy should be further assessed with a bronchial provocation test. Methacholine sensitivity is defined as the percent concentration that produces a 20% decrease in FEV1 below baseline denoted PC20. In general, the individual with a PC20 < 4 mg/ml has a strong probability of having asthma.

Chest Radiography

Chest radiography for occupational screening is increasingly uncommon, mainly because of the low yield of abnormal findings, but most aeromedical agencies still require chest radiography as part of the initial medical examination for flying fitness. Developmental skeletal abnormalities, mostly trivial but sometimes important (kyphoscoliosis) and cardiovascular disorders (coarctation and other forms of coronary heart disease: CHD) are additional reasons for routine radiography. Bronchopulmonary abnormalities include single or multiple opacities, sometimes calcified, cysts, bullae, basal shadows (bronchiectasis, sequestration), apical infiltration, or hilar enlargement. Although a few (healed varicella) of these abnormalities are acceptable in the presence of normal respiratory function, most require detailed investigation and specialist advice on fitness for selection. Many minor, healed, or nonprogressive conditions that have no effect on respiratory function are compatible with acceptance for a private pilot's licence (PPL). Because of the stresses of military flying, the great cost of flying training, and the career expectations of both military and professional civil aviation, few candidates with respiratory diagnoses are acceptable for these occupations.

Ventilation, Perfusion, Gas Exchange, and +Gz

Lung function is significantly affected by gravitational forces (67). Both ventilation and perfusion distribution are markedly gravity-dependent. Even under normal +1G conditions, matching of ventilation and perfusion and, hence, gas exchange is less than ideal.

Gravitational forces distort lung architecture with the elastic lung being stretched at the apices and compressed at the bases. Because of the weight of the lung within the thoracic cavity, the pleural pressure increases down the gravitational gradient so that different parts of the lung operate on different portions of the pressure-volume curve, creating regional differences in ventilation distribution. The result is that under normal +1Gz conditions through most of the vital capacity range, dependent lung regions operate on the steeper part of the pressure-volume curve and are better ventilated. An exception to this occurs at low lung volumes when airway closure occurs in dependent lung regions and the ventilation gradient is reversed.

Partly because of the relatively low pressures in the right ventricle and pulmonary circulation, lung blood flow is likewise affected by gravity with perfusion increasing down the gravitational gradient. Increasing gravitational forces directs blood flow progressively to lower lung zones.

Under normal circumstances in dependent regions perfusion exceeds ventilation creating venous admixture and arterial desaturation. In superior regions, ventilation exceeds perfusion contributing to wasted ventilation or alveolar dead space.

Increased gravitational-inertial forces greatly magnify and distort these regional differences. At +5Gz airways at the base of the lung are closed and lung apices are at the flat top portion of the pressure volume curve and receive little ventilation. Most ventilation takes place in central segments at the hilar area. Lung perfusion, conversely, primarily flows through the lung bases where airways are mostly closed, which results in greatly increased venous admixture and increasing arterial desaturation (See Chapter 9).

Lung architecture and function are increasingly stressed and distorted with progressive gravitational-inertial forces and may well prove to be the limiting factor in human tolerance in this environment (68).

Acceleration atelectasis occurs in fighter aircrew who breathe high inspired concentrations of oxygen while engaging in sustained high G maneuvers, such as air combat. The increased gravitational forces induce airway closure at lung bases and the oxygen is rapidly absorbed from air spaces distal to the closed airways producing atelectasis. G-suit inflation is a contributing factor by causing a central shift of blood promoting small airway closure. Symptoms include cough, chest tightness, and a dyspneic sensation. Chest radiography shows atelectasis at lung base(s). Aircrew should not be returned to flying duty until resolution is complete, usually over two to three days.

Diseases that cause small airway dysfunction, such as reactive airway disease or early chronic obstructive pulmonary disease, may be expected to accentuate regional inequalities related to increasing gravitational-inertial forces and predispose to acceleration atelectasis.

Asthma in Aircrew

Asthma is characterized by airway inflammation and increased bronchial reactivity. Reactive airway disease and bronchial hyperreactivity are also used to describe asthmatic individuals, although bronchial hyperresponsiveness should not be considered synonymous with asthma; not all individuals with bronchial hyperresponsiveness have or ever will have asthma. Symptoms of asthma are characteristically variable and include wheezing, variable dyspnea, a sensation of chest tightness and cough. The latter may be the prominent symptom of asthma.

Recently, the primary role of the inflammatory response in asthma has been more clearly defined, with bronchospasm and wheezing occurring as a result of the inflammation (69). Treatment directed towards reducing the inflammation is considered a key element in control of asthma. The asthmatic response (inflammation/bronchospasm) can be triggered by a variety of different stimuli as outlined in Table 15.9.

Table 15.9.
Triggers of Asthmatic Response

- Allergens
- Occupational sensitizers
- Respiratory infections
- Additives—food, beverages
- Drugs—β-blockers, NSAIDs
- Cigarette smoke
- GI reflux
- Exercise
- Cold air
- Air pollution
- Emotional stress

An asthmatic individual exposed to an environmental trigger frequently shows a dual-phase response: an immediate bronchoconstrictor response followed several hours later by an asthmatic response. The delayed response is characterized by bronchial inflammation and is less responsive to bronchodilator therapy, which may be an important consideration in aircrew.

Epidemiology/Natural History

Asthma occurs in about 5% of the general population. The incidence and severity of asthma are rising in most developed countries, and, of particular concern, mortality is increasing despite, and possibly because of, increasing use of antiasthmatic medications. Evidence is accumulating that the increasing death rate may be due to increased use of β-agonists that may adversely affect the function of mast cells in modulating the late asthmatic response.

Although childhood asthma may remit in adulthood, this is far from being universal. Natural history studies have demonstrated that almost half of children with even mild asthmatic symptoms have further wheezing episodes later in life; the probability is higher for children with more frequent or severe childhood asthma. This information is of particular concern in selecting applicants for aircrew because many asthmatics may be completely asymptomatic and have a normal examination between episodes.

Asthma has a wide spectrum of severity, from mild, intermittent symptoms requiring only infrequent inhaled bronchodilators to chronic, severe symptoms requiring daily inhaled and systemic medications. One of the challenges for aviation medicine practitioners is to accurately assess the severity of asthma in trained aircrew to facilitate a rationale for aeromedical disposition.

Aeromedical Concerns

Asthma is of concern in the aviation environment for a number of reasons, which are detailed

Table 15.10.
Aeromedical Concerns

- Acute incapacitation due to bronchospasm
- Performance degradation due to mild bronchospasm, hypoxia
- Side-effects of medications
- Lung rupture with rapid cabin depressurization
                    Military Aircrew
- Acceleration atelectasis in fast jet aircrew
- Inability to wear protective equipment for extended periods

in Table 15.10. Acute bronchospasm on the flight deck may be acutely incapacitating or, if mild, impair performance through distraction or by causing mild hypoxia. Medications, including inhaled β-agonists, may produce undesirable side effects. In fast jet aircrew, asthma may destabilize small airways predisposing these people to acceleration atelectasis and increasing ventilation-perfusion mismatch and hypoxia. Asthmatic symptoms in military aircrew may seriously limit their capacity to wear protective equipment, such as chemical defense ensembles. The possibility of a pulmonary overpressure event with lung rupture in the event of rapid cabin depressurization or during aeromedical training is an additional concern.

Screening Aircrew Candidates for Asthma

Because of the capricious nature of asthma, which may require removal from flying duties, and the high cost of training aircrew, it is important to select out candidates with asthma. Although the history is important, previous symptoms of wheezing may be unintentionally or deliberately omitted by candidates. It may be helpful to obtain a signed questionnaire inquiring about previous wheezing or persistent respiratory symptoms in childhood, including cough, about other atopic symptoms, such as hay fever or eczema symptoms, and about a familial history of atopy or asthma.

A multiple-antigen radio-immunoassay (RAST) test may be helpful in identifying individuals with significant atopy who then may be further investigated for bronchial hyperreactiv-

ity. One commercially available kit has been tested and found to have a sensitivity of 98% and a specificity of 77%. Some aeromedical agencies reject outright any candidate with a history of childhood asthma; the recurrence of asthmatic symptoms in about half of such individuals later in life supports such a standard. In many countries, further evaluation and demonstration of pulmonary dysfunction or bronchial hyperresponsiveness may also be required.

Routine spirometry may show mild expiratory airflow limitation but may well be normal in mild asthmatics during symptom-free intervals. An increase in flow rates of 20% or greater after bronchodilator inhalation even with normal baseline flow rates is highly suggestive of increased bronchomotor tone. Lung volume measurements may show hyperinflation with increased functional residual capacity; the diffusing capacity may be increased.

Airway reactivity can be objectively assessed by means of a bronchial provocation test with methacholine or histamine. These tests have been standardized and provide an objective measure of the individual's airway reactivity at that time. However, airway reactivity varies depending on a number of factors, and normal airway reactivity on bronchial provocation testing does not preclude the possibility of future asthma (false-negative tests). Viral respiratory infections increase bronchial reactivity and may produce false-positive tests.

Final disposition requires an overall assessment of the clinical history and objective testing of atopy and pulmonary function, including bronchial provocation.

Asthma in Trained Aircrew

The diagnosis of "asthma" in an experienced aircrew is generally alarming to aeromedical authorities and presents a challenge to aeromedical clinicians to quantify the severity of the asthma accurately. Accurate information as to triggering stimuli and treatment requirements, including whether ER treatment was required, must be obtained. Investigations, including objective assessment of atopy (skin prick testing or RAST), airway function through pulmonary function tests, and reactivity to bronchial challenge, are important in the overall assessment. Generally, it is difficult to develop a clear picture of the severity of reactive airway disease on an initial assessment, and a final disposition should be delayed for at least six months. In general, aircrew should be grounded during this period of observation.

Treatment

Treatment should be aimed at removing or avoiding any provoking environmental stimuli such as pets, feather/down clothing or bedding or other irritants identified by skin prick testing or RAST. Smoking cessation is a top priority for aircrew who develop asthmatic symptoms; airway reactivity will decrease with smoking cessation and may return to normal.

Pharmacologic treatment should be aimed at aggressively reducing and controlling inflammation with inhaled steroids and cromolyn sodium. The side effects of these classes of inhaled medications are minimal and are not of aeromedical concern, although high doses of high-potency, inhaled steroids may suppress the hypothalamic-pituitary-adrenal axis. Cromolyn can reduce both the immediate and delayed asthmatic response, while inhaled steroids are effective only against the late asthmatic response.

Inhaled β-agonists produce adrenergic side effects and generally are not approved for flight deck aircrew. Requirement for acute bronchodilator treatment suggests a degree of airway reactivity unacceptable in flight deck aircrew.

Systemic medications, including theophylline, steroids, or β-agonists, are generally not compatible with flying duties.

Aeromedical Disposition

On initial presentation of asthmatic symptoms, aircrew should be grounded while investigations are carried out, treatment initiated, and a sufficient period of time for observation allowed, generally several months. Aircrew with mild asthma that can be controlled with inhaled steroids or cromolyn with normal pulmonary function and normal or mildly increased airway reactivity on bronchial provocation testing while on these medications generally may be safely returned to flying. Occasional use of an inhaled β-agonist (e.g., salbutamol) as the only treatment may also be acceptable provided airway reactivity is normal or near-normal. An exception is in military fighter operations where small airway instability promotes ventilation-perfusion mismatch and acceleration atelectasis.

Chronic Obstructive Pulmonary Disease

Chronic obstructive pulmonary disease (COPD) remains a common cause of illness and death in many Western countries and is an increasing problem in developing nations. In the United States, COPD is the fifth most common cause of death, accounting for 57,000 deaths annually. In Europe, chronic bronchitis became known as the "British disease" and despite a slowly declining incidence, still causes 15,000 deaths per year in the United Kingdom; 10% of all illness-related absence is due to COPD. Even in countries with severe industrial atmospheric pollution and poor social conditions, tobacco smoking, especially of cigarettes, is responsible for most COPD. In the United States, more than four of five deaths from COPD are attributable to cigarette smoking. British doctors who smoked an average of a pack of cigarettes daily were 25 times more likely to die of COPD than their nonsmoking colleagues.

For these and other reasons, tobacco smoking is now strongly discouraged by air force and civilian aviation authorities. Some airlines recruit exclusively from nonsmokers, a policy which, although economically sound, may encourage concealment and be attacked as discriminatory. In many countries, cigarette smoking is in decline, especially in young people with university qualifications who are highly represented among aircrew candidates. Unfortunately, young women, who are increasingly recruited to both

military and civil flying, have not reduced cigarette smoking. More women may now smoke
and be less likely to quit than are men. Cigarette
marketing in many developing countries is both
aggressive and successful. It is likely, therefore,
that cigarette-related diseases common in Western countries will increase in aircrew from developing nations.

Clinically evident COPD is, fortunately, rare
among aircrew. Early, small airway disease may
be detected in high-risk patients (i.e., smokers)
with pulmonary function testing as described
earlier.

Chronic bronchitis and emphysema are two
disease states most often associated with COPD.
Chronic bronchitis is defined as the production
of mucoid sputum on most days for at least three
months during two consecutive years. However,
many cigarette-smoking aircrew are little incon-
venienced by these seemingly minor symptoms,
which they may ignore or attribute to catarrh or
allergy. Emphysema, defined pathologically as
a permanent, abnormal enlargement of the air
spaces (acini) distal to the terminal bronchioles,
is rarely apparent in its early stages. Exertional
dyspnea, the cardinal symptom, is often attributed initially to overweight or general lack of
physical fitness. Dyspnea sufficient to interfere
with daily activities indicates advanced disease,
which rarely occurs in aircrew. Similarly, abnormal physical signs (barrel chest, reduced air
entry, reduced cardiac and hepatic dullness to
percussion) and radiologic abnormalities (narrow mediastinum, flattened diaphragm, transra-
diant lung fields and cysts) are features of late
disease.

The effect of COPD, however mild, is increased by the conditions of flight. Even in mild
disease, cough may be distracting or interfere
with voice communication, thus prejudicing
flying safety particularly at the critical stages of
taxiing, take-off, approach, and landing. Rarely,
cough syncope may cause complete incapacity.
Impaired ventilation of parts of the lung, causing
ventilation-perfusion mismatch, may be of little
consequence at sea level but cause appreciable

hypoxemia at altitude. The exaggerated consequences of sudden decompression could tip the
balance against successful recovery of the aircraft in an emergency. A cigarette smoker, even
without lung disease, is disadvantaged by the up
to 10% of circulating hemoglobin being bound
as carboxyhemoglobin and unavailable for oxygen transport. Smokers are more prone than nonsmokers to acute respiratory infections and are
more likely to fly while requiring medication.
Smokers are prone to many other diseases, some
of which (e.g., CAD) are direct threats to flying
safety. Heavy smokers run a greater risk of accidents and injury.

The educational background of most candidates for aircrew selection ensures that only a
minority will be smokers; selection policy may
reduce the proportion further. The health value
of persuading trained aircrew to quit smoking
cannot be exaggerated. Measures may include
education, persuasion, peer and family pressure,
smoking cessation clinics (group therapy), nicotine chewing gum or transdermal patches, fiscal
(tax), and legislative measures (smoking confined to designated areas or banned in public and
on airplanes).

Aircrew with symptoms or signs of COPD or
with abnormal spirometry require further investigation, including, when possible, the single-
breath nitrogen test, which is sensitive in the
detection of small airway disease (increased
closing volume), and the Heliox test, in which
inhalation of a low-density gas mixture (oxygen
and helium) confirms that ventilatory obstruction is due to small airway narrowing. Exercise
testing, when possible with oximetry, or measuring blood gases in an altitude chamber, may
show abnormal desaturation. In mild or early
cases, particularly in heavy smokers, remarkable
improvement may be seen with smoking cessation, best combined with general health measures, such as a daily aerobic exercise program
and weight reduction. Under these circumstances, aircrew with mild, early disease may be
able to return to unrestricted flying duties subject
to specialist review. Well-established COPD

rarely shows appreciable improvement, and remorseless deterioration in respiratory function at a greater than physiologic rate is the rule. Permanent grounding is usually necessary.

Spontaneous Pneumothorax, Cysts and Bullae

Spontaneous pneumothorax is defined as the presence of air in the pleural cavity without apparent cause. Underlying pulmonary disease (e.g., cancer or tuberculosis) may cause a spontaneous pneumothorax, but most cases in aircrew show no such cause. Most victims are tall, thin, healthy young men who present with the sudden onset of lateralized chest pain, often pleuritic. Simultaneous bilateral pneumothoraces (2.5% of all patients), hemothorax, and tension pneumothorax—all of which are life-threatening complications—fortunately are rare.

The incidence of spontaneous pneumothorax is 4.7 per 100,000 per year, but concentration of cases among healthy young men means that a disproportionately higher frequency occurs in the aircrew population. The effects of altitude are adverse; the volume of the pneumothorax increases in accordance with Boyle's law. Documented patients with spontaneous pneumothorax in flight (70) or in altitude chambers (71) suggest that decreased ambient pressure may precipitate an attack in a predisposed individual.

The underlying lesion is usually a subpleural bleb, commonly at the lung apex, that ruptures and allows the negative intrathoracic pressure to suck air into the pleural space. Though the defect is usually small and heals spontaneously, recurrence is common; the risk increases from 30% after a first attack to 80% after a third attack. Most recurrences occur within two years of the preceding episode, but a few occur much later. Standard methods of treatment for the acute illness appear not to affect the chances of recurrence.

Because of this risk, candidates for flying training who give a history of spontaneous pneumothorax, however remote, are rejected by some

air forces. Elsewhere, an arbitrary period of freedom from recurrence is required for selection. Trained aircrew who suffer a spontaneous pneumothorax must be grounded. A long period (two years) of observation on the ground is rarely acceptable. Pleurodesis, with talc or silver nitrate solution, causes appreciable disability and may fail to prevent recurrence. Thoracotomy with excision or oversewing of pulmonary blebs with as complete as possible stripping of the parietal pleura is surprisingly well tolerated and gives excellent long-term results. Most aircrew so treated can return to flying duties within three months and require no specialist follow-up. Rarely, a bilateral procedure is required. Recently, thoracoscopy with local surgery to the apices has been reported but long-term results are unknown.

Cysts and bullae are circumscribed single or multiple air-filled spaces within the lungs. By convention, any such lesion may be called a cyst, while the term ''bulla'' refers to a clear space one centimeter or more in diameter, surrounded radiologically by a fine hairline border. Though numerous etiologies exist, most lesions in aircrew are single, unilateral bullae detected on routine radiography. A few patients have early emphysema, but most have no apparent lung or other disease. The importance of the lesion depends on whether it communicates with the bronchial airways, in which case ascent to altitude causes no problems, or whether it is closed, in which case it will expand and may cause pain or even rupture in flight with potentially disastrous results (pneumothorax or interstitial emphysema). It may be possible to establish radiologically that a cyst or bulla does not enlarge during a chamber ride. When any doubt exists, it is safer to proceed to surgical excision. Surgery may be required for any lesion that shows progressive enlargement on successive radiographs. A few patients with medium-sized bullae have significantly impaired respiratory function, raising fears of generalized COPD, but regain completely normal function after surgery.

Surgical excision may be required to establish

a definite tissue diagnosis of some cysts. Cavities remaining after successful drug treatment of pulmonary tuberculosis are best excised, for the reasons given above and also because apparently viable tubercle bacilli are often detected by microscopy in such supposedly healed lesions.

Sarcoidosis

Sarcoidosis is a granulomatous disease of uncertain etiology. Characteristics of the disease are its bewildering variety of clinical manifestations and course. Almost any tissue in the body may be affected. Many patients in hospital practice show multisystem disease and follow a chronic or relapsing course with uncertain benefit from steroid or other treatment. By contrast, in previously healthy young people, the disease is often benign and remits apparently completely and permanently. Aircrew are usually diagnosed either because of an acute illness with erythema nodosum, florid arthropathy (mainly of medium and large lower-limb joints), fever and systemic upset, or because routine chest radiography shows bilateral hilar lymphnode enlargement in an ostensibly healthy person. On inquiry, many patients in this latter group admit to minor "bronchitic" symptoms, productive cough and wheezing, and sometimes to feelings of generally impaired health for a few weeks or more.

For reasons explained later, an aviator with suspected sarcoidosis should be grounded at once and not returned to flying duties until all evidence of the disease has remitted and the requirements of a standard protocol have been satisfied. The diagnosis of hilar lymphodenopathy involves exclusion of tuberculosis, other rarer infections, lymphoma, and other malignant diseases. There is usually little difficulty, particularly as these other diseases rarely if ever show the tendency to spontaneous improvement seen in sarcoidosis. A tissue sample obtained by either bronchial biopsy or Kveim test is commonly diagnostic. In the erythema nodosum syndrome, angiotensin-converting enzyme levels are often elevated, declining in recovery. Bilat-

eral upper- and mid-zone pulmonary involvement, often asymmetrical, seen as soft mottling or increased bronchovascular markings on radiography, is common in both types of disease and usually resolves along with hilar adenopathy. More extensive or progressive, persistent pulmonary shadowing is an adverse prognostic feature and is fortunately uncommon.

Presentation as disease of other systems (e.g., hepatic, neurologic, dermatologic, or ophthalmic) usually implies a less favorable prognosis, as does hypercalcemia. Many patients require systemic steroid treatment which precludes most types of flying duty irrespective of the extent of the disease which may itself cause disqualifying disabilities.

The main cause for concern in aircrew, however, remains involvement of the heart by the sarcoid process. Sarcoid granulomas may be found in any part of the heart, including valve leaflets, chordae tendineae, conduction system, or pericardium. Usually, involvement is patchy and often the disease is clinically silent. However, a wide variety of cardiac presentations are documented, including rhythm disturbances (ectopic beats, atrial, junctional and ventricular tachycardias), blocks (e.g., RBBB or LBBB, various degrees of atrioventricular blocks, including Stokes-Adams attacks), and a dilated cardiomyopathic picture. The frequency of cardiac involvement is uncertain. Fleming, a British cardiologist who has made a lifetime study of the disease, reported 300 cases including 138 deaths (72). Though rhythm disorders were the commonest presentation, 61% showed some degree of heart block, which was complete (third degree) in 26% of patients. Other authors found that, of patients diagnosed during life and confirmed postmortem as having cardiac sarcoidosis, sudden death has occurred in two-thirds and congestive heart failure in an additional one-quarter. Some patients have precordial pain that may simulate angina pectoris, and sarcoidosis is a cause of regional ventricular wall-motion abnormalities. Wall thinning, akinesia, and even cardiac aneurysm formation show a predilection for the upper interventricular septum and left ventricular free wall, the cardiac apex being commonly spared. Thallium scans may be abnormal even when coronary angiography is normal. However, granulomatous sarcoid vasculitis may affect the coronary arteries.

Evidence of complete healing is rare in cardiac sarcoidosis, and complications, including sudden death, may occur many years after initial diagnosis.

Management of aircrew with apparently recovered sarcoidosis concentrates on the exclusion of cardiac disease. An initial period of one year of nonflying is usual; this may have to be extended when slow resolution occurs (e.g., hilar node enlargement). An extensive noninvasive cardiac work-up is undertaken following apparent complete recovery. Investigations include 12-lead, 24-hour ambulatory (Holter) and maximal exercise stress ECG, echocardiography, and various isotopic scans (thallium, gallium, MUGA). Unfortunately, the large number of tests makes it likely that one or more will show a nonspecific finding common in healthy young people, such as minor atrioventricular conduction prolongation (first-degree heart block) or an intraventricular conduction delay. Further cardiologic assessment, including invasive procedures, may be necessary. Unfortunately, because of the patchy nature of the disease, endomyocardial biopsy is rather insensitive in diagnosis.

Negative results allow return to flying, although activities are usually restricted (i.e., individual may be unfit for solo operations). After one year without evidence of disease recurrence and following a second, noninvasive cardiologic work-up, return to unrestricted flying duties is usually allowed. Thereafter, specialist follow-up is repeated at some arbitrary interval (every two to three years) for the rest of the individual's flying career. A definite diagnosis of cardiac sarcoidosis, however, mandates permanent disqualification from flying duties.

The experience of the Royal Air Force (RAF) and USAF with this policy has been generally favorable. It seems that both the acute erythema nodosum syndrome and isolated hilar lymphadenopathy are normally benign, usually self-limiting forms of the disease. Ninety percent of RAF patients have been able to return to unrestricted flying duties, and the USAF experience of much larger numbers has been almost as good. Any relaxation of present restrictions would depend on marked improvement in the detection and/or treatment of cardiac sarcoidosis.

Because present methods of diagnosing cardiac sarcoidosis are insensitive, and because long-term prognosis and forecasting of relapse are impossible, candidates for military flying training who have histories of sarcoidosis are unlikely to be selected. An applicant for a commercial flying licence with a remote history of a benign type of sarcoidosis may be acceptable if the individual were to have recovered rapidly, has been disease-free for longer than two years and no evidence of persistence, recurrence, or cardiac involvement were to exist on full clinical and laboratory assessment. A private pilot's license may be granted on somewhat less stringent criteria.

ACKNOWLEDGMENTS

The authors are indebted to George M. McGranahan, M.D., Paul V. Celio, M.D., William C. Wood, M.D. and Samuel B. Parker, M.D., whose invaluable contributions and thoughts from the first edition have been carried forward.

This chapter is dedicated to the memory of Maj. Gwynne Neufeld, USAFR (MS), a co-author of the first edition chapter.

REFERENCES

1. Mallory GK, White PD, Salcedo-Salgar J. The speed of healing of myocardial infarction: a study of the pathologic anatomy in seventy-two cases. Am Heart J 1939; 18:647–671.
2. Kragel AH, Reddy SG, Wittes JT, Roberts WC. Morphometric analysis of the composition of atherosclerotic plaques in the four major epicardial coronary arteries in acute myocardial infarction and sudden coronary death. Circulation 1989;80:1747–1756.

3. Strong JP, Solberg LA, Restrepo C. Atherosclerosis in persons with coronary heart disease. Lab Invest 1968; 18:527–537.

4. Epstein SE, Quyyumi AA, Bonow RO. Myocardial ischemia—silent or symptomatic. N Engl J Med 1988; 318:1038–1043.

5. DeWood MA, Spores J, Notske R, Mouser LT, Burroughs R, Golden MS, Lang HT. Prevalence of total coronary occlusion during the early hours of transmural myocardial infarction. N Engl J Med 1980;303: 897–902.

6. Spain DM, Bradess VA, Mohr C. Coronary atherosclerosis as a cause of unexpected and unexplained death: an autopsy study from 1949–1959. JAMA 1960;174: 384–388.

7. Ragland KE, Selvin S, Merrill D. The onset of decline in ischemic heart disease mortality in the United States. Am J Epidemiol 1988;127:516–531.

8. Higgins M, Thom T. Trends in CHD in the United States. Int J Epidemiol 1989;18(Suppl 1):S58-S66.

9. Chronic disease reports: mortality trends—United States, 1979–1986. MMWR 1989;38:189–191.

10. MacDorman MF, Hudson BL. Advance report of final mortality statistics, 1989. Monthly Vital Stats Report 1992;40(Suppl 2):17–17.

11. McCall NJ, Wick RL Jr, Brawley WL, Berger BT. A survey of blood lipid levels in airline pilot applicants. Aviat Space Environ Med 1992;63:533–537.

12. Enos WF, Holmes RH, Beger J. Coronary disease among United States soldiers killed in action in Korea. JAMA 1953;152:1090.

13. McNammara JJ, Molot MA, Stremple JF, Cutting RT. Coronary artery disease in combat casualties in Vietnam. JAMA 1971;216:1185.

14. Doyle JT, Kannel WB, McNamara PM, Quickenton P, Gordon T. Factors related to suddenness of death from coronary disease: combined Albany-Framingham studies. Am J Cardiol 1976;37:1073–1078.

15. Kannel WB, Feinleib M, Dawber TR. The unrecognized myocardial infarction: fourteen-year follow-up experience in the Framingham Study. Geriatrics 1970;25: 75–87.

16. Kannel WB, Abbott RD. Incidence and prognosis of unrecognized myocardial infarction: an update on the Framingham Study. N Engl J Med 1984;311: 1144–1147.

17. Kannel WB, Schatzkin A. Sudden death: lessons from subsets in population studies. J Am Coll Cardiol 1985; 5:141B-149B.

18. Rosenman RH, Friedman M, Jenkins CD, Straus R, Wurm M, Kositchek R. Recurring and fatal myocardial infarction in the Western Collaborative Group Study. Am J Cardiol 1967;19:771–775.

19. Lindberg HA, Berkson DM, Stamler J, Poindexter A. Totally asymptomatic myocardial infarction: an estimate of its incidence in the living population. Arch Intern Med 1960;5:628–633.

20. Rentrop KP, Thornton JC, Feit F, Van Buskirk M. Determinants and protective potential of coronary arterial

21. Hackett D, Verwilghen J, Davies G, Maseri A. Coronary stenoses before and after acute myocardial infarction. Am J Cardiol 1989;63:1517–1518.

22. Thrombolysis in myocardial infarction (TIMI) trial: phase I findings. N Engl J Med 1985;312:932–936.

23. Proudfit WL, Bruschke AVG, Sones FM Jr. Clinical course of patients with normal or slightly or moderately abnormal coronary arteriograms: 10-year follow-up of 521 patients. Circulation 1980;62:712–717.

24. Kemp HG, Kronmal RA, Vlietstra RE, Frye RL. Seven year survival of patients with normal or near normal coronary arteriograms: a CASS Registry study. J Am Coll Cardiol 1986;7:479–483.

25. Klag MJ, Ford DE, Mead LA, Jiang HE, Whelton PK, Liang KY, Levine DM. Serum cholesterol in young men and subsequent cardiovascular disease. N Engl J Med 1993;328:313–318.

26. Clark DA, Tolan GD, Johnson R, Hickman JR, Jackson WG, McGranahan G. The West Point study: 40 years of followup. Aviat Space Environ Med 1994;65(5 suppl): A71-A74.

27. Stokes J III, Dawber TR. The "silent coronary": the frequency and clinical characteristics of unrecognized myocardial infarction in the Framingham study. Ann Intern Med 1959;50:1359–1369.

28. Clemmensen P, Grande P, Saunamaki K, Wagner NB, Startt-Selvester RH, Wagner GS. A comparison of electrocardiographic QRS changes and two-dimensional echocardiographic left ventricular wall motion score pre-discharge and in the fourth year following first acute myocardial infarction. J Electrocardiol 1992;25(suppl): 1–2.

29. Willems JL, Abreu-Lima C, Arnaud P, Van Bemmel JH, Brohet C, Degani R, Denis B, Gehring J, Graham I, Van Herpen G, Machado H, Macfarlane PW, Michaelis J, Moulopoulos SD, Rubel P, Zywietz C. The diagnostic performance of computer programs for the interpretation of electrocardiograms. N Engl J Med 1991; 325:1767–1773.

30. Blanke H, Cohen M, Schlueter GU, Karsch KR, Rentrop KP. Electrocardiographic and coronary arteriographic correlations during acute myocardial infarction. Am J Cardiol 1984;54:249–255.

31. Durrer D, Van Dam RT, Freud GE, Janse MJ, Meijler FL, Arzbaecher RC. Total excitation of the isolated human heart. Circulation 1970;41:899–912.

32. Hurd HP II, Starling MR, Crawford MH, Dlabal PW, O'Rourke RA. Comparative accuracy of electrocardiographic and vectorcardiographic criteria for inferior myocardial infarction. Circulation 1981;63:1025–1029.

33. McHenry PL, O'Donnell J, Morrs SN, Jordan JJ. The abnormal exercise electrocardiogram in apparently healthy men: a predictor of angina pectoris as an initial coronary event during long-term follow-up. Circulation 1984;70:547–551.

34. Hopkirk JAC, Uhl GS, Hickman JR, Fischer J. The magnitude of ST segment depression and predictive accu-

collaterals as assessed by an angioplasty model. Am J Cardiol 1988;61:677–684.

racy of exercise testing in asymptomatic men. Circulation 1980;62:268.

35. Wolthuis RA, Froelicher VF, Fischer J, Noguera I, Davis G, Stewart A, Triebwasser JM. New practical treadmill protocol for clinical use. Am J Cardiol 1977; 39:697–700.

36. Froelicher VF, Thomas MM, Pillow C, Lancaster MC. Epidemiologic study of symptomatic men screened by maximal treatment testing for latent coronary artery disease. Am J Cardiol 1974;34:770.

37. Loecker TH, Schwartz RS, Cotta CW, Hickman JR. Fluoroscopic coronary artery calcification and associated coronary disease in asymptomatic young men. J Am Coll Cardiol 1992;19:1167–1172.

38. Detrano R, Markovic D, Simpfendorfer C, Franco I, Hollman J, Grigera F, Stewart W, Ratcliff N, Salcedo EE, Leatherman J. Digital subtraction fluoroscopy: a new method of detecting coronary calcifications with improved sensitivity for the prediction of coronary disease. Circulation 1985;71:725–732.

39. Agatston AS, Janowitz WR, Hildner FJ, Zusmer NR, Viamonte M Jr, Detrano R. Quantification of coronary artery calcium using ultrafast computed tomography. J Am Coll Cardiol 1990;15:827–832.

40. Agatston AS, Janowitz WR, Aizawa N, Gasso J, Hildner FJ, Viamonte M Jr, Prineas R. Quantification of coronary calcium reflects the angiographic extent of coronary artery disease. Circulation 1991;84(Suppl):II-159.

41. Breen JF, Sheedy PF II, Schwartz RS, Stanson AW, Kaufmann RB, Moll PP, Rumberger JA. Coronary artery calcification detected with ultrafast CT as an indication of coronary artery disease. Radiology 1992;185: 435–439.

42. McGranahan GM, Hickman JR, Uhl GS, Montgomery MA, Triebwasser JH. Minimal coronary artery disease and continuation of flying status. Aviat Space Environ Med 1983;54:548–550.

43. McGranahan GM, Munson RA, Celio PV. The natural history of minimal coronary artery disease in US air force aviators. Aviat Space Environ Med 1993;64:442.

44. Chaitman BR, Davis KB, Dodge HT, Fisher LD, Pettinger M, Holmes DR, Kaiser GC, CASS participants. "Should airline pilots be eligible to resume active flight status after coronary bypass surgery?" A CASS Registry study. J Am Coll Cardiol 1986;8:P1318–1324.

45. Celio PV. Disposition for coronary artery disease. Advisory Group for Aerospace Research and Development (NATO). Springfield: National Technical Information Service (NTIS), 1993.

46. Newman WP III, Freedman DS, Voors AW, Gard PD, Srinivasan SR, Cresanta JL, Williamson GD, Webber LS, Berenson GS. Relation of serum lipoprotein levels and systolic blood pressure to early atherosclerosis. The Bogalusa heart study. N Engl J Med 1986;314:138–144.

47. Hickman JR. Coronary risk factors in aerospace medicine. Advisory Group for Aerospace Research and Development (NATO). Report No. 758. Springfield: National Technical Information Service (NTIS),1987.

48. Kruyer WB. Primary prevention of coronary heart disease. Advisory group for aerospace research and development (NATO). Springfield: National Technical Information Service (NTIS), 1993.

49. Lancaster MC, Ord JW. The USAF central electrocardiographic library. U.S. Air Force Med. Service Dig 1972;23:8–10.

50. Batchelor AJ, Kruyer WB, Hickman JR. Ventricular ectopy in totally symptom-free subjects with defined coronary anatomy. Am Heart J 1989;117:1265–70.

51. Celio PV. Aeromedical disposition of electrocardiographic findings in aircrew. Advisory group for aerospace research and development (NATO). Springfield: National Technical Information Service (NTIS), 1993.

52. Richardson LA, Celio PV, Kruyer WB, Besich WJ, Hickman JR. The aeromedical implications of supraventricular tachycardia. Aviat Space Environ Med, In press.

53. Lancaster MC, Schechter E, Massing GK. Acquired complete right bundle branch block without overt cardiac disease: clinical and hemodynamic study of 37 patients. Am J Cardiol 1972;30:32.

54. Canaveris G, Halpern MS. Intraventricular conduction disturbances in flying personnel: incomplete right bundle branch block. Aviat Space Environ Med 1988;59: 960–964.

55. Wehrly DJ. Historic aeromedical perspective on left bundle branch block. Aviat Space Environ Med 1986; 57:462–5.

56. Canaveris G, Halpern MS, Elizari MV. Intraventricular conduction disturbances in civilian flying personnel: left anterior hemiblock. Aviat Space Environ Med 1992;63: 292–298.

57. Tamura T, Komatsu C, Asukata I, Yamamoto K, Hokari M. Time course and clinical significance of marked left axis deviation in airline pilots. Aviat Space Environ Med 1991;62:683–686.

58. Krivisky M, Aberbouch L, Shochat I, Ribak J, Tamir A, Froom P. Left anterior hemiblock in otherwise healthy pilots. Aviat Space Environ Med 1988;59:651–652.

59. Eighth Bethesda Conference of the American College of Cardiology. Cardiovascular problems associated with aviation safety. Am J Cardiol 1975;36:573–628.

60. Kruyer WP, Schwartz RS. Valvular and congenital heart disease in the aviator. Advisory group for aerospace research and development (NATO). Report No. 758. Springfield: National Technical Information Service (NTIS), 1993.

61. Engel PJ, Alpert BL, Hickman JR. The nature and prevalence of the abnormal exercise electrocardiogram in mitral valve prolapse. Am Heart J 1979;98:716–724.

62. Collins R, Peto R, MacMahon S, Herbert P, Fiebach NH, Eberlein KA, Godwin J, Qizilbash N, Taylor JO, Hennekens CH. Blood pressure, stroke, and coronary heart disease: part 2, short term reductions in blood pressure: overview of randomized drug trials in their epidemiological context. Lancet 1990;335:827–838.

63. Roberts WC, McAllister HA, Ferrans VJ. Sarcoidosis of the heart: a clinicopathologic study of 35 necropsy patients (group I) and review of 78 previously described necropsy patients (group II). Ann J Med 1977;63:86.

64. Celio PV, Munson RAV. History of sarcoidosis in USAF aviators. Aviat Space Environ Med 1993;64:43.
65. Berend N. Tests of small airway function. Semin Resp Med 1983;4:214–223.
66. Cockroft DW, Killian DN, Mellor JJA, Hargreave FE. Bronchial reactivity to inhaled antihistamine: a method and clinical survey. Clin Allergy 1977;7:235–43.
67. Glaister DH. Effect of acceleration. In: West JB, ed. Regional differences in the lung. New York: Academic Press, 1977;323–379.
68. Wood EH, Hoffman EA. The lungs, ''Achilles' heel''

of air breathers in changing gravitational-inertial force environments. Physiologist 1984;27:47–48.
69. Snapper JR. Inflammation and airway function: the asthma syndrome. Am Rev Resp Dis 1990;141:531–33.
70. Rayman RB. Sudden incapacitation in flight 1 Jan 1966–30 Nov 1971. Aerosp Med 1973;44:953–955.
71. Voge VM, Anthracite R. Spontaneous pneumothorax in the USAF aircrew population: a retrospective study. Aviat Space Environ Med 1966;57:939–949.
72. Fleming HA. Sarcoid heart disease. Br Med J 1986;292:1095–1096.

Chapter 16

Ophthalmology in Aerospace Medicine

Thomas J. Tredici

And God said, "Let there be light."

Genesis 1:3

Vision has always held a dominant place in the attributes necessary for flying. This was recognized by early pioneers, such as Drs. William Wilmer and Conrad Berens, who established the first laboratory to study the visual problems of the flyer in 1918 at the Air Service Medical Research Laboratory at Mineola, Long Island, New York (1). This almost total dependence on vision is evident today as astronauts have reported the necessity of vision for orientation in space.

Vision occurs peripherally at the eye and centrally in brain. In the eye, the retina receives electromagnetic energy (photons) and, through a photochemical reaction, converts it into electrical signals. These nervous impulses are relayed to the occipital area of brain, where the signals are processed and interpreted as vision.

APPLIED ANATOMY AND PHYSIOLOGY

Embryology

The eye develops from neural and surface ectoderm and mesoderm. The neural ectoderm eventually develops into the retina, ciliary epithelium, the sphincter and dilator muscles, and the pigment layer of the iris. The surface ectoderm becomes the epithelial lining of the cornea, conjunctiva, and lids and their glands and also forms the lens. The mesoderm gives rise to all the permanent and transitory blood vessels, the sclera, sheath of the optic nerve, ciliary muscle stroma and endothelium of the cornea, stroma of the iris, and the extrinsic muscles of the eye.

Orbit

The bony orbits develop so as to afford both protection and support of the globe while allowing it maximum exposure for vision. The bony orbit is shaped like a quadrilateral pyramid, which allows the cornea and conjunctiva to be exposed anteriorly and tapers down to the openings located at the apex. In an adult, the medial walls of the orbit are parallel and the lateral walls make an angle of 90° with each other. The posterior openings allow the cranial nerves and blood vessels from the brain to communicate with the eye, which is acting as an external sensor, gathering information and relaying it along neural paths for final processing in the central nervous system. All of the extraocular muscles except for the inferior oblique muscle originate from a fibrous ring, the annulus of Zinn, which is located at the orbital apex and in close approximation to the optic nerve. Thus, inflammation of the optic nerve (retrobulbar neuritis) may, at times, manifest as pain on motion of the eye. Fractures of the orbital floor, so-called blowout fractures, may cause double vision, especially in upward gaze. The thinnest bones are in the medial wall, and orbital cellulitis may ensue secondary to a

519

fracture of these delicate bones, creating a communication with the ethmoid sinuses or nasal cavity. Hemorrhage into the orbit following an injury may displace the globe, causing proptosis, immobility, and ensuing diplopia. The orbit also contains Tenon's capsule, which acts as an articular socket. The remainder of the orbit is completely filled with fat pads so that an accumulation of fluid in the body (edema) shows around the eyes as puffy lids, whereas the opposite (dehydration and/or starvation) causes the eyes to sink deeply into the orbit.

Globe

The globe measures approximately 25 mm in diameter. It has three coats. The two outer layers, the sclera and uveal coats, are involved with support, protection, and nutrition. The inner coat, the retina, contains the light-sensitive elements. The eye can be considered an external sensor, converting and then relaying signals to an internally located computer. The eye is beautifully developed to concentrate electromagnetic energy, or photons, onto the light-, or photon-, sensitive retina. The wavelength of electromagnetic energy is, designated in nanometers (1-billionth of a meter; m $\times$ 10^{-9}). Another, older designation was millimicrons. A narrow band within the electromagnetic spectrum from 400 to 760 nm is absorbed by pigments in the retina; a photochemical reaction occurs, and this chemical activity is converted into electrical energy, which is transmitted through the retina and the optic nerve onto the occipital area of the central nervous system, where these signals are interpreted as vision.

The sclera is the tough outer fibrous coat, which is composed of collagen bundles laced in an irregular fashion. The extraocular muscle tendons are continuous with the sclera and merge into it. The sclera has a radius of approximately 12 mm. The sclera has an anterior bulge, the cornea, which measures approximately 12 mm in diameter. The cornea has a shorter radius, measuring only 7.5 mm. The transition zone be-

tween the opaque sclera and the clear cornea is known as the limbus. Most surgical procedures for entering the anterior segment of the eye are done at the limbus. The sclera is thinnest (0.3 mm) under the insertion of the muscle tendons and is thickest (1.0 mm) at the posterior pole (Fig. 16.1).

The cornea is composed of collagen fibers similar to those found in the sclera. The cornea is transparent to visible radiation. Absorption by the cornea becomes apparent and increases steeply in the long ultraviolet range at about 370 nm. At 300 nm, only 25% of the incident radiation is transmitted through the cornea, and at 290 nm, a mere 2% of the radiation is transmitted into the inner eye. Corneal transparency is enhanced by its structural composition, including the following: collagen fibers that extend in regular layers of parallel fibers; action of the endothelial cell pump mechanism, which keeps the cornea continuously dehydrated; and no blood vessels or pigmented cells are present in the corneal stroma. The cornea is thinnest in the center (0.6 mm) and thickens toward the edge (0.8 mm). The oxygen that is supplied to and metabolized in the cornea is derived from three sources: the aqueous humor, the perilimbal vascular supply, and the tear film bathing the epithelial cells. The oxygen supply to the epithelium is primarily derived directly from the atmosphere as it is absorbed by the tear layer and passed directly into the epithelial cells. Capping this oxygen source, as by placing some types of contact lenses over the cornea, reduces the oxygen tension at the corneal epithelium. The oxygen tension is reduced as an aviator achieves high altitude; this is one of the reasons why contact lenses should be thoroughly evaluated before being fitted on aviation personnel.

As shown in Figure 16.2, the eye is approximately a 60-diopter (D) refracting system. Because it separates elements of the greatest difference in indices of refraction (air/cornea), the cornea is the most powerful component in the ocular refracting system. Approximately 45 D of the total refraction is due to the cornea, and 15 D is due to the unaccommodated lens. Because

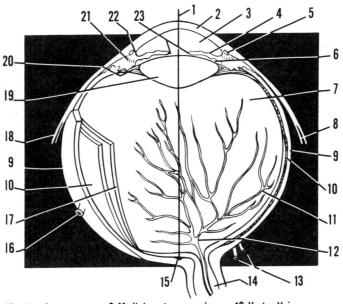

1. Visual axis
2. Cornea
3. Anterior Chamber
4. Iris
5. Schlemm's canal
6. Posterior chamber
7. Vitreous

8. Medial rectus muscie
9. Sclera
10. Choroid
11. Retinal   vessels
12. Central retinal vessels
13. Ciliary artery & nerve
14. Optic nerve
15. Fovea centralis

16. Vortex Vein
17. Retina
18. Lateral rectus muscle
19. Lens
20. Ciliary zonule
21. Ciliary muscle
22. Angle of anterior chamber
23. Pupil

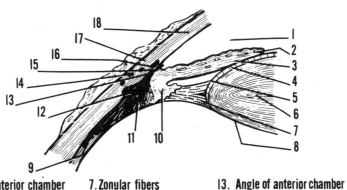

1. Anterior chamber
2. Iris sphincter muscle
3. Iris dilator muscle
4. Lens epithelium
5. Anterior lens capsule
6. Lens nucleus

7. Zonular fibers
8. Posterior lens capsule
9. Ciliary epithelium
10. Ciliary muscle (Circular)
11. Ciliary muscle (Radial)
12. Ciliary muscle (Meridional)

13. Angle of anterior chamber
14. Aqueous vein
15. Trabecular meshwork
16. Canal of Schlemm
17. Sclera
18. Corneal stroma

Figure 16.1. Anatomy of the eye.

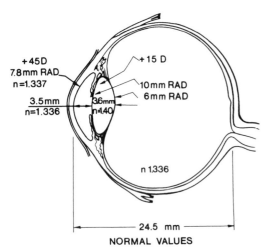

NORMAL VALUES

Figure 16.2. The normal values for the optical properties of the eye (RAD = radius; D = diopter; n = index of refraction.)

small changes in the cornea's radius can cause substantial changes in refraction, attempts are often made at altering the corneal curvature to change the refraction, such as by the use of contact lenses (orthokeratology) or the newer surgical procedures (e.g., radial keratotomy), and, more recently, by excimer laser lamellar keratectomy, also known as photorefractive keratectomy (PRK).

The uvea lie inside of the scleral coat. The uvea is the pigmented vascular portion of the eye and consists of the choroid posteriorly and the iris and ciliary body anteriorly. The uveal tract contains melanin pigment. Anteriorly, the iris color is a function of the degree of pigmentation. For instance, brown eyes are heavily pigmented, whereas blue or green eyes have a rather sparsely pigmented iris. The outer half of the retina is nourished by the choroid's abundant vascular supply. Anteriorly, the choroid, along with the anterior extensions of the retina, becomes the ciliary body. The ciliary body is composed of smooth muscle laying in circular, longitudinal, and radial directions. More than 70 ciliary processes are formed that extend centrally toward the lens. The ciliary muscle, innervated by the parasympathetic nervous system, supplies the contractile forces that are necessary for accommodation, which allows one to see

clearly close up. Aqueous humor is produced by diffusion and secretion in the epithelium of the ciliary processes. This aqueous humor is derived from blood plasma. Only one-one thousandth as much protein is manifest in the aqueous as in the blood. The iris is a thin, circular disk that controls the amount of light entering the eye and affects the depth-of-field of the eye's optical system. The iris divides the anterior segment into an anterior and posterior chamber. The aqueous, formed in the ciliary processes, enters the posterior chamber, bathes the lens, flows through the pupillary opening into the anterior chamber, continues through the trabecular meshwork, where it meets sufficient resistance to keep the intraocular pressure at 10–22 mm Hg, continues into Schlemm's canal, and then flows into the aqueous veins and returns to the general circulation. The pupil is controlled by a delicate balance of the sympathetic and parasympathetic tone of the autonomic nervous system. The sympathetic system innervates the dilator of the iris while the parasympathetic system innervates the sphincter. This mechanism regulates the amount of light entering the eye, which is proportional to the square of the pupillary diameter. In the brightest daytime illumination, the pupil can constrict down to 1.5 mm and open to 8 mm in diameter in darkness. In the aviator's environment at altitude, even a 1.5-mm wide pupil will allow excess light to enter the eye for comfort; therefore, filters in the form of sunglasses can reduce the ambient illumination to a comfortable level. In darkness, even with an 8-mm wide pupil, sufficient light may not be sufficient to stimulate the retinal receptors. Waiting 30 minutes in darkness, however, allows another mechanism, adaptation, to be triggered. Adaptation is a retinal mechanism that increases the light sensitivity many thousand times and is discussed in more detail in the section entitled "Night (Scotopic) Vision" later in this chapter.

Lens

The lens is approximately 9 mm in diameter and 4 mm in thickness in its unaccommodated state.

Its anterior radius is approximately 10 mm, whereas the posterior radius is shorter (6 mm). The lens is held in place by zonular fibers. These zonular fibers are inserted into the lens capsule and into the valleys between the ciliary processes on the ciliary body. In young individuals, the lens is quite malleable. Its elastic capsule deforms the lens to view near objects clearly. When accommodation takes place, an increase in refractive power is manifest on the lens as it becomes more spherical. This is accomplished by constriction of the circular muscle of the ciliary body through parasympathetic innervation. The zonular fibers slacken, and the inherent elasticity of the lens capsule allows it to become more spherical and thus increase its diopteric power. In the young individual, this can be as much as 15 D over the amount of refractive power in the resting state of the lens. At age 40, approximately 5 D of accommodative power remain, and when this amount drops to 4 D, the individual is considered to be presbyopic. Actually, most reading is done at 0.33 m, where it is necessary to exert 3 D to see clearly. One must, however, maintain a 20–25% reserve of accommodation; otherwise, presbyopic symptoms will ensue. By age 65, only 1 D of accommodative power remains. The stimulus for accommodation is probably the blurred retinal image; however, chromatic aberration may play a substantial role in one's ability to focus rapidly. Monochromatic light systems, such as red cockpit lighting, work against this aspect of accommodative adjustment, and, perhaps much more importantly, monochromatic red light is focused 1–1.25 D behind the retina, in essence making the individual hypermetropic or more presbyopic. This extra accommodative requirement increases the difficulty for individuals who are farsighted or are early presbyopes. Therefore, from the visual system standpoint, it is a good thing that red cockpit lighting has almost disappeared. Low-level white light is much more effective for seeing in the cockpit, and, provided its intensity is kept low, the degradation of night vision is minimal. The reason that red light is focused

behind the retina and monochromatic blue is focused in front of the retina is because of chromatic aberration in the optical system of the eye. The eye is in focus for monochromatic yellow only, being hypermetropic for red and myopic for blue (2).

Retina

The retina is the innermost photosensitive layer and is protected and nourished by the sclera and choroid (Fig. 16.3). The outer half of the retina, from the inner nuclear layer out, is nourished by the choroid. From the internuclear layer to the inner limiting membrane, the retina is nourished by the retinal vasculature. Nutrients leave the choriocapillaris in the choroid, pass through Bruch's membrane, which separates the choroid from the retina, and into the single layer of the pigment epithelium. The tips of the receptors, the rods and cones, are nestled in between these cells, and all metabolites of the outer retina pass through the retinal pigment epithelium. The neurosensory retina consists of 10 layers. The light-sensitive elements are the rods and cones. The rods serve vision at low levels of illumination (scotopic vision), whereas the cones are effective both for medium and high levels of illumination (mesopic and photopic vision) and for color vision. The cones are mainly concentrated in the fovea centralis, where the density has been measured at 47,000 cones/mm^2. Fifteen degrees temporal to the optic disk lays the center of an avascular area known as the macula, as shown in Figure 16.4. The macular area is 1.5 mm in diameter and subtends 5° at the nodal point. The fovea centralis, where form vision is most acute, measures approximately 0.3 mm in diameter and subtends an arc of 54 minutes, or approximately 1°. In the center of this 1°, visual acuity can be as high as 20/10, whereas at the edge of the macula, or 2.5° from the center of the fovea, the visual acuity already has dropped to 20/50 (Fig. 16.4). This is why central serous retinopathy or a foveal macular burn is such a devastating condition for the aviator. The other retinal

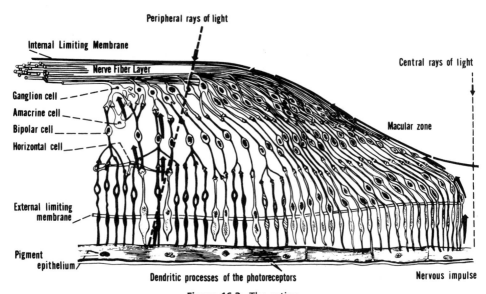

Figure 16.3. The retina.

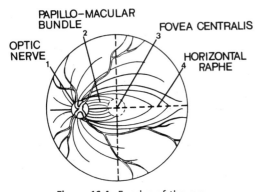

Figure 16.4. Fundus of the eye.

system, the rod receptors, are mainly useful in low illuminations because they are more sensitive than the cones and are better at motion detection. The rods reach a maximum density in the retina at 15–20° from the fovea centralis; therefore, looking 15° off-center maximizes one's scotopic vision. Rod receptors contain the photo pigment rhodopsin, which has its maximum sensitivity at 510 nm. The maximum sensitivity of a light-adapted human eye is at 555 nm. This change in luminosity function of the human eye is called the Purkinje shift (Fig. 16.8).

To facilitate color vision, the cones have three different photosensitive pigments, one absorbing primarily in the blue wavelength at 445 nm, one in the green wavelength at 535 nm, and one in the red wavelength at 570 nm. Absorption at these wavelengths in varying amounts gives the human eye its color vision capabilities (3). All the retinal nerve fibers combine into the optic nerve and leave the globe at the disk. No receptors are manifest here; thus, a functional "blind spot" is formed. The optic disk, or blind spot, is located 15° nasal from the fovea and covers an area 7° in height and 5° in width. Because one blind spot is covered by the functioning retina of the other eye, we are unaware of its existence unless the visual field is being mapped. The optic nerves extend through the optic foramina, decussate at the chiasma, and continue as optic tracts to the lateral geniculate body. From the lateral geniculate body, the optic radiations fan out over the temporal and parietal lobes, eventually reaching the occipital lobe and concentrating in the posterior calcarine fissure of Brodmann's area 17. Decussation of the nerve fibers allows us to have corresponding points in each retina, which facilitates stereoscopic vision, the highest order of depth perception obtainable.

The vitreous, a clear, colorless, gellike structure, fills the posterior four-fifths of the globe. The vitreous is firmly attached to the ciliary epithelium in the area of the ora serrata and surrounding the optic disk. The vitreous is composed of 99.6% water, with proteins and salt comprising the remainder. The proteins are important because they form a scaffolding. These fine fibrils are composed of collagen. The spaces between the fibrils are filled with hyaluronic acid and form the molecular network in the vitreous. The complaint of vitreous floaters is universal and usually is innocuous. Floaters are probably due to collapse of the protein/collagen scaffolding, which causes thickening and casts a shadow on the retina. More ominous floaters, which must be investigated at once, are often referred to as a "shower" of floaters; these floaters are probably red blood cells following a hemorrhage into the vitreous. The complaint of a dark floating membrane that may obscure vision should be investigated for the possibility of a retinal detachment.

Adnexa

The adnexa of the eye are the extraocular muscles, the eyelids, and the lacrimal apparatus (Fig. 16.5). Six extraocular muscles are attached to each globe, and because of the strong desire for fusion and the maintenance of single binocular vision, both foveas are maintained on the object of regard by both reflex and voluntary action. This is done by the yoke muscles of each eye, which are driven by Hering's law of equal and simultaneous innervation to each yoke muscle. If a breakdown were to occur in either the nervous arc organization or in the actual muscles themselves, binocularity would break down and strabismus and diplopia would ensue. The elevators of the globe are the superior recti and inferior oblique muscles. The depressors are the inferior recti and superior oblique muscles, and the horizontal rotators are the medial and lateral recti muscles. The actions of the muscles are described with the eye in the primary position of gaze (Fig. 16.24). The actions of these muscles change, however, depending on the position of the globe. In the eye examination for flying, the flight surgeon should be able to discern the difference between a tropia or strabismus (manifest deviation of the eyes) and a phoria or heterophoria, which is a latent deviation that becomes manifest only when fusion is interrupted by an opaque occluder, Maddox rod, or prism.

The corneal epithelium is covered by a thin, three-layered, precorneal tear film. The thin, outer, oily layer is derived from the meibomian glands of the tarsal plate. The middle aqueous layer is derived from the lacrimal glands, and the inner mucoid layer arises from the goblet cells of the conjunctiva. The external oily layer helps to retard evaporation of the tears and produces a smooth and regular anterior optical surface to the cornea. Ordinarily, a large part of the tear film evaporates each minute, with only the remainder passing through the lacrimal passages. This evaporation causes the tears to become slightly hypertonic, producing an osmotic flow of water from the anterior chamber through the cornea to the tear film. The lacrimal gland is situated in a bony fossa of the frontal bone just posterior to the superior and temporal rim of the orbit. It secretes the aqueous portion of the precorneal tear film layer. Accessory lacrimal glands, located in the conjunctiva, also can secrete tears. The drainage system for the tears consists of a small punctum, or opening, in the innermost edge of the upper and lower lids. These openings lead into a common canaliculus, then into the lacrimal sac, and finally into the nasolacrimal canals exiting under the inferior turbinate in the nose. Obstruction in any part of this system prevents normal drainage from the conjunctival sac, and a chronic conjunctivitis and dacryocystitis can result. Excess tearing interferes with an aviator's visual capabilities; a dry eye due to lack of tears also interferes with visual efficiency.

The eyelids provide protection for the cornea and the remainder of the eye by reflexive, involuntary closing. The lids blink involuntarily six

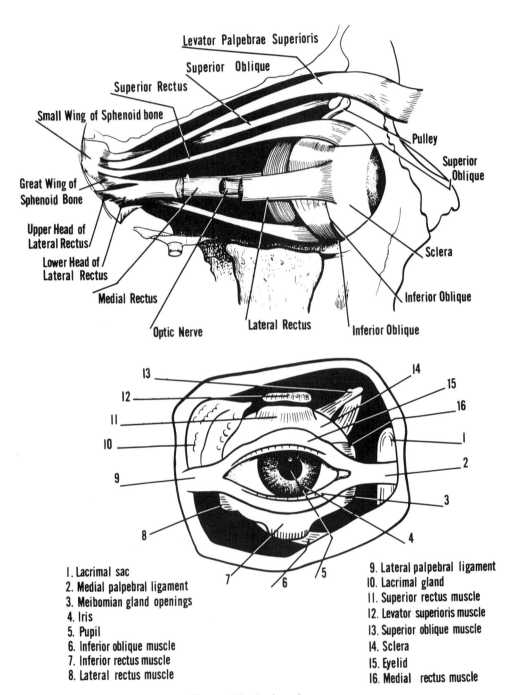

Figure 16.5. Ocular adnexa.

1. Lacrimal sac
2. Medial palpebral ligament
3. Meibomian gland openings
4. Iris
5. Pupil
6. Inferior oblique muscle
7. Inferior rectus muscle
8. Lateral rectus muscle
9. Lateral palpebral ligament
10. Lacrimal gland
11. Superior rectus muscle
12. Levator superioris muscle
13. Superior oblique muscle
14. Sclera
15. Eyelid
16. Medial rectus muscle

to eight times per minute, thus evenly distributing and smoothing the precorneal tear film to enhance the optical qualities of the cornea. The eyelids are closed by action of the orbicularis oculi muscle, which is innervated by the seventh cranial nerve, and are opened by the levator palpebrae superioris muscles, which are innervated by the oculomotor nerve (III cranial nerve), assisted by Müller's muscle, which is innervated by the sympathetic nervous system. Thus, pilots on long and exhausting missions may begin to have a droopy, sleepy look because of a lack or reduction in sympathetic flow to Müller's muscle. The lids are composed of four layers: the thin outer skin, which is the thinnest on the body and contains no subcutaneous fat; the muscle layer, which is formed by the orbicularis oculi muscle; the tarsal plate, which is a fibrous plate lending shape to the lids and inside of which lay the meibomian glands that secrete the oily portion of the precorneal tear film; and the conjunctiva, which is inside the lid and proximal to the cornea. The oily secretion of the tarsal glands is also spread over the lid edges, and when the lids are tightly closed, a watertight seal is formed. The lids have an abundant vascular supply such that they heal quite rapidly even when severely injured. The ducts of the meibomian gland are located at the inner edge of the ducts from the glands of Moll, and the hair follicles are on the outer, or skin, edge of the lid. When the duct of the meibomian gland becomes occluded, the oily secretion remains in the tarsal plate, forming a small granuloma or chalazion. This "lump" in the lid usually will have to be removed surgically. It also should be differentiated from the hordeolum, or stye, which is an infection of the hair follicle and usually can be differentiated from the chalazion because the stye is red and painful and responds to heat and antibiotics. These are relatively minor afflictions, but in the aviator, it is important to determine whether the chalazion is applying pressure to the cornea, thus causing astigmatism and distortion of vision or whether the stye is interfering with optical appliances and headgear.

VISUAL PRINCIPLES

Vision is essential in all phases of flying and is most important in the identification of distant objects and in perceiving details of shape and color. The visual sense also allows the judgment of distances and gauging of movements in the visual field. In flying modern aircraft and spacecraft, near vision is also exceedingly important because it is absolutely necessary to be able to read the instrument panel, radio dials, charts, visual displays, and maps. At night, even though one's vision is reduced, one still must rely on vision to safely fly the aircraft.

Physical Stimuli

The electromagnetic spectrum extends from the extremely short cosmic rays with wavelengths on the order of 10^{-16} m to the long radiowaves several kilometers in length (Fig. 16.6). The part of the spectrum that stimulates the retina is known as visible light and extends from 380 nm (violet) to about 760 nm (red). A nanometer is a millionth of a millimeter, or 1×10^{-9} m. Adjacent portions of the spectrum, although not visible, affect the eye and are, therefore, of interest. Wavelengths of 380 nm and shorter, down to 180 nm, are known as ultraviolet or abiotic rays. Exposure of the eyes to this portion of the electromagnetic spectrum produces ocular tissue damage; the severity of the damage depends on the intensity and duration of exposure. Wavelengths longer than 760 nm, up to the microwaves, are known as infrared or heat rays. These rays, too, may cause ocular tissue damage, depending on the intensity and exposure time. The light intensity in extraterrestrial space above 30,000 m is approximately 13,600 footcandle (ft-c). At 3000 m on a clear day, the light intensity is about 12,000 ft-c and approximately 10,000 ft-c at sea level. Water vapor, dust particles, and air in the atmosphere absorb some of the sun's light; in addition, selective absorption occurs. Ultraviolet light shorter than 200 nm is absorbed by dissociated oxygen. Ultraviolet

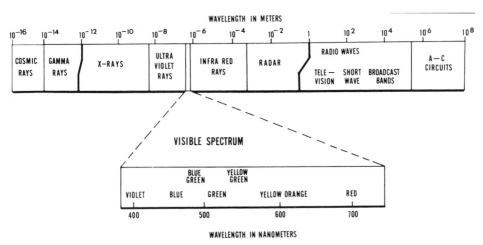

Figure 16.6. Electromagnetic spectrum.

light 200–300 nm is absorbed by the ozone layers in the atmosphere; this is fortunate because wavelengths 200–300 nm are the most damaging to the eye. These wavelengths produce the actinic keratoconjunctivitis that welders suffer when they fail to wear protective lenses. These wavelengths of 200–300 nm are no problem until an altitude of approximately 40,000 m is reached. This is about the height of the second ozone layer. Above this altitude, these ultraviolet wavelengths must be considered. Recent work done in the space program shows that the most abiotic rays have a wavelength of 270 nm (4). They must be filtered by protective visors, or they will severely limit the time that can be spent in extravehicular space activities. The rays that reach the earth, therefore, are 300–2100 nm in wavelength, with an intensity varying between 10,000 ft-c at ground level to about 13,000 ft-c at presently attainable altitudes.

Visual Functions

The visual apparatus, stimulated by light, primarily must perform three basic functions. It must be able to perceive an object by the detection of light emitted or reflected from it; this is known as light discrimination. Second, it must be able to perceive the details of an object; this is known as visual acuity. Third, it must allow

one to judge distances from objects and to perceive movement in the field of vision. These latter two functions combined are known as spatial discrimination. Obviously, all of these functions are perceived simultaneously; however, in this chapter, they will be discussed separately. Light discrimination consists of brightness sensitivity, which is the ability to detect a dim light; brightness discrimination, which is the ability to detect a change or difference in the brightness of light sources; and color discrimination, which is the ability to detect colors. As noted in Figure 16.7, when the illumination is below a certain intensity, approximately 10^{-6} log ml, the eye does not respond and only total darkness is seen. As the level of illumination increases, one begins to see shapes and objects; this is rod or scotopic vision. At best, this vision is on the order of 20/200 to 20/400 in scope. As illumination increases, such as with snow in full moonlight of 10^{-2} log mL, the threshold for the cones is reached, and this is known as mesopic vision; here, both rods and cones are functioning. A further increase in illumination (such as with white paper under 100 ft-c, equivalent to approximately 10^2 log mL, causes the cones alone to be functional; this is known as photopic vision. The cones are now sensitive to color, and minute details can be appreciated. Increasing the illumination beyond 10^2 log mL does little to enhance

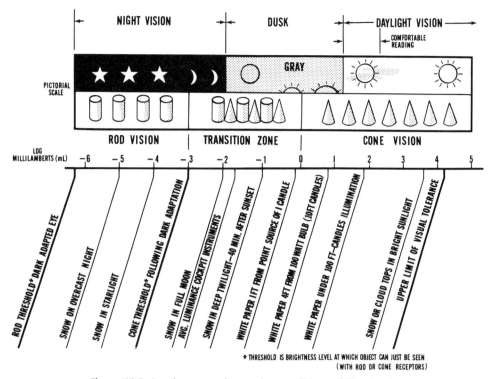

Figure 16.7. Luminance under varying conditions of illumination.

visual efficiency. The upper limit of tolerance for normal vision is 10^4–10^5 log mL of luminance. This would be equivalent to staring at the sun or at the detonation of a nuclear weapon. The eye can adapt to this tremendous range of illumination because of the dual system of rods and cones in the retina. The rods contain the photosensitive pigment rodopsin and are sensitive to minute quantities of light energy. They are also sensitive to motion but not to color. The cones contain photosensitive pigments with maximum absorption at 445 nm (blue), 535 nm (green), and 570 nm (red). The cones must have much more light energy than the rods to be stimulated; however, the cones can perceive fine detail and discriminate colors.

The three psychologic components to color are hue, saturation, and brightness. Hue is the component denoted by naming a color, such as red, yellow, or orange. This is closely related to the wavelength of the light. Saturation refers to adding white light to the pure color so as to de-

crease the saturation of this color. For instance, a spectral red becomes pink when it is mixed with white light. The hue is still red, but its saturation has now been decreased. Finally, brightness relates to the amount of luminous flux reaching the eye. In essence, a source of high intensity or luminance seems brightly colored, for example, bright red or bright yellow, whereas a source of low intensity or luminance appears dark or dull-colored (3).

At night or under low levels of illumination, the fovea, containing all cones, becomes a relative blind spot. Therefore, best vision is attained at night by looking 10–15° off-center to utilize the part of the retina containing both cones and rods. As is noted in the dark adaptation curve (Fig. 16.11), the cones adapt quickly, taking six to eight minutes; however, the rods are much slower in adapting, requiring another 20–30 minutes in the dark. Rods and cones also have different peak sensitivities. The relative luminosity curves of photopic and scotopic vision

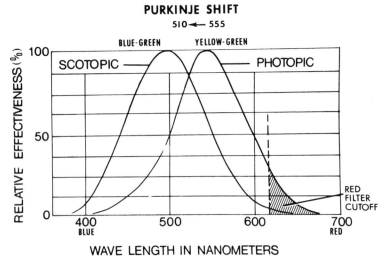

Figure 16.8. Luminosity curves for scotopic (rod) and photopic (cone) vision.

show that scotopic vision (rod function) peaks at 510 nm, whereas photopic vision (cone function) peaks at 555 nm, as shown in Figure 16.8. The difference in these peak sensitivities is the basis of the Purkinje shift. The luminosity curves also show why red filter goggles with a cutoff at 610 nm allow the cones to receive enough light for the individual to function, while greatly reducing the light to the rods and allowing dark adaptation to take place.

The second of the basic functions, visual acuity, is the ability to see small objects, to distinguish separate details, or to detect changing contours. This is usually measured in terms of the reciprocal of the visual angle subtended by the detail. Central (foveal) visual acuity is high, whereas peripheral visual acuity is poor, < 20/200. The retinal distribution pattern of rods and cones causes this difference in visual acuity, as shown in Figure 16.9. The cones are dense in the foveal and macular areas and even have a 1:1 nerve fiber-to-brain relationship in the fovea, whereas images outside of the macular area lose detail, becoming worse in the peripheral retina. In certain areas of the peripheral retina, many hundreds of rods may be connected to a single nerve fiber. This is an excellent system for picking up a minimum of light energy or

detecting motion but poor for perceiving detail. Visual acuity is influenced by the refractive state of the eye. Visual acuity can be separated into four basic types: minimum visible, which is the ability to see a point source of light, with intensity determining whether it can be seen or not; minimum perceptible, which is the ability to see small objects against a plain background, where size (the angle subtended) and contrast become the determining factors; minimum separable, which is the ability to see objects as separate when close together (also known as two-point discrimination); and minimum distinguishable, which is the form sense, usually measured on the Landolt C or Snellen charts and resolving one minute of arc break in the C or thickness in letters at 20/20 visual acuity.

A new form of testing visual resolving power is by the use of contrast sensitivity and gratings (Fig. 16.10). The most useful form for visual testing is the sine form. The use of this sinusoidal form allows the ready application of a powerful mathematical tool, the Fourier transform. A sine grating of 30 cycles/degree visual angle may be compared with one minute of visual angle or 20/20 Snellen equivalent. A contrast sensitivity plot shows that the human visual system is most sensitive in the area of 2–4 cycles/degree (5). This

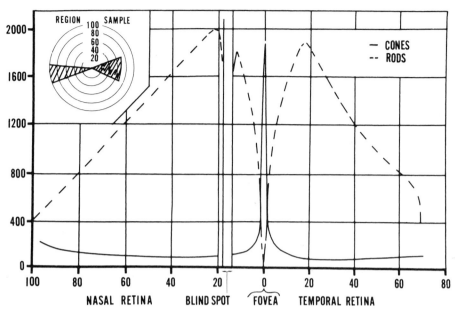

Figure 16.9. Rod and cone density in the retina. (Adapted from Chapanis, RN: Vision in military aviation. Wright Aeronautical Development Center. Wright Field: Technical Report 58–399, 1958.)

method of testing may show reduced contrast sensitivity in conditions such as amblyopia, multiple sclerosis, optic neuritis, cataract, and possibly glaucoma. As yet, this test has not shown any distinct advantage in the testing and screening of aircrew, who are already subjected to an adequate battery of vision tests.

Presently, this testing procedure has more value in the examination and evaluation of aircrew with ocular disease, unexplained visual loss, and research purposes (6).

The third important visual function necessary for aerospace flight is depth perception. This is the judging of distance and the perception of motion in the visual field. Distance judgment, or depth perception, is the ability to judge absolute distance or, more commonly, the relative distance of two or more objects. It is aided by conscious and subconscious cues learned from experience, such as aerial perspective, relative motion, relative size, distribution of light and shadow, overlapping contours, and, perhaps the most important of these monocular factors, motion parallax.

The binocular factors of convergence and stereopsis also are involved in this process. Stereopsis, caused by the disparity of images on the retina of the two eyes, is the most important factor in judging the distance of near objects. In flying aircraft, however, maximum practical limit of stereopsis is believed to be only 200 m.

Vision is a complex physiologic and psychologic process that necessitates a decoding or interpretation of signals coming from the sensor (the eye) to the brain. Environmental stresses may disrupt the delicate physiologic balance necessary for maintaining clear vision and are discussed in ensuing sections.

VISION IN THE AEROSPACE ENVIRONMENT

The aviator and astronaut function in a hostile environment. In this section the effects of this environment on the eye and vision are discussed. Some of the factors affecting vision include hypoxia, decompression, glare, high-speed acceleration, and, if one were to proceed into space, excessive electromagnetic energy, zero gravity, and other factors. All of these factors can

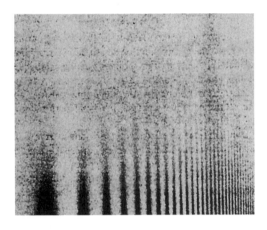

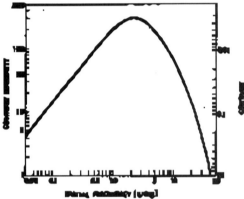

Figure 16.10. Contrast-sensitivity function. Upper half of figure: viewing, the sine gratings shows the effect of contrast and spatial frequency on visual resolution. Lower half of figure: normal contrast-sensitivity curve.

degrade vision and, therefore, one's ability to perform duties at the most effective level possible.

Environment and the Eye

Hypoxia

Vision is the first of the special senses to be altered by a lack of oxygen, as evidenced by diminished night vision. The extraocular muscles become weakened and incoordinated and the range of accommodation is decreased, causing blurring of near vision and difficulty in carrying out near visual tasks. From sea level to 3000 m is known as the indifferent zone because ordinary daytime vision is unaffected up to this altitude; however, slight impairment of night vision occurs such that all combat crews flying at night should use oxygen equipment from the ground up. From 3000–5000 m is the zone of adaptation. Some impairment of visual function occurs; however, this impairment can be overcome sufficiently for duties to be performed. At this altitude, retinal vessels become darker and cyanotic, arterioles show a compensatory increase of 10–20% in diameter, retinal blood volume increases up to four times, retinal arteriolar pressure, along with systemic blood pressure, increases slightly, the pupil constricts, and, at 5000 m, a loss of approximately 40% in night vision occurs. Accommodation and convergence decrease, and one's ability to overcome heterophorias decreases. All of these changes can return to normal when the flyer returns to ground level or uses oxygen. Physiologic compensatory reactions enable flyers to perform normal tasks unless they remain at this altitude for long periods without oxygen. The zone of inadequate compensation is 5000–8000 m, so-called because the physiologic processes can no longer compensate for the lack of oxygen. The visual disturbance described above becomes more severe, with reaction time and response to visual stimuli becoming sluggish. Heterophorias can no longer be compensated for and become heterotropias with double vision. Accommodation and convergence are so weakened as to cause blurred vision and diplopia. Night vision is most seriously impaired. Once again, if one were not subjected to too long a stay at this altitude, all changes would be reversed by the use of oxygen or a return to sea level. Above 8000 m is the zone of decompensation, or lethal altitude. Circulatory collapse occurs, with loss of vision and consciousness, and permanent damage to the retina and/or brain may result from the lack of circulation and hypoxia. Commercial aircraft and other aircraft with pressurized cabins maintain cabin-equivalent pressures of 2500 m. None of the aforementioned visual effects are felt at this altitude except for an almost immeasurable effect on night vision. For smokers, the altitude zones can be considerably lower due to the effects of carbon monoxide (7).

Reduced Barometric Pressure

Decompression sickness is a disturbance that affects the flyer as a result of reduced barometric pressure. Infrequently with decompression sickness, a transitory visual defect consisting of homonymous scotoma or even hemianopia may occur, followed by headache that closely resembles migraine. Even more rarely, the aviator may be afflicted by transitory hemiplegia, monoplegia, aphasia, and disorientation. In rare cases, permanent visual impairment occurs.

Visual Environment

The aviator's visual environment is constantly changing. One travels from night to day, from sunlight to shadow, from well-structured scenes to empty visual fields. Fortunately, the eye is quite adaptable, functioning in light levels from 1×10^{-6} log mL to 1×10^5 log mL. For example, the brightness of the full sun on a cloud is approximately 6×10^3 log mL, snow in full moonlight is 1×10^{-2} log mL, and snow in starlight is 1×10^{-4} log mL. As higher altitudes are attained, the sky darkens, being lighter at the horizon and darker at the zenith. This reverses what is considered normal light distribution, creating a bright view below and darkness above. At high altitudes, less haze is evident and the sun's rays are much more intense, so that 13,600 ft-c of illumination occurs at 30,000 m. A higher proportion of ultraviolet rays are also found at this altitude. For each kilometer (3300 ft) increase in altitude, ultraviolet radiation increases by approximately 6%. Glass sunglasses decrease the intensity of light and protect against ultraviolet radiation as well. Plastic spectacle lenses must have attenuators in the plastic to filter out ultraviolet radiation. New materials, however, such as polycarbonate, being used in the windscreens of modern aircraft substantially reduce the amount of ultraviolet radiation that enters the cockpit. This material cuts off most of the ultraviolet light below 380 nm. The aviator's vision is also affected by the lack of detail in the sky at altitude. This empty field, or space myopia, causes a decrement in his visual capabilities. Finally, changes occur in the appearance of sunlight and areas of shadow. Areas in shadow are illuminated by scattered light, but less light scatter and brighter sunlight occur at high altitude, so that the contrast between the sunlit and shadowed areas increases.

Visibility

Much of modern flying is done in the cockpit. This necessitates good near vision and is dependent on having an adequate amount of visual accommodation. In spite of instruments and radar scopes, one must still see outside the cockpit to land and take off, fly formation, navigate, and, especially, watch for other aircraft. Multiple related factors allow the aviator to see objects in the environment: (1) the size of the target, which is relative to its distance; (2) the luminance or overall brightness; (3) the degree of retinal adaptation; (4) the brightness and color contrast between the target and background; (5) the position of the target in the visual field; (6) the focus of the eye; (7) the length of time the object is seen; and (8) atmospheric attenuation.

The visibility of an object depends mostly on its size and contrast with the background. In daylight, with the best of contrast (a black object on a white background), an object would be seen at near the threshold of visual acuity, subtending 0.5 minute of arc, or the equivalent of 20/10 vision. A speck of light against a black background, such as a star, can be seen even when it is much smaller and obviously at enormous distances; however, this example is not a function of visual acuity but only of light perception. A star appears bigger because it is brighter not because it subtends a larger visual angle. The visibility of objects is lost as the contrast is reduced between the object and its background. In such a case, the object, now with lower contrast, must be much larger or nearer before it can be seen. In conditions of haze or mist, such a marked loss of contrast exists that even a large object may not be seen at all. Newly emerging testing techniques (contrast sensitivity function tests) hold promise for the possible identification of individuals whose systems function more effectively at lower contrast thresholds. The visibility factors outlined above are, to a certain extent, interrelated, so that a reduction in one may be compensated for by an increase in one of the others. For instance, an object may be so small or so far away that it is just below the threshold of visibility. It may be made visible by an increased illumination or by improving the contrast between it and its background or both. In other instances, the object may be better perceived when more time is spent viewing it.

Targets in the periphery of the visual field must be proportionally larger to be seen. To get maximum visibility, the target will have to be seen within 1° of fixation (fovea). When the object in the peripheral field is moving, it is easier to detect.

One final factor capable of degrading target acquisition is empty field or space myopia. Older theories explained that the resting state of the eye was one of zero accommodation. Recently, more sophisticated testing techniques (laser optometer) show that in some individuals, the resting state of the eye is actually one in which a small amount of accommodation is exerted, thus defocusing the eye for distance vision. In the so-called resting states, these individuals have 0.75–1.00 D of myopia, thus degrading their distance visual acuity because their resting focus is 1–1.5 m distant from the eye. This is said to occur in both emmetropic and myopic individuals. Moderately farsighted individuals (hypermetropes), however, may find that this accommodative tonus is actually advantageous and that their distance vision perhaps may be enhanced. In bright daylight, the small pupil produced compensates somewhat for the space myopia by increasing the depth of field; however, a better method of overcoming this induced myopia is to fix on a distant object. Actually, anything more distant than 15–18 m helps to relax the accommodation sufficiently to im-

prove the distance visual acuity. Night myopia, which is similar to empty field and space myopia and is only worse at times, is discussed in the following section on night vision.

Night (Scotopic) Vision

Night vision is extremely important in aviation. It is quite different from day or photopic vision. The eyes must be used differently at night for the aviator to gain maximum usefulness of vision. The aviator must understand the principles of night vision and must practice using the eyes at night to gain efficient night vision.

All parts of the retina are not alike in their reaction to light. A small, central area containing only cones is responsible for maximum visual acuity and for color discrimination, but it fails to operate under low intensities of illumination. This is the fovea, the area with which one reads and where one focuses objects in the direct line of vision. It gives us central vision, which is useful in high and moderate illumination (photopic and mesopic conditions).

In the remaining peripheral area, both the rod-type and cone-type receptors are present. The peripheral retina is capable of less acute visual perception and of only poor color determination, but it functions under low illumination or scotopic conditions. According to the widely accepted duplicity theory of vision, the human eye is an eye within an eye. Central vision requires light of about 1×10^{-3} log mL intensity or greater. Bright moonlight gives about 1×10^{-2} log mL. Hence, in light that is less intense than moonlight, little central vision is evident. Peripheral vision requires only one-thousandth as great an intensity 1×10^{-6} log mL or more. On a dark, starlit night, the individual sees only with the peripheral area of the retina. This explains why pilots often complain that they are able to see an aircraft at night only to have it disappear when they look directly at it. To keep an object in sight at night, one must learn to look off to the side at about a 10 to 15° angle. When the light intensity is between 1×10^{-3} and $10°$

log mL, both the rods and cones are functioning, and mesopic vision occurs (Fig. 16.7).

Individuals can determine which type of vision they are using by noting whether they have color sense. The cones perceive all colors. Rods pick up colors only as shades of gray. Most of the cones are in the central area of the retina, so that if color were recognized at night, one would have central vision; however, if everything were to appear in shades of gray, one would only have peripheral or rod vision.

Dark adaptation is the process by which the eye adjusts for maximum efficiency in low illumination. It is commonly experienced when one first enters a theater or walks into darkness from a brightly lit room. The central area of the retina dark-adapts in about six to eight minutes, but this part of the retina is useless for night vision. The peripheral area dark-adapts in about 20 to 30 minutes, although further slight adaptation continues over a period of two days (Fig. 16.11). This peripheral area is not sensitive to dark-red light (630 nm or longer in wavelength). Such light is not perceived even as gray, so dark adaptation occurs in the periphery in dark-red light as though no light existed. This characteristic is fortunate because, by wearing red, light-tight goggles before a flight, pilots can read or rest in a brightly lit room while the peripheral areas of their retinas are dark-adapting.

Dark adaptation is an independent process in each eye. It is slow to develop in the dark and is quickly lost in the light. The aircrew must be so familiar with the location of their equipment and controls that lights are unnecessary for making adjustments in flight. The aviator should avoid gazing at exhaust stacks or any other bright light sources. When using light at night in the plane, such as in reading instruments, maps, or charts, as little light as possible should be employed and for as brief a time as possible, and red light should be used; however, red lighting does create problems, such as accommodative fatigue and reduction of color perception. Thus, red light is no longer favored for cockpit visual activities. When an individual who is exposed to bright light closes one eye, the closed eye remains dark-adapted, even though the exposed retina has been bleached.

Dark adaptation also depends on an adequate supply of vitamin A in the diet. Vitamin A is found in vegetables that are green or were green at some stage of development, such as lettuce, carrots, cabbage, peaches, tomatoes, green peas, and bananas. Other sources of vitamin A include milk, eggs, butter, cheese, and liver. A deficient diet or an illness that decreases the vitamin A supply impairs night vision and a return to normal vision may take several months, even when large doses of vitamin A are ingested. Excessive vitamin A ingestion, such as in taking large doses of vitamin capsules, is worthless to a normal person. Various drugs also have been studied and have not been found to improve a normal person's dark adaptation.

Under conditions of low-intensity illumination, the peripheral area of the eye is most sensitive to green light and is least sensitive to red light; both colors are perceived as shades of gray, of course, but green light is picked up readily, whereas red light is spotted with difficulty. If a red light with a wavelength of 630 nm or longer were used at an intensity that made it just visible to the central area of the eye, the individual could dark-adapt in 20–30 minutes and have acute vision of the cones available. An observer cannot see this light with peripheral vision, and can spot it with central vision only when fortunate enough to look directly at it. The red warning light on the airplane wing has so

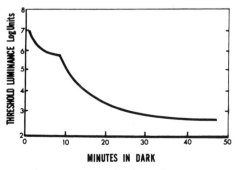

Figure 16.11. Dark-adaptation curve.

much yellow and shortwave red that it easily can be seen at night.

Because of the central blind spot under low illumination, one should not look directly at the objects one needs to see but rather to one side of the object. This seems unnatural, and some practice is required to perfect this technique. The eyes also should not be held in a fixed position at night. The use of a scanning technique with intermittent stops at points of fixation is best for night observation. Objects are seen only by contrast at night; that is, they are either lighter or darker than their surroundings. Ordinarily, aircraft can be seen better when they are above and silhouetted against the sky. Contrast is reduced by fog, haze, and dirty or scratched windshields or goggles. For this reason, goggles, spectacles, and windshields should be scrupulously cleaned for night operation. Reflection of light from instruments on the surfaces also reduces the ability to sight planes at night.

An emmetropic or myopic observer has a shift toward myopia under conditions of reduced illumination. This shift is believed to be due to the spherical aberration of the eye and to involuntary accommodation exerted. This myopia is no different from the previously discussed space myopia. Individuals vary but may have 0.75–1.25 D of increased myopia which, in turn, indicates a decrease in functional visual ability.

Without supplemental oxygen, the average percentage decrease in night vision capability is 5% at 1100 m altitude, 18% at 2800 m, 35% at 4000 m, and a 50% decrease in night vision capability at 5000 m altitude without supplemental oxygen. Oxygen lack, fatigue, and excessive smoking all reduce the ability to see well at night. Oxygen should be used from the time of takeoff for maximum visual acuity. Fatigue should be prevented, insofar as possible, by obtaining adequate sleep prior to flying. Hypoxia resulting from carbon monoxide poisoning affects brightness discrimination and dark adaptation in the same way as altitude-induced hypoxia. As an example, 5% saturation with carbon monoxide has the same effect as flying at 3000

m without oxygen. Smoking three cigarettes before a flight may cause a carbon monoxide saturation of 4%, with an effect on visual sensitivity equal to an altitude of 2800 m or a 15–18% decrease in night vision.

The rules for the most effective use of night vision by pilots include the following:

1. Eat a diet with adequate vitamin A;
2. Become dark-adapted before takeoff;
3. Avoid bright exterior or cockpit light. Make any exposure to light as brief as possible and use light of as low intensity as possible. Close one eye when exposed to a bright light source;
4. Look 10–15° off to one side of objects viewed;
5. Develop a scanning technique to search the sky;
6. In wartime situations, make use of contrast. Fly below an enemy when over dark ground and fly above when over snow, sand, or white clouds;
7. Keep goggles, spectacles, and windshield clean;
8. Use oxygen from takeoff because hypoxia reduces night vision (Fig. 16.12).

During World War II, much work was done on the use of red cockpit illumination. The use of a red light having a wavelength greater than 630 nm illuminating the cockpit is desirable from the viewpoint of dark adaptation. The intent was to retain the greatest rod sensitivity possible while permitting an effective illumination for foveal vision; however, with the increasing use of electronic devices for navigation as well as for enemy aircraft and target detection, the importance of the pilot's visual efficiency inside the cockpit has increased markedly. Therefore, low-intensity white cockpit lighting is presently advocated because it affords a more natural visual environment within the aircraft without degrading the color of objects that are not self-luminous. The disadvantage of the previously used red lighting caused red markings on aerial

THE EYE IN NIGHT VISION

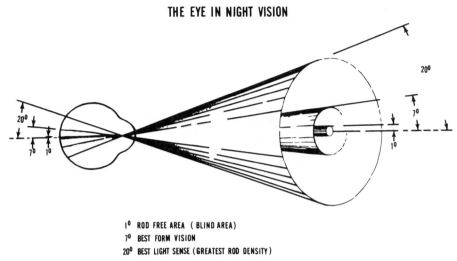

1⁰ ROD FREE AREA (BLIND AREA)
7⁰ BEST FORM VISION
20⁰ BEST LIGHT SENSE (GREATEST ROD DENSITY)

Figure 16.12. Zones of sensitivity for night vision.

maps to be invisible when viewed in this light. Red light also tends to create or worsen near-point blur in prepresbyopic, presbyopic, and, at times, hypermetropic pilots. Because of the chromatic aberration of the eye, humans are hypermetropic for red (8).

Ultraviolet light has been used for cockpit illumination and has a disconcerting side effect if it were to become reflected directly into the eye. These radiations produce a fluorescence of the crystalline lens in the eye, giving the pilot a sensation that he is flying in a fog. Properly adjusting the ultraviolet lamps and reducing their intensity can overcome this fluorescence problem to some degree. Radiations from these lamps are not injurious to the eyes because, even at highest intensity, they are still far below the threshold for affecting the corneal epithelium.

During World War II, the problem of night vision was studied intensively by numerous scientists, but no single, satisfactory test of night vision was developed. The USAF did develop the radium plaque night-vision tester, which is a self-illuminating Landolt C target; however, because it contains radium, it is rarely used today (9).

At present, the best test of night vision is the Goldmann-Weekers Dark Adaptometer. This in-strument is capable of determining the dark-adaptation curve of an individual with great detail and accuracy. It obviously is not something that should be done on everyone because it is time-consuming, the apparatus is expensive, and only research institutions and larger clinics have it available. With this instrument, one can establish the threshold of night vision in an individual. The testing results in the familiar dark-adaptation curve (Fig. 16.11).

The most direct way of protecting and enhancing night vision is by adapting in the dark or wearing red goggles for at least 30 minutes and maintaining an adequate intake of vitamin A.

NIGHT-VISION GOGGLES

Modern technology has also introduced night-vision goggles (NVGs), which enhance vision at night over and above that possible by the naked eye (Fig. 16.13). Presently available NVGs can intensify ambient light to about one-thousand times (1000×). Several electrooptical devices are available to improve vision at night, including NVG and forward-looking infrared (FLIR) systems. Most NVG systems are helmet-mounted and look like binoculars. To make objects and landscape visible at night, NVGs

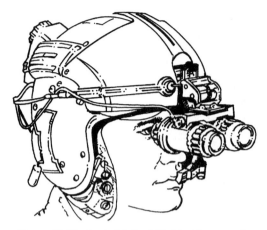

Figure 16.13. Anvis (III-Gen) Night-vision goggle.

usually employ two image-intensifier tubes to amplify or intensify low levels of reflected and emitted ambient light. Image-intensifier tubes are sensitive to some visible and short-wave infrared (IR) radiation, but a minimum amount of ambient light is needed to excite the green phosphor screen and produce visible images.

The NVG-intensified image resembles a black-and-white television image except that it is in shades of green instead of in shades of gray, due to the selected display phosphor. The image that is seen by the aircrew member is not a direct view, but an image displayed on a phosphor screen. The NVG system is analogous to using a microphone, amplifier, and speaker to amplify a faint sound and make it audible. In both cases, some of the "natural fidelity" may be lost in the amplification process.

NVGs enhance night vision over unaided scotopic vision; however, they do have significant limitations. The performance limitations include visual acuity of about 20/40 at best, a field of view of 40° or less, degraded depth perception, little or no stereopsis, and a different spectral sensitivity than the human eye. Thus, training and experience with NVGs is critically important for flying safety (See Chapter 22).

An FLIR device consists of a cockpit-or helmet-mounted video monitor that displays picture from an internal IR sensor that is usually fixed forward (i.e., slaved to the nose of the airplane).

These sensors are sensitive to the long wavelength IR (thermal) and provide excellent resolution. IR sensors can detect radiation in either the 3,000–5,000 nm or the 8,000–12,000 nm spectral range. An FLIR must have thermal radiation available, but many objects radiate measurable amounts of IR energy in the spectral range.

ELECTROOPTICAL DESIGN

A brief description of the operating principles of NVGs will make it easier to understand their workings and limitations. Ambient light entering the intensifier tubes is focused by an objective lens onto a photocathode. The schematic diagram of an intensifier tube is presented in Figure 16.14. When photons of ambient light strike the photocathode, which is sensitive to visible and near-IR radiation, electrons are released, creating a cascading effect. The number of electrons released from the photocathode is proportional to the number of photons striking it. The electrons are then accelerated and multiplied by a microchannel plate which acts like a large array of photomicromultiplier tubes. The microchannel plate, about the size of a nickel, guides the accelerated electrons to a phosphor screen which produces an intensified light image. The light amplification is referred to as the gain of the device. The gain is the ratio of the light delivered to the eye by the phosphor screen to the light striking the objective lens. Modern NVGs have a gain of 400–1,000.

NVGs do *not* turn night into day. Although pilots are usually impressed the first time they look through NVGs, many complaints occur the first time they fly with them. Although it is true that visual function with NVGs is impressively enhanced over scotopic function in many ways, NVG performance is inferior compared to normal photopic function. The degradation in visual performance that NVGs impose must be emphasized to aircrew.

Much more detailed information on NVGs, operational issues, environmental considerations, and fitting techniques is explained in the

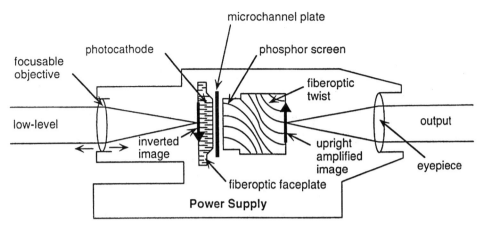

Figure 16.14. Photocathode tube schematic.

publication, "Night Vision Manual for the Flight Surgeon" by Miller and Tredici (10).

Spatial Discrimination, Stereopsis, and Depth Perception

In aviation, it is important to accurately localize in three-dimensional space. When this cannot be done, one becomes spatially disoriented, a marked hazard to the flyer. Under $+1\,G_z$ acceleration, one orients to the earth by proprioceptive impulses from various parts of the body, from receptors in the semicircular canals and vestibular apparatus, and with the strongest cue to orientation, the visual system. Linear and angular accelerations are capable of producing spatial disorientation, especially when outside visual reference is excluded; however, when adequate external visual references are available, spatial disorientation usually does not occur. The pilot's ability to resist spatial disorientation, then, is greatly enhanced by adequate visual references and is diminished by mental stress. The visual cues to the perception of depth are both monocular and binocular. The monocular cues are learned, and some investigators believe that they can be improved by study and training. These cues, however, are the ones that can be the most easily tricked by illusions. Conversely, stereopsis, which is the most important binocular cue, is innate and inescapable. When flyers have this capability, it remains with them, even when the learned cues are sparse, such as at night, under conditions of low visibility, and in unfamiliar surroundings. Unfortunately for flyers, however, the maximum range at which their stereoscopic vision is useful is only up to 200 m. This is not to imply that stereopsis is required in flying an aircraft because numerous individuals who lack stereopsis still make good aviators; however, when the pilot does have stereopsis, so much the better. Therefore, stereoscopic testing procedures should be retained in the flight examination. The stereoscopic test for flying is probably the single most revealing component of the visual examination. Individuals who pass the stereoscopic test down to 15–20 seconds of arc must, of necessity, have well-functioning visual systems. They must have two eyes that are equally balanced: visual acuities must be excellent to attain this kind of arc disparity; they must have normal retinal correspondence; and their motility status must be functioning normally in at least the straight-ahead position. In essence, even if stereopsis had nothing to do with flying, retaining the stereopsis portion of the ophthalmologic examination is wise.

Depth Perception (Spatial Localization)

Depth perception is the mental projection onto visual space of a perceived object in real space.

Correlation of the real object in real space with that projected in visual space results in accurate depth perception. Both monocular and binocular cues to depth perception exist.

The monocular cues are as follows:

1. Size of the retinal image (size constancy)—being able to judge the known and comparative size of objects is an important cue;
2. Motion parallax—the relative speed of motion of images across the retina. Objects nearer than fixation move against the observer's motion, distant objects move in the same direction as the observer's motion;
3. Interposition—one object obscured from vision by another;
4. Texture or gradient—detail loss at increasing distances;
5. Linear perspective—parallel lines converging at distance;
6. Apparent foreshortening—for example, a circle appears as an ellipse at an angle;
7. Illumination perspective—light sources usually are assumed to be from above;
8. Aerial perspective—distant objects appear more bluish and hazy than do near objects.

The binocular cues are as follows:

1. Convergence—the value of this cue is questionable and is generally used only for near distances;
2. Accommodation—also useful only for near distances;
3. Stereopsis—this is the visual appreciation of three dimensions during binocular vision, occurring during fusion of signals from slightly disparate retinal points, which are disparate enough to stimulate stereopsis but not so disparate as to cause diplopia.

The two most important monocular factors for flying are considered to be motion parallax and size of the retinal images. All monocular cues are derived from experience and are subject to

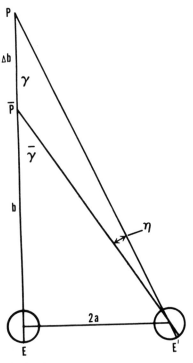

Figure 16.15. Linear stereoscopic depth interval. The eyes fixate point $\bar{P}$; Δb is the linear stereoscopic interval; 2a is the interpupillary distance; b is the fixation distance; $\bar{\gamma}$ is the binocular parallax angle for point $\bar{P}$; γ is the binocular parallax angle for point P; and E and E^1 are the right and left eye, respectively.

interpretation. Stereopsis is believed to be the most important binocular cue and is based on a physiologic process that is innate and inescapable. Like visual acuity, stereopsis can be graded and is known as stereo acuity, which is measured in seconds of arc of disparity. In administering the various tests of stereopsis, the finer the stereoscopic angle is, the fewer the seconds of arc disparity are appreciated (Fig. 16.15).

The limiting distance for stereopsis is shown in the following equation as b_1. The interpupillary distance is 2a and the threshold disparity is n_t:

$$b_1 = \frac{2a}{n_1} \tag{1}$$

The limiting distance varies directly as the interpupillary distance and inversely as the stereopsis threshold (stereo acuity). Theoretically, the limiting distance of stereopsis is about 1300 m; however, for all practical purposes, stereopsis is not reliable beyond 200 m (11).

Stereopsis occasionally is called depth perception and is measured by several different instruments. One can measure stereopsis for near distances, on the Verhoeff depth-perception apparatus, where stereo acuity is measured at 1 m without special optical devices. Stereopsis for near distances also can be measured by the Wirt (Titmus) circles. In this case, the eyes are dissociated with polarizing lenses. Stereoscopic vision for distance is measured in testing devices, such as the Bausch and Lomb Ortho-Rater, Titmus, Keystone or Optec instruments. Using these instruments, separate images are presented to each eye, and lenses in the instruments project the images to 6.1 m or infinity. In essence, these are tests of stereoscopic vision for distance, and many examiners are not aware that in some motility disturbances, such as microstrabismus, the candidate may have normal stereoscopic vision (depth perception) for near but not for distance or vice versa.

Color Vision

In 1920, Drs. William Wilmer and Conrad Berens noted in their article, "The Eye in Aviation," (1) that the proper recognition of colors plays an important part in the success of all types of flyers. Can this still be said today? One would have to answer "yes" because a quick glance at what is required in the form of color discrimination by pilots and aircrew, both military and civilian, indicates that this is true. For instance, aviators and aircrew must be able to identify colored light signals, such as navigation lights, airport beacons, approach lights, runway lights, taxi strips, biscuit gun, Aldis lamp, and the various colors on the instrument panel, as well as the colors of various reflecting surfaces such as flags, panels, smoke, and flares. It is important to be able to identify colors used on maps and charts and, especially in the military, for ascer-

taining the subtle color differences in terrain. Modern aircraft use color extensively in their electronic flight information systems. Under certain conditions, such as in bright daylight, the color contrast of the displays may be degraded. All of this now places more emphasis on the aviator having normal color vision than in the past. Therefore, even though flyers use largely form vision in the performance of their tasks, color vision is a bonus that increases efficiency without demanding much further conscious effort.

Individuals with normal color vision can be identified with near certainty by using pseudoisochromatic plates, which screens normal and abnormal color vision. Another point to be considered, however, is that flying is done predominantly by males, and nearly 8.5% of all males are color-defective. Only 0.5% of females are color-defective. Congenital color vision defects are inherited as a sex-linked recessive trait. Approximately 3% of males with defective color vision fall into a category that is classified as mild, and these individuals have been shown to be safe for aviation duties. The problem is to separate this 3% of men from the 5.5–6% of individuals with moderate-to-severe color-vision deficiencies who are considered unsafe in the aviation environment. At present, this separation can best be done by lantern tests, such as the USAF School of Aerospace Medicine's Color Threshold Tester (CTT), which was devised by Dr. Louise Sloan at Randolph Field in Texas during World War II; however, because of the unavailability of certain Wratten filters, the USAF has removed it from use as a test instrument. Test results done in the past when the instrument was in use are still considered accurate, reliable, and valid. Another lantern that can accomplish this test is the United States Navy Farnsworth lantern. Other more definitive tests of color vision are the 15-hue and 100-hue Farnsworth tests, the Nagel Anomaloscope, and more recently devised tests. The flight surgeon and aeromedical examiner, however, need not go beyond the pseudoisochromatic plate test and perhaps one lantern test. One must point out here, however, that the pseudoisochromatic plate test, whether it be Ishihara, American Optical, Dvorine, or Richmond, must be illuminated with light of proper Kelvin temperature. The most commonly used light is the MacBeth light, which has a temperature of about 6000°K (12).

According to the Young-Helmholtz theory of color vision, three classes of cones are present in the macula. These cones absorb light with peak sensitivities of 445 nm (blue), 535 nm (green), and 570 nm (red), as shown in Figure 16.16. Any color of the spectrum may be constituted with varying combinations of these three primary colors, and when all three colors are stimulated, the color perceived is white. Individuals with defective color vision inherit their conditions. The most severe deficiency is known as monochromatism, a complete absence of color sensation. There are, perhaps, only 1:100,000 such individuals in the general population, with central visual acuities in the 20/200 range, and it is doubtful that they will enter aviation. Individuals with dichromatism constitute 2–3% of the males, and they recognize only two distinct hues. These individuals require only two primary colors to match all hues. The types are protanopia (1% of males, whose only color sen-

sations are blue and yellow and who confuse reds with greens and blue-greens), deuteranopia (also 1% of males, whose only color sensations are blue and yellow and who confuse purple with green), and tritanopia (exceedingly rare, only red and green are perceived).

The vast majority of individuals with defective-color vision are anomalous trichromats. They recognize three distinct hues but have a weakness in one of the hues. Protanomaly, constituting 1% of the males, means red-weak, and these individuals require more red stimulation than normal people to acquire a color match. Deuteranomaly, affecting 5% of males, means green-weak, and these individuals need more green stimulation than normal people to acquire a color match. Tritanomaly, a condition in which more blue stimulation is required to obtain a color match, is exceedingly rare. The pseudoisochromatic plates will screen out all of these anomalous types. The 3% of individuals with mild defective-color vision will be anomalous trichromats and can be identified by various color lantern testing procedures (Table 16.1).

Color vision defects can also be acquired. They are, at least early in the disease, not bilateral as are the congenital defects. These acquired color-vision defects can be brought on by diseases and conditions of the cones in the retina, the optic nerve, and, occasionally, by brain injury. Some of the causes are central serous retinopathy; drug and toxic poisoning, such as by lead, tobacco, or alcohol; diseases of the central nervous system, such as multiple sclerosis; and brain injuries. One simple test that all examiners

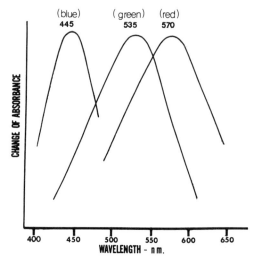

Figure 16.16. Cone-photosensitive pigments. Maximum absorption wavelengths.

Table 16.1.
Incidence of Color-Vision Deficiency

Males	Percent	Females	Percent
Protanopia	1.0	Protanopia	—
Deuteranopia	1.4	Deuteranomaly }	
Protanomaly	0.78	Protanomaly }	0.4
Deuteranomaly	4.6	Deuteranomaly	—
Total*	8.0	Total*	0.4

* Monochromatism occurs in 1/100,000 individuals.

can use to separate the acquired color deficiency from the congenital deficiency (besides a good history) is to examine each eye separately when screening with the pseudoisochromatic color vision plates.

For a long time, designers have thought about engineering the necessity for color vision out of flying. Shape, size, numbers, configurations, and lights would be used rather than color itself. At first, this sounds like a good idea, but it appears to be exceedingly expensive, and tests have proved that it is actually much less efficient than the use of color in a coding system.

A new filter technique has been developed to "cure" color-vision defects. It is the "X-chrome lens," a red, 15–20% transmitting-filter contact lens that is worn on only one eye. The lens has been touted as the device to put individuals with defective color vision into the cockpit; however, recent scientific evaluations have shown that disadvantages to this approach may be more significant than the fact that some individuals wearing this lens can actually pass the pseudoisochromatic plate test. This device has not made the individual's color vision normal; one still may not be able to identify colors in the real world in which the aviator performs and usually will fail the lantern tests (13).

AIRCRAFT/ENGINEERING FACTORS

G Force (Gravity)

The visual system is profoundly affected in high-speed flight by acceleration (G forces), vibration, and a normal lag in human visual perception. On earth, the human body is constantly affected by gravity, and this force is termed 1 G. In flight, the speed, acceleration, and changes in direction can increase the amount and direction of this G force. These G effects are discussed in much more detail in Chapter 9; however, G forces have significant effects on the aviator's vision, and these effects will be discussed here. In flight, the aviator encounters linear acceleration, such as in catapult takeoff, aircraft carrier

landings, ditching, and high-speed bailout. Radial acceleration is encountered in banks, turns, and pullouts from dives, loops, and rolls. Angular acceleration occurs in spins, in storms, and in tumbling following bailout from aircraft. It is the $+G_z$ acceleration that mainly concerns pilots, especially those in high-speed aircraft. When $+G_z$ are being pulled, the quantity of blood returning to the heart is diminished. The heart continues to beat, but diminution of the volume of systolic blood reduces the cardiac output, lowers the arterial tension, and causes a decrease in pressure. Figure 16.17 shows that with increasing G forces, a point will be reached when arterial pressure in the ophthalmic artery no longer exceeds intraocular pressure. It is at this point that visual function is definitely impaired and blackout ensues. However, sufficient perfusion pressure exists in the remainder of the central nervous system so that unconsciousness does not occur until the increasing G force further decreases the arterial pressure and the resulting pressure in the central nervous system is zero. On average, the pilot begins to lose peripheral vision at $+3.5$ to $+4.5$ G_z. Blackout, or a complete loss of vision, occurs at $+4$ to $+5.5$ G_z. Hearing, however, persists and orientation remains. From $+4.5$ to $+6$ G_z the pilot loses consciousness. These are only average values, and they vary depending on the rapidity of onset of the G forces and the physical condition of

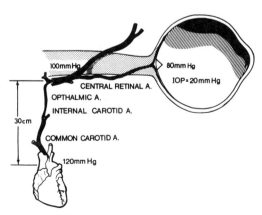

Figure 16.17. Normal arterial blood pressures from the heart to the eye.

the aviator. In the recent past, training, certain maneuvers, and protective clothing enabled the aviator to reach $+8$ to $+9$ G_z and maintain efficiency for longer periods. These factors entail improving one's physical condition, tensing of muscles, performing maneuvers, such as the M-1, and wearing improved anti-G suits. G-force protection could be further enhanced if reclining, tilting seats were available.

Negative G forces are not often encountered. If these forces were prolonged, however, they would result in congestion of the blood vessels of the upper part of the body, leading to a violent headache. Visually, a so-called "red out" may occur. The actual cause of this phenomenon is still unknown; it may be due to looking through a congested lower lid, which then acts as a filter. At high speeds, in order to maintain functional vision, one must maintain a radius of turn large enough so as not to cause excessive G loading. Table 16.2 shows the radii of high-speed aircraft turns that produce $+6$ G forces. For example, at a speed of 3200 kph, pilots could not make a turn in a circle smaller than 27 km in diameter or they would black out unless performing the aforementioned protective maneuvers and were wearing good anti-G suits. Figure 16.18 shows the effects of acceleration and time on vision.

Table 16.2.
Radii of High-Speed Aircraft Turns Producing $+6$ G Forces

Kilometers Per Hour	Number of Meters
400	209
1200	1,882
1600	3,395
3200	13,597

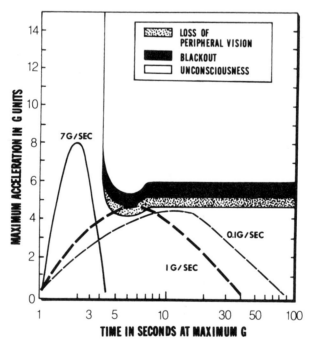

ACCELERATION AND TIME AT MAXIMUM G REQUIRED TO PRODUCE VISUAL SYMPTOMS AND UNCONSCIOUSNESS. CURVES SHOWING DIFFERENT RATES OF G DEVELOPMENT ARE GIVEN TO SHOW THE IMPORTANCE OF THIS PARAMETER FOR THE OCCURRENCE OF PERIPHERAL VISION AND BLACKOUT.

Figure 16.18. Visual effects produced by various $+G_z$ environments.

Vibration

Vibration causes blurred vision and thus reduces the visual efficiency of the aviator. Studies have shown that during vertical sinusoidal vibrations at frequencies above 15 Hz, visual acuity is degraded. Particularly degrading to vision have been the frequency bands in the ranges of 25–40 and 60–90 Hz. When vibration cannot be avoided, its effect on visual performance can be reduced somewhat by the proper design of the visual instruments, displays, and printed materials, and an increase in their illumination and contrast.

Lag in Visual Perception

The length of time between an event and when the person sees the event depends on two factors: the length of time required for light to reach the eye and the conduction time in the visual pathways and brain tracts. Because of the speed of light, the interval between the event and the eye is an unimportant factor, but the lag in the visual mechanism is appreciable and, at supersonic speeds, turns out to be an important factor. This is demonstrated in Figure 16.19. Pilots flying at 1000 kph see aircraft in their peripheral vision; they have traveled 28 m before the images are transmitted from the retina to the brain. They travel 300 m before they consciously recognize it. They travel more than 1 km before they have decided whether to climb, descend, or bank. They travel nearly 1.5 km before they can change their flight path. At 3000 kph, speeds that can be attained in advanced fighter aircraft, all of these distances are tripled. The times noted here are probably absolute minimums and are

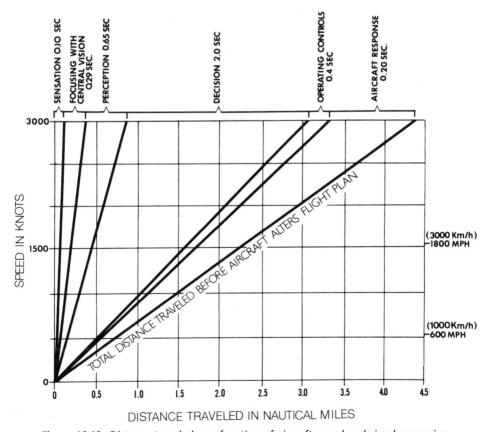

Figure 16.19. Distance traveled as a function of aircraft speed and visual processing.

not reducible by any mechanical or electronic ingenuity solely because they are unchanging characteristics of the human eye, mind, muscle, and nervous system. Conversely, the distance traveled at each interval will undoubtedly increase as the speed of new-generation aircraft increases. Further, one must also be aware that anything that would interfere with the pilot's vision, whether a structural component of the aircraft, the windscreen, his clothing, his spectacles, haze, or grayout induced by G forces, could greatly stretch out the time required to perceive and recognize an event. Pilots must not only identify the object as an aircraft, but they must also decide whether it is a friend or foe. The recognition time will then probably stretch out to perhaps 1.5 seconds, and duration time would probably be in the 4- to 8-second range rather than the 2 seconds indicated in the chart. A pilot may fly blind for thousands of feet while performing such simple operations as glancing at an instrument. At 1000 kph, vision outside the aircraft is interrupted for nearly 1 km. At 3000 kph, vision is interrupted for 2 km. In shifting sight from outside the aircraft to the instrument panel and back, the accommodation time (the time required for the eyes to focus on the instrument), becomes important. Accommodation and relaxation take up a total of 1 second, or 1 km at 3000 kph (14). This is an important factor for the aging pilot who is losing the ability to accommodate. Recognition of the instruments consumes a good deal more than 0.8 second if they were poorly designed or poorly lit. Likewise, if the sky were bright and the panel dim,

the pilot would first have to adapt to the dim light in the cockpit, then readapt to the brightness outside. One can do little to speed up these times. All of this shows that the modern pilot, especially in fighter aircraft, must be given the best design possible in illuminated cockpit instruments. Skimping in this area is unwise because a decrease in the pilot's visual efficiency does not allow for taking advantage of an otherwise superbly designed and powered aircraft.

Aircraft Windscreens

The pilot must, of necessity, look through several layers of transparent materials. One must look through the wind-screen. One also may be using a visor, and, if one were ametropic, spectacles would have to be worn. Vision through these multiple transparencies may be distorted; therefore, it is imperative that the transparencies have a minimum amount of distortion and that the pilot should use as few as possible (Fig. 16.20). Aircraft windscreens are shaped for aerodynamic reasons, and at times these designs are not compatible with the requirements of good visibility. When only flat panels of glass were used in aircraft windscreens, the problems of distortion and multiple images were minimal. Newer aircraft demand compound shapes that can only be fabricated in plastic, and flying high-speed aircraft at low altitudes has introduced another peril: bird strikes. The combination of the aircraft and bird speeds can easily fracture any glass windscreen, necessitating multiple layers of new-generation plastic, such as polycarbon-

Figure 16.20. Different transparencies that may be interposed between a pilot and the world outside the aircraft.

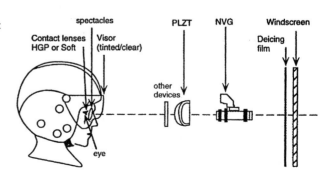

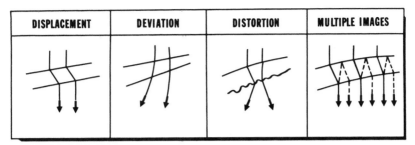

Figure 16.21. Windscreen optical effects.

ate, to withstand the impact created by bird strikes. This, however, has introduced another problem. Because the plastic windscreens are made of multiple layers of the material, a reflection of the image occurs at each layer, and these multiple images can become annoying and contribute to confusing visual effects for the pilot. Light rays striking the windscreen can be displaced, deviated, or distorted, or can cause multiple images, as shown in Figure 16.21. Refracted light is displaced but remains parallel to the incident light. Deviations occur when the refracted light travels at an angle to the incident light, and distortion is relative deviation among numerous refracted rays. The false projection in displacement is so small that it can be ignored. In deviation, however, a larger false projection occurs, whereas distortion causes a misshapen appearance of the objects viewed. Displacement alone occurs only in plain parallel panels and is greater with an increased angle of incidence and an increased thickness of the panel. Deviation occurs when the panel is wedged (in other words, is shaped like a prism) and increases with the angle of incidence and thickness of the transparency and with a decrease in the radius of the curvature. Distortion occurs in irregular, wedged, and curved panels, and it increases with the irregularity of the panel and the angle of incidence, thickness of the glass or plastic, decrease in its radius of curvature, and increase in the distance of the observer from the transparency. Optically, a flat, thin glass or plastic would be the most desirable from the visual standpoint. For the reasons mentioned previously, however,

curved, thick, and laminated transparencies are a necessity in today's aircraft. In the final design, a compromise has to be made between the aerodynamic, optical, and stress considerations (15).

AVIATOR SELECTION—VISUAL STANDARDS

The visual selection of individuals for flying careers, the steps that need to be taken to maintain vision at peak efficiency, and the protection of the eyes from hazards that may affect the peak efficiency of the aviator's vision are discussed in this section. It cannot be denied that vision is the most important sense needed to fly an aircraft or spacecraft. In the early days of scarf, helmet, goggles, and open cockpit, good distance vision was by far most important. With the advent of closed cockpits and cluttered instrument panels, both distance and near vision became absolutely necessary. In modern closed aircraft, flying with spectacles is now acceptable when the refractive error is not too extreme. In military flying, especially in the new advanced fighters, however, spectacles are still a nuisance and, at times, are a definite disadvantage, because of the following:

1. They are uncomfortable on long missions;
2. High G forces may dislodge them;
3. A reduction of light transmission occurs through any transparency;
4. One more transparency is necessary to look through;
5. A limitation of the visual field occurs;

6. Spectacles have a tendency to fog;
7. They give annoying light reflections at night;
8. They are particularly difficult to integrate with other personal equipment;
9. High-refractive powers may cause aberrations and distortions of the image;
10. High-myopic corrections reduce the image size on the retina.

Selection of Candidates for Flying

The techniques used for the visual selection of candidates for flying should not be absolutely restrictive as to eliminate major segments of the population. Different visual demands are required for the aviator, depending on the mission and aircraft. All missions do not require maximum visual capabilities. The examination techniques should be able to select those who have the ability to do the following:

1. Discriminate small, distant objects, as detected by:
   Visual acuity tests for distance;
   Stereoscopic/depth perception tests (confirmatory);
2. Appreciate the relationships between self/aircraft/other objects and the earth, as detected partially by:
   Stereoscopic/depth perception tests;
   Motility-red lens tests;
3. Distinguish small objects as near, as detected by:
   Near visual acuity tests;
   Accommodation tests;
4. Distinguish colors, as detected by:
   Pseudoisochromatic plate tests, Farnsworth lantern, United States Navy and USAF;
   Other color testing lanterns;
5. Distinguish objects in the peripheral field, as detected by:
   Confrontation test;
   Perimeter and tangent screen tests;
6. Vision with reduced illumination, as detected

by:
   History;
   Goldmann adaptometer;
   Contrast sensitivity function test;
7. Use both eyes simultaneously and fuse the images, as detected by:
   Stereoscopic/depth perception tests;
   Cover test;
   Red lens test;
   Heterophoria tests;
8. Perform previous function with eyes rotated in various directions, as detected by:
   Cover test;
   Heterophoria test;
   Red lens test;
   Near point of convergence;;
9. Maintain all of these functions throughout a flying career, as detected by:
   Passing all previous testing procedures;
   Ophthalmologic/fundus examination that reveals a disease-degeneration-free ocular status.

Newer techniques will examine visual function in even greater depth, including contrast sensitivity function measurements, the dark focus examination, dynamic visual acuity tests, analysis of visual processing, electroretinography, electrooculography, and visual-evoked responses. At present, these are mainly laboratory studies. Should these tests be more widely used in the visual examination, they would create more new data to be considered. At present, one would be hard put to decide how all this information would correlate with the performance of such a complex task as flying.

Examination Techniques

History

One should attempt to elicit a complete ocular history from the patient. This would include any ocular disease, injury, medication, operations, loss of vision, double vision, and/or use of glasses or contact lenses. It also would be useful to get a family history of any ocular disorders, especially a history of glaucoma, night blindness, crossed eyes, cataracts, or color blindness.

Equipment for Ocular Examination

The following equipment will save time and make it easier to perform the ocular examination:

1. A flashlight and a second flashlight with a bare bulb that can be used as a point source of light;
2. A distance target, which can be the flashlight with the point source of light;
3. A near target, such as a tongue depressor with a small letter printed on it;
4. Ophthalmoscope;
5. Prisms to measure phorias and tropias if one were not using a vision screener;
6. An occluder;
7. A millimeter scale or a Prince rule;
8. A loupe that magnifies approximately $2\times$.

General Eye Examination

External Examination

The orbits are examined for any abnormality or asymmetry; exophthalmus or enophthalmus is noted. The eyes are then observed for any gross motility disorders or nystagmus. The presence of any tearing or discharge is noted. The lids are examined for symmetry and the presence of any ptosis. Lashes are observed and any inversion or eversion of the lids noted. Inflammation, cysts, or tumors of the lids and margins can quickly be discerned. The palpebral and bulbar conjunctivas can then be examined by everting the upper lid and depressing the lower lid. Here, one looks for hyperemia, injection, discharge, tumors, or pigmentation.

With the use of a flashlight, the pupils are examined. At this time, it should be noted whether any contact lenses are worn. Soft-contact lenses are more difficult to detect, and it may be necessary to use the magnification of the loupe, or better yet a slit lamp, to see them. The pupils are examined for size, symmetry, po-

sition, and reaction (i.e., reaction to the light—direct, consensual, and accommodative). The Marcus Gunn pupillary sign is an extremely valuable indication of an optic nerve or retinal lesion. It is present when pupillary response to light is greater consensually than on direct stimulation, and it is elicited by the swinging light test. For instance, with the light shining in the right eye, the right pupil reacts directly and the left pupil consensually; when the light is swung to the left eye, the left pupil reacts directly and the right pupil consensually. If an incomplete lesion were present in the right optic nerve, the right pupil would dilate somewhat when the light is switched back to the right from the left eye, that is, the consensual light response is greater than the direct light response. This indicates a positive Marcus Gunn pupillary sign.

The ocular examination is completed by observing the corneas, anterior chambers, irides, and as much of the lenses as possible with the flashlight and loupe. The corneas should be free of opacities and vascularization. With experience, the depth of the anterior chambers can be estimated, the irides observed for any cysts, tumors, or unusual pigmentation, and the lenses observed for opacities.

CORNEAL TOPOGRAPHY

With the advent of refractive surgery, especially radial keratotomy (RK) and photorefractive keratectomy (PRK), more advanced types of corneal examination and measurement have developed, allowing the examiner to know whether these procedures have been performed on the eye. Computer-assisted video keratography (corneal topography) has evolved as an instrument to accurately evaluate the status of the anterior corneal curvature (16). Early keratoconus can now be more readily diagnosed, and contact lens fitting is enhanced by having this more accurate corneal curvature data.

Visual Acuity/Refractive Errors

At 6 m, the entire letter on the 20/20 line subtends the visual angle of five minutes of arc. As shown in Figure 16.22, each component of the letter subtends one minute of arc, so that 20/20 indicates that at 6 m this individual can identify the component parts of the test letters. Vision should be tested in each eye separately, first without spectacles and then with spectacle correction. When they have below-normal visual acuity without correction and have no spectacles, patients may be tested with a pinhole of 2–2.5 mm in diameter. An improvement in visual acuity signifies that the subnormal vision is most likely due to a refractive error. If visual acuity were not to improve, most likely an opacity in the cornea or lens or a defect in the retina or optic nerve is present. If spectacles were used but did not improve the patient's visual acuity

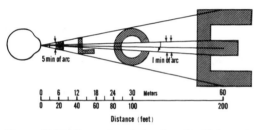

Figure 16.22. Geometry of visual acuity. (Adapted from Adler FH: Physiology of the eye: clinical application. St. Louis: C.V. Mosby Co., 1970.)

to 20/20, the pinhole test also can be used over the spectacles. An improvement in vision signifies that a change in the patient's prescription is indicated. Figure 16.23 shows the approximate visual acuity for spherical refractive errors up to +4 (hypermetropia) or −4 D (myopia).

Refractive errors are only rarely due to disease processes. They are mainly a mismatch between the diopteric power of the refractive system of the eye and the length of the globe. With a close match of these components, the individual is nearly or actually emmetropic. A mismatch can lead to hypermetropia (farsightedness) when the globe is too short for the refractive power, or the individual can be myopic (nearsighted) when the diopteric power of the refractive surfaces is too strong; therefore, the eye is relatively too long. The third and most common aberration is astigmatism. This is most often due to an asphericity of the cornea; that is, one meridian of the cornea has a higher diopteric power or is more curved than a second meridian located at 90° from it. The rays of light passing through an astigmatic eye form a path known as Sturm's conoid. This form of astigmatism is known as regular astigmatism and can be corrected by cylindric and spherocylinder lenses. Occasionally,

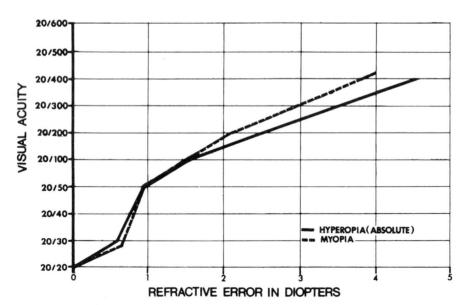

Figure 16.23. Visual acuity as a function of refractive error.

an eye is encountered that has irregular astigmatism; in this case, the astigmatism's maximum and minimum powers are not at 90°, and this form of astigmatism can only be corrected by contact lenses. The hard contact lens can uniquely correct this deficiency because the tear film layer beneath the contact lens fills in the irregularities of the astigmatic cornea. If the candidate's vision were worse than 20/20, refraction should be required. A cycloplegic refraction is preferable because it totally relaxes the accommodation and thus yields the true and total refractive error. This especially helps to delineate the refractive errors in hypermetropes because these young, farsighted individuals obscure the total amount of their error by exerting an accommodative effort, which corrects some part of the spherical error; however, accommodation does not help to correct a myopic error. In fact, accommodation increases myopia and makes the refractive error even worse. Astigmatic individuals may not be able to see clearly at either near or far distances. Only a cylinder or spherocylinder or contact lens correction can clear their vision. Accommodation may be of some help in mildly astigmatic individuals by shifting Sturm's conoid on the retina to the circle of least confusion. As is the case with the hypermetropic individual, however, this takes ciliary muscle effort, and symptoms of fatigue and blurred vision would ensue if the refractive error were not corrected.

To see clearly at near distances, the diopteric power of the crystalline lens must be increased an appropriate amount for the distance of the object seen. After the age of 45, most individuals do not retain sufficient accommodation to see clearly at reading distances of 33–35 cm. This condition is known as presbyopia and must be corrected by plus lenses when one wishes to be able to read at near distances.

Distant visual acuity can be examined in a 6-m lane with an eye chart or a projector chart. A smaller room, such as a 3- to 4-m room, can be used with reverse charts and mirrors. Perhaps the best way for a flight surgeon or aeromedical

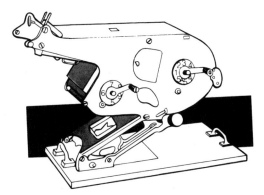

Figure 16.24. Vision screener used to assess visual function.

examiner to check the visual acuity and other visual functions as well is by using a vision screener, such as the one shown in Figure 16.24. These instruments conveniently check a patient's distance and near visual acuities, phorias, and stereopsis. Without a screener, near vision also can be examined with a near vision test card held at 33–35 cm as per the instructions on the card. Each eye is tested separately.

Accommodation is tested in each eye separately using a Prince rule or its equivalent. One must be aware that when the patient has a refractive error, accommodation is tested through the spectacles. Should patients be presbyopic and wearing bifocals or trifocals, they must be tested only through the upper, or distance, part of the spectacles and not through the bifocal or trifocal. Allowing the patient to look through the bifocal portion alters the test and adds accommodative amplitude equal to the value of the strength of the bifocal. Figure 16.25 shows that accommodation normally decreases with age at an almost constant rate. It becomes manifest at about age 45 because most reading materials subtend a visual angle that is too small to see if held much beyond 0.3 m from the eye.

Motility

Normal ocular motility is expected in individuals who will be controlling aircraft. Diplopia or loss of stereopsis at a critical phase in flight could be devastating. The physician looks for straight eyes in the primary position of gaze and ensures that they remain so when taken into the six cardinal positions of gaze, as shown in Figure 16.26. As discussed earlier in this chapter, the six extraocular muscles rotate the eyes into infinite positions of gaze by the use of the yoke muscles operating under Hering's law of equal and simultaneous innervation to each yoke muscle. The yoke muscles and their actions are shown in Figure 16.27. A manifest deviation of the eyes is known as a tropia and usually can be observed by inspection and quantitated by the Hirschberg test, that is, observing the position of the corneal light reflex in the deviating versus the fixing eye, as shown in Figure 16.28. A phoria, conversely, is a latent deviation. It is only present when fusion (binocular viewing) is interrupted, such as by an occluder, a Maddox rod, or a red lens placed over one eye. Tropias are

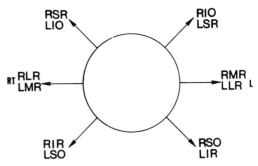

Figure 16.27. Yoke muscles.

present in approximately 3% of the population, whereas phorias are present in nearly 100% of the population, meaning that, in essence, a phoria is normal unless it is extreme. It measures the resting state of the eyes. The eyes can be deviated inward, which is an esotropia or esophoria; deviated outward, which is an exotropia or exophoria; or deviated upward or downward, signifying hyper- or hypotropia or phoria.

An individual with a tropia (strabismus) may be seeing double, suppressing the vision in the deviated eye, or the eye may be amblyopic, with ensuing poor vision in that eye. Because almost all individuals have a phoria, it is not of too great a concern unless it is excessive. If the phoria were excessive, a large neuromuscular effort would be required to maintain fusion and, therefore, single binocular vision. Any added stress may cause a breakdown of fusion, thus leading to diplopia and loss of stereopsis. Hypoxia and fatigue are common stresses to the aviator that can alter phorias; this is the principal reason for taking phoria measurements as part of the visual

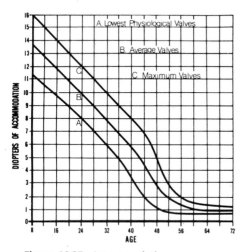

Figure 16.25. Accommodation-age curve.

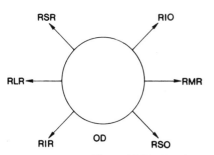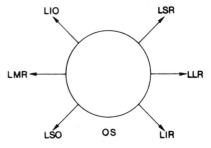

Figure 16.26. Muscle actions in the cardinal positions of gaze.

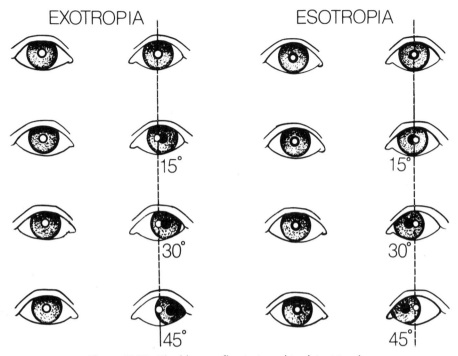

Figure 16.28. Hirschberg reflex test used to detect tropias.

examination for flying. The easiest way for an aeromedical examiner to accurately measure phorias is by use of a vision screener. Ophthalmologists and optometrists mainly use a Maddox rod, occluder, and prisms in the eye lane to detect and measure phorias. As has already been mentioned, the Hirschberg (inspection) test delineates a large-angle tropia. Small-angle tropias can only be detected by the cover test.

In doing the cover test, one uses an opaque occluder and has the patient fixate on a target at distance or one held at near while the examiner observes the position of the eyes. The right eye is covered and the left eye observed; if the left eye moves, it must not have been fixing, and the patient has a left tropia. This can be esotropia, exotropia, or hypertropia. Should the examiner cover the right eye and, while observing the uncovered left eye, note that the left eye does not move, the examiner would then cover the left eye and observe the uncovered right eye. If the right eye moves, it signifies a tropia; if the right eye does not move, no tropia exists because both

right and left eyes were fixing on the target. If no tropia were noted on the cover test, the examiner could proceed to the alternate cover test in which the right eye is covered and then the left eye, and then back to the right eye, and back to the left eye, and so on. The examiner observes the uncovered eye. If movement occurs to take up fixation on the target because the eye was deviated (phoric) under cover, this constitutes a phoria. Movement outward means the eye was in, or esophoric; movement inward means the eye was out, or exophoric. Should no movement of the uncovered observed eye occur, the examiner has noted a rare case of no phoria, or orthophoria.

The near point of convergence is also important in this examination because it too is influenced by hypoxia and fatigue. The near point has a tendency to recede under these conditions. Normally, the near point of convergence is 100–120 mm from the eye, but in military aviators, the near point of convergence is expected to be 70 mm or less. The Prince rule can be used to do this test. A small, dim light or a small test target is brought forward along the rule until the patient breaks fusion and sees double. Simultaneously, the examiner notes that one of the eyes deviates out. A measurement at that point is the near point of convergence and should be within acceptable limits.

When the examiner notes nystagmus, whether it be pendular or rotary, when occluding an eye, the patient should be to an ophthalmologist for a complete evaluation.

Color Vision

The pseudoisochromatic plate test differentiates between individuals with normal color vision and those with defective color vision. Approximately 8.5% of the male population fails this test. Approximately one-third of these individuals can be classified as having only mild color deficiencies and are considered safe for flying. The other two-thirds, those with moderate and severe color deficiencies, are considered hazardous in the flying environment. The plates most commonly used are Ishihara, Dvorine, American Optical, and Richmond. All of these must be administered with the proper illumination of approximately 6000° K temperature. These tests are best administered under the MacBeth lamp. Ordinary tungsten lighting will increase the pass rate for some people with defective color vision, especially those with deuteranomaly (green-weak). The Dvorine and American Optical tests consist of 14 plates and one demonstration plate. Ten or more correct responses are necessary for the patient to be considered as having normal color vision. The USAF and the Federal Aviation Administration (FAA) utilize various color lanterns to test those who fail the pseudoisochromatic plate test. In the past, the USAF used the School of Aerospace Medicine Color Threshold Tester, in which eight different colors with eight different intensities are presented to the patient. A passing score of 50 or better of the 64 available colors identified the individual with mildly defective color vision who would be eligible for aviation duties. The

test was given in a darkened room at a 3-m distance. The USAF has discontinued the test because the Wratten filters could not be supplied. Past tests done on the lantern are still valid. The Farnsworth color lantern is presently used in place of the CTT. The United States Navy Farnsworth color lantern consists of nine presentations of two colored lights each, for a total of 18 colors. This test can be administered under room illumination or in a darkened room, also at a 3-m distance. If any errors were made on the first test, the patient would be retested twice. An average of more than one error for both series of nine color pairs is a failing score. The Farnsworth panel D-15 is a reliable, readily available, color vision test that fails dichromats and severely anomalous trichromats, while allowing mild and moderate anomalous trichromats and normals to pass.

Stereopsis/Depth Perception

Tests of binocular vision given to aviators are usually referred to as depth perception tests. In reality, they are tests of stereopsis, one component in the perception of depth. Visual screeners, such as the Bausch and Lomb, Titmus, Keystone, or OPTEC with excellent test slides quantify stereopsis down to as fine as 15 seconds of arc. Military flyers are expected to have stereopsis of at least 25 seconds of arc disparity. These tests, done in visual screeners, are at optical infinity; therefore, they are distance tests. Near tests of stereopsis are also available, such as the Verhoeff, with its three bars of varying width. This test is administered at 1 m without any special optical devices. The patient should be wearing spectacles, when needed, to correct for distance, and the patient must have no failures in the eight presentations to pass the Verhoeff depth perception test. This equals approximately 32 seconds of arc disparity. Another commonly used near-stereoscopic test is the Wirt. This test necessitates using polarizing glasses but has the disadvantage of only going to 40 seconds of arc disparity. Normal room illumination is used for all three stereo tests.

Field of Vision

Aeromedical examiners need only do confrontation fields, which compare the monocular field of the examiner and the patient. Any aberration in this field examination or history of neurologic disease or increase in intraocular pressure necessitates that a more precise perimetric study be done on a tangent screen or perimeter. Perimeters, such as the Goldmann hemispheric, have been the standard since the late 1950s. However, over the past decade, automated static threshold perimetry is becoming the new standard for evaluating the visual field, especially in patients with glaucoma. The Humphrey and Octopus models are the most popular. The extent of normal visual fields is shown in Figure 16.29.

Night Vision

Night vision is not routinely tested unless indicated by history. If a history of difficulty in seeing at night were elicited, dark adaptometry would be indicated. This test must be accomplished by referring the patient to a center that has an adaptometer.

Intraocular Pressures

Glaucoma is a disease of maturity. Most of the glaucoma seen in aircrew members is of the open-angle variety, which is rarely found in individuals below the age of 40. The intraocular pressure measurements need only be done in individuals 35 years of age or older. If, however, a family history of glaucoma were to exist, intraocular pressure measurements should be done at any age. Yet, recently more patients with "pigmentary glaucoma" are being diagnosed. This is an open-angle type of glaucoma with pigment derived from the iris, causing a blockage of the trabecular meshwork (17). These individuals, who are usually mildly myopic, are first noted to have pigmentary dispersion syndrome, with a worsening of the condition to pigmentary glaucoma. The USAF now screens aviators for an increase in intraocular pressure beginning at age 29 and at each complete physical thereafter. Schiøtz (indentation) tonometry is most readily available for the aeromedical examiner. Applanation tonometry is an excellent technique; however, this takes more practice and requires the availability of an expensive slit lamp. In any case, the results are comparable regardless of which instrument is used. Space-age technology has brought us the air or puff tonometer. It also gives reliable results in experienced hands. Any intraocular pressures consistently over 22 mm Hg should be referred for a full glaucoma workup. Most of these individuals will be found to have only intraocular hypertension; that is, they will show an increase in intraocular pressure without any field loss or disk cupping. This condition generally requires no treatment; however, these individuals must be followed carefully at regular intervals, such as every three to six months, with intraocular pressure measurements, ophthalmoscopy, and visual field examinations. If their conditions were to deteriorate, as indicated by scotomas in the visual field or abnormal cup-to-disk ratios, treatment would be indicated and consultation should be sought from an ophthalmologist immediately.

Internal Examination

The final part of the examination for flying is an examination of the clear media and fundus

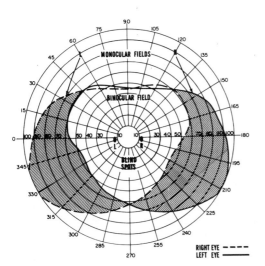

Figure 16.29. Normal visual fields.

of the eye. To get a good look at the fundus, the pupils should be dilated. In light-colored irides, two drops of 2.5% phenylephrine will suffice to dilate the pupil without altering the accommodation. With a darker-colored iris, a short-acting cycloplegic agent will probably have to be added to dilate the pupil sufficiently to view the fundus. One drop of 1% cyclopentolate or 1% tropicamide along with one drop of 2.5% phenylephrine will dilate the pupil for several hours. The examiner views the patient's right fundus with the right eye, then switches the direct ophthalmoscope to the left eye to view the patient's left fundus. A +6- or +8-D lens is rotated in the ophthalmoscope, and the red reflex is visualized at about 15 cm from the eye and examined for opacities, streaks, or any other alterations. If any of these conditions were noted, the patient should probably be referred for a consultation.

Moving closer to the pupil and simultaneously reducing the power of the plus lens, at some point near the zero power—when the patient and examiner have only minimal refractive errors—the optic disk and vessels of the fundus come into view (Fig. 16.30). If they were not seen until high-powered minus lenses were rotated into the ophthalmoscope, the patient's refraction could be estimated. In this case, the patient would be myopic. If it were to take plus lenses to view the patient's fundus, hypermetropia would be diagnosed. The examiner now views the optic disk and cup and estimates the cup-to-disk ratio. Then one looks at the arterioles and veins as they leave the optic nerve in

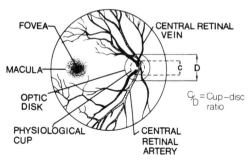

Figure 16.30. Normal fundus details.

all four quadrants. Finally, the examiner looks at the macula and fovea. Normal fundus details are shown in Figure 16.30. If the examiner were to have trouble locating the fovea, the patient should be asked to look at the ophthalmoscope light, and this area will be brought into view by the patient as fixation occurs on the light. Individuals with fundus abnormalities should be referred to an ophthalmologist for diagnosis and possible treatment.

MAINTENANCE OF VISION

Individuals preparing for a lifelong career in aviation should have a thorough ophthalmologic examination. For a military flying career, long-term prediction of the health of the visual system is extremely important because it is expected that the aviator will serve for at least 20 years. Examiners should strive to select individuals with excellent visual capabilities who are up to the visual demands of the duties to be performed. The selection of individuals with disease-free visual systems will go a long way toward assuring a 20 + year flying career. Periodic reexaminations will aid in maintaining a disease-free ocular system. Proper nutrition is vital to the maintenance of the visual system. Vitamin A is necessary for night vision and to aid in the production of visual pigments, whereas the water-soluble B vitamins protect against nutritional amblyopia. Protection from physical forces in daily activites, sports, and in the aircraft is important. Protection from excess electromagnetic energy is also a necessity. This energy can be an occupational hazard encountered in aviation. If ocular disease or injury were found, proper, timely, and correct treatment would speed recovery. This treatment should be followed by a reevaluation to consider the degree of impairment, if any, and its possible effects on the aviator's flying efficiency. Finally, the aeromedical examiner or flight surgeon should educate all aircrew in the proper use and care of their eyes and vision.

Many drugs are used to diagnose and treat

ocular conditions. Most of these drugs should be left to the use of the ophthalmologist; however, the aeromedical examiner should have a basic knowledge of the action of certain commonly used drugs on the eye. The eye is an excellent field to observe the pharmacodynamics of the autonomic nervous system. Both the sympathetic and parasympathetic parts of the autonomic nervous system innervate the pupil and ciliary body. The dilator muscle of the pupil is innervated by the sympathetic nervous system, and the sphincter is innervated by the parasympathetic nervous system. The ciliary muscle involved in accommodation is innervated by the parasympathetic nervous system. Some common ophthalmic drugs and their actions are summarized in Table 16.3.

The aeromedical examiner should consult an ophthalmologist when atropine or steroid preparations are to be prescribed. Finally, one should never prescribe ocular anesthetic agents for use by the patient.

Conditions Affecting the Aviator's Vision

Once selected with a disease-free visual system, the aviator usually remains so for several decades except for minor refractive changes and the universal onset of presbyopia in the fifth decade of life. Young flyers, especially those who do not use spectacles, may become victims of ocular trauma. Ocular trauma can be devastating to a flying career. Aeromedical examiners should warn their patients to use protective goggles or impact-resistant spectacles for all sports in which a high-speed missile may be involved, such as handball, tennis, squash, and hockey.

Table 16.3.
Common Ophthalmic Drugs

Dilate Pupil	
Adrenergic (Sympathomimetic; Dilating, Direct-acting)	Anticholinergic (Parasympatholytic; Competitive Antagonists to Acetylcholine)
Epinephrine (alpha and beta)	Atropine
Norepinephrine (alpha)	Scopolamine
Phenylephrine (alpha)	Homatropine
Isoproterenol (beta)	Cyclopentolate
Timolol (beta-blocking)	Tropicamide

Constrict Pupil—Cholinergic (Parasympathomimetic)	
Direct-acting	Indirect-acting (Anticholinesterase)
Pilocarpine	Edrophonium
Carbachol	Isofluorophosphate (DFP)
Methacholine	Echothiophate

Drug	Concentration	Begin Effect	Duration
Pilocarpine	0.5 to 6%	15 minutes	4–6 hours
Tetracaine (Pontocaine)	0.25 to 0.5%	1 minute	15 minutes
Proparacaine (Ophthaine)	0.5%	30 seconds	10 minutes
Lidocaine (Xylocaine)	1%, 2%	5 minutes	3–4 hours
Phenylephrine (Neo-Synephrine)	2.5%, 10%	10 minutes	2 hours
Atropine	0.5 to 2%	2 hours	7–14 days
Homatropine	2 to 5%	30 minutes	6 hours
Cyclopentolate (Cyclogyl)	0.5%, 1%, 2%	15–30 minutes	24 hours
Tropicamide (Mydriacyl)	0.5%, 1%	15–20 minutes	2–3 hours

Injuries to the eye should be referred at once for definitive diagnosis and treatment. In the older aviators, glaucoma or intraocular hypertension (preglaucoma) is often encountered. With the latest medical philosophy on when treatment for glaucoma should be instituted and with new medications that do not secondarily affect vision, one need not fear the effects of glaucoma on a flyer's career. Observation and the treatment regimen pioneered at the USAF School of Aerospace Medicine (USAFSAM) have kept 95% of these Air Force patients on flying status for a full career (18). Those individuals with intraocular hypertension (intraocular pressure > 22 mm Hg but < 30 mm Hg, without field defects) are observed at regular intervals without treatment. Those individuals with glaucoma (> 30 mm Hg or with visual field or optic disk changes at any pressure) are treated with either levo-epinephrine or β-blocker eye drops with remarkable success without creating secondary visual aberrations. Recently, the laser has also been used to treat glaucomatous conditions. For instance, trabeculoplasty is now often used for open-angle glaucoma treatment. Microscopic laser burns are placed in the trabecular meshwork. This enhances the outflow of aqueous and may eliminate the need for ocular medications. In the more rare, narrow-angle glaucoma, the laser can be used to create an iridotomy. Previously, this necessitated surgical iridectomy. Both of these procedures are used in USAF aviators, allowing them to return to full flying duties.

Retinal disorders also are seen in the younger patients. Central serous retinopathy, an edema of the macula of unknown origin, plays havoc with a pilot's stereopsis/depth perception. Fortunately, 97% of these afflicted individuals recovered and were returned to full flight status as noted in a recent review of USAF aviators with this condition (19). Older flyers may develop macular degeneration that may eventually end their flying careers because presently no effective treatment exists.

A small number of flyers may develop keratoconus or irregular astigmatism, but many of these individuals can be returned to full flight status by the proper fitting of hard-contact lenses. A recent article showed that 82% of USAF aviators with a diagnosis of keratoconus were returned to full flight status (20).

A fair number of individuals suffer from migraine, but only a few flyers complain of it to the aeromedical examiner. The most significant aspect of this condition for flying personnel is developing a central scotoma during an attack or becoming incapacitated by the headache that may follow.

Cataracts commonly are seen in the older flying population or as a result of ocular trauma. If the opacity were dense enough, it would affect vision and, therefore, a flyer's career. Modern surgical procedures and operative or postoperative optical correction by either an intraocular lens placed into the eye at surgery or by a contact lens fitted after surgery should allow many individuals to pass the visual examination and return to flying. Recent data shows that this procedure is quite successful, even in military aviators. In 52 eyes with intraocular lenses, 96% attained 20/20 visual acuity and 86% were returned to full flight status, three being grounded for nonophthalmologic disease and three for ocular complications. The longest follow-up in these patients has been eight years (21).

Correction of Refractive Errors

Standard Techniques

Refraction is a procedure used to determine the lens power needed to correct a patient to emmetropia. The refractive error can be estimated by retinoscopy, which is usually done following the use of cycloplegic eye drops. A manifest or subjective refraction is done with lenses, crossed cylinders, or astigmatic dials, and a third and common way of calculating the refractive error is with a lensometer, which measures the patient's present spectacle correction. If spectacles were to correct the patient's vision to 20/20, nothing further would need to be done concerning the refraction. The aviator's distance

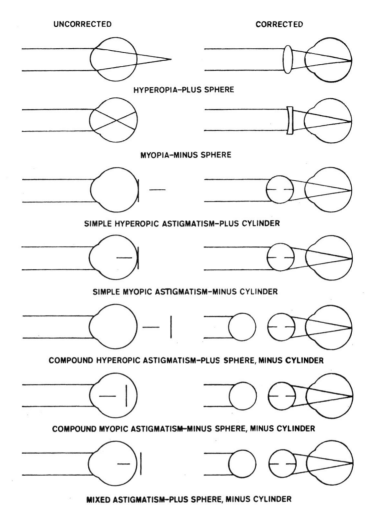

UNCORRECTED   CORRECTED

HYPEROPIA–PLUS SPHERE

MYOPIA–MINUS SPHERE

SIMPLE HYPEROPIC ASTIGMATISM–PLUS CYLINDER

SIMPLE MYOPIC ASTIGMATISM–MINUS CYLINDER

COMPOUND HYPEROPIC ASTIGMATISM–PLUS SPHERE, MINUS CYLINDER

COMPOUND MYOPIC ASTIGMATISM–MINUS SPHERE, MINUS CYLINDER

MIXED ASTIGMATISM–PLUS SPHERE, MINUS CYLINDER

Figure 16.31. Refractive errors and corrective lenses.

refraction changes little during the ages of 20s and 30s. After the age of 40, even though the error for distance may remain static, a correction for early presbyopia is often necessary. Spherical plus lenses correct the deficient accommodation. Once presbyopia has commenced, the patient needs to be reexamined every two years to maintain clear, comfortable near vision. A half-eye spectacle will suffice for the patient with no error in distance vision, but bifocals will be needed to correct the error in those who also require a correction for distance. Figure 16.31 depicts all the refractive errors except presbyopia. Lenses used to correct each type of error also are shown.

The use of contact lenses to correct refractive errors began about 35 years ago. They have found acceptance in civilian aviation and since 1989 have also been used in military aviation.

After a formidable research effort, the USAF now allows its aviators to use soft-contact lenses in place of spectacles. A limited number of tested soft-contact lenses are approved for use. Flyers with astigmatism over 0.75 diopters are fitted with toric soft lenses. The major problem encountered has been the dry cockpit environment. To date, the USAF Soft Contact Lens Program has been a success (22). Hard lenses are made of polymethyline-thacrylate (PMMA) and soft contact lenses of hydroxyethylmethacrylate

(HEMA) and silicone plastics. The hard lenses are used in a limited manner by the military to correct visual defects, such as irregular astigmatism, keratoconus, and aphakia. The soft contact lens is more comfortable to wear, less time is needed for adaptation, and the soft lens rarely alters the corneal curvature. Soft lenses, however, do have a significant drawback for aviators in that they cannot correct astigmatism of over 1 D. In certain individuals, hard lenses may temporarily or permanently mold the cornea to a different refractive status or curvature. This could fortuitously improve the vision or it could lead to corneal warpage and degrade visual acuity.

New Techniques for Refractive Error Correction

In the preceding discussion, it was stated that hard contact lenses could mold the cornea and alter the refractive error. About two decades ago, some practitioners attempted purposefully to alter the corneal contour with contact lenses in the hope that it would improve the vision to where no contact lenses or spectacles would be necessary. This procedure is called orthokeratology (to straighten the cornea). Evaluation of the technique has shown that in some instances, corneas will change contours, usually flattening, reducing the myopia while one is wearing the lenses. On removal of the lenses, however, most corneas revert to their original curvatures and refractive errors in several weeks' time. Occasionally, this procedure results in a permanent increase in "with the rule" astigmatism, and in rare cases the cornea may warp so that the condition cannot be distinguished from keratoconus. Orthokeratology can alter the corneal curvature, but the procedure is highly unpredictable and is not permanent (23).

Refractive Surgery

Over the past 15 years, a rediscovered technique to alter the refractive status of myopic individuals has been employed. It is a surgical procedure

called radial keratotomy. Radial K, as it is known, involves making four, eight or 16 radial incisions in the corneal stroma down to the depth of Descemet's membrane, reaching radially to the limbus, and sparing a central 3- or 4-mm pupil. On healing, the cornea flattens in the center, thus altering the radius of curvature in that area and hopefully decreasing the myopia sufficiently to render the patient emmetropic. Just as in orthokeratology, this procedure is unpredictable; however, radial K is much more permanent (24). Pilot aspirants willingly undergo this procedure in an attempt to pass entrance examinations. Presently, the USAF is not accepting individuals who have had this surgery because of the unpredictability of results, frequently noted fluctuations in visual acuity, an increased susceptibility to glare, and, primarily, because the long-term (10–15 years) status of the corneal integrity is as yet not known.

For the past decade, a new form of refractive surgery has been in development. This is excimer laser photorefractive keratectomy (PRK). The excimer, at 193 nm wavelength, is in the ultraviolet part of the electromagnetic spectrum. It ablates a thin layer of the central cornea, creating a new anterior surface curvature, thus altering the refractive power of the cornea. Presently, it is being used mainly for the correction of myopia. It works best on myopia of low degree (-1.00 diopter to -3.00 diopters). High myopia (-6.00 to -8.00 diopters) shows more complications. Federal Drug Administration (FDA) clinical trials and foreign reports show that 60–90% of low myopes obtain 20/40 or better visual acuity following this laser surgery. Accuracy to within ± 1.00 diopter varied between 65% and 90%. In most cases, low myopia had better results (25). The procedure seems to be about equal to RK in correcting myopia, without the weakening effect of the surgical incisions of RK. However, all is not rosy for PRK either. Discussing only the aeromedical implications, complications such as haloes and glare at night when the pupil dilates and a decrease can be noticed in sharpness of vision in many cases due to the haze present postoperatively. Predictability for aviation is still a problem. If one were corrected to within the ± 1.00 diopter accuracy, the 20/20 uncorrected visual acuity desired for a pilot would not be met. Finally, the possibility of a regression of the corrections two to six months or longer after the surgery exists. Aviation candidates should be aware that visual standards have changed markedly in the recent past. No longer is 20/20 uncorrected visual acuity, with a maximum refractive error of only -0.25 diopters of myopia the standard. Now a candidate can qualify for USAF flight training with as low as 20/70 uncorrected visual acuity and a maximum of -1.50 diopter of spherical equivalent of myopia corrected by spectacles or contact lenses.

Although PRK has been approved by the FDA, the military services will undoubtedly study all aspects of this vision-correcting procedure before coming to a decision as to its possible acceptance for military aviators.

PROTECTION OF VISION

Ocular Protective Materials

Since June, 1972, all spectacle lenses used in the United States have had to be impact-resistant by a Federal Drug Administration (FDA) ruling. Impact-resistant does not mean that they are unbreakable, just that a glass lens must withstand a $\frac{5}{8}$-in diameter steel ball dropped on it from a 50-in height. Glass lenses are hardened to withstand the drop-ball test by heat or chemical tempering.

A plastic, allyldiglycol carbonate (CR-39) lens also may be used in place of glass. A new, space-age, transparent plastic polycarbonate (Lexan) is being used in helmet-mounted visors and as a cockpit transparency that is strong enough to withstand bird strikes. Bird strikes are hazardous to low-flying, high-speed aircraft. The combination of a multilayered polycarbonate windshield and a visor of similar material for the aviator's helmet has markedly improved

the protection against this lethal hazard. A dual-visor system, one clear and one tinted, allows for maximum protection under all flight conditions. Polycarbonate lenses are now available in all forms to correct refractive errors. For sports and occupational activities, this material (Lexan) can be used as a protective goggle over ordinary spectacles, or polycarbonate lenses can be placed directly into spectacle frames, thus correcting the visual acuity and protecting the eyes. This material also has a secondary benefit in that it protects against ultraviolet light. It begins to transmit at 385 nm, blocking all shorter wavelengths. However, one drawback to this near-perfect lens material exists: it is susceptible to scratching (26).

Filters and Sunglasses

The extent and effects of electromagnetic energy (light) on the eye have been previously discussed. As noted, light intensities in the aviation environment can be up to 30% higher than on earth. Abiotic ultraviolet radiation (200–295 nm) is filtered by the atmosphere but does begin to become significant at high altitudes. Ultraviolet radiation 300–400 nm, which is abundant on earth, is now reputed to have some damaging effect on the human lens following long-term, chronic exposure. Infrared radiation above 760 nm is a contributor to solar and nuclear retinal burns. Sunlight falling on the earth is comprised of 58% infrared energy (760–2100 nm), 40% visible light (400–760 nm), and only 2% ultraviolet radiation (295–400 nm). At high altitude, ultraviolet radiation may be as high 4–6% and makes up 8–10% of the solar energy spectrum in space. Sunglasses can protect the aviator from excessive and harmful electromagnetic energy.

The ideal sunglasses for the aviator should do the following:

1. Correct refractive errors and presbyopia;
2. Protect against physical energy (wind or foreign objects);
3. Reduce overall light intensity;

4. Transmit all visible energy but attenuate ultraviolet and infrared radiation;
5. Not distort colors;
6. Not interfere with stereopsis (depth perception);
7. Be compatible with headgear and flying equipment;
8. Be rugged, inexpensive, and need minimal care.

Five types of sunglasses are now in common use: colored filters, neutral filters, reflecting filters, polarizing filters, and photochromic filters. They all allow only a certain percentage of the total amount of incident light to get through to the eye but produce this effect in different manners. The colored, neutral, polarizing, and photochromic filters achieve this effect by absorbing some of the light and allowing the rest to pass. Spectral filtering is achieved in glass lenses by adding specific chemicals to the melt, producing a through-and-through tint. The anterior surface of the glass lens also may only be tinted, but this method is subject to scratching. Plastic lenses are usually dipped into dyes to produce their filtering effect.

Colored filters have the disadvantage of altering the color of viewed objects and may possibly reduce color discrimination of color-vision-deficient persons.

Neutral filters adequately reduce the amount of light. Mainly, they do not distort colors and most will adequately eliminate excessive infrared and ultraviolet radiation.

Reflecting filters can be coated uniformly. They eliminate the ultraviolet and infrared energy; however, this type of coating scratches and peels easily and gives a greenish tint to objects.

Polarizing filters reduce glare off water or highways. For the aviator, they can cause a problem, such as blind spots in windshields and canopies, due to stress polarization of the canopy matching that in the spectacles. Plastic polarized filters scratch easily and, when laminated in glass, are expensive and heavy.

Photochromic filters (variable light transmis-

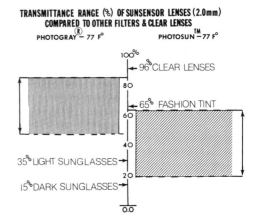

Figure 16.32. Effectiveness of various tints of lenses in reducing light transmission.

sion) are photodynamic lenses that vary in intensity in response to the ultraviolet content of the incident light. Some flyers may find the darkest density sufficient; however, for military use, the range of transmission variation is not adequate. The darker lenses remain too dark in the "open" state, and the lighter lenses are not dark enough at their maximum density (27). Their cycling time was found to be slow, and the density is less in hot and low-ultraviolet environments, such as inside automobiles or cockpits, where the light must traverse another transparency. This is shown in Figure 16.32, which also compares these lenses with other filters.

Selection of Sunglasses for the Aviator

The lens material should be CR-39 or polycarbonate plastic or impact-resistant glass. After much experimentation, it was finally decided that a 15% transmitting lens was probably the best all-around compromise for use by the aviator. Some individuals prefer a 25% transmitting lens for daily use (e.g., driving or sports) but switch to the 15% transmitting lens for aviation use. The lens should have a fairly flat curve in the visible energy range but attenuate the ultraviolet and infrared radiation. An ideal transmission curve is shown in Figure 16.33.

This type of lens allows a fairly equal amount of all spectral colors to pass through, and it will

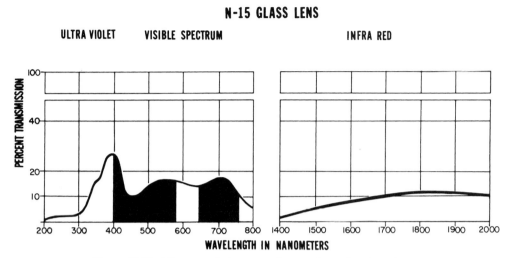

Figure 16.33. Idle transmission curve for sunglasses for the aviator.

not distort the color of the overall scene. The difference in overall transmission between the two spectacle lenses should not be >10%; otherwise, this difference in density will induce the Pulfrich effect which, in turn, may affect stereoscopic vision and depth perception. When sufficient overall light intensity is present, such as in daylight, visual acuity through neutral density, 15% transmitting lenses will be as good as in the eye lane without filters. Under low-light levels, such as at dawn or evening and on dark cloudy days, sunglasses reduce both contrast sensitivity and central visual acuity and, therefore, should be removed. Much has been said concerning certain filter lenses known as ''blue blockers.'' They cut out all of the ultraviolet and blue portion of the spectrum. Cutting out any of the colors in the spectrum is not desirable in aviation. The aviator's ''neutral density'' sunglass lenses allow all colors through and effectively reduce ultraviolet light as well.

Under extraordinary conditions, electromagnetic energy may reach such a magnitude that ordinary protective devices will not be adequate. Such tremendous amounts of energy can be released during a nuclear detonation or packaged in a laser beam that protection of the eye against these energy sources is a must; otherwise, permanent injury to the eye will ensue (28).

Nuclear Flash Protection

In spite of the fact that the possible use of nuclear weapons has been dramatically reduced, they are still available; therefore, the material to follow has more than an historical interest.

The eye is more susceptible to injury from nuclear explosions at far greater distances than any other organ or tissue of the body. When a pupil of a given size is exposed to a nuclear detonation at a given distance, it will result in a certain amount of energy being distributed over the image on the retina. When one doubles the distance from the detonation, the amount of energy passing through the same size pupil will be only one-fourth as great. The image area on the retina, however, will be only one-fourth as large; therefore, the energy per unit area will remain constant irrespective of the distance from the detonation except for the attenuation due to the atmosphere and ocular media. The potential danger of flashblindness and chorioretinal burns resulting from viewing nuclear fireballs remains a concern to aircrew members and thus has created new problems for the flight surgeon.

During daylight, with high-ambient illumination and through a small pupillary diameter, the retinal burn and flashblindness problems are greatly diminished. At night, with a large pupil, protection is a must. Many different ideas for eye protection have been advocated. Fixed-density filters, either on the pilot or the windscreen, electromechanical and electrooptical goggles, explosive lens filters, and phototropic devices have been developed. The sum total of all this work is that a 2% transmission-fixed filter, gold-plated visor gives adequate protection against retinal burns and reduces flashblindness to manageable proportions during daylight. This filter, however, cannot be used at night. Another aid, a readily available countermeasure to flashblindness, day or night, is the ability to raise instrument panel illumination by auxiliary panel lighting to 125 ft-c. This increased illumination significantly reduces visual recovery time. The ideal ''omni'' protector against nuclear flash is still being sought. The most recently developed material for protecting against nuclear flash is a transparent ferroelectroceramic material (lead lanthanum zirconate titanate, PLZT) placed between crossed polarizers, as shown in Figure 16.34, reacts to the light energy of detonation within 50–100 milliseconds, reaching an optical density of three. Its biggest drawback is that in its open state, it transmits only 20% of the light. It may also be of interest that the 2%-transmitting gold-plated visor, developed at the USAF SAM for protection of aircrew against the flash of enemy nuclear weapons, was never used for that purpose. Instead, it was used as the outermost visor by astronauts in the peaceful exploration of the moon and space.

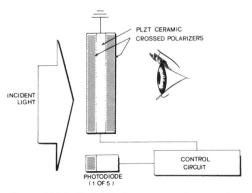

Figure 16.34. Flash-blindness-protective goggles.

Laser Eye Protection

Lasers (light amplification by stimulated emission of radiation) produce monochromatic, coherent, collimated light. The laser beam diverges little, so that the energy of the beam decreases only minimally with increasing distance from the source. Laser energy is capable of severely injuring tissue in the eye that absorbs the beam energy. If a sufficiently powerful carbon dioxide laser (10.6 mm) were to strike the eye, it could severely injure the cornea. Argon (480 nm), ruby (693 nm), and neodymium (1060 nm) lasers can injure the retina and choroid because they absorb these wavelengths. Lasers have now been classified by the American National Standards Institute standard Z-136.1 as follows:

Class I—nonhazardous
Class II—safe lasers, but may produce retinal injury when looked at for long periods of time
Class III—medium-power, medium-risk lasers
Class IV—high-risk lasers, potentially hazardous by both direct and specular reflected beams (29)

The military applications of lasers are increasing in the areas of target ranging and illumination. Pilots themselves are not usually at hazard from their own laser beams, but technicians and others working with such instruments should wear protective goggles or visors with an optical density that is considered safe at the laser wavelength being employed. It is possible that the laser itself may be used as a weapon. Here it would be helpful if one knew the threat and used a visor filter to protect from that waveband. Ideally, an agile filter would be in the open state but close down when struck by the laser beam. Unfortunately, this type of protection is as yet not available. The medical management of laser eye injuries is fully covered in a USAFSAM technical report, TR-88–21 (30). Injuries to the external eye, cornea, and lids can be treated. Retinal injuries affect vision, depending on the energy density absorbed by the retina and, more importantly, the location of the injury on the retina. A direct hit to the fovea markedly reduces central vision and is permanent, with little recovery of function. Other safety factors also should be considered, such as educating the worker in laser safety, not looking at the laser beam, examining for reflective materials in the laboratory or shop, posting warning signs, and operating a laser in well-lit rooms when possible (small pupils). Laser-safe working distances, the selection of protective materials, and safety programs are becoming quite complicated and involved for the flight surgeon to manage alone. One should have help from a bioenvironmental engineer or health physicist when possible.

The flight surgeon or aeromedical examiner, however, is responsible for setting up and performing ocular surveillance programs. Minimally, the examiner should give laser workers complete ocular examinations before they begin their assignments or employment. This should include a distance and near-central visual acuity examination, both corrected and uncorrected, an Amsler grid examination, and an ophthalmoscopic examination of the fundus, with special attention to the fovea (any anomalies of the fundus should be meticulously recorded). A similar examination should be performed at the termination of the assignment or employment. Annual ocular examinations are not considered necessary; however, anyone working with lasers who has an ocular complaint or claims to have been injured by a laser should be examined and the complaint evaluated (31).

As stated at the beginning of this chapter, vision plays the most important role in data-gathering for humans; anything affecting vision is significant for the aviator. The flight surgeon and aeromedical examiner who care for aviators and attempt to increase their effectiveness should pay special attention to the vision and visual systems of aviators.

Instantaneous, clear vision assures us of receiving uncluttered and accurate visual data into our mental computers. The integrating and processing of this information after its reception is in the domain of the central nervous system and is enhanced by training and education of the aviator. If inaccurate or incomplete visual information were received, however, we would almost be assured of failing to perform the task. With the time element for decision-making becoming ever-shorter in modern aviation, there is added impetus to look carefully at the visual system.

This chapter examined the physical, physiologic, medical, and bioengineering aspects of vision. With visual selection and enhancement by visual aids, the aviator's visual range has been extended, thus giving more time for reaction and decision-making. After selecting aviators with exceptional visual capabilities, it is important to employ the techniques for maintaining and protecting their vision and visual apparatus so that they enjoy full flying careers. Ophthalmology and the other visual sciences are now complex, scientific specialties. This chapter, however, has attempted to give information and data in a manner that is understandable and useful for all physicians.

REFERENCES

1. Wilmer WH, Berens C. The eye in aviation. In: Office of the Director of Air Service. Aviation medicine in the Army Expeditionary Forces (AEF). Washington D.C.: Government Printing Office, 1920.
2. Duke-Elder SS. System of ophthalmology, volume V: ophthalmic optics and refraction. London: Henry Kimpton, 1970;81.
3. Moses RA, Hart WA Jr. Adler's physiology of the eye: clinical applications. St. Louis: C.V. Mosby Co., 1987; 561–582.
4. Pitts DG, Tredici TJ. The effects of ultraviolet on the eye. Am Ind Hyg Assoc J 1971;32:235.
5. Campbell FW, Maffei L. Contrast and spatial frequency. Sci Am 1974;240:30–38.
6. Editorial: Making sense of contrast sensitivity testing—has its time come? Arch Ophthalmol 1987;105: 627–629.
7. Randel HW ed. Aerospace medicine, 2nd ed. Baltimore: Williams & Wilkins Co., 1972;594–595.
8. Aircraft Instrument and Cockpit Lighting by Red or White Light. Conference Proceedings. Advisory Group for Aerospace Research and Development (AGARD)/ North Atlantic Treaty Organization (NATO), Springfield: 1967.
9. Mims JL III, Tredici TJ. Evaluation of the Landolt ring plaque night vision tester. Aerosp Med 1973;44: 304–307.

10. Miller RE II, Tredici TJ. Night vision manual for the flight surgeon. AL-SR-1992–0002, August, 1992.
11. Pitts DG. Visual illusions and aircraft accidents. SAM-TR-67–28, United States School of Aerospace Medicine, Brooks Air Force Base, Texas: 1967.
12. Procedures for Testing Color Vision. Report of Working Group No. 41, Committee on Vision, National Research Council, National Academy of Sciences. Washington D.C.: National Academy Press, 1981.
13. Welsh KW, Vaughan JA, Rasmussen PG. Aeromedical implications of the X-chrome lens for improving color vision deficiencies. Aviat Space Environ Med 1979;50: 249.
14. Wulfeck JW, et al. Vision in military aviation. WADC Technical Report 58–399, Wright Air Development Center, Wright-Patterson AFB, Ohio: 1958.
15. Provines WF, Kislin B, Tredici TJ. Multiple images in the F/FB-111 aircraft windshield: their generation, spatial localization, and recording. SAM-TR-77–32, United States Air Force School of Aerospace Medicine, Brooks Air Force Base, Texas: 1977.
16. Sanders DR, Koch DD. An atlas of corneal topography. Thorofare: Slack, Inc., 1993.
17. Peters DR, Green RP Jr. The pigmentary dispersion disorder in USAF aviators. Aviat Space Environ Med 1992; 63:1049–1053.
18. Tredici TJ. Screening and management of glaucoma in flying personnel. Milit Med 1980;145:1.
19. Green RP Jr, Carlson DW, Dieckert JP, Tredici TJ. Central serous chorioretinopathy in US Air Force aviators: a review. Aviat Space Environ Med 1988;59:1170–1175.
20. Carlson DW, Green RP Jr. The career impact of keratoconus on Air Force aviators. AJO 1991;112:557–561.
21. Tredici TJ, Stern C, Burroughs J, Ivan DJ. Poster: cataract surgery in USAF pilots. American Academy of Ophthalmology annual meeting. Atlanta: 1995.
22. Dennis RJ, Apsey DA, Ivan DJ. Aircrew soft contact lens wear: a survey of USAF eye care professionals. Aviat Space Environ Med 1993;64:1044–1047.
23. Tredici TJ. Role of orthokeratology: a perspective. Ophthalmology 1979;86:698.
24. Rowsey JJ, Balyeat HD. Preliminary results and complications of radial keratotomy. AJO 1982;93:437.
25. Diamond S. Excimer laser photorefractive keratectomy (PRK) for myopia—present status: aerospace considerations. Aviat Space Environ Med 1995;66:690–693.
26. Miller D. Optics and refraction. New York: Gower Medical Publishers, 1991;10–13.
27. Welsh KW, Miller JW, Shacklett DE. An acceptability study of photochromiclenses. Optometric Weekly 1976; 21:16–21.
28. Byrnes JA, Brown DVL, Rose HW, Cibis PA. Chorioretinal burns produced by an atomic flash. Arch Ophthalmol 1956;55:351.
29. American National Standards for the Safe Use of Lasers. ANSI Z136. 1–1976, New York: American National Standards Institute, 1976.
30. Green RP Jr, Cartledge RM, Chaney FE, Menendez AR. Medical management of combat laser eye energies. USAFSAM-TR-88–21, 1988.
31. Air Force Occupational Safety and Health (AFOSH) Standard 161–10, Health Hazards Control Laser Radiation. Washington D.C.: Department of the Air Force, 1980;23–24.

Chapter 17

Otolaryngology in Aerospace Medicine

C. Thomas Yarington, Jr.,

H. H. Hanna

If God had intended for man to fly, He would have provided him with wings.

Anonymous

In this chapter, otolaryngologic abnormalities related to aerospace medicine are considered under the major headings of examination, clinical conditions, and implications of surgical procedures. Only anatomic and physiologic considerations pertinent to flying are discussed. General aspects of assessment of hearing and vestibular function are presented. Clinical conditions directly related to flying are essentially limited to those entities that result from the mechanical effects that exposure to environments of changing barometric pressures has on gases trapped in various cavities of the head. Barodontalgia is included, although the precise mechanism of symptom production is not known and trapped gases may be involved. Abnormalities not directly related to flying but having aeromedical significance are discussed, as are the aeromedical implications of otologic and rhinologic surgical procedures.

EXAMINATION

Anatomic and Physiologic Considerations Pertinent to Flying

External Auditory Canal

The size and configuration of the external auditory canals vary considerably from person to person and even from one side to the other in the same individual. In general, the canal proceeds medially in a slightly anterior and superior fashion and at about its midpoint inclines somewhat inferiorly to reach the eardrum. This configuration is the basis for the need to pull the pinna posteriorly and somewhat superiorly to facilitate visualization of the eardrum. Some individuals have essentially a straight outer ear canal, and in others the apparent hump inferiorly is quite marked (Figure 17.1). In many individuals, a bony prominence anteriorly overhangs the anterior portion of the annulus of the eardrum (Figure 17.2). One of the primary aeromedical considerations is that the external auditory canal configuration be compatible with earplugs. Experience showed that the majority of aircrew can be fitted; however, it is not uncommon for an individual to require different sized plugs for the ear canals. The disparity is usually no greater than one size difference. The experience at the United States Air Force School of Aerospace Medicine (USAFSAM) has been that approximately 14% of candidates for such ear protection require a different size plug in each ear. An equally significant aeromedical consideration is that the examiner must be able to visualize a sufficient amount of the eardrum to be able to

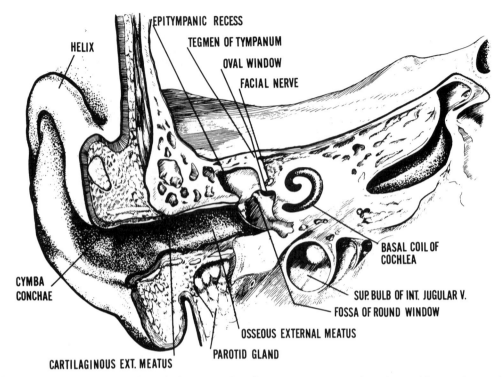

Figure 17.1. Curved section through the external auditory meatus, tympanic cavity, cochlea, and pyramidal part of the temporalbone, right side. (From: Jackson C, Jackson CL. Diseases of the nose, throat and ear. Philadelphia: W.B. Saunders, 1959.)

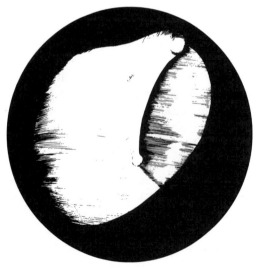

Figure 17.2. Normal right ear drum showing the bony prominence (anterior canal wall) overhanging the anterior portion of the annulus.

check for satisfactory performance of the Valsalva maneuver and for the presence of significant findings on the eardrum (e.g., manifestation of acute barotitis media or ear block).

The Valsalva maneuver is one way to ventilate the middle ear cavities unphysiologically. The individual inhales, closes the nose with thumb and index finger on the nasal alae, and then exhales with the mouth closed. Positive pressure quickly builds up in the nasopharynx. The exhalation effort is augmented until the pressure in the nasopharynx becomes great enough to open the eustachian tubes and ventilate the middle ear spaces. When air enters the middle ear, the eardrum moves laterally and remains distended for a while. Ventilation of one or both ears is readily perceived by the patient, who will generally mention that one or both ears "popped." The physician can verify ventilation of the middle ear by observing the eardrum while the patient performs the Valsalva maneuver.

Exostoses and osteomas occur in the inner half or bony portion of the outer ear canal. Exostoses are much more common and usually present as smooth, rounded, bony prominences of varying sizes along one or both of the suture lines joining the tympanic portion of the temporal bone to the squama and mastoid posteriorly and the squama and zygomatic process portion anteriorly. In rare cases, exostoses attain sufficient size to preclude adequate visualization of the eardrum and may also limit access to the eardrum (e.g., cleaning and medicating the ear canal as in acute otitis externa). When exostoses are large enough to be clinically significant, surgical removal is indicated. An osteoma has the same clinical significance as exostoses; however, these benign tumors are much less frequent.

Middle Ear Cavity

The primary aeromedical consideration of the middle ear cavity is its role in barotrauma. In this consideration, the middle ear should be regarded as a rigid-walled cavity, even though its lateral partition, the tympanic membrane, is a thin structure normally consisting of an external layer of thin skin, an intermediate layer of elastic tissue, and an inner mucosal layer. As long as the eardrum remains intact, however, it is not capable of distending enough to accommodate any appreciable amount of pressure and thus functions as a rigid wall. The amount of pressure change (either positive or relatively negative) that the normal eardrum tolerates varies; however, any time the pressure differential exceeds 100 mm Hg the eardrum may rupture.

Eustachian Tube

The eustachian tube extends from the lateral wall of the nasopharynx to the anteroinferior part of the middle ear space. It has two primary functions: (1) to ventilate the middle ear space; and (2) to drain the middle ear space. The primary aeromedical consideration is the role that the eu-

stachian plays in the ventilation of the middle ear. The posterior third of the eustachian tube is a bony channel that is always open; the anterior two-thirds is a membranocartilaginous structure that is normally closed and opens physically only with swallowing, yawning, or working the lower jaw—any action that causes the tensor veli palatini and levator veli palatini muscles to contract. The action of the tensor veli palatini muscle is more important in opening the auditory tube than the levator veli palatini muscle (Figure 17.3). The structure of the anterior two-thirds of the eustachian tube is such that it functions essentially as a one-way flutter valve. The luman of the tube is a vertical slit that is normally closed (Figure 17.4). Air under pressure in the middle ear space readily passes through to the nasopharynx, but if the air pressure in the tym-

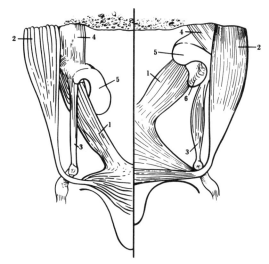

Figure 17.3. The action of the tubal muscles. On the left side of the figure the tube is at rest, and on the right side of the figure the tube is illustrated during swallowing. The levator veli palatini (1) pulls the soft palate up, back, and lateral to help close the nasopharynx and to elevate and help rotate the tubal cartilage (5). Forward rotation is checked by the superior tubal ligament (4). Medial fibers of the tensor veli palatini (3) pull the hook of the cartilage (5) downward and dilate the tubal lumen (6), thus opening it. Lateral fibers of the tensor (2) tense and elevate the soft palate. (From: Proctor B. Anatomy of the eustachian tube. Arch Otolaryngol 1973;97:6.)

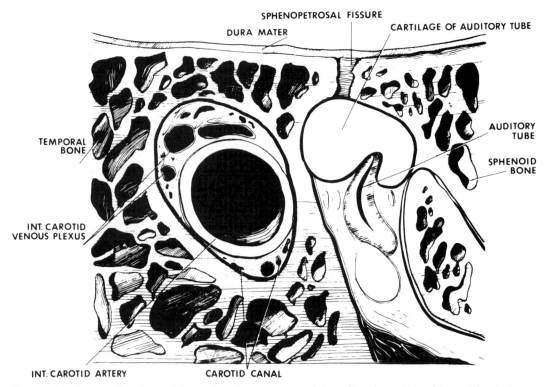

Figure 17.4. Cross section through the cartilaginous portion of the left auditory tube. (From: Sobotta J, Figge FH. Atlas of human anatomy, vol. 3. New York: Hafner Press, 1974; 185.)

panic cavity were less than the pressure in the nasopharynx, the eustachian tube would remain closed unless it were opened physiologically or by one of the unphysiologic maneuvers (e.g., Valsalva maneuver or politzerization).

Nasal Cavity

In humans, the nasal cavity is the preferred route for inspired air, and the nose performs three basic functions in preparing inspired air for the lungs: cleansing, humidification, and warming. Cleansing is accomplished by two means. Larger particles are screened by the vibrissae, or hairs, in the anterior nares, and smaller particles, including bacteria, are trapped on the mucous blanket and swept by ciliary action posteriorly into the nasopharynx and then into the "common gutter," or oral pharynx. Inspired air is humidified, when necessary, by mucus which is largely provided by glands located in the middle turbinates. If warming were

required, this would be accomplished by the inferior turbinates, or "radiators," which contain many submucosal venous sinusoids. These turbinates enlarge when subjected to cold air, thus reducing the airway and providing for longer contact of the air with the turbinates. This mechanism is the basis for nasal stuffiness commonly noted when one leaves a warm house in the wintertime and encounters the cold outside air. These functions of humidification and warming are under autonomic control; in essence, the amount of mucus in the nose and the size of the turbinates, primarily the inferior turbinate, vary constantly in response to the degree of dryness and temperature of the inspired air.

Adequacy of the nasal airways is critical in flying; any significant obstruction can result in an inability or decreased ability to conduct ventilation via the preferred route with loss of the cleansing, humidifying, and warming actions of the nose. Adequate nasal airways become even more important when oxygen is required for any appreciable period because oxygen in aircraft systems is dry. When aircrew resort to mouth breathing, the air is humidified at the expense of oral, pharyngeal, and laryngeal mucosa, which can rapidly lead to dryness and irritation in these areas, as well as thickened residual secretions. Adequate nasal airways also are required for optimum ventilation of the paranasal sinuses and middle ear cavities.

Paranasal Sinuses

The paranasal sinuses are rigid-walled cavities that communicate with the nasal cavity by way of ostia. These openings must be patent when the cavities are subjected to changing barometric pressures or abnormal conditions may be produced within the sinus, usually a relatively negative pressure, which can lead to pathologic changes. Normal pressure changes across sinus ostia are small, and considerable time is required for air in one of the larger sinuses to be replaced. With this relatively inefficient ventilation, it is critical for the sinus ostium to be unobstructed, particularly when unphysiologic pressure changes are encountered.

The normal sinus lining is a thin, ciliated mucoperiosteum. Mucus glands are normally limited to the region of the ostium. Drainage is affected by both ciliary action and gravity in the frontal, ethmoid, and sphenoid sinuses; in the maxillary sinus, the location of the ostium is high on the medial wall, creating a "water bottle" effect, and drainage is dependent on ciliary action. In all of the sinuses, ciliary streaming always leads to the ostium. A sinus canal renews its mucous coat in 5–10 minutes; the journey from the farthest corner of the most distant sinus to the pharynx takes about 20 minutes. Patency of the ostium is also critical for adequate clearing of secretions from the sinus cavity.

The close proximity of the roots of the maxillary dentition, particularly the molars, to the floor of the maxillary sinus may have aeromedical significance. Development of a relatively negative pressure in a maxillary sinus during descent from altitude may be interpreted as being of dental origin. Conversely, a pathologic process in a maxillary molar tooth (e.g., pulpitis and periapical abscess) may extend to the sinus cavity.

Pharynx

The pharynx can be divided into the nasopharynx, oropharynx, and hypopharynx (or laryngopharynx). The most aeromedically significant part is the nasopharynx because it contains the pharyngeal end of the eustachian tube in its lateral wall. The mucosa of the nasopharynx contains a significant amount of lymphoid tissue, which may respond to viral and bacterial invaders and lead to edema, which can compromise tubal function.

The velopharyngeal sphincter, which closes off the nasopharynx from the oropharynx, is also significant in flight. Competency of this sphincter is essential for proper deglutition and speech. Normal function of this mechanism also is required for accomplishment of politzerization, an unphysiologic means for ventilating the middle ear space.

Larynx

The larynx has respiratory sphincteric (protective), and phonatory functions. The main respiratory effect is the valvular action provided by variation in the size of the glottis. This influences intraalveolar pressures and the interchange of oxygen and carbon dioxide. Sphincteric actions include protection against the aspiration of food and fluids, as the larynx is closed during the second stage of deglutition; tussive and expectorative functions, as the cough reflex requires tight closure of the larynx; and fixation of the chest for effective movement of the shoulder girdle and for efficient action of the abdominal muscles. In its phonatory role, vibration of the vocal cords generates sound, which is modified into speech by certain supra laryngeal articulators, mainly the lips, teeth, and tongue. Production of a voice that is adequate for radio communication is essential, and any laryngeal abnormality that affects this capability is aeromedically significant.

Functional Assessments

Hearing

The hearing of aircrew presenting for aeromedical evaluation should be assessed both clinically and audiometrically.

The clinical evaluation of hearing should consist of physician observation of the patient, with attention to any obvious difficulty in communicating. When the patient is referred for hearing loss, the examiner may wish to deliberately vary the intensity of speech and to note the effect of depriving the patient of visualization of the examiner's lips while talking. This may reveal considerable dependence of the patient on lipreading. During examination of the patient, tuning-fork tests should be done. These should consist of the Rinne test (comparison of air conduction with bone conduction) and the Weber test (test for lateralization with the fork placed in the midline). A 512-Hz tuning fork should be used. Results of the fork tests should be correlated with audiometric findings.

Audiometry should be performed by an audiologist or a fully-trained technician utilizing a sound-attenuated booth and equipment that is in proper calibration. All patients should have as a minimum evaluation the determination of thresholds for pure-tone, air-conducted stimuli at the following frequencies (Hz): 250, 500, 1000, 2000, 3000, 4000, 5000, 6000, and 8000. When significant hearing loss occurs at 1000 and/or 2000 Hz, then a 1500-Hz evaluation also should be done. The threshold for bone-conducted sound should be determined for any frequency from 250 through 4000 Hz in which the air-conduction (AC) threshold is not within normal limits (up to 25 dB at any frequency). When significant loss occurs by AC in one or both ears, the bone-conduction (BC) thresholds can be utilized to determine whether the loss is conductive, sensorineural, or combined. If the BC thresholds were, in general, equal to the AC

thresholds, the hearing loss would be sensorineural; if the BC thresholds were within normal limits, the hearing loss would be conductive. In a combined loss, the BC thresholds manifest somewhere between normal and the AC thresholds. In most aircrew, pure-tone audiometry is adequate for the clinical evaluation of hearing loss, including determinations made for hearing conservation purposes. When indicated, additional audiometric procedures may be accomplished; these include speech audiometry, impedance audiometry, various so-called "site-of-lesion" tests intended to aid the clinician in differentiating an end-organ or hair-cell lesion from a nerve-fiber lesion, and certain special procedures, such as auditory brainstem responses (ABR). A detailed discussion of all of these additional procedures is beyond the scope of this chapter; however, the procedures that are utilized most frequently at USAFSAM are mentioned.

Speech auditory should probably be requested for any patient with a significant pure-tone deficit, particularly when the pure-tone loss is unilateral. Speech audiometry consists of the speech reception threshold (SRT), which is determined with a suitable list of tape-recorded bisyllabic, vowel-rich words, and the discrimination score, which is determined with a suitable list of tape-recorded phonetically balanced (PB), consonant-rich words. The SRT is expressed in decibels and usually should correlate within 5-10 dB with puretone threshold average for the primary speech frequencies (500, 1000, and 2000 Hz). The discrimination score is expressed in percentage; the patient is given 50 words, and 2% is deducted for each word that is not repeated correctly. These words are presented at an intensity level well above the pure-tone threshold to minimize any sound transmission factors and determine, as accurately as possible, the true cochlear reserve. In general, patients with normal hearing, conductive loss, and mild sensorineural loss have good discrimination, which is defined as 90% or better. With cochlear impairment, the discrimination score decreases as involvement of the speech range increases. An individual with high-tone loss only may have good discrimination. Lesions that involve the eighth cranial nerve usually produce more severe decrements in discrimination than do cochlear abnormalities. Impedance audiometry primarily measures the functional compliance of the sound-conducting mechanism in the middle ear (middle ear transformer or impedance-matching mechanism). Because this instrument can demonstrate sudden changes in impedance of the middle ear mechanism, contraction of the stapedial muscle, the ''stapedial reflex,'' in response to an appropriate stimulus can be recorded along with the intensity of the stimulus that is required to elicit the reflex. The acoustic reflex is normally present and can be elicited by stimuli below 100 dB in intensity. The most useful frequencies are 500, 100, and 2000 Hz. The acoustic reflex is absent in conductive losses, which usually are easily determined; however, the acoustic reflex also may be absent or its threshold may be elevated or it may exhibit abnormal decay when a lesion involves the eighth cranial nerve. Accordingly, the acoustic reflex may be useful in evaluating patients with unilateral findings that suggest nerve involvement.

A number of ''site-of-lesion'' tests are available to the clinician who may be confronted with the need to determine whether hearing loss and other otologic manifestations (e.g., tinnitus) are due to involvement of the inner ear (cochlear) or to some pathologic process of the eighth cranial nerve (neural). Most of the tests are based on demonstrating the presence or absence of a phenomenon that is known to be either cochlear or neural in origin. One cochlear manifestation that may be employed is recruitment. Recruitment may be demonstrated in suitable patients by the alternate binaural loudness balance test. A neural manifestation that can be utilized in the differential diagnosis is the phenomenon of adaptation or tone decay, which may be demonstrated by several tests; the version generally preferred at present is the suprathreshold adaptation test, originally described by Jerger and Jerger (1).

This version involves stressing the auditory system with intensity and has been shown to be more reliable than threshold techniques. Other tests are based on the difference limen phenomenon—the smallest difference in intensity that can be perceived by the patient; the test most commonly used is the short-increment sensitivity index. Individuals with cochlear disorders are able to hear 1-dB changes in intensity, whereas a person with normal hearing or a neural lesion usually cannot detect these changes in intensity. Another test that is useful in differential auditory diagnosis is based on the observation that the ability to discriminate PB words may breakdown at high-intensity levels in the presence of a nerve lesion. Such a patient may score well at 40 dB above threshold but do significantly poorer when the intensity is increased. This decrease in discrimination is referred to as the ''rollover'' phenomenon; that is, at high intensity levels, the discrimination score rolls over to a lower level. This test is usually called the performance-intensity functions for phonetically balanced words. As emphasized by Jerger and Jerger, it is wise to obtain a battery of tests rather than to rely on any one test (1).

A special audiometric procedure developed in the mid 1960s by Jewett et al. is based on recording waveforms that are produced centrally during the first 10 milliseconds after exposure to a suitable auditory stimulus, such as a click (2). Because this electrical activity is of low voltage and is projected against ongoing brain activity, an averaging computer is required to record these ABRs. A wave pattern is produced that consists of waves I-VII; however, the most clinically useful parameters are the intraaural waves I-V interval and the interaural wave V latency difference. Lesions involving the eighth cranial nerve, usually acoustic neuromas, may produce prolongation of intervals I-V, which also may produce a significant increase in interaural wave V latency. ABR has proved to be a useful procedure in otolaryngology, primarily in the evaluation of unilateral otologic findings that suggest a cerebellopontine angle lesion. In any single patient, the test battery employed should be determined by consultation with an otolaryngologist.

Vestibular Function

Vestibular function usually is not specifically evaluated unless the patient has a history of vertigo or relates a complaint suggestive of an abnormality in the vestibular system. If assessment of vestibular function were indicated, it should be accomplished both clinically and by appropriate tests.

The clinical evaluation of vestibular function should include observing the patient for the presence of spontaneous nystagmus and testing for positional nystagmus. The Dix-Hallpike maneuver should be performed while the physician observes the patient's eyes for nystagmus. This maneuver is the combination of a definite stimulus and the assumption of a certain head position. The patient, who is sitting up on the examining table, is briskly placed in the supine position with head lowered about 30° below the horizontal plane and rotated so that one ear is down. After allowing the patient to rest for five minutes, the stimulus is repeated with the head rotated to the opposite side. A ''typical'' response is characterized by a brief, latent period of a few seconds, followed by rotary or horizontal-rotary nystagmus, which is accompanied by subjective vertigo. The nystagmus and vertigo also are brief, usually lasting 5–10 seconds. When nystagmus and vertigo occur, the stimulus should be repeated after a one-minute rest, and the response will be reduced or absent, which confirms that it is fatigable. An ''atypical'' response is the production of nystagmus without one or more of the other features. In a normal individual, this maneuver produces neither nystagmus nor vertigo. A typical response is indicative of an end-organ or peripheral abnormality; an atypical response is a nonspecific finding.

The cranial nerves should be checked and coordination and balance assessed. The inability to walk in tandem fashion is usually indicative of a cerebellar disorder but also may be seen in unilateral labyrinthine disease. In the Romberg test, the patient stands erect with feet together and arms at the sides, and with the eyes closed, eliminating visual input; the test can result in two of the three orientation mechanisms becoming inoperative. When the patient falls, disturbance of proprioception exists due to dorsal column involvement. The ''sharpened Romberg'' test, in which the patient's feet are placed in tandem rather than side-to-side, is a significant modification of the Romberg test (3). This modified test is more sensitive and may be positive in labyrinthine abnormalities.

Vestibular function testing should be as complete as possible. When facilities permit only a simple cold-water caloric test, this should be done. Ideally, appraisal of the status of the vestibular system by calorization should include both cold and warm stimuli, the bithermal technique, and the results should be recorded by electronystagmography (ENG). The suppressive effect of visual fixation can be eliminated by recording with the patient's eyes closed. In addition to caloric stimulation, the ENG usually records for ocular dysmetria and visual tracking, gaze nystagmus, spontaneous nystagmus, optokinetic nystagmus, positional nystagmus, response to the Dix-Hallpike maneuvers, and fixation suppression of calorically-induced nystagmus. Responses to caloric stimulation are hand-scored and then converted to percentages of unilateral weakness and directional preponderance according to the method described by Jongkees and Philipzoon (4).

At USAFSAM, vestibular function testing includes stimulating the system physiologically with harmonic or sinusoidal acceleration at frequencies of 0.1–0.16 Hz, one octave apart, at a maximum velocity of 50 degrees/sec. Eye movement analysis yields primary measures of phase and left-right asymmetry, or labyrinthine preponderance (5).

It is important for the clinician to keep vestibular function tests in their proper perspective. Vestibular function studies, regardless of how elaborate the equipment may be, do not make diagnoses; they may provide the physician with findings that must then be correlated with the patient's history and physical examination in an effort to make as specific a diagnosis as possible. Either unilateral labyrinthine weakness or no response is a significant finding and usually indicates a peripheral abnormality. Directional preponderance is a nonspecific finding that may not be clinically significant. Vestibular, spontaneous nystagmus and positional nystagmus are nonspecific findings. The "typical" Dix-Hallpike response is consistent with a peripheral disorder, but an atypical response is nonspecific. Calibration overshoot, abnormal visual pursuit or tracking, gaze nystagmus, optokinetic asymmetry, and failure of fixation suppression usually indicate a central abnormality. Phase shifts in response to harmonic acceleration cannot identify unilateral involvement; in general, peripheral abnormalities cause shifts at the low end (0.1Hz) of the stimulus spectrum; central involvements can cause shifts at both low and high frequencies or even across the entire spectrum. Harmonic labyrinthine preponderance may be toward the involved side (irritative) or away from the involved side (depressed). Neuromas consistently show the picture of depression; with central abnormalities, the preponderance is usually the depressed type and is greater at the higher frequencies.

CLINICAL CONDITIONS

Conditions Related to Flight Environment

External Otitic Barotrauma

The term, external otitic barotrauma refers to injury to the lining of the external ear canal due to the creation of an airtight space between an object in the outer ear canal and the eardrum. Earplugs, such as those used for protection against aircraft noise, tightly impacted cerumen, or any other foreign material may produce a seal in the ear canal and entrap air. During descent, the pressure of this entrapped air may become relatively negative with respect to ambient pressure. Because of this mechanical effect, the outer layer of epithelium of the tympanic membrane and/or that of the inner aspect of the external canal wall may be sucked away from the underlying tissue to form hemorrhagic areas beneath the epithelium. If these areas were to become large enough, hemorrhagic bullae may be formed. The primary manifestation is pain and is most likely due to stripping of the epithelium from the underlying bone. Small subepithelial hemorrhages usually require no specific treatment. When large hemorrhagic bullae have formed, recovery is more rapid when the blood is evacuated with a syringe and needle or by means of a small incision.

No one should be subjected to barometric pressure changes when the external auditory canal is completely obstructed in any manner. Earplugs and similar devices should be vented in some manner to permit pressure equalization to take place, or some provision for rapid removal should be made such as a loop of string through the tab on an earplug that is long enough to be accessible to the aircrew with the helmet in place. Various earplugs have been worn by military personnel during flight operations in various aircraft for several years. Experience has shown that in most aircrew, these earplugs do not form an airtight seal in the ear canal because in the overwhelming majority of instances, external otitic barotrauma does not occur, even with rapid descents. This fact was verified by a study at USAFSAM that was conducted in an altitude chamber (6). External otitic barotrauma has occurred occasionally, and even these relatively rare instances can be prevented when the aircrew are alert and respond to the early symptoms of barotrauma. It is not necessary to remove the plug completely; all that is required is that the plug be moved laterally enough to break the seal.

Barotitis Media (Aerotitis Media)

Barotitis media can be defined as an acute or chronic traumatic inflammation in the middle ear space that is produced by a pressure differential between the air in the tympanic cavity and mastoid air cells and that of the surrounding atmosphere. A classic description of this entity was published by Armstrong and Heim in 1937 (7). The middle ear space in this context should be regarded as a rigid-walled cavity that communicates with nasopharynx by way of the eustachian tube, which acts essentially as a one-way flutter valve that favors the release of pressure from the middle ear to the nasopharynx but not the reverse. Ascent produces a relatively positive pressure in the tympanic cavity as the pressure of the atmosphere becomes progressively less. This positive pressure usually is readily equalized because the air can pass easily through the eustachian tube to the nasopharynx. The pressure change is greater at lower altitudes because the air is denser. This relatively positive pressure in the middle ear may be perceived by the individual as a slight fullness in the ear, which usually can be relieved readily by swallowing. On descent, however, a different situation exists. The eustachian tube remains closed unless actively opened by muscle action or high positive pressure in the nasopharynx. When the eustachian tube opens, any existing pressure differential is immediately equalized. If the tube were not to open regularly during descent, a pressure differential may develop. If this pressure differential were to reach 80–90 mm Hg, the small muscles of the soft palate could not overcome it, and either reascent or an unphysiologic maneuver would be necessary to open the tube.

Barotitis media, which is frequently referred to as an "ear block," results from failure of ventilation of the middle ear space on changing from low- to high-atmospheric pressure—that is, descent. The most common cause is swelling of the nasopharyngeal end of the eustachian tube, which is usually due to acute upper respiratory tract infection. Edema secondary to allergic rhinitis may be an etiologic factor. Ignorance of the necessity for swallowing at frequent intervals during descent in an aircraft also may be a significant contributory factor. Most individuals engaged in diving receive adequate indoctrination before actual operation, whereas many individuals who fly, particularly those who do so in commercial aircraft, may not be properly indoctrinated. The ability to recognize the early pressure changes incident to beginning descent and to adjust the intervals between swallowing to meet the demands of the rate of descent comes only with flying experience; however, preflight indoctrination is certainly valuable.

The rate of descent is also a significant factor. This fact has been recognized for many years by commercial airlines; their descent rates are usually quite gradual, generally < 400 mpm (1200 fpm), whereas descent rates in military aircraft are often much greater, frequently several thousand fpm. The use of oxygen during flight increases the likelihood of barotrauma because oxygen delivered from an aircraft's oxygen system is usually quite dry and may irritate the mucosa of the upper respiratory tract. The absorption of oxygen by the middle ear and mastoid mucosa also contributes to the relatively negative pressure in those cavities. When oxygen absorption is the primary factor in the development of a pressure differential, the term, delayed barotitis media may be used. Personnel who fly in jet aircraft that are equipped with a system that delivers 100% oxygen throughout the flight are most likely to develop this type of ear block. The absorption of 100% oxygen, however, usually must be combined with the infrequency of swallowing that occurs during sleep to produce a pressure differential sufficient to cause symptoms. Individuals who operate aircraft equipped with this type of oxygen system are aware of this possibility and will try to keep their ears well ventilated following the termination of a flight. However, if a flight were completed in the late evening hours or during the night and the individual would retire a short time later, a significant pressure differential may develop during sleep because of the combined factors of oxygen absorption and infrequent swallowing. Once the pressure differential develops, the situation is similar to that which occurs due to failure of ventilation of the eustachian tube. Sleeping during descent in an aircraft can lead to an ear block, again due to the infrequency of swallowing while asleep.

Pathologic changes in the middle ear vary with the magnitude of the pressure differential between the tympanic cavity and the ambient air pressure and with the length of time the pressure alteration acts on the tissues before equalization takes place. For practical purposes, the pressure differential results in a partial vacuum in the middle ear space that produces retraction of the tympanic membrane and engorgement of the blood vessels in the eardrum and middle ear mucosa. In mild ear blocks, pathologic changes may be limited to these effects. When the pressure differential is great enough and persists long enough, a transudate usually forms, which may be serous, serosanguineous, or even hemorrhagic. In rare cases, with the development of a severe pressure differential, the eardrum may rupture, the break usually occurring in the weakest area or in an area previously damaged by an earlier pathologic process. Formation of a transudate is the more frequent occurrence. Once fluid accumulates in the middle ear space, tension on the eustachian tube is relieved; this is followed by reinflation of the middle ear space, manifested by bubbling, and eventual resolution of the process.

Symptoms also vary with the magnitude of the pressure differential and the speed with which it develops. In minimal barotrauma, symptoms usually are limited to mild ear pain, a feeling of fullness in the ear, and mild conductive-type hearing loss. A low-pitched tinnitus may be noted. With this category of involvement, symptoms usually disappear fairly quickly and completely soon after the middle ear space is ventilated. With moderate degrees of pressure differential, all symptoms are increased in intensity. If a transudate were to occur, the patient may notice sensations due to fluid movement as the head position is changed or during the act of swallowing. In severe barotrauma, particularly when the pressure differential develops relatively quickly, the pain may be so great that it is incapacitating. The hearing loss usually will be greater and the tinnitus louder.

Vertigo may be experienced with severe barotrauma; this is uncommon but significant because it may be disabling. The precise mechanism for the production of vertigo by reduced pressure in the middle ear is not known; the labyrinth is evidently stimulated by the pressure change that is applied to the oval and round windows. If the tympanic membrane were to rupture, pain and other symptoms usually would subside quickly. Clinical findings also vary with the degree of pressure change and the length of time the condition has been present when the patient is seen. Development of a relatively negative pressure in the middle ear space produces retraction of the eardrum, with prominence of the short process of the malleus and what is referred to as ''foreshortening'' of its long process. Vascular engorgement produces injection and hyperemia of the eardrum, which is most marked peripherally and along the long process of the malleus. Hemorrhagic areas may be seen in the eardrum, again most likely along the long process of the malleus or in the drum periphery. These tiny hemorrhages also occur throughout the middle ear mucosa but usually cannot be seen. The formation of a transudate may be manifested by a middle ear that is full of serous fluid or by an air-fluid interface in the form of a relatively straight line (that shifts with changes in head position) or by bubbles. A hemorrhagic transudate produces a hemotympanum. Perforation of the tympanic membrane may occur at any point, usually at the weakest area in the eardrum and possibly at the site of an earlier perforation or an atrophic scar.

The usual audiometric finding is a conductive-type hearing loss. In the earlier stages, before any transudate develops, the low frequencies are primarily affected due to increased stiffness of the conduction system. When transudation occurs, stiffness is lessened and, the mass of the conduction system is increased, which is reflected in less involvement of the lower frequencies and increased involvement of the higher tones. This hearing loss is usually mild, unless hemorrhage occurs in the tympanic cavity, which can produce a greater loss. Fork tests are consistent with conductive hearing loss.

The diagnosis in most patients should not be difficult and is based primarily on a history of pain and hearing loss developing during or immediately following descent in an aircraft. Retraction of the tympanic membranae and tiny hemorrhages into the substance of the eardrum, as well as serous or perhaps serosanguineous fluid in the middle ear space, aid in establishing the diagnosis. The differential diagnosis should include serous otitis media, acute and chronic otitis media, external otitis, and myringitis bullosa. An adequate history of barotrauma and characteristic eardrum findings should aid in differentiating barotitis media from other entities.

Therapeutic measures should be divided into two general categories: (1) in-flight measures that can be employed by aircrew; and (2) therapeutic measures that the physician may employ when one examines an individual who has sustained an ear block.

The primary in-flight measure is the performance of the Valsalva maneuver as soon as a feeling of fullness is noted in either ear. When the individual has a nasal decongestant (such as 0.25% phenylephrine or Neo-Synephrine®), the nose should be sprayed. This procedures is best accomplished by spraying each side initially and then applying a second spray a few minutes after the initial application has had time to take effect. The second application has a better chance of reaching the nasopharyngeal area and shrinking the mucosa around the tubal orifice. If the ear could not be ventilated by the Valsalva maneuver, a return to higher altitude should be conducted promptly when operational conditions permit. The ear should then be ventilated and a gradual descent conducted while the individual performs the Valsalva maneuver frequently.

When aircrew present to the clinician with ear block, management should be based on the clinical findings. If no evidence of transudation were

to exist, an attempt should be made to ventilate the ear. Politzerization usually will be required because the Valsalva maneuver will be effective; otherwise, the individual would not have developed an ear block. Either the Politzer bag or a source of compressed air may be used. The nose should be sprayed well with a decongestant solution; maximum shrinkage of the mucosa should be attained. For the bag method, the olive tip is placed in one nostril, the nose is compressed between the physician's fingers, and the patient is then instructed to say "kick, kick, kick" while the bag is squeezed, thereby increasing the pressure in the nasopharyngeal cavity to the point at which the eustachian tube is opened and the middle ear space ventilated. If compressed air were used, the pressure would be turned down to 4–5 psi, and a suitable empty spray bottle that takes a nasal tip, such as a DeVilbiss nebulizer, is used to deliver air to the patient's nose. It may be necessary to increase the pressure gradually several times until air enters the middle ear; however, the pressure should not be > 5–6 psi. When politzerization cannot be accomplished at this pressure level, it is not likely that increasing the pressure further will result in success. If the ear could not be ventilated by having the patient say "kick, kick, kick," the procedure may be repeated while having the patient swallow a small amount of water during the application of the air. An effort must be made to synchronize delivery of the air with the second phase of deglutition, at which time the velopharyngeal sphincter is closed. The patient can be relied on to verify that the middle ear has ben inflated. When necessary, however, the physician can use a Toynbee tube to auscultate the involved ear while air is blown into the nasal cavity. If air were to enter the middle ear in any significant quantity, it usually would be heard. When desired, one physician may apply the air to the nasal cavity while another physician observes the eardrum directly for evidence of ventilation.

Successful inflation of the ear does not necessarily indicate immediate resolution of the ear block. When significant trauma to the eustachian tube occurs, simply ventilating the ear will not reverse the process. The one type of ear block in which ventilating the ear may effectively terminate the process is a delayed ear block due to oxygen absorption from the middle ear space because, in this variety of ear block, little or no trauma has occurred to the eustachian tube. If politzerization were initially successful, it may be necessary to repeat this procedure for several days until eustachian tube adequacy were reestablished.

When transudation into the middle ear space has occurred by the time the patient is first seen, no attempt should be made to ventilate the ear. The formation of fluid usually eliminates any persisting pressure differential and relieves any pain, and the patient's primary complaint will be the feeling of fullness in the ear and mild hearing loss. The patient should be started on conservative therapy, consisting of both topical and systemic decongestants. It is a good practice to combine the systemic decongestant with an antihistamine. When the eustachian tube begins to open, as manifested by bubbles behind the eardrum, resolution of the process may be hastened by politzerization. As soon as the patient can perform the Valsalva maneuver, however, politzerization can be discontinued.

Regardless of the condition in which the patient presents for treatment, therapy must be continued until the process has completely subsided and the eustachian tube and middle ear function normally. It is imperative that aircrew be grounded for this period and that they not be returned to flying duties prematurely.

Hemotympanum should be managed conservatively. Considerable time, up to several weeks, may be required for blood to clear from the middle ear space. Myringotomy should be avoided if possible. The only absolute indication for myringotomy would be the need for an aircrew member to return immediately to flying duties for some compelling operational reason. Myringotomy does not restore the eustachian tube to functional status, but it will open the

middle ear space and prevent further trauma to the eustachian tube and relieve ear symptoms.

Perforation of the tympanic membrane should be treated conservatively. The ear should be kept dry and the patient followed on an outpatient basis. If healing were not well under way by the end of two weeks, local measures, such as cauterizing the margins and installing a paper patch, should be considered and would probably require referral to an otolaryngologist.

It cannot be overemphasized that the management of barotitis media is essentially conservative. Mucous membrane of the upper respiratory tract is delicate and nothing should be done to possibly augment existing trauma. Catheterization of the eustachian tube orifice is never indicated. This procedure would only further traumatize the eustachian tube and undoubtedly prolong the disorder.

Recurrent barotitis media is essentially the problem of chronic eustachian tube obstruction, which is usually secondary to a pathologic process in either the nose or nasopharynx. The most common causes are hypertrophic lymphoid tissue in the nasopharynx, allergic rhinitis, and chronic sinusitis. Lymphoid tissue deposited submucosally along the anterior two-thirds of the eustachian tube (Gerlach's tonsil) may be hyperplastic. Occasionally, deflection of the nasal septum may be a significant factor. Treatment should be directed at the primary problem and may be either medical or surgical. In an occasional patient, no apparent cause for chronic eustachian tube obstruction can be found, and hyperplastic submucosal lymphoid tissue along the anterior two-thirds of the tube may be suspected.

Alternobaric Vertigo

Alternobaric, or pressure, vertigo should be regarded as a type of barotrauma in which symptoms result from the effect of expansion of trapped gases within the middle ear space. The precise mechanism by which vertigo is produced is not known; however, the role of positive pressure in the middle ear is generally accepted. The production of vertigo implies stimulation of the vestibular system, probably through an intact oval window. The increase in pressure due to failure to ventilate the middle ear on ascent is gradual and, in most instances, is not enough to produce vertigo; however, the addition of a sudden pressure increment caused by the performance of a forceful Valsalva maneuver can be sufficient for vestibular stimulation. Minimal residual eustachian tube edema secondary to a resolving upper respiratory tract infection can make ventilation of the ears on ascent difficult, requiring a more forceful Valsalva maneuver than is usually necessary.

Alternobaric vertigo is probably fairly common in pilots of high-performance jet aircraft capable of a rapid rate of ascent. The role that pressure change plays is corroborated by the higher incidence of alternobaric vertigo in divers because pressure changes are much greater in an aqueous media. In 1957, Jones reported an incidence of 10% in 190 pilots (8); in 1966, Lundgren and Malm reported an incidence of 17% in 108 pilots (9). The understandable reluctance of pilots to report symptoms of this type makes it reasonable to assume that this entity is more common than is generally realized.

In most instances, the history is fairly typical. The aircrew, most often a pilot flying a high-performance jet aircraft, usually relates the sudden onset of vertigo following the performance of a forceful Valsalva maneuver to relieve a feeling of fullness in one or both ears. This vertigo usually occurs on ascent, but it has been described on descent following a particularly forceful Valsalva maneuver (10). Vertigo is characteristically brief, ordinarily lasting a few seconds. The individual usually feels normal as soon as the vertigo clears. Whether this brief episode of vertigo actually compromises flight safety is determined by the operational circumstances and the experience of the individual concerned, but that it is capable of so doing is obvious.

The management of alternobaric vertigo is essentially prevention. This implies a continual process of education for aircrew in which the common nature and hazard potential of this condition are emphasized. The admonition not to fly with a cold cannot be overemphasized. It is reasonably safe to assume that the most common reason for having difficulty ventilating the middle ear is residual eustachian tube involvement from an acute upper respiratory tract infection. Aircrew most likely to encounter this condition should be advised to clear their ears more frequently during climb-out and avoid the necessity for a forceful Valsalva maneuver.

The aeromedical significance of alternobaric vertigo is obvious; it is capable of producing sudden incapacity in flight. The fact that it may be of brief duration should neither negate its significance, nor assume that it may not occur at a critical time in flight. In the operation of high-performance, fighter-type jet aircraft, all aspects of flight are critical, and several seconds are sufficient for an unsafe operational condition to develop. That alternobaric vertigo is relatively common must be realized by pilots and should be emphasized on a continuing basis by flight surgeons.

Barodontalgia

Barodontalgia, or aerodontalgia, is a toothache that is provoked by exposure to changing barometric pressures (during actual or simulated flight).

In 1937, Drefus first reported pain in a tooth that occurred in flight at 1800 m (5,500 ft) (11); he later relieved this pain by pulpectomy. In World War II, many episodes of odontalgia occurred during flight and were referred to as aerodontalgia. It was relatively uncommon, 1–2% in most series, but in many instances was severe enough to compromise the mission success. Barodontalgia, the preferred term at present, has persisted as an aeromedical problem, although the incidence has remained low (e.g., < 1% of altitude chamber reactions, as shown in Table 17.1).

The precise mechanism for pain production in barodontalgia has not been determined; how-

Table 17.1.
Distribution of Altitude Chamber Reactions (%)

Symptom	52,113 United States Air Force Trainees—1964	49,603 United States Air Force Trainees—1965
Aerotitis	8.730	8.660
Abdominal gas pain	1.960	1.850
Aerosinusitis	1.590	1.860
Bends	0.310	0.300
Barodontalgia	0.230	0.300
Chokes	0.003	0.008
Neurologic symptoms	0.002	0.000
Other	0.780	0.670
Total	13.605	13.648

From: Flight Surgeons Guide, Air Force Pamphlet 161–18. Department of the Air Force, Washington, DC: U.S. Government Printing Office, 1968.

ever, exposure to reduced atmospheric pressure is obviously a significant factor. This exposure to reduced barometric pressure is evidently a precipitating factor, with disease of the pulp the primary cause. Pressure changes do not elicit pain in teeth with normal pulps, regardless of whether the tooth is intact, carious, or restored. In his classic review on the effects of changes in barometric pressure, Adler classified symptoms as due either to trapped gases or evolved gases, and he placed barodontalgia in the trapped-gas category primarily because symptoms frequently appear at altitudes well below those considered necessary to produce evolved gases (12). Orban and Rithey concluded that the mechanism had to be liberation and expansion of gases from the blood and tissue fluids (13); however, they were able to demonstrate empty, bubble-like spaces in only 6 of 75 teeth that they studied. Air trapped under restorations has been suspected of producing tooth pain, but experimentally produced air bubbles under dental restorations followed by exposure to reduced barometric pressure did not result in symptoms. Other possible factors have been considered. Studies found that low temperatures were not significant and eliminated radial acceleration as a possible factor. Also, detrimental effects from the use of oxygen in flight have not been identified. Pulp disease appears to be the significant dental factor, and the initiation of symptoms is

probably due to a circulatory disturbance. The pulp organ is unique in that it is encapsulated in a nonyielding structure. It contains a complicated vascular system, including metarterioles and precapillaries. Circulation to the pulp is a delicate and sensitive system, which can be injured by tooth trauma. For reasons not fully understood at present, a damaged pulp can react to reduced atmospheric pressure and produce pain. This reaction appears to involve edema, which can lead to necrosis. In some patients, gas may form by the action of enzymes on necrotic pulp tissue.

Strohaver advocated the differentiation of barodontalgia into direct and indirect types (14). In the direct variety, reduced atmospheric pressure contributes to a direct effect on a given tooth; in the indirect type, dental pain is secondary to stimulation of the superior alveolar nerves by maxillary barosinusitis. Direct barodontalgia is generally manifested by moderate-to-severe pain, which usually develops during ascent and is well localized, with the patient frequently able to identify the involved tooth, whereas indirect barodontalgia is a dull, poorly defined pain that involves the posterior maxillary teeth and develops during descent.

Certain generalities may be useful in establishing the diagnosis of direct barodontalgia. Posterior teeth are more frequently involved than anterior teeth, and maxillary teeth are affected more often than mandibular teeth. Teeth with amalgam restorations are more likely to be involved than unrestored teeth, and recently restored teeth are particularly susceptible. The character of the pain is useful in determining whether the pulp involvement is acute or chronic; however, in an individual patient, this degree of diagnostic precision may not be possible. When pain occurs during descent, indirect barodontalgia due to barosinusitis should be strongly suspected. The patient should be asked which tooth or teeth are suspected, and then the physician should inquire about the approximate age of any restorations in the suspected area, as well as any history of previously unprovoked pain and any sensitivity to heat, cold, sweets, or pressure.

Examination should include the estimation of the age of restorations in the suspected area, exploration for caries or defective restorations, percussion of any suspected tooth, and the patient's response to application of electrical stimulation and/or ice and heat. Appropriate radiographs of the suspected teeth should be obtained, with the understanding that a negative radiograph does not rule out pulpitis.

Management should include the removal of any restorations that are clinically or radiographically defective. Any carious lesions should be curetted, with particular attention paid to exposed pulp horns. Zinc oxide and eugenol base may be useful if the pulpal condition were reversible. If irreversible pulpitis were found, endodontic treatment should be conducted, or the tooth should be extracted. Reexposure to altitude in a chamber can be employed to confirm a doubtful diagnosis or to determine the effectiveness of therapy. If indirect barodontalgia were diagnosed, the patient should be referred to an aeromedical specialist for treatment.

Strohaver reported that the incidence of barodontalgia has apparently decreased since World War II, possibly due to better dental care for flyers and improvements in cockpit and passenger compartment conditions (particularly pressurization) (14). To date, barodontalgia has not

been a problem in space flight because astronauts operate in a pressurized cabin and are not exposed to the spectrum of pressure changes that are encountered in flights in military aircraft. Direct barodontalgia can be largely prevented by high-quality dental care, with an emphasis on the slow and careful treatment of cavities and the routine use of a cavity varnish. Pulp-capping materials should be employed in deep preparations due to the possibility of a nonbleeding pulp exposure. Occlusion should be perfected until it is not self-damaging. Flying duties should be restricted for 48–72 hours after dental treatment involving deep restorations to allow time for dental pulp to stabilize. Obviously, regular dental examinations are essential for aircrew; any dental problem that may predispose the crew member to barodontalgia should be corrected and the development of symptoms prevented.

Barosinusitis

Barosinusitis can be defined as an acute or chronic inflammation of one or more of the paranasal sinuses produced by the development of a pressure difference, usually negative, between the air in the sinus cavity and that of the surrounding atmosphere.

In 1878, Burt documented the experience of Cezanne, who had noted bleeding from the nose and throat in his employees doing caisson work. The first detailed description of sinus barotrauma was made by Marchoux and Nepper in 1919; they described the results of their experiments in a decompression chamber and applied their conclusions to the operation of aircraft. They pointed out the increasing likelihood of this problem as pilots approach runways, at which time they require maximum use of their faculties to accomplish safe landings. In the mid 1940s, Campbell published several reports on the effects of barotraumatic changes on the sinuses, including his demonstration of the formation of submucosal hematomas in the frontal sinuses of dogs.

The USAF chamber flight data in Table 17.1 show the relative incidence of barosinusitis. According to these data, barosinusitis is much less common than barotitis media, the latter occurring four to five times as often. This general incidence is confirmed by the frequency with which each occurs in flight operations.

A paranasal sinus is a rigid-walled cavity that directly or indirectly communicates with the nasal cavity or nasopharynx by way of an ostium. During ascent, air in such a cavity moves out by way of the ostium until equilibrium is attained at altitude. During descent, air moves back into the sinus cavity until equilibrium is again reached at the earth's surface. This movement of air out and back into the sinus cavity is not perceived and does not produce any symptoms. Abnormal conditions may alter or even prevent this free flow of air from the sinus and produce symptoms and pathologic changes. The larger sinuses are more often involved than are the smaller ones. Sinuses having small-caliber tubal structures as exits, such as the frontal sinus with its nasofrontal duct, are more likely to be involved than are sinuses with relatively larger orifices. The frontal sinuses are most often involved, with the maxillary sinuses next. Involvement of the ethmoid and sphenoid sinuses is possible but rarely seen.

The free movement of air out of and back into a paranasal sinus may be impeded or blocked by pus or mucopurulent material covering its ostium or by redundant tissue or an anatomic deformity. When mucopurulent material covers the ostium of the sinus, the relatively positive pressure that develops during ascent can cause air in the sinus to bubble through the exudate, and no symptoms will result. On descent, however, the development of a relatively negative pressure within the sinus cavity may suck the material into the sinus ostium and sinus cavity. In the case of the frontal sinus, with its rather long and frequently tortuous nasofrontal duct, thick mucopurulent material can obstruct the duct and create a sinus block. Mucopurulent material also can contaminate the sinus cavity and result in a purulent sinusitis. When an ostium of a sinus is obstructed by swollen or redundant tissue or by

an anatomic deformity, a one-way flap or ball valve may be produced. During ascent, the flow of air out of the sinus cavity pushes the "valve" away from the opening, and the pressure equalizes at altitude. On descent, however, the relatively negative pressure inside the sinus pulls the tissue into the ostium, forming an airtight seal and producing a sinus block.

The production of a relatively negative pressure inside a sinus cavity results in space-filling phenomena. The most common of these are swelling of the mucous membranes and/or transudation of fluid either into the cavity of the sinus or beneath the sinus mucosa. When sufficient space is filled to equalize the pressure differential, the valve mechanism is released and recovery begins. In mild-to-moderate degrees of sinus barotrauma, vascular engorgement and generalized submucosal edema occur. With more severe trauma, mucosal detachment and submucosal hematoma may develop.

The symptoms of barosinusitis are usually proportional to its severity and may vary from a mild feeling of fullness in or around the involved sinus to excruciating pain. Pain can develop suddenly and be incapacitating. The pain is believed to be produced by the submucosal accumulation of blood dissecting the mucoperiosteum from the underlying bone. Some tenderness over the involved sinus and some bloody discharge from the nose may occur.

Sinus barotrauma should be differentiated from acute purulent sinusitis. A history of pain over one or more of the paranasal sinuses during or shortly after exposure to a barometric pressure change usually simplifies the differential diagnosis. In more severe cases, the patient usually describes the onset of pain as quite sudden and severe. In less severe cases, the pain may be described by the patient as having developed slowly after return to ground level. Exacerbation of symptoms after a return to ground level may be due to an increase in the relatively negative pressure within the sinus following the absorption of oxygen from the air trapped in the sinus (because oxygen is readily absorbed transmucosally). Bleeding from the nose during or after exposure to barotrauma strongly suggests sinus involvement.

Radiographs are the most valuable diagnostic aid. The standard sinus radiographic series in most institutions consist of Waters, lateral, and submentovertex projections. Radiographs do not differentiate any contributory forms of preexisting disease or an anatomic abnormality from the results of barotrauma. The usual finding is mucosal thickening, which may be localized or so generalized and severe that it simply produces an opaque sinus. An air-fluid level also may be demonstrated. These are nonspecific findings that must be correlated with the history. If hematoma were present, it would usually be found in the frontal sinus and would present as an oval density varying from a few millimeters in diameter to practically complete occupancy of the sinus cavity. Hematomas may be single or multiple, unilateral or bilateral.

In milder cases, the involvement is usually self-limited, with resolution taking place within a few hours to a few days. In the more severe cases, the clinical course may run from a few days to as long as a few weeks. Complete resorption of a submucosal hematoma may take several weeks. If secondary infection were to occur, severe, purulent sinusitis may result from the lower resistance of the traumatized tissues and/or the excellent culture medium afforded by the transudate in the sinus cavity. This transudate, whether it is serous or serosanguineous, is usually sufficiently space-filling to relieve the pressure differential, thereby releasing the flap or ball valve and alleviating pain.

Treatment should begin at the first sign of barosinusitis and consists of returning to the altitude at which the block occurred, spraying the nose well with a decongestant solution and then slowly descending to ground level. This treatment may or may not be possible depending on operational conditions and may not be feasible in a combat situation. If the patient were first examined at ground level, an altitude chamber may be available at some installations in which the patient could be returned to altitude. From a practical standpoint, this procedure is rarely necessary. Active treatment is usually limited to those procedures that relieve pain, promote drainage from the sinus cavity, and offer protection from infection. Oral analgesics usually are sufficient. The patient's nasal mucosa should be thoroughly decongested with a topical agent, and be given a supply of the same along with a systemic decongestant. The application of heat, preferably in the form of hot packs, is usually helpful. When the maxillary sinuses are involved and significant pain persists, any relatively negative pressure in the sinus cavity can be promptly relieved by cannulating the sinus cavity. This procedure should be done through the canine fossa or inferior meatus; the region of the natural ostium should not be instrumented. Cannulation of the frontal sinus is not recommended; when the frontal sinus must be entered, it should be by an external approach. An adequate course of an appropriate antibiotic can be prescribed to prevent secondary infection.

In most patients, barosinusitis can be managed conservatively, and uneventful recovery is the rule. It is imperative that a patient remain grounded until fully recovered and nose and paranasal sinuses are functioning normally. A simulated flight in an altitude chamber may be required when any doubt exists as to whether the crew member is fully recovered and ready to return to flying duties.

The most important preventive measure that should be emphasized by physicians on a continuing basis is that aircrew should not fly when they have upper respiratory tract infections. Any intranasal condition that could affect ventilation of the paranasal sinuses should be corrected, such as a significant septal deviation or presence of nasal polyps.

Total cabin pressurization would prevent the occurrence of barotrauma; however, this cannot be anticipated in the foreseeable future. Partial pressurization decreases the rapidity of the fluctuations of barometric pressure, as well as their magnitude. The cabin altitude of commercial aircraft usually does not exceed 2700 m (8200 ft); consequently, little barosinusitis is experienced in commercial aviation. In military aviation, pressurization is used primarily to increase performance parameters. Obviously, in military operations, aircrew are subjected to greater barometric pressure changes because military aircraft are capable of much greater rates of ascent and descent.

Abnormalities with Aeromedical Significance

Otitis Externa

The acute, diffuse variety of otitis externa is most common and usually results from wetting the outer ear canal. Sufficient pain and tenderness may exist to preclude wearing a helmet or headset until the involvement has cleared. The use of earplugs and earmuffs also will not be possible in the presence of inflammation of the external auditory canal.

In a crewmember with recurrent otitis externa, an effective preventive measure is to dehydrate the outer ear canal after each wetting from swimming, shampooing, or showering with a solution of ethyl alcohol (95% is best, but 70% is usually adequate and is more readily available) mixed with a mild acetic vehicle, such as 1% acetic acid.

Perforation of the Tympanic Membrane

The tympanic membrane is the most important part of the middle ear mechanical transformer, which largely compensates for the impedance to sound that is created by an air-fluid interface due to air in the middle ear and fluid in the inner ear. This impedance-matching mechanism essentially offsets this loss of energy, and its primary factor is the ratio of the area of the tympanic membrane to the area of the footplate of the stapes (approximately 14:1). Sound is concentrated at the oval window. The eardrum also is part of the preferential route for the conduction of sound to the oval window. This is essential for maintaining proper phase relations which are necessary for adequate stimulation of the organ of Corti in the cochlea. Obviously, an intact tympanic membrane is essential for the optimum accomplishment of these functions.

The tympanic membrane also seals the middle ear from the external auditory canal which, in turn, communicates with the external environment. Perforation of the eardrum makes the middle ear vulnerable to contamination by way of the external ear canal and can lead to infection of the middle ear, which may be recurrent or even become chronic. A crew member's performance can be compromised, particularly during operations in the field. Tympanostomy tubes have the same implications as other perforations. These tubes provide a bypass for a malfunctioning eustachian tube, but this temporary measure is unacceptable as a definitive solution for tubal incompetence. A tympanostomy tube may become obstructed, displaced, or the route for contamination of the middle ear. These are unacceptable risks for flying personnel. The primary tubal problem must be resolved and continuity of the eardrum restored for the crew member to continue on active flying status.

Vertigo

Vertigo has great aeromedical significance because it is capable of producing sudden incapacity that can compromise flight safety. Obviously, the flight surgeon must differentiate pathologic vertigo from spatial disorientation, or "pilot's vertigo," and alternobaric vertigo. A detailed history is the physician's best tool for accomplishing this differentiation.

Pathologic vertigo involves a false perception of movement or orientation in space. Vertigo is usually due to a peripheral vestibular abnormality, but it may be central in origin, which increases the likelihood that a serious condition is present.

Peripheral vertiginous entities include Ménière disease, benign positional vertigo, labyrinthitis (toxic, serous, and infectious), posttraumatic vertigo, and perilymph fistulas. Cerebellopontine angle lesions rarely produce

typical vertigo because the lesion is slow-grow-
ing and central compensation develops as the
end organ is deafferentated by the enlarging
mass. Central causes of vertigo include vertebro-
basilar insufficiency, vascular accidents, multiple sclerosis, epilepsy, migraine, neoplasms, and
head injury.

The primary aeromedical implication of vertigo is the possibility of recurrence with sudden
incapacitation. When the patient's history and
findings are reasonably consistent with a fairly
well-known entity, disposition can be made with
some confidence (15). A crew member with Ménière disease should be permanently grounded
because recurrence of vertigo is probable, and
the interval between episodes is unpredictable.
Conversely, one with viral involvement of the
vestibular system, either viral labyrinth or vestibular neuronitis, can be returned to flying duties following full recovery. If benign positional
vertigo or posttraumatic vertigo were suspected,
a period of observation may be helpful in deciding whether a return to flying duties should be
recommended. If a perilymph fistula were confirmed by tympanotomy and the leak were
sealed with clearing of the vertigo, return to
flying duties could be considered, although the
crew member should probably be regarded as a
greater risk for recurrence than nonflying personnel. All central causes of vertigo should be
considered disqualification from flying duties
except for certain head injuries, after which return to flying duties may be possible following
an adequate period of observation provided no
neurologic symptoms exist.

Anosmia

Inability to perceive odors has obvious safety
implications in that various substances, such as
fuel vapors, lubricants, or smoke, may be present
in the aircraft and go unnoticed by the pilot or
other aircrew. This may be less significant in
aircraft where an oxygen mask is worn throughout the flight because the aircrew would probably note only odorants in the oxygen system. In
bomber and cargo aircraft, where crew members
do not wear oxygen masks throughout the flight,
olfactory capability is a significant alerting
mechanism, and the loss of this sense through
injury or disease will affect flying safety. An
individual who notes a diminution in the ability
to smell or the complete loss of the faculty
should receive a thorough medical evaluation to
elucidate the causative factors and determine
whether the abnormality is amenable to treatment. The impact of any persisting olfactory impairment on the patient's aircrew status should
be determined.

Allergic Rhinitis

Allergic rhinitis is a common medical problem that can make a person more liable to barotrauma because nasal congestion and discharge
are frequent manifestations. Antihistamines are
effective in many patients with nasal allergy;
however, because sedation is a common side effect, aircrew should be cautioned about the regular use of these drugs. New-generation antihistamines markedly reduce the sedation side effect
and may be considered for treatment. Any crew
member with significant allergic rhinitis should
probably have an allergy evaluation; if significant sensitivities were found, the patient could
be started on a hyposensitization program that
is compatible with the continuation on flying
status. Another therapeutic option that can now
be considered is the inhalation of an intranasal
steroid. The indicated agent is beclomethasone
dipropionate; in the one range recommended for
intranasal use, no significant depression of adrenal function has been noted (16). This agent may
be useful in the control of symptoms in certain
patients with nasal allergy. Patients with allergic
rhinitis should be strongly advised to avoid the
use of intranasal decongestants because dependence on one of these preparations may ensue,
with the development of rhinitis medicamentosa,
which would clearly indicate disqualification
from flying duties.

Nasal Polyposis

The presence of nasal polyps clearly makes a
person more vulnerable to sinus barotrauma and

should be regarded as disqualifying for flying until the polyps are removed and any contributory condition is controlled. In some patients, polyps are secondary to allergic rhinitis; however, in many patients, no relationship between nasal allergy and nasal polyps can be found. Evaluation of a patient with nasal polyposis should include CT scans of the paranasal sinuses because ethmoid and/or maxillary sinus involvement also may be present. Small polyps may regress with medical management, the control of allergies, or a short course of a systemic or intranasal steroid; however, large polyps usually require surgical removal. Any coexisting sinus involvement also should be appropriately treated. The importance of adequate follow-up must be appreciated; nasal polyps have a strong potential for recurrence, and subsequent removal or removals may be required.

Vasomotor Rhinitis

Vasomotor rhinitis should be regarded as an autonomic dysfunction in that the basic mechanism consists of accentuation or exaggeration of normal vasomotor and secretomotor activity. A sympathetic-parasympathetic imbalance results, with peripheral vasodilatation, edema, and hypersecretion. The most common etiologic factor is stress; therefore, the vulnerability of aircrew in the highly demanding flight environment is obvious. In some individuals, physical factors of the environment (e.g., temperature and humidity changes) may be operative. Most patients complain of nasal congestion or rhinorrhea or a combination of the two symptoms. Shifting nasal obstruction is characteristic of this disorder; typically, one side of the nose is obstructed for varying periods. Nasal drainage is usually described as clear or mucoid; it may be primarily posterior (postnasal drip) or anterior (frequent nose-blowing) or both. Various therapeutic measures may be tried depending on the primary symptom and its severity. Antihistamines and systemic decongestants may be beneficial, but the use of these drugs may require grounding of the aircrew member. Patients with vasomotor rhinitis frequently employ topical decongestants, which are readily available over-the-counter, and may develop rhinitis medicamentosa. Steroids are effective; topical steroids are preferred, and beclomethasone dipropionate is the drug of choice. In some patients, the careful intermittent use of this preparation may be beneficial. Most patients must simply learn to live with their nasal problems. This "reality therapy" is accepted much better when it is presented with a detailed explanation of normal nasal physiology and the aberrations present in vasomotor rhinitis (17).

Vasomotor rhinitis should be regarded as possibly disqualifying for flying duties unless it is mild and unlikely to limit flying activities. As indicated above, the possibility of interference with ventilation of the paranasal sinuses should be considered, as well as the propensity for self-medication with topical decongestants and the increased likelihood of developing rhinitis medicamentosa. When treatment is successful and significantly improves nasal function and the therapy is compatible with flying duties, aircrew duty may be resumed. Fortunately, most patients with vasomotor rhinitis have mild symptoms that can be tolerated without specific treatment other than explanation and reassurance.

Acute Sinusitis

Generally, acute sinusitis is an acute medical problem that requires grounding until the condition has cleared. Many patients regard headache as a manifestation of sinusitis; however, localized pain and tenderness are more reliable indicators of paranasal sinus inflammation. The importance of obtaining appropriate radiographs in the evaluation of an individual with sinus complaints cannot be overemphasized (18); radiographs are the most valuable diagnostic modality and should always be requested, not only for immediate diagnosis but also a basis for follow-up.

At USAFSAM, a routine Water's radiographic projection was performed on everyone presenting for aeromedical evaluation and a 4%

incidence of asymptomatic maxillary sinusitis was found (19). The same incidence was found in a nonflying control group; therefore, this condition is not related to flying, per se. It was concluded that in many individuals, maxillary sinusitis often occurs asymptomatically and evidently resolves without specific therapy. It also was concluded, however, that if relatively asymptomatic maxillary sinusitis were demonstrated radiographically in an aircrew member, appropriate treatment should be instituted and resolution confirmed by follow-up radiographs because normal function of the paranasal sinuses would be essential in flying. Therapy should include an adequate course of an appropriate antibiotic and both topical and systemic decongestants. In choosing an antibiotic or chemotherapeutic agent, the physician should consider that the bacteria most frequently causing acute sinusitis are the pneumococcus, Hemophilus influenzae, and various anaerobic bacteria (20). Good therapeutic agents include ampicillin or amoxicillin, erythromycin-sulfisoxazole, trimethoprim-sulfamethoxazole, and cefaclor.

The maxillary sinus is most frequently involved by an inflammatory process, followed by frontal sinusitis, whereas ethmoid and sphenoid sinus involvement is relatively uncommon. Most patients with maxillary sinusitis can be treated on an outpatient basis; however, in an individual with frontal sinusitis, the possibility of significant complications warrants consideration of hospitalization unless resolution is prompt (21). In all patients diagnosed with paranasal sinusitis, treatment should be followed by radiographic reevaluation to ensure resolution; those patients with conditions that are not resolved by appropriate medical measures should be considered for surgical intervention before being returned to flying duties.

Laryngitis

The primary aeromedical implication of laryngitis is impairment of the crew member's ability to communicate effectively by radio, intercom, or against background noise in aircraft

compartments, thus creating a significant hazard for the afflicted crew member, as well as other crew members.

Acute laryngitis is usually viral in etiology, and laryngeal involvement is frequently associated with other signs of acute upper respiratory tract infection. Treatment consists of resting the voice and symptomatic measures for the accompanying upper respiratory tract infection. The importance of voice rest should be emphasized to ensure compliance and preclude prolonged grounding. Whispering should be prohibited. Smoking also should be discontinued during the period of voice rest. If the patient were not to respond promptly to these measures, referral to an otolaryngologist for further evaluation would be mandatory. Obviously, chronic or recurring hoarseness should be promptly evaluated by an otolaryngologist.

The management of acute airway problems secondary to inflammation or foreign-body obstruction in aircrew who are isolated for long periods is important. Laryngeal intubation requires special equipment and training in its use. An instrument has been devised for use by relatively inexperienced individuals, and intubation training should be considered for aircrew who may be subjected to long-term isolation, as in space operations (22).

Maxillofacial Trauma

Maxillofacial trauma may constitute a significant problem in air evacuation. Flight crews must be knowledgeable in the care of patients with injuries in this area (23). The possibility of injury to the cervical spine should be considered and evaluated with an appropriate radiograph. Adequate initial measures, including tracheotomy for control of the airway, and essential inflight maintenance of the airway are paramount (24). The treatment of fractures usually can be deferred to the specialty center; however, if the teeth were placed in interdental fixation, rubber bands should be used rather than wire, and the patient must be provided with scissors for the prompt release of the fixation in the event that vomiting ensues.

IMPLICATIONS OF SURGICAL PROCEDURES

Otologic Implications

Mastoidectomy and Tympanoplasty

Persistent perforations of the tympanic membrane should be closed to protect the middle ear from external contamination via the outer ear canal. This is the primary aeromedical implication of a type I tympanoplasty or myringoplasty. This premise assumes more significance when the aircrew member does not have medical care readily available and may be exposed to potential extrinsic hazards, as in combat situations involving bailout or ditching and water survival. A persistent perforation, including tympanotomy tubes, should not be regarded as an acceptable solution for an aircrew member with compromised eustachian tube function; a flyer should be able to ventilate the middle ear adequately with an intact eardrum under the stresses of flying.

Other types of tympanoplasty and mastoid procedures may be considered collectively from an aeromedical point of view, excluding auditory acuity (which should be assessed separately) and violation of the oval window area. The primary consideration is that any air-containing space must communicate with the nasopharynx through openings that are adequate to assure pressure equalization under the stresses imposed by flying, with no positive-pressure buildup during ascent and no relatively negative-pressure development during descent. In addition to no air-conditioning pockets without adequate openings, a sufficiently functional eustachian tube is important. The resolution of this condition can be assessed with a medical altitude chamber flight postoperatively after allowing adequate time for the maximum contraction of scar tissue; six months is advisable, assuming that the ear is dry.

Any surgical procedures on the middle ear/ mastoid area must not involve the oval window area if continuation of flying status were a consideration. Any surgical activity in the oval window area can increase the likelihood of perilymph fistula formation, with the possibility of acute vertigo and sudden incapacitation.

Stapedectomy

Stapes procedures, stapedectomy being the most common, are directed precisely at the oval window area and, as indicated above, result in a situation in which the likelihood of the spontaneous formation of a perilymph fistula is increased. Following removal of the stapes, the oval window is sealed by a thin membrane. Considerable accumulated experience has established that this membrane is more vulnerable to stresses than is the stapedial footplate with its annular ligament. These stresses may be applied from within (explosive), in the form of surges of increased cerebral spinal fluid pressure transmitted via the cochlear aqueduct, or from the middle ear side (implosive) due to changes in air pressure in the middle ear (25). Perilymph fistulas are now known to develop in apparently normal individuals (26); therefore, the increased likelihood of this significant complication occurring following stapedectomy is apparent. Obviously, this consideration becomes even more pertinent when the aircrew member is operating a modern, high-performance jet aircraft.

Removal of Acoustive Neuromas

The acoustic neuroma is a benign tumor; therefore, if one were completely removed without any significant complications other than hearing loss, the situation would be essentially analogous to a "one-eared" pilot, and continuation of flying duties is possible when a good seal is obtained without any postoperative cerebrospinal fluid leak. The individual will compensate for the loss of the labyrinth; the hearing loss usually will be total and permanent. USAFSAM established a precedent for returning pilots with severe-to-total hearing loss in one ear to flying duties, assuming that no significant facial weakness resulted to compromise eye function or the wearing of an oxygen mask.

Rhinologic Implications

Nasal Septoplasty and Rhinoplasty

Nasal septoplasty can result in significant improvement of nasal airway patency. Because adequate airways are a requisite for flying duties, any significant septal deflection should be corrected as soon as possible. In a candidate for pilot training, this correction should be done prior to beginning training. If the examining physician were uncertain as to the functional significance of any intranasal abnormality, the patient should be referred to an otolaryngologist for evaluation and recommendations.

Rhinoplasty primarily is a cosmetic procedure; however, reduction of a nasal hump or correction of some other significant abnormality of the external nose can result in a better fit for an oxygen mask.

Nasal Polypectomy

As previously indicated, nasal polyps may be disqualifying for flying due to the increased likelihood of sinus barotrauma. However, adequate removal of polyps qualifies an individual for return to flying duties. The frequent association of nasal polyps with allergic rhinitis also should be considered. In addition, the importance of adequate follow-up cannot be overemphasized. Nasal polyps have a strong tendency to recur, and follow-up by an otolaryngologist is essential to determine whether the treatment regimen is effective. If recurrence were noted, the aircrew member should again be advised that the polyps should be removed and any medical management reappraised.

Sinus Surgery

Current otolaryngologic opinion strongly supports a conservative approach to sinus surgery. Radical procedures with meticulous removal of all mucosa are avoided except in ablation of the frontal sinus for chronic, recurrent infection. Because the maxillary sinus is most frequently involved by inflammatory processes, it is the sinus usually involved in aeromedical considerations. The value of the creation of an antrostomy in the inferior meatus should be fully appreciated. This procedure frequently is curative for recurrent or chronic maxillary sinusitis, and it has no limiting effect on an individual's ability to fly. This opening can be made transnasally, but many surgeons prefer a sublabial antrostomy (Caldwell-Luc) approach for better visualization of the sinus cavity and the creation of a large, competent, and permanent nasoantral window. Endoscopic surgery is rapidly replacing the above procedures.

The frontal sinus is most frequently involved in barosinusitis, and this condition requires consideration of procedures designed to improve ventilation of this sinus. Unfortunately, any procedure that involves enlarging the nasofrontal communication predisposes patients to late cicatrization, with reduction or closure of the nasofrontal duct. A conservative procedure that should be considered is removal of the intersinus septum (creating a common cavity) for recurrent, unilateral, frontal barosinusitis. For recurrent, bilateral, frontal barosinusitis, total obliteration of the frontal sinuses can be done; however, ablation of every vestige of mucosa is essential to preclude repneumatization of the sinus. This surgery is extensive for continuation on flying status and is usually performed for persistent frontal sinus infection. Several procedures for long-term maintenance of frontal duct patency, as well as endoscopic sinus procedures, are currently under study for long-term results.

REFERENCES

1. Jerger J, Jerger S. A simplified tone decay test. Arch Otolaryngol 1975;102:403–407.
2. Jewett DL, Romano MN, Williston JS. Human auditory evoked potentials: possible brain stem components detected on the scalp. Science 1970;167:1517–1518.
3. Fregly AR. Handbook of sensory physiology, Vol. VI, Part 2. Berlin: Springer-Verlag, 1974.

4. Jongkees LBW, Philipzoon AJ. Electronystagmography. Acta Otolaryngol 1963;189(Suppl):1–111.
5. Wolfe JW, Engelken EJ, Kos CM. Low-frequency harmonic acceleration as a test of labyrinthine function: basic methods and illustrative cases. Trans Am Acad Ophthalmol Otolaryngol 1978;86:130–154.
6. Stork RL, Gasaway DC. Evaluation of V-51R and EAR™ earplugs for use in flight. USAFSAM-TR-77–1. United States Air Force School of Aerospace Medicine, Brooks Air Force Base, Texas, 1977.
7. Armstrong HG, Heim JW. The effect of flight on the middle ear. JAMA 1937;109:417.
8. Jones GM. Review of current problems associated with disorientation in man-controlled flight. Flying Personnel Research Committee 1021. Great Britain: Royal Air Force, 1957 (restricted).
9. Lundgren CEG, Malm LU. Alternobaric vertigo among pilots. Aerospace Med 1966;37:178.
10. Brown FM. Vertigo due to increased middle ear pressure: six-year experience of the Aeromedical Consultation Service. Aerosp Med 1971;42:999.
11. Drefus H. "Les dents des aviateurs." L'Odontolgie 1937;75:612-613.
12. Adler HF. Dysbarism. USAFSAM Aeromedical Review 1964;1–64:6.
13. Orban B, Ritchey BT. Toothache under conditions simulating high-altitude flight. J Am Dent Assoc 1945;32:145.
14. Strohaver RA. Aerodontalgia: dental pain during flight. Med Serv Dig 1972;23:35.
15. Lindeman RC. Acute labyrinthine disorders. Otolaryngol Clin North Am 1979;12:357–387.
16. Harris DM, et al. The effect of intranasal beclomethasone dipropionate on adrenal function. Clin Allergy 1974;4:291–294.
17. Pogorel BSL. Vasomotor rhinitis and nasal dyspnea. ENT 1977;56:261–272.
18. Yarington CT Jr. Emergency problems involving sinusitis. Aviat Space Environ Med 1979;50:80–82.
19. Hanna HH. Asymptomatic sinus disease in aircrew members. Aerosp Med 1974;45:77–81.
20. Gwaltney JM Jr, Sydnor AS Jr, Saude MA. Etiology and antimicrobial treatment of acute sinusitis. Ann Otolaryngol Rhinol Laryngol 1981;90(Suppl 84):68–71.
21. Yarington CT Jr. Sinusitis as an emergency. Otolaryngol Clin North Am 1979;12:447–454.
22. LeJeune FE Jr. Laryngeal problems in space travel. Aviat Space Environ Med 1978;49:1347–1349.
23. Yarington CT Jr. The initial evaluation in maxillofacial trauma. Otolaryngol Clin North Am 1979;12:293–301.
24. Linscott MS, Horton WC. Management of upper airway obstruction. Otolaryngol Clin North Am 1979;12:351–373.
25. Goodhill V. Traumatic fistulae. J Laryngol Otolaryngol 1980;94:123–128.
26. Fee GA. Traumatic perilymphatic fistulas. Arch Otolaryngol 1968;88:477–480.

Chapter 18

Neuropsychiatry in Aerospace Medicine

David R. Jones, Marc S. Katchen,

John C. Patterson,

and Michael Rea

For a pilot, flying is never dangerous, for a man must be a little bit insane or under the press of duty to willingly remain in a position that he truly considers dangerous. Airplanes occasionally crash, pilots are occasionally killed, but flying is not dangerous, it is interesting.

Richard Bach, *Stranger to the Ground*

Aeromedical practitioners have a specific approach to the selection and care of flyers that differs from conventional health care delivery. Their focus on health maintenance applies to psychiatric as well as somatic concerns. An operational flight surgeon must deal with the mental aspects of aviators' health when deciding who is qualified for flight training. The physician must assess the adequacy of psychologic defenses against anxiety about the natural dangers of flying and must decide when to ground and when to restore flying duties. Much of our information in this field derives from military sources and is worth reviewing.

Specific mental health factors were not considered in the earliest pilot selection standards. A directive from the Surgeon General of the United States Army in 1912 did not mention psychiatric matters, although it did call for the rejection of any applicant with such psychophysiologic afflictions as chronic digestive disturbances, constipation, or "intestinal disorders

tending to produce dizziness, headache, or to impair vision." The United States Naval letter issued later that year echoed these prohibitions, adding that "any candidate whose condition shows that he is inclined to any excess that may disturb his mental balance or to alcoholism should be rejected (1)."

Flight surgeons quickly recognized the importance of psychologic influences on a flyer's performance. One of the first textbooks of aviation medicine contained nine chapters. Two, entitled "The Psychology of Aviation" and "The Aero-Neuroses," were devoted to mental and emotional matters (2). "The Aero-Neuroses" dealt with the problem that we now call "fear of flying," which the author ascribed either to the strain of learning to fly or to involvement in an aircraft accident. "Nervous breakdowns have been noted since the early days of flying," he wrote only 15 years after the Wright brothers first flew. "In fact, they may be classed as an occupational neurosis (in) a comparatively new occupation, namely: flying.''

Aircraft have come far, but flyers enclosed in titanium alloy are much the same as those borne on wings of fabric. Aeromedical practitioners understand the need for selection criteria that consider motivation as well as ability. Flyers are sought who are not merely sound of mind but who also have coping skills suited to the particular stresses and dangers of flight. It is known that adults are not unchanging in their adaptation to the stresses of life, but that time and experience alter their methods of responding to such stresses. Thus, the understanding of the psychologic makeup of the successful aviator must include considerations of personality style, motivation to fly, ability to fly, and adult personality growth patterns.

Once selected and trained, the flyer faces not only the stresses of aviation but also the normal stresses of everyday life. Wings on the chest do not protect against acute stress reactions, psychophysiologic disorders, or depression. The skilled physician must be prepared to recognize a variety of psychopathologic disorders and to make the required judgements about when to fly and when to ground. Psychiatric treatment may exceed the capabilities of many aeromedical physicians, just as may ophthalmologic or orthopedic treatment, but few mental health professionals can judge as well as the personal aeromedical practitioner when an aviator is ready to return to unrestricted flying duties.

Aeromedical practitioners in civilian practice face particular challenges in regard to mental health. Unlike their military counterparts, who function within a unitary health care system, civilian physicians may not have easy access to complete medical records. Psychiatric or stress symptoms occurring in flying or nonflying job environments may not easily be brought to the physician's attention by supervisors or colleagues. The many informal contacts, and even the opportunity to care for the flyers' families, may not be practical or possible. Thus, civilian practitioners must develop a sharp clinical in-

stinct for indirect and nonverbal clues to disorders arising from stress or from psychiatric symptoms, especially those with clear aeromedical implications.

This chapter discusses the psychiatric aspects of aerospace medicine, the aeromedical aspects of psychiatry, and the neurologic function of the aviator.

PROFILE OF THE AVIATOR

Everyone knows what a military pilot is like: steely-eyed, granite-jawed, an overgrown adolescent who can party til 4 A.M., slip into a clean flight suit, and show up at 6 A.M. ready to ''kick the tires, light the fires, brief on Guard, and the first one in the air gets the lead!'' A stereotype about the personalities of aviators exists, to say the least, but flyers are quite diversified. Some, for example, are women. Still, something is distinctive in the way a successful aviator deals with life, an intangible factor that the experienced flight surgeon recognizes. Civilian pilots are even more diverse, yet have an essential sameness about them. Acknowledging the difficulty of capturing this essence in words, we will discuss some aspects of the ''normal'' aviator.

Personality

Personality describes the ways that people interact with situations and other people. These adaptations are generally developed by midadolescence and tend to change slowly, if at all, through the years. For example, the neat and careful teenager is likely to be neat and careful all his life.

It is likely that no occupation has attracted as many studies of its participants as has flying. Beaven mentioned control of the imagination, confidence, patience, and especially a strong motivation to fly as important characteristics of successful aviators during World War I (1). Christy described the balance necessary between various factors such as rigidity and flexibility (3). In other words, the flyer should be careful about such things as necessary checklists but also should be able to deal imaginatively with unforeseen situations or emergencies. As Christy pointed out, a good pilot who is mature, well-motivated, and self-confident would probably succeed in any chosen profession or undertaking.

Fine and Hartman studied 50 successful military pilots in detail, using both psychiatric and psychological data (4). They defined the "modal military pilot," contrasting these characteristics with flyers known to have failed and with characteristics reported in astronauts (Table 18.1). A similar report refers to the typical United States Air Force (USAF) aviator as possessing an above-average intelligence, a matter-of-fact

view of life, and a preference for action over introspection in dealing with stress (5). This latter finding is of particular importance because exaggeration of such tendency may lead a pilot who is frustrated to act out these frustrations in inappropriate ways (drinking or impulsive physical action) rather than thinking the problem through in a deliberate manner.

A study of 105 superior jet pilots noted that they had a particular self-confidence, desire for challenge and success, and strong identification with their fathers, many of whom were also military flyers. These energetic and optimistic pilots tended to be firstborn or eldest sons. They tended to make life choices on a consciously rational basis, being willing to take risks only when a

Table 18.1.
Adaptive Personality Traits in Flyers

Conditions for Expected Failure or Adaptation (Grounding or Patient Status)	Typical Adult Adjustment (Modal Military Pilot)	Conditions for Expected Superior Adaptation (the Test Pilot or Astronaut)
Failure to succeed at a goal	Alloplastic; self-sufficient; short-range goal	More ambitiousness with success
Restriction from flying; retirement	Achievement; novelty; responsibility	Opportunity for a life-style that synthesizes these needs
Ambiguous situations (particularly social); inconsistency of background with current task	Terse; direct; nonintellectual; emotionally avoidant	Exceptional consistency of background and task
Less well-endowed intellectually or physically	Bright-normal intelligence; perceptual, motor skills, courage, and energy	Outstanding endowment; better social or economic conditions while growing up
Physical illness; instability of background while growing up; neurotic predisposition	Excellent physical health; lack of neurotic symptoms	Freedom from neurotic conflict
Insoluble personality conflict at work	Unconflicted relationships with men	Work with teams of similar job-oriented men
Too much emotional stimulation; failure in family stability	Anxiety when too close to women	Marriage to self-contained women; good family functioning; easily explained absences from home
Unavoidable confrontation with inner emotional life	Relative inflexibility for drive reduction	Better capacity for emotional introspection
Irresponsibility or lack of social sanctions for hostility	Well-controlled unconscious hostility; tendency to act out	A nonhostile but aggressive assignment
Exceptionally strong limitations	Self-image; creative; intellectual limitations	Advanced education; a broader range of interests
Unavoidable confrontation with self-limitations	Low tolerance for personal imperfections	Much recognition and approval for lifelong success

Adapted from Fine PM, Harman BO: Psychiatric strengths and weaknesses of typical air force pilots. USAFSAM Technical Report 68-121. United States Air Force School of Aerospace Medicine, Brooks Air Force Base, Texas, 1968; 131–168.

consideration of the odds led to a high chance of successful outcome. They were curious, restless, involved in many projects, and had high-energy levels. They made friendships easily, but these relationships were rarely deep or intense. They preferred not to be dependent on other people, but to keep interpersonal distance (6).

The new flight surgeon quickly begins to realize the diversity of personalities represented among successful pilots. Nevertheless, an appreciation of their similarities begins to emerge. With experience, a flight surgeon is able to recognize whether a given individual thinks and acts like a flyer, a clinical instinct that is particularly valuable in assessing applicants for flight training. This perception is especially true in the case of military aviators, upon whom most of the data in the literature are based.

Motivation

Successful flyers have been identified as intelligent, energetic, competent, action-oriented men and women whose obsessive-compulsive personality style is usually flexible enough to adapt to novel situations. What motivates such a person to fly?

Motivation is the psychic force or energy that moves a person to satisfy a yearning or to attain a goal. Although the distinction may be a bit artificial, it is useful to consider these two aspects of motivation as the emotional component and the cognitive component.

Emotional Component

Most studies of the emotional aspects of flying motivation have been conducted in the context of the treatment of fear of flying. Bond worked with flyers of the Eighth Air Force in World War II and noted that his patients' flying careers seemed to be based on deep-seated aggressive urges, with the aircraft perceived as a symbol of power that became an extension of the self (7). Pilots speak of feeling as if "the plane is a part of me" when describing the point at which flying becomes a natural action. As

with riding a bicycle, this ability, once achieved, is never lost. Pilots who return to the cockpit after a 10-year absence find that their hands "remember" what to do.

Human infants, like the young of other mammals, are born with an instinctive fear of falling. Children overcome this fear through life experiences, such as learning to walk, playing on swings, climbing trees and engaging in other activities that increase confidence in their ability to control their environment. A child's pleasure in mastering the body and environment may extend into powerful fantasies of flying, which is perceived as the ultimate freedom and mastery. Mythical figures from Apollo, to Peter Pan, to Superman have had the power of flight. Modern children learn at a young age that this power is available to them through the airplane. In their classic book, *Men Under Stress*, Grinker and Spiegel described "this super toy, this powerful snorting but impatient machine" that enables a human to escape the usual limitations of time and space (8). Those who interview prospective student pilots frequently hear, "I've wanted to fly for as long as I can remember;" that is, since before five years of age. Such an expression of a lifelong dream of flying signals a strong, deep-seated, and emotional attraction to flight.

An unhealthy or neurotic motivation to fly may have equally deep roots. A need to compete with or to overcome symbolically a father figure through such an aggressive activity carries with it the unconscious risk of danger should the effort succeed: such individuals may become increasingly anxious as they move toward the attainment of their goals. Others may have a neurotic need to prove themselves by undertaking dangerous activities. Such unhealthy motivational roots should be considered during the selection process and is discussed further in the section on examination.

Cognitive Component

In contrast to those who have wanted to fly all their lives, many applicants express their interest in less emotional and more practical terms, such as, "As long as I was coming into the Air Force through ROTC (Reserve Officer's Training Corps), I thought I might as well try to be a pilot, since they get promoted faster." Frequently, the genesis of interest in such people is the result of conscious, logical decisions made in mid or late adolescence, when career choices are considered. A career in aviation offers concrete rewards: the pay is good, the working conditions are reasonably pleasant, prestige is attached to such a career, and one certainly travels. In the military, the flyer has distinct career advantages over the nonflyers. Such realistic elements are a definite consideration and must not be ignored in search for purely subconscious factors.

For example, some men applied for USAF ROTC in the early 1970s to avoid being drafted from college into the Army and then applied for flying training to enhance their careers in the Air Force. Although this primary motivation to fly was purely cognitive, some of these men decided to stay in the Air Force until retirement and have had wholly successful flying careers.

Ability

Along with motivation, the other neuropsychologic characteristic of a good pilot is the ability to handle aircraft. This ability requires a central nervous system free of significant injuries or disease. Flying today is a complex activity and requires at least normal intelligence. In fact, USAF flying personnel have intelligence quotients that average 123. Intelligence alone is not enough, however; the aviators also must possess good manual dexterity, finely-tuned organization of perceptual inputs, ability to attend to important stimuli selectively and to disregard those judged to be extraneous, and the ability to reason quickly and clearly, especially when under acute stress (9). Much research effort has been put into the development of psychological and performance tests that will measure these abilities, research that continues to this day. In general, tests of ability will have been given to candidates for

military aviation before they ever see the flight surgeon, and those individuals who fail these tests already have been eliminated for further consideration. No such tests are given to the civilian applicant, and it is left to the instructor pilot to weed out those who are so clumsy, inflexible, or ruminative in their responses to the sudden demands of aircraft control that they are unable to adapt to the novel situations that confront them. The application of flying skills must be flexible, rapid, decisive, and correct; nothing less will do.

Normal Adult Growth Patterns

Once selected and trained, flyers' attitudes toward flying may change. Young aviators generally have a total preoccupation with their newfound skills. No matter what the original topic of their conversation, it ends with flying. Any lingering fears generally have been overcome by the sheer delight of mastery of the sky. Youthful enthusiasm, along with denial of the actual dangers, leads to a period when the new pilot may be dangerous because of inexperience and a failure to recognize all the hazards that may occur. New factors may also intervene. Young pilots may be married by their late 20s and may have children. Responsibilities grow, and other interests compete with aviation for their attention and energy. Some fellow aviators have been killed in crashes, and every pilot has had a close call or two. The truth of the adage—"there are old pilots, and there are bold pilots, but there are no old bold pilots"—becomes clear.

During their 30s, flyers generally become increasingly conservative, priding themselves on their professional approach to flying. Physical health is generally good; a strong background of experiences has developed, and the more cautious approach to the demands of the aircraft shows that youthful recklessness has been left behind. As time passes, other interests—career, promotion, family, preparation for years to be spent in areas not involving flying—may surpass the once all-consuming interest in flying.

Should physical illness cause grounding, aviators in their mid 40s and beyond may greet the news with less disappointment than would their younger colleagues.

MENTAL HEALTH SELECTION STANDARDS

Philosophy

The greater the number of standards used for selection to a job, or the more rigorous those standards are, the smaller the number of people who can meet them. Aeromedical standards generally pertain to one or more of the following three factors: (a) maintaining the health and safety of the individual aviator; (b) flying safety; and (c) competent and dependable accomplishment of flight. Because failing to meet a standard removes a person from competition for that job, justifying the use of that standard must include the concept of fairness, and of equal opportunity. Valid mental health standards for selection of flyers, then, must themselves meet the metastandards of safety, health, dependability, competence, and fairness. Of course, the ultimate arbiter of the validity of any aviation medical standards is a flyer's career-long inflight performance.

Validation

Mental health standards, like other medical and operational standards for aviators, have developed by evolution. The historic justifications for some of these standards have been lost, if they ever were explicit, and so the aerospace medicine establishment today must either adhere to anonymously written traditional standards, periodically rejustify them, or revise them. Bureaucratic inertia being what it is, the burden of proof is upon the one who wishes to revise the standards. This makes it difficult to apply new information or techniques to the dynamic process of selecting new flyers, maintaining the health of those already selected, and validating the criteria used to ground those who develop

difficulties and to later restore their flying privileges.

Refining standards is hard enough in the technically-oriented field of aerospace cardiology, and it has been even more difficult in evaluating the mental fitness of aviation candidates, generally a subjective process. Part of this difficulty is due to the intermingling of research ethics with clinical ethics, which can result in refusal of aviation managers to approve or fund studies because of concern that information may be discovered about their flyers which could possibly be seen as deleterious, and thus serve as a basis for criticism or legal action in case of a later mishap. Lack of assured confidentiality can also inhibit aviators from volunteering as subjects due to fear of the possible loss of flying status because of findings incidental to the research. Informed consent necessary in such research means that flyers must be told of these career risks. In order to avoid later legal problems, some investigators have gone to the extreme of storing the results of mental health research in a different country from the one where the investigation was done, so as to avoid the possibility that research data could be subject to subpoena.

Working with mental health standards, however, has been somewhat simplified by the recent development of more objective criteria for psychiatric diagnosis, which allow the examiner reasonable and reproducible means of establishing major psychiatric diagnoses (10). No authority would consider a person with a psychotic disorder to be either safe or dependable, and such a person should not be allowed to fly. Conditions formerly known as neurotic (e.g., phobias, generalized anxiety disorders, functional amnesias) are generally considered disqualifying by most licensing agencies on the basis of their interference with safe and effective flying. Drug and alcohol abuse are obviously dangerous. However, policies are not so easily established in other diagnostic areas (e.g., those involving personality disorders). Some of the most difficult aeromedical decisions concern the amount of disturbed behavior in a flyer necessary to diagnose a disqualifying personality disorder. When the misbehaving or maladaptive flyer is not found to be medically disqualified, then administrative, not medical, authorities should take necessary corrective or disciplinary action. Some regulatory agencies do not regard personality disorders as disqualifying, and deal only with the observed behavior, but the decisions remain difficult (See below, Personality Disorders).

EXAMINATION TECHNIQUES

Psychiatric assessment of candidates for flying training should address two issues: freedom from significant psychiatric disease, and quality of motivation to fly: in other words, who *can* fly, and who *wants to* fly. Just as an efficient stethoscopic examination rules out the disqualifying murmurs, an efficient psychiatric interview should rule out disqualifying mental conditions. However, a mental fitness evaluation should also establish that the motivation to fly is healthy (or at least not unhealthy). The first aim, assuring freedom from mental illness, is conducted by examiners in both the civil and the military sectors of the United States. The second, defining the quality of mental health, is explicitly addressed in the United States military by the Adaptability Rating for Military Aviation (ARMA) used by the Army and Air Force, and by the Navy's concept of aeronautical adaptability. This factor is not addressed in civil aviation.

The psychological aspects of the selection of prospective student pilots generally involve matters of innate ability and motivation. Tests assessing the ability to learn to fly are usually not considered part of the medical examination, except in the rare instances where the inability is due to a neuropsychological deficit, such as dyslexia. Some aeromedical examiners, however, are charged with the responsibility of assessing the quality of the motivation of the would-be pilot. Because all of the information in the literature, and most of the clinical experience, concerns male military applicants, this section deals

mainly with their assessments. Similar data on applicants for civilian training and on female applicants are almost nonexistent, or at least unreported.

The part of the United States Federal Aviation Administration (FAA) regulations dealing with psychiatric standards makes no reference to an applicant's motivation to fly, but addresses only psychiatric diseases, and alterations of consciousness. This approach is appropriate because most civilian pilots are able to stop flying whenever their motivation or interest wanes. However, the aeromedical examiner should be alert to evidence of a desire to fly arising from pathologic roots, such as counterphobic urges, which may lead to dangerous flying habits. These tendencies are identified below.

The military requires a more detailed evaluation of psychologic factors. In each branch of the service, regulations require a psychiatric-style interview to evaluate the applicant's emotional stability and to assess motivation. This evaluation is in addition to any inquiry concerning significant psychopathologic conditions and requires the examiner not just to assure that nothing negative is present, but to make an affirmative statement about the applicant. The United States Navy refers to this as ''the psychiatric examination.'' The United States Army and Air Force label this specialized interview the ''ARMA.''

Initial Interview

First, the examiner must identify those applicants with frank psychopathology. Table 18.2 compares the psychiatric standards of the three United States military services and the FAA. Recall that the services have already applied basic psychiatric standards to all who enter the military, and that these stricter psychiatric standards for flying are in addition to the basic requirements.

Many of the additional flying standards may not appear at first glance to have any direct bearing on an individual's fitness to fly. For

Table 18.2.
Comparison of Military and Civilian Psychiatric Standards

Psychological Factor	United States Army	United States Navy	United States Air Force	Federal Aviation Administration
Psychosis	+[a]	+	+	+
Personality disorder	+	+	+	+
Specific symptoms[b]	+	+	+[c]	0
Substance abuse	+	+	+	+
Psychotropic medications	0	0	0	+
Adjustment reactions	+	0	+	0
Examiner's judgment	+	+	+	+
Fear of flying[d]	+	0	+	0

[a] + means a disqualifying finding.

[b] Includes enuresis, somnambulism, nightmares, severe insomnia, tics, habit spasms, stammering, or psychogenic amnesia.

[c] Original examination only; thereafter, a reason for administrative grounding unless a symptom of a psychiatric disease is present.

[d] Administrative action taken unless fear is a part of psychiatric disease.

example, enuresis or somnambulism would not seem pertinent in choosing a pilot who is presumably awake in the cockpit. Such symptoms, however, may herald significant psychopathology, or may be the only evidence of an unsuspected seizure disorder. Similarly, prolonged nervous tics (nail-biting, hair-eating, or habitual grimacing) may lead the astute examiner to discover a history of substantial psychiatric or neurologic pathology. Few would argue against the significance of such findings.

Mental Status Evaluation

The aeromedical examiner should be familiar with some specific and fairly formal method of mental status evaluation, which is the psychiatric equivalent of a general physical examination. Just as one performs a physical examination in an accustomed order (e.g., head and scalp, ears, eyes, fundi, nose, mouth and throat, thyroid, lymph nodes), one must also examine specific elements of the mental processes, and an orderly process—a checklist—should be established and followed. (For more details about this system, as well as the means by which each element may be tested, see the chapter on the AMSIT by Fuller in Leon (11).)

AMSIT

I. Appearance:
   A. Apparent age, sex, identifying features.
   B. Dress, grooming, hygiene, obvious symptoms, distress.
   C. Manner of relating to examiner—usual for an applicant?
   D. Amount of psychomotor activity.
   E. Obvious evidence of emotion: tremulous, sweating, wrinkled brow.
   F. Mannerisms or activities: gestures, posture, stereotypes, tics.
   G. Attention: distractibility, self-absorption.
   H. Speech: coherence, relevance, spontaneity, pressure, volume, affectation, slurring, stammering, pathologic constructions.

II. Mood and Affect:
   A. Mood (the overall emotional tone): neutral, depressed, elated, anxious, angry.
   B. Affect (emotional changes): range, appropriateness, intensity, rate of change, relation to examiner.

III. Sensorium:
   A. Orientation (time, place, person, situation).
   B. Memory (immediate, recent, remote).
   C. Concentration, attention.

IV. Intellectual Function:
    A. General fund of information.
    B. Vocabulary, grammar.
    C. Complexity of concepts.
    D. Present function, compared to the capacity indicated by history.
V. Thought:
    A. Process: coherence, goal direction, loose associations, pathology.
    B. Content: major themes, special preoccupations, delusions, false perceptions (e.g., hallucinations, depersonalization, body image distortion).
    C. Abstracting ability: similarities and differences, proverbs.
    D. Judgment: social (by history, observed); formal (specific questions).
    E. Insight: idea of self and situation, expectations of others.

Obviously, this entire process is not applied to every would-be pilot. For instance, clinical signs of disturbance of sensorium rarely are found in aviators or applicants. However, the subtleties of appearance (e.g., facial expression, tone of voice) may reveal more than the content of the interview. Thus, when the examiner has the clinical sense that something is amiss, this methodical check of the evaluee's mental status serves to define the nature of the problem.

The assessment of motivation requires different clinical skills, those of directive and nondirective interviewing. These skills cannot be taught in a textbook, but must be learned in contacts with real applicants, preferably under some supervision at first. The art is one of gently helping an applicant who is by nature action-oriented to discuss feelings and fears. At times, direct questions are in order: "Has there been anyone in your family who is as interested in flying as you are?" At other times, indirect methods apply: the understanding nod that elicits more detail, the timely "Can you tell me more about that?" A good source for further discussion of these methods is the section on interview techniques in *The Psychiatric Interview in Clinical Practice* (12).

ARMA: Adaptability Rating for Military Aviation

This process has been discussed elsewhere at length (13). By nature a subjective procedure, the ARMA has never been demonstrated to be a valid and reproducible means of evaluating the quality of a person's motivation to fly. Nevertheless, some applicants want to fly for reasons that are not sound, and aeromedical examiners need a method to screen them out. When the general principles underlying the approaches given here are understood, one or more may be adapted to the particular circumstances of the examiner.

Flying differs from other forms of transportation in that humans instinctively fear heights. Aviation involves real danger, and everyone who flies must deal with that fear, consciously or unconsciously. Military flying is more dangerous than civilian flying. Fighters are more dangerous than transports. Night flying is more dangerous than day flying. Flying in combat introduces even more dangers. One may reasonably assume that the basic, healthy way to deal with such fears is not to volunteer to fly in the first place. The examiner, therefore, must determine how the applicant copes with the real dangers of flight.

Early flight surgeons gave rigidly structured interviews, seeking the answers to about 40 specific questions (e.g., United States Army Air Force's "Flight Surgeon's Handbook," April 20, 1942; pp. 49–51). Modern techniques call for a more flexible approach, allowing the examiner to follow promising leads.

The examiner may conduct a brief interview during the pauses in the physical examination; for example, when the examinee is getting undressed and dressed, or onto and off the examining table. This type of interview involves natural, conversational questions, such as: "How did you get interested in flying?" "What aircraft have you flown in?" "Where did you fly?"

"With whom?" "How did you like it?" "Has anyone in your family been an aviator?" The examiner will make further inquiries into role models, their experiences, combat experiences, or accidents. Many eldest sons take up their fathers' occupations, and aviation is no exception. Successful pilots tend to be eldest sons, frequently with military family backgrounds. When the examiner suspects undue parental pressure, he or she should inquire what the applicant would do if turned down for pilot training, and look for the energy involved in the answer—is there real interest in another career? Or has the applicant never even considered the possibility of nonselection?

Evaluate the applicant's interest in daring, slightly dangerous pursuits or hobbies: martial arts, skydiving, motorcycle racing, or similar activities. Does the individual seem to have a need for risk, to prove the lack of fear? Some have a psychologically overdetermined urge to prove themselves by activities that are counterphobic. Such flawed motivation may fail when the individual faces the realities of flying training. The examiner should not forget the need for discipline involved in aviation today.

What else has the evaluee done in life? Future successes may be foretold from past successes: the ability to set a goal and achieve it, the ability to stick to a difficult project, the ability to use both mind and body under stress, or the ability to work cooperatively and yet to depend on oneself.

"What do you think about the dangers of flying?" Some will answer, "I never thought about it." Respond, "Now that I mention it, what do you think?" Most will answer to the effect that one can get killed driving, or crossing the street. Point out that this is true, but that flying is an additional danger, not a substitute. The next layer of defense generally involves "It's not really all that dangerous," with comments about check rides, safety procedures, redundant systems, boldface checklist items, ejection seats, and parachutes. Point out that all these, and more, are true, yet good flyers get

killed every year. The third layer of defense is usually "I don't care—it won't happen to me," or "I want to fly anyway." These layers of denial, rationalization, and (at times) magical thinking are the norm, the defenses that most flyers use.

If the candidate were being evaluated for possible combat flying, one should ask about feelings concerning the possibility of killing others in a war. Most would-be military pilots have not thought much about this subject, and regard air-to-air combat as an abstraction, hitting a target. Be careful of the evaluee who expresses pleasure at the prospect of killing another person. One should ask follow-up questions about how aggression has been handled in the past. Begin with inquiries about fights in school: were weapons used (e.g., rocks, sticks). Was serious injury caused? How is anger expressed now toward family, peers, subordinates, or strangers? Look for evidence of violent fantasies. Consider psychiatric consultation when any indications exist of aggressive or antisocial personality disorders, or of frankly paranoid processes.

From this point, the examiner may easily ask about the candidate's family background. Be alert to the father's expectations; some sons, especially eldest sons, may want to fly in response to the father's desires, particularly if the father were an active or retired military aviator. Such motivation is not necessarily flawed, but one should look carefully to see whether the applicant is truly interested in flying, or merely reflecting the father's desires. A good question to ask is: "What will you do if you get turned down for flight training?" One young man, the son of an Air Force colonel, relaxed, smiled broadly, and told the examiner with great animation about his real interest, music.

History can be reviewed lightly. One should examine past interests, achievements, and tendencies toward activity or passivity. Has the applicant followed through on projects, or quit at the first resistance? Worked after school? What sort of social life does the applicant have? Was the family discipline abusive, strict, loving, or lax? What sort of trouble has the applicant been in? ("What's the worst thing that ever happened to you? How did you handle it?")

Throughout, one should observe the candidate for poise, especially when challenged. Most are a little tense at first, but can loosen up and engage the examiner in adult conversation. One study of the ARMA found two specific correlations of the interview with later flying success: past history of positive achievements, and social poise during the interview (14). Be alert for nervous habits that emerge in the stress of the conversation: scratching, wiggling around, tics, speech disturbances, blushing, poor eye contact, or mumbling. Can the examiner "see" the evaluee in an aviation setting, among peers? Does the conversation feel like one that may be held with an actual pilot? The more experience the examiner has with successful aviators, the more he or she may depend upon that experience to indicate whether the examinee has the right blend of intelligence, energy, judgment, audacity, and independence to be a flyer.

Astute examiners are aware of their own reactions to applicants. Such perceptions can help decide on suitability to fly. One should beware of identifying too closely with a candidate. ("How could I disappoint such a nice person?") This impulse may reflect the dependency needs of the applicant that elicit such protective feelings. Similarly, one should not disqualify an applicant who is somewhat negative about the examination when this really represents a healthy, independent spirit. In moderation, this is an asset for a pilot, a quality with which every experienced flight surgeon is familiar.

Some busy examiners have the applicants fill out a personal history questionnaire that may be used as an introduction to the individual. Reviewing this form, and augmenting its items with a few pertinent questions, may save time and enable the examiner to get right to the heart of the matter. However, this process depends upon the examiner not becoming too attached to the form and neglecting the interview. As noted below, no one has reported a stand-alone questionnaire that can distinguish between sound and faulty motivation.

The flying training experience itself may serve as a selection process, although this is expensive and may be dangerous. Some agencies use introductory flight-training program in light, simple, safe, and inexpensive-to-operate aircraft to identify the hopelessly inept and those with poor motivation. Instructors should know what to look for in terms of student attitudes and behavior. They should maintain close liaison with a flight surgeon so as to identify quickly any lack of healthy motivation.

EVALUATION BY CONSULTANTS

Psychiatric Interview

When an aeromedical examiner encounters significant psychiatric signs or symptoms in a flyer or prospective flyer, that flyer may be referred for an evaluation to a mental health professional: a psychiatrist or a clinical psychologist. Generally, psychiatrists are concerned with the detection and diagnosis of frank psychopathological conditions. Aeromedical practitioners must carefully explain to the consultant the need to assess such matters as the health of the candidate's motivation to fly, or to examine an applicant with such symptoms as persistent somnambulism for underlying psychiatric disorders. Not all mental health professionals are fully aware of the purposes and parameters of flight physical examinations, and the wise aeromedical examiner takes the time and makes the effort to ensure that the consultant understands the purpose of the referral.

Consultants unused to dealing with flyers or prospective flyers may encounter difficulties, especially when the flyer has never been interviewed in this context before. Some consultants may err on the side of overdiagnosis, resulting in unnecessary disqualification, and others on the side of underestimating the possible effect of symptoms on flying safety. Two additional elements that differ a bit from those associated with the ordinary patient should also be avoided, as they feed into the tendencies to over- or underdiagnose.

First, most flyers dislike being interviewed by mental health professionals. By nature, flyers like to be in control of situations; in fact, this element of control is one reason they have chosen their profession. Thus, they are uncomfortable in a setting where they are not in control, where they do not know the rules, where they perceive their license to fly—and, at times, their livelihood—to be at risk. In a mental health interview, their future depends upon a person whose professional capabilities may be unknown to them, and who, they fear, may not understand the implications of the decisions to be made. Fliers' reactions to such situations vary with individuals and circumstances, but a few patterns are commonly seen.

One such pattern is for the flyer to attempt to bluff through the interview as if nothing at all were the matter. Greeting the examiner with a confident smile and a firm handshake, the flyer assures the examiner that he (let us assume a male flyer) is glad to be there, that he has heard good things about the examiner, and that he welcomes the opportunity to set the record straight. It has all been some sort of misunderstanding, and he is sure that the examiner will find him fit to fly.

Another approach is for the flyer to "stonewall it," to profess surprise at being in the office of a mental health professional, and to have no idea why he was sent there. This goes beyond repression and denial, as it is fairly conscious, and may represent an attempt to discern what the examiner knows, or if the examiner has already decided anything. Such flyers will do what they can to put the examiner to the test, a process that may prove unsettling to an interviewer who is used to being treated with some deference.

Some flyers are angry at being evaluated, and make no attempt to conceal their displeasure. Others do attempt to do so, but in such a passive-aggressive way that they elicit anger from all with whom they come in contact. This process may, in fact, have some clinical usefulness because a flyer who angers the people who have the power to deny him the right to fly is exhibiting self-defeating and inappropriate behavior. Such actions and attitudes may reflect the very processes that led to the request for evaluation in the first place.

Obviously, some flyers are in true mental or emotional distress, and acknowledge their need for help. A few even display enough insight to state that what they need is to get well; that flying is a secondary consideration at present.

The aeromedical examiner may help the mental health consultant in several ways. First, and most helpful in establishing rapport, the consultant should know something about flying, a subject about which the aeromedical examiner can furnish some information. One should never bluff, but a basic understanding of the principles of flight, the vocabulary, the outlines of typical flying careers, and (best of all) some personal experience beyond that of having been a passenger on an airliner helps to break the ice. One should also have enough confidence in the interview situation that one avoids any hint of a power struggle with the flyer over control of the interview. A consultant who is also a pilot should not fall into the error of relating "as one pilot to another," but should retain the "provider and patient" roles. Professional confidence and a calm and assured mien does much to establish and maintain a proper relationship.

Another useful technique is to frankly acknowledge the situation the flyer faces. After a few introductory moments of greetings and a question about the nature of the reason for referral, one inquires how the flyer feels about being referred. If he were to profess pleasure and interest at the prospect of a psychiatric interview, and if he were to appear outwardly free of disabling symptoms, it may be useful to lean back in the chair, look at him for a moment, and say something along the lines of "Really? If I had to go to the office of a stranger who held the key to my entire future in his hands, and I didn't know the rules, I'd be trying to figure out what he wanted and how to give it to him so I could get out of there with as little damage as possible."

At this, many flyers will laugh, lean back and cross their legs. They know that you know how important this is to them, and you have demonstrated that you know your business: you know how they feel.

The second pitfall is a bit more subtle. Some interviewers tend to over-identify with the flyer, and may begin to adopt a flyer's view of the proceedings. The interviewer may begin to believe that this interview is among the worst things that have ever happened to the flyer, and that any outcome other than "observation only; no diagnosis" will ruin the flyer's career. Thus, the interviewer may identify clinically significant symptoms, such as those of anxiety or depression, yet underdiagnose the flyer's condition out of sympathy (or, more technically put, out of excessive countertransferential identification with the flyer). This process may do real harm. For example, in one instance a clear major depression was diagnosed as situational anxiety, and treated with benzodiazepines. This simply prolonged and deepened the depressive symptoms, which persisted until the depression was correctly labeled and treated with antidepressant medication, with immediate improvement of symptoms.

A complete consultation report to the aeromedical examiner should reflect the following: a clear understanding of the reason the flyer was referred; a statement of the genesis of the flyer's interest in the profession; a review of pertinent familial, developmental, and social factors; a mental status examination; a summary; a diagnosis (if applicable); and clear and reasoned comments concerning disposition and recommendations. Such a complete evaluation and report is particularly necessary when the examination must be sent forward to a military or civil agency for approval.

CLINICAL PSYCHOLOGICAL AND NEUROPSYCHOLOGICAL TESTING

Psychometric Techniques

Early in military aviation, psychologists were asked to improve pilot selection with psycholog-

ical tests, to be used in addition to flight surgeons' interviews (15). In many civil and military aviation programs, psychological evaluation remains a major component in the selection process. Much later, psychological evaluation and testing became important in decisions involving retention of aviators, and questions of suitability to fly. Historically, such tests have been more useful in evaluating ability and stable personality features than motivation; therefore, the ideal test has yet to be developed. Below, psychological selection issues are reviewed and then clinical psychological testing of flyers, with particular emphasis on questions involving retention on flying status, or return to flying after being grounded.

Selection

Psychological evaluation for selection can be divided into two areas: select-out and select-in. Select-out evaluation refers to identifying an individual's undesirable or pathological characteristics that may be incompatible with flying. Here, psychological evaluation is used in much the same way as it is used to answer questions about returning to flying duties or retention in the military; looking for pathognomonic signs, psychiatric diagnoses, or even subtle, cognitive and personality factors that may result in the applicant's failure to learn to fly.

Select-in psychological tests identify highly desirable cognitive, personality, and emotional features that predict successful flying training and flying careers. Though this research is not as well developed as select-out testing, a person who possesses positive and strong qualities in each of these categories is likely to succeed in flying training and in a flying career as long as these characteristics remain stable. All of these characteristics may be necessary for a flyer, but high levels of all three are not absolutely required; two may compensate for deficiencies in the third. For instance, a person with less ability but with high motivation and adequate psychological stability may be successful as a pilot.

Thus, some variability among the three characteristics may be acceptable, though clearly a point would be reached at which no amount of motivation and stability could overcome inadequate ability. Examiners often see people with inadequacies in one or more of these areas, which may account for their failure to learn to fly. Ability and stability may contribute to "who can fly," while motivation characterizes "who wants to fly."

The United States military has had some limited experience with psychological assessment in aviator selection, but other military and commercial organizations have for many years routinely used such assessments (e.g., Japan Air Lines, Lufthansa, Northwest Airlines, and the air forces of Norway, Germany and Israel).

Return to Flying Duties

In addition to the selection of potential flyers, as noted above, the other aeromedical application of psychological testing is in the clinical evaluation of aviators. Usually the psychologist is faced with a question about return to flying duties, such as following a head injury, an anxiety disorder, or a suicide attempt. The total psychological evaluation process involves two components: the clinical interview and psychological testing.

The clinical psychological interview involves taking a history, determining current functioning, assessing the motivation and adaptability to fly, and performing a mental status evaluation; all of this information results in an impressionistic description of the aviator's status, similar to the psychiatric interview described earlier. Psychological testing involves two types: neuropsychological tests, and tests of personality and psychological adjustment. Neuropsychological tests evaluate brain functioning: memory, attention, concentration, information processing, and language (16). These tests involve visual, auditory, tactile, and kinesthetic stimuli; they are based on right or wrong answers and actual performance, and they are often timed. The Halsted-

Reitan Neuropsychological Test Battery is the best known and most widely used assessment battery in this area of functioning (17). These tests have clinical norms that have been developed mostly from hospital databases, though some aeromedical centers have developed their own norms specifically for aviators. The neuropsychological tests evaluate such referral conditions as closed-head injury, memory change, aging, issues of inadequate training or upgrade performance, and flying deficiency.

Tests of personality and psychological adjustment comprise the second category used to evaluate flyers. These tests measure both the longstanding personality structure of an individual and his or her current psychological adjustment. Examples include the Minnesota Multiphase Personality Inventory (MMPI), the NEO Personality Inventory (NEO-PI), and various sentence-completion tests. Such tests measure anxiety, depression and energy level, as well as self-concept, personality style and traits, and psychological defenses. They generally use questionnaires that are usually self-administered and not timed, and that have no right or wrong answers. Examples of aeromedical referral questions appropriate for personality tests include alcohol or drug abuse, somatization, stress reactions, and malingering in relation to fitness to fly.

Interview and test techniques each have strengths and weaknesses. An interview is uniquely helpful for a self-referred flyer with specific and acknowledged complaints or problems. However, it can lack objectivity, has no norms for comparing results across different groups of people, and can suffer from issues of transference and countertransference, especially with aviators or other occupational groups whose jobs depend upon the interview results. Thus, psychological subtleties may be missed. Psychological tests, conversely, are normal and standardized, thereby providing objectivity, offering uniform questions to all evaluees, and giving detailed coverage of all areas important to psychological functioning. However, testing may be quite time-consuming, and the results may be misinterpreted when not compared to aviators' norms. Further, examiners without aeromedical experience may miss critical, subtle, aeromedically relevant interpretations, or they may overinterpret aeromedically insignificant findings. For these reasons, psychological tests are best used in combination with the clinical interview.

In summary, psychological evaluation is best used in the context of the full aeromedical evaluation, and should include both a clinical interview and psychological testing as critical components of the full psychological evaluation of the aviator.

MAINTAINING MENTAL HEALTH

Aerospace Psychology

As noted above, psychologists have been involved with aviation from its earliest days. Their numbers include human factors specialists, cognitive psychologists, educational and training psychologists, and experimental psychologists. They provide useful aeromedical information in such areas as fatigue, vision, and cockpit design. The aerospace clinical psychologist provides clinical evaluation as discussed above, but can also provide preventive and treatment services as well.

The clinical psychologist is well suited to provide programs in mental health prevention, maintenance, enhancement, and augmentation (18). As noted by Unger in the Foreword and DeHart in the preface to the first edition of this text, aerospace medicine is specifically concerned with preventive medicine and health maintenance. Psychologists can provide consultation and education to aviators about health compliance behaviors, such as smoking cessation, weight loss and control, and exercise discipline. They may assist in other areas of health and well-being, such as mishap aftercare, marital communication, parenting skills, and stress management. Obviously, effectiveness in such

work requires credibility with the aviator that comes from training and experience, as well as a bit of persuasiveness and the capacity to tolerate and enjoy working with a somewhat resistant and skeptical group. The value of such efforts is apparent when one considers that flyers' personalities and coping skills generally are more congruent with elements of action and danger than with interpersonal relationships, a fact that is considered at length below.

Cockpit Resource Management

A specific application of psychological enhancement, education, and augmentation is cockpit resource management (CRM). NASA and various commercial airlines have been pioneers in this area of study and training (Chapter 30). In an excellent, comprehensive review, Orlady and Foushee reported that CRM developed in response to the findings that many aviation mishaps were traced to human factors or "pilot error," and that many of the human factors discovered could not be explained by "stick and rudder" deficits. Rather, the problems emanated from "decision-making, crew coordination, command, leadership, and communication skills (19)." Others add problem-solving, task management, and workload distribution as the focus of crew performance problems, rather than inadequate resources, skill, or ability (20). These authors found that recency, familiarity, and crew position influenced these variables, pointing to the complexity of research in this area.

Most agree that CRM is an important concept that can yield excellent results. Issues of optimal training methods, length of training effectiveness, crew resistance to training, the recalcitrant or failed student, and outcome measurements remain controversial subjects and are open to further investigation. Thus, specific research projects and training programs were developed to study these problems and specifically to educate aviators in not "stick and rudder" topics, but in operationally critical ones.

CLINICAL CONDITIONS OF CONCERN

Fear of Flying

Fear of flying is a term coined during World War II that originally referred to the mixtures of fear and anxiety seen in the combat theaters. In the USAF today, the term, fear of flying, connotes unreasonable fear or anxiety that develops in trained aviators who are free of other emotional symptoms. Thus, fear of flying is a symptom and not a disease.

Fear, the emotion we feel in the face of real and immediate danger, is the emotional equivalent of pain. Both fear and pain warn us to withdraw from danger: fear at the instinctive level and pain at the somatic reflex level. A conscious act of will can overcome both fear and pain, at least for awhile. For example, individuals may be fearful about their first dives from high boards, and yet they conquer their fears and dive, discovering that the danger is not as real as they believed. Most individuals can also learn to control their reactions to the pain of injections and tolerate needles in their flesh with some degree of equanimity.

The primitive fear of falling has been overcome in most, if not all, military aviators. The initial physical examination and its accompanying inquiry into the prospective pilot's perceptions of the dangers of flying have, it is hoped, eliminated those with pathologic or inadequate defenses against these dangers. Those remaining should react to this perception with the usual mix of denial, rationalization, and healthy fantasy.

Once flight training begins, fantasies about flight become realities. A few student pilots may drop out of flight training because they cannot maintain their defenses against the dangers of flight that are real and immediate. Their fear may take many forms: as an overt apprehension that interferes with the progress of training; as a disabling psychophysiologic symptom, such as headache or airsickness; or as rationalized, self-initiated elimination in which applicants simply declare that they were not cut out to be pilots.

In the USAF, such fear openly expressed during flight training is grounds for disqualification under the heading "manifestations of apprehension." This disqualification is handled in a nonpunitive manner, with the student pilot generally being disenrolled from training and reassigned to a nonflying position. Civilian student pilots, of course, may merely stop their lessons.

Once flyers complete flying training, it is assumed that they have successfully adapted to flying and have demonstrated healthy, mature defenses against whatever instinctive or primitive anxieties may be aroused by flying. From this point on, the USAF handles openly expressed fear of flying in a different manner. An aviator who admits to disabling anxiety about flying is evaluated for any psychiatric disease. If none is found, the flyer is declared physically and mentally fit to fly and then must meet an administrative flying evaluation board for disposition. This disposition may be as mild as reassignment to a nonflying job or as severe as a recommendation for dismissal from the service. A previously well-adapted aviator who becomes fearful thus has an additional conflict to face that arises from the knowledge that the Air Force may take punitive administrative action when fears are openly admitted. In addition, organizational pressure and peer pressure may be exerted in such a flyer to continue flying and to overcome fears alone.

United States Army flight surgeons handle aviators who become fearful about flying in much the same way. The United States Navy takes a somewhat different approach. Such flyers may be evaluated at the naval Aviation Medicine Institute at Pensacola, Florida. When no overt mental illness is detected and the aviator affirms the fear of flying, and when this fear is not amenable to treatment, he is designated physically disqualified but not aeronautically adapted. Thus identified, the flyer is reassigned to nonflying duties.

The military flight surgeon may be caught in the middle between an aviator who wants to stop flying and the organization that requires him to continue. The briefly worded regulation is clear and apparently inflexible, reducing fear of flying to a single decision: Is the disposition to be medical or administrative? In fact, the circumstances of various flying situations and the complexities of human emotions and behavior interact so that every case of fear of flying seems unique to the flight surgeon who must deal with it. Perhaps the simplest instance would be the flyer who develops a pure phobia to flight, a straight-forward medical diagnosis. This condition is distinguished by its free-floating, primitive anxiety, which is generally considered unreasonable, its symbolic nature, and its ego-dystonicity, the psychiatric term that means that the aviator dislikes the fear and wants to be rid of it.

For example, an F-4 weapons systems operator became increasingly anxious about low-level flying, although he could handle any other sort of flying without difficulty. His anxiety was heightened if the pilot were younger than he. He finally became so anxious that he found himself holding on to his ejection handle while flying low-level missions, at which point he reported to his flight surgeon. It became apparent that the anxiety about flying with a younger pilot symbolized his need to perceive the pilot as a father figure, which was not possible when the pilot was younger than he. His symptoms were egodystonic in that he hated his feeling of fear and wanted to be rid of it so that he could enjoy flying. Such phobias can be treated by behavioral means, such as systematic desensitization, in which the flyer first learns to relax on cue and then is exposed to progressively closer contact with the feared situation within brief periods. Such a flyer, once cured of the phobia, may be given a waiver and returned to full flying duties, as happened in this instance.

Other aviators may become acutely fearful after a brush with death or the loss of a friend in an aircraft accident. In such situations, some flyers may be returned to flying by an aeromedical practitioner who uses a crisis intervention approach, giving the aviator a chance to express feelings of anger, sadness, and guilt openly in an accepting environment, mutually exploring the realities of the situation, and helping the flyer to rethink the decision to fly or not. It is our impression, although we have no hard data, that the success or the failure of the flight surgeon or therapist in this situation may depend on the strength of the flyer's subconscious motivation and whether it originated in an early, primitive joy of mastery or arose from a later, less emotional, and more cognitive decision that "flying looks like a good career." Certainly, other current stressful factors, such as family or work problems, may contribute to the feeling of apprehension about flight. When these factors can be identified and successfully treated, the situational anxiety may subside and the flyer will return to the cockpit.

One is most likely to be able to help such a flyer conquer anxieties and return to flying when he perceives this as a desirable outcome. One may form a therapeutic alliance with a fearful flyer who wants to be rid of the fears but not with a fearful flyer who does not want to be helped. The physician should help the flyer determine what is wrong and explore all possible solutions. Insisting that the aviator work toward a return to flying duties puts one in an adversarial position and is likely to fail. When the flyer agrees that the fear is a problem that needs exploration, examining that fear and looking for possible solutions are acceptable therapeutic goals. Once these things are done, the question of whether that aviator should fly again may be considered. When the flyer is not interested in exploring the symptom, however, and when no mental or physical disease is present that would be disqualifying, one may return the flyer to the squadron as physically and mentally fit to fly, with a recommendation for appropriate administrative action. This problem seems to be unique to military flying because civilian aviators may simply quit whenever they wish.

Some of the most difficult situations arise when the anxieties manifest themselves, not as conscious fear of flying, but as psychosomatic symptoms. In such instances, the aviator will ask for help with the symptoms that prevent him from flying. He will not have any anxiety about flying itself but will discuss the symptoms mainly in terms of their preventing him from flying. Of course he wants to fly, he says, but these headaches (or abdominal pains or low back pains) bother him so much in flight that he is not safe. Most aeromedical practitioners take a purely somatic approach at first, ruling out specific illnesses. Finding no physical explanation for the symptoms, the physician may then begin to consider that anxiety about flying is the basis for the problem. Three observations may help to identify the unconscious anxiety. First, the flyer tends to describe symptoms in terms of their effects on his flying. The experienced flight surgeon quickly notices the difference in emphasis from that of usual flyers, who tend to minimize this aspect of their illnesses. A clear difference exists between a flyer who comes in complaining about backache and a flyer who comes in repeatedly complaining that the backache is so severe that he won't be able to fly today. Second, the aviator may express no particular anxiety about the possible illness causing symptoms. One pilot expressed: "I only worry about having the headaches when I'm flying." He was not concerned that his severe headaches may signal some underlying illness. Third, one may ask a flyer: "Will you fly if (or "when," to be more positive) we get rid of the headaches?" The unconflicted flyer, without hesitation, responds in the affirmative. The aviator who is conflicted about flying pauses, equivocates, or otherwise signals reluctance, either verbally or nonverbally. When this question was put to the pilot with headaches, he paused, and finally answered "yes" in an unenthusiastic tone. When told that he did not look happy about this, he replied that he was not, repeating that he was worried about the effect of headaches on his flying. Although the flight surgeon may be sure that basic anxiety about flying exists in such instances, the flyer is not conscious of it and will deny it. A medical disqualification based on the

symptoms may be the most suitable disposition on refractory cases.

Fear of flying may present a somewhat different problem among nonmilitary, professional flyers. It is generally regarded as basically a medical problem and may even be grounds for disability retirement action when it is severe enough and is not responsive to psychotherapeutic intervention. Although an individual presenting with fear of flying may have some symptoms that are basically those of anxiety, one must not overlook the role of some secondary gain factor in intensifying the symptoms or in complicating the therapeutic process. Financial recompense and the chance to move from flying into fields of endeavor perceived as more attractive may be powerful gain factors, both in the military and in civilian life.

No problem in aviation medicine is more difficult to deal with than fear of flying. The flight surgeon who can deal with it gracefully is a master of the art.

Adjustment Disorders

An operational aeromedical practitioner probably sees more adjustment disorders (stress reactions) than any other sort of mental health-related condition. These disorders vary considerably in the mode of presentation and in intensity and may occur in response to any sort of life stress. An event that one person accepts with equanimity may be dreadfully upsetting to another, the difference depending on the adequacy of coping mechanisms and particular vulnerabilities. Clearly, adjustment disorders may affect any sort of flyer: civilian, commercial, or military.

The fourth edition of the Diagnostic and Statistical Manual of Mental Disorders (DSM-IV) defines an adjustment disorder as "the development of clinically significant emotional or behavioral symptoms in response to an identifiable psychosocial stressor or stressors." By strict definition, such a disorder should be a departure from the individual's usual response to life stresses. The reaction occurs within three months of the stress and results in either social or occupational impairment or in symptoms beyond those ordinarily seen in such situations. Stressors may, of course, occur in groups (''a run of bad luck'') or may be recurrent.

Adjustment disorders may take several forms. Depressive symptoms may predominate in one form, symptoms of anxiety in another. Some individuals, especially the young or the immature, may act out their distress by abusing alcohol, fighting, reckless driving, or flying violations. Others may become withdrawn. Obviously, some individuals may show a mixture of these symptoms.

Depressive symptoms may include disturbances in sleeping patterns or appetite. Self-esteem may be diminished, and the flyer may report feeling ''down'' or ''blue.'' Inquiry usually reveals lack of energy or initiative, loss of usual sexual interest, and perhaps an increase in minor physical complaints. Feelings of guilt (justified or unjustified), irritability, pessimism, or helplessness also may be revealed. One should always inquire after suicidal ideas or equivalent thinking (''I'd just like to chuck it all in,'' or ''I'd like to get in a car and drive away—I don't care where'').

Symptoms of anxiety are somewhat different; the flyer may report feeling uneasy or fearful, with no clear idea why. Autonomic symptoms may predominate: pounding heart, air hunger, dry mouth, digestive upset, tremulousness, or a lump in the throat. In some instances, attacks of real dread may occur, as though an indefinable but fearful ''something'' were about to happen. These panic attacks may be intense enough to be disabling.

Some aviators are particularly apt to react to stress with inappropriate actions. Alcohol abuse is likely to be involved: ''I was so upset I just went out and got loaded.'' Most of us are familiar with the person who acts out his emotions behind the wheel of an automobile. The alert clinician listens carefully to aviators who report that a fellow flyer is flying poorly—taking chances, not as sharp, not up to the usual standards. Knowledge of a recent life stress in such instances should lead to an interview with the flyer involved, either in a formal medical setting or informally. The flyer who takes out his feelings on his aircraft is an accident looking for a place to happen.

Management of adjustment disorders is fairly simple in some instances, but the help of a mental health professional may be needed in other situations. An accurate review of recent life events usually uncovers the stressor: family disruption, job stress, financial reversal, sexual complaint, or other recent change. Once the stressor is acknowledged, the physician may explore the flyer's reaction to it, explaining the connection with the symptoms if the flyer were not already aware of it. Stressful life experiences happen to everyone; the ways one copes with stressful situations determine whether the outcome is adaptive or maladaptive.

Some aeromedical physicians are comfortable exploring with the flyer the means used to cope with the crisis, explaining what is happening and strengthening healthy coping mechanisms. A nonjudgmental and sympathetic listener who encourages the patient to express feelings, is reassuring, provides explanations, and gives realistic advice may be all that is necessary in some milder cases. Grounding the flyer may be in order, especially when symptoms are distracting. Medications should be used sparingly, if it all, and should be directed at clear target symptoms for a brief time only. The use of the benzodiazepines (Valium® or Librium®) for depressive symptoms should be strictly avoided because these antianxiety agents make depressions worse. When a flyer's situational reaction calls for medication, consultation with a psychiatrist is desirable.

Chronic- or Delayed-stress Reactions

Posttraumatic stress disorders may be acute, beginning within six months of trauma and lasting less than six months, chronic, lasting more than six months, or delayed, occurring more than six months after trauma. Such trauma is defined as an event that is psychologically damaging and is beyond the range of everyday human experiences: aircraft accidents, combat, natural or manmade disasters, rape, torture, or severe captivity or hostage experiences. The disorder evoked may include reliving the experience through flashbacks (brief dissociative states) or through nightmares. Emotional numbing may occur in response to real world situations, such as the inability to experience joy, pleasure, or intimacy. The individual may lose the ability to use concentration or memory fully, may have a hyperalert startle response, may feel guilty about surviving, or feel irrational anger at those who did not survive. Other reactions include irritability, insomnia, and difficulty in attending to the ordinary affairs of life. Symptoms may be intensified by exposure to events that are reminders of the trauma. Thus, survivors of an air disaster may become unbearably anxious when required to fly again. Conventional wisdom dictates that a person who has had a terrifying experience should face the circumstances of that experience again as quickly as possible to give the lie to the fantasy that the trauma will inevitably recur. One flyer who had escaped death in a crash by the merest of margins remarked after his next flight: "The thing I was most afraid of was that I'd be afraid. As soon as I took off and found that I wasn't afraid, I relaxed." This works in many instances but not in all. When such disorders do occur, they should be treated by mental health professionals.

Anniversary reactions are more common in flyers than in the population at large (21). Marsh and Perry reported anniversary phenomena in 11 of 360 carefully investigated aeromedical psychiatric consultation patients (22). Characteristically, the flyer reports symptoms of depression or anxiety with no obvious connection to recent life events. Careful inquiry into the patient's history may yield a traumatic event occurring almost exactly 1, 2, 5, 10, or 20 years previously. Alternately, some tragic event—usually death—happened to a signicant person of the same age as the flyer's present age. At times, the event may be repressed, and the history is only elicited from another family member. Several times we explained this concept to a flyer and asked him to check with other family members; he returned to report, with some emotion, that he had forgotten the death of a person who was important to him and he didn't know why he had forgotten. Such an emotional response almost certainly indicates psychological paydirt: the traumatic event that is buried because it was too painful to bear, the emotion surfacing a year or more later as free-floating anxiety or depression. Deaths of friends in aircraft accidents may well be handled in this manner, repressed because they are too threatening. Usually, simple explanation and the chance for the patient to express his feelings are sufficient treatment. Psychiatric consultation should be sought when symptoms persist.

Substance Abuse

Substance abuse is an exceedingly complex question and was discussed in Chapter 14, "Aircrew Health Care Maintenance." Aviators may abuse alcohol in response to stress, especially because it is somewhat sanctioned by others in the flying milieu. About one of six civil aircraft accidents involves alcohol abuse. Pursch has written humorously and realistically about the social situations that are used to excuse drinking: births, deaths, arrivals, departures, promotions, passovers, and so on (23). Alcohol abuse complicates many psychiatric conditions and must be carefully assessed in every situation.

We offer the following general counsel: nothing excuses alcohol abuse. It is maladaptive behavior that may quickly become an addicting disease. Alcoholics Anonymous (AA) has the best record in dealing with alcohol abuse. As the aviator participates in AA (or other rehabilitation activities), he must be put on notice that one recurrence will end his flying career. This rule must be enforced. Some individuals do not believe this policy and test the system. Their fate—certain and unmistakable dismissal—lets others know that the rules are enforced. This procedure is the successful industrial approach: offer help and do not tolerate alcohol-degraded performances.

Drug abuse is simply not compatible with flying. More details are available regarding support to the airlines in Chapter 25.

Personality Disorders

Personality disorders are particular traits or styles of interaction with others that are so marked, so maladaptive, or so lacking in flexibility that the individual suffers personal distress or is significantly impaired in social interactions or occupational functioning. This distress or impairment may begin in adolescence and generally continues throughout the adult years, perhaps diminishing in late middle age. People with personality disorders are frequently regarded as eccentric, difficult to get along with, or merely unpleasant, without a diagnostic label being considered. The maladaptive features that mark the individual's relationships with others should be considered diagnostic of a true disorder when they are found to be typical of function in many areas of life over a period of years, rather than being found only in circumscribed relationships or on a temporary basis.

These personality traits may be unpleasant to the individual, traits that he wishes to be rid of, or they may be regarded as adaptive and useful, even in the face of evidence to the contrary. Treatment is particularly difficult in this latter instance because the individual is comfortable with this method of relating to others and sees no reason to change. Such traits are called ego-syntonic. Traits regarded as undesirable by the individuals are called ego-dystonic. It follows that a therapist has a better chance of forming a therapeutic alliance with an individual whose symptoms are ego-dystonic than with one whose symptoms are ego-syntonic and who generally

has been referred for treatment somewhat against his will.

Those personality disorders likely to be encountered in flyers are discussed in the following sections. A fuller discussion may be found in any standard psychiatric text or in the DSM-IV.

Paranoid Personality Disorder

The behavior of the individual with a paranoid personality disorder is marked by a thorough mistrust of others, a continuing and unjustified suspiciousness, and an unusual sensitivity to real or imagined slights. Suspicions are maintained even in the face of evidence that would convince an ordinary person that they are groundless. These people are alert for threats, tend to avoid blame for anything, and are regarded by those who know them as secretive, jealous, and thoroughly unpleasant. They argue, are always alert for the slightest insult, exaggerate disagreements, counterattack with vigor, are prone to legal action, and are quick to criticize but unable to accept criticism. They are uncompromising, hostile, stubborn, and do poorly in cooperative efforts. Such individuals are not psychotic; that is, they do not harbor underlying delusional systems or have hallucinations. They may adapt poorly to the enforced closeness of a military squadron. Such people are distinctly different from the usual aviator, who is more friendly, comfortable to converse with, and sociable. Treatment is difficult because these individuals are threatened by the closeness necessary in a therapeutic relationship.

Narcissistic Personality Disorder

The person with a narcissistic personality disorder has an inappropriate sense of self-importance and a continuing need to be the center of attention. An unrealistic overestimation of personal abilities may exist, which is particularly dangerous in the flying environment. Ambitions and fantasies of achievement may be unrealistic and may be pursued with inappropriate energy and an insensitivity to the needs of others, who may be exploited and devalued. Thus, ''the great one'' expects others to smooth his way and to provide instant admiration while receiving nothing in return. Self-esteem, although overblown, is likely to be fragile under stress. A major failure, perceived or real, may lead to a significant depression that requires therapeutic intervention. Most successful flyers have narcissistic traits of independence, self-assuredness, and a sense of being able to handle anything, but not to the degree of arrogance and insensitivity displayed by people with a narcissistic personality disorder.

Antisocial Personality Disorder

Antisocial personality disorder has been known in the past as ''sociopathic,'' ''psychopathic'' or ''antisocial character and behavior disorder.'' Its onset in midadolescence heralds a lifetime of conflict with authority, lying, cheating, sexual promiscuity, and substance abuse. It is much more common in males and may arise in part from a chaotic childhood. Some evidence indicates that genetic influences also are important. A history of truancy, serious misbehavior in school, delinquency, fighting, lying, sexual misconduct, theft, vandalism, lack of responsible function as a parent, inability to work consistently, lack of acceptance of social norms, impulsivity, recklessness, or daring behavior should arouse the suspicion of the concerned flight surgeon. Such people may be superficially charming but are constantly in trouble. As flyers, their lack of dependable, predictable, and safe behavior, their impulsivity, their willingness to lie about anything, and their abuse of others makes them poor risks to complete mission assignments safely. This condition is essentially untreatable.

Borderline Personality Disorder

As its name implies, the borderline personality disorder is difficult to diagnose because it represents instability in several areas, presenting different aspects at different times. The individual may vary between idealizing friendship and baseless rage, leading to shifting interpersonal

conflicts. Moody and uncertain, such a person has difficulty with loneliness and boredom. Brief episodes of frank psychosis may occur. The individual lacks a firm sense of identity and has difficulty maintaining consistency in relationships with others. Suicidal gestures or irrational, self-mutilating actions may occur. Although such persons may be chosen for flight training, it is unlikely that they could maintain the consistent high level of performance and the close interactions with the instructors necessary to complete the training.

Compulsive Personality Disorder

Individuals with a compulsive personality disorder find it difficult to relate warmly to others. Their superficial perfectionism, expressed as careful planning, list-making, and scheduling, actually interferes with the accomplishment of tasks. Stubbornly insistent on ''doing it my way,'' their moralistic dedication to their work excludes pleasure from leisure activities or cooperative relationships. Indecision is another indication; such people may be so afraid of making a mistake that they become immobilized by choices and are unable to establish realistic priorities. Like those with borderline personality disorders, these individuals are unlikely to succeed in the trying environment of flight training. Those who do succeed may have increasing difficulty in using compulsive behavior to control their anxiety, especially in the sometimes unpredictable world of the flyer. Decompensation, if it were to occur, may take the form of depression, phobias, or panic attacks.

Passive-aggressive Personality Disorder

This personality pattern was dropped from DSM-IV as a diagnosable condition (10). However this pattern may be recognized. Such individuals express their resistance to the desires of others through covert opposition, such as stubbornness, forgetfulness, chronic tardiness, poor work, inefficiency, or dawdling. This behavior frequently elicits anger and frustration in associates, both in the occupational arena and in social settings. The frustrating behavior continues in spite of counseling, persuasion, or threats. Because it expresses hidden aggression, this behavior may be particularly disruptive in a group or organizational setting. In the flying environment, such a personality structure may be expressed as a pattern of ineffective performance accompanied by inadequate excuses, grumbling, and obstructionism, with "the other guy" always blamed for the flyer's own shortcomings.

Psychophysiologic Disorders

Regardless of specialty, every physician is aware of the influences that psychological factors have on somatic diseases. Far from being "all in your head," these conditions may involve the body to a life threatening degree. For example, asthmatic attacks may be lethal. Regional enteritis and ulcerative colitis are somatic conditions that are clearly affected by environmental stimuli mediated through emotions. Some patients affected by such ailments are aware of the connection between life stress and physical symptoms; other patients remain forever skeptical. Two psychosomatic complaints are of particular interest to the aeromedical practitioner: syncope and airsickness.

Syncope

Loss of consciousness in a flyer may have immediate and fatal consequences at worst. Because loss of consciousness is a neurologic event, the central nervous system must be carefully evaluated. The cause also may be of cardiac origin, such as an embolus or arrhythmia. Less dangerous, at least from a general health point of view, are those losses of consciousness ascribed to acute and self-limited loss of blood pressure, which are called vasovagal syncope, or "fainting." Psychological factors also may be associated with low G tolerance.

Sledge and Boydstun reviewed the pertinent literature as it applies to aerospace medicine and presented their own analysis of 24 patients seen at the United States Air Force School of Aerospace Medicine (USAFSAM) for vasovagal syncope (24). Upon investigating the life circumstances of these patients and comparing them with nonsyncopal controls, these authors found that those who had fainted reported considerably more difficulty in their work situation and less job satisfaction than those who had not fainted. Further, the events immediately preceding the fainting episode almost always involved some sort of threat, physical or social, against which the flyer believed he was unable to defend himself. Unable to fight or flee, the flyer became totally helpless by losing consciousness, thus, in a sense, giving up to the threat.

Classically, such events occur when the flyer has blood drawn, undergoes a minor surgical procedure, such as electrodesiccation of a wart, or is required to see a motion picture about first aid. These circumstances are so commonplace that "fainting at the sight of blood" is a cliché. Tense social circumstances are not as commonly acknowledged, but may be found in many instances of vasovagal syncope.

For example, a high-ranking officer was entertaining an even higher-ranking guest in his home. He had served oysters and had eaten one that he found was bad, too late to avoid swallowing it. Later, engaging his guest in a farewell conversation at the door, he felt nauseated. He did not want to excuse himself to vomit so near the end of the evening because his guest was only moments from leaving. Fighting back the nausea, he became weak and sweaty, and then fainted.

In this instance, the flyer felt bound by social amenities not to acknowledge his strong visceral urges, but was helpless to stop them. A less-inhibited individual would have stated the truth of the matter and excused himself.

In a different example, a flyer was watching a training film on first aid when he became aware of strong defecatory urges. He fought them back because he was seated in the middle of the row and did not want to inconvenience everyone by crowding past to go to the bathroom. Finally, as the urges became stronger, he stood up to go to the bathroom and fainted. Later, he related that he had been upset by the sight of blood since he had seen his father castrating pigs. He had fainted twice before, each time in circumstances where he had felt the need to use the bathroom and was ashamed to admit it: once in class and once in the Air Force examination station where he had been told not to urinate until he got to the laboratory. This flyer had a strong sense of personal danger when confronted with blood. He also was extremely inhibited about his excretory functions. The combination of defecatory urges and of seeing blood was, for him, a uniquely intolerable threat.

In such cases, no immediate threat to flying safety exists, as long as the flyer can take action when threatened. It is possible to teach flyers to avoid the feeling of powerlessness by showing them alternative behaviors. For example, such individuals may learn to demand to be allowed to lie down before blood is drawn. Simply knowing that they do not have to put themselves passively into the hands of the technician, but that they retain power over the situation by controlling some aspect of it, may be enough to alleviate the perceived threat.

Theoretically, such a flyer may be exposed to blood in the cockpit if a fellow flyer were struck by a bird coming through the windscreen or by shell fragments in a combat situation. This situation would pose no syncopal hazard because of the urgent need for corrective action in either circumstance. No feeling of enforced passivity would occur and no psychological need to "leave the scene" through syncope would be needed. We discussed with several syncope patients how they felt and reacted to real and bloody accidents; each time, the flyer was able to cope with the situation through action, and did not faint.

Hyperventilation

Anxiety in flyers may be expressed through hyperventilation, which may occur in any aircraft at any time. This is a major concern in the pilots of single-seat high-performance jet air-

craft who experience the onset of "feeling bad" at altitude. The disconcerted flyer, seeking to identify the source of the symptoms, must distinguish between hypoxia, hyperventilation, and toxic fumes in the cockpit, and react appropriately in a situation that has manifested itself through a significant alteration in cognition. Paradoxically, the pilot who realizes that his or her thinking is acutely diminished is required to think clearly in order to respond correctly. The usual procedure in such cases is to follow rote instruction, something like "Go to 100% oxygen (isolates flyer from possible toxic gases in cockpit), take three deep breaths (to relieve possible hypoxia), and control your breathing (to diminish possible hyperventilation)."

Other considerations must be addressed in an episode of inflight hyperventilation, in addition to just getting the aircraft back safely. One of the most distressing aspects of such an occurrence is the pilot's perception of loss of control. Unable to explain why it happened or to predict when it may recur, the aviator feels at the mercy of an unknown danger. The flyer's new uncertainty about physical fitness is added to the unexpressed anxiety that caused the hyperventilation initially, and the flyer may well decide not to fly "until you guarantee that it will never happen again." In vain, the flight surgeon may point out that the physical evaluation has demonstrated no disease process, or offer to the skeptical aviator a careful explanation of the changes in blood gases resulting from hyperventilation. The flight surgeon must avoid the trap of looking for just one more test to "prove" that nothing is wrong with the flyer. The more extensive the evaluation, the more the anxious aviator may become convinced that: "Something really must be wrong, or else you wouldn't be doing all these tests."

Many aviators respond well to the flight surgeon's confidant reassurance. The flight surgeon, convinced that no significant underlying pathology exists, must become direct: the incident was caused by hyperventilation, and hyperventilation can be controlled. One should ask the flyer to show his or her method of respiratory control, and almost invariably a demonstration is given of how to increase the respiratory depth while maintaining a normal respiratory rate, thereby increasing the minute volume and aggravating the problem. One effective way to teach ''control'' of respiratory depth and rate is to have the flyer breathe through the nose (nostrils serve as flow-limiting valves) and to make each exhalation four times as long as the inhalation in order to limit respiratory rate (e.g., one second to inhale, four seconds to exhale; two seconds to inhale, eight seconds to exhale). By limiting the depth and rate of respiration, minute volume is controlled.

The flyer will learn the technique, and may give intellectual approval to the new knowledge, yet may continue to refuse to fly. ''You don't know what it was like up there.'' The flight surgeon can preempt the flyer's position: ''I know you don't believe me; I wouldn't believe me either, not until I knew it would work by trying it out.'' One should instruct the flyer to fly as a passenger with a trusted pilot (in another aircraft type, if necessary), and to try to hyperventilate in flight while using the control technique. Having tried to hyperventilate and failed, confidence increases, and the flyer may be convinced that even if hyperventilation were to occur again, he or she would not be a helpless victim; an effective and dependable countermove has been provided. No longer at the mercy of the unknown, the flyer has added one more emergency procedure to the long list that each pilot accumulates during a flying career.

If the procedure were to fail, or if the aviator were to refuse this suggestion, a more serious underlying process may be involved, and the aviator would need a thorough mental health evaluation.

Airsickness

Airsickness is a complex interdisciplinary subject, already discussed from the neurosensory point of view in Chapter 11. Psychological elements clearly enter into instances in which the chronically airsick student aviator does not accommodate after continued exposure to flying. Some military student pilots become so conditioned by repeated airsickness that they are nauseated on the ground by the smell of jet fuel or the smell of the compounds used to clean their oxygen masks or even by the sight of the aircraft on the flight line. They become so anxious about the possibility of getting sick again and washing out of flight training that the anxiety itself contributes to airsickness. This sort of anxiety also may affect civilian student pilots.

Several treatments are available to airsick student pilots. Two medication combinations may be tried: dextroamphetamine 5 mg and scopolamine 0.5 mg orally 1 hr before flight or promethazine hydrochloride (Phenergan®) 25 mg, and ephedrine 25 mg orally 1 hr before flight. It is wise to try the first dose on the ground to guard against any idiosyncratic reaction that may pose a danger in the air. These combinations must be used only when the student pilot is accompanied by an instructor pilot. If one of the combination of medications were to effectively control the symptoms, the student flyer may be able to accommodate to the novel and conflicting sensory inputs of flight after about six flights and would then no longer need the medication.

A recent addition to the therapeutic possibilities is the behind-the-ear disk of 0.2 mg of scopolamine (Transderm-V®), which leaks into the circulation over three days, possibly furnishing protection against motion sickness. It is reported to produce fewer side effects and to be about as effective as oral medication. This treatment has not been systematically tested in military flyers as of this writing.

USAFSAM tested a biofeedback-mediated behavioral modification procedure for selected, highly motivated flyers with chronic airsickness. This intense course of therapy was given two hours per day for two weeks. Flyers were given cross-coupled biaxial Coriolis stimulation by a revolving, tilting chair while electronically monitoring surface skin temperature and sweat rate.

In lay terms, they were taught to remain warm and dry instead of becoming cold and clammy.

Of 53 flyers who had been grounded for chronic severe airsickness and who were treated with this technique, 42 (79%) returned to full flying duties and were still successfully flying at two-year follow-up, three (6%) were partially successful, and eight (15%) were unsuccessful. The disadvantages of this technique—the special equipment required and its time-intensive nature—prevented its wide adoption (25). Similar work by Giles and Lochridge using a Bárány chair as the stimulus has also been successful, especially when used early in undergraduate pilot training, and without grounding the student pilots involved (26). Cowings et al. suggested the possible application of autogenic techniques to avoid space sickness encountered by many astronauts in their first few days in microgravity (27).

Anxiety Disorders

Approximately 2–4% of the general population suffers from a clinically significant anxiety disorder at some time. This group of disorders includes anxiety either as the primary symptom or as a feeling experienced in specific situations. In the older literature, these disorders are referred to as neuroses or neurotic reactions. Phobic disorders, anxiety states, obsessive-compulsive disorders, and stress disorders are included in this category.

Phobic Disorders

Phobic disorders are characterized by primitive anxiety experienced as fear of a situation or object. This feeling is recognized by the person as excessive or irrational, and it is ego-dystonic (i.e., the flyer would like to be rid of it). These elements were discussed in the earlier section entitled "Fear of Flying." One such condition is agoraphobia, the fear of being alone or in public places where a panic attack or other incapacitation may leave one helpless. This fear usually results in increasingly restricted activities. An-

other condition is social phobia, a fear of situations that could potentially expose one to public ridicule, such as fear of public speaking. A variety of simple phobias concern common objects or situations, such as cats, snakes, heights, darkness, or cockroaches. In each case, the individual realizes that the anxiety is groundless or exaggerated, but the anxiety seems to be beyond cognitive control. When flying situations or aircraft are the objects of phobia, the treatment may be complicated by the fact that true dangers are involved, and the therapist must acknowledge them. Nevertheless, even the most risky military flying is believed to be reasonably safe by those involved in it, or they would not continue. As the quotation at the beginning of this chapter observes, they find it interesting.

Much of the general public, however, finds flying more frightening than interesting. Various surveys indicate that 15–20% of the American public is somewhat afraid to fly, if not clinically phobic about aircraft. For those dedicated non-flyers who wish to overcome their fear of airline flying, a number of behavior modification programs are available, some sponsored by commercial airlines (28).

Panic disorders are attacks of pure terror occurring without reason in otherwise unremarkable circumstances not involving physical exertion or any true danger. No specific stimulus may be identified, as would be possible with a phobic disorder. Somatic symptoms may include dyspnea, palpitations, sensation of choking, dizziness, vasomotor flushing or chills, trembling, or sweating. A fear of going crazy or behaving uncontrollably also may be present. Physical causes should be considered, such as hormonal or endocrine disturbances. In studies of patients with anxiety or panic disorders, 40% were found to have mitral valve prolapse, a percentage out of proportion to the 5–7% of individuals found to have this condition in the general population (29). The reason for this association is not known, but may involve an inborn dysautonomia. Such attacks occurring in flight would interfere considerably with a pilot's ability to fly safely.

Obsessive-compulsive Disorders

Many flyers, particularly navigators, are informally referred to as being obsessive or compulsive. Such traits may be quite adaptive in flying, especially where adherence to standard procedures or checklists helps to maintain safe flight conditions. Obsessive-compulsive disorders are a grotesque magnification of these useful human characteristics. Obsessions are persistent, recurrent impulses, ideas, or images that the individual experiences as involuntary and nonsensical, if not outright alien to one's way of life. They may be violent or sexual in nature. Compulsions are behaviors that are repeated in a purposeful way while serving no useful purpose. Omitting these rituals results in intolerable tension or anxiety, even when it is not clear what evil may befall the sufferer in consequence. These rituals may distress or effectively cripple the individual, and yet they must be carried out: a common example is washing one's hands dozens of times each day to avoid dirt. Flyers may experience mild anxiety when they do not recheck an item once or twice, but they rarely become neurotically obsessed with elements of flight. Such strange urges and behavior are obviously incompatible with safe flying.

Affective Disorders

Affective disorders also could be termed disorders of mood and include both depression and pathologic elation (mania). Because depression is a reasonable human reaction to a variety of circumstances, most physicians are already familiar with it.

Depression

In this spectrum of psychiatric disorders, the physician is most likely to encounter depressive symptoms, especially presenting as minor physical complaints that persist or bother the patient in a medically inexplicable way. Faced with a flyer whose headaches, backaches, dizziness, or malaise seems to have no physical basis, especially in an individual whose past record reveals no physical complaints or who has previously been stoic in the face of real illness or injury, the prudent aeromedical practitioner will inquire about changes in patterns of sleeping, eating, sexual desire, and general mood. Perceived difficulty with concentration and memory, loss of usual self-assuredness, an unaccustomed sense of despair about the future, or an unreasonable sense of guilt or worthlessness are positive indications of depression. Psychiatric consultation and treatment are necessary. Full-blown depression may be associated clearly with a significant loss in a person's life, or it may occur for no obvious reason. Symptoms may include a change in eating habits: most depressed individuals lose their appetites and some grossly overeat. The flyer may complain of multiple vague or minor physical problems or symptoms. A loss of sleep or oversleeping may be a means of escaping the painful world. Activity may be slowed down or speeded up in an agitated way; usual activities seem joyless and uninteresting, and the individual may cry easily. Sexual drive may be considerably diminished, and the person feels unable to concentrate or to remember with the usual clarity. Unjustified feelings of guilt, remorse, worthlessness, sinfulness, and self-reproach appear. Escapist thinking ("I just want to get away from it all") or frank suicidal ideation may be expressed. In depressions of psychotic proportion, delusions of things done or not done, if true, would cause the feelings the sufferer has. In such instances, behavior may become bizarre or neglectful.

It is important to remember that many physicians do not distinguish clearly between the symptoms of anxiety and those of depression. In some people, clinical depressions include an overlay of anxiety and agitation, and the underlying depression may not be recognized. If symptoms of anxiety were treated with the benzodiazepines (e.g., Valium®, Librium®, Dalmane®, Ativan®), the depression may worsen.

When they are used in such patients, medications should include antidepressants, given in proper doses for a proper length of time by a physician skilled in their use.

Suicide

Suicidal potential should be considered when dealing with any patient who has emotional complaints, especially when depressive features are present. The vegetative signs of depression should alert the aeromedical practitioner to the possibility of suicide: disturbed sleeping or eating patterns; loss of memory, concentration, or energy; diminished libido; or loss of enjoyment of life. Some demographic information may help in assessing the potential for suicide in a given individual. Suicide is more likely in those who are unmarried, older, Protestant, homosexual, of a lower socioeconomic class, who have insomnia, abuse alcohol, live alone, or are unemployed. Individuals who have recently lost someone close are more at risk, as are those who have had a relative or a close friend commit suicide (role model). Although women attempt suicide about twice as often as men, men succeed twice as often as women.

Among aviators, the incidence of suicide and attempted suicide is low (30). Few estimates are even available, suggesting that aviator suicide does not warrant study. However, as with other aeromedical disorders, "the special problem for the pilot, of course, is that subtle errors on his part can have large consequences (31)." Even less frequent is the use of the aircraft as the instrument of suicide, a special consideration that is discussed below. The more troubling problem with suicide among aviators is the duration and severity of perturbation preceding the actual self-destructive act. In some groups, precipitating stresses have been found to exist and to grow for several years (J.C. Patterson, unpublished data). Such stress is commonly based on problems in an intimate relationship—60–80% of the time—and is usually found in flyers in mid-career, about age 30. Alcohol is often involved, as are factors of depression and anger. Attempt-

ers are more likely to appear to be impulsive than are completers. As in other groups studied, aviators who attempt suicide unsuccessfully do so more frequently by overdosing with drugs, while completers are more likely to use more lethal means, such as carbon monoxide or a firearm.

A flyer who has a deteriorating intimate relationship, along with signs, such as a significant change in mood or sociability, or development of tardiness or procrastination over several weeks, may warrant special monitoring and specific expressions of concern and support. Suicide has been extensively studied (32). In summary, one should be as watchful for suicidal potential in a depressed flyer as in any depressed person.

Suicide by Aircraft

One factor sets flyers aside in considering their potential for self-destruction: the availability of the aircraft as an instrument (33). Suicide by aircraft is unusual, but by no means unknown. A case report of such a suicide in the early 1970s reviewed the literature to that point (34), and other instances have occurred subsequently. Circumstances vary: some mishaps in which self-destruction has been alleged or proved have involved depressed persons who wished to leave their families large amounts of insurance, at times when they were under great personal financial stress. Others have involved religious delusions. Some have involved persons who stole aircraft and then could not handle them. Some have involved subintentional self-destructive tendencies, such as one in which the flyer flew dangerously and foolishly, daring death in a "Russian Roulette" manner; liquor may be involved in some such instances (D.R. Jones, unpublished data).

Because many such cases in general aviation rapidly involve litigation, it may be difficult to investigate them as evenhandedly as in the military, where legal immunity and the absence of liability issues may allow witnesses more latitude. It may also be difficult to distinguish medically between a death that occurred because of intentional action and one resulting from foolhardiness, inattention, or neglect. In such a field as aircraft accident investigation, which attends to such elusive elements as distraction, longing to be home, "get-home-itis," sensory overload, fatigue, or external sources of stress, the additional psychological factors, such as depression, romantic misadventures, financial strain, feelings of hopelessness or guilt, and others made matters much more difficult. The diagnosis of suicide by aircraft must begin with the recognition that such things occur, and the question should be raised not only by the circumstances of the mishap, but also by clinically significant recent events in the victim's life. As is true elsewhere in medicine, nothing replaces a good history.

Mania (Bipolar Affective Disorder)

Manic episodes are not as commonly encountered and, because the individual may well find these episodes pleasant, they may be first reported by someone else. The mood of the manic individual is elated or elevated or may be predominantly irritable. Symptoms may include tireless activity with no time or need for sleeping, eating, or ordinary activities; overweening self-esteem may manifest, as well as involvement in multiple, novel, and often unwise activities. These endeavors may have a strong potential for personal or financial disaster, which the individual does not recognize. The elation may have an infectious quality to it but may quickly turn to unwarranted anger when the person is thwarted. Incessant planning and activity may occur in business, social, religious, political, and sexual ventures, accompanied by inappropriate sociability; for example, telephone calls made to anyone in the world at any hour. Grandiosity may predominate: spree-spending, dangerous driving, flamboyant or intrusive behavior, loud and pressured speech, and incessant joking. Flight of ideas may occur, with easy distractibility, sometimes internally generated, so that the individual appears to interrupt himself, causing disorganized speech and even incoherence.

No one would fail to recognize such mania in full bloom. The hypomanic states are less extreme and may be perceived as great good spirits occurring in a person who is usually more reserved. One's clinical suspicions should be aroused by pressured speech and behavior, decreased sleeping, inflated self-esteem, loss of usual inhibitions, heedless hypersexuality, physical restlessness, irritability, and inappropriate actions representing a change from usual behavior.

Occurring alternately and severely, mania and depression comprise the disorders formerly known as manic-depressive and now termed bipolar affective disorder. In a lesser degree, without disordered thinking, such a condition is termed a cyclothymic disorder.

Psychotic Disorders

Disordered thinking is the hallmark of psychotic disorders: examples are hallucinations (false perceptions), delusions (real perceptions misinterpreted because of false beliefs), bizarre thinking, autistic or idiosyncratic patterns of pseudologic, and loose associations. Regardless of its cause, functional psychotic thinking that occurs in the absence of toxic or metabolic causes is generally cause for permanent disqualification from flying. Functional causes include schizophrenia, bipolar affective disorder, paranoia (irrational grandiosity or ideas of reference), or an acute situational reaction of psychotic proportions.

Organic psychoses may result from a wide variety of causes, including neoplasms, injuries, toxins, drugs, alcohol, metabolic or endocrine disorders, or infections. The existence of an organic brain disorder requires removal from flying status. Return to flying depends on a variety of factors, but the flyer should be clearly safe to fly and free of any specific risk of recurrence, seizure disorder, or significant neurologic dysfunction before such action is taken. About the only psychotic conditions allowing such returns are those due to temporary and reversible infections, or toxic or metabolic causes.

TREATMENT AND REHABILITATION

Psychotherapy

Simply listing some of the treatment modalities available to people with emotional disorders gives the aeromedical practitioner a feeling for the bewildering variety of choices for the flyer who needs help. Treatment may be given individually or in groups. The therapist may be a psychiatrist, psychologist, social worker, or clergyman. Treatment may be provided by a classic psychoanalyst—from one of many schools, including Freudian, Jungian, or Adlerian—or by a psychodynamic psychotherapist. Behavior modification, transactional analysis, gestalt therapy, biofeedback, rational-emotive therapy, family therapy, and marital therapy may be employed, as well as the newer fringe therapies: rolfing, est, primal screaming, or rebirthing. Few psychiatrists can speak authoritatively about all of these therapies. In such matters, the referring physician is best served by contacting local professional associations or societies and by talking with trusted colleagues. One certainly must help the patient avoid unethical practitioners and charlatans.

One must also consider the goals of therapy. The psychiatric consultant who is asked to evaluate a person's fitness to fly may well be faced with a defensive, somewhat hostile patient who wishes only to be cleared for flying status. The goal of the therapist may be to help the patient reach a better adaptation to life, whereas the goal of the flyer may be to return to flying. These goals may not always coincide, especially when the patient sees the therapist as an impediment to flying, a person who is denying the sought-after goal. Such issues should be settled early in the therapeutic process; it may be best to have the therapist be someone other than the psychiatric consultant who evaluates flying status.

Medications

Psychotropic medications are not compatible with active flying duties, both because of their primary and secondary effects and because any flyer whose emotional distress requires medication should not fly until that distress is relieved.

Antianxiety Medications

The benzodiazepines are widely used to allay anxiety and also as sedatives. Two commonly used compounds are diazepam (Valium®) and chlordiazepoxide (Librium®). Both may be given orally or intravenously; intramuscular administration should be avoided because the lipid solubility of these drugs leads to unpredictable absorption rates and uneven therapeutic effects. The biologic half-life of diazepam is 20–50 hours, and the half-life of chlordiazepoxide is 6–30 hours; therefore, several days should be allowed after completion of a course of medication before flying is resumed. These medications should not be used in patients who have symptoms of depression along with anxiety because they may deepen depression. Flurazepam (Dalmane®) is widely used for nocturnal sedation. The half-life of its active metabolite may extend to 65 hours; therefore, repeated doses have a cumulative effect. Temazepam (Restoril®) has a half-life of about eight hours; these drugs may be desirable when quick clearance is desired.

Antidepressant Medications

Tricyclic antidepressants are the medications most commonly used to treat depression. In general, these medications must be taken for about two weeks at a therapeutic level before clinical effects are noted. The side effects, mainly anticholinergic and sedative, begin immediately and thus tend to interfere with compliance because the patient initially feels even worse than before treatment. Desipramine (Norpramin®, Pertofrane®) has the fewest anticholinergic effects. If no antidepressant effect were noted after three weeks, blood levels of the primary drug and its metabolites should be obtained to assure adequacy of the dosage. Tricyclic antidepressants should be used with care in patients with known cardiac disease, and potentially suicidal patients should be given only two to three days of medication at one time. Cumulative experience with tricyclic antidepressants has led some authorities to allow flyers to return to the cockpit on such medications when they have been stable on them for several years without demonstrable side effects, and when they have become depressed attempting to discontinue them. Obviously such exceptions require close medical follow-up for side effects or recurrent depression, as well as the intelligent, motivated, and well-informed cooperation of the aviator. As clinicians gain experience with new antidepressant agents (e.g., Trazadone [Desaryl®], bupropion, [Wellbutrin®], fluoxetine [Prozac®]) and those being developed, the same policies may be cautiously applied to some patients taking them as well.

Another major antidepressant group is the monamine oxidase inhibitors [MAOIs]. These are powerful medications and should be employed only by those skilled in their use. Patients receiving these drugs should be carefully instructed to avoid foods containing tyramine because ingestion of such foods and absorption of tyramine, a catacholamine precursor, may lead to a hypertensive crisis. Such crises also may result from the concomitant use of sympathetic amines, such as ephedrine, phenylephrine (Neo-Synephrine®), or phenylpropanolamine (Propadrine®), frequently used in over-the-counter medications. Such a hypertensive crisis may be treated with a slow, intravenous infusion of phentolamine [Regitine®]. This potential for hypertensive crisis precludes consideration of an aviator to obtain a waiver to return to cockpit duties while taking this class of medication, regardless of duration or stability of the clinical course.

Neuroleptics or Major Tranquilizers

Neuroleptic drugs or major tranquilizers now include several families, including the aliphatic, piperidine, and piperazine phenothiazines, with which many physicians are already familiar, thioxanthine derivatives, butyrophenones, and some of the newer agents. Physicians who need to use these medications generally become familiar with one member of each group; intragroup differences are minor. Because the clinical indications for these medications usually include psychotic thinking or a major emotional disturbance, their use in a flyer should automatically indicate grounding and a psychiatric consultation.

Lithium Carbonate

Lithium carbonate is primarily used to treat bipolar affective disorders, usually manic in nature, and may be of some use in a subgroup of schizophrenic patients. Management requires a careful attention to blood levels, sodium intake, and the state of hydration and should be undertaken only by a physician experienced in such measures. Toxic effects may involve the cardiac, renal, or central nervous systems. Physicians requiring detailed data should consult the current psychopharmaceutic literature.

Behavioral Techniques

Behavior therapy is based on experimental observations of animal and human behavior and on modifications of those human behaviors that therapist and patient agree are causing problems. Feelings and thoughts also may be changed when behavior is modified.

Psychotherapists today have a variety of behavioral techniques available. Many of these techniques are discussed superficially in lay magazines and popular psychologically-oriented paperback books. Thus trivialized, they sound so simple that the casual reader may feel like an instant expert. Anyone who has approached a true psychopathologic condition this simplistically has probably encountered a maze of hidden agendas and subconscious resistances that seemed utterly inexplicable. Several of these techniques, however, may be useful in treating some of the problems an aeromedical practitioner may face, and these methods are discussed briefly in the following sections. They should not be undertaken by those unskilled in their application.

Relaxation

Perhaps the most familiar relaxation training was developed by Jacobson (35). This technique consists of strongly contracting various groups of muscles and then slowly relaxing them so that, by contrasting the contracted and the relaxed feelings, patients learn to relax even further. With training and practice, patients may learn to become relaxed rapidly, simply by willing themselves to do so. Other techniques involve the visual imagery of quiet scenes, repeating relaxing phrases, and abdominal breathing techniques.

Biofeedback

Biofeedback uses electronic monitoring to give the patient digital or analog information about physical states that are otherwise only dimly perceived. Frontalis muscle tension, fingertip sweat rate, and peripheral skin temperature are frequently measured in this manner. With instantaneous information about any changes, the patient can learn by trial and error to control these functions and thus lower the state of autonomic arousal. This technique is frequently helpful in avoiding tension or vascular headaches, aborting airsickness, controlling other disorders of muscle tension, and enhancing relaxation.

Systemic Desensitization

Systemic desensitization was made popular by Wolpe (36). This method consists of learning a relaxation technique and then applying that technique while being gradually, but progressively, exposed to a phobically feared object or situation. This method has been successfully incorporated into the treatment of flying phobias in would-be airline passengers and also has been used in a few military flyers with success. The patient must be motivated to change because this

therapy requires close and intelligent cooperation between therapist and patient.

SPECIAL SUBJECTS

Astronaut Selection

The medical process of astronaut selection has always been challenging. Mental health challenges begin with the factors mentioned previously in the selection of aviators. These are magnified by the large number of applicants for the few positions available, and are complicated by the lack of measurable outcome factors against which to validate the original selection process. Given the consequences of a mistake, the selection process is daunting; still, it must be done, even in the face of insufficient information and under the bright light of public scrutiny.

How do we know that the right person has been selected to fly in space? Until recently, the only positive outcome criterion available was successful mission completion, but no objective criteria were available as to how successful a given astronaut had been on a given mission. An unsuccessful mission did not mean that the wrong person had been selected, although that was a possibility. No measures were available concerning the quality of an astronaut's performance, or his or her suitability for the work. Medical authorities were not sure whether they had to select the preeminent applicant ''best qualified'', or one who was simply competent ''fully qualified''. ''The Right Stuff'' became a chic phrase for the indefinable aspects of the classic astronaut spirit, but its components were never translated from author Tom Wolfe's artistry into standard psychological terms. Two factors, in our opinion, contributed to this gap.

The first was the very natural desire of the astronauts themselves, individually and collectively, to maintain their privacy. Most people are cautious about disclosing personal psychological information, and the makeup of ''the right stuff'' includes both a particular disinclination to concern oneself with emotional insight, and a strong desire to control one's own destiny. Psychological information threatened both tendencies: it involved "mystical information" about oneself that one could barely understand, yet which could result in losing out on selection for a mission or, worst of all, in being removed from the competition for reasons beyond one's control. Mental health professionals of all types, then, were best avoided, when possible, and were given minimum information "damage control" when contact was unavoidable. In this, astronauts were much like other professional flyers, but with more clout.

The second reason for the dearth of psychological information was the NASA's desire to present the American public with a spotless group. "America needs heroes" meant that information that might be interpreted as reflecting poorly on the public image of the group was not welcome: the fact that mental health evaluations may help to avoid selection of the kinds of people who would behave in potentially embarrassing ways was perhaps not fully appreciated.

Eventually, however, new developments eroded institutional resistance. Although the original groups of American astronauts were made up mostly of test pilots, all of whom were white males, the advent of nonpilot space crew members (e.g., mission specialists) diluted group homogeneity. Selection of female space crew members, and those of other nations, cultures, and ethnic backgrounds, introduced new personality factors. Plans for long duration missions made it clear that revised standards and selection procedures were necessary. Plainly put, one would have concerns about the group dynamics of a three-year Mars mission in which crew members were all fighter pilots.

After much discussion, a system evolved under the direction of NASA physician Patricia A. Santy, M.D., that divided the mental health aspects of NASA selection into two parts, dubbed "select-out" and "select-in" (P.A. Santy, personal communication). These terms are used much as was discussed earlier in this chapter: "select-out" refers to the process that assures the absence of psychopathology. To this end, a structured interview was derived from research and clinical experience that methodically ruled out significant psychopathology and personality disorders, in addition to examining (as well as can be done, considering the lack of deeper psychodynamic understanding) the nature of the applicant's desire to travel in space. The structured interview was adapted from Endicott's Schedule for Affective Disorders and Schizophrenia, also involving lifetime issues and an anxiety component, and from the Personality Assessment Schedule, developed by Tyrer in the United Kingdom to investigate personality traits and possible disorders. This interview, lasting up to four hours, is performed by psychiatrists and psychologists skilled in working with aviators, and is standardized to some extent by the rotation of observers through the interview rooms. About four hours of psychological tests, some standardized to flyer norms, are administered separately. The final decision on psychological fitness is made by all examiners, meeting together to consider the information on each candidate presented by that candidate's specific examiner. The final recommendation, the only information transmitted to the selection board, is a simple "qualified" or "disqualified."

Select-in designates the process whereby an individual, once in the astronaut corps, is assigned to a mission, trains for it, and flies it. The mental health portion of this process includes a separate and confidential evaluation made at selection, plus later assessments that are kept separate from NASA records in order not to influence subsequent outcomes. These are to be compared against performance criteria developed from astronaut self-appraisals, management assessments, and other relatively objective criteria. The data are scored, so that one person's results may be compared with another's. The products of the select-in evaluation and the later appraisals then are available as "outcome criteria" against which to assess the original selection process. Once this process is completed, investigators have a much better idea which aspects of the mental health selection process correlate with actual, measured success in space flight, especially long-duration missions. The process may also contribute to our understanding of group dynamics, which will play such an important role in establishing a lunar base, and in traveling to Mars and back. As results are validated, they are then fed back into further refinement of selection procedures, to simplify and concentrate the process.

This is an ambitious and sensitive project which, if successful, will also provide much-needed objective information about the larger process of selection of flyers in all areas of aviation.

Marriage and Family Issues

Much is written about the need for flyers to function under stressful conditions, and about ways to defend against stressful effects by lessening the numbers of stressors, lowering each stressor's level, and raising flyers' defenses. The clinical experience of veteran aeromedical practitioners and the aerospace medical literature attest to the value of a healthy family relationship as support to a flyer (37). Conversely, undue family stress may have a devastating effect upon flying performance. In fact, an experienced aviator's acquired phobic fear of flying almost never derives from the flying milieu, but instead may usually be traced to interpersonal stresses within personal relationships (38). Thus, when an experienced pilot presents with an inexplicable, recent increase in free-floating anxiety, or an uncontrollable fear about some factor affecting flight (e.g., thunderstorms, flying at altitude, sitting in the passenger compartment), the aeromedical practitioner should take a careful social history involving the status of the flyer's parental and marital family relationships. One should especially examine changes that occurred just before the onset of the present symptoms or the recent, intolerable exacerbation of previously controllable fears about flying; consider possible anniversary reactions as well.

As noted in the section on fear of flying,

symptoms arising from aviation accidents or near-misses are easily identified by the flyer: cause and effect are clearly related. Cause and effect may not be as clear, however, when the flyer reacts to family-related problems. Confusion may arise if the family-based fears were attached (cathected) onto actual threats to flying safety, such as thunderstorms. These fears may become phobic in proportion, so that the flyer cannot stop obsessing about them. Such instances reflect the cathexis of intolerable intrapersonal anxiety upon a preexisting, generally rational fear of a true hazard: sensible pilots fear thunderstorms, and stay out of them when possible. However, mentally fit pilots do not lose sleep for three days, obsessing and worrying about whether they may encounter a thunderstorm on their next flight, becoming consumed with anxiety during flight about the possibility that one may develop near the destination airport. Thus, if an experienced flyer were to become crippled by anxiety about an aviation hazard that previously elicited only healthy respect, one should look to family dynamics for the cause.

Factors of independence, self-sufficiency, authority, responsibility, and decisiveness, which are adaptive for a pilot, may translate into maladaptive features within a marriage. The male pilot—no comparable data exists about female flyers—may be seen by his wife or partner as nonfeeling, noncommunicative, demanding, perfectionistic, and autocratic, a man who responds to others' emotional distress with intellectualized and distant arguments, who doesn't know or care how she feels, and who regards honest emotional expression as illogical, demeaning, and unworthy. He, conversely, may portray her as moody, unpredictable, easily upset, hard to understand, and unappreciative of the stresses under which he works. Alcohol abuse may contribute to the problem (he drinks because she nags, and she nags because he drinks). An excellent review of spousal factors in pilot stress underlines the strength of such stressors in the aviator's life, and notes the value of recognizing the contributions that spouses may make to flying safety (39). Each partner should be aware of the effects that a flying career may have on their relationship, and vice versa, and of the ways that such effects may be constructively managed in both arenas.

Preventive measures may be made available by management, operational authorities, medical departments, pilot associations, or unions. Briefings and presentations to spouses, group support systems (especially within the military), easy access to knowledgeable medical and mental health professionals, and, when necessary, counseling programs all help to control stress-related effects.

Female Flyers

Women were involved in aviation from the beginning. The first woman to fly was Madame Thible of France, who flew in one of the Montgolfier balloons in the 18th century, and the first woman to be licensed as a pilot was Elise Deroche, in 1910 (40). The first woman licensed in the United States was Harriet Quimby, and such well-known pilots as Bessie Coleman and Margaret and Katherine Stinson soon followed. Ruth Law Oliver set several altitude and distance records in 1916, and Ruth Nichols later established more than 35 aviation records. The many accomplishments of such pioneer aviators as Jacqueline Cochran and Amelia Earhart are justly famous (41).

Although American women flew in a number of paramilitary organizations during and after World War II, it wasn't until 1976 that they began routinely flying as military pilots in the USAF, a change that grew out of the women's liberation movement. USAF mental health standards were not gender-specific, and so were not affected by the new policy. However, many social changes and novel interpersonal interactions resulted from the presence of female flyers in previously all-male domains. Inevitably, some of these pressures were manifested psychiatrically, and were summarized in 1983 in a review of patients referred to USAFSAM (42).

During a six-year period, USAFSAM evaluated 3669 males and 34 females. Most of the men were active flyers, although a few (numbers unknown) were not. Of the women, two were pilots (one from another service), five were student pilots, two were student pilot applicants, three were space flight applicants, one was a flight nurse, and four were enlisted: three ground controllers and one altitude-chamber technician. Thus, only six (one pilot, five students) could be said to have come from the 175 or so women flying as primary USAF aircrew or trainees at the time. The men came from a pool of over 40,000 total aircrew.

Of those referred to USAFSAM, 570 (15%) of the men and 17 (50%) of the women received psychiatric evaluations. Of the 570 men, 203 (36%) were grounded; of the 17 women, 8 (47%) were grounded. However, only two (12%) of the women were grounded for psychiatric reasons; the other six were grounded for medical reasons: EEG abnormality, syncope, visual problems, hyperthyroidism, decompression sickness, and airsickness. Comparable information was not compiled for the men.

At least one useful clinical observation was made as a part of these evaluations, however. The two psychiatric groundings of women derived directly from reactions to sexual issues: divorce and a later rape in one instance, and depression based on pre-Air Force sexual molestation in the other. Interviews with the other female pilots revealed less blatant gender-related issues. For instance, one female student pilot, the only woman in her class in a geographically isolated location, had no other women with whom to socialize, and became wary of forming friendships with her male classmates because of their frequent and unwelcome sexual advances. She was thus deprived of the morale-building peer support that strengthened and reassured her male counterparts.

Two women reported that they felt their (male) instructors did not demand the same performance levels of them as of their male classmates, and they feared that their grades were better than their actual proficiency, which led to some anxiety about flying. One woman, a student pilot who became hypoglycemic and then hyperventilated in flight, received outright harassment from her commander, who regarded her as a "hysterical woman." (She went on to graduate and to fly successfully as a tanker pilot.) Those who evaluated these women at USAF-SAM found them to be, like their male counterparts, varied in their abilities, in their motivation, and in their emotional resiliency. The lesson learned from the review was that women in aviation are under all the same stresses as men, to which are added those relating to their gender. "The behavior of male military flyers toward their female counterparts is at times prejudicial, at times exploitive, at times patronizing, and at times frankly sexual. Flight surgeons, supervisors and instructors will benefit from an awareness of some of the subtleties encountered when these age-old relationships are introduced into the arena of military aviation (42)."

Labor-management Issues

Deregulation of the United States commercial airlines led to numerous changes, involving mergers, corporate takeovers, bankruptcy procedures, strikes, lockouts, job insecurity, and a variety of labor-management difficulties. Such events would be upsetting in any industry, and their effects on cockpit aircrew members became a legitimate aviation safety concern. In simple terms, can such life changes cause stress-related effects, including poor morale, sleep disturbances, somatic complaints, anger, and depression, all of which may dispose an aviator to accident-prone behavior? If this were true, what would be the responsibility of the aerospace medicine practitioner?

Girodo reported on 24 pilots involved in a two-year labor-management dispute that had included layoffs and callbacks, strikes, strike-breaking, mixed union and nonunion crews, demotions, and other stress-producing situations (43). Gathering data from psychometric test data and semistructured interviews, he concluded that

"while some pilots (9 of 38: 24%) experienced the kind of psychological distress that should have prevented them from assuming flying duties, others (29 of 38: 76%) seemed to function quite well." However, in a comparable study, Little et al. found that pilots employed by an airline with a history of corporate instability reported significantly more symptoms of stress and depression than those employed by more stable airlines (44).

Ideally, labor-management dissension, corporate takeovers, and similar disputes would be settled without aircrew becoming so emotionally involved. Life is not ideal, however, and flyers also differ in their vulnerability to such stressors. Although aircrew members are generally fairly adaptable, those who develop clinical, stress-related symptoms of depression, anxiety, or anger should be evaluated by an aeromedical practitioner who may request knowledgeable mental health consultation when indicated. Significant psychopathology should be treated as it would be in ordinary circumstances.

Should a flyer behave irresponsibly under such circumstances, ample safeguards may be provided by the presence of other crew members and the many cross-checks already available: standard procedures, air traffic control, aircraft warning systems, and the like. If a given crew member were to consciously undertake dangerous activities, such as noncooperation with other crew members or sabotage, such behavior should be dealt with either therapeutically or administratively, as appropriate. Heightened scrutiny, through government or company check rides, union Professional Standards Committees, the Employee Assistance Program and/or psychotherapy, is available. Angry feelings may be constructively handled by standard stress management techniques: recognition, ventilation, and making conscious decisions about expressing them through socially acceptable and positive channels.

Mishaps and Psychological Management

When a mishap occurs, the primary concern is with the physical rescue and recovery of those involved. Evidence is mounting, however, that emotional and psychological adjustments to a mishap can be crucial to a victim's later recovery (45, 46). Relatively straightforward aftercare principles have been tested in a variety of disaster scenarios, and such stressors as identification of victims, and such responses as specific intervention strategies are now key concepts in psychological aftercare.

All classes of disaster victims should be considered. Taylor identified six (46). The primary victims are those directly involved, such as aviators dying in or surviving an aircraft mishap. Secondary victims include family members of the mishap victims. Members of entire flying organizations (squadrons, other pilots based together) may also become secondary victims of the mishaps in which their friends suffered or died (47). Tertiary victims may include professional rescuers, such as paramedics, firefighters, and police. Research suggests that 35% of this group may be at risk in a single mishap, when workers' abilities to meet the demands of the situation with adaptive coping skills are overcome (48, 49). At the fourth level are victims in the general community: supervisors, managers, and other leaders who may feel, or be seen as, in some way responsible for the mishap. The fifth level includes emotionally unstable people who may overidentify with the mishap or the actual victims, and the sixth level victims are those who were not actually involved, but who might have been: those who "just missed being on the aircraft," for example.

Particular attention should be paid to the third level, or rescuer, victims, because they may not be considered as such and, no doubt, may have strong personal prohibitions against accepting help. Professional rescue workers are likely to have a great deal of experience with disaster and thus have often built psychological protection for themselves against the negative effects of their work. However, they must undergo various unusual stresses, such as body handling, exhausting work schedules, personal danger, and seeing peers injured or killed in rescue work;

they often feel responsible for life-and-death decisions and outcomes even though, realistically, they could do little. Understanding the cumulative effects of such experiences may explain why a rescue worker, after years of feeling no special negative emotional effects, may finally have a marked stress reaction to a specific mishap. Perhaps something occurs that has personal meaning to the rescue worker, or is particularly gruesome, and precipitates a reaction. Because of this possibility, a disaster aftercare plan should be offered to such workers, using techniques of education and ventilation, as it is available to other classes of victims.

Providing such services to all victims can be important to their future stability and productivity (50). Although many of those exposed to the mishap do not experience significant emotional reactions, those who do may find them disabling. They may report fatigue, sleep disturbances, nightmares, gastrointestinal upsets, and increased alcohol use. They may experience social withdrawal, symptoms of anxiety or depression, emotional lability, disturbances of memory and cognition, and intrusive thoughts or flashbacks. The goal of the postmishap evaluation and intervention should be to identify such victims and to work with them so as to attend to the emotional reactions and return them to normality as soon as possible.

The specific interventions tend to be relatively simple, but are quite specific in terms of effectiveness (51). Such victims may need to recognize and express their observations and feelings. Many respond fully to expressions of interest and concern, while others may angrily deny their mishap-related problems and reject any offer of help. On occasion, these strong deniers are the ones who later show significant emotional distress. Much of the immediate postmishap psychological intervention may be accomplished in a group setting, so that one or two care providers can reach a large number of victims simultaneously. It is best to keep the various classes of victims mentioned above separate because their needs are different and, indeed, their training and experience with mishaps are different.

The first level of intervention is education. The victims should understand that humans have natural emotional reactions to experiences that are physically or emotionally traumatic. Victims should know that the range of reactions includes the symptoms noted above. They should be warned further about the danger of self-medication with increasing amounts of alcohol or drugs. In the second stage of intervention, victims are encouraged to describe their experiences, to ventilate. Depending on the reaction of a particular victim, some may actually relive the experience, but most describe what they saw, heard, and felt. "Telling the story" seems to be important, and requires only a sympathetic listening ear and an occasional open-ended question to encourage the victim to continue with the story.

Most victims respond well to education and brief ventilation, with no need for further care. Some, however, do not do well, and can be identified during the first two stages of intervention as needing further help. The third phase of intervention is applied to these few, who are approached separately and offered more specific care on scheduled follow-up visits. When these victims need specific therapy, they may be referred to mental health care providers, with telephone contact made in a few days to ensure that each has been seen, and that needs are met.

This model of progressive intervention is relatively simple, but it helps the victims understand that normal reactions may be somatic, psychological, or both. They should be reassured that such reactions tend to resolve with time, and that specific help can be sought to help deal with such feelings. Ventilation seems to help relieve the emotional tension caused by the mishap, and the idea of care and concern may be extremely efficacious in rapidly returning the victims to normal functioning.

Mishap aftercare for the various levels of victims is fairly simple and cost-effective. When victims are given only physical examinations and somatic treatment, longer periods of dysfunction, distress, and low productivity may occur. Few victims experience crippling, emotional reactions to mishaps, but, as with other areas of aerospace medicine, preventing rare occurrences of severe problems with significant consequences is preferable to waiting for psychological distress to occur before attempting therapy. Mishap aftercare provides significant prevention at small expense of resources, compared with the cost of definitive psychotherapy for established pathological reactions.

COMBAT FLYING

Considering the movies, books, and anecdotes arising from combat flying, one may recall Robert E. Lee's remark to General James Longstreet at the battle of Fredericksburg: "It is well that war is so terrible—we should grow too fond of it!" Solo aerial combat is probably second only to knightly jousting as a source of romantic fantasy. As judged from personal accounts, it is exhilarating but exhausting and is as wearing in its own way as warfare on the ground. Certainly, chronic fatigue and stresses caused by combat flying in bombers and transports have been investigated by several psychiatric authorities.

The books by Bond (7) and Grinker and Spiegel (8) about their experiences in World War II are basic texts for anyone interested in anything deeper than a superficial discussion of the topic. One must keep in mind that the flyers of those days were usually quite young; high school graduates or college students who volunteered either from patriotic motives or to avoid being drafted into the ground forces. They were given relatively brief training and were quickly sent into combat. Missions were not necessarily undertaken in an area of air superiority, and, especially in bombers, casualties might be hundreds per mission. Gann described the "over the Hump" operation of transports in the Himalayas, when 32 men were lost on four crashes during one routine day of noncombat flying (52).

Such heavy losses did not occur in the United States forces in Korea or in Vietnam, but the descriptions of the war of combat flying are similar. Sleep disturbances, nightmares, anxiety symptoms, irritability, loss of sense of humor, social withdrawal, and other changes from the usual personality are the hallmarks of incipient battle fatigue in both aviators and soldiers. Irregular work-rest-sleep schedules add circadian upset to the mental strain of facing death daily and to the physical fatigue intrinsic in any flying schedule. The flight surgeon who has to support a flying unit in a combat issue can do a number of things to help lessen, or at least delay, the attrition of flyers from battle fatigue.

Environmental Factors

Basic amenities must be as well provided as possible. Sleeping facilities should be quiet and somewhat removed from the flight line. These quarters should be soundproofed and climate-controlled, so that flyers' sleep may be undisturbed. When flying operations are going on around-the-clock, as they frequently do, good sleeping quarters are particularly important. Meals should be nourishing, attractive, and easily obtained at any hour. The flyer should have easy access to showering facilities and to a source of clean laundry. Attention of base authorities to matters such as these is not only important in the physical comfort of the flyer but also serves as tangible evidence of the unity with which the base supports the combat mission. "Nothing's too good for our boys in combat, and that's what we give 'em" was a sarcastic tag line heard in Vietnam whenever another shortage occurred. Like much gallows humor, it disclosed true feelings about the perceived lack of support. Nonflyers complained about night-patrol pilots sleeping in air-conditioned and soundproofed quarters, but pilots who could not sleep in the daytime because of heat and noise were certainly less ready to fly night missions. This attention to physical comfort was not coddling; it was good common sense.

Personal Factors

Today's military flyers, as noted previously, tend to be older, better educated, and more experienced as a group than those written about by past authors. If combat experience in Vietnam or the Gulf War offers any indication, most would approach combat situations with the attitude that the USAF refers to as "professional:" that they are there to do the job for which they have been trained. Identification with a unit regarded as competent and professional is an important factor in overcoming feelings of personal inadequacy in a combat situation. Studies of infantry soldiers identified the feeling that "I am the only one who is frightened" as contributing to battle fatigue in that the individual feels that he alone has the cognitive and autonomic sensations of fear. Frank discussion of these feelings by the flight surgeon or, more to the point, by the squadron commander help to allay the perception of any individual that he is the only frightened person in a band of heroes. The clear message should be that it is normal to be aware of one's fear and that the unit tolerates such fears without question as long as the individual performs his duties. Stated simply, it is acceptable to feel fear and to talk about fear, but it is not acceptable to act afraid in combat.

Battle fatigue is based on true physical fatigue, as well as on the struggle between the natural instinct to avoid danger and the will to face it in order to do one's duty. Thus, those responsible for scheduling flights should provide time for sleep; four hours of uninterrupted sleep per 24 hours is the irreducible minimum (53). Flyers should have one to two days off every week or two and a longer break every few months, when possible. Experienced flight surgeons in previous wars and in Vietnam concurred in the observation that flyers on a rest-and-recreation (R and R) break get much recreation and little rest; it is a good idea to have one to two days off the flying schedule after the flyer returns from R and R to allow him to catch up on sleep before he resumes flying. This and associated subjects have been thoroughly discussed in a Technical Report from USAFSAM (54).

Alcohol consumption generally increases in a combat zone. One can preach about it endlessly, but unit discipline is probably the strongest weapon in avoiding situations of excessive drinking and too-short rest periods before flying. Otherwise, the old rule of ''12 hours between bottle and throttle'' is extremely hard to enforce. Although it is not always sufficient aeromedically, it does have the virtue of being easy to remember. The flight surgeon should help the squadron and flight commanders establish such a rule as a strict squadron tradition, enforced by peer pressure as well as by fiat. How much is too much? Since normal sleep patterns are disturbed by alcohol, flyers may be counseled to keep their alcohol intake below the level that causes sleep changes, as a simple personal measure.

The brain and mind occupy the same part of the body. A disorder occurring anywhere in the body, in peace or in war, may have major mental health implications; therefore, the distinction between neurologic and psychiatric disease is basically artificial. Alcoholism has psychic and somatic components, as do sudden loss of consciousness, epilepsy, brain injury, fatigue, and multiple sclerosis.

The wise aeromedical physician keeps mental health factors in mind when dealing with conditions labeled neurologic, and will keep organic factors in mind when dealing with conditions labeled psychiatric.

AEROSPACE NEUROLOGY

Introduction

Aerospace neurology applies the tools of clinical neurology, including the neurologic examination, neuroimaging, neuropsychological and electrophysiologic testing, to define aeromedically-significant disease. Progressive, degenerative diseases of the musculoskeletal or central

nervous system (CNS), either idiopathic or hereditary, are reviewed in standard neurology textbooks and are obvious in their deleterious effect on fitness to fly. The scope of aerospace neurology is to identify the gray area between aeromedically-significant illness and aeromedically-benign conditions.

An illness or reasonable threat of illness that can adversely affect flight or personal safety is thus defined as aeromedically significant. Rather than enumerating diseases, it is more useful to follow general rules to decide which are aeromedically significant. This process eliminates the need for establishing a specific diagnosis, and allows the aeromedical practitioner to view the flyer's problem in the context of the flying environment. Simply stated, we want to determine whether a flyer can fly safely and effectively, regardless of the disorder. Aeromedically significant disease is therefore present when: (a) the process occurs suddenly or unpredictably and is or may be incapacitating; (b) it progresses at an unpredictable rate; or (c) it has the potential to interfere with flight safety. (Marc S. Katchen, personal communication.)

New technologies, including the routine use of MRI, add a new dimension to aerospace neurologic evaluations because of their ability to identify subclinical disease, as in the evaluation of multiple sclerosis (MS), and decompression sickness (55). Clinical application of single-photon emission computed tomography (SPECT) and positron emission tomography (PET) scans, respectively, allow dynamic cerebral blood flow and metabolic mapping of CNS function.

Electrophysiologic measurements with brainstem auditory evoked responses (BAER), visual evoked response (VER), and somatosensory evoked potential (SEP) are routinely used in the clinical setting, and recently were applied as measures of neurologic dysfunction under toxic or hyperbaric conditions (56). Cognitive evoked potentials (CEP) are used to find a measure for human performance capacity and limitations. The expanded function of EEG using spectral analysis (brain mapping) is applied to problems, such as G-induced loss of consciousness (G-LOC).

Research efforts in aerospace neurology must be guided toward identifying the earliest form of clinical disease and predicting its course before the patient shows persistent signs of the disease. This end of the disease spectrum is rarely dealt with in routine clinical research. The age of populations tested, the end points used, and the severity of illness studied by clinical investigators are usually well beyond the gray areas where aeromedical significance begins. One should keep in mind that aerospace neurology is a part of occupational medicine. Every illness, no matter how clinically benign, must be considered in the context of the job requirements and the environment of the workplace.

New problems arise in which information about the many problems of the disease are still unknown. This is occurring with acquired immune deficiency syndrome (AIDS), caused by human immunodeficiency virus (HIV) infection. The known stages of the disease range from serologically-positive asymptomatic patients to those with overwhelming opportunistic infections. Although controversy exists over the neuropsychologic deficits in the HIV-positive person (57, 58), these tests are not scored against aircrew norms. The emphasis on environmental conditions, speed of information processing, and motor output make the aerospace environment an area in which extrapolation of ground-based data cannot be assumed. In addition, careful follow-up is necessary to determine progression of disease. The early use of antiviral agents in asymptomatic patients with low T-cell counts may make it necessary to consider such medications for waivers for flying duties. However, the no-waiver policies of the USAF and United States Navy have been published (59, 60).

Electrophysiology and Neuroimaging

The electroencephalograph (EEG) was first used as a selection tool for pilot candidates during World War II. This application of the new technology was abandoned after it failed to predict successful pilot candidates. In the 1960s and 1970s, several studies screened cadets' EEGs at the United States Naval Academy and the United States Air Force Academy (61, 62). The yield of abnormalities was low, and the predictive value for future seizures was questionable. In addition, many "abnormal" wave patterns have since been revealed to be normal variants. The USAF and United States Navy have stopped using the EEG as a screening tool for pilot candidates. In some other air forces, EEG is used to screen only for true epileptiform discharges. The fact that those denied training slots may never have seizures is accepted because the risk of an in-flight seizure is considered great enough to justify the program.

Brain mapping has been made possible by applying computer transformations of EEG waveforms. At present, clinical applications are limited and should be restricted to those with expertise in EEG, and the limitations of the EEG brain-mapping procedure, according to the American Academy of Neurology (63). Research is underway linking brain mapping to neuropsychological testing, or to specific stressors, with the hopes to identify "fingerprint" wave patterns that give insights into how the brain works and reacts. One application of brain mapping or spectral analysis of waveforms is currently being evaluated in the period just before G-LOC.

Evoked potentials are electrophysiologic measurements linked to specific stimuli, which use computer averaging of resultant waveforms recorded over the scalp. Evoked potentials routinely used in clinical practice include VER, BAER, and SER. Their development, and the details of how they are performed, can be found in standard textbooks of electrophysiology. The measurements recorded include the time from the stimulus until the wave appears (latency), its polarity (negative or positive), and its amplitude. Typically, these tests are used in diseases in which white matter tracts are involved, such as multiple sclerosis; trauma to the peripheral nerves (e.g., brachial plexus injury); or during surgical procedures of the peripheral nerves, spinal cord, or brainstem structures. Recently, several groups tried to apply the evoked potentials as a measure of injury to the CNS under conditions of stress, such as hyperbarism.

Cognitive evoked potentials (CEPs) are similar to those described above, except that the stimuli involve mental activity instead of passive stimulation. The best known CEP wave generated is the P300 (positive polarity, 300 msec latency), although other waveforms are being evaluated by researchers. The significance of the CEP is its potential as a measuring tool for human cognitive performance. CEP would be used as a measure or predictor of impaired cognitive functioning under different stressors, such as hyperbarism, hypoxia, or workload stress.

Magnetic resonance imaging (MRI) applies the principles used in analyzing chemical compounds (nuclear magnetic resonance) to humans, using computer reconstructions. The images give details of brain, brainstem, and spinal cord not possible by CT. It can identify multiple sclerosis plaques, infiltrating tumors, or ischemic damage not seen on CT. Its role and drawbacks are discussed below in the section on "Multiple Sclerosis and Optic Neuritis." In addition, areas of abnormal signals were found after decompression sickness where CNS injury was not yet suspected (55).

Single proton emission computed tomography (SPECT) has moved from its role as a research tool into clinical practice. Using specific radionuclides, it can measure cerebral blood flow or metabolic activity. The stability of radionuclides may allow for metabolic and flow measurements minutes to hours after a G-LOC, hypobaric injury, or head trauma, and opens future possibilities for investigation in those areas.

Optic Neuritis and Multiple Sclerosis

The search for subclinical manifestations of disease is best exemplified by the uncertain relationship between optic neuritis and multiple sclerosis. Depending on the studies reviewed, 15–80% of patients who develop optic neuritis

go on to develop multiple sclerosis. The diagnosis of multiple sclerosis depends on the history, neurologic signs, and confirmatory laboratory support (MRI, cerebral spinal fluid analysis, evoked potential studies). In aerospace neurology, one cannot wait for the natural history of the illness to present itself. Any tests that would predict the course of the patient's future illness would be of great benefit. MRI is the "gold standard" for finding multiple sclerosis plaques in brain, brainstem and spinal cord. Although sensitive, it is not specific, and the results must be interpreted with respect to the clinical findings.

From these factors arise the uncertainty about whether clinical optical neuritis plus an MRI consistent with multiple sclerosis is sufficient to diagnose definite multiple sclerosis. A multicenter, nationwide study is in progress to answer this question. Until this study is completed, no pathognomonic markers are known to be specific for multiple sclerosis. The aeromedical practitioner must diagnose this based on currently accepted standards for diagnosing multiple sclerosis while keeping informed on this rapidly developing field (64).

MRI used with and without contrast material has been suggested as a marker of active blood-brain barrier disruption, implying ongoing plaque development (65). Further studies of optic neuritis patients with serial MRI scans, looking for a marker of active disease, are underway. If a consistent pattern emerges, it will have a great effect upon both selection and retention standards for flying crew members.

Headache

Headache is the second leading cause of days lost from work in the United States. The cost of treatment plus lost production and work days is calculated at $40–60 billion per year. Headache was recently reclassified to give more specific criteria for each type of headache and facial pain (66).

Headaches have specific aeromedical implications. Of the United States population, ages 20–40, 20% have headaches (range: 10–60%);

therefore, a significant number of aircrew and support personnel will suffer from headaches. The important questions are: What types of headaches interfere with flight safety? Can such headaches be effectively controlled? Aircraft accidents have been documented as being caused by inflight headaches, and so the characteristics of the different headaches that can interfere with flight safety must be considered. These characteristics include the severity of the pain (Is it incapacitating?) and neurologic deficits that precede, accompany, or follow the actual headache (e.g., aphasia, visual loss, confusion). Incapacitation can accompany a headache of any type: sinus, muscle contraction, or vascular (migraine, cluster). Neurologic deficits are usually part of vascular-type headaches.

Any headache that recurs, is unpredictable with no discernable triggers, and is incapacitating or has neurologic sequelae presents a possible threat to flight safety. Allowable treatment for headaches may modify this statement. Military and civilian aeromedical authorities vary in the medications they consider safe to use while flying. With these concerns specified, the more common types of headaches may be considered.

Vascular headaches include migraine and cluster headaches. Migraines are more common in females after age 13. The new classification system divides migraines into seven distinct categories distinguished by: (a) presence and (b) type of aura, (c) any retinal or (d) ophthalmic symptoms, (e) childhood onset, (f) complicated by stroke, or (g) not otherwise specified. Separate from this category are specific vascular headaches distinguished by their triggers, such as exertional headaches or coital headaches. The importance of accurate characterization is that once the diagnosis is established, the question of acceptable and effective treatment needs to be addressed. When an identifiable trigger can be found (e.g., foods, specific maneuvers, such as anti-G straining, or specific activities, such as weight-lifting), headaches can be avoided by eliminating the trigger activity. Otherwise, medical control is required. This is divided into acute

and prophylactic treatment. Acute management includes ergot derivatives and similar vasoactive compounds or nonsteroidal anti-inflammatory agents that are taken at the earliest sign of aura or headache. Some of these compounds can cause sedation. Newer intramuscular preparations, such as dihydroergotamine (DHE), are used for acute management, but this would not be suitable for inflight use. Prophylactic treatment includes β-adrenergic blockers, calcium channel blockers, antihistamine and anti-serotonergics (Periactin®), tricyclic antidepressants, and anti-convulsants. Each type of medication has its own side effects, and the flyer should be monitored for these.

Cluster headaches predominate in males, with a peak about age 20–40. The quality of the pain is usually severe, hemicranial, and periodic. These headaches occur suddenly and can be accompanied by unilateral conjunctival injection and nasal lacrimation. Although medications used for both prophylaxis and acute treatment of migraines can be applied to cluster headaches, the results are not always as satisfactory. In addition, acute management with nasal 100% oxygen at 6 L/min is sometimes effective. Prophylaxis with lithium carbonate can also be tried.

Tension headaches are identified by the quality of the pain. The new classification divides tension-type headaches into episodic or chronic categories, both with or without muscle contraction components. The most important aeromedical factors are that tension headaches may involve nausea or photophobia, and can be incapacitating. The chronic type requires at least 15 days of headaches per month, for six months, for diagnosis.

This brief introduction stresses the importance of identifying the type of headache and any possible triggers through careful history-taking, which will guide diagnostic testing and aeromedical decision-making.

Head Injury

This chapter addresses only closed-head trauma. The risk of seizures and permanent disability after open-head trauma are well reviewed by Caveness et al. in their postwar follow-up studies (67, 68) and, in general, this risk removes aircrew members from future flying duties.

Aeromedically significant problems secondary to closed-head trauma can be divided into three categories: (a) permanent neurologic deficits, (b) risk of sudden incapacitation, and (c) postconcussive or posttraumatic syndrome.

The first category represents permanent deficits, such as loss of motor function, impaired cognitive function, or language dysfunction (aphasias). The second category includes those at risk for posttraumatic seizures. These can be divided into groups: impact (immediate), early, and late. Impact seizures occur at the instant of trauma and are not considered to be a risk factor for future seizures. Early posttraumatic seizures, which occur one to three weeks after injury, are considered a significant indication of possible future seizures. Late, posttraumatic seizures usually occur one to three months after head injury, but can occur several years later.

The aeromedical question is not whether early or late seizures will help predict a future seizure, because the risk at that point is already aeromedically significant. The unanswered question is how long should a seizure-free interval be after mild, moderate, or severe closed-head injury before the risk of posttraumatic seizures is acceptably low.

The classic work on posttraumatic seizures by Jennett (69) established guidelines for the definition of closed-head injury and its risk of seizures. Refinement of these guidelines was needed, especially in mild-to-moderate closed-head injury. In 1979, a panel discussing the neurological conditions associated with aviation safety addressed the problem, but did not develop specific guidelines from the then-known literature. They did state that "new seizure cases level off after one year, and beyond two to three years, new cases are rare but do occur (70)." They also addressed the role of EEG and stated "the EEG is firm diagnostic confirmation when it shows a paroxysmal abnormality that correlates with the attack

patterns. Less specific abnormalities are of no diagnostic aid." Deymeer and Leviton assessed the posttraumatic seizure literature up to 1985, and found only two reports with control groups (71); only one involved an adult population. Annegers et al. divided the severity of closed head injury into several categories (72): severe—brain contusion, intracerebral or intracranial hematoma, or longer than 24 hours of unconsciousness or posttraumatic amnesia; moderate—skull fracture or 30 minutes to 24 hours of unconsciousness or posttraumatic amnesia; and mild—< 30 minutes of unconsciousness or posttraumatic amnesia. These patients were followed and their relative risks for seizures reported at one and five years.

At one year, the mild head trauma group's risk of seizure was equal to that of the controls. The moderate group's risk was 0.6% at one year and 1.6% at five years. The severe group's risk was 7.1% and 13.3%, respectively. This work leaves some question as to the safest minimum length of observation required before returning to flying duties after moderate head injury, because of the two data points of one and five years. These are statistics based on a population that is not exposed to a high-stress environment, such as that of aviators, which includes chronic fatigue, circadian rhythm changes, intermittent hypoxic or hypobaric conditions, sleep-cycle alterations, or sleep deprivation. Similar studies using military patients would be more directly applicable. Because of this, more conservative guidelines may be needed.

Head trauma evaluation can be divided into acute, subacute, and follow-up periods. Acute management is well described in textbooks of neurology or emergency medicine. Subacute management requires careful observation during the first several days after head injury, watching for signs of a delayed subdural hematoma or intracerebral contusion (e.g., any focal neurologic deficit). Any suggestion of these complications requires an urgent CT. Follow-up is essential, to observe for possible symptoms of posttraumatic syndrome. This is a constellation of symptoms that includes poor concentration, increased irritability, headaches, vertigo, and behavioral changes that can follow mild-to-moderate head trauma. Careful contact with the injured aviator, as well as the family, and (when applicable) fellow crew members may be necessary to discover these problems.

The full spectrum of possible effects of mild head trauma on information processing is under increasing scrutiny. Neuropsychological tests may discover deficits in "asymptomatic" patients who may prove dangerous in the flying environment. In the future, cognitive evoked potential testing may help in developing an objective measure of the extent and effects of mild closed-head injury.

Syncope

Establishing the appropriate diagnosis in a flyer who lost consciousness demands a careful history, both from the involved individual and from any eye witnesses. Identification of any disorder that could be recurrent, such as seizures, has obvious implications for flight safety.

Benign forms of syncope are well documented, such as those triggered by such identifiable stimuli as venipuncture, emotional upset, micturition, or sudden pain. In general, these do not presage future loss of consciousness. However, when a pattern of recurrent syncope from a specific and unavoidable stressor is established, then this may become a risk to flight safety.

Evaluations become more involved when loss of consciousness is unexplainable. Special attention should be placed on reports given by trained medical personnel who arrive on the scene, and on the vital signs recorded close to the event. Initial blood chemistries may indicate disturbances, such as hypoglycemia, anemia, or dehydration. Blood pressure and heart rate may indicate the autonomic discharges often seen after seizures. Distinguishing between primary seizures, metabolic or withdrawal seizures, or convulsive syncope may be impossible without proper witnesses or appropriate tests performed soon after the event. When no identifiable event

or abnormal test is evident, then an evaluation for unexplained loss of consciousness is warranted. Even with complete evaluations, up to half of syncopal patients go undiagnosed (73). Remember that most published studies on syncope originate from ER or inpatient hospital studies, and that such patient populations reflect a cross-section of age and general health different from the flying population.

The extent of the workup necessary for syncope is debated (74).

An initial history, physical examination, blood chemistries (including glucose and electrolytes), and ECG are the usual first steps. The history should inquire about syncopal triggers, such as pain, anxiety, micturition, or orthostatic symptoms. A checklist of historical questions, signs, and symptoms may be found in Table 18.3. The type of tests and extent of testing are guided by the initial history, examination, and findings.

A cardiac examination usually includes Holter monitoring for 24–48 hours, or a Memory Trace Ambulatory ECG Recorder. The latter allows monitoring without leads or connecting wires. It is placed over the precordium during an event or recurrence of symptoms. The recording is played back to a monitoring facility by telephone. When indicated by symptoms, further cardiac evaluation may include an echocardiogram, treadmill stress tests, or electrophysiologic studies.

When the history suggests a possible seizure in the differential diagnosis, an EEG in both the awake and sleep-deprived states should be obtained. It is important to emphasize that the EEG can be normal in an individual who has a seizure disorder. A 24-hour ambulatory EEG is useful in evaluation of seizures.

Neuroimaging, by either CT or MRI, is indicated when seizures are a consideration, or when syncope is associated with a sudden, severe headache. In the latter case, a lumbar puncture is also indicated if neuroimaging were normal, in order to rule out subarachnoid hemorrhage.

In summary, the literature suggests that the

Table 18.3.
Suggested Worksheet for Syncope in Aviators

History from Patient	
Within One Week	Within Minutes of Event
Cold symptoms	Injection
Family with cold/flu	Micturating
symptoms	High G stress
Excessive alcohol intake	Bowel movement
Dieting with weight loss	Valsalva maneuver
GI symptoms	Threatened
Flu symptoms	Emotional shock
Depression	Running
Insomnia	Change to vertical position
Over-the-counter	Exercise
medications	Coughing
Sleep deprived	Vaccination
Recent travel	Hyperventilating
Emotional event (death/	Blood drawn
divorce)	Questioning
Party with alcohol	Sitting

Prodrome	
Lightheadedness	Tiredness
Tinnitus	Nausea and/or vomiting
Olfactory aura	Sweating
Seeing stars	Feeling ill
Vertigo	Visual aura
Hot flashes	Headache
Hearing loss	Other

Vital Statistics	
Age ___ Sex ___ Pulses ___	Regular/Irregular BP ___/___

History from Witnesses	
Position at time of	Horizontal
syncope:	Vertical
	Inclined
Time unconsciousness	
Time till coherent:	
Atypical findings:	Head injury
	Tonic-clonic movements
	Urinary incontinence
	Tongue biting

majority of syncopal patients are either the result of vasodepressor episodes, or go undiagnosed. The extent of the investigations performed is guided by the history and physical examination, initial laboratory results, and the necessity of establishing an absolute diagnosis. In aerospace medicine, where the latter is important, one can see that laboratory results do not always provide the answers. Many judgments are made on his-

torical data alone. Long-term, prospective follow-up studies with consistent histories and evaluations are needed to differentiate benign from potentially hazardous forms of syncope.

NEUROCHEMISTRY OF JET LAG

Jet lag is a syndrome of general malaise frequently experienced after transmeridian jet travel across multiple time zones. The syndrome is characterized by disruption of sleep, increased fatigue, decreased attention and vigilance, and certain gastrointestinal disturbances (75). The severity and duration of symptoms vary substantially among individuals and increase with the transmeridian distance traveled. Eastward flights usually require a longer period of adjustment than westward flights of comparable distance. Although the psychophysical manifestations of jet lag amount to little more than temporary discomfort for most holiday travelers, the impaired performance associated with the syndrome could limit the effectiveness of military operations involving rapid transmeridian deployment of forces.

The phenomenon of jet lag occurs as a result of the abrupt phase-shift of the environmental light-dark (LD) cycle relative to that of the brain's endogenous circadian clock. This clock, which is located in the suprachiasmatic nuclei (SCN) of the hypothalmus, is responsible for the generation and synchronization of many circadian physiologic and behavioral rhythms, including the sleep-wake cycle. Normally, our circadian rhythms are entrained to (synchronized with) the environmental LD cycle. Entrainment occurs as a result of the interaction of light with the retina. The entraining photic information is conveyed to the SCN via a direct pathway, the retinohypothalamic tract. After rapid relocation to a new time zone, reentrainment of clock-driven rhythms occurs slowly. For example, after a six-hour eastward flight, as many as 10 days may be required before the body's physiologic rhythms achieve synchrony with the new LD cycle (76). During this period, the physiologic processes synchronized by the clock, including sleep, body temperature, hormone secretion, and gastrointestinal activity, are no longer coordinated. It is this state of "internal desynchronization" that is responsible for the sense of malaise that characterizes jet lag.

Recently, several strategies aimed at alleviating the effects of jet lag have been explored. Most of these approaches attempt to exploit potentially entraining natural and pharmacologic cues to cause rapid reentrainment of the circadian clock.

Bright light

As discussed above, light is the most effective environmental influence (Zeitgeber) capable of entraining human circadian rhythms. Under certain conditions, exposure to bright (> 2500 lux) light can "reset" the human circadian clock (77). Both phase advances (setting forward) and phase delays (setting back) of the circadian clock are possible (78). Wever reported that circadian rhythms of patients re-entrained more rapidly after a six-hour phase delay when the light intensity was increased from 300 to 3000 lux (79). This finding is consistent with other reports (76, 77), indicating that the subjective effects of jet lag are reduced when patients were encouraged to spend more time in the bright sunlight after arrival. These observations led Daan and Lewy to propose that programmed bright-light exposure may be used to reset the clock in advance of transmeridian travel, as well as to increase the rate of reentrainment after arrival (80). Despite some degree of success (79, 80), this approach has received little attention from the military aerospace community. However, programmed bright-light exposure facilities may soon become available on commercial intercontinental flights.

Melatonin

Melatonin is an indoleamine hormone that is produced in the pineal gland and, to a lesser extent, in the retina. In mammals, the production and release of melatonin by the pineal is regulated by the SCN circadian clock. Melatonin levels in blood begin to rise at twilight and decrease abruptly at the first light of dawn. Thus, the period of time that melatonin levels are elevated in the blood represents the length of the night. As the days grow shorter, the length of the melatonin peak increases, signaling the approach of winter and initiating the physiologic and behavioral adjustments necessary to ensure the survival of seasonal mammals as environmental conditions change.

Although the role of pineal melatonin in seasonal species is well established, the function of the hormone in humans remains unknown. Recent observations suggest that melatonin may play a role in the etiology of a relatively common form of mild depression called seasonal affective disorder (SAD), also known as winter depression (81). Large doses of melatonin have been reported to cause sedation, further suggesting that the hormone may be active in the human SCN.

Melatonin receptors have been detected in the SCN of rodents and humans, suggesting that the indoleamine may participate in feedback regulation of the human circadian timing system (82, 83). In support of this proposal, Redman et al. (84) and Cassone et al. (85) reported that daily melatonin injections are capable of entraining the free-running activity rhythm in rats. Further, exogenous melatonin increases the rate of reentrainment of circadian rhythms in the rat after phase shifts (86) or inversion of the LD cycle (87).

In light of these observations, it seemed reasonable to evaluate the usefulness of melatonin and related indoleamines in the treatment of circadian desynchrony associated with jet lag. Arendt et al. were the first to report the results of a controlled study of the effects of programmed melatonin administration on the subjective effects of jet lag (88, 89). Melatonin was effective in reducing both the severity and duration of jet lag symptoms when administered for two days prior to departure through seven days after arrival of a westward flight across nine time zones. Petrie et al. reported similar results (90).

Although melatonin appears to offer great potential as a treatment for jet lag in humans, more work is needed to perfect the treatment regimen and to characterize possible side effects of the drug. It is likely that the sedative effects of melatonin, as well as the possibility of melatonin-induced depression in sensitive individuals, will limit the usefulness of this compound in treating jet lag. Synthetic analogs of melatonin with selective effects on the circadian timing system are currently under development (91). Ultimately, the use of melatonin-related compounds in combination with an appropriate bright-light exposure regimen may provide the most effective treatment for human jet lag.

Benzodiazepines

The use of short-acting benzodiazepines, such as triazolam, to treat jet lag has recently been proposed (92). Benzodiazepines have been reported to induce phase alterations of the free-running activity rhythm in hamsters (93), and to increase the rate of reentrainment of the activity rhythm after an abrupt phase shift of the light-dark cycle. However, at least some of the effects of these compounds on the rodent circadian timing system appear to be indirect, and dependent upon an acute effect of the drugs on locomotor activity. At present, no study of the effects of short-acting benzodiazepines on the jet lag syndrome has been reported.

REFERENCES

1. Beaven CL. A chronological history of aviation medicine. The School of Aviation Medicine. Randolph Air Force Base, Texas, 1939.
2. Anderson HG. The medical and surgical aspects of aviation. London: Oxford University Press, 1919.
3. Christy RL. Personality factors in selection of flight proficiency. Aviat Space Environ Med 1975;46:309–311.
4. Fine PM, Hartman BO. Psychiatric strengths and weaknesses of typical air force pilots. SAM Technical Report 68–121. United States Air Force School of Aerospace Medicine, Brooks Air Force Base, Texas, 1968; 131–168.
5. Jennings CL. The use of normative data in the psychological evaluation of flying personnel. In: Perry CJG, ed. Psychiatry in aerospace medicine, vol. 4. International Psychiatry Clinics. Boston: Little, Brown and Co., 1967; 37–52.
6. Reinhart RF. The outstanding jet pilot. Am J Psychiatry 1970;127:732–735.
7. Bond DD. The love and fear of flying. New York: International Universities Press, Inc., 1952.
8. Grinker RR, Spiegel JA. Men under stress. Philadelphia: Blakiston, 1945.
9. Sledge WH. Aerospace psychiatry. In: Kaplan HI, Freedman AM, Sadock BJ, eds. Comprehensive textbook of psychiatry, 3rd ed. Baltimore: Williams & Wilkins Co., 1980; 2902–2914.
10. American Psychiatric Association. Diagnostic and statistical manual of mental disorders. 4th ed. Washington DC: American Psychiatric Association, 1994.
11. Leon RL. Psychiatric interviewing: a primer, 2nd ed. New York: Elsevier/Science Publishing, 1989.
12. McKinnon RA, Michels R. The psychiatric interview in clinical practice. Philadelphia: W.B. Saunders Co., 1971.
13. Mills JG, Jones DR. The adaptability rating for military aeronautics: an historical perspective of a continuing problem. Aviat Space Environ Med 1984;55:558–562.
14. Rafferty JA, Deemer WI Jr. Statistical evaluation of the experimental adaptability rating for military aeronautics (ARMA) of World War II. United States Air Force School of Aviation Medicine, Randolph Air Force Base, Texas. Project No. 21–02–097, Report No. 1, Aug. 1948, and Report No. 2 (Factor Analysis), Aug 1949.
15. Henman VAC. Air service tests of aptitude for flying. J Appl Physiol 1919;3:103–109.
16. Banich MT, Stokes A, Elledge VC. Neuropsychological screening of aviators: a review. Aviat Space Environ Med 1989;60:361–366.
17. Reitan RM, Wolfson D. The Halsted-Reitan neuropsychological test battery, theory and clinical interpretation. Tucson: Neuropsychology Press, 1985.
18. Senechal PK, Traweek AC. The aviation psychology program at RAF Upper Hayford. Aviat Space Environ Med 1988;59:973–975.
19. Orlady HW, Foushee HC, eds. Proceedings of a NASA/MAC workshop: cockpit resource management training. Washington DC: NASA Conf. Pub. 2455, 1986.
20. Kanki BG, Foushee HC. Communication as a group process mediator of aircraft performance. Aviat Space Environ Med 1989;60:402–10.
21. Perry CJG. Psychiatric support for man in space. In: Perry CJG, ed. Psychiatry in aerospace medicine, vol 4. International psychiatry clinics. Boston, Little, Brown and Co., 1967; 197–222.
22. Marsh RW, Perry CJG. Anniversary reactions in military aviators. Aviat Space Environ Med 1977;48:61–64.
23. Pursch JA. Alcohol in aviation: a problem of attitudes. Aerospace Med 1974;45:318–321.
24. Sledge WH, Boydstun JA. Vasovagal syncope in aircrew: psychosocial aspects. J Nerv Ment Dis 1979;167:114–124.

25. Jones DR, Levy RL, Gardner L, Marsh RW, Patterson JC. Self-control of psychophysiologic response to motion stress: using biofeedback to treat airsickness. Aviat Space Environ Med 1985;56:1152–7.

26. Giles DA, Lochridge GK. Behavioral airsickness management program for student pilots. Aviat Space Environ Med 1985;56:991–4.

27. Cowings PS, Billingham J, Toscano WB. Learned control of multiple autonomic responses to compensate for the debilitating effects of motion sickness. Ther Psychomatic Med 1977;4:318–323.

28. Forgione AG, Bauer FM. Fearless flying. Boston: Houghton Mifflin Co., 1980.

29. Kantor JS, Zitrin CM, Zeldis SM. Mitral valve prolapse syndrome in agotaphobic patients. Am J Psychiatry 1980;137:467–469.

30. McDowell CP. Suicide among active duty USAF members: 1980–1989. Washington: HQ USAF OBI, April 1990.

31. Green RG. Stress and accidents. Aviat Space Environ Med 1985;56:638–41.

32. Shneidman E. Definition of suicide. New York: Wiley, 1985.

33. Gibbons HL, Plechus JL, Mohler SR. Consideration of volitional acts in aircraft accident investigation. Aerosp Med 1967;38:1057–1059.

34. Jones DR. Suicide by aircraft. Aviat Space Environ Med 1977;48:454–9.

35. Jacobson C. Progressive relaxation. Chicago: University of Chicago Press, 1938.

36. Wolpe J. The practice of behavior therapy, 2nd ed. New York: Pergamon Press, Inc., 1973.

37. Raschmann J, Patterson JC, Schofield G. A retrospective study of marital discord in pilots: the USAFSAM experience. Aviat Space Environ Med 1990;61:1145–8.

38. Jones DR. Flying and danger, joy and fear. Aviat Space Environ Med 1986;57:131–6.

39. Karlins M, Koh F, McCully L. The spousal factor in pilot stress. Aviat Space Environ Med 1989;60:1112–5.

40. Taylor JWR, Munson K, eds. History of aviation. New York: Crown Publishers, 1978.

41. Josephy AM, ed. The American heritage history of flight. New York: American Heritage Publishing Company, 1962.

42. Jones DR. Psychiatric assessment of female fliers at the U.S. Air Force School of Aerospace Medicine (USAFSAM). Aviat Space Environ Med 1983;54:929–31.

43. Girodo M. The psychological health and stress of pilots in a labor dispute. Aviat Space Environ Med 1988;59:505–10.

44. Little LF, Gaffney IC, Rosen KH, Bender MM. Corporate instability is related to airline pilots' stress symptoms. Aviat Space Environ Med 1990;61:977–82.

45. Bartone PT, Ursano RJ, Wright KM, Ingraham LH. The impact of a military air disaster on the health of assistance workers. J Nerv Ment Dis 1989;177:317–28.

46. Taylor AJW. A taxonomy of disasters and their victims. J Psychosom Res 1987;31:535–44.

47. Slagle DA, Reichman M, Rodenhauser P, Knoedler D,

48. Davis CL. Community psychological effects following a non-fatal aircraft accident. Aviat Space Environ Med 1990;61:879–86.

48. Miles SM, Demi AS, Mostyn-Aker P. Rescue workers' reactions following the Hyatt hotel disaster. Death Educ 1984;8:315–31.

49. Taylor AJW, Frazer AG. The stress of post-disaster body handling and victim identification work. J Human Stress 1982;8:4–12.

50. Hartsough DM, Meyers DG. Disaster, work, and mental health: prevention and control of stress on workers. Rockville: NIMH, 1985.

51. Mitchell JT. When disaster strikes: the critical incident stress debriefing process. J Emerg Med Svcs 1983;8:36–9.

52. Gann EK. Fate is the hunter. New York: Simon and Schuster, 1961; 265–271.

53. Haslam DR. The military performance of soldiers in sustained operations. Aviat Space Environ Med 1984;55:216–21.

54. Jones DR. U.S. Air Force combat psychiatry. Brooks AFB, TX, USAFSAM Technical Report TR-85–83, January 1986.

55. Levin HS, Norcross K, Amparo EG, Guinto FC Jr. Neurobehavioral and magnetic resonance imaging findings in two cases of decompression sickness. Aviat Space Environ Med 1989;60:1204.

56. Vaernes RJ, Hammerberg D. Evoked potentials and other CNS reactions during a heliox dive to 360 MSW. Aviat Space Environ Med 1989;60:550–557.

57. Grant I, et al. Evidence for early central nervous system involvement in the acquired immunodeficiency syndrome (AIDS) and other human immunodeficiency virus (HIV) infections. Ann Intern Med 1987;107:828.

58. Miller EN, et al. Neuropsychological performance in H.I.V. infected homosexual men: the multicenter AIDS cohort study (MACS). Neurology 1990;40:197.

59. DeHart RM. Air Force HIV policy. Aviat Space Environ Med 1988;59:685.

60. Clark JB. Policy considerations of human immunodeficiency virus (HIV) infections in U.S. Navy Aviation personnel. Aviat Space Environ Med 1990;61:165.

61. Merren MD, Letourneau DJ. Experience with electroencephalography in student naval personnel, 1961–1971: a preliminary report. Aerosp Med 1973;44:1302.

62. Richter P, et al. Electroencephalograms of 2, 947 United States Air Force Academy cadets. Aerosp Med 1971;42:1011.

63. Van denNoart S, et al. Assessment. EEG brain mapping. Neurology 1989;39:1100.

64. Poser CM, et al. New diagnostic criteria for multiple sclerosis: guidelines for research protocols. Ann Neurol 1983;13:277.

65. Miller DH, et al. Serial gadolinium enhanced magnetic resonance imaging in multiple sclerosis. Brain 1988;111:927.

66. Oleson J, et al. Classification and diagnostic criteria for headache disorders, cranial neuralgia and facial pain. Cephalgia 1988;8:1.

67. Caveness WF, et al. Incidence of post traumatic epilepsy in Korean veterans as compared with those from World War I and World War II. J Neurosurg 1962;19:122.

68. Caveness WF, et al. The nature of post traumatic epilepsy. J Neurosurg 1979;50:545.

69. Jennett B. Epilepsy after non-missile head injuries, 2nd ed. London: Heinemann Medical Books, 1975.

70. Doege TC. Neurological and neurosurgical conditions associated with aviation safety. Arch Neurol 1979;36:1.

71. Daymeer F, Leviton A. Post traumatic seizures: an assessment of the epidemiologic literature. Cent Nerv Syst Trauma 1985;2:33.

72. Annegers JF, Hauser WA, Kurland LT. Seizures after head trauma: a population study. Neurology 1980;30:683–689.

73. Kappor WN, et al. A prospective evaluation and followup of patients with syncope. N Engl J Med 1983;309:197.

74. Mozes B, Confino-Cohen R, Walkin H. Cost-effectiveness of in-hospital evaluation of patients with syncope. Israel J Med Sci 1988;24:302.

75. Moore-Ede MC. Jet lag, shift work, and maladaptation. News Physiol Sci 1986;1:156–160.

76. Klein KE, Wegmann HM. The resynchronization of human circadian rhythms after transmeridian flights as a result of direction and mode of activity. In: Scheving LE, Halberg F, Pauly JE, eds. Chronobiology. Tokyo: Igaju 1974; 564–570.

77. Czeisler CA, Allan JS, Strogatz SH, Ronda JM, Sanchez R, Rios CD, Freitag WO, Richardson GS, Kronauer RE. Bright light resets the human circadian pacemaker independent of the timing of the sleep-wake cycle. Science 1986;233:667–671.

78. DeCoursey PJ. Daily light sensitivity in a rodent. Science 1960;131:33–35.

79. Wever RA. Use of light to treat jet lag: differential effects of normal and bright artificial light on human circadian rhythms. Ann NY Acad Sci 1985;453:282–304.

80. Daan S, Lewy AJ. Scheduled exposure to daylight: a strategy to reduce ''jet lag'' following transmeridian flight. Psychopharmacol Bull 1984;20:566–568.

81. Lewy AJ, Sack RL, Singer CM. Melatonin, light and chronobiological disorders. In: Everad D, Clark S, eds. Photoperiodism, melatonin and the pineal. London: Pitman, 1985; 231–252.

82. Duncan MJ, Takahashi JS, Dubocovich ML. 2 (125I)-Iodomelatonin binding sites in hamster brain membranes: pharmacological characteristics and regional distribution. Endocrinology 1988;122:1825–1833.

83. Reppert SM, Weaver DW, Rivkees SA, Stopa EG. Putative melatonin receptors in a human biological clock. Science 1988;242:78–81.

84. Redman JR, Armstrong SM, Ng KT. Free-running rhythms in the rat: entrainment by melatonin. Science 1983;219:1089–1091.

85. Cassone VM, Chesworth MJ, Armstrong SM. Dose-dependent entrainment of rat circadian rhythms by daily injection of melatonin. J Biol Rhythms 1986;1:219–229.

86. Armstrong SM, Cassone VM, Chesworth MJ, Redman JR, Short RV. Synchronization of mammalian circadian rhythms by melatonin. In: Wurtman RJ, Waldhauser FJ, eds. Melatonin in humans: proceedings of the First International Conference on Melatonin in Humans. Neural Tranmission 1986;21(Suppl):375–396.

87. Murakami N, Hayafuji C, Sasaki Y, Yamazuki JM, Takahashi K. Melatonin accelerates the reentrainment of the circadian adrenocortical rhythm in inverted illumination cycle. Neuroendocrinology 1983;36:385–391.

88. Arendt J, Aldhous M, Marks V. Alleviation to jet lag by melatonin: preliminary results of a controlled double blind trial. BMJ 1986;292:1170.

89. Arendt J, Aldhous M, English J, Marks V, Arendt JH. Some effects of jet-lag and their alleviation by melatonin. Ergonomics 1987;30:1379–1393.

90. Petrie K, Conaglen JV, Thompson L, Chamberlain K. Effect of melatonin on jet lag after long haul flights. BMJ 1989;298:705–707.

91. Dubocovich ML. Luzindole (N-0774): a novel melatonin antagonist. 1988;246:902–910.

92. Turek FW, van Reeth O. Altering the mammalian circadian clock with short-acting benzodiazepine, triazolam. Trends Neurosci 1989; 11:535–541.

93. Turek FW, Losee-Olsen S. A benzodiazepine used in the treatment of insomnia phase-shifts of the mammalian circadian clock. Nature 1986;321:167–168.

Chapter 19

Additional Medical and Surgical Conditions of Aeromedical Concern

Royce Moser, Jr

The secret of the care of the patient is in caring for the patient.

Francis W. Peabody, M.D.

The physician evaluating individuals with the conditions discussed in this chapter needs to apply the same basic criteria for qualification for flying duties which were used for the conditions considered in other chapters in this text. In essence, these criteria are that there be no hazard to an individual's health, to flying safety, or to mission completion when that person participates in flight activities. All three considerations are of concern for military and commercial crews and passengers, but the first two are of primary interest in general aviation.

In determining whether these criteria are met, the practitioner has to consider both the significance of the underlying condition and the effects of any required medication or other treatment. Tragedies have occurred when flight surgeons concentrated on only one of these two factors. For example, a practitioner caring for a pilot was primarily concerned about possible side effects of a prescribed medication and did not fully consider compromises due to the medical problem itself. Because the medication produced no demonstrable side effects and was, therefore, believed to be "safe" for the flyer, the physician qualified the pilot to fly. Although the medication did not produce any problems, it only partly alleviated the symptoms. The pilot was distracted by the residual symptoms during a critical phase of flight and a fatal crash resulted. Of course, the physician caring for flyers must also determine whether a medication may produce a hazard if the patient were qualified for flight while taking the drug. Allowing a person to fly with a minor problem that is not expected to cause difficulties, while prescribing medication with side effects, such as drowsiness or similar unacceptable sequelae, can obviously set the stage for disaster. The following discussion of some of the more typical conditions aerospace medicine practitioners will evaluate illustrates applications of these criteria and principles. The discussion cannot, of course, be all-inclusive, but it should assist the practitioner in managing patients with other medical and surgical conditions of aeromedical significance.

HEMATOLOGIC CONSIDERATIONS

Oxygen Transport

As was discussed more extensively in Chapter 5, oxygen is carried in the blood in physical solution and in combination with hemoglobin. The amount of oxygen in solution depends on Henry's Law. At 38°C and an arterial oxygen pressure of 102 mm Hg, each 100 ml of blood carries 0.306 ml of dissolved oxygen. Of far more significance is the amount of oxygen carried by hemoglobin. Each gram of normal hemoglobin combines with 1.34 ml of oxygen. Thus, when a person has 15 g/dL of hemoglobin, each 100 ml of blood theoretically could carry 20 ml of oxygen (1.34 × 15) through the hemoglobin mechanism. Due to the admixture of fully saturated blood coming from the lungs with undersaturated blood which passed through anatomic or physiologic dead spaces in the lungs, arterial blood is approximately 97% saturated. As a result, the amount of oxygen carried by 15 g of hemoglobin is closer to 19 ml/100 ml of blood.

At the tissue level, 5–6 ml/dL of oxygen are consumed at rest. The returning venous blood is approximately 75% saturated with oxygen, and the venous P_{O_2} is 40 mm Hg. Because of the shape of the oxygen dissociation curve, even slight reductions in the P_{O_2} at the tissue level results in the release of significant additional oxygen; therefore, a reserve does exist to meet additional demands for oxygen.

Due to its significance in oxygen transport, any reduction in the effective hemoglobin concentration of either a crew member or passenger is of aeromedical concern. This reduction may, of course, be due to actual blood loss, as in the case of acute or chronic hemorrhage. Reduction also may effectively occur when available hemoglobin, even when present in ''normal'' concentrations, is not able to carry the usual amount of oxygen. Carbon monoxide exposure is one such situation. Because of the greater affinity of carbon monoxide for the hemoglobin molecule, small amounts of inhaled carbon monoxide can prevent the normal transport of oxygen in an individual with a normal hemoglobin concentration who is inspiring air with a normal P_{O_2}. In other instances, a hemoglobin abnormality may prevent the red blood cells from carrying a normal amount of oxygen. Again, an effective anemia exists even though the hemoglobin concentration may be within normal limits.

Aeromedical Concerns in the Anemic Patient

Whatever the cause, a reduction in effective hemoglobin concentration can significantly affect the amount of oxygen available for tissue metabolism. When, for example, hemoglobin is reduced to approximately half the normal value at 7 mg/dL, only 9.4 ml/dL of oxygen is carried by hemoglobin if the blood were fully saturated. Even if tissue P_{O_2} level decreases to 30 mm Hg, only 40%, or approximately 3.8 ml/dL of oxygen, is released to the tissues. If the body's oxygen requirement were to remain constant, cardiac output would have to increase, in accordance with the Fick principle, to meet the body's oxygen demand. Although such compensatory mechanisms can offset significant hemoglobin reductions, the reserve remaining to compensate for any additional demands is reduced. With exercise or heavy physical work, the oxygen requirement may increase twentyfold. In an individual who is compromised by anemia, sufficient additional compensatory reserves may not be present, and the exertion may precipitate abrupt onset of symptoms. If inspired P_{O_2} were reduced at the same time exertion requirements were to occur, the situation could rapidly become critical. Obviously, just such a situation could occur in an anemic crew member during rapid decompression.

Because of the importance of compensatory mechanisms, the aerospace medicine practitioner evaluating an anemic patient who is contemplating a commercial flight must determine whether pathologic processes are affecting those compensatory capabilities. It also should be noted that patients with chronic anemias are more likely to have adjusted to reduced hemoglobin than are patients with acute anemias with similar hemoglobin levels. In general, an individual who is asymptomatic during mild exertion at ground level, such as climbing one flight of stairs, does not experience symptoms during a routine flight in a commercial aircraft (1). If the passenger's compensatory capabilities were significantly compromised, however, the relatively slight reductions in P_{O_2} that occur in commercial flights could produce symptoms.

In developing recommendations for an anemic traveler, the physician should consider both the duration of exposure and the cabin altitude. Prolonged exposure to reduced P_{O_2} increases the probability that the anemic patient, who is marginally compensated, will develop symptoms. Should the anemic patient smoke cigarettes during a flight, the oxygen-carrying capacity of hemoglobin may be reduced by as much as 15% due to the inhaled carbon monoxide (2). The practitioner also must note that the provision of supplemental oxygen in flight to prevent or control symptoms may be progressively more difficult the longer the flight. Unless additional arrangements are made prior to the flight, many airlines can provide only a limited supply of oxygen. This supply may not be sufficient for continuous use during a long flight. In advising the patient or flight attendants whether and when to use supplemental oxygen, the physician should emphasize that cyanosis may not be a reliable indication of significant hypoxia in an anemic patient. Approximately 6 g/dL of hemoglobin must be deoxygenated for cyanosis to be manifest. In some anemic patients, it may not be possible to recognize cyanosis because all oxygen cannot be removed from hemoglobin, even though the tissues may be hypoxic. As a result, several grams of hemoglobin per deciliter remain oxygenated, and sufficient deoxygenated hemoglobin may not be present to produce cyanosis.

Sickle Cell Disease and Trait

Naturally, the physician providing a recommendation concerning flying also is concerned with determining the cause of the anemia. Ascertaining the cause is essential to providing proper therapy and making an informed recommendation regarding flying. In one particular hemoglobinopathy, sickle hemoglobin (Hb-S), the differential diagnosis is of particular concern to the flight surgeon because exposure to reduced P_{O_2} can directly affect the ability of the red blood cells to carry oxygen. Sickle hemoglobin is due to alterations of β polypeptide chains of the hemoglobin molecule. Individuals with hemoglo-

bin mixtures SS, SC, S-thal, SD, and SF have sickle cell disease. Those heterozygous people who have Hb-S and a normal hemoglobin (A, A_2) have the sickle cell trait. In sickle cell disease, the patient demonstrates hemolytic anemia and, particularly during intercurrent infections, may experience hemolytic crises and tissue infarctions. When the blood P_{O_2} of patients with sickle cell disease decreases to below approximately 60 mm Hg, erythrocytes become deformed in a rigid, sickle shape. The loss in elasticity prevents these cells from passing through some blood vessels, producing an effective increase in viscosity. As the viscosity increases, the blood flow is reduced further, increased hypoxia results, and more cells sickle. This vicious circle produces more blood vessel blockage and tissue infarction and crises (3).

Because the alveolar P_{O_2} at 3048 m (10,000 ft) is approximately 60 mm Hg, and the tissue level would be below this level at even lower altitudes, some physicians do not recommend passenger flight for patients with sickle cell disease unless oxygen is readily available. Because of the risk of a hemolytic crisis on altitude exposure, individuals with sickle cell disease should not be qualified for crew member duties.

In contrast to sickle cell disease, the individual with the sickle cell trait may be asymptomatic. Overall life expectancy is the same as that for Hb-AA individuals, and Hb-AS erythrocytes do not sickle until the oxygen tension is much lower than that required for Hb-SS erythrocytes. Although a recommendation regarding flying can be made with some assurance for patients with sickle cell disease, the situation is much more complicated for a patient with sickle cell trait. Hemolytic crises and even sudden death have been reported in individuals with the sickle cell trait who were exposed to relatively low altitudes (4,5). Investigators often reported the onset of symptoms after a period of exertion at altitude. Many of these reports, however, are anecdotal in nature and not all included hemoglobin electrophoretic studies to confirm the presence of Hb-S. In some patients, other hemoglobin abnormalities were present as well as Hb-S. Although some investigators recommended that no individual with the sickle cell trait fly, a national study group noted that such individuals should not be restricted from flight duties unless they were a pilot or copilot (6).

A number of countries accept individuals with the sickle cell trait for both commercial and military flight duties. Until 1981, the United States military restricted people with the sickle cell trait from flight training, service as an aircrew member, or attendance at the Air Force Academy in Colorado Springs, CO. The latter restriction was because the facility is located at over 1524 m (5000 ft), and symptoms had been reported after exertion at field training sites at comparable altitudes (4,5). In 1981, this policy was changed, and individuals with the sickle cell trait can now be qualified to attend the Air Force Academy. In addition, candidates with the sickle cell trait can be accepted for flight training according to standards established by the services. Simultaneously, a program was developed for the medical monitoring of Air Force individuals with the sickle cell trait in an effort to provide a definitive answer concerning any possible complications caused by altitude exposure. Monitoring has not revealed any in-flight or altitude chamber incidents in Air Force flyers with sickle cell trait (7). However, considerable controversy continues regarding the significance of the risk from altitude exposure, and some argue against individuals with sickle cell trait performing crew member duties (8,9,10).

GASTROINTESTINAL DISORDERS

Gastroenteritis

Gastroenteritis is a frequent problem of both crews and passengers. It has been cited as a leading cause of inflight incapacitation in aircrew (11). Fortunately, the incapacitation is usually not so abrupt that the crew member cannot either pass the controls to another crew member or land before symptoms reach their peak. Prevention is of paramount importance, and both crews and passengers will benefit by considering and applying the basic principles of sanitation. One of the most common afflictions of travelers is the so-called "travelers' diarrhea." The consumption of raw vegetables in salads, undercooked meat or fish, or shellfish is associated with particularly high attack rates of this malady. Although a variety of agents have been implicated in this condition, strains of enterotoxigenic Escherichia coli are a leading cause (12). Other organisms often implicated include Giardia lamblia, Campylobacter jejuni, Salmonella species, and some viruses. Less frequently, more virulent pathogens, such as Entamoeba histolytic or Shigella species, are the causative agents. Agents used in treatment of travelers' diarrhea include bismuth subsalicylate (Pepto Bismol®), loperamide, diphenoxylate, trimethoprim-sulfamethoxazole, doxycycline, and ciprofloxarin (12). Antimotility agents should not be used when the patient has a high fever or blood in the stool. Their use may prolong the duration of some episodes and increase the risk of complications. Trimethoprim-sulfamethoxazole, trimethoprim alone, doxycycline, and bismuth subsalicylate have been shown to be effective in preventing travelers' diarrhea (12). Some question the use of these agents as prophylaxis, however, because their use may change the intestinal flora and increase susceptibility to more serious invasive enteric pathogens or produce undesirable side effects. Such considerations underscore the necessity for proper hygiene as the first line of defense against the onset of travelers' diarrhea.

In evaluating a patient with diarrhea symptoms, it is imperative that the practitioner obtain an adequate history, including travel and diet history. It is, of course, possible to return from another country to the residence country during the incubation period of a serious gastroenteritis infection. For example, one patient examined in consultation developed diarrhea several days after his return from the Far East. He was treated symptomatically through two recurrences over a four-week period by a practitioner who neglected to obtain a history of either the recent travel or the fact that the patient had consumed fresh salads and seafood when in another country. While being treated with diphenoxylate hydrochloride, the patient collapsed and became semicomatose. He responded to intensive life-support measures, and subsequent evaluation disclosed systemic Entamoeba histolytic infection, with three separate liver abscesses. After prolonged therapy, the patient eventually resumed normal activities. The development of the serious complications, however, could perhaps have been prevented by early recognition of the fact that the patient was at increased risk as a result of his recent sojourn in other countries.

Peptic Ulcer

Peptic ulcer disease is seen frequently by the aeromedical practitioner. Crew members who respond to treatment can be considered for return to flying duty. In considering return to flying recommendations, the practitioner must ensure that the patient is aware of both the possibility and manifestations of recurrence and complications. The possibility of gastrointestinal hemorrhage due to ulcer disease is of particular aeromedical concern. Hemorrhage may present, of course, as the initial manifestation of disease in up to 25% of patients. It also may pose a hazard to the flyer who has been treated for ulcer disease with a previous bleeding episode because of the significant risk of a recurrent bleeding episode. In addition to the fact that serious bleeding may occur without warning symptoms, the chance of incapacitation is increased in a flyer who works in even the slightly hypoxic environment of commercial flight. If the flyer were required to perform stressful duties or were exposed to low ambient Po_2 during an emergency, the chances of incapacitation would be further increased. Changes in stool color, weakness, palpitations, or any other symptoms suggesting a bleeding episode should prompt the patient with a history of ulcer disease to seek immediate attention from the flight surgeon if the counseling

and education efforts of the aeromedical practitioner were effective.

It has become clear that peptic ulcer disease most commonly reflects infection with Helicobacter pylori or use of aspirin or other nonsteroidal anti-inflammatory agents. As cure of H. pylori infection decreases recurrence rates and facilitates healing, antibiotic therapy is indicated for all such ulcer patients. To date, no optimal simple antibiotic regimen has yet emerged. Treatment with Proton pump inhibitors (PPIs) is the most effective means of healing peptic ulcers. In addition to healing a higher proportion of ulcer than H_2-receptor antagonist, PPIs provide faster healing and relief of symptoms. Eradication of H. Pylori infection is more effective than maintenance therapy with an antisecretory agent in reducing the rate of recurrence of peptic ulcers initially healed using antisecretory therapy. For routine clinical practice, the highly sensitive and specific rapid urease test remains the most useful diagnostic approach. Once diagnosed, a 1–2 week treatment with the combination of PPI and two anti-microbial agents achieves eradication of the peptic ulcer with a response rate in excess of 90% (13,14).

Gastrointestinal Hemorrhage

Gastrointestinal hemorrhage in a flyer poses a challenging problem for the aerospace medicine physician. In addition to managing the acute problem, the practitioner must make every effort to determine the site of bleeding. Endoscopic examination during the bleeding episode has been particularly valuable in making this determination. When the practitioner can demonstrate that bleeding is from gastritis due to excessive alcohol ingestion or the use of medications, such as aspirin, it presumably is possible to prevent recurrence by avoiding such insults. With appropriate patient cooperation, it would then be possible to recommend a return to flying duties.

If the bleeding source were a peptic ulcer, however, the picture would be more complex. In such situations, the practitioner has to determine whether the individual is likely to have a recurrence. Various authorities have reported different rates of recurrence of gastrointestinal bleeding in individuals who have had a prior bleeding episode due to peptic ulcer disease. For example, the reported recurrence rate of bleeding for medically treated patients ranges approximately 8–51% and 4–27% for surgically-treated patients (7). The success rate among different surgical modalities varies as well, and the lower recurrence rate, 4–10%, has been reported for patients treated by vagotomy and pyloroplasty (7). Although controversy does exist, such findings indicate that surgery may be appropriate for pilots who have bled from a peptic ulcer before unrestricted qualification for flying duties is recommended. Naturally, an appropriate period of observation after surgery is necessary to evaluate the effectiveness of this treatment before recommending a return to flying duties. If a crew member were restricted to transport or similar aircraft, some agencies may consider waiver for return to flying status without surgery when the following occur:

1. the source of bleeding was positively identified by endoscopy;
2. the patient is free of symptoms;
3. healing, as demonstrated by endoscopy is without residual spasm, irritability, or duodenitis;
4. no continuing need for medications;
5. neither specialized nor frequent feedings are required;
6. no evidence of cirrhosis, esophageal varices, neoplasm, erosive gastritis, hiatal hernia and esophagitis, familial telangiectasia, or other complicating gastrointestinal conditions exist;
7. the flyer demonstrates understanding of the factors that affect recurrence and complications; and
8. no bleeding has occurred during a six-month observation period (15).

Hiatal Hernia and Gastroesophageal Reflux

Hiatal hernia disease may be either symptomatic or an incidental finding detected in conjunction with other evaluations. Symptoms due to gastroesophageal reflux may occur without demonstrable hiatal hernia disease, as well as in association with the condition. Evaluation may include esophageal pH measurements, esophageal endoscopic examinations, esophageal motility and manometry studies, and radiographic examinations. In evaluating such patients, it is imperative that the practitioner rule out more serious causes of symptoms, especially cardiac disease. When, after such an evaluation, symptoms are attributable to gastroesophageal reflux, either with or without hiatal hernia disease, it may be possible to control the symptoms completely with standard treatment procedures, such as smaller meals, no food three hours before retiring, avoidance of aggravating foods and alcohol, weight loss, and elevating the head of the bed. Patients who respond completely with no recurrence on such a program can be recommended for flying duties. In more severe cases, long-term medication therapy, including antacids, bethanechol, or H_2-receptor antagonists may be necessary. In chronic reflux esophagitis, surgery may have to be considered. Patients requiring chronic therapy to control symptoms usually cannot be recommended for military aircrew duties (15). Over-the-counter availability of H_2 receptor antagonists may reduce physician oversight of chronic esophagitis. If symptoms were controlled, these individuals could fly as passengers. As an item of interest, United States Air Force (USAF) crew members with hiatal hernia disease used to undergo altitude chamber flights before being qualified for flying duties to determine whether gas was being trapped in the hernia. No significant trapping was observed, and altitude chamber exposure is no longer required as part of the evaluation of crew members with this condition.

Irritable Bowel Syndrome and Functional Diarrhea

Patients with chronic or intermittent constipation or diarrhea may require extensive treatment programs. Specific diagnosis is often difficult, and treatment may not be completely successful. Individuals with functional diarrhea or irritable bowel syndrome may actually be manifesting a specific food intolerance. When this particular agent can be identified and removed from the diet, it is possible that such individuals may be able to return to flying duties. In other instances, periodic treatment with agents to expand stool bulk may be successful in preventing or controlling symptoms. If such programs were not successful, however, or if follow-up were to reveal worsening of the condition, these patients may have to be removed from crew member duties due to the incapacitating nature of the problem. Removal may also be necessary when the symptoms can be controlled but require such agents as tricyclic antidepressants or other compounds that may produce undesirable side effects. Ability of patients with these conditions to fly as passengers depends on the current status of the disease and response to therapy.

Inflammatory Bowel Disease

Individuals with Crohn disease or ulcerative colitis may undergo extensive evaluation and treatment before a definitive diagnosis is made. Although these individuals can safely fly as passengers when these conditions are in remission or have responded to therapy, such patients generally cannot perform duties as a crew member. Regrettably, a symptom free period of months or even years does not indicate that the individual will be free of problems while flying (7). The long-duty hours, schedule disruptions, unusual foods, and other physiologic stresses that flight crews experience may be associated with exacerbations in individuals whose conditions were previously considered to be under control. Exacerbations could not only jeopardize flying safety and mission completion but, if they were to occur at a foreign location without adequate medical aid, could also present a threat to the individual. Because of such considerations, crew members with either Crohn disease or ulcerative colitis are usually permanently suspended from flying duties in some military services (15).

Hemorrhoids

As in other occupations with prolonged sitting, disruption of sleeping and eating schedules, dehydration, poor nutrition, and similar stresses, flying appears to be particularly associated with hemorrhoids. It also appears possible that exposure to G forces may aggravate any tendency toward this condition. Although standard treatment procedures are appropriate for an acute problem, a definitive program to increase the bulk in the diet and hydration may be necessary on a long-term basis to preclude the recurrence of this condition. As in the other medical conditions previously considered, it is essential that the practitioner conduct the necessary evaluation to ensure that symptoms, including any bleeding, are due only to a benign condition and not to a more serious condition, such as an underlying malignant tumor.

Other Gastrointestinal Considerations

Patients who have recently undergone intestinal surgery may experience significant pain due to trapped gas when exposed to reduced atmospheric pressures. In addition, sutures could rupture on exposure to such reduced pressures. In accordance with Boyle's Law, appropriately modified to reflect the fact that gases in the body are saturated with water, intestinal gases can expand over 50% at an altitude of 3048 m (10,000 ft) and over 100% at an altitude of 5468 m (18,000 ft). Passengers recovering from intestinal surgery usually should not fly for two weeks after surgery, and those individuals with a history of gastrointestinal hemorrhage should defer flying for three weeks after surgery. With respect to returning crew members to duty who have undergone abdominal surgery, time recommendations vary depending on the practitioner. In general, crew members are restricted from duty until wound healing is complete and full functional return of the affected area has occurred.

Patients with ileostomies and colostomies may fly as passengers after healing is complete. Patients, however, should take extra bags with them when flying because the expansions in the intestinal tract at altitude can produce significantly increased flow and require more frequent bag changes.

Patients with rare symptoms due to diverticulosis or diverticulitis, or who have undergone colectomy for recurrent diverticulitis, can be considered for flying duties (7). Qualification for flying requires that the patient be asymptomatic or require treatment only rarely. Any treatment must be compatible with flying activities and no significant concerns exist regarding flying safety or mission completion.

GENITOURINARY DISORDERS

Renal Lithiases

Urinary calculi are a significant problem for aviators and passengers. Although such calculi are responsible for approximately one hospital admission per 1000 individuals per year in the United States, the true incidence is considerably higher. Dehydration is associated with prolonged flights, and requirements to perform crew duties in hot environments can further aggravate dehydration. As a result, the incidence of stone formation may be increased by flight operations. Although some stones can pass with minimal symptoms, others produce severe pain, which can rapidly become incapacitating. Whether in a crew member or a passenger, the abrupt onset of such pain due to stone passage may require diversion to the nearest air field with medical facilities. The situation can rapidly become critical if the condition were to occur in a single pilot of an aircraft.

On occasion, asymptomatic calculi are incidentally discovered in a crew member during routine evaluation. In such circumstances, the aviator's physician has to determine whether the individual should be qualified for continued flying duties. In the USAF, the presence of a retained calculus in the parenchyma or a calyceal diverticulum can be considered for unrestricted flying duties when metabolic and renal studies are normal. If the stone were in a papillary duct or more distal portion of the collecting system, the flyer could be considered for waiver if the individual were restricted to tanker, transport, or bomber aircraft (15).

In some situations, stone removal is warranted due to medical considerations. After extracorporeal shock-wave lithotripsy or other therapy appropriate for the type of stone present, waiver for flying duties may be considered depending on results of metabolic and renal studies.

Proteinuria

Although most individuals excrete < 50 mg of protein every 24 hours, some normal people pass considerably more after exercise or prolonged standing. Individuals in this latter category who apply for commercial or military flight training can pose a management problem for the aeromedical practitioner. Although proteinuria may only represent benign orthostatic proteinuria, it may be the manifestation of significant kidney disease. When no significant excretion of protein occurs during a prolonged period of bedrest, urinalysis is otherwise normal, and both renal function and anatomy are normal, the practitioner may recommend qualification. Because proteinuria possibly represents early kidney disease, even though all the qualifying criteria are met, long-term annual follow-up is warranted.

OBSTETRIC-GYNECOLOGIC CONSIDERATIONS

Pregnancy

For a number of years, physicians were hesitant to recommend that a pregnant woman fly as either a passenger or crew member. Although part of this hesitancy was due to concerns about possible complications during the flight, much of the reluctance was because of fears that hypoxia may produce malformations of the fetus or cause abortions. It has subsequently been determined that the fetus normally lives in an environment where the arterial partial pressure of oxygen is much reduced from that of an adult. The fetus is able to tolerate this environment because fetal oxyhemoglobin is able to deliver all necessary oxygen to the developing tissues. Thus, the normal fetus at sea level has a P_{O_2} of 32 mm Hg in its umbilical cord arterial blood and 10.6 mm Hg in the cord venous blood (16). This is in sharp contrast to the P_{O_2} of approximately 100 mm Hg in the arterial blood of the mother and of 40 mm Hg in the mother's venous circulation. When the mother is breathing a P_{O_2} equivalent to 2438 m (8,000 ft), her arterial P_{O_2} decreases to 64 mm Hg, but the fetal P_{O_2} decreases only from 32 to 25.6 mm Hg. Even at this level, the maternal arterial oxygen saturation is still approximately 90%. Further assisting fetal circulation in the delivery of oxygen during such mild hypoxic stress is the fact that the oxygen dissociation curve for fetal hemoglobin differs from that for mature hemoglobin. As a result, fetal hemoglobin is more fully saturated at lower P_{O_2} levels than is the mother's (16). Also, with the change in pH resulting from any hypoxic stress, the dissociation curve shifts to increase oxygen delivery. Thus, the fetus appears able to withstand the hypoxia of a commercial flight (17,18). This impression is confirmed by studies of pregnant women during routine commercial flights. Investigators found that the flights posed no hazard for the mother or the fetus in uncomplicated pregnancies (18). Although it has been suggested that pregnant flight attendants are at increased risk of spontaneous fetal loss, recent investigations indicated that the risk is no greater than that of other employed women (19). These results are consistent with studies of pregnant women residing at altitude which suggest that mortality rates of infants born

at high altitude do not differ from those born at lower altitudes (20). Some studies indicated infants born of mothers living at altitude have lower birth weights than do infants born to mothers residing at low altitudes (20), but other investigators reported that birth weights at high altitude are essentially normal for gestational age (21).

Pregnancy is associated with increased incidence of superficial and deep thrombophlebitis. Consequently, some authorities recommended that pregnant flyers request the less cramped aisle seat and walk 15 minutes approximately every hour (17).

Different gestation times have been recommended for the cessation of flight duties by a pregnant crew member. Some reports have recommended that commercial crew members terminate flying at the thirteenth week, with 20 weeks of gestation as the limit for flight duties (16). Others would permit flying until the 26th week (22). Recommendations regarding crew member duties are based both on concern over the ability to perform necessary duties and the increased possibility of injury due to the unavailability of adequate restraint systems, particularly during an emergency situation.

With respect to pregnant passengers, authorities also vary in their recommendations. Some experts rely on the judgment of the patient's own physician. Other authorities believe that pregnant passengers generally should not be accepted on flights when they are beyond the 35th or 36th week of gestation (1,17). However, obstetrical patients greater than 34 weeks gestation are moved within the USAF aeromedical system without problems (23). Both the duration of the flight and possibility for care at an enroute stop must be considered in providing a recommendation for a patient during the later stages of pregnancy. After delivery, the mother should experience no difficulties when flying as soon as she is stable and feels she can tolerate the trip. However, due to time needed for lung maturation, term infants should not fly until two to seven days after birth (1). Time may have to be extended for a premature infant.

Increasing concern exists regarding the effects of passive smoke on pregnant and nonpregnant women. Although smoking is now prohibited on most United States flights, it is still permitted on longer-duration flights where exposure may be even more significant. Studies of relatively short-duration flights (approximately four hours) measured passive exposure to nicotine by personal monitors and urinary nicotine level determinations. Both nonsmoking flight attendants and passengers in some "nonsmoking" seats had measurable exposures (24).

Menstrual Cycle

Groups of flight attendants in different airlines have been studied in an effort to determine whether flying significantly affects the menstrual cycle. Irregular flight schedules, shifts in circadian rhythm, diet changes, and similar events could reasonably be expected to have an impact on the psychophysiologic factors affecting the menstrual cycle. Although these studies have demonstrated various changes in the cycles of some attendants, it has not always been possible to relate these changes solely to flight activities. One study demonstrated increased irregularity and dysmenorrhea in flight attendants when they first began flying (25). With increased flight experience (six years in the referenced study), however, these disorders tended to subside and the cycles to return to normal. This improvement was not due to age changes because individuals who ceased flying again experienced increased irregularity. These findings led the investigators to postulate that flight duties in themselves had less effect than did the stress associated with a job change—in this instance either beginning or ceasing work as a flight attendant.

Studies also suggested that flight attendants flying transmeridian routes are prone to having irregular menstrual cycles (26). In general, the irregularity consisted of prolonged cycles, and

the investigators noted the possibility that the changes were due to disruption of the circadian rhythm. Investigators used isolation units to study the effects of time-zone changes on stewardesses. They could not demonstrate consistent changes in the group exposed to time-zone changes, when compared with a control group.

Flight attendants on another airline noted changes in their menstrual cycles after they began flight duties (27). Thirty-nine percent reported either the development of menstrual disorders or aggravation of previous disorders as they commenced flight duties. The most frequent problems encountered were hyperpolymenorrhea, dysmenorrhea, or increased irregularity. Neither age nor sexual activity appeared to influence the development of or increase in menstrual disorders. The investigators also found that a large proportion of these women, 38%, experienced pelvic discomfort or congestion after prolonged flights, which could perhaps be attributed to the prolonged times the attendants spend upright or seated.

Although various studies of the effects of flying on the menstrual cycle demonstrated changes associated with flying, it is difficult to relate the changes to flying, per se. Investigators emphasized the need for further research to delineate the causes and mechanisms of observed changes in the menstrual cycle. Overall, it would appear that the changes reflect the impact of the demands and stresses associated with flight duties on the delicately balanced hormonal system involved in menstrual cycles. As may be expected, the impact apparently subsides as the individual adjusts to these demands. At present, no clear evidence indicates that flying duties produce any long-lasting, adverse effects on the menstrual cycle of crew members.

Acceleration Forces

USAF female crew members participated in acceleration studies on centrifuges for a number of years. An incidental observation during these studies stated that exposure to forces up to $+9G_z$ neither produced uterine problems, nor caused adverse effects on menstruation. Isolated instances of stress incontinence were reported in some patients during high G loads and with anti-G suit inflation. Because pregnant women were excluded from these studies, it is not possible to define any possible deleterious effects of acceleration forces in this group.

ENDOCRINE AND METABOLIC ABNORMALITIES

Diabetes Mellitus

The spectrum of diabetes mellitus can extend from mild abnormalities of glucose metabolism detected only on blood screening examinations to severe forms requiring intensive long-term therapy to prevent episodes of coma and even death. Due to the threat of hypoglycemic reactions, complications due to dehydration, disruption of meal schedules, circadian rhythm shifts, and similar factors, an individual requiring daily supplemental insulin cannot be qualified for flight duties. However, people with milder forms of the disease may be able to perform flying duties safely. Similarly, some passengers with diabetes mellitus may experience no difficulty during long fights, whereas flying may place other diabetics in a life-threatening situation.

Before considering recommendations for such individuals any further, it is perhaps appropriate to stress the necessity of confirming the diagnosis in crew members with milder forms of the disease prior to recommending qualification or disqualification. Glycosuria only indicates the need for further evaluation and is not diagnostic. The standard test for evaluating the condition is the glucose tolerance test, but it also can be a misleading diagnostic tool. Although the need for effective carbohydrate loading (e.g., 150–200 g of carbohydrate for at least three days before the test) has been documented (28), glucose tolerance testing may be accomplished without such preparation. Of particular concern

to the aerospace medicine practitioner is the fact that an "abnormal" determination may be a false-positive result. Further evaluation could disclose that the abnormal result was due to fasting, some other physiologic factor, or a different disease state.

Unless detected, a false-positive determination can result in a recommendation for disqualification for flying duties that can affect an individual's career and job opportunities for life. For example, on rare occasions, combat military crew members have been unnecessarily disqualified for a period of weeks because of a false-positive glucose tolerance test. Proper investigation, including a repeat glucose tolerance test after appropriate carbohydrate loading, revealed the spurious nature of the first determination, and the flyers were returned to duties.

Some individuals with definite glucose abnormalities can be considered for a return to flying duties. Criteria for return to flying duties can include absence of evidence of end-organ disease, evidence of ketoacidosis, signs or symptoms of hyperglycemia or hypoglycemia, or use of any medication, including oral hypoglycemic agents. Some organizations allow consideration of the use of oral antidiabetic agents if their use were compatible with safe aircraft operation or air-traffic-control duties. Final decision in such instances is left to the appropriate national or military organization.

In some countries, the return of flyers using such agents is generally restricted to selected cases involving private pilots or air-traffic controllers. In such situations, it should be recalled that a number of other agents, including some antiinflammatories, antihypertensives, and antibiotics can potentiate the effects of hypoglycemic agents. These interactions can increase the risk of significant side effects.

It should be noted that it is possible to return elevated blood glucose levels of some patients to an acceptable level through a weight reduction program alone. Some may argue that individuals with an elevated glucose tolerance test have an increased tendency toward diabetes, and any deficiency in preparation for the test or weight elevation merely unmasked this tendency. Although it is appropriate to follow such patients to rule out the subsequent development of diabetes, it is not necessary to suspend trained aviators when subsequent tests disclose no abnormalities. One of the more satisfying aspects of the practice of aerospace medicine is watching a previously disqualified crew member attain acceptable blood glucose levels solely through weight control. Although they require periodic follow-up to ensure that they do not develop more significant glucose elevations, such aviators returned to flying status benefit both themselves and their operational organization.

In considering candidates for crew member training, both family history and current status are significant. A family history of diabetes in both parents places an individual in a prediabetic group at increased risk of developing diabetes. Intermittent glycosuria with abnormalities on glucose tolerance testing may place the patient in a "latent" or "chemical" diabetes category. These applicants also may have an increased chance of developing diabetes. Consequently, it may be appropriate to disqualify such individuals for military or commercial training rather than to place them in an expensive training program for a career that has a higher-than-average risk of being terminated due to a medical disqualification. Applicants for private pilot training could be qualified with appropriate follow-up by the examiner.

Although the use of insulin generally precludes an individual from crew member duties, numerous airline passengers do require this therapy. These individuals may tolerate even long flights without problems. A required diabetic diet can be obtained on many airlines, and the passenger can carry the necessary insulin on the flight. Irregular meal schedules, fatigue, circadian rhythm shifts, difficulty in obtaining proper medical care for many medical problems, emotional stresses, and similar factors associated with flying can affect insulin requirements and dosage schedules. Compounding the problem

are difficulties replacing medication, syringes, or needles that are damaged or lost in baggage transfer. Because of these factors, it is recommended that diabetic patients consult their physicians before undertaking air travel to ensure that necessary adjustments to the dosage schedule are planned and any required arrangements for medication replacement are made.

Thyroid Disorders

Thyroid disorders can be similar to diabetes mellitus in presenting difficult diagnostic challenges to the practitioner. Certainly, tests for L-thyroxine (T4), 3,5,3-triiodo-L-thyroxine (T3), thyroid-stimulating hormone (thyrotropin, or TSH), the binding globulins, and other aspects of thyroid function have markedly assisted in the diagnosis of abnormalities. The manifestation of disease can be varied, however, and so many complaints can be attributed to any demonstrated abnormality that the physician faces a significant challenge in considering and then diagnosing the disorder, particularly in its earlier or milder forms.

Once the abnormality has been diagnosed and appropriately treated, the tests used to diagnose the condition are also of marked benefit in determining whether an aviator can return to flying duties. A patient with hyperthyroidism can be considered for a return to flying activities when treatment has produced a euthyroid status, as determined by appropriate endocrine studies, and no evidence of end-organ disease exists. In addition to cardiovascular effects, ophthalmopathy, myopathic problems, and central nervous system disorders are of particular concern in evaluating a flyer with hyperthyroidism.

Treatment of hyperthyroidism may result in clinical hypothyroidism. Whether spontaneous or as the result of hyperthyroidism therapy, adult-onset hypothyroidism does not necessarily require permanent suspension from flying duties when treatment has produced a euthyroid condition. Again, the practitioner must ascertain whether any evidence of cardiovascular or other end-organ disease exists. If no complicating factors were present and the patient were to attain a euthyroid condition, a recommendation to return to flying duty may be considered. The use of long-term thyroid therapy does not preclude a return to flying duties. Naturally, in either situation, the practitioner must observe the patient for a sufficient period to ensure that a stable euthyroid status has been achieved and that no side effects from any required thyroid replacement therapy occur. Depending on the circumstances involved, this observation period may last several months to over a year.

Gout

Elevated uric acid levels may be associated with the typical symptoms of gout or may be detected fortuitously during a routine screening examination. Although the patient may present with a uric acid renal stone, the more usual manifestation is acute arthritis, typically in the first metatarsophalangeal joint. Because gout may involve multiple joints, as in rheumatoid arthritis, radiographic examinations may not be diagnostic. Uric acid levels also can be misleading, and the detection of negatively birefringent monosodium urate crystals in joint fluid is considered to be the hallmark of the disease. The aerospace medicine physician must not only be concerned with the diagnostic challenge of this condition but also determine what treatment program is appropriate for the patient with symptoms, as well as for the individual who has only elevated serum uric acid levels. Additionally, the presence of conditions frequently associated with elevated uric acid, such as sarcoid, hypertension, diabetes, renal disease, and malignancies must be considered. If the patient were an aviator, the physician could then make the appropriate aeromedical recommendation.

An elevated uric acid level may be due either to the overproduction or underexcretion of uric acid. This distinction is of more than academic interest because it can play a significant role in determining which type of therapeutic agent to use when treatment is indicated. Making the distinction is complicated by the fact that some commonly prescribed therapeutic agents can affect serum acid levels. Thus, aspirin in small doses, the chlorothiazides, other diuretics, acute alcohol ingestion, and ethambutol reduces renal excretion of uric acid. If such factors were excluded, a patient could be considered an overproducer when > 600 mg/day of uric acid is excreted after a five-day period of restriction of dietary purines (29). These patients can be treated by attempting to inhibit uric acid production with an agent, such as allopurinol. The majority of patients with elevated uric acid levels are underexcreters. These individuals can be managed with a uricosuric agent, such as probenecid, unless renal function is impaired with a creatine clearance < 80 ml/min, tophaceous tophi are present, the patient excretes > 700 mg/day of uric acid on a regular diet, or uric acid nephrolithiasis occurs (29).

Although the above treatment programs can be effective in caring for symptomatic patients with elevated uric acid levels, a number of individuals with asymptomatic hyperuricemia do not require therapy. In evaluating these patients, it is first necessary to ensure that the finding is not due to medication or underlying conditions, such as malignancy. Once such etiologic possibilities are excluded, the examiner must then consider whether treatment is warranted. Considerable controversy exists, but the treatment of asymptomatic elevations of uric acid may be deferred unless; symptoms occur; the patient has a strong family history of renal disease, renal lithiasis, or gout; or the patient excretes > 1000 mg/day of uric acid (29). It should be noted that some patients with asymptomatic, elevated uric acid levels who meet the criteria for treatment may respond to simple dietary control and weight loss.

If treatment with medication were initiated in a patient with either symptomatic or asymptomatic uric acid elevations, a return to flying duties should be deferred until a response to the treatment, as well as the absence of side effects, is demonstrated. Once the uric acid level is controlled and no evidence of gout complications or undesirable effects from any required medication exists, the physician may recommend a return to flying duties. If the elevation were an incidental finding in an asymptomatic patient and none of the criteria for treatment were to exist, the examiner may recommend continued flying duties.

MALIGNANT TUMORS

General Considerations

Many individuals with histories of malignant tumor can fly safely as passengers or crew members. Others could pose a serious risk to themselves or others, even though no evidence of a tumor recurrence exists. The aerospace medicine physician must consider a number of factors in attempting to decide between the alternative recommendations concerning flying. Some items that have proved to be valuable in developing an appropriate recommendation for a particular patient are considered in the following sections.

Tumor Classification

The more virulent forms of a tumor may place the individual at increased risk of recurrence. Because the more aggressive neoplasms may express themselves sooner, however, the physician may be able to categorize a recurrence free patient as "cured" sooner than would be possible if the tumor were not so virulent. Thus, it may be appropriate to recommend a return to flying duties sooner for the patient with a history of a more serious type of malignancy than for the patient with a less serious form. Such action would reflect the fact that if the patient were to survive, the risk of recurrence would decrease to an acceptable level faster than it would for a more slowly growing tumor, where a more prolonged period of observation would be necessary to rule out recurrence.

Staging at Diagnosis

Spread of the tumor beyond the primary site obviously increases the risk of recurrence. For many tumors, however, local extension does not carry the severe prognosis that evidence of spread to more distant sites does. Microstaging also may provide information of value in defining the risk of recurrence.

Method of Treatment

Once the type and staging of a malignant tumor are known, it is usually possible to define the expected effectiveness of the particular treatment regimen that was applied. In evaluating the patient, it is important to consider not only the effect of the treatment of the malignancy but also the impact on the physical and mental functioning of the patient. Radionecrosis, hormone imbalance, restricted use of an extremity, or similar results from therapy have the potential to restrict the patient from crew member duties as completely as recurrence of the malignancy.

Current Therapy

The flight surgeon evaluating a crew member for a possible return to status after treatment of a malignant tumor must evaluate the current therapy. Both the effectiveness of the therapy and the existence of any side effects have to be ascertained. Therapy may include long-term or periodic chemotherapy, as well as medication to compensate for the necessary side effects of treatment. For example, hormone therapy may be required permanently after testicular, thyroid, or ovarian surgery. It may be possible to return the patient to flying duties on chronic maintenance therapy when no deleterious side effects occurred and the therapy restored the individual to an essentially normal state.

Probability of Recurrence

Overall, the risk of recurrence decreases as the time without recurrence increases. It is difficult, however, to use standard mortality tables to determine the earliest point when the risk of recurrence becomes an acceptable level to recommend flying duties. Conrad et al. analyzed USAF experience regarding cancer treatment and survival in an effort to provide information the flight surgeon could use to recommend return to flying (30–32). These investigators evaluated a series of Air Force patients with malignant tumors to develop techniques to help predict the chance of tumor recurrence. One technique is the hazard function. This technique defines the risk of developing a recurrence within the immediate future for all individuals who have survived to the beginning of a given time period. This is not the percentage of the entire patient population but only of that proportion who had been recurrence free until the start of a given time period. The examiner can apply this information as a hazard rate to predict when the risk of recurrence becomes acceptable to recommend return to flying. The physician could, for example, decide that an acceptable hazard rate was 5%, which indicates that only one patient in 20 who has survived recurrence free to that point in time will develop a recurrence. Using hazard function information for that specific malignancy, the practitioner can determine how long a period of time is required before the patient reaches an acceptable level of risk. These techniques are more useful than the usual survival rates because survival rates include patients with recurrences who are still alive. Consequently, survival rates cannot be used to predict recurrences. Hazard function information also can be used to predict the onset of symptomatic recurrence in conditions where the disease, although not cured, is in remission for a prolonged period.

Hodgkin's disease is one such condition. In some forms of the disease, a patient may be symptom free for several years after therapy with a risk of symptomatic recurrence of < 5%. In later years, the risk of recurrence increases, and the individual may require increased monitoring to detect new activity. Although the patient may have to be disqualified if a symptomatic recurrence were to occur, the flight surgeon

could have safely allowed the aviator to fly during earlier, low-risk years.

Site of Recurrence

The physician also needs to determine whether a recurrence will be heralded by warning signs or symptoms or whether the first indication of complication may be abrupt incapacitation. Obviously, aeromedical disposition would be different if a significant risk of sudden incapacitation were to exist than would be the case if gradual progression were to occur. Even a recurrence hazard rate of < 5% may be unacceptable for tumors where the initial sign of spread is a seizure or other form of abrupt incapacitation. Lung carcinoma, for example, is the most common metastatic tumor of the brain, and the physician may choose to defer a return to flying duties for these patients even after the recurrence risk was less than would otherwise be acceptable.

Current Physical and Mental Status

A person who is treated for a life-threatening malignancy may experience long-lasting mental, as well as physical, effects. A residual physical defect can be evaluated in the same manner as it would be in an individual without a history of malignant tumor. The evaluation of mental trauma and effects is more difficult. Many patients experience the same acute emotional trauma at the initial diagnosis as do patients with confirmed terminal illnesses. Subsequent to the psychological trauma resulting from the diagnosis, the patient undergoes the strain of waiting for the results of studies for metastasis. Then the patient awaits the outcome of the treatment program. Throughout these periods, the patient is continually concerned about whether a new symptom or finding represents recurrence. Changed relationships with family members or friends can add to the stress. In some patients, the emotional aspects can be overwhelming, even in the absence of objective evidence of recurrence. Such stresses can result in drastic action, and an ''accidental death'' in a patient with a known or suspected recurrence may actually be suicide. Because of such considerations, it is imperative that the physician ascertain both the mental and physical stability of a patient being considered for a return to flying duties. Even passengers should be similarly evaluated because disaster could result if a patient with actual or only suspected extension of a malignancy decided to take drastic action during a flight. (See also the subsequent discussion of AIDS.)

Specific Tumors

Germinal Cell Tumors of the Testes

Germinal cell tumors of the testes are among the more common malignant tumors in older males in the military. Conrad et al. analyzed 552 patients with such tumors and determined the hazard rate for different combinations of type, stage, and treatment (32). For example, the hazard rate for recurrence decreases to < 5% after one year for teratocarcinoma (Dixon-Moore type IV) stage A (tumor confined to testis and adnexa). Depending on the function of the other testis, lifelong testosterone replacement therapy may be necessary. Treatment may include lymphadenectomy, which can produce varying degrees of lymphedema. Should a teratocarcinoma of this type and stage recur, it would not be expected to produce incapacitation. Considering these factors, a recurrence free patient with type IV, stage A tumor seen one year after definitive treatment could be considered for a return to flying duties. For many testicular tumors, advances in radiotherapy and chemotherapy now offer cure rates approaching 100%. Return of patients with a history of treatment of such a tumor would be contingent on the absence of significant lymphedema or any other physical problem, serum hormone studies demonstrating adequate testosterone replacement, and appropriate mental status.

Melanoma

Melanoma demonstrates the need to evaluate the possibility of abrupt incapacitation. Moseley et al. evaluated 712 patients with this disease (33). Lesions were classified according to body site and staged to reflect spread from the primary site. When possible, microstaging using the techniques of Clark and Breslow was accomplished. Melanoma is known to metastasize to brain, doing so in approximately one-third of patients. Brain, however, is not always the first site of metastasis in this malignancy. These investigators found that brain was the first site of recurrence in only 8% of state III (disseminated melanoma) patients. In addition, the metastasis presented as a catastrophic event, such as a stroke or seizure, in only 1.6% of stage III patients. The risk of a catastrophic event decreased to 0.6% for the entire group of patients. Conrad et al. studied 604 patients with melanoma; 184 had recurrent disease (30). Thirty-one percent of these patients had brain metastasis, and central nervous system symptoms were the first evidence of recurrence in 7% of 184 patients with recurrent disease. No catastrophic event occurred without prior symptoms in this study. The hazard rate for recurrence varied with tumor location and staging. For example, the hazard rate decreased to < 5% in three years for head or neck lesions with negative lymph nodes but did not reach this level for five years for lesions on the trunk with negative lymph nodes. Considering the results of such studies, it is possible, when no other physical or mental contraindications exist, to recommend a return to flying duties for selected patients with histories of melanoma in spite of the possibility of metastasis to brain. Because of such possibilities, close follow-up of these patients is indicated. When a patient has extensive disease, it may be appropriate to recommend against even passenger flight because of seizure risk.

ORTHOPEDIC DISORDERS

Fractures, Sprains, and Dislocations

Although passengers can fly with an arm or leg cast, crew members must be able to perform their functions unencumbered. Further, they usually must have normal function of the musculoskeletal system to accomplish the myriad of tasks involved in flight activities. In general, a crew member who has experienced an orthopedic injury should not be qualified for a return to flight duties until the injured part has regained essentially normal motion and muscle strength. In addition, no residual discomfort or pain should be present at rest or during exertion that could restrict required activity. For example, a pilot may have a normal range of motion after an ankle injury but be unable to apply necessary brake pressure due to residual pain. A flight attendant with apparently normal range of arm motion may not be able to operate emergency equipment because of residual muscle weakness or pain restriction. Such examples emphasize the need to ensure that the crew member with a "healed" injury is in fact fully qualified for a return to duty. They also demonstrate the need for the aerospace medicine physician to have detailed knowledge of the crew member's duties in order to make appropriate recommendations.

In still other instances, some obvious residual defect in strength or motion exists in spite of excellent care. Again, the evaluating examiner needs to have sufficient knowledge of the crew member's tasks to determine whether return to flying is appropriate. In evaluating patients with and without residual defects, the physician may find it beneficial to evaluate the patient in the actual workplace. Monitoring a patient throughout a simulated flight has uncovered previously unsuspected problems that could compromise flying safety or the individual's well-being.

Another consideration in evaluating a postinjury patient is whether any predisposition to further injury exists in the flight environment. For example, a patient seen at the Aeromedical Consultation Center of USAFSAM had experienced a cervical spine fracture during a dive into a pool. He received prompt attention, and the paralysis he initially experienced due to spinal cord compression gradually subsided. He eventually regained essentially normal function and applied for flight training. The healing process, however, had resulted in marked angulation of the cervical spine. If the applicant were to participate in operational flying and had to eject, the possibility existed that the ejection forces could produce a fracture and even transection of the spinal cord. Consequently, even though his musculoskeletal function was acceptable, the individual had to be disqualified for military flight duties.

A similar concern about the possibility of increased risk of reinjury was studied in crew members who had experienced a compression fracture during an ejection and then subsequently had to eject again (34). In open ejection-seat aircraft, the T-10 to L-2 vertebrae are most frequently injured, usually as a compression fracture, during ejection. The compression fractures typically heal without difficulty, and the flyers return to flying duties. The review of crew members with this history who were involved in a subsequent ejection did not reveal any increased risk of additional fractures during later ejection.

Back Pain

One of the more frequent conditions evaluated in family practice is back pain, and this problem is common to flyers, as well. Prolonged sitting, on occasion in seats without properly designed support, may cause initial or recurrent low-back pain in passengers or crew members. The problem may be aggravated further for aircrew who have to wear personal equipment, including parachutes, and remain strapped in place throughout a long flight. These and similar stresses result in frequent patient visits to the flight surgeon for the evaluation and treatment of back pain.

In evaluating a complaint of back pain, the examiner must, of course, rule out such disorders as renal lithiasis or malignant tumors. In some patients, the physician may detect significant disk disease, which can only be corrected by surgery. In most patients, however, the symptoms are due to mechanical derangement of the spine, often caused by faulty sitting or standing posture or improper use of the back at work. Obesity and lack of exercise also may contribute to mechanical symptoms. The evaluation and treatment of this group may be complicated by the very studies obtained to rule out a more serious cause. For example, lumbosacral spine radiographs may demonstrate degenerative changes. Both the physician and the patient may then attribute the symptoms to these changes. It is known, however, that similar changes are present in large proportion of otherwise normal individuals without any history of back pain. Consequently, it is possible that the changes seen in a particular patient are unrelated to the symptoms of that patient. Such possibilities are of concern in the long-term management of the patient. Acute symptoms may respond promptly to a standard treatment program, including bedrest with a firm mattress or bed board, heat, analgesics, antiinflammatories, muscle relaxants, or appropriate exercises. When the patient and practitioner believe that the symptoms are the inevitable consequence of back disease, they may believe that future episodes cannot be prevented. If, however, the practitioner were to decide all or most of the symptoms have a muscular etiology, the patient could be strongly encouraged to begin a program of regular low-back exercises and proper use of the back in an effort to prevent a recurrence of the pain. A similar situation exists for those patients who have had surgery for an actual herniated nucleus pulposus or other spine disorder. Again, these patients may naturally attribute any subsequent back pain to the earlier surgery. As a result, they do not begin a program that may be successful in preventing future symptoms.

Back pain also may be a vexing problem for the practitioner because of the well-recognized fact that a patient may consciously or subconsciously use the complaint to avoid an unpleasant duty, for compensation, or for some other reason. This can result either in complaints when no symptoms actually exist or in exaggerations of the amount of discomfort present. The astute physician may be able to demonstrate the emotional or malingering basis of the complaints. Techniques, such as accomplishing straight-leg raising without pain by extending the legs while the patient is seated, may convince both the physician and the patient that no further treatment is required. In other situations, particularly when the actual symptoms are exaggerated, demonstrating the actual cause of the pain is more difficult. Numerous evaluations and consultations may be necessary before a final, appropriate disposition is accomplished.

Scoliosis

Scoliosis is an abnormal lateral curvature of the spine, with an associated lack of normal thoracic spine flexibility. The resultant change in the structure of the spine affects the response of the spine to both static and dynamic loads. As noted in the discussion of ejection injuries, the dynamics of force application have to be evaluated in an individual who is exposed to the stresses of flight. With increasing lateral curvature, the risk of symptoms and injury are increased when the individual is exposed to ejection or other high G forces. For example, one aviator with scoliosis experienced incapacitating back pain while experiencing 6.5 G in an F-4E aircraft. The pilot in the rear seat took control and landed. The patient could not exit the aircraft and had to be lifted from it by rescue personnel. The pain was at the point of maximum curvature of the spine where old degenerative changes were present. Because of concern about the possibility of such incapacitation, current USAF directives preclude flying duties for an individual with more than 20° of scoliosis as measured by the Cobb method.

Spondylolysis and Spondylolisthesis

Spondylolysis and spondylolisthesis appear to be manifestations of a fracture or cleft in the pars interarticularis of the vertebrae. In spondylolysis, no concomitant vertebral slippage occurs. In spondylolisthesis, the vertebral body involved slips anteriorly on the vertebral body inferior to the affected vertebral body. These defects appear to reduce the ability of the spine to withstand the application of mechanical force. An increased incidence of back pain has been reported in patients with spondylolysis, and high G forces may produce symptoms in an individual with spondylolisthesis. Flyers with recurrent symptoms and requirements for chronic medication should not continue to fly. Flyers with rare symptoms may be able to continue flying when they do not have the potential for exposure to high G forces, either during typical mission profiles or during ejections (35,36).

Other Spinal Problems

Other conditions, such as Scheuermann disease (rigid kyphotic deformity of the lower thoracic spine), spondylosis deformans (occurrence of bony protuberances on the upper or lower ridges of vertebral bodies), Klippel-Fiel syndrome (fusion and deformities of the cervical vertebrae), significant spinal trauma, and similar conditions also affect the ability of the spine to tolerate increased G forces. As a result, individuals with these conditions should be considered for disqualification for flying duties when they will be in situations where they may be exposed to increased G forces (37).

Thrombophlebitis and Deep Venous Thrombosis

Although deep venous thrombosis and pulmonary emboli have been reported after long-duration flights, the reports are anecdotal and do not permit calculation of actual incidence. A study of 53 healthy individuals traveling nonstop from Amsterdam to Tokyo was accomplished using 125 I fibrongen leg scanning techniques. None of the individuals was found to have any venous abnormalities when evaluated after the flight (38). As previously discussed, pregnant flyers are at increased risk of these problems, and exer-

cise every hour during long-duration flights has been recommended.

On occasion, the flight surgeon may evaluate a patient with symptoms of thrombosis or thrombophlebitis. Studies such as impedance plethysmography, Doppler flow studies, labeled fibrinogen scanning, and duplex ultrasonography can assist in making the diagnosis. Once the condition is treated and resolved, return to flying status depends on the type of duties performed and the probability of recurrence (39). Studies of crew members with deep venous thrombosis suggested that the flyer can be safely returned to duty if evaluation were to confirm the following: a small risk of recurrence, use of antiembolic therapy were not required, and the flyer were not a crew member in a high-performance aircraft or required to sit immobile for prolonged periods (7).

AIDS

No evidence suggests that the human immunodeficiency virus (HIV) can be transmitted in workplace environments where no contact with blood, tissue, or body fluids occurs. Feces, nasal secretions, sputum, sweat, tears, and vomitus do not pose a hazard unless blood is present (40). Regardless of transmission risk, however, knowledge that a coworker is HIV-positive can create significant problems among workers. Further, the high fatality rate, lack of curative treatment, and absence of human vaccine create concerns and fears not associated with other communicable diseases. These concerns can significantly affect both coworkers and the individual who is infected with HIV.

Similarly, a crew member who is HIV-positive presents important challenges for the aeromedical physician. Of particular concern are studies that demonstrate marked increase in the risk of suicide in patients with AIDS. These findings are not unexpected because suicide rates have been shown to be higher in persons with other chronic or life-threatening illnesses. However, the magnitude of the increased risk has underscored the problem presented by patients with HIV infections. For example, one investigation found that the risk of suicide in men, ages 20–59, with AIDS was 36 times the risk in men of the same age who did not have AIDS (41). Numerous factors may contribute to this increased risk, including social stigma of the illness, loss of family support, impact of knowing that no effective cure or way to prevent fatal results exists, financial problems due to loss of health insurance and major medical costs, and loss of friends or lovers, in some instances due to AIDS itself. Additionally, the diagnosis is associated with depression, psychosis, dementia, and other neuropsychiatric conditions (42). In essence, an HIV-positive person faces a combination of stressors that are unique, and the increased suicide risk may reflect the continuing impact of these stressors.

The risk of suicide, combined with the increasing recognition that dementia or other neuropsychiatric conditions may be early manifestations of infection, pose serious dilemmas for the aerospace medicine physician. Some government directives require that an individual with AIDS be treated the same as any other handicapped individual and provided employment as long as the patient can perform necessary duties. A flight deck crew member or flight attendant who is HIV-positive may be physically able to accomplish all desired tasks and pose no risk of infection to other flight crew members or passengers. However, because of the possibility of serious neuropsychiatric problems and their impacts, the same individual may pose a safety risk to others in the flight environment. Detailed examination, including mental status and suicide evaluation, combined with close follow-up, may enable the examining physician to develop appropriate recommendations regarding flying status. However, because of concerns about suicide and dementia, some airlines have adopted the policy that HIV-positive crew members are permanently restricted from performing flying duties. Since October 1985, U.S. military pilots have been tested for the presence of HIV anti-

body and grounded if found positive. In May 1991, the Executive Council of the Aerospace Medical Association approved a position statement that supports testing of pilots for infection by HIV and maintains that individuals confirmed to be infected should be found medically disqualified for flying duties (43). The Federal Aviation Administration requires all pilots to obtain a medical certification and when a diagnosis of AIDS is made, a denial of the medical permit will occur. In a recent case involving two commercial airline pilots, this policy was challenged. Although both pilots were HIV positive, neither demonstrated the progression of their disease to AIDS. At the time of this writing, the case is still in litigation (44).

Sarcoidosis

In the past, aerospace medicine physicians usually recommended a return to flying duties for crew members who had sarcoidosis, provided certain criteria were met. These criteria included resolution, or at least prolonged stability, of pulmonary adenopathy or infiltrates, normal pulmonary function studies, and the absence of any requirement for medications. As it became apparent that myocardial and neurologic involvement occurred, it also became necessary to modify evaluation procedures and criteria for recommendations for return to flying status (45).

Sarcoid involvement of the heart has been reported in up to 27% of autopsies of patients with sarcoidosis (46). A review of military pilots with documented sarcoidosis resulted in suspected involvement of the heart in one-third of individuals (45). Of particular concern to the aerospace medicine physician is the fact that such involvement can lead to conduction disturbances, arrhythmias, and sudden death. Sudden death may occur in up to two-thirds of patients with myocardial sarcoidosis (47,48). Such high frequencies are found primarily in patients with more severe cardiac involvement who, as a result, usually had a history of cardiac symptoms. An increased incidence of arrhythmias and conduction disturbances, however, has been reported in patients whose myocardial involvement could only be demonstrated histologically (46). The significance of myocardial sarcoidosis was demonstrated in a USAF crew member who was found to have pulmonary sarcoidosis during a routine periodic examination. Before evaluation of the condition could be completed, he abruptly collapsed at his home and died. Autopsy studies demonstrated previously unrecognized sarcoidosis of the heart, and this condition was considered to be the cause of death.

Neurologic involvement also has been reported in sarcoidosis. Studies suggest that such involvement, although uncommon, is not the rare event once supposed. Although only limited autopsy studies are available, and both peripheral and central nervous system involvement are grouped together, it appears that the nervous system may be involved in up to 5% of patients with sarcoidosis (49). Of particular concern is the fact that neurologic abnormalities may be the first manifestation of the disease. Further, in those patients with neurologic symptoms, the more critical central nervous system involvement tends to occur early in the disease, whereas peripheral involvement is more often seen later in chronic conditions.

Because of the increased concern regarding sarcoidosis, USAF aviators who had previously been granted a waiver for sarcoidosis were reevaluated. Of the first 34 flyers reevaluated, six (18%) were diagnosed as having myocardial sarcoidosis. This frequency was in agreement with that reported in the literature (13–27%). The diagnosis of cardiac involvement was based primarily on a persistent filling defect on resting and exercise thallium scintigraphy. Two of six patients also had defects on the gallium-67 citrate scans that matched those of the thallium-fixed defect. None of the six patients had cardiac symptoms, and it is noteworthy that only two patients still had bilateral hilar adenopathy. This finding is in accord with the suggestion by some authors that patients with myocardial involvement may not show other evidence of persistent

or active disease (47). Of concern is the fact that one individual so evaluated had normal scans 58 months after the sarcoidosis initially was diagnosed. One year later (approximately 70 months after the initial diagnosis), both his gallium and thallium scans were positive. Such findings have resulted in the recommendation for annual evaluations for any flyer with a history of sarcoidosis.

In most instances, patients with sarcoidosis which is manifest only by asymptomatic hilar lymphadenopathy will clear within two years. In some individuals, activity will persist, placing these patients in a chronic category.

Flyers with complete remission of sarcoid symptoms can be considered for return to flying duties. Because of the natural history of the disease, some aeromedical specialists recommend deferring such consideration for two years after the diagnosis is established or one year after all medication has been stopped and no evidence of disease activity has occurred. Evaluation must be structured to help assure that no ongoing process or residua exists which could produce sudden incapacitation.

In addition to a complete examination incorporating standard sarcoid pulmonary studies, evaluation should include appropriate neurologic and cardiac studies. Cardiovascular studies may include resting and ambulatory ECGs, exercise tolerance testing, echocardiography, thallium scintigraphy, and gallium-67 citrate studies.

Patients with the following should not be cleared for aircrew duties (7,48):

1. Evidence of active disease
2. Presence of chronic disease, including bone or skin sarcoidosis or posterior uveitis secondary to sarcoidosis
3. Evidence of myocardial involvement
4. Evidence of central nervous system involvement
5. Presence of persistent widespread pulmonary residuals, including cysts and bullae.

Because of the natural history of sarcoidosis, periodic follow-up is recommended for flyers who have been cleared for return to flying duties.

Dermatitis

Dermatitis is one of the leading causes of loss of time in industrial workers, and flyers may be affected similarly by skin disorders. Aviators may be exposed to dehydration during flight and then have to cope with increased temperatures, excessive humidity, and resultant marked perspiration during ground operations. Life support and personal equipment, such as oxygen masks or parachute straps, can initiate skin reactions or further irritate an involved area of the skin. Prolonged operations with disruption of personal hygiene, can set the stage for infection or other aggravation of an otherwise easily managed dermatologic problem. These complications may make diagnosis particularly difficult in spite of the usual scrapings, cultures, and other diagnostic procedures. As a result, appropriate therapy may be delayed. Of equal concern, dermatologic manifestations of an underlying systemic disorder may be so modified that the physician fails to diagnose the true cause of the skin condition. For example, aviators may be treated for a stubborn skin ailment over a period of months by different practitioners. Therapeutic failures may repeatedly be ascribed to aggravation resulting from flight operations before the actual cause, such as underlying diabetes mellitus, is diagnosed. Exposure to a variety of often exotic agents also may complicate diagnostic or therapeutic efforts. Many hours were expended in attempting to determine why flight attendants on one particular overwater commercial flight repeatedly developed unusual dermatitis. Only after prolonged study was it found that the reactions were due to chemicals in the life vests the attendants used for demonstrations at the start of the flight.

In addition to making the diagnostic problem more difficult, flight duties also may foil treatment efforts or delay healing of the skin problem. The aggravating environmental factors and hygiene difficulties that made diagnosis a problem may likewise adversely affect therapy. In some instances, cure is possible only when the individual is removed from flight duties until healing is complete. Unfortunately, when the aviator has a chronic skin problem, such suspension may be for a prolonged period. In more severe situations, the crew member may have to be permanently disqualified from flight duties.

Systemic therapy may be indicated for some conditions, and in many instances medication can be prescribed without prolonged disqualification from flying duties. Tetracycline may have to be used for a long period to treat severe acne. It is usually possible to recommend a return to flying duties for crew members receiving this medication after an appropriate observation period, approximately five weeks, to rule out significant side effects.

In other situations, however, systemic medications may not be compatible with flying duties. It is usually appropriate to disqualify individuals on systemic steroid therapy from flying. This action not only helps to prevent the onset of a complication at an enroute stop where only limited medical care may be available but also ensures that the physician will be able to evaluate the therapeutic response at the desired time. Systemic medications for fungal skin conditions also can preclude flight duties. Significant side effects, including fatigue, dizziness, mental confusion, and impairment of performance of routine duties may occur with some agents. Such effects obviously could be a significant hazard for an aviator, and it would be appropriate to disqualify crew members for flight duties while taking such agents.

SUMMARY

As mentioned at the start of this chapter, it is not possible to consider all the medical conditions that can occur in flyers. It also should be recognized that the recommendations for even those conditions discussed cannot be considered absolute. The rapid progress in medicine will undoubtedly produce significant changes in the management of many conditions in the near future. The selected disorders are, however, representative of the more common problems that develop in aviators, and the principles of aerospace medicine used in evaluating and caring for patients with these conditions apply also in other medical and surgical circumstances. Through the application of these principles, aerospace medicine physicians can develop appropriate treatment programs, including recommendations regarding flying, for the flyers they serve.

REFERENCES

1. Green RL, Mooney SE. Carriage of invalid passengers by civil airlines. In: Ernsting J, King P, eds. Aviation medicine, 2nd ed. London: Butterworths, 1988.
2. Scott V. Anemia and airline flight duties. Aviat Space Environ Med 1975;46:830–835.
3. McKenzie JM. Evaluation of the hazards of sickle cell trait in aviation. Aviat Space Environ Med 1977;48: 753–762.
4. Sears DA. The morbidity of sickle cell trait, a review of the literature. Am J Med 1978;64:1021–1036.
5. Diggs LW. The sickle cell trait in relation to the training and assignment of duties in the Armed Forces: III. hyposthenuria, hematuria, sudden death, rhabdomyolysis, and acute tubular necrosis. Aviat Space Environ Med 1984;55:358–364.
6. Diggs LW. The sickle cell trait in relation to the training and assignment of duties in the Armed Forces: I. policies, observations, and studies. Aviat Space Environ Med 1984;55:180–185.
7. Rayman RB. Internal medicine. In: Rayman RB, ed. Clinical aviation medicine, 2nd ed. Philadelphia: Lea and Febiger, 1990.
8. Diggs LW. The sickle cell trait in relation to the training and assignment of duties in the Armed Forces: IV. considerations and recommendations. Aviat Space Environ Med 1984;55:487–492.
9. Voge RM, Rosado NR, Contiguglia JJ. Sickle cell anemia trait in the military aircrew population. Aviat Space Environ Med 1991;62:1099–1102.
10. James CM. Sickle cell trait and military service. J Nav Med Serv 1990;76:9–13.
11. Buley LE. Incidence, causes, and results of airline pilot incapacitation while on duty. Aerospace Med 1969;40: 64–70.
12. Consensus Conference. Travelers' diarrhea. JAMA 1988;253:2700–2704.
13. Soll AH. Medical treatment of peptic ulcer disease. JAMA 1996;275:622–629.
14. Hunt RH, Malfertheiner P, Yeomans ND, et al. Critical issues in the pathophysiology and management of peptic ulcer disease. Eur J Gastroenterol Hepatol 1995;7: 685–699.
15. Air Force Regulation 160–43. Medical Examination and Medical Standards, No. 160–43. Washington, D.C.: United States Air Force Headquarters. 1986, (including change 7, October 1989).
16. Scholter P. Pregnant stewardess—should she fly? Aviat Space Environ Med 1976;47:77–81.
17. Barry M, Bia F. Pregnancy and travel. JAMA 1989;261: 728–731.
18. Huch R, Baumann H, Fallenstein F, et al. Physiologic changes in pregnant women and their fetuses during jet air travel. Am J Obstet Gynecol 1986;154:996–1000.
19. Daniell WE, Vaughan TL, Millies BA. Pregnancy outcomes among female flight attendants. Aviat Space Environ Med 1990 (In press).
20. Unger C, Weiser JK, McCullough RE, et al. Altitude, low birth weight, and infant mortality in Colorado. JAMA 1988;259:3427–3432.
21. Cotton EK, Hiestand M, Philbin GK, Simmons M. Re-evaluation of birth weights at high altitude—study of babies born to mothers living at an altitude at 3100 meters. Am J Obstet Gyncol 1980;138:220–222.
22. Rayman RB. Genitourinary. In: Rayman RB, ed. Clinical aviation medicine, 2nd ed. Philadelphia: Lea and Febiger, 1990.
23. Connor SB, Leons TJ. U.S. Air Force aeromedical evaluation of obstetric patients in Europe. Aviat Space Environ Med 1995;66:1090–1093.
24. Mattson ME, Boyd G, Byar D, et al. Passive smoking on commercial airline flights. JAMA 1989;261:867–872.
25. Cameron RG. Effect of flying on the menstrual function of air hostesses. Aerospace Med 1969;40:1020–1023.
26. Preston FS, Baterman SC, Short RV, Wilkinson RT. Effects of flying and of time changes on menstrual cycle length and on performance in airline stewardesses. Aerospace Med 1973;44:438–443.
27. Iglesias R, Terres A, Chavarria A. Disorders of the menstrual cycle in airline stewardesses. Aviat Space Environ Med 1980;51:518–520.
28. Cahill GF Jr, Arky RA, Perlman AJ. Diabetes mellitus. In: Rubenstein E, Federman DD, eds. Scientific american medicine. New York: Scientific American, 1988.
29. Kelley WN, Palella TD. Gout and other disorders of purine metabolism. In: Braunwald E, et al. Harrison's principles of internal medicine, 11th ed. New York: McGraw-Hill Rock Co., 1987.
30. Conrad FG, Rossing RG, Allen MF, Bales HR Jr. Hazard rate of recurrence in patients with malignant melanoma. Aerospace Med 1971;42:1219–1225.
31. Conrad FG, Allen MF, Bales HR Jr, Rossing RG. Hazard rate of symptomatic recurrence in Hodgkin's disease. Aerospace Med 1972;43:1020–1023.
32. Conrad FG, Bales HR Jr, Allen MF, Rossing RG. Hazard rate of recurrence in germinal cell tumors of the testis. Aerospace Med 1972;43:893–897.
33. Moseley HS, Nizze A, Morton DL. Disseminated melanoma presenting as a catastrophic event. Aviat Space Environ Med 1978;49:1342–1346.

34. Smelsey SO. Study of pilots who have made multiple ejections. Aerospace Med 1970;41:563–566.

35. Rayman RB. Orthopedics. In: Rayman RB, ed. Clinical aviation medicine, 2nd ed. Philadelphia: Lea and Febiger, 1990.

36. Froom P, Ribak J, Tendler Y, Cyjon A, et al. Spondylolisthesis in pilots: a follow-up study. Aviat Space Environ Med 1987;58:588–589.

37. Schall DG. Non-ejection cervical spine injuries due to + Gz in high performance aircraft. Aviat Space Environ Med 1989;60:445–456.

38. ten Cate JW, Buller HR, van Royen E, Kamps J, et al. Incidence of deep venous thrombosis (DVT) during long non-stop air flights. Aviat Space Environ Med 1990;61: 485.

39. Steinhauser RP, Stewart JC. Deep venous thrombosis in the military pilot. Aviat Space Environ Med 1989; 60:1096–1098.

40. Centers for Disease Control. Update: universal precautions for prevention of transmission of human immunodeficiency virus. Hepatitis B virus, and other bloodborne pathogens in health-care settings. MMWR 1988;37: 377–382,387–388.

41. Marzuk PM, Tierny H, Tardiff K, Gross EM, et al. Increased risk of suicide in persons with AIDS. JAMA 1988;259:1333–1337.

42. Clark JB. Policy considerations of human immunodeficiency virus (HIV) in U.S. naval aviation personnel. Aviat Space Environ Med 1990;61:165–168.

43. Pitt HO, Pagano MA, Garau MA. HIV-encephalopathy: should we await a catastrophe before screening? Aviat Space Environ Med 1994;65:70–73.

44. AIDS Clearinghouse. Two pilots seek reinstatement because they had HIV, not AIDS. AIDS Policy Law. 1995; 10:5–6.

45. Pettyjohn FS, Spoor DH, Buckendorf WA. Sarcoid and the heart—an aeromedical risk. Aviat Space Environ Med 1978;48:955–958.

46. Silverman KJ, Hutchins GM, Bulkley BH. Cardiac sarcoid: a clinicopathologic study of 84 unselected patients with systemic sarcoidosis. Circulation 1978;58: 1204–1211.

47. Roberts WC, McAllister HA Jr, Ferrnas VJ. Sarcoidosis of the heart: a clinicopathologic study of 35 necropsy patients (group 1) and review of 78 previously described necropsy patients (group 11). Am J Med 1977;63: 86–107.

48. Hopkirk JAC. Respiratory diseases. In: Ernsting J, King P, eds. Aviation medicine, 2nd ed. London: Butterworths, 1988.

49. Delaney P. Neurologic manifestations in sarcoidosis, review of the literature, with a report of 23 cases. Ann Intern Med 1977;87:336–345.

Chapter 20

The Passenger and the Patient in Flight

Kenneth R. Hart

Aeromedical evacuation presents no problem as long as one remembers that man is adapted for life at or near sea level.

A. Johnson, Jr.

The airplane has revolutionized virtually all aspects of life. In the past quarter century aircraft travel has created a bit of revolution or at least major evolution in the transportation of patients by air. The ubiquity of air travel has generated questions for passengers and their physicians regarding the medical safety of this method of transportation. This chapter will provide principles and guidelines to physicians and flight surgeons regarding both the air transport of the patient and medical advice to the traveling public.

THE FLIGHT ENVIRONMENT

The flight environment is physically and physiologically different from man's normal habitat. These differences and their clinicopathologic implications make flying a challenge and sometimes a threat to the passenger and patient (1,2,3).

Accelerative and Decelerative Forces

Accelerative and decelerative forces normally encountered in takeoff, landing, and maneuvers in general aviation and commercial aircraft are of no significance to the healthy individual other than the anxiety they may produce. For the seated passenger, these forces are either directed perpendicular to the abdomen and back or are head-to-foot force vectors of low magnitude produced in turns and are well tolerated. In a prone or supine patient, however, the landing and takeoff forces are in the long axis of the body and may become very significant (4). In the patient whose head is toward the front of the aircraft and who has an unstable or compromised circulation, venous pooling on takeoff can cause a significant decrease in cardiac output. The aircraft attitude on climb-out further aggravates this condition as a consequence of the acceleration vector and the steep climb angle, thus creating a sustained reverse Trendelenburg's position. Since few if any negative physiologic changes occur during the landing phase, it has become an accepted rule to position the patient with his head toward the rear of the aircraft. If there is any doubt about a given patient's sensitivity to this mild, sustained, headward acceleration, it can easily be countered by elevating the head and trunk.

Changes in Barometric Pressure

Barometric pressure decreases with increasing altitudes above sea level. The most familiar result of this change is "popping" or "clearing" of the ears, which equalizes the middle ear pressure. Gas volume expands as pressure decreases

(Boyle's Law), doubling at 5500 m (18,000 ft), where the pressure is halved. At cabin altitudes normally encountered in pressurized aircraft and in most unpressurized aircraft flights, these pressure/volume changes are not of great importance as long as air-containing body cavities are ventilated.

Barotrauma of the middle ear and paranasal sinuses is covered in detail in Chapter 17, "Otolaryngology in Aerospace Medicine," and only a few additional comments will be made here. The eustachian tube, normally closed, is readily opened by pharyngeal muscle action. Valsalva's maneuver or autoinflation will add active air pressure to this muscle action and is used by many experienced flyers. However, a "point of no return" can be reached, even with normal anatomy, at which the negative pressure in the middle ear cannot be overcome with maneuvers, and ear block or barotitis ensues. Flying with an upper respiratory tract infection is the usual cause of barotitis. Sleeping while descending is a common cause of barotitis because the sleeper does not readily sense the building ear pressure and does not naturally swallow as often as when awake. Nursing infants should be fed or encouraged to suck on a pacifier to stimulate swallowing; chewing gum is adequate for most older children.

Topical vasoconstrictors and antihistamine/decongestant medications are advised when flying with an upper respiratory tract infection, or when chronic obstruction cannot be avoided. Persons who use nasal drops or sprays should be advised to use their medication 15 to 30 minutes before descent and definitely not wait for the first sensation of middle ear obstruction. "Before descent" deserves an additional caution: these preventive measures should be used when the cabin pressure starts to rise, an event that commonly occurs on commercial airline flights before actual aircraft descent begins.

If ear block develops in the passenger or patient, the immediate use of topical vasoconstrictor may be of benefit and is worth trying. Many airline attendants and flight nurses are taught

polterization, forcing air into the middle ear with an external air pressure source while the patient swallows. This can be done using a rubber bulb designed for this purpose (Politzer bag), a bag-mask respirator, or, on most commercial aircraft, an emergency oxygen bottle-mask assembly. A common recommendation has been to ascend to an altitude above that at which the block occurred. Although sound, this is often impractical and may even be a safety problem with crowded airways and controlled airspace. A comatose, disoriented, psychotic, or uncooperative patient may require elective myringotomy before flight if transport by air is unavoidable.

The normal intestinal tract is relatively tolerant of gas expansion, and discomfort can be relieved by expelling flatus. Below 3000 m (10,000 ft) flight or cabin altitude, this gas expansion usually is not a problem unless compounded by gas-producing foods or gastrointestinal disorders. Normal abdominal gas expansion may cause considerable discomfort in the pregnant passenger, particularly in the last trimester of pregnancy.

Trapped gas anywhere in the body is a major problem and can have disastrous or fatal consequences. Disease, trauma, an invasive procedure, or surgery may cause trapped gas. In addition to gas trapped within the body, gas may be trapped around the body, as in pneumatic splints. Other pneumatic medical devices that may produce problems include cuffed endotracheal tubes, balloon bladder catheters, and aortic balloons. Such trapped gas must be eliminated, vented, or otherwise compensated for by pressurized cabin atmospheres that would minimize pressure changes. Certain specific conditions will be covered in more detail later in this chapter.

Hypoxia

The atmosphere contains 20.94% oxygen, and the absolute amount contained is a function of total atmospheric pressure. As one ascends to

3000 m (10,000 ft), the partial pressure of oxygen falls. For all practical purposes, this is the range of primary importance to passengers and patients. Pressurized aircraft rarely fly at altitudes that produce a cabin pressure altitude higher than the equivalent of 3000 m (10,000 ft), and the majority of unpressurized aircraft fly below that level. Physiologically, the body can compensate for altitudes of 3000 to 5000 m (10,000 to 15,000 ft) for a limited period of time. Above 5000 m (15,000 ft), supplemental oxygen always should be used.

The term "indifferent stage" often is used to describe the hypoxia that may occur at altitudes up to 3000 m (10000 ft), but many individuals are not indifferent at all. Deeper respirations may be felt, particularly while in light sleep, and breathlessness may be noted on mild exertion such as walking to and from the lavatory in a commercial aircraft. Frequent flyers are accustomed to these sensations, but airline personnel and physicians must remember that not everyone is a veteran flyer. The first-time or occasional flyer generally has some degree of anxiety about flying. This anxiety may be aggravated by mild symptoms of hypoxia and result in a distinctly uncomfortable, uneasy, or frankly agitated passenger or patient.

Compensatory mechanisms called into play in the presence of hypoxia include increased respiratory rate and volume, elevated heart rate and cardiac output, and the oxygen-hemoglobin transport characteristics often referred to simply as the oxyhemoglobin dissociation curve. Any condition that interferes with one or more of these compensatory mechanisms make the person more sensitive to any decrease in oxygen tension.

Known disease in a passenger or patient must be considered and allowances made or precautions taken if necessary. For example, the patient with coronary artery disease and exertional angina should be specifically cautioned about avoiding exertion on the aircraft. This precaution appears obvious but should be further translated or expanded to include the restriction of fluid intake (particularly alcohol) to minimize required trips to the aircraft lavatory. Of equal significance to known disease is the threat of unknown disease; subclinical and compensated pulmonary or cardiovascular disease or undiagnosed gastrointestinal bleeding with secondary anemia are examples.

Pressurized Cabins, Altitude Restrictions, and Oxygenation

All aircraft with pressurized cabins can maintain a certain pressure differential. This varies with each specific aircraft model and is determined by the engineering design of the pressurization system. A sea-level or ambient ground-level cabin altitude can be maintained up to the flight level at which the maximum pressure differential of the system is equalled. Above the flight level, cabin pressure will rise as a function of the inside to outside pressure differential (ΔP).

Because airframes, pumps, valves, and seals age and wear, each airframe loses some pressurization capability with time. The actual or effective ΔP will thus be less than the predicted or original design capability. This difference generally is negligible, however.

The United States Air Force C-9A (DC-9) can maintain a sea-level cabin altitude to about 5500 m (18,000 ft) (Fig. 20.1). This is typical of a large jet aircraft in commercial use, as well as executive jet aircraft. This capability is not indicative of the cabin altitude to be expected in normal flight profiles. Today, civil and military transport aircraft fit a profile that is determined by multiple considerations of distance, the best

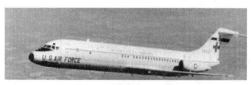

Figure 20.1. Air Force C-9A transport. This aeromedical evacuation aircraft, a modification of a civilian airliner, is specifically designed to meet Air Force patient-carrying responsibilities (official United States Air Force photo).

performance altitude, en-route weather, passenger comfort, aircraft safety, and optimum fuel economy. Pressurization systems consume energy and, therefore, are part of the total fuel costs. An aircraft capable of maintaining a 1,300 m (4,000 ft) cabin altitude at 11,300 m (37,000 ft) altitude with a maximum cabin pressure differential may actually be flown with a ΔP that results in a 2,300 m (8,000 ft) cabin altitude at that same flight altitude.

Medical recommendations for cabin altitude restrictions must be based on what a patient needs and how to meet these needs with a combination of supplemental oxygen and cabin altitude restriction. Unnecessarily extreme restrictions force the aircraft to be flown at lower flight levels, thus putting the aircraft into bad weather and turbulance that otherwise could be avoided, increasing fuel consumption and flight time by virtue of slower airspeeds, and perhaps requiring an en-route fuel stop, which extends the total mission time.

Misuses or abuses of the physician-recommended cabin altitude restriction are common. A patient who is adequately oxygenated in Denver, Colorado (1,700 m or 5,500 ft) or Albuquerque, New Mexico (2,000 m or 6,500 ft) does not need

a sea-level cabin on a flight to San Antonio, Texas but may well require a restriction to not exceed the cabin altitude of the point of origin.

A common problem that illustrates this fact regularly occurred in the western Pacific with an emergency air evacuation request to move a neonate from the United States Army Hospital at Seoul, South Korea to the neonatal intensive care unit at Tripler General Hospital on Oahu, Hawaii. Often, this request included a sea-level cabin restriction. If an infant requires 100% inspired oxygen at ground level for adequate oxygenation, this request is appropriate. A C-141 can make this move with a sea-level cabin; however it requires a flight altitude of 5,400 to 6,100 m (18,000 to 21,000 ft) resulting in slower speeds, increased fuel consumption and an added travel time of nearly two hours (Fig. 20.2). While the C-141B has inflight refueling capability, only under extreme circumstances will the aircraft be refueled with patients on board. This well-intended sea-level cabin restriction may then affect the patient and the attendants by virtue of the extra landing and takeoff required for refueling as well as the added total travel time, which can be as much as 5 hours.

In several years' experience with the United

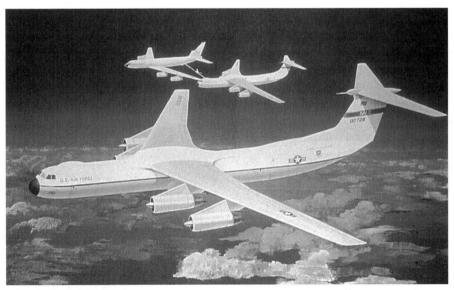

Figure 20.2. Airforce C-141 transport. This aircraft can be retrofitted for aeromedical evacuation missions (official US Airforce photo).

States Air Force worldwide aeromedical evacuation system, a 1,700 to 2,000 m (5,500 to 6,500 ft) cabin altitude restriction proved to be a magic number that ensured patient safety with a minimum impact on flight planning considerations in most cases. This rule of thumb was arrived at by assuming that ill patients do not have the same compensatory capabilities or tolerance to mild hypoxia as the healthy passenger because of obvious conditions such as anemia, cardiac disease, or pulmonary insufficiency. This assumption also was felt to be rational for anyone who was acutely or chronically ill. This empiric limit also correlates well with the conclusions of investigators at the British Royal Air Force Institute of Aviation Medicine after more than 20 years of experimental work (5).

Another fairly obvious rule of thumb arrived at by experience is "when in doubt, add supplemental oxygen." A fraction of inspired O_2 (F_{IO_2}) of 30 to 40% with a cabin altitude of 1,700 to 2,000 m (5,500 to 6,500 ft) allows for some leaks or losses in the delivery to the patient and still gives the patient a sea-level equivalent alveolar oxygen concentration.

The sine qua non in all difficult moves is a physician or flight surgeon who understands both the clinical needs of the patient and the capabilities and limitations of the aircraft as a consultant to the originating physician and balancing these often divergent factors.

Apprehension and Anxiety

Many individuals experience real apprehension or anxiety about flying. Some people are simply afraid to fly and, if they have the freedom to choose other options, either do not travel or use surface transportation. A widely known individual in this category is the former professional football coach and now television sports telecaster, John Madden. The majority of individuals do not have this freedom to choose an alternative method and are forced to fly because of various circumstances, such as the urgent need to travel a considerable distance in a short period of time,

when occupational situations allow no other alternative. The plentiful statistics that testify to the safety of both general aviation and commercial aircraft travel do not make as strong an impression as the sensational news coverage attending a major aircraft accident.

Airline personnel are trained to recognize, expect, and deal with the anxious passenger. Doctors must not forget that patients also may be afraid to fly. Reassurance is of great benefit, but some passengers or patients with significant anxiety may require medication.

It is difficult to recommend any particular drug because the choices are wide and individual response is highly variable. Today, many people who become airsick easily are aware of this and know those medications that are effective for them. A recent addition to the wide spectrum of available drugs is transdermal scopolamine. Dramamine, Bonamine, dextroamphetamine-scopolamine combination, and others are effective, as are the classic antihistamines and a variety of tranquilizer preparations.

METHODS OF TRANSPORT

A variety of aircraft are in use world-wide for the movement of passengers and patients. Aircraft types generally can be viewed as a single-engine and multi-engine, pressurized and unpressurized, and fixed-wing and rotary-wing. Single-engine and twin-engine unpressurized aircraft make up the largest group of general aviation aircraft; however, the number of executive and commuter, multi-engine, pressurized aircraft is increasing significantly. Rotary-wing aircraft (helicopters) are usually unpressurized; however, a new growth segment of the industry is the pressurized, "executive," turbine-powered helicopter. Commercial aircraft or those used in scheduled airline service are almost exclusively large, multi-engine, pressurized, turboprop or purejet aircraft.

Larger aircraft are less affected by turbulence, are less noisy, and the pressurized cabin offers significant comfort advantages to the passenger and the patient in the control of both cabin altitude and temperature. Features present in scheduled airline travel generally may apply to charter and airtaxi operations, with the exception that the amenities are fewer, and in some instances there may be no cabin attendant.

Commercial Airline Transportation

A paucity of data is available on the frequency and variety of passenger medical problems in commercial aircraft. Many anecdotal observations and experiences are well known to frequent travelers. Chapter 25, which discusses airline medical operations, provides some information for civil aviation. It also should be noted that there is only a limited system for reporting such data in military aviation.

The advent of jet aircraft that fly above most turbulence has greatly decreased the problems of airsickness, but it still occurs. Clinical problems of a more serious nature than airsickness also occur on commercial airlines and run the gamut from anxiety to heart attack and sudden death. Among the 450 million domestic air travelers per year it has been estimated there will be 3,000 inflight medical emergencies. The inflight national death rate was recently determined by one study to be 91 per 1 billion passengers (6).

A recently instituted Federal Aviation Administration (FAA) regulation now requires enhanced medical kits on board all aircraft capable of carrying 30 or more passengers. Contents of the kit are listed in Table 20.1. A published report of a review of the one year's experience with the enhanced kits revealed them to be extremely useful in some cases of life saving (6). This, combined with the frequent availability of health care providers among the passenger population, lowering morbidity and mortality associated with the emergencies may prove to be quite significant. Cabin attendants on commercial aircraft, while trained to recognize and cope with common maladies, have minimal medical emergency training (6).

Table 20.1.
Contents of Required Emergency Medical Kit

Component	Number
Sphygmomanometer	1
Stethoscope	1
Airways, oropharyngeal (3 sizes)	3
Syringes (sizes necessary to administer required drugs)	4
Needles (sizes necessary to administer required drugs)	6
50% Dextrose injection, 50 cc	1
Epinephrine 1:1000, single dose ampule or equivalent	2
Diphenhydramine HCl injection, single dose ampule or equivalent	2
Nitroglycerin tablets	10
Basic instructions for use of the drugs in the kit	1

Anderson JM. Medical News and perspectives: Emergency Medical Kits to be required cargo on commercial airlines. But will they fill the bill? JAMA 1986;256:167–169.

Passenger Accommodations

Major air carriers and airports are well equipped to accommodate the elderly, disabled, or ill passenger with a variety of assistance for transportation within the airport terminal and getting on and off an airplane. The cardinal rule here is plan ahead. If forewarned, airlines can make provisions, but last-minute "shows at the gate" with a passenger requiring total boarding assistance may result in a missed flight.

Many patients are transported by scheduled commercial airlines and, again, preparation and advanced notice are mandatory. A common airline practice is to accommodate stretcher patients in the first-class section by removing two to four seats (one or two seat pairs). This practice usually results, not unexpectedly, in a basic billing or fare scheduled based on four first-class seats.

Most commercial carriers are neither willing nor logistically able to transport a patient who requires extensive medical paraphernalia such as drainage tubes and bottles, suction, or electronic equipment (intravenous pumps and cardiac monitors). Nor are airlines required to carry a patient who might be considered offensive to other passengers. Virtually none have onboard therapeutic oxygen systems, but many airlines can provide or accept a carry-on oxygen supply if arranged well in advance. The FAA has stringent rules regarding oxygen bottles and other carry-on medical equipment, and individual airlines may have rules of their own. It is best to assume that there will be no preexisting clinical capability, and lead time will be needed to make everything work. (Don't forget connecting airline flights!)

Military Aeromedical Evacuation

The frequently cited first use of aeromedical evacuation was in 1870, during the siege of Paris, when casualties were evacuated by balloon (2,3). However, this has been questioned by the French General Berqeret who has stated that an evacuation of patients by balloon never occurred in 1870–1871 (7). The United States Army Air Corps used aircraft equipped to evacuate casualties in World War I, but an organized military patient air evacuation system did not exist until midway through World War II. The "air evac" value of the helicopter first became evident during the Korean War and was further expanded and widely utilized in southeast Asia. The United States Air Force short-haul and long-haul fixed-wing air evacuation system likewise expanded during these same years, and in 1975, the United States Air Force Military Airlift Command became the single manager for aeromedical evacuation for the Department of Defense. By charter and doctrine, the ground combat forces retain responsibility for battlefield evacuation.

In 1943, 173,500 sick and wounded were evacuated from overseas to the United States; in 1944, 545,000 were transported, and at war's end in 1945, the rate reached 1 million/year. The deaths during transport decreased throughout this period from 6/100,000 individuals in 1943 to 1.5/100,000 persons in 1945 (8).

The death rate for wounded in World War I who lived long enough to get medical care was

8.5%. During World War II, this rate dropped to 4%; during the Korean War, this rate was approximately 2%, and during the Vietnam War, this rate was 1% (8,9).

All improvements in the mortality rate cannot be attributed solely to air evacuation because many major advances were made in medical and surgical care, but rapid transportation by air with effective medical care en route certainly was a major factor. Not quantitative but perhaps even more important is the fact that the air evacuation system prevented overloading of the medical care facilities in the war theater.

Aircraft

Military air evacuation techniques always have been based on the inherent logistic facts of wartime that aircraft flying cargo (bombs and bullets) to the war zones are what must be used to evacuate patients on their return trip, or backhaul. Consequently, various systems or subsystems of medical personnel and medical equipment have been designed to refit the cargo aircraft for its air evac role. The C-131A Samaritan, introduced into service in 1954, was the first single-purpose aircraft in the United States Air Force inventory for aeromedical transportation, with built-in patient care features such as a therapeutic oxygen supply. This was followed in 1968 by the acquisition of the McDonnell-Douglas C-9A, which was totally designed as a single-purpose air evac aircraft.

Today, the United States Military Airlift Command operates an extensive worldwide network of people and aircraft providing peacetime routine and emergency movement of patients within and between overseas areas and the United State (Fig. 20.3). Medical policy and management are exercised from the United States Air Force Surgeon General through the Command Surgeon, Military Airlift Command to the Deputy Commander for Aeromedical Services, 375th Aeromedical Airlift Wing (AAW), which is headquartered at Scott Air Force Base in Illinois.

This structure includes two United States-

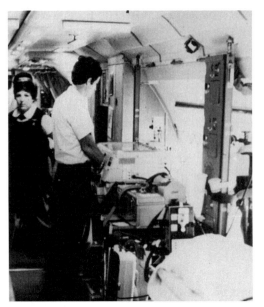

Figure 20.3. Patient management aboard the C-9A transport. A flight nurse is attending a premature infant being carried in a portable incubator (official United States Air Force photo).

based and two overseas-based squadrons of medical personnel and over 30 similar units of the Air Force Reserve and Air National Guard. This system operates regularly in peacetime, providing a necessary service to the military personnel of all the services stationed around the world. The primary reason for these peacetime operations is to provide the training and experience necessary to maintain a wartime capability. The system is capable of responding to national and international catastrophes on a moment's notice, as with the Jonestown, Guyana massacre and the Lebanon terrorists' attack on the peacekeeping forces.

The aircraft utilized in this Air Force system are the McDonnell-Douglas C-9A within the Pacific and European theaters and the CONUS and Lockheed C-141B for the strategic or long-haul routes between overseas and the United States. The C-21 Learjet, a recent addition to the air evac fleet, is being used with some frequency for emergency situations. The backbone of the tactical wartime system, the Lockheed C-130,

continues to provide support in some areas and some circumstances.

Other military air evac operations include the United States Army Military Assistance in Safety and Traffic (MAST) helicopter units and elements of the Aerospace Rescue and Recovery Service.

Policy and Doctrine

The United States Department of Defense (DOD) is prohibited by law from competing with private industry, and this fundamental precept underlies the existing DOD and Air Force rules on the use of the military air evacuation resources in response to the many civil requests for assistance. A key determination to be made in every case is whether civilian commercial air ambulance service is available and adequate. If it is available and adequate, policy and public law dictate that these civilian resources should be used instead of the military. Genuine medical need and not merely convenience also must be present.

When a civilian or non-DOD beneficiary is moved in the military aeromedical evacuation system, reimbursement is generally required. Depending on the circumstances, the actual dollar amount arrived at may be based on actual flying hour costs or more often, a fare basis. In the latter case, the standard use, assuming the passenger is in a stretcher or litter patient, is the previously mentioned commercial airline system of charging four first-class fares; to avoid the competition rules, the government billing then adds $1.00.

These recurring requests for military assistance are not easily dealt with because other considerations come into play. Is the commercial air ambulance service available and adequate in terms of equipment, personnel, and aircraft capability and adequate in timeliness? Also, while the request for air evacuation may meet all the necessary criteria, is the patient stable enough to withstand the move? These are frequently judgmental issues without clear black and white definitions and/or answers. The requestor is frequently dismayed or even outraged that such questions and deliberation are involved.

Air Ambulance Service

The air ambulance industry has grown exponentially in the past decade. This growth has been driven by a number of factors. The military experience in general and in southeast Asia in particular demonstrated the value of rapid air transport of the injured to definitive care facilities. Advances in medical care, with the concentration of centers of expertise such as in neonatology and trauma centers, created a greater need for safe transportation. The United States Army MAST program probably provided the single most important stimulus to community helicopter air ambulance service. Through agreement with the Department of Transportation and the Health and Human Services, MAST continues to play a major role in assisting local communities that do not otherwise have such services available. In addition to immediate air rescue for trauma victims, MAST now has an interhospital transfer system that is also available to those local communities where the need can be demonstrated. Australia, a land of vast distances and a scattered population, probably deserves the credit for being the leader in integrating the airplane into the health care delivery system by taking routine and emergency health care to the patients as well as using aeromedical transportation to transfer patients to centers of care.

Today, there are many first-rate private air ambulance companies as well as community-operated systems. There are also individuals who equate "air ambulance" to nothing more than having an airtaxi operator's license and an airplane.

Standards

In the United States at present, there are no federally mandated air ambulance standards. FAA regulations to date remain limited to aircraft safety and it appears unlikely those regulations will be expanded to include, within the purview of that agency, the essential aspects of emergency medical systems and patient care. Relative to federal assistance with respect to the medical systems of air ambulance, guidelines have been published by the Department of Transportation. These guidelines, while helpful, are not legally binding (10). Fourteen states have enacted rules and regulations that apply to air ambulances operating within their respective borders. Much variation exists among the standards, however, and must be based on the ground ambulance concept.

The air ambulance industry has not stood still, however. Major first-line companies have banded together and set a "standard" by precept and example, most notably the Association of North American Air Ambulances. In addition, standards established by the American Society of Hospital Based Air Medical Services (ASHBEAMS) in 1982, now the Association of Air Medical Services (AAMS), and standards published by the National Flight Nurses Association in 1986, remain in existence. However, there has been no structured accrediting process that would encourage agreement on national standards. With this concern, and after a comprehensive review addressing issues surrounding safety, quality assurance, standardization and reimbursement, the AAMS has taken the initiative to develop a commission to accredit air medical services. That organization has invited a number of relevant sponsors and has made extensive progress in forming the commission (11).

The air ambulance industry and the educated professional community remain firm in their convictions, and demand for high quality standards may prove to be the most effective of all. If not, the increasing number of related court cases may become the greater influence in setting standards for the air ambulance industry.

Type of Aircraft

Many air ambulance systems utilize the helicopter primarily for local area services and generally are limited to a 1-hour flying time radius

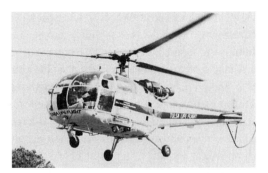

Figure 20.4. A community helicopter ambulance used for emergency patient transport.

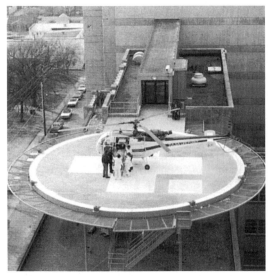

Figure 20.5. A patient being transferred from the Tulsa Life Flight helicopter to Hillcrest Medical Center in Tulsa, Oklahoma. Frequently, hospitals have built helipads on or immediately adjacent to the medical facility to expedite patient transfer.

of operations (Figs. 20.4 and 20.5). This can translate to a 100 to 200 mile radius of coverage. Virtually all of these helicopters are unpressurized aircraft simply because of the costs and mission profiles.

Helicopter transport of accident victims to hospitals can reduce patient mortality rates to less than half of those reported for similarly injured patients who are transported by ground ambulance. When similar injuries are considered, the airlifted patient experiences a 25% lower mortality rate. To achieve such spectacu-

lar results, it is imperative that the equipment and personnel delivered by helicopter and accompanying the patient to the hospital are appropriately trained for this demanding task. Further, appropriate continuation of care must be guaranteed at the receiving institution if the use of the helicopter is to achieve its optimum potential.

Fixed-wing aircraft in air ambulance services are as varied as they are in general aviation. Many short-haul systems utilize single-engine or twin-engine unpressurized aircraft, and, again, costs are primary considerations to the operator. The geography of the terrain also may dictate light aircraft with short takeoff and landing capabilities such as the intermountain western United States, Alaska, and Australia, where landing strips are often short, rough, and surrounded by natural obstacles. At the other end of the spectrum is the company offering coast-to-coast service in pressurized jet aircraft, the Lear jet being a common example.

Costs

Local community systems and some regional services are primarily driven by community and government subsidization. For example, some companies are transporting patients on a space available basis using their corporate jets. With these "Angel Flights" the costs are absorbed by the company. Consequently, the ultimate cost to the patient may range from nothing to a fee based on partial operating costs to a charge based solely on economics, that is, operating costs plus some amount of profit (12,13).

The cost to the patient will certainly vary depending on the sophistication of the system, the number of attendants required and the patient's needs for special medical equipment. This could be a few hundred dollars for a local-area helicopter mission to thousands of dollars for coast-to-coast jet air ambulance service.

Medical Attendants

Medical attendants should be provided by the air ambulance operator. In the major companies, these are often highly trained intensive care unit or coronary care unit nurses who have had additional training in flight physiology and patient care in the air. Major companies also will have full-time or consultant physicians who are both clinically expert and can fulfill the flight surgeon's role.

ASSISTING THE PATIENT

General Consideration

There are few, if any, absolute contraindications to moving a patient by air. Patients with acute myocardial infarction, pneumothorax, cerebral air embolism, and central nervous system dysbarism can be moved relatively safely with proper planning, personnel, medical equipment, and the right aircraft.

Improvements in medical care, somewhat synonymous with increasing technologic sophistication, also relate to the centralization of advanced medical institutions. This raises the demand for more patient transfers because the standards of care rise and the centers capable of meeting these higher standards are fewer and farther apart, for example, neonatal intensive care units, and organ transplant centers.

The major questions that must be faced and answered included: Is the risk to the patient in being transferred less than the risk of not being moved? Is the patient adequately stabilized? Are the benefits of the move real, and do they justify the clinical and fiscal costs? Is the move medically necessary or being driven by nonmedical or emotional concerns or the family's concerns?

These considerations may seem elementary, but one anecdotal experience stands out that will illustrate the importance of some of these questions. The patient was a 13-year-old girl who had sustained 90 to 95% second- and third-degree burns and had pulmonary complications. The Air Force was asked to move her from a major, well-staffed general hospital to a burn center in the Midwest. Part of the attending physician's rationale was that although her chances for survival were not good, she had the best

chance in a burn center. She was hypotensive, had little renal output, and, with the pulmonary burns, could not be adequately oxygenated in spite of all the best measures. After a consultation with the attending physician, the receiving physician, the air evac physician, and a physician in the United States Army Burn Center, there was general agreement that an immediate move was not medically indicated nor was it in the best interest of the patient. A transfer would be planned if and when the patient could be stabilized.

The attending physician needs to be cautious when faced with pressures or demands to transfer a patient for essentially nonmedical reasons. An example is the tourist who has a myocardial infarction while on a vacation trip, and the family wants the patient moved back home. Perhaps the move can be arranged with minimal risk, but even minimal risk may not be justifiable when the care required and being provided is the same in Honolulu, Hawaii as in Milwaukee, Wisconsin.

Transport Concerns

Mode of Transport
The mode of transport is generally dictated by what is locally available because there are many air ambulance companies with regional, national, and even international capabilities. In general, a patient will need at least the same provisions for care en route as is being provided at the hospital of origin such as oxygen, suction, intravenous tubes, and drainage bottles. Likewise, the medical attendant requirements will be at least as demanding.

A small, general aviation, unpressurized aircraft may be adequate in terms of distance and weather en route, but medical attendant and medical equipment requirements may dictate a larger aircraft. If cardiopulmonary resuscitation (CPR) is a potential en-route emergency, this will require an aircraft with adequate cabin room (13). The medical indications for a transfer also may dictate speed and a long-distance flight.

These conditions usually will mean utilizing a commercial air ambulance company that has larger jet aircraft.

Equipment

If a commercial air ambulance is being used, all equipment needs must be made known to the operator and the equipment's availability and suitability verified. If the originating hospital is providing equipment, special care and effort must be taken to ensure that the equipment will work on the airplane. Most aircraft have 28 V direct current and 110 V/400 Hz power, but 120 V/60 Hz power, which most hospital-based equipment requires, is a rarity. If battery-powered equipment is used, the power supply must be sufficient for the entire trip. Spare batteries are generally a good idea and are absolutely essential if needed for critical life-support equipment.

The amount of oxygen required should be calculated and then doubled. Plastic intravenous bags should be used instead of glass bottles, which can become hazardous missiles in turbulence. Pressure pumps or intravenous infusion pumps should be available because most aircraft cabins do not have sufficient height for adequate gravity flow.

A valid rule or approach to planning is to assume that ''Murphy's Law'' will be functioning. Every possible contingency must be thought of and accounted for in supplies and equipment: ''if you might need it, take it.'' This approach includes having all potentially necessary connections and adapters for such items as ventilators (13,14,15).

Coordination

The receiving hospital and attending physician must be fully aware of the evacuation plan and be prepared. Ground transport at origin and destination must be available and adequate to fully support the patient, equipment, and transport team. If the attendants who accompany the patient are not going the full route, that is, to the receiving hospital, the originating and receiving

physicians and the air ambulance must make sure before the fact that all needed preparations have been made.

Records

All pertinent records should travel with the patient. In addition, there must be adequate documentation of the en route phase—a complete record of treatment given and medication used.

CONSIDERATIONS FOR THE AEROMEDICAL TRANSFER OF PATIENTS WITH SPECIFIC CONDITIONS

Cardiovascular Disease

As has been indicated earlier, all care and treatment considerations that were needed at the hospital of origin are needed during transport. Whether the patient has a myocardial infarction, valvular heart disease, or some other cardiovascular disorder, if oxygen was required on the ground, it will be needed in the air, and the percentage of supplemental oxygen should be increased or ''titrated'' upward to give the same oxygen concentration at the en-route cabin altitude that was used at the originating hospital. If the patient did not require supplemental oxygen, adding it should be strongly considered, particularly if the cabin altitude will be above 1,400 m (4,500 ft).

If there is any question of cardiopulmonary resuscitation being required en route, the patient should be placed on a CPR board before the flight. This will be uncomfortable for the patient, but having it in place will pay handsome dividends if CPR is needed. The medical attendant should be qualified to treat cardiac arrhythmias and have the necessary medication to control this condition.

Pulmonary Disease

Untreated pneumothorax is an absolute contraindication to movement by aircraft unless there is no respiratory compromise and cabin altitude can be maintained at the ambient altitude of the point of origin. By far, the safest approach is to insert a chest tube. All chest tubes should have a Heimlich valve or other one-way valve assembly to prevent the retrograde flow of air into the chest.

Chest tubes should not be removed just before flight. Otherwise, evacuation should be delayed 72 hours after removal if possible, and a chest radiograph should be obtained 24 hours prior to flight. Glass-bottle drainage systems should be replaced with unbreakable plastic containers. Systems for this purpose are commercially available.

Chronic obstructive pulmonary disease patients require careful individual evaluation, with a tailoring of altitude and supplemental oxygen to maintain preflight conditions.

The transport of adults with acute respiratory failure is a major undertaking and is encountered more frequently today because of the recognition that specialized respiratory intensive care centers can greatly reduce morbidity and mortality. This type of move is best managed by a highly trained and experienced team (15). The physical space needs of such a team generally require a relatively large aircraft. Adequate stabilization of the patient prior to movement is of absolute importance. The cuffs of endotracheal tubes should be filled with normal saline to avoid problems associated with an inflated cuff during ambient air pressure changes. Given an adequately prepared and stabilized patient, blood gases en route are generally not needed (14).

Anemia

The patient who is acutely anemic because of hemorrhage or hemolysis will require the continuation of blood transfusions en route as well as supplemental oxygen. Many chronically anemic patients are moved by air, and generally do well if their hemoglobin is 8.5 g/dL or higher. Supplemental oxygen may be required in these patients, particularly on long flights or on flights

with a cabin altitude above 1,400 m (4,500 ft). In patients with hemoglobin values below 8.5 g/dL, supplemental oxygen should be used routinely. Patients with sickle cell disease should be maintained on an F_{IO_2} equal to that of their point of origin.

Burns

The two single most important considerations in the burn patient are adequate assessment and stabilization (15). Assessment is critical because resuscitation formulas are based on percentage of total body surface and the depth of burn. This calculation, in turn, determines the volume of fluids to be given in the first 24 hours and becomes a critical factor in stabilization. Commonly, the extent of burn in adults is overestimated, leading to overhydration and incipient or even frank cardiac failure and pulmonary edema. Infants and children are just as frequently underestimated as to the extent of burn. The presence or absence of pulmonary burn is likewise all-important, and all too often the survivable surface is fatal because of pulmonary burn. A preflight chest radiograph is important as part of the assessment regarding pulmonary burn and particularly important if a subclavian line has been put in or attempted because of the risk of pneumothorax.

Stabilization includes adequate airway patency, ventilation, and oxygenation, as well as adequate fluid resuscitation. In addition to intravenous lines, the patient should have a nasogastric tube in place because gastric distension and ileus are common.

Gastrointestinal Concerns

The special considerations regarding gastrointestinal conditions relate to trapped gas and gas expansion with altitude. Anxious patients tend to swallow air. This action could predispose to nausea and vomiting, which is not desirable in a patient with recent gastrointestinal surgery. Following abdominal surgery, pockets of air may remain in the abdominal cavity. For this reason, a general recommendation is that patients not be transported by air until 24 to 48 hours after the surgery.

Trapped gas in an ileus, hernia, or volvulus can expand, producing pain, and also may compromise the circulation in the bowel. For this reason, it may be prudent to delay the transport of patients who have had bowel anastomoses until intestinal motility has returned. When these conditions are present or if there is any doubt, a nasogastric tube with suction is indicated. Colostomy patients need to be advised to expect more frequent bowel movements because of gas expansion and be provided with extra bags.

Orthopedic Situations

As a general rule, all casts should be bivalved, unless, in the opinion of the attending orthopedic surgeon, bivalving would jeopardize the fracture. This is not necessary in the case of an injury in which sufficient time has elapsed to be confident of no vascular compromise from wound edema. Some still remain skeptical regarding tissue swelling at altitude and the need for bivalved casts. There is, however, a dramatic and tragic illustrative case report in the literature, where this phenomenon led to bilateral leg amputation in a child who was transported by commercial airliner from the United States to South America on the sixth postoperative day (3).

Swinging weights for traction are dangerous in an aircraft because the weights are potential missiles and, even if restrained, can bounce in turbulence and produce painful and possibly damaging jerks on the limb. A relatively simple solution is a bungee cord traction or spring tension. Air splints should not be used because of gas expansion. A newer type of "apneumatic" splint is available that is filled with plastic pellet material, molded to the limb, and becomes essentially rigid when evacuated. This should not be a hazard from gas expansion; however, some air will remain, will expand, and may weaken or lessen the rigidity.

Stryker frames are recommended for spine fractures and spinal cord injury patients. The "Wedge Stryker" should not be used because it cannot be secured to the floor of the aircraft with standard tie-down spacing; the "modified wedge" is acceptable. Stryker frames also should be shipped as a complete unit because not all parts are interchangeable with other frames.

Vibration in the aircraft can be particularly disturbing to the fracture patient, and this is especially true in helicopters. The frequency and amplitude characteristics of helicopter vibrations are distinctly different and can potentially cause fracture movement and displacement. In the case of vascular injury and repair, casts should be windowed over the site of the repair in addition to being bivalved. This windowing will allow immediate access to the repair site in the event of a hemorrhage.

Neurologic Concerns

Patients with increased intracranial pressure and cerebral edema should be given supplemental oxygen to eliminate even the mild hypoxia present at reduced altitude. Cabin altitude should not exceed 2,000 m (6,500 ft). Brain injury patients may be exceedingly sensitive to footward acceleration on takeoff if transported with their head toward the front of the aircraft. If at all possible, these patients should be positioned with their head toward the rear.

Intracranial air is potentially disastrous regardless of whether it is from a penetrating injury, surgery, or diagnostic studies. If such a patient must be moved, a pressurized aircraft is necessary, and the cabin altitude should not exceed the ambient field level pressure at the point of origin. The presence of a cerebrospinal fluid leak from the nose or the ear is sometimes a contraindication to air transportation. The primary concern is that cerebrospinal fluid will be forced out on ascent and air and bacteria will be forced into the cranial vault on descent. One solution is a pressurized cabin and maintaining the cabin altitude at the altitude of the point of origin. That solution is ''no solution'' if the patient is being moved from high altitude to low altitude, for example, from Colorado Springs, Colorado to San Antonio, Texas. In that instance, the attending physicians must be made aware of the aeromedical concerns and make the final decision.

Those with seizure disorders must also be managed with special consideration relative to the inflight environment. Theoretically, mild hypoxia may precipitate seizures in the susceptible and supplemental oxygen to maintain ground-level equivalent will eliminate this risk. Also, the photic stimulated seizure in those with the disorder is well known, however, with appropriate shielding, particularly in propeller and rotary wing aircraft, this phenomenon can be prevented.

Psychiatric Situations

Psychiatric patients are just as prone to anxiety about flying as nonpsychiatric patients; consequently, sedative or tranquilizing medications should be ordered for flight if indicated. Any patient who required locked-ward precautions prior to transport would be moved as a stretcher patient, be specifically sedated or otherwise medicated for the flight, and be restrained.

Physicians and air evac personnel tend to be reluctant to insist on patient restraints, but this is misplaced sympathy. A violent patient on an airplane can have serious or even disastrous consequences in an incredibly short period of time. Subduing a violent patient is difficult in the best of times and places, and an aircraft in flight is the worst time and place.

Air Embolism and Decompression Sickness

Patients with air embolism or decompression sickness, whether from diving, flying, or surgical misadventure, are ''trapped gas time bombs.'' They may be disastrously ill, and air transportation is frequently called on to move

the patient to a hyperbaric treatment facility. The two important aeromedical concerns are 100% oxygen en route and cabin altitude control.

The 100% oxygen establishes a P_{O_2} differential to encourage nitrogen washout and may aid ischemic areas throughout the body. This is, of course, no substitute for compression therapy. A pressurized aircraft is mandatory unless faced with a short-distance move in an unpressurized aircraft that is immediately available versus a wait of several hours for a suitable pressurized aircraft. If faced with this dilemma, consultation with an expert in hyperbaric medicine should be obtained. The ideal situation is a pressurized aircraft that can maintain point-of-origin or destination field level pressure, whichever is lower.

High-Risk Pregnancy

Early identification of the high-risk pregnancy and elective transfer is clearly the best for mother, child, and the transport system (17). Unfortunately, the pregnancy may not be high risk until the membranes rupture prematurely or there is early onset of labor. There is also a reluctance on the part of many women to accept an early elective transfer because of the impact on the family unit.

If there is no active labor or other complicating factors, the transfer of the high-risk obstetric patient presents little in the way of problems and is of no particular risk to the mother or the infant. A cabin altitude restriction to 1,600 m (5,000 ft) may be recommended to avoid uncomfortable abdominal gas distension in an abdomen already filled with a uterus. If there is any question of placental insufficiency, supplemental oxygen should be considered.

If there is active labor, therapeutic efforts to stop or delay the labor should be used unless otherwise contraindicated, and a physician should accompany the patient (16). An obstetric delivery pack should be included along with any special equipment required by the physician.

Neonates

Neonatal transport has become a highly specialized type of patient evacuation by ground and air. The necessity of such transport has been driven by the development of neonatal intensive care units and the recognition that these units can significantly decrease infant morbidity and mortality.

The approach used in the United States Air Force aeromedical evacuation systems is similar to that found in many metropolitan areas in the United States and in other countries: first moving the neonatal transfer team to the patient for optimum assessment and stabilization and then transfer of the infant on a controlled-environment life-support system (18,19).

All factors in the transport of critically ill neonates are vital, and the two most important factors are temperature control and adequate oxygenation. These factors present significant difficulties if special transfer units are not available. A standard hospital incubator is better than no incubator at all and can be aided by keeping the aircraft cabin at as high a temperature as possible.

An aircraft with a pressurized cabin is preferred both for better temperature control and to minimize barometric pressure changes. Cabin altitude restrictions should be carefully determined based on the infant's oxygen requirements and the opposing factors related to the flight itself, that is, the minimum safe altitude for the route of flight, the aircraft's pressurization capability, and time, distance and fuel requirements.

Absolute assurance of compatibility must exist between the equipment needed and the aircraft used, as well as the availability and sufficiency of oxygen and electrical power. Equal attention must be given to the same factors in the transportation links at each end of the total move, from hospital to aircraft and aircraft to neonatal intensive care unit (18,19).

FUTURE PROSPECTS

Some vision of the future can be realized based simply on today's numerous related evolving initiatives. Those efforts directed to the enhancement of air evacuation systems in response to increasing needs is certain to increase specialization and sophistication in terms of our future technologic capability.

The Civil Reserve Air Fleet (CRAF) concept presently being developed will utilize specially designed equipment and "ship sets" to rapidly convert commercial MD-80s and Boeing 767s for military aeromedical evacuation during wartime. The concept as well as the technology that has evolved from the design are already influencing presently developing air evacuation systems. Similarly, development of equipment, supplies, and medical technology for space flight has and will continue to have a lasting impact on our operational inflight medical capabilities. Community short-haul systems will proliferate, particularly in metropolitan areas driven by centralized trauma units, neonatal intensive care units, and other specialty units, and city growth that outstrips surface road capacities. As these commercial ventures grow, they will create a larger market for specialized medical equipment designed for aeromedical use rather than fixed hospital use. This market exists today and will increase. This same market demand will see more specialized aircraft designs with built-in patient care features. Lastly, there will be a market for well trained aeromedical physicians, nurses, and technicians whose abilities as well have been enhanced with these rapid and dramatic developments.

ACKNOWLEDGMENT

In the first edition this chapter was authored by Daniel H. Spoor, M.D., M.P.H.

REFERENCES

1. Johnson A Jr. Treatise on aeromedical evacuation: I. Administration and some medical considerations. Aviat Space Environ Med 1977;48:546–549.

2. Johnson A Jr. Treatise on aeromedical evacuation: II. Some surgical considerations. Aviat Space Environ Med 1977;48:550–554.
3. Parsons CJ, Bobechko WP. Aeromedical transports: Its hidden problems. Can Med Assoc J 1982;126:237.
4. Reddick EJ. Aeromedical evacuation. Am Fam Phys 1977;16:154–159.
5. Ernsting J. The 10th annual Harry G. Armstrong lecture: Prevention of hypoxia—acceptable compromises. Aviat Space Environ Med 1978;49:495–502.
6. Cottrell JJ, Callaghan JT, Kohn GM. In-flight medical emergencies. One year of experience with the enhanced medical kits. JAMA, 1989;262:1653–1656.
7. Evard E. Letter to the editor. Aviat Space Environ Med 1989;60:472.
8. Department of the Air Force. Office of the Surgeon General. Concise history of the United States Air Force aeromedical evacuation system. Washington, D.C.: Government Printing Office, 1976;626–850/379.
9. McNeil, EL. Airborne care of the ill and injured. New York: Springer-Verlag, 1983.
10. Bare, WW. Air ambulance standards for Association of North American Air Ambulances. 116 West Church Road, Blackwood, New Jersey, 08012: Association of North American Air Ambulances, 1982.
11. Pozzi, E. Maintaining the highest standards. J Air Med Transport 1990;7:133–138.
12. Cooper MA, Klippel AP, Seymour JA. A hospital-based helicopter service: Will it fly? Ann Emerg Med 1980; 9:451–455.
13. Gilligan JE, McCleave D, Nicholson B. Retrieval of the critically ill in South Australia: A coordinated approach. Med J Aust 1977;2:849–852.
14. Safar P, Esposito G, and Benson DM. Ambulance design and equipment for mobile intensive care. Arch Surg 1971;102: 163–168.
15. Harless KW, Morris AH, Cengiz M. Civilian ground and air transport of adults with acute respiratory failure. JAMA, 240:361–365, 1978.
16. Pruitt BA Jr. The burn patient: I. Initial care. Curr Prob Surg 1979;16(4):1–55.
17. Brown FB. The management of high-risk obstetric transfer patients. Obstet Gynecol 1978;51:674–676.
18. Colton JS, Pickering DE, Colton CA. Evaluation of a life-support module used for air transport of critically ill infants. Aviat Space Environ Med 1978;50: 177.
19. Roy RN, Kitchen WH. NETS: A new system for neonatal transport. Med J Aust 1977;2:855.

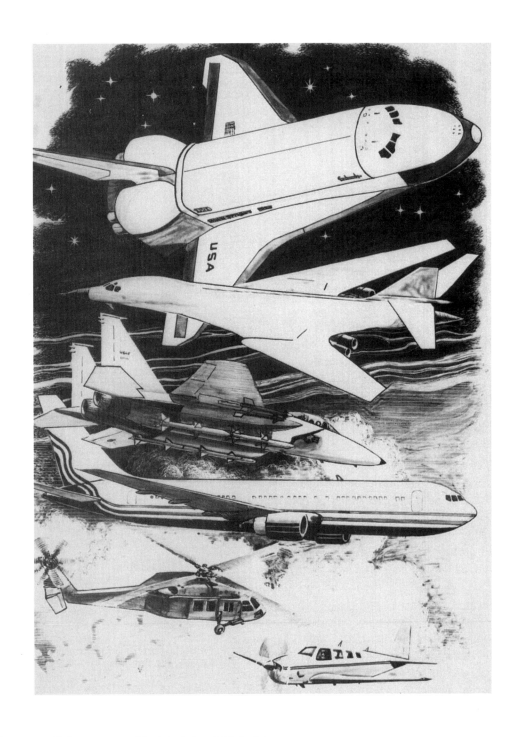

SECTION IV

Operational Aerospace Medicine

Supporting the flyer normally requires more than an office consultation. The physician who is unaware from observation and personal experience of the joy, demands, and stress of flying is ill prepared to deal professionally with the full spectrum of aeromedical issues. For the flight medical examiner or flight surgeon, the halls of the hospital become the runways of the airport. The excitement and tension of the surgical suite has its counterpoint in the exhilaration of flight, and the expectation of the delivery room is paralleled in each new experience that reaches beyond terra firma.

Like an expensive diamond, flying has many facets. Whether vocational or avocational, an airman is normally challenged by only a portion of the flight envelope. The pilot may never need worry about hypoxia while flying an ultra light or alternatively may be faced with all the demands placed on her flying skill and physiologic limitations when orbiting the earth.

Flight operations vary greatly depending on the purpose of the flight; however, the physician needs to be knowledgeable about those operational activities which are to be supported. Private flying ranges from soaring in a sail plane to flying high-performance jet aircraft. Commercial aviation may include agricultural flying, cargo transport, air ambulance activities, and of course, passenger services, ranging from the small commuter airlines to international air carriers. Aerospace operations are of international scope and require an international organization to coordinate and facilitate cross border flight operations.

Military operations provide the greatest professional challenge to the flight surgeon because all aspects of this specialty come into play. Each branch of the armed forces has unique features as part of its air operations, and these features are delineated in the appropriate chapters.

Human engineering, ergonomics, and flight deck management are important considerations for safe flight operations. When an aircraft incident occurs, search and rescue and aircraft accident investigation activities commence.

Although the numbers of individuals fortunate enough to go into space are small, the interest is great, and the physician lucky enough to work in the space program is frequently involved in the scientific frontier of aerospace operations.

Recommended Readings

Air Forces Institute of Pathology. Aerospace pathology for the flight surgeon. Washington, DC: US Printing Office, 1986.

Boff KR, Lincoln JE, eds. Engineering data compendium. Human perception and performance. Wright-Patterson, AFB, OH, Armstrong Aeromedical Research Laboratory, 1988.

Crowley JS, ed. United States Army aviation handbook. 3rd ed. The Society of US Army Flight Surgeons, Fort Rucker, AL, 1993.

Famer E. Human resource management in aviation. Brookfield,UT: Auebury Technical, 1991.

Mekjavic IB, Banister EW, Morrison JB, eds. Environmental ergonomics sustaining human performance in harsh environments. Philadelphia: Taylor and Francis, 1988.

Nicogossian AE, Hunton CL, Pool SL. Space physiology and medicine. 3rd ed. Lea and Febiger, Philadelphia, 1994.

O'Hare D, Roscoe S. Flightdeck performance, the human factor. Ames, IA: Iowa State University Press, 1990.

Weiner EL, Kanki BG, Helmreich RL, eds. Cockpit resource management. San Diego: Academic Press, 1993.

Chapter 21

Aerospace Medicine in the United States Air Force

Warren L. Carpenter and

Kenneth R. Hart

In the future, the limitations for optimal use of air and space may not be imposed by mechanical systems but by the physiological systems of man.

Harry C. Armstrong

The United States Air Force's (USAF) aerospace medicine program began with World War I. The high loss rate of American pilots in Europe caused General Pershing to direct a medical board to travel to France to study and define contributing medical problems and to draft recommendations for their correction. These recommendations formed the rationale for the establishment of an aviation medicine program; to provide trained military surgeons to implement and conduct this program, a school for flight surgeons was established in 1918. The first 50 flight surgeons were authorized by the Army in that same year. Central to many of the recommendations were three elements: (a) aviator selection criteria; (b) health maintenance specific to the needs of the aviator; and (c) the development of aircrew protective equipment. These three elements remain vital constituents of today's Air Force aerospace medical program.

The 396,000 active duty men and women of the Air Force form a key element of our national defense posture. Of the 26,500 aircrew officers, 19,500 are pilots. Assigned to support these and other aircrew personnel are over 500 flight surgeons, 100 of whom are certified specialists in aerospace medicine. The USAF program has the largest professional commitment to aerospace medicine found in the western world.

AIR FORCE MISSION

In the pursuit of our nation's defense, the USAF has a vital, diverse, and challenging role. It maintains a strategic warfare deterrent by operating two legs of our nation's triad — long-range bombers (Figure 21.1, Figure 21.3) and intercontinental ballistic missiles (ICBMs) — and provides military ground forces with air superiority and tactical air-to-ground frontline support capability. The Air Force operates a massive airlift force capable of transporting men and equipment worldwide. It also commands a broad space program, including operational manned space systems. Table 21.1 summarizes the type and number of active Air Force aircraft.

TRAINING MISSION

Each year, 1800–2200 young men and women enter undergraduate pilot training. A smaller

687

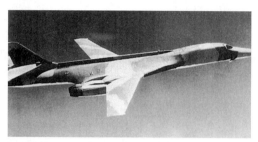

Figure 21.1. B-1B "Lancer." The Air Force's latest operational strategic bomber which assumed the penetration mission from the vintage B-52 (official USAF photo).

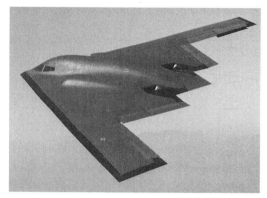

Figure 21.3. B-2 "Spirit" Advanced Technology Bomber. The product of a highly successful research and development program to develop a long-range, low-observable nuclear/conventional capable bomber (official USAF photo).

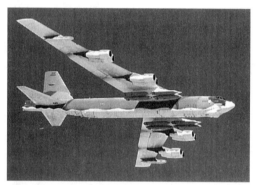

Figure 21.2. B-52 "Stratofortress." The mainstay of the Triad's strategic bomber leg for more than a quarter of a century (official USAF photo).

Table 21.1.
Number and Type of USAF Aircraft (1994)

Type of Aircraft	Number
Bomber	178
Tanker	332
Fighter/attack	1817
Reconnaissance	137
Cargo	734
Airborne warning/C3I	71
Helicopter	135
Trainer	1205
Special operations	136
Total USAF Active-Duty	4745
National Guard	1596
Air Force Reserve	468
Total available aircraft	6809

Table 21.2.
Applicants for Undergraduate Flight Training and Medical Qualifications

Year	1987	1988	1989
Number of applicants	6527	5305	5453
Medically qualified	5613	4722	4677
Granted medical waiver	244	242	218

number of individuals begin navigator instruction. Each of these students undergoes a preliminary flight physical examination and takes a written test to evaluate flying aptitude.

The physical examination is conducted by a flight surgeon. Unique to this examination is an extensive interview to assess the motivation and suitability of the candidate for aircrew training. The flight surgeon pursues the reasons why the candidate desires a flying career. During these inquiries, physicians assess the psychosocial development of the candidate and focus attention on any history of susceptibility to motion sickness or episodes of unconsciousness. The physical standards for entry into pilot training are among the most demanding in the Air Force.

Table 21.2 illustrates that in the initial selection process approximately 13% of applicants are disqualified. Unusually qualified candidates

who have only minor medical defects may be granted a medical waiver to permit further processing for possible selection for aircrew duty. Over the years, the medical reasons for disqualification have remained essentially the same. Historically, impaired vision and refractive

Table 21.3.
Medical Attrition of Undergraduate Pilot Trainees (UPT)

	1986	1987	1988	1989
UPT	2085	2088	1891	1931
Medical attrition	74	87	68	62

errors accounted for the greatest percentage of disqualifications. Other causes included allergic and vasomotor rhinitis, excessive and substandard height, history of unconsciousness, and immature psychosocial development evident during the interview.

The rationale for the attention given the physical examination becomes clear when one realizes that the cost of undergraduate pilot training is over $308,000 per student. Thus, to select an individual who is later eliminated for medical reasons is not only devastating emotionally to the individual but costly to the taxpayer.

One of the initial courses given students is physiologic training. This is an introduction to the stresses of flight and to the hazardous environment in which they will be working. Important features of this training are the opportunities provided the student to experience the effects of hypoxia, gravity-induced loss of consciousness (G-LOC), spatial disorientation, and situational awareness. The symptoms of hypoxia and their sequence of occurrence tend to be reproducible and unique to each student. The flight surgeon provides numerous hours of lectures and has the opportunity to interact with the students.

During the year of training, a percentage of students are medically disqualified and fail to complete training. These numbers are small and reflect the excellence of the medical selection process in identifying medical defects prior to the student selection for training. Table 21.3 reviews the medical attrition rate for undergraduate pilot training for four consecutive years beginning in 1986. Chronic airsickness leads the specific causes for disqualification, followed by visual defects, dysfunction of the eustachian tube, allergic and vasomotor rhinitis, and disorders of the musculoskeletal system. Sports injuries and motor vehicle accidents are the primary reasons for musculoskeletal disorders occurring during training. In undergraduate flight training, medical attrition for all causes averages 3.6% of the total number of students who receive training.

Students experiencing problems with airsickness may request assistance from the flight surgeon. It is the physician's responsibility to evaluate the problem thoroughly. Should there be no underlying cause other than the flight environment, the flight surgeon provides reassurance and, if necessary, supervises the limited use of medication for a prescribed period to permit adaptation. Should they fail to overcome symptoms, students are eliminated from training.

In the past, upon completion of primary training, the pilot or navigator was selected to enter training for a specific type of aircraft. The aircraft designation was most often based upon airmanship, with little consideration given to medical factors. Modern aircraft — with their increased speed, high G-loading, and cockpit complexities — place demands on the pilot for increased cognitive abilities, strict crew discipline, and rapid adaptability to stress. As such, aviation life sciences inputs have become increasingly important in matching the pilot to the aircraft. Recognizing this, the USAF has instituted a system of Specialized Undergraduate Pilot Training (SUPT), whereby an individual is classified into one of two "tracks" prior to entering flying training. One track leads to pilotage of fighter/bomber type aircraft and the other to tanker/transport. The decision regarding which track an applicant pursues is determined following a battery of evaluations, which includes a physical examination, psychomotor testing, various psychological questionnaires, personal interviews, anthropometrics, and an assessment of the applicant's motivation. Should an individual be eliminated from training in one track, limited opportunity to cross to the other would exist.

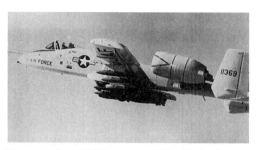

Figure 21.4. A-10 "Thunderbolt II" attack aircraft. This airplane was principally designed as an anti-tank and close air support aircraft (official USAF photo).

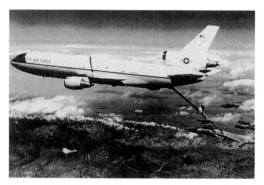

Figure 21.6. KC-10 "Extender" refueling an F-15 "Eagle" (official USAF photo).

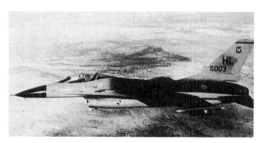

Figure 21.5. F-16 "Fighting Falcon" fighter aircraft. This aircraft was designed as both an air-superiority tactical fighter and close air support attached aircraft (official USAF photo).

The attributes needed by a pilot flying a low-level, highly maneuverable A-10 mission (Figure 21.4) or a high-speed, air-to-air "dog fight" F-16 profile (Figure 21.5) are different from those required of the pilot on a long-duration, tedious B-52 bomber mission or a short-haul, repetitive C-130 cargo flight. For example, visual correction may be tolerable in a cargo aircraft but could reduce the combat edge for a tactical mission. Asymptomatic mitral valve prolapse may be of little concern in selecting KC-135 copilots, but could result in serious cardiac arrhythmia when pulling G forces while maneuvering after a weapons delivery run in an A-10 or F-16. The flight surgeon, through professional training and operational experience, can make significant contributions in matching the person to the aircraft. The attributes that can be assessed biomedically are potentially as significant as airmanship or intellect.

AIRLIFT MISSION

The airlift mission is the rapid transportation of military personnel and equipment anywhere on the globe. Strategic airlift employs large aircraft, such as the C-141, C-5, C-17 and KC-10 (Figure 21.6), flying intercontinental, transoceanic, long-duration flights. The tactical element uses smaller cargo aircraft, such as the C-130 or C-23, conducting in-country, short-haul flights. The type of mission defines the aeromedical problems and issues to be addressed by the flight surgeon.

In the strategic airlift scenario, the crew is faced with fatigue, boredom, noise, circadian rhythm desynchronization, inflight feeding, and dietary disruption. The tactical airlift operation may involve numerous flights daily, often to poorly equipped airfields under marginal landing conditions with minimal hygienic standards, fatigue, environmental extremes, and noise. Use of the chemical defense protection suit may be required if the crew were in a combat area. The suit may compromise crew performance significantly and increase physiologic and psychological stress.

TACTICAL MISSION

Military tactical airpower has two fundamental mission elements: assuring air superiority and providing air-to-ground interdiction and frontline support. The flight surgeon must be prepared to address the effects of the combined stressors that are inherent in the high-performance aircraft environment and that tend to reduce pilot effectiveness. High acceleration with rapid onset and extended duration can be exceptionally fatiguing and has the potential to impair vision and induce loss of consciousness. Sensory data inputs from inside and outside the cockpit have the potential for cognitive overload. Thermal extremes are common, and the intense threat from air-defense systems appropriately produces anxiety.

RECONNAISSANCE MISSION

The collection, assimilation, interpretation and transmission of information is essential to all military operations. Operating above the Armstrong line (20km or 61,000 ft), the high-flying U-2 and TR-1 aircraft are but one element of a series of related programs used for these purposes. For about 30 years, U-2 aircraft performed strategic reconnaissance missions, as well as important nonmilitary photographic roles. The TR-1, a derivative of the U-2, is the airborne platform for the Tactical Reconnaissance System and is designed to provide theater commanders with a nearly real-time comprehensive picture of the battlefield situation. Flying at altitudes in excess of 21,340 m (70,000 ft) necessitates that the solo pilot wear a full-pressure suit, often for periods exceeding 12 hours. This, in conjunction with an oxygen prebreathing period for denitrogenation purposes, the complexities of the mission profile, a confining cockpit environment, problems with inflight "tube meals," and water intake and egress are adversities with which the pilot must contend. In addition, waste products must be disposed of without undue pilot inconvenience or interference. At this altitude, concerns about radiation exposure exist. Further, pilots occasionally experience the break-off phenomena.

The flight surgeon and aeromedical team supporting these complex missions must be cogni-

zant of these problems and others in order to prevent combined physiologic and psychological stressors from degrading the crew member's ability to operate these demanding aircraft.

Strategic Mission

The Air Force's strategic mission is accomplished from both airborne platforms and subterranean facilities. The B-1B, B-52, and FB-111 constitute the major elements of the airborne strategic force. When declared operational, the long-range B-2, Advanced Technology Bomber (ATB), will provide a major improvement in capability by operating across the full spectrum of conflict and complement the B-1 in responsibility for penetration roles. The B-52 will then become an air-launched cruise missile carrier, and the FB-111 will transition to theater operations with the tactical forces. The nature of the mission frequently requires aircrew to be on flightline alert for immediate deployment. This procedure contributes to stress, which becomes amplified when airborne. The flight surgeon, participating as an aircrew member, becomes intimately aware of these factors and the effects on the crew. Low-level, long-duration flights, involving precise navigation, frequent refueling, and constant threat in a combat environment are concerns for aeromedical support of these aircrew.

Missile crews in underground launch facilities also have specific stressors with which they must cope. Because of similarities in operational factors, missile crew medical support is the responsibility of the aerospace medical service. Boredom, isolation, and noise, as well as the possibility of radiation and toxic exposures, are some of the factors with which the flight surgeon must be prepared to cope.

Military Man in Space

The Air Force Space Command is the executive agent for the Air Force military man-in-space (MMIS) mission. Specific responsibilities and functions appropriate to the military organizations are well defined and heavily weighted toward operational utility. Responsibilities in command and control, surveillance and observation, and testing and evaluation of military systems aboard the Space Shuttle have become continuing activities for the MMIS community. Flight surgeons supporting this mission must be trained and well versed in the art and science of aviation medicine. In addition, they must be professionally competent in space medicine. They are prepared to assist their crews in coping with the space adaptation syndrome (space sickness), problems of ergonomics and human engineering, galactic and solar radiation, cardiovascular and muscle deconditioning, bone demineralization, and the many problems involved with extravehicular activity.

AIR FORCE AEROSPACE MEDICINE PROGRAM

USAF directives define succinctly the objectives of the aerospace medical program to be the promotion and maintenance of the physical and mental health of Air Force personnel and other persons for whom the Air Force is responsible. These objectives are to be attained by the application of principles of flight medicine, environmental health, and bioenvironmental engineering. The flight surgeon is charged with the primary responsibility for the conduct of this program. The physician is the coordinator of the team of specialists involved. In the USAF, the operational systems that the flight surgeon supports include aircraft, missiles, and space vehicles.

Flight Medicine

Within the USAF environment, flight medicine is that branch of healthcare that is responsible for the medical aspects of the selection and maintenance of flying personnel. The population served by this discipline is not limited to aircrew members but frequently involves all personnel who are directly involved in the support of aerospace operations, including all flying personnel, missile crew members, and air-traffic-controller personnel. Many flight medicine clinics expand their medical role by incorporating other individuals, such as maintenance personnel, who support operational activities. It is also essential for the flight surgeon to become the "family physician" to the dependents of flying personnel.

The flight surgeon's responsibility is broad and includes a variety of activities integral to the maintenance of the health of flying personnel. These activities include providing periodic flight physical examinations, supporting flying safety activities, ensuring crew effectiveness, providing medical training regarding self-care, conducting periodic aeromedical indoctrination on the hazardous environment of flight, actively participating in the squadron's flying activities or joining a crew in a missile launch facility, conducting a variety of medicomilitary activities, and encouraging participation in prospective healthcare programs. To accomplish these activities, the flight surgeon must spend a considerable amount of time outside the office. As in the case of any practicing physician, the flight surgeon must make ward rounds, but in this context the ward becomes the flight line, control tower, or missile launch facility.

Another major and important responsibility for the primary flight surgeon involves the aeromedical disposition process. The process is outlined as three levels of care. Primary care involves the initial evaluation by the base or primary flight surgeon who evaluates the crew member for medical care or routine periodic evaluation. Secondary care or evaluation by the consultant begins when the primary flight surgeon refers the crew member to an aeromedical specialist. The next level or tertiary care may be required and involves referral of the crew member for an extensive evaluation at the Aeromedical Consultation Service of the Armstrong Laboratory at Brooks Air Force Base. Each of these levels is addressed in more detail throughout this chapter.

Aeromedical Disposition

The aeromedical disposition process begins when the applicant applies for flight training. When selected to participate in aerial flight, the individual has successfully completed the first element of a career-long physical assessment process. Subsequently, the aircrew member receives periodic physical examinations varying in frequency and detail depending on duties as a crew member. Normally, these assessments find the crew member in excellent health, but occasionally medical abnormalities are revealed that require further evaluation and illnesses are experienced requiring intervention by the medical team. The disposition of these medical problems, whether found on physical examination or presented as a clinical problem, must be evaluated with regard to job performance and safety.

Primary Care: Evaluation by Flight Surgeon

When a crew member presents for medical treatment or evaluation, the flight surgeon must decide whether the medical findings will jeopardize health, flying safety, or mission completion. Within the Air Force, it is normal practice to remove individuals from flight duties when they experience acute illnesses, sustain injuries, or require medication. During the periodic physical assessment, changes in examination findings may exceed acceptable norms. In such patients, the flight surgeon must make a disposition regarding the patient's ability to continue flying. In the vast majority of cases, the crew member is grounded only temporarily to allow sufficient time for the acute illness to subside or to clarify the significance of an abnormal physical finding.

Procedurally, flight surgeons do not actually ground anyone. They serve as consultants and staff officers to flying unit commanders and provide recommendations that the individual be removed from flying status for a period of time. Such recommendations are rarely ignored.

Once crew members have recovered from acute illnesses, they return to the flight surgeon for reassessment and clearance to return to flying. Likewise, if the physical examination were to reveal minor abnormality outside the range routinely permitted for that physical condition, the flight surgeon would request a waiver for the medical problem from higher headquarters. In both cases, the flyer is returned to duty. Periodically, the flight surgeon is faced with a disease or physical finding requiring the assistance of consultants.

Secondary Care: Evaluation by Consultant

Acute illnesses are a potential for serious sequelae. Physical findings necessitating more refined evaluation require the flight surgeon to turn to professional colleagues for consultation. Such consultative services may be available at the local medical facility, or they may require the crew member to go to a large, regional hospital or medical center for more extensive evaluation. From the aeromedical point of view, the evaluations have two goals. The first goal is to ensure that the medical problem is not complicated by engaging in aerial flight, and the second goal is to ensure that the medical condition will not compromise flying safety. With these two goals in mind, the flight surgeon arranges for the consultation and necessary evaluation.

The consultant's primary role is to evaluate the medical condition and to provide a diagnosis. The consultant physician may recommend appropriate treatment or determine the frequency and scope of further evaluation. It is not the consultant's role to define the impact of the medical condition on the flying career of the individual. This remains the province of the unit flight surgeon who is directly responsible for the medical support of the crew member.

Tertiary Care: Evaluation by Aeromedical Consultation Service

Once the consultant's evaluation is complete, the flight surgeon initiates the appropriate disposition action, returning the person to aeronautical duties, requesting waiver for an established medical condition, or advising the flyer of the incompatibility of the medical condition with continued flying. Periodically, the base flight surgeon requests evaluation and consultation from the Aeromedical Consultation Service of Armstrong Laboratory. The service and process of this disposition process is detailed in the section describing the activities of the Armstrong Laboratory.

In the USAF, flight surgeons must be physically qualified to participate in aerial flight. When possible, the flight surgeon is expected to fly frequently as a crew member in the primary aircraft of the squadron. When multiseat aircraft are not available, the flight surgeon conducts flying activities in designated support aircraft.

For 35 years, the USAF has conducted a pilot-physician program. These physicians, who are qualified both as operationally-current pilots and flight surgeons, have made significant contributions to advancing aerospace medicine. Currently, 5–10 physicians fly as operationally-qualified military pilots. Their activities are deeply involved with flying safety, aircraft accident investigation, medical consultation to aircraft systems project offices for new aircraft, and evaluation of problems involving human-machine interfaces. Past experience has shown that one to two exmilitary pilots rejoin the Air Force as physicians each year. From this pool, the cadre of pilot-physicians is drawn to meet high-priority Air Force requirements.

Public Health

Within the aerospace medicine program context, public health is concerned with preventive medicine, public health, and health education. Responsibilities for this phase of the aerospace medical program rest with flight surgeons and environmental health officers. This function, in its broadest sense, has as its concern the health of the community. The immunization status of the population on the base, including the military work force as well as the civilian employees and dependents, is an area of interest. The public health control of communicable disease, such as influenza, hepatitis, and disease endemic in other parts of the world, is a responsibility of this program. In consonance with this, the Public Health Office becomes actively involved in international activities as a monitor of quarantine programs associated with movement of materiel across international borders. The wholesomeness of food brought on base for service military personnel, its preparation, and its storage are important considerations. Issues of hygiene in public facilities, barber and beauty shops, and food service concessions receive attention under this program.

The role of appropriate health education to encourage effective preventive health practices is a part of environmental health. Programs are conducted not only in the medical and dental facilities but also in educational and recreational facilities throughout the base. Special courses are conducted periodically to assist in weight control, physical fitness, smoking cessation, and nutrition.

The objective of the USAF occupational medicine program is to protect occupationally-exposed personnel, both military and civilian, from health hazards in their working environment. The department assists in the placement of personnel in occupations that the individual can perform effectively without endangering the worker or others. Such placement advice is provided after due consideration of all the physical, clinical, and emotional capabilities of the employee. The flight surgeon or occupational medicine specialist provides guidelines for physiologic monitoring of exposure to adverse environmental factors, reviews hazard assessments, establishes a diagnosis and makes disposition in occupational illnesses, and works closely with other components of the aerospace medical team toward optimizing the working environment for the occupational employee.

Bioenvironmental Engineering

Working closely with the physician is the bioenvironmental engineer (BEE), whose primary responsibility is conducting the nonclinical portion of the occupational medicine program. The BEE supervises health and environmental quality of the work environment and the implementation of controls for hazard abatement. It is the BEE's responsibility to establish and conduct industrial hygiene and environmental monitoring programs to assess compliance with federal, state, and local standards. To this end, the BEE is the Air Force's compliance officer for these legislated programs, which typically include all compliance and testing elements required by state health and environmental protection agencies. Recent legislation in air quality, hazardous materials, asbestos control, and drinking water has markedly increased the importance of this program in the Air Force. This department also maintains surveillance and compliance of potable water supplies and waste disposal systems. Engineering expertise is most needed in responding to accidents that could pose significant health hazards to the base and community.

Other Disciplines

Although not considered organizational elements, aerospace physiology, aerospace nursing, and aeromedical evacuation remain significant members of the flight medicine team.

These disciplines, as well as others to be described, represent a broad spectrum of services that collectively comprise a complex range of activities that involve aeromedically-related research and development, medical care, environmental and occupational health, and preventive medicine.

Through a multiplicity of evolutionary changes, the education, training, and research involving these disciplines have become integrated within two organizations, the USAF School of Aerospace Medicine and the Armstrong Laboratory. Both organizations are under the management of Human Systems Center at Brooks Air Force Base. The establishment of two separate institutions at Brooks Air Force Base represents a recent change in the long standing organizational structure that once included only the School of Aerospace Medicine as the center of national and international preeminence for Aerospace Medicine research and education. This most recent change was conceived and implemented in consideration of progress and the necessity to react to the demands of further requirements.

Remodeling for Change

Throughout their 75-year evolution, the USAF School of Aerospace Medicine and the Armstrong Laboratory not only have had to realign themselves to changing technology, but in so doing they have influenced the course of that technology, as seen in today's explosive advances in the aviation and space medical environments. The institutional flexibility and vision in responding to ever-changing challenges have been built on the foresight of its founders and fostered by the fresh thinking required to maintain its continuing focus on science and academics. In the many organizational changes of the past 75 years, the academic and research programs have addressed the many disciplines necessary to support the functional environment of the aviation and aerospace systems of their day. The needs which drive those environments and systems have sustained the institutions in which many of us have worked for more than 30 years.

All who have taken part in this impressive heritage can look with pride upon the products of our institution. In 1917, our aeromedical research laboratory became a separate academic institution. This change, undertaken during a perceived decline in research needs, set the stage for a series of fluctuations in mission priorities between academics and research. Although integration was maintained conceptually, the two activities have been physically separated and rejoined several times since the 1930s as a result of meeting new demands and in response to expanding technologic needs. Although the model of integration of the worlds of academic, clinical and research efforts still holds true today, the geometric proliferation of aerospace medical technology continues to strain conceptual boundaries, forcing more explicit redefinition of scientific and academic goals and objectives. The need exists once more to readjust the organization and the philosophy of the USAF aerospace medicine program to meet the changing demands of the future.

The latest readjustment was influenced, in part, by trends in an academic world that stress the importance of a structured learning environment to enhance not only basic knowledge but, notably, to foster performance. Education, as an applied science, became an integral factor in the adjustments to government-mandated resource limitations and the growing technologic environment. Organizational roles and needs of the future must be redefined more clearly, and resources currently available to meet those needs must be identified and applied before looking to new discoveries. Clearly, our roles will inevitably become more distinct and specialized as current realities displace cherished traditions of the past. Most specifically, we are faced with the paradox of broadened demands, limited resources, and increasing expectations for precision.

The most recent, and perhaps the most significant, change in the chronology of the USAF aerospace medical program has been precipitated by the current evolving (and somewhat bewildering) milieu of science and technology, a milieu that required reorganization and revision of management. Refinement and consolidation are the key terms that apply; their necessity is apparent when one considers the constraints of resources in the face of expanding and overlapping areas of organizational activity. The terms also apply in defining our scientific, clinical, technologic, and educational efforts. Although the structural changes within the Human Systems Center (HSC) began in December, 1990, their implementation continues today. The wisdom of similar changes in the past has been proved historically; therefore, we can project into the future our perception of a current need for change.

All the many laboratory functions of HSC, which included such activities as Aeromedical Clinical Sciences, Crew Technology, Armstrong Aeromedical Research Laboratory, have been combined into a multicentered but well defined Armstrong Laboratory. The consolidated laboratory joins with HSC's Human Systems Program Office to ease the translation of laboratory technology into operational systems. A preeminent agency in aeromedical life sciences, Armstrong Laboratory, with the Human Systems Program Office, provides a smooth science-to-system flow, ensuring that people remain the central focus in aerospace systems. The base of academic knowledge for this system's development lies within the newly-defined USAF School of Aerospace Medicine. With this mission, the USAF School of Aerospace Medicine emerges solidly as the academic arm of the Human Systems Center vision, and the premier institution for aerospace medical education for the USAF Medical Service.

The school's academic status, enhanced through expanded and refined curricular content, and its association of faculty appointments and medical center affiliations, recalls clearly the university concept envisioned more than 40 years ago by Major General Harry G. Armstrong. Whether Armstrong's concept of the synergism of clinical medicine, research, and academics has remained intact through the recent organizational realignment remains to be proven.

It is important to recognize the concept of integration and consolidation as we review the organizational and functional aspects of each of the scientific, technologic, and educational elements of the new organization.

USAF SCHOOL OF AEROSPACE MEDICINE

Postgraduate Medical Education in Aerospace Medicine

Within the United States, the Air Force is the largest employer of professionally- and paraprofessionally-trained personnel in the field of aerospace medicine. To meet the demand for quality-trained professionals, the USAF conducts an extensive program in postgraduate education in the field of aerospace medicine. The scope of the program ranges from a primary course to a residency program for physicians, and includes education and training for nurses and medical technicians in aeromedical evacuation, training for scientific personnel in the environmental hazards of flight, and training for engineers in the assessment of the environment.

The Primary Course in Aerospace Medicine

Three times per year, approximately 110 physicians arrive at the USAF School of Aerospace Medicine (USAFSAM) at Brooks Air Force Base, Texas, to begin their indoctrination and professional education as Air Force flight surgeons (Figure 21-7). In the seven weeks that they remain at USAFSAM, they are exposed to and participate in lectures, seminars, and workshops. They receive training in aircraft egress, accident investigation, disaster response, triage, altitude chamber indoctrination, principles of survival, and an indoctrination flight in an Air Force jet trainer. The clinical skills of these physicians are sharpened in those areas of particular interest to aerospace medicine, such as ophthalmology, otolaryngology, psychiatry, and internal medicine. Throughout the course, one principle is stressed: an effective flight surgeon is above all

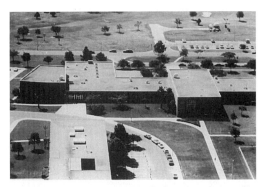

Figure 21.7. The USAF School of Aerospace Medicine, Brooks Air Force Base, Texas (official USAF photo).

an excellent physician. The training is devoted to the extra attention necessary to meet and solve the special problems of the flyer.

The training and practice in aerospace medicine involves three functional areas. The first area addresses flight and missile medicine, the most unique area for the majority of physicians coming into the field. The prospective flight surgeon must learn the processes of applying medical standards to the initial selection and follow-up evaluation of aircrew members. As in most phases of medicine, periodic examinations must be used to detect unexpected disease and to prevent the onset or progression of chronic ailments. Emphasis is placed on the careful evaluation of minor complaints to maintain pilots in peak mental and physical health for optimal performance in their flying duties. The second functional area receiving emphasis is the application of clinical medical specialties in the fields of otolaryngology, ophthalmology, internal medicine and its subspecialties, neurology, and psychiatry. Each has significant contributions to make in its area of expertise in relation to the health maintenance of the flyer. The third functional area is the broad concept of environmental health. This concept involves the review of classic public health principles and the establishment of an appreciation of the responsibilities of occupational medicine. The various techniques of evaluating occupational hazards are discussed and the concept of protective measures introduced.

Successful completion of the primary course permits the physician to wear the wings of a flight surgeon. Not all flight surgeons are assigned to primary duty in support of flyers or to operational flying units. Career Air Force physicians are encouraged to take the primary course in aerospace medicine to enable them to better support the Air Force mission regardless of their normal clinical and professional responsibilities. Since the conclusion of World War II, approximately 22,000 physicians have received primary aerospace medical training in the USAF.

Specialty of Aerospace Medicine

The specialist in aerospace medicine has made the career decision to receive extensive formal training in the field. The USAF has requirements for over 100 aerospace medicine specialists. To satisfy these requirements, the Air Force conducts the largest aerospace medicine residency program in the western world. Each year, 20–25 physicians enter the program. These Residents in Aerospace Medicine (RAM) are men and women who have had operational experience as flight surgeons and have now selected more extensive education in the field. The Air Force program also trains military physicians from other services, applicants from other federal agencies, and medical officers from allied nations. For convenience of management, the residency is divided into three phases.

Phase 1 is an academic year normally conducted at a university department of public health and leads to a master's degree in public health (MPH). The completion of this year ensures that the flight surgeon receives appropriate postgraduate education in epidemiology, biostatistics, healthcare administration, and environmental health. These studies provide the RAM with a strong foundation on which to base future contributions to the field of aerospace medicine.

Phase 2 is conducted at USAFSAM. The RAM receives an extensive ground school and indoctrination program in an Air Force jet trainer and actively participates in the evaluation and disposition of problem aeromedical cases involving aircrew. The RAM participates in site visits to numerous operational USAF bases, industrial and manufacturing complexes, space training and launch facilities, and research institutions. The RAM also has the opportunity to pursue individual interests through rotational study periods within various research and investigational agencies at Armstrong Laboratory.

Because of the increased emphasis on the role of the RAM in space, emergency, occupational, and clinical preventive medicines, and in order to serve the Air Force's needs into the 21st Century, an extensive and comprehensive review of the residency program was made in 1990 in terms of mission redefinition, validated personnel requirements, and curriculum revision. As a result of this study, a curriculum was developed and approved for a Phase 3 program in Aerospace Medicine. The first residency class entered the third year in 1993.

Phase 3 consists of 12 months of practical experience in preventive and occupational medicine. Three months of preventive medicine training provides the resident experiences at city and state health departments through rotations in each of the program areas of responsibilities. Four months are dedicated to industrial occupational medicine at both military and civilian facilities where large occupational medicine departments are monitoring workplace hazards and addressing employee health concerns. Four additional months are spent at a referral medical center, where the residents concentrate their studies in those clinical areas that are of particular interest to the occupational medicine physician: orthopedics, dermatology, neurology, pulmonary medicine, allergy, or immunology. The remaining month is an elective in occupational medicine. Following this additional year of training, the resident is able to manage the entire aerospace medicine program which includes flight medicine, preventive and occupational medicine issues, and programs at military installations that protect the environment, workplace, and worker.

Additional Professional Education and Training

To ensure that the broadest application of all aspects of aerospace medicine are applied to the aerospace medicine program, all other team members also are trained at USAFSAM.

Hyperbaric Medicine

Management of patients with air embolism occurring in aircraft or altitude chambers led the Air Force to initiate a hyperbaric medicine program. Located at key bases around the world, the Air Force has positioned small, one-patient hyperbaric chambers to be available, when needed, for the management of aviators' bends. These chambers are also used to deliver oxygen under hyperbaric conditions as a treatment method for specific medical conditions. Technicians, physicians, and nurses are trained in hyperbaric medicine to operate these chambers and may expand their training via a one-year hyperbaric medicine fellowship program at USAFSAM. With growing awareness in the medical community of the benefits of hyperbaric oxygen therapy, the Air Force has constructed hyperbaric centers at its medical treatment facilities at Travis and Wright-Patterson Air Force Bases. The training program at USAFSAM is geared to provide an experienced cadre of professionals and technicians to operate these chambers

Aeromedical Evacuation

Each year approximately 300 nurses and technicians receive training in the management of patients to be transported in the Air Force international aeromedical evacuation system. Key to the training of these aeromedical crews is knowledge of the environmental factors of flight. Aircraft, such as the C-9, are designed for aeromedical evacuation, although they can not be considered true flying hospitals. Similarly, the C141 and C-130 cargo aircraft can be converted to provide backhaul aeromedical evacuation. Thus, all these aircraft are patient transportation systems and, although they may be sophisticated in their capabilities to support patients, they are nevertheless aircraft that generate acceleration forces, atmospheric pressure changes, noise, and temperature and humidity variations. These medical crews receive extensive training in the management of patients in such an environment.

Aerospace Physiology Training

Within the Air Force, the aerospace physiology training officer is the individual principally responsible for the indoctrination of student aircrew in the discipline of altitude and acceleration physiology. The training of these officers and

the technicians who support them is conducted at USAFSAM.

Bioenvironmental Engineering

Bioenvironmental engineers receive formal, postgraduate training in environmental engineering, environmental assessment, hazard abatement, industrial hygiene, and employee protection at both USAFSAM and civilian universities. In addition, these graduate engineers receive extensive firsthand experience as part of the educational program.

Preventive Medicine Residencies

Similar to the RAM program, other physicians may receive postgraduate training in general preventive medicine and occupational medicine at the Uniformed Services University of the Health Service (USUHS) and through sponsorship in civilian institutions. These separate residency programs are conducted to satisfy Air Force requirements. The programs draw on the enormous potential for worldwide teaching experience in these fields that is available to the Department of Defense.

Allied Officer Training

Many of the courses described in the previous sections are attended by allied officers from throughout the free world. An advanced course in aerospace medicine for allied medical officers is offered yearly by the Air Force. This six-month course is attended by 10–20 highly selected medical officers from friendly nations throughout the world. This course is designed to provide the knowledge and experience necessary for flight surgeons to return to their own countries and become leaders in aerospace medicine. The course has many parallels to the USAFSAM portion of the RAM program previously described. It is usual for the senior leadership of a nation's Air Force medical department to be drawn from graduates of this program.

ARMSTRONG LABORATORY

For over 50 years the USAF has had two institutions that have been key to the quality of its aerospace medicine program. The Armstrong Aerospace Medical Research Laboratory (AAMRL) at Wright-Patterson Air Force Base, Ohio (WPAFB), was founded prior to World War II and has maintained continuing research programs in aerospace human factors. The School of Aerospace Medicine (USAFSAM) at Brooks Air Force Base, Texas, has maintained its preeminence in the fields of education, clinical evaluation, and research.

However, as a result of the recent changes previously described, the clinical and research activities that were managed within USAFSAM and AAMRL were placed under the management of the Armstrong Laboratory. These two institutions, Armstrong Laboratory and USAF School of Aerospace Medicine, are now under a single organization for management and program direction: the Human Systems Center.

Armstrong Laboratory— Wright-Patterson Air Force Base

Founded in 1935, the Aero Medical Laboratory was chartered to resolve protective equipment deficiencies for aircrew flying open-cockpit aircraft. In 1985, this laboratory was renamed Armstrong Aerospace Medical Research Laboratory (AAMRL) in honor of its founder, Major General Harry G. Armstrong. Although still located at WPAFB, the laboratory has become an integrated element of the newly formed Armstrong Laboratory. Through the years, AAMRL has continued to conduct biomedical and behavioral research to define the limits of human tolerance and to assure that humans can perform under the environmental stresses associated with aerospace operations. These activities are directed toward the advancement of technology in physiologic tolerance of the aircrew member to the effects of acceleration, noise, vibration, and toxic hazards; human-machine integration and protection requirements have been major long-term activities.

The staff of more that 270 scientists, engineers, and technicians at AAMRL are currently involved in research organized in three primary disciplines: (a) biodynamics and bioengineering as it relates to protecting USAF personnel against environmental injury associated with aerospace operations; (b) human engineering studies aimed at learning more about physical and mental performance capabilities as an element in modern complex systems; and (c) toxic hazards.

Biodynamic and Bioengineering Research

Mechanical forces are imposed on crewmembers in their day-to-day operations conducted by the USAF. These forces include sustained and transient acceleration and deceleration, aerodynamic deceleration, vibration, impact, and noise. For successful mission accomplishment, it is essential that the effects of the forces be controlled to acceptable levels in terms of human tolerance and safety. Research objectives in the areas of noise and direct mechanical forces emphasize effective performance and safety in the operational flight environment. Another application of biodynamics technology is in the reduction of morbidity and mortality resulting from ejection from disabled high-performance aircraft.

Noise produced in the Air Force environment impairs performance and can affect health. Voice communication problems are critical in tactical air operations. Research is ongoing to reduce these difficulties. The objective is to establish specifications and parameters that ensure voice communications effectiveness in high noise level environments. For the communities surrounding air bases, noise as an environmental quality issue becomes a concern. Technology has been developed by AAMRL to permit Air Force organizations to satisfy environmental noise assessment requirements stemming from the National Environmental Policy Act of 1973. Appropriate noise assessment technology must also be available to meet the requirements of the Air Installation Compatible Use Zone (AICUZ) program.

The AAMRL provides the Air Force expertise

in the bioeffects of mechanical force resulting from impact or alternating force fields (vibration). The research and development activities are typically associated with performance enhancement, crew comfort, and safety. With the use of the dynamic environment simulator, a multidimensional centrifuge, the laboratory conducts complex, real time simulations of air-to-air and air-to-surface combat engagements to define the effects of acceleration on pilot performance. Research is then directed toward developing technologies to reduce performance decrements.

The AAMRL represents a national resource with regard to both its scientific expertise and its sophisticated flight environment simulation devices. Organizations, such as the Department of Transportation and the National Aeronautics and Space Administration turn to this laboratory for support of their research requirements. The laboratory also accommodates both Army and Navy aeromedical research needs.

Human Engineering

The demands of modern warfare, particularly against numerically superior forces, require that Air Force research and development departments design systems and equipment for maximum effectiveness. The human operator is often simultaneously the critical component and the limiting factor of manned systems. High-performance aircraft, low-level, high-speed flight, high-density threat environments, and task saturation combine to provide a severe challenge to effective human-system performance. This challenge necessitates the development of revolutionary methods of reconnaissance, target acquisition, rapid data processing, decision-making, and effective command and control. The AAMRL conducts a major program to develop the technology for advanced visual display systems. These efforts concentrate on display and control systems that optimize the interface of systems operators to flight control, navigation, and command and control systems. This work has enhanced pilot capabilities through the development of head-up and head-down display

systems. Other aspects of this research address the critical questions of systems automation: that is, the allocation of decision making and control functions to the operator or to the onboard computer, the types of display information, stress effects, workload control, effective human communications, and appropriate human-machine interaction. Critical to evaluating the effectiveness of the application of these technologies is the development of methods to quantify the workload imposed on the aircraft operator. Both subjective and objective methods are under development to improve the ability to quantify workload and, more significantly, to prevent overload.

Toxicology

The research program in toxicology is designed to identify and quantify toxic hazards created by chemical agents characteristic of advanced Air Force systems and operations. Safe exposure criteria are developed for toxic chemicals that have the potential to cause adverse effects on personnel and the environment. Advanced analytic techniques are employed to study the environmental impact of these compounds and to clarify the modes of toxic action of a compound in biologic systems. The data derived from these studies provide guidance to Air Force product developers and users to ensure safe operations. Efforts continue to evaluate a number of new in vitro and in vivo screening methods for compounds with mutagenic, teratogenic, and oncogenic potential. Major studies concentrated on hydrazine, jet fuels, metallic slurries, new hydraulic fluids, tributyltin paints for ships, carbon-carbon fibers, and tracer substances used to identify leaks in gas masks.

Armstrong Laboratory—Brooks Air Force Base, Texas

From its origin to support medical requirements for the fledgling Aviation Section in the United States Army Signal Corps in World War I, to its ongoing research supporting the space shuttle orbiter, the USAFSAM and now the Armstrong Laboratory are the oldest continuously operating units in the USAF and have been at the forefront of aerospace medical research and development. As noted previously, the institutions fulfilled and continue to fulfill clinical aerospace medical practice and education missions, in addition to its research and development role. This execution of Air Force programs in research and development, education, and medical support in these institutions have been highly successful because of the synergistic effect and cross utilization of the professional staff. Clinicians involved in aeromedical assessment of problem medical cases still fulfill a significant teaching role in the educational program. Epidemiologists not only teach but define research requirements to be pursued by other elements of the institutions. Training of flight nurses and technicians in aeromedical evacuation delineated shortfalls in patient support requiring the research and development of new equipment. The Armstrong Laboratory research and development program is divided into three disciplinary categories.

Clinical Sciences

The value to the Air Force of highly skilled aircrew members increases in direct proportion to the increasing complexity and cost of new aeronautic and space systems. It is critical, therefore, that accurate and specific medical selection criteria be applied in choosing candidates for flight training, that the best possible medical care be given to the fully trained aircrew member, and that prevention of disease and the refinement of medical retention criteria be optimized to increase the career life expectancy or ''cockpit longevity'' of the Air Force flyer. The process of evaluating an aircrew member in the Aeromedical Consultation Service contributes to a growing data base enabling the clinical specialist, with increasing precision, to establish the significance of a medical finding to aerospace flight. Crucial to much of the effort conducted in this research program is the differentiation of normal from abnormal findings in asymptom-

atic, generally healthy aircrew. It has become clear that medical findings in this population may have a different significance from that related to hospital treatment populations.

Research is conducted and techniques developed to enhance aircrew performance. Biofeedback has been successfully employed in the treatment of those suffering from chronic airsickness. Visual corrective devices that are compatible with the aerospace environment have been developed; the acceptance of the use of soft contact lenses by aircrew of high-performance aircraft is such an effort. Research is ongoing to identify the psychophysiologic characteristics that may predict pilot performance in high-performance aircraft. This research contributes to the criteria for the selection of pilots for specific types of flight vehicles and missions.

Aeromedical Consultation Service

The Aeromedical Consultation Service at the Armstrong Laboratory was established to bring together experts in the major clinical specialties for the purpose of making recommendations regarding flyers whose aeromedical disposition is in question. Each year, 700–850 aircrew members, predominantly pilots, are evaluated by the Aeromedical Consultation Service. Historically, in 70% of patients, the result has been a recommendation for a return to flying duties. The vast majority of those individuals arriving for evaluation are assigned duties not involving flying (DNIF) at the time of evaluation. These evaluations, or the tertiary care previously discussed, enables the Air Force to retain the invaluable experience of more senior aviators and to avoid the enormous cost that otherwise would have been incurred in training replacements.

The consultation center is staffed primarily by specialists with flight surgeon experience. It is common to have physicians professionally qualified both in aerospace medicine and in a clinical specialty assisting in the assessment of those being evaluated. To ensure the emphasis on aerospace medicine and the integrity of the operational flight medicine concept, each patient is assigned to a flight surgeon who serves as a personal physician during the evaluation. Evaluations are extensive and take approximately one week to conduct. Problems most frequently seen are related to the cardiovascular system, central nervous system, and visual system. Consequently, these are the strongest departments in the consultation center.

Not all patients are initially referred by their base flight surgeon. Some referrals are requested by the consultation center as a result of preliminary evaluations. This request occurs most commonly in the area of cardiology, because the USAF Central ECG Library reviews and maintains a record of every ECG performed on aircrew members throughout the world. This valuable database is a one-of-a-kind resource for the epidemiology of various abnormalities and their predictive values. Abnormalities revealed by these tracings may require further evaluation and, consequently, the consultation center may request that the aircrew member be sent for an in-depth assessment.

Once the evaluation is complete, an aeromedical summary is prepared and forwarded to the base flight surgeon, who is responsible for the primary care of the aircrew member. It then becomes the flight surgeon's responsibility to determine the necessary action for disposition of the patient. Because of the significant nature of the majority of patients seen by the consultation center, waiver from higher headquarters, including the Office of the Surgeon General, is frequently necessary.

Disposition by Waiver

When it has been determined that the event or the medical condition, although normally disqualifying, would not compromise the health of the individual or flying safety, the flight surgeon may initiate action requesting a waiver. It remains the flight surgeon's responsibility to determine whether the condition of the patient is compatible with flying duties and to submit the appropriate waiver request. In many cases, the Major Air Command Surgeon has the authority to approve a waiver for a history of an event or medical condition. For potentially serious problems, the Air Force Surgeon General is the exclusive waiver authority. Crew members who are medically disqualified, but receive waivers for the disqualification, frequently are required to undergo periodic special medical assessments.

Within the USAF, the waiver policy is dynamic. It changes with improvements in diagnostic capabilities resulting from advancements in medical technology and the prognostic estimations of modern epidemiology. For many years, it was Air Force policy that a pilot must be medically qualified to fly any aircraft in the Air Force inventory. A major change has occurred in the medical waiver policy for flying personnel. Now waivers are issued in four major categories: (a) aircrew member who is universally assignable; (b) aircrew member is limited to tanker, transport, bomber, and mission support aircraft for reasons of low tolerance to acceleration or essential presence of a second pilot; (c) aircrew member who is limited to flying non-ejection seat aircraft; and (d) aircrew member for whom specific limitations are described.

By broadening the waiver window, the Air Force can expect to save \$95–100 million annually by avoiding the replacement training costs for aircrew members who otherwise would have been lost from duty. This new waiver policy increases the responsibility of the flight surgeon to make the proper aeromedical disposition.

Not all personnel receive a waiver for their disqualifying medical problems. Table 21.4 lists the causes for medical disqualification of pilots and navigators for 1980 to 1981 for which the Surgeon General has records, representing approximately 60% of those aircrew disqualified. Although these data are dated, no significant change has occurred over the past decade.

Advanced Crew Technology

Research programs under this discipline are pursued to ensure the protection, readiness, and effective utilization of aircrew in advanced and

Table 21.4.
Causes for Medical Disqualification of USAF Pilots and Navigators for Two Years, 1980 to 1981[a]

Diseases	Age Groups			Totals	Percentage
	20–29	30–39	40+		
Coronary artery disease	0	2	29	31	10%
Hypertension	0	7	23	30	10%
Degenerative spine disease	3	2	15	20	7%
Diabetes mellitus	0	6	8	14	5%
Asthma	3	4	6	14	5%
Headaches (migraine, other)	5	2	6	12	4%
Arrhythmias	1	4	5	11	4%
Abnormal ECG/EFF (treadmill)	0	0	10	10	3%
Peptic ulcer disease	3	0	5	8	3%
Syncope	1	4	3	8	3%
Alcoholism	0	3	5	8	3%
Obesity	2	2	4	8	3%
Abnormal EEG/seizure disorder	3	3	1	7	2%
Allergic rhinitis	5	1	1	7	2%
Sarcoidosis	2	4	0	6	2%
Ulcerative colitis	4	1	0	5	2%
Melanoma	2	1	1	4	1%
Peripheral neuropathy	1	1	2	4	1%
Chronic sinusitis	1	2	1	4	1%
Personality disorder	3	1	0	4	1%
Subtotal	36	50	125	214	71%
Other diseases	14	35	41	90	29%
Total	53	85	166	304	100%

[a] Data abstracted from the USAF medical waiver file by R. C. Whitton.

future aeronautics and space systems. The multistress environment of flight is simulated by the use of altitude chambers, thermal-stress generating devices, motion-based flight simulators, and a human centrifuge. Advanced lifesupport systems, including onboard oxygen generating systems (OBOGS), breathing and filtration masks, acceleration protection equipment, altitude protection systems, and personal thermal-stress protection systems are products of research and development efforts.

The objective of another research program is the prevention of aircraft accidents caused by human error. A database has been generated that includes actual accidents, near mishaps, and data concerning flight systems and operations. This database is structured to provide the ability to analyze actual accidents and to predict situations that could lead to accidents plus the capability to control and eliminate human factor related accidents.

Medical systems requirements for safe and effective transportation of patients by air in peacetime and wartime require research, development and operational testing of new airborne medical equipment. This is accomplished in advanced aircrew technology research and development programs.

Radiation Technology

The biologic effects of all forms of electromagnetic radiation, including lasers, radio frequency emitters, directed energy beams, and sources of ionizing radiation are addressed by this disciplinary effort. Technology documents define personnel hazard assessments, safe separation distances, performance estimates, and nuclear radiation hazard environments. Research is conducted to determine the bioeffects of both continuous wave versus pulsed radio frequency radiation generated by radar systems. Biologic dosimetric methods, the effects of electromagnetic radiation, and the mathematical modeling of the environmental impact of various energy generators are other important elements of this research.

In the future, the Air Force's operational commitment will continue to be shared by aeronautic and space systems. Hardware technology will continue to impose greater demands on the operator, in terms of environmental stresses, performance and integration of cognitive information processing, decision making and systems control. The USAF aerospace medical program will continue to be expected to meet the challenges: to select quality flight crew members, to ensure their protection inflight, to optimize their interactions with flight vehicle systems, and to maintain and extend their professional longevity.

Chapter 22

Army Aviation Medicine

Glenn W. Mitchell,

N. Bruce Chase,

Robert J. Kreutzmann

The helicopter has now changed the nature of warfare.
MG Rudolph Ostovich, III

During the last five decades, rotary wing aircraft have expanded the operational capabilities of both military and civil aviation. Although this chapter focuses primarily on helicopters used by the US Army, the principles discussed readily apply to other services and other nations. Helicopters are formidable weapons systems when configured as military gunships, yet they also save many lives each day when employed as medical evacuation vehicles. Helicopters may be used to carry troops into battle, thrill sight-seeing tourists, report urban traffic advisories, or interdict drug smuggling. They have been designed and/or modified to move heavy cargo, spray crops, and fight forest fires. Tilt rotor aircraft currently in final development blur the distinctions between fixed and rotary wing aircraft. For the foreseeable future, helicopters will continue to expand their roles in both military and civil flight applications due to versatility, improving capability, and decreasing cost of operation.

The United States Army has the world's greatest number and variety of helicopters, except perhaps for the former Soviet Union's forces. In 1990, 94% of the Army's nearly 9000 aircraft were helicopters, and the percentage increases as the size of today's Army shrinks. Its Aviation Medicine Program, therefore, must focus on the support of rotary wing flight operations. Although similarities exist, there are also major differences between high-performance, fixed-wing flight operations and the demanding nap-of-the-earth and air-to-air flight envelopes flown by the Army aviator, especially when performed under cover of darkness with night-vision goggles. Army flight surgeons and their staffs must conduct effective Aviation Medicine Programs during times of both peace and war to support the Army's physically and psychologically demanding flight programs.

ARMY AVIATION HISTORY

The early history of Army aviation and its aeromedical support is shared with the United States Air Force (USAF). Other sources cover its many details, but a brief overview sets the stage for what United States Army Aviation and Aviation Medicine have become today.

The United States became the first country to contract for a military airplane when the Signal Corps called for bids in December, 1907. According to official records, the Army took delivery of its first complete airplane, a Wright Type B Flyer, on August 2, 1909, and produced its own aviator, Lieutenant Frederick E. Humphreys, on October 6, 1909, when he soloed in that airplane. Another early Army airplane was reputed to have been made from 4468 lbs of salvage obtained from an aircraft crashed by the Wright brothers and sold to the Army for $1500. It was received in 17 boxes at the Wells Fargo Offices in San Antonio, Texas on February 3, 1910 and subsequently assembled and flown by LT Benjamin D. Foulois on March 2, 1910 at Fort Sam Houston, Texas. By 1914 the Army's "1st Aero Squadron" had grown to six aircraft. The first military use of these aircraft occurred during General Pershing's expedition against Pancho Villa in Mexico.

Airplanes made by several manufacturers were used extensively during WWI. At first they were employed to adjust artillery fires, but friendly hand waves between enemy pilots were soon replaced by dueling handguns. It was not long until machine guns and aerial dogfights involving whole flights ushered in air-to-air combat. Between the First and Second World Wars larger, faster, more heavily armed war planes appeared on the scene and challenged man's physiologic limits. Aviation assets during this era were known first as the Army Air Corps (1926) or Army Air Forces (AAF) (1941) until a USAF was established in 1947.

During the war, however, planners recognized the need for small observation and utility aircraft in the direct support of ground forces. On June 6, 1942, the War Department approved fixed-wing aviation, separate from the Army Air Forces, for use as spotters for field artillery. The first mission began November 9, 1942, when three L-4 Grasshoppers (Piper Cubs) were launched from the USS Ranger to adjust artillery fire in North Africa. All three aircraft were lost on that mission, largely due to friendly fire (1). Subsequent missions by L-4 and L-5 aircraft included adjustment of artillery and naval fire, reconnaissance, photography, message drop and pickup, medical evacuation, guiding patrols through dense jungles, supply of isolated units, and courier missions (2). These missions de-

manded durable, inexpensive aircraft with a short, unimproved field capability. The potential for using helicopters in these roles had been recognized earlier, but rotary wing technology was still in its infancy. In the interim, the military relied instead upon versions of small, single-engine commercial fixed-wing aircraft. After reaching a peak of over 3000 fixed-wing aircraft in the mid 1960s, the Army steadily replaced them with helicopters and in 1996, Army fixed-wing aircraft numbered < 400.

The Army funded research in helicopter design beginning in the 1920s. However, the first United States military helicopter flight did not take place until April 20, 1942, when Igor Sikorsky demonstrated his prototype helicopter. By January 1943, the YR-4B helicopter was undergoing tests as an air ambulance. Procurement and deployment followed, and on April 23, 1944, the first helicopter combat medical evacuation was performed by LT Carter Harmon in Burma (3). One hundred thirty-four R-4s were purchased for observation, reconnaissance, and medical evacuation. In spite of the advantages of rotary wing flight, the exploitation of helicopters progressed slowly due to low airspeed, limited payload and range, and greater maintenance requirements. As these limitations were overcome, use of helicopters grew. During the Korean Conflict, helicopters were known primarily for their medical evacuation role, but their use for observation, movement of personnel and supplies, and other purposes also grew steadily.

The military use of the helicopter came of age in Vietnam. This was due in large measure to the turbine powered engine, typified by the UH-1 Iroquois manufactured by Bell Helicopter. First designated the HU-1, its nickname became "Huey." It became known throughout the world by its characteristic sound in flight. This aircraft eventually exceeded the production record of all other aircraft in the history of aviation and became an ubiquitous symbol of rotary wing flight. Its great success was due largely to the greater reliability, lift capability, and lowered maintenance requirement of its turbine engine. Army aviation medicine takes great pride in the fact that this aircraft was initially developed under contract with the Army Surgeon General as an air ambulance.

Its advantages over contemporary helicopters led to its rapid adoption for many other military and civilian missions. In Vietnam, helicopters moved the vast majority of troops, supplies, patients, and equipment as well as seeing extensive service as gunships outfitted with rockets, grenade launchers and mini-guns. By overflying impassable terrain and landing at unimproved sites, (or even hovering where necessary) helicopters dramatically reduced response time from days to minutes for resupply, evacuation, and other missions, clearly proving the versatility and military importance of this platform. Today, every combat division is now heavily dependent upon rotary wing aviation for firepower, mobility, and power projection.

Each new helicopter and mission brought new challenges to the aeromedical community. New dimensions of physical, physiologic, and psychological stresses encountered as a result of evolving technologies and military strategies demanded an increasingly sophisticated aviation medicine program to help the aircrew deal with the aviation environment. Progress in countering these challenges has been remarkable, with accident rates going down as mission demands have increased (Fig. 22.1).

ARMY AVIATION MEDICINE HISTORY

The light fixed-wing aircraft assigned to field artillery units during World War II did not have organic aeromedical support. When the Army Air Forces converted into the USAF, most Army flight surgeons were transferred to this new service. In 1950, former AAF flight surgeon Lieutenant Colonel Rollie M. Harrison, stationed at Fort Sill, Oklahoma, was the only practicing aviation medical officer left in the Army. Most Army artillery aircrew depended upon generalists or AAF/USAF flight surgeons for their support.

Medical problems encountered early in the Korean Conflict by Army aviation units in forward areas underscored the need for organic aviation medicine support. In March, 1951, Major Spurgeon H. Neel (now Major General ret.) became the first Army physician to complete the Air Force basic aviation medicine course at Randolph Air Force Base, Texas (4). Next assigned to Korea, he played a major role in conversion of ad hoc line USAF and Marine aeromedical evacuation programs into an organized medical system. The concepts put into practice by MG Neel in Korea are still in use today, including subordination of evacuation assets to medical control, training of Army Medical Department (AMEDD) officers as medical evacuation pilots, and forward medical stabilization of injured soldiers when possible.

The growing importance of Army aviation led to reestablishment of an aviation medicine section in the Office of the Army Surgeon General on November 6, 1952 and to the institutionalization of Army aeromedical policy. Army Regulation 40–110, 12 November 1952, reestablished medical standards for Army pilots. The Army began an aviation medicine training program in 1953 at the Medical Field Service School at Fort Sam Houston, Texas, but this program was short-lived due to reduced funding after the Korean Conflict. By 1954, aviation medicine was officially recognized by the assignment of a separate military occupational specialty code for its practitioners. Completion of a recognized course in aviation medicine was a requirement for the new designation of Aviation Medical Officer.

In 1954, Army flight training moved from Fort Sill to the new Army Aviation School at Fort Rucker, Alabama. Colonel William H. Byrne became the Aviation School Surgeon in 1955 and developed programs to minimize aviator fatigue. During the same year, flight status for aviation medical officers was authorized. By September 1955, 28 Army aviation medical officers were practicing aviation medicine. Distinctive flight surgeon wings were authorized in 1956, and in the next five years, 150 Army flight

Accident Rates for US Army Helicopters
per 100,000 Flying Hours During FY73-90

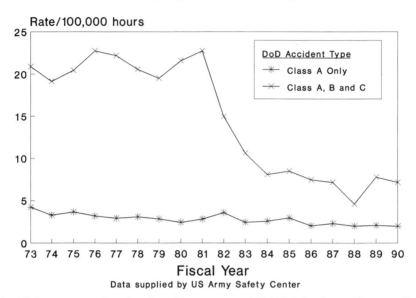

Figure 22.1. US Army rotary wing aircraft accident rates per 100,000 flying hours (data supplied by US Army Safety Center).

surgeons were trained, mostly by the USAF, with seven or eight per year trained by the Navy. Beginning with then-LTC Spurgeon Neel in 1956, experienced short course Army flight surgeons were selected for and trained in the USAF Aerospace Medicine Residency Program.

The 1960s saw continued growth of the Aviation Medicine Program. The formation of the US Army Aeromedical Research Unit (later Laboratory) at Fort Rucker, Alabama on July 6, 1962 under LTC John D. Lawson was a significant milestone. Then, in 1964, the Army again began training its own flight surgeons when the Department of Aeromedical Education and Training (DAET) was established under Colonel Spurgeon Neel as a department of the Army Aviation School. Over 130 flight surgeons per year graduated from 1966 through 1969 in support of the Vietnam Conflict.

The 1970s evidenced both growth and accomplishment. In January 1970 MAJ William Caput completed the first Army Flight Surgeon's Manual and provided two volumes of information

on both classic aeromedical subjects and Army unique aspects of flight medicine. In April, 1974 COL James E. Hertzog took command of the newly established US Army Aeromedical Center at Fort Rucker and consolidated the functions of Lyster Army Community Hospital and the Army Aeromedical Activity (AAMA). The Aeromedical Activity consisted of DAET, the worldwide mission of aircrew medical standards from the Office of the Surgeon General, and the local mission of rescue and aeromedical evacuation (FLATIRON or "always hot"). Tangible illustrations of Army aviation medicine's accomplishments during the 1970s also include the installation of the Army's only training hypobaric chamber at Hanchey Army Airfield in 1973, the testing of a molecular sieve oxygen generator for aviation, COL(ret) Burt Kaplan's invention of the MAST trousers, and Joseph Haley's development (with Harry Robertson) of a crashworthy helicopter fuel system.

The 1980s began auspiciously with the addition of flight training in the Army TH-55 helicopter through solo proficiency to the Basic Army Flight Surgeon's Course. This gave the new flight surgeon the valuable perspective of an aviator rather than a passenger. Between 1983 and 1984, a new multi-million dollar Army Aeromedical Center (USAAMC) was constructed at Fort Rucker. In 1984, the Academy of Health Sciences (now the Army Medical Department Center and School) and the Aeromedical Center formed the United States Army School of Aviation Medicine (USASAM) at Fort Rucker with responsibility for teaching aeromedical topics to aviation students as well as physicians, physician assistants, and other health care providers. Other highlights included the installation of the Army's only clinical hyperbaric chamber at USAAMC in 1986, construction of the new Aeromedical Research Laboratory (USAARL) in 1982, and formation of the Aeromedical Epidemiology Data Register (AEDR) in 1983.

ARMY AVIATION TODAY

Personnel, Equipment, and Missions

For many years, aviation personnel were drawn from Infantry, Armor, Artillery, Transportation, Military Intelligence, and the Medical Service Corps. This challenged the flight surgeon with the medical management of personnel of widely divergent training, experience, and philosophy. On April 12, 1983, the Army formed a separate Aviation Branch incorporating all aviation personnel except those in the Medical Service Corps. By 1990, the total aviation assets of the Army exceeded 8800 aircraft, along with nearly 24,000 pilots and 23,000 enlisted aircrew. Army Aviation today is an important combat arms branch having missions of air assault with movement of large combat units rapidly on the battlefield, close air support, resupply, air-to-air combat, special operations, command and control, armed reconnaissance, and deep interdiction into enemy rear areas. Army aviation is a highly lethal, mobile, flexible, and efficient combat force.

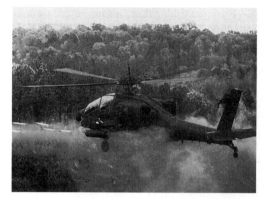

Figure 22.2. US Army AH-64A Apache attack helicopter (official United States Army photo).

The Army's newest helicopter gunship, the AH-64A Apache (Figure 22.2), because of its flight envelope and advanced avionics, gave the Army control of night combat and proved itself in the 1991 Desert Storm War in Saudi Arabia and Iraq. Its advanced electro-optical and weapons systems, high cost, potential for task overload of its crew, and physiologic and psychological demands from the monocular helmet-mounted display amplified the importance of aeromedical support. The next Army aircraft to be fielded is the light attack helicopter (AH-65 "Comanche") and will add significant flexibility and firepower to the Combat Army Aviation Team. Deployable weapons bays quickly convert from stealthy scout (weapons retracted but ready) to powerful gunship with Hellfire, Stinger/TACAWS and HYDRA-70 missiles as well as a 2-barrel 20mm Gatling gun. Helmet-mounted control systems now being developed for this aircraft include two monocular displays with different images presented to each eye.

Tactical Aeromedical Evacuation

The first Table of Organization and Equipment for an aeromedical evacuation unit was published in August, 1952, with seven officers, twenty-one enlisted, and five helicopters. This marked the beginning of the only dedicated aeromedical evacuation capability in any armed force in the world. Other military forces provide aeromedical evacuation, but this function competes with other mission demands for the limited aviation assets available. Helicopter ambulances grew to a peak of 140 in Vietnam and were widely known by their adopted call sign DUST-OFF. From May, 1962 to March, 1973, approximately 900,000 patients were evacuated. By May, 1966 hoists were installed in most medical evacuation helicopters to evacuate casualties from locations where landing was impossible, and approximately 8,000 hoist evacuations were made by the end of the conflict.

Statistics from Vietnam confirm that aeromedical evacuation in combat is high risk duty. Flying an unarmed, single aircraft with an immediate response mission in a hostile environment, air ambulance crew losses were 3.3 times greater than all other helicopter missions. Most hazardous was the hoist mission, which was seven times as likely to be hit as a nonhoist mission.

The helicopter air ambulance has decreased the time required to move a casualty from point of injury to a medical treatment facility. This has contributed significantly to increased survival rates. The current medical evacuation support for a division of 16,000–18,000 personnel is an air ambulance company with 15 UH-60A (Blackhawk) aircraft and 130 officers and enlisted soldiers.

Military Helicopters in Other Nations

In many nations all military aircraft are under the operational control of, or are located organizationally within, the Air Force of that nation. This is probably more a result of the total size of the forces involved rather than any lack of importance assigned to having tactical air mobility available to ground forces; the necessity of dedicated, readily available vertical lift capability is fully appreciated by all the forces involved. The full spectrum of helicopter missions, ranging from tank killer to medical evacuation, is found in military forces worldwide. In most nations, however, only a relatively small number

of rotary wing military aircraft and associated aircrew exist. A partial survey of the availability of such assets among NATO nations in 1990, for example, showed a range of 57–1322 helicopters and 84–2000 pilots per nation. (NBC, unpublished data.)

AEROMEDICAL CONCERNS OF ROTARY WING FLIGHT

From the beginning, the helicopter introduced new and unique aeromedical challenges. Unlike fixed-wing aircraft, most helicopters are unstable, and must be under active control during all phases of flight. Until the UH-60A Blackhawk, few helicopters had automatic piloting equipment or flight directors which reduce pilot work load. Army helicopter pilots often fly extended hours during challenging nap-of-the-earth (NOE) flight profiles, using night-vision goggles, enduring climatic extremes, and carrying out difficult tactical missions. All of these are highly important for the physician dealing with problems of aircrew fatigue. Helicopters as weapons platforms are relatively new to warfare, and present unique psychologic stresses. Army aviation, formerly in a combat support role, is now a full-fledged combat arms branch and a high-priority target of the enemy.

Vision

Almost from the dawn of aviation, good visual abilities were recognized as critical to successful flight. The earliest aeromedical standards (WWI) included both ocular health and visual function requirements. Because early rotary-wing aviators were initially fixed-wing qualified, the selection and retention vision standards were identical. Changes to vision standards have been made only recently. Although these changes have been relatively minor, more significant changes—to include functional clinical tests having greater predictive value, such as contrast sensitivity and visual evoked potentials—can be expected as understanding of the visual demands of helicopter operations increases.

Helicopter flight places unique demands on the vision of a rotary-wing aviator. Operations in and out of unimproved landing sites, without sophisticated electronic aids, impose a greater burden on individual decision making. The threat of ground contact is much more immediate; confined area, slope, and pinnacle landings demand valid distance judgments to determine clearance and closure. New weapon threats and tactics restrict the flight envelope. The rotary-wing aviator conducting terrain-following or NOE flights operates at very low altitudes, frequently below treetop level. The physical world at low altitude has a different perspective; navigation is much more difficult, and the aviator must rely on visual input and learn to interpret terrain features. The information provided by the moving flow of images across the peripheral retina has greater significance in estimating airspeed at these low levels. The aviator must constantly clear the airspace for obstacle avoidance. Detection of wires is so difficult and the threat of wire strikes so prevalent that hardware has been installed on most aircraft to either detect wires in the flight path or to cut them if they are contacted. However, none of the new systems is completely successful and aviators must depend primarily on the fidelity of their own visual systems.

The requirement for all-weather, day and night operational capability has provided the impetus for major advancements in light amplification systems. In the early 1970s, Army aviation adopted ''second-generation'' AN/PVS-5 night-vision goggles which had been developed for the infantry. These were mounted to the flight helmet and used as the primary means to acquire visual information so that flights could be conducted during darkness down to quarter moon levels. The United States Army Aeromedical Research Laboratory (USAARL) designed a modification to the full face goggle to allow much of it to be removed and provide a ''look

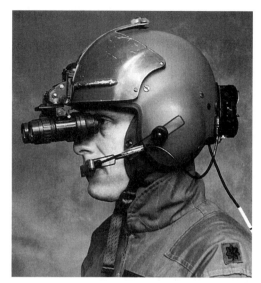

Figure 22.3. Aviator night vision imaging system (ANVIS) night vision goggles (official United States Army photo).

under'' capability for peripheral target detection and reading aircraft instruments.

More recently, the aviation night-vision imaging system (ANVIS) was developed specifically for aviation (Fig. 22.3). The principal improvement in these new systems is the third generation light amplification tube with enhanced sensitivity and extended range to the near infrared region. The ANVIS allows operations down to starlight levels. Although night-vision devices have increased the hours during which flight operations can be conducted, they do not turn night into day. Visual acuity with high-contrast targets varies from 20/40 to 20/60, depending on ambient illumination. For targets having contrasts more realistic for the flight environment, acuity with goggles may be as low as 20/70 to 20/120. Field-of-view is restricted to 40 degrees, and both stereopsis and color vision are essentially eliminated (5).

Thus, aviators using night-vision devices must operate with visual information quite different from the normal daytime unaided input (6). Operations involving night vision devices require different flight rules. Preflight planning and coordination become vital for mission safety

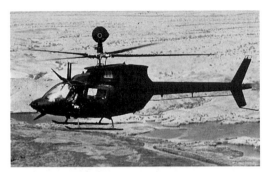

Figure 22.4. OH-58D Scout helicopter with mast-mounted sight and wire strike protection system (official United States Army photo).

and success. Aviators must be trained to know the capabilities and deficiencies of the devices, and, most importantly, must know that constant scanning using head movements to clear airspace is absolutely essential to compensate for the reduced field-of-view.

Another family of night vision devices in the cockpit is based on infrared imaging technology. Forward-looking infrared (FLIR) systems are in use on OH-58D and AH-64A helicopters (Fig. 22.4). The AH-64A is the newest Army aircraft and has direct view magnifying optics, stabilized sights, and day TV, as well as FLIR. Superimposed on the imagery are symbols and numbers representing various flight parameters, including altitude, attitude, airspeed, heading, and engine torque. This combined video picture is presented to the pilot via a helmet-mounted display (HMD) (Fig. 22.5). Because the HMD is monocular, in front of the right eye, the AH-64A aviator is never binocular during flight. During the development of the AH-64A, serious questions developed over whether a left-eye dominant pilot could learn to attend to a right-eye display. In fact, evidence linking sighting dominance with handedness and cognitive ability exists, including tracking ability and rifle marksmanship. However, this small amount of research is far from compelling, and the HMD was produced to fit the right-eyed majority.

Probably a more troublesome phenomenon is binocular rivalry, which occurs when the eyes receive dissimilar input. This ocular conflict is resolved by the brain by suppressing one of the images. The Apache sighting system presents the eyes with a multitude of dissimilar stimuli: color, resolution, field-of-view, movement, and brightness. Pilots report difficulty making the necessary switches of attention between the eyes, particularly as a mission progresses. For example, the relatively bright and compelling green phosphor in front of the right eye can make it difficult to attend to a darker visual scene in front of the left eye. Conversely, when bright city lights are in view, it may be difficult to shift attention to the right eye. It may be hard to read instruments or maps inside the cockpit, because the HMD eye ''sees'' through the instrument panel or floor of the aircraft, continuously presenting a conflicting outside view. Attending to the unaided eye may be difficult if the symbols presented to the right eye are moving or jittering. Some pilots resort to flying for periods with one

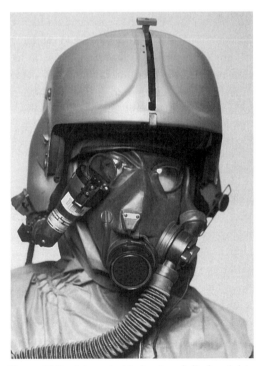

Figure 22.5. Integrated helmet and display sight system (IHADSS) and M-43 protective mask for the AH-64A Apache attack helicopter (official United States Army photo).

eye closed, an extremely fatiguing and danger-ous endeavor. The published user surveys gener-ally agree that the problems of binocular rivalry tend to ease with practice, but under conditions of a long, fatiguing mission, particularly when system problems occur (e.g., focus, flicker, FLIR), rivalry is a recurrent pilot stressor.

An obvious disadvantage of a monocular dis-play like the HMD is the complete loss of stere-opsis (visual appreciation of three dimensions during binocular vision). Stereopsis is believed to be particularly important in tactical helicopter flying because the terrain is invariably within the 200 M (620 feet) limit of stereo vision. Aviators using monocular pilotage systems can improve their nonstereo depth perception with training, although the degraded acuity inherent in these systems will adversely affect the perception of even monocular depth cues to some extent. An-other challenge to normal vision by the AH-64A visionic system is presented by the location of the sensors in a pod on the front of the aircraft. Thus, although the helmet-mounted viewing screen is placed close to the right eye, it is as if that eye were removed and positioned in the pod on the front of the aircraft. The oculocentric po-sition from which all distance and directional judgments are made is located three feet below and nine feet forward from the aviator. Exten-sive training is essential to compensate.

Development programs are underway to field new devices which protect the aviator's eyes from lasers, chemical exposure, and nuclear flash. Integrating the aviator with the various protective devices and the new electrooptical de-vices which provide visual input has become quite difficult. For example, traditional correc-tion of refractive errors using spectacles is no longer viable when using certain equipment combinations. Disposable long-wearing soft-contact lenses have been developed, fielded, and demonstrated to be effective in actual combat. Exploration of other options continues.

Although new technical advances are provid-ing better protection or extending operational ca-pabilities into areas not previously possible, the physiology of the aviator has not changed. Tech-nical advances or enhanced capability often are accompanied by compromise. The flight sur-geon must maintain awareness of new equip-ment introduced into the cockpit to ensure that the aviator is not physiologically compromised to an unacceptable limit.

Hearing and Noise Protection

Balloonists and glider enthusiasts are the only aeronauts for whom silence is golden. For oth-ers, the absence of sound in the aerial environ-ment is ominous. But the sounds of engines, transmissions, and rotors are excessive and facil-itate detection by an enemy. Noise generated by most rotary-wing aircraft is the combined effect of engine, transmission, and rotor-blade activity. Each aircraft may have a particular part or sys-tem that generates the majority of noise at each crew site. Noise spectra for many aircraft not only exceed the damage risk criteria by a wide margin but can exceed the limits of hearing pro-tective devices and communications systems.

Helicopter noise can be reduced at its source by improving gear design (i.e., use of polished helical gears), shrouds to enclose noisy compo-nents, and insulation. Acoustic blankets are used inside most helicopters. However, individual protection is the primary method of protecting the aircrew, and the SPH-4 and new SPH-4B helmets plus well-fitted V-51R or disposable plastic foam earplugs provide excellent protec-tion. Research in phase-canceling ear phones holds considerable promise of active noise re-duction, and new helmets under develop-ment—such as the integrated aircrew hel-met—should provide improved attenuation.

Disorientation and Simulator Sickness

Disorientation
Disorientation is always a troublesome problem of aviation, and is aggravated by three charac-teristics of helicopter flight: hovering flight in all directions, low-level flight with reduced visibil-

ity, and the inherent instability of the helicopter platform. Flight operations at night, under marginal weather conditions, with limited instruments, with night-vision goggles or with helmet-mounted displays, increase the risk of disorientation.

Fixed-wing aircraft may cause disorientation by unexpected induced motions from physiologic illusions, turbulence, poor handling, or complicated inflight maneuvers; but these do not compare to the helicopter's additional, innate ability to travel side ways, rearward, or vertically. These motions cause relatively few problems under good conditions but are significant when visual cues are reduced. Most flight instruments used on helicopters were designed for fixed-wing aircraft and respond poorly to helicopter maneuvering at low speeds. Disorientation also can occur when helicopters are hovered over snow, sand, or loose dirt that is picked up by the rotor wash, leading to loss of visual reference ("white-out" or "brown-out"). The sudden change to instrument references, combined with the unreliability of both human sensory perception and instruments during hovering, can lead to disorientation and accidents.

New horizontal situation indicators and video displays have been developed and may help alleviate this problem. However, simpler strategies such as aircrew education, avoidance of the situation, and aircraft stability augmentation systems (including an automatic hover mode) hold the greatest promise for reducing this problem. Strong aeromedical and aviation training programs remain the most important defensive measures for disorientation. Increased emphasis on night missions and the development of helicopter air-to-air combat doctrine will increase the challenge to the flight surgeon with new physiologic, perceptual, and behavioral effects, including disorientation not previously experienced by Army aircrew.

Simulator Sickness

The increasingly high cost of aviation training and the risk of accidents make simulation attractive, especially when the cost of firing sophisticated weapons is added. Lack of realism has detracted from simulation, but as fidelity has increased, so has "simulator sickness." This syndrome is manifested by physiologic discomfort in the simulator which does not occur when the same maneuvers are flown in the actual aircraft. The classic motion sickness symptoms of stomach awareness, nausea, and vomiting occur, but drowsiness, headache, eye strain, vertigo, and ataxia may also be present. The latter two symptoms may occur as flashback phenomena hours later and without warning. Like motion sickness in real aircraft, simulator sickness may result in negative effects on training as users adopt otherwise inappropriate strategies to avoid unpleasant experiences; for example, using less than the full capabilities of the simulator. Infrequently, residual effects or flashbacks can compromise actual aircraft flight, operation of ground vehicles, or sleep.

Although several theories have been proposed to explain this phenomenon, the neural mismatch theory is the most accepted. This theory ascribes the symptoms to discrepancies among motion cues delivered by multiple sensory inputs, or to differences between expected and perceived sensory input. The theory postulates that vestibular, visual, and kinesthetic inputs to a neural referencing network are compared to expected results, based on either experience or some innate neural standard. In most real life situations, the expected and the experienced correlate; therefore, no mismatch exists. Significant conflict encountered in the simulator, however, causes simulator sickness. The disparities may be due, for example, to delayed response of the simulator compared to real aircraft, or to lack of sustained movement of the simulator in any one axis compared to that occurring in an aircraft.

The Army has a strong interest in simulator sickness because it occurs with higher incidence in rotary wing simulators. The greater yaw, rearward flight, and low level flight profile of helicopters make high demands on visual simulators and produce the greatest incidence of symptoms.

Pilots new to the simulator and those with considerable flight time in the actual aircraft are particularly susceptible. Concurrent medical or physiological conditions, such as fatigue, dehydration and upper respiratory infections, have been associated with increased incidence of the syndrome. Some reports indicate that while most affected aviators report diminishing symptoms as they accumulate time in simulators, there is a concomitant increase in postsimulator ataxia.

Treatment of simulator sickness is controversial. Pilots should first be reassured that simulator sickness alone is not disqualifying, and then concurrent medical conditions must be ruled out. Frequent, short-duration, minimal maneuver simulator flights with progressive increases in both duration and complexity is the most ''natural'' method of adaptation. This strategy works well, but may be impractical for a tightly scheduled simulator. Pharmacologic therapy is not recommended.

The Aviation Environment

Military helicopters traditionally are equipped with minimal environmental control systems and little or no cabin insulation. As a result, aircrew are often subjected to environmental temperature extremes that affect comfort, endurance, performance, and safety. The tactical environment presents many additional challenges.

The Operational Environment

Army aviation medicine faces the challenge of supporting worldwide air, ground, and sea operations. Army aviation is deployed around the world where it provides for fire power, inspection of troops, logistical support, observation of enemy movements, evacuation of the sick and wounded, and other missions. Personnel are exposed to environmental extremes, exotic diseases, parasitic infestations, high terrestrial elevation, chemical and toxic agents, noise, vibration, circadian dysynchrony, and other stresses. Army aircrew, including the flight sur-

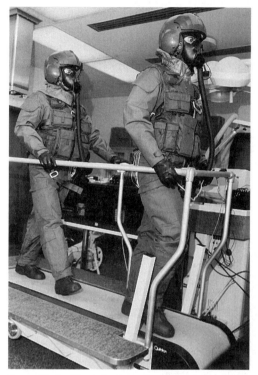

Figure 22.6. Physiologic testing of US Army aviators in the aircrew uniform integrated battlefield (AUIB) chemical defense ensemble (official United States Army photo).

geon, usually share living conditions with ground soldiers and are subject to the same diseases and environmental hardships. Flight conditions include everything from wearing bulky chemical protective gear during NOE flight in a tropical rain forest to night flight in isolated and distant mountain terrain during bitter cold arctic winters or the harsh desert of the Middle East (Fig. 22.6). The Army aviators must know the limitations of their aircraft and themselves under these highly varied conditions. Crew endurance varies widely under this wide range of conditions, and the flight surgeon must be very knowledgeable in this area.

Advances in technology and the associated communication, navigation, target acquisition, and weapons system management have increased aviator workload. The effective use of sophisticated optical equipment requires exceptional visual acuity and ocular motility. NOE flight with night-vision goggles under adverse weather conditions demands the utmost levels of skill, training, and mental acuity. The burdens of chemical, toxic, and laser protective equipment add further to the combined stresses the Army aviator endures.

Army flight surgeons must enhance human dimensions to the fullest by carefully integrating the principles of preventive, occupational, behavioral, and clinical medicine. The flight surgeon must apply these principles to the aviator's environment and equipment and to the total threat the aviator faces, ranging from disease to enemy attack. The flight surgeon's knowledge of scientific, medical, aviation, and military disciplines must be applied throughout a total mission spectrum to achieve peacetime readiness and combat effectiveness. To this end, flight surgeons must be observant, inquisitive, action-oriented, and in concert with their units, staffs, and professionals of many other disciplines.

Hot Weather Flying

The climb to altitude in fixed-wing aircraft brings welcome relief in hot climates, but the non-air-conditioned helicopter flying near the ground subjects aircrew to significant, often inescapable heat stress. On a sunny day, expansive aircraft canopies designed to maximize visibility add to the heat load via the "greenhouse effect." The olive-drab flight helmet, fire-resistant flight suit and gloves cover virtually all of the aviator's skin surface, severely limiting evaporative and convective heat loss. The problem is compounded by the addition of other life-support equipment, such as the survival vest and body armor. Heat stress is especially critical when the aviator must wear chemical protective gear.

Army flight surgeons must constantly stress to aviators the importance of preventive measures in hot weather. Scheduled mandatory water intake is one method used by aviation units during hot weather operations to avoid dehydration. Some modern, closed-cockpit helicopters (e.g., AH-1S and AH-64A) have effec-

tive air-conditioning systems, but often these are primarily intended to cool the avionics and computers. Above a critical temperature, for example, the AH-64A pilot is instructed to divert all cooled air away from the cockpit directly to the avionics bays. Personal cooling systems are being developed that either circulate cold liquid within a special garment or blow cooled air over the aviator's skin. The latter is preferred as it promotes evaporation of perspiration, avoiding a cold-wet sensation, and is logistically simpler (7). Because it is likely that the helicopter combat mission of the future will still be at NOE altitudes, these technologic solutions to the heat stress problem are considered essential, even though cost, weight, and power consumption are formidable obstacles to operational use.

Cold Weather Operations

The Army aviator often must fly with cold-weather clothing designed to be worn on the ground. Vapor barrier arctic boots are too large for anti-torque pedals, arctic mittens are too bulky to operate small switches, and large parkas interfere with movement, vision, and emergency egress. Although it is hazardous to fly in isolated winter climates without adequate winter clothing, the bulky nature of such clothing can compromise the fine control movements necessary for safe flight. Experience, education, and patience are all required for winter operations while better solutions are sought.

Cold environmental temperatures present many other operational challenges for the deployed aviation unit. Oil seals may crack and leak, requiring increased maintenance. This is exceedingly difficult except in heated hangars, which are not available in the tactical environment. Cold temperatures may triple the time to accomplish even the simplest maintenance work. Super cooled fuel is a cold injury hazard if in contact with exposed skin. Even mild hypothermia can result in psychological degradation and apathy, leading to impaired flight performance and maintenance errors. Dehydration is a hazard when cold weather conditions interfere with proper fluid intake. Cold weather operations must always include the prospect of winter survival. The flight surgeon must be especially observant for signs of difficulty in those personnel involved in winter operations, and must assist in training for cold weather survival.

Vibration

The most recognized symbol of Army aviation has been the UH-1 "Huey" helicopter. A well known Huey hallmark is the low-frequency (5.4Hz) vibration of the semirigid, two-blade rotor system (8). Other helicopters produce vibration of 2–35 Hz at up to 0.35 G. This range encompasses the resonant frequency of many body structures and is potentially injurious depending on intensity and duration. Disturbances in dynamic visual acuity, speech, and fine motor coordination have been reported when the vibration is near the resonant frequency of the affected body structure (Chapter 8).

Most pilots adapt to the acute effects and only consider it a nuisance. However, there is controversy about long-term effects near the resonant frequency of the spinal system (4–5 Hz). Some researchers believe that back pain and premature intervertebral disc disease may result from chronic exposure (9). Others relate back problems to the forced posture one must assume to operate most helicopters. In any case, the high prevalence of back pain in helicopter pilots has been well documented. It is less clear whether there is a higher incidence of intervertebral disc disease or other spinal pathology in other helicopter crew members. The problem of pregnancy and vibration has also been raised recently. USAARL is currently investigating some of these relationships.

The vibration spectrum of a helicopter is influenced by the number of blades in its main rotor system. In the past, most Army helicopters had two-blade systems. Newer helicopters have four or more blades, with changes in vibration patterns and vertical amplitudes. These aircraft are less likely to cause problems because their dominant frequencies generally do not coincide with the natural frequency of important body structures and the amplitudes are less than in two-blade systems.

Rotary-wing Aircraft Accidents

The flight characteristics of helicopters result in accident considerations very different from fixed-wing aircraft.

Inflight Escape

A major concern in rotary-wing flight is inflight escape from disabled aircraft. Current doctrine requires Army helicopters to fly at NOE altitudes which severely limits time available to initiate an escape. The hazard posed by the proximity of the rotor system further complicates the use of ejection or extraction systems. Several rocket extraction and ejection systems which employ rotor system jettison have been designed but have not been deemed practical for the Army flight environment. Consequently, the future of these systems is uncertain. The penalties in useful load, cost, possibility of malfunction, and inherent dangers of aircrew ejection or blade jettison in the proximity of other aircraft offsets many of the potential advantages. For the foreseeable future, the "ride-it-in" philosophy will likely prevail in helicopter aviation. This underscores the need for structural crash worthiness, effective personal protective equipment, and auto-rotation capability. This approach also has the added advantage of limiting damage to the helicopter and its cargo (10,11).

Midair Collisions

The maneuverability of the helicopter in all directions and aircraft density in many tactical scenarios increase the risk of midair collisions. The tips of most rotor blades move at tangential velocities approaching Mach 1; contact with other structures usually results in blade damage, causing intense vibration incompatible with aerodynamic or structural integrity. Fatality rates due to midair collisions are high. Many midair accidents occur in good daylight visibility or at night with night-vision devices. The flight surgeon and safety officer must continually concentrate on problems of channeled attention, limitations of peripheral vision, and the value of effective visual scanning. The educational effort must also extend to air traffic control personnel.

Crash Injury Effects

In contrast to the typical longitudinal crash pattern of fixed-wing aircraft, helicopters tend to impact vertically at lower forward velocities. Rotor blades, transmissions and other high mass items may separate from the helicopter, but more frequently enter the cabin or cockpit, causing serious injury or death. As in fixed-wing crashes, fire is a major source of injury in helicopters not equipped with crashworthy fuel systems.

Injury Patterns

In survivable crashes, injury patterns reflect the primarily vertical orientation of the crash acceleration vector ($+Gz$). In the US Army, approximately 60% of all injuries in survivable helicopter crashes are due to collapse of structure into occupied spaces, intrusion of high mass items, flailing of torso, head and extremities, or a combination of these. Another 12% of injuries are attributed to excessive vertical acceleration forces. Despite universal usage of flight helmets, the head is the most frequently injured body region. Head injury accounts for 26% of major injuries in survivable crashes and was the cause of death in over 55% of fatalities in survivable crashes. Injuries to the spine account for almost 18% of major injuries and are a significant source of disability for survivors. Upper and lower extremity injuries are frequently encountered, but tend to be less significant than head or spine injuries (12).

Emphasis on crashworthy design has changed injury patterns (13,14). Crashworthy fuel systems have all but eliminated thermal injury as a cause of death in survivable crashes. Energy absorbing landing gear and load-limiting seats in the UH-60A and AH-64A appear to be very successful in reducing spinal injury. Increased tie-down strength of transmissions and changes in rotor systems have almost eliminated rotor intrusion as a cause of injury. Future efforts to reduce injury in helicopter crashes will have to concentrate on methods to prevent collapse of structure into occupied areas and improved methods of preventing flail injuries to the head, torso and extremities. USAARL is exploring crash-activated inflatable restraint systems (air bags) to prevent flailing injuries.

Postcrash Fires

For years, the postcrash fire was one of the greatest causes of fatality and disability in otherwise survivable accidents. The thin aluminum skins or impregnated cloth of helicopter fuel cells ruptured easily, resulting in a large fuel vapor cloud which ignited rapidly on contact with hot engine components, sparks, or electrical sources. The resulting 1150°C inferno allowed only a few critical seconds for uninjured aircrew to escape. The combination of thermally resistant flight clothing (polyamide flight suits and gloves), leather boots, and helmets with face visors greatly improved the chances of escaping a postcrash fire without serious burn injuries. Research performed at USAARL was critical to the development of biodynamic standards for the protective helmet and the fire-resistant materials (Nomex®) used by Army aircrew.

Crashworthy Fuel Systems. A major thrust by USAARL in the 1960s was to find a suitable postcrash fire prevention system for helicopters. Although fuel solidification, breakaway fuel tanks, honeycomb tank fillers, and ignition-inserting methods were evaluated, neoprene-impregnated nylon cloth tanks with breakaway valves proved to offer the most economical and effective protection. This was demonstrated in 1967, when a UH-1 with nylon tanks and breakaway valves was crashed by remote control, resulting in no fuel spillage or subsequent fire. Crashworthy fuel cell retrofit of the Army helicopter fleet (along with installation in new aircraft) began in the early 1970s and is now complete. As accident data of aircraft with the new crashworthy systems were analyzed, results exceeded all expectations (15). Survivable crashes through 1990 showed a thermal injury and fatality rate of near zero compared to 40% in helicopters having conventional systems. This success illustrates the need for the combined efforts of aeromedical and aeronautical engineering disciplines.

Helmets (Figure 22.7)

Since September 17, 1908, when Lieutenant Thomas Selfridge tragically made aviation history as the first aircraft accident fatality, the importance of head protection in aviation has been recognized. Head injuries have repeatedly been shown to be the most common fatal injury in potentially survivable helicopter accidents. Reasons include the forward location of the engine and transmission assemblies, high vertical G-forces, and the tendency for helicopters to spin and roll during the crash sequence. Introduced in 1970, the SPH-4 flight helmet is essential life-

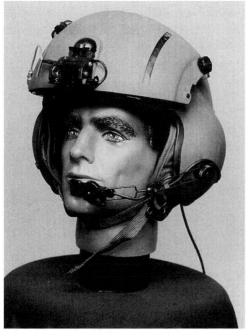

Figure 22.7. Current US Army SPH-4B helmet (official United States Army photo).

support equipment in Army aviation. However, estimated helmet use in some civilian helicopter fleets is low. Data from the US Army Safety Center show that the SPH-4 reduces the likelihood of serious and fatal head injuries in severe (Class A) helicopter accidents which were at least partially survivable by 3.8 and 6.3 times, respectively, compared to occupants not wearing a helmet (16,17). A new version, the SPH-4B, with a Kevlar shell, dual visors, crushable earcups, and night-vision goggle mounts was introduced in the early 1990s. Changes improve ballistic and crash protection, hearing and eye protection, and comfort. All personnel regularly participating in helicopter flight, civilian or military, should be equipped with protective helmets.

THE ARMY AVIATION MEDICINE PROGRAM

The Army Aviation Medicine Program is the responsibility of the Army Surgeon General, who oversees aeromedical programs, policies, and directives and provides technical advice to the Army on matters of aviation medicine. The Program has operational, educational, research, and other components implemented at levels from Department of the Army to small flight detachments. Application of aircrew medical standards, education of flight surgeons, aeromedical research, and clinical care of the flyer are all integral components of the Program. The approximately 24,000 officers, 25,000 enlisted personnel, 1250 civilians, and 9000 aircraft at nearly 100 locations worldwide which make up the Aviation Branch comprise by far the Army's most expensive personnel and equipment. The branch functions as one of the army's most effective combat arms and is possibly the operational area with the greatest potential for major disaster. Although the unit level practice of the flight surgeon is the keystone of aeromedical support to Army Aviation, the supporting areas of policy development, research, and education, are also essential elements of Army aviation medicine.

Aeromedical Education and Training

Army aeromedical education and training is provided by the US Army School of Aviation Medicine (USASAM), at Fort Rucker, Alabama. The proponent for aeromedical education is the Commandant, Army Medical Department Center and School, who receives advice from the Surgeon General's Aviation Medicine Consultant and the Dean, USASAM.

Aeromedical training is provided to medical and aviation personnel with specific inflight responsibilities. Training for medical personnel includes the Army Flight Surgeon Primary Course, the Flight Medical Aidman Course, and the Essential Medical Training for Army Medical Department Aviators Course. Training for aviation personnel is provided to initial entry student pilots, pilots in advanced transition or refresher training, aviation safety officers, artillery and aeroscout observers, and precommand course attendees.

Aeromedical Training for Medical Personnel

The Army Flight Surgeon Primary Course (AFSPC) provides initial training for commissioned medical corps officers (physicians and physician assistants) volunteering for aviation medicine duty (18). The course is six weeks of intensive classroom, clinical, flight line, and field environment training. The objective is to prepare medical officers for duty with aviation battalions and brigades, where they provide primary medical care for aviation personnel and their families, serve as special staff officers to the brigade or battalion commander and supervise other medical personnel. To prepare the flight surgeon students for success in the many roles they will encounter operationally, the AFSPC concentrates on providing those skills necessary to integrate previously acquired medi-

cal knowledge into a capability for effective aeromedical decision making. Students learn aeromedical decision making to become advocates for the aviation commander (and the mission) in addition to acting as the patient's advocate.

Training concentrates on defining the scope of aviation medicine and the administrative infrastructure of the Army aviation medicine program. Aeromedical standards for aviation service are thoroughly explored, including methods for aeromedical evaluation of aviators or flight training applicants. Familiarization with virtually all facets of the Army aviation branch missions, organization, and equipment is provided. Physiologic effects of the flight environment including atmospherics, acceleration, heat, cold, night, aviation life support equipment, oxygen systems, and aviation toxicology are studied in detail as they relate to mission needs and effect on aviator performance. The aeromedical approach to commonly encountered clinical problems in aviation medicine, including psychiatry, cardiology, ophthalmology, and otolaryngology, is another major instructional module. The flight surgeon's role in unit safety programs, mishap prevention, and accident investigation with emphasis on human factors is stressed. Finally, a set of practical skills is taught: how to supervise medical subordinates, plan medical support for military operations, and prepare, organize, and deliver military briefings.

Each year the Army Medical Department supports three career flight surgeons for residency training in aerospace medicine. This training may be completed in accredited civilian or military (United States Air Force or US Navy) programs. Continuing aeromedical education for Army flight surgeons is by the annual Army Operational Aeromedical Problems Course sponsored by USASAM each spring. This one week conference provides updated administrative information, refresher training in a variety of operational topics, and insights into evolving medical and aviation doctrine. Additional continuing education comes in regular newsletters from the

Surgeon General's Aviation Medicine Consultant; the Director, Army Aeromedical Activity; and the Newsletter of the Society of US Army Flight Surgeons. Video teleconferencing is also used.

Aeromedical Training for Aircrew Personnel

Aviators attending courses at the United States Army Aviation Center (USAAVNC) are given initial or refresher training in aeromedical subjects at USASAM using lecture and participatory methods. The instruction is to develop an awareness of scientific and medical information necessary for individual health promotion, safety of flight, mission completion, and preventive medicine to assure health readiness. Basic aeromedical information is presented to the initial student pilots prior to their first flight. A 22-hour academic annex is taught during their first week of flight training. The instruction emphasizes how various factors in the environment constrain or degrade performance (19).

Flight students learn the effects of altitude through experiencing these effects in an altitude chamber. The demonstrations include pressure changes, hypoxia, and changes in night and color vision. Self imposed stress and its effect on aviator performance is another important block of instruction. Noise as a serious problem in Army aviation is dealt with by educating the aviator on its origins, its physiologic effects, and how to combat it. Acceleration instruction acquaints the aviator with the effects of high- and low-magnitude acceleration in flight. The students are also shown how this knowledge may be applied for use in crash injury protection.

A most important module involves spatial disorientation and illusions of flight. The role of the perceptual apparatus in maintaining orientation in flight is presented in the context of several types of disorientation. Conflicting neurosensory information is experienced briefly in the Barany chair, while several visual illusions are demonstrated in the night-vision classroom.

Formal night-vision training is presented just before the student begins night flight and night vision goggle training. The student acquires a knowledge of the anatomy, physiology, and limitations of the visual process. Practical exercises in the night-vision classroom teach night scanning techniques, night-vision constraints, and degradation of aviator performance.

Refresher aeromedical training for Army aviators is required annually during unit training and is usually provided by the unit flight surgeon. Most aviators return to the Army Aviation Center for graduate flight training or refresher training during their careers. During these periods aeromedical update and refresher training is included in the program of instruction.

AIRCREW MEDICAL STANDARDS

Medical Classification of Army Aircrew

The standards for medical fitness for flying duty are in Army Regulation 40–501 and in USAAMC Aeromedical Policy Letters. These are under constant review and evolution to reflect the current standard of aeromedical care (20).

Initial applicants for aviator training come under Class 1 standards for Warrant Officers and Class 1A standards for Commissioned Officers. The medical standards for both classes are the same, except that vision standards for Class 1 are more strict.

Class 2 standards apply to rated Army aviators, military and civilian. Class 2F applies to flight surgeons. The medical standards for these classes are the same except the vision standards for Class 2 are more strict.

Class 3 standards apply to aircrew who do not control Army aircraft, including crew chiefs, gunners, flight medics, aerial observers, maintenance aircrew, and altitude chamber technicians. Standards for Class 3 are the same as Class 2 except the vision standards for Class 2 are more strict.

Class 4 standards apply to air traffic controllers, military and civilian. Standards are similar to the FAA Air Traffic Control Specialists Health Program.

Medical Examination of Army Aircrew

Initial applicants for Army aviation training of all Classes undergo comprehensive flying duty medical examinations every eighteen months until training begins. The causes for medical disqualification of student pilots are shown in Table 22.1.

Trained Army aircrew under 40 years of age in Classes 2, 2F, 2S, 3, and 4, undergo a comprehensive history and physical examination every five years. In the interim years, a limited history and physical screening focuses on detection of common aeromedical disqualifications. After age 40, comprehensive examinations occur every three years until age 50 (when they are required annually). The findings of these examinations lead to preventive medicine interventions and additional occupationally based medical investigations as required.

Table 22.1.
Medical Eliminations of US Army Student Pilots: 1986 to 1989

Concealed medical history	70
Refractive error	54
Allergic rhinitis	43
Orthopedic, arms and legs	36
Psychiatric disorders	35
Migraine headaches	35
Hearing loss	34
Orthopedic, back	19
Ocular motility disorder	15
Color vision	13
Depth perception	12
Cardiovascular	12
Middle ear disorders	12
Drug and alcohol abuse	11
Head injury	10
Anthropometrics	8
Gastrointestinal disorders	6
Inguinal hernia	5
Genitourinary disorders	5
Syncope	4
Motion sickness, chronic	4
Asthma	3
Other miscellaneous diseases	24

Reports of all classes of aircrew, except Class 3 locally waiverable conditions, are reviewed by the attending flight surgeon and then forwarded for review by an appointed Regional Flight Surgeon or centrally at the US Army Aeromedical Activity (USAAMA). Data from these examinations are entered into the computerized Aeromedical Epidemiological Data Repository (AEDR), maintained jointly by the USAAMC and USAARL. Qualified examinations are returned to the attending flight surgeon. Disqualified examinations are referred for further aeromedical consultation as described below.

Reports of Class 3 aircrew are evaluated by the local flight surgeon, who determines if the aircrew are qualified or disqualified and recommends disposition to the local aviation commander or are referred for further aeromedical consultation as described below.

Aeromedical Consultation

After an initial evaluation by the attending flight surgeon and regional consultants, the case histories of partially waiverable disqualified aircrew of all classes, except Class 3 locally waiverable conditions, are referred to an aerospace medicine specialist at the Aeromedical Consultation Service, USAAMA. An Aeromedical Board, composed of aerospace medicine specialists, convenes and makes a recommendation for waiver or suspension from flying duties through the Commander, USAAMC to the aircrew's waiver authority at the Army Personnel Command or Army National Guard Bureau. Annual renewal of the waiver is often contingent upon a prescribed follow-up evaluation and/or specific inflight restrictions. The Aeromedical Board refers complex or precedent cases to the Aeromedical Consultant's Advisory Panel (ACAP) for further consideration. This panel is composed of aerospace medicine specialists, senior flight surgeons with various medical specialty backgrounds, and senior Army aviators. ACAP recommendations are then forwarded to the Commander, USAAMC.

Selected patients are referred for more comprehensive evaluations at Lyster Army Community Hospital, Fort Rucker, or the Ellingson Aeromedical Consultation Service at Brooks Air Force Base. Both of these facilities are supported by experienced aerospace medicine clinicians and researchers. The Army Aviation Center, Fort Rucker, provides senior standardization and instructor pilots in any Army aircraft or aircraft simulator to perform inflight evaluations of medically disqualified aircrew when questions of waiverability lend themselves to performance testing.

The Army Aeromedical Consultation Service manages a computerized, prospective Waiver and Suspense File of all disqualified aircrew referred for consultation. The cases in this database are archived on microfiche, and the database is cross-referenced with flight physical data in the AEDR. These databases are utilized by the staff of USAAMA in conducting retrospective and prospective epidemiologic studies that directly impact on the formulation of aeromedical dispositions, policy, and standards. The causes for medical suspension from flying duty and medical disqualifications that can be waivered are shown in Tables 22.2 and 22.3.

Operational Aviation Medicine

Army Aviation Medicine is preventive in concept, environmental in nature, and military in orientation. Under guidance from the Army Surgeon General, the USAAMC, and major commands of the Army, flight surgeons establish local aviation medicine programs tailored to the specific needs of the supported population.

Unit Level Programs

The practice of aviation medicine at unit level is designed to promote health, prevent illness, enhance performance and combat capability, and prevent the loss of life and property. Unlike the sister services, the Army flight surgeon is often supported in daily practice by an aeromedical physician assistant (APA). Because disper-

Table 22.2.
Suspension Issued for 320 US Army Aviators During 1989

Cardiovascular		170
Abnormal electrocardiogram	90	
Coronary artery disease	22	
Hypertension	14	
Myocardial infarction	7	
Psychosocial		93
DSM-III-R diagnoses	45	
Unsatisfactory ARMA	22	
Alcohol abuse/dependence	18	
Marijuana/cocaine abuse	9	
Orthopedic/rheumatologic		54
Pregnancy		31
Neurologic		32
Gastrointestinal		25
Ear, nose, and throat		22
Pulmonary		13
Ophthalmologic		9
Oncologic		8
Renal stone		5
Diabetes mellitus		5

Table 22.3.
Waivers Granted to 1280 Army Aviators During 1989

Ophthalmologic		428
Presbyopia	198	
Myopia	148	
Ocular hypertension	15	
Cardiovascular		350
Abnormal electrocardiogram	220	
Coronary artery disease	15	
Hypertension	85	
Hearing loss		302
Orthopedic/rheumatologic		255
Herniated disc	35	
Ear, nose, and throat		130
Allergic rhinitis	101	
Genitourinary		88
Renal stone	51	
Gastrointestinal		86
Psychosocial		64
Alcohol abuse/dependence	33	
DSM-III-R diagnoses	31	
Neurologic		37
Oncologic		30
Endocrinologic		27
Pulmonary		22
Dermatologic		20
Hematologic		17

sion of aviation assets results in many small units being supported by a single flight surgeon, the APA not only is a valuable assistant but may be the only immediate source of aeromedical support in the absence of the flight surgeon. This may occur not only during leave and temporary duty but when part of the unit deploys or goes on exercises. Except for the APA and at locations such as Fort Rucker and Fort Campbell, where aviation assets are concentrated, Army flight surgeons often practice alone as compared to their Air Force and Navy colleagues. The latter usually practice under the supervision of a more experienced, more highly trained Chief of Aerospace Medicine or carrier Senior Medical Officer. However, many Army specialists have previously been unit flight surgeons and function in a supportive role for new unit flight surgeons.

Within the operational structure of the Army, flight surgeons are assigned to aviation brigades and groups in divisions and corps, and to Air Cavalry, Special Forces, and other unique field units with aviation assets. The majority of these unit level flight surgeons have completed only one year of postgraduate medical education and six weeks of training in aviation medicine. Flight surgeons usually operate a clinic close to their unit on the flight line, when possible. This clinic is supported with personnel, consultation, and logistics by an area Army hospital. To support small units and detachments not authorized organic medical support, flight surgeons are assigned to nearby hospitals or clinics. Since the aviation medicine requirement may be less than full time, many of these are fully trained in other specialties and conduct aviation medicine programs on a part time basis.

Flight surgeons support their units through occupational and preventive medicine, clinical care, and staff responsibilities. Their duties include: routine medical care for aviation personnel, with particular attention to significant aviation medical problems; the annual flight physical, or flying duty medical examination (FDME); a general preventive and occupational

medicine program to maintain and promote health and safety; support of the aviation safety program to include presentations at safety meetings and participation in aircraft mishap investigations; serving as a special staff officer to the unit commander as primary medical advisor in matters pertaining to medical care and medical planning; and providing aeromedical advice to the hospital commander, aeromedical evacuation units, and others related to or supporting the local aviation medicine program.

Whether examining an applicant for flight school or assessing an aviator for continuation of flight duties, the ability of flight surgeons to accomplish this appropriately depends greatly on their understanding of the aviation unit mission and how the individual aviator functions within this environment. The daily practice of aviation medicine relies on flight surgeons participating as integral members of the units they support. The flight surgeon provides for direct medical support of the aviation unit when deployed or during field exercises. Monthly requirements for flight time enable them to observe their patient population within the work environment and to personally experience on a recurring basis the hazards and hardships of military aviation.

High Level Assignments

Division, Major Command, and other high-level assignments are filled by Army flight surgeons who are residency trained in the specialty of aerospace medicine. This usually includes those combat divisions which are heavily dependent upon aviation, such as air mobile and air cavalry, along with commands such as US Army Europe, US Army Safety Center, USAAMC, USASAM, USAAMA, USAARL, and others. These specialists in aerospace medicine make aeromedical policy, determine fitness for flying duty, conduct aeromedical research, and act in consultant and advisory roles. Many also serve in executive medicine positions, such as major command surgeons or hospital commanders.

Aeromedical Epidemiology Data Register

Centralization of Flying Duty Medical Examination (FDME) review at the USAAMC in 1974 provided the potential for a wealth of aeromedical epidemiological information. The implementation of computerization made such data accessible for review and analysis. The Aeromedical Epidemiology Data Register (AEDR) was jointly established by USAARL and the USAAMC to contain all Army initial entry and Class 2 flight physicals as well as medical waiver, suspension, and flight training information.

This data base is the oldest and largest of its kind, containing currently more than 160,000 records representing information on more than 60,000 aircrew members since 1986.

The AEDR facilitates the establishment of aircrew selection and retention standards, provides anthropometric data for the design of crew stations and personal protective equipment, and provides a means of studying disease and health trends in aviation personnel and the relationship between health status and flight training performance.

Major research applications for these data have included analysis of medical attrition (21), analysis of the relationship between smoking and flight performance, development of selection criteria for specific cockpits, development of visual standards for visionic systems, contact lenses, helmet sizing and other anthropometric requirements, and analysis of the prevalence of specific medical conditions or episodes in the Army aviator population. As the size of the data base grows, it will become an ever more valuable tool for aeromedical epidemiology.

Aviation Medicine Research

Army aeromedical research is primarily conducted by USAARL. The laboratory has addressed a multitude of medical problems in the aviation and airborne (parachute) environment and, since 1977, has also conducted research in nonaviation areas, such as artillery blast overpressure, weapon impact noise, and combat vehicle crew performance.

Studies in the aviation environment have included development of biomedical criteria for helmets and flight clothing, inflight and simulator studies of performance under a variety of environmental and pharmacologic stresses, noise protection, aircraft visibility enhancement, operational dynamic visual acuity, protective eye wear, contact lenses in operational environments, effects of rotary wing flying on the vertebral column, circadian dysynchrony and its pharmacologic intervention, and the performance effects of chemical agents and antidotes.

Other efforts have included biomedical aspects of aircraft cockpits and aircrew anthropometry, onboard oxygen generating systems, medical aspects of collision avoidance systems, psychologic and physiologic aspects of sustained performance, rotor down wash effects, and pharmacologic enhancement of performance.

USAARL is currently (1993) staffed with about 80 military and 70 civilian personnel. Approximately 30 scientists conduct original research in a wide variety of areas in support of the Army's ground, airborne, and aviation soldiers. USAARL's state-of-the-art facilities feature an environmentally controlled UH-60/ simulator for studies of interactions among such factors as workload, cockpit environment, clothing, fatigue, and medications (Fig. 22.8).

Army Hyperbaric Medicine

Aviation Medicine has taken the lead in establishing clinical hyperbaric medicine in the Army. The Army's first clinical hyperbaric chamber is co-located with the altitude chamber at the USAAMC. Patients have been treated for decompression sickness since 1986. Routine clinical treatments for other accepted hyperbaric indications were first performed in 1987 (Chapter 7). The Army has trained a pool of hyperbaric

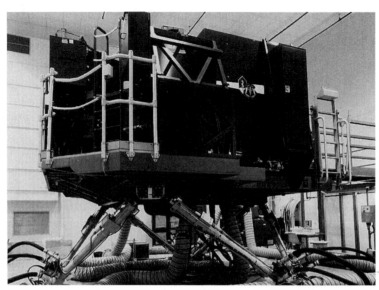

Figure 22.8. US Army aeromedical research laboratory's UH-60A Blackhawk research flight simulator with environmental control and real-time physiologic and flight performance monitoring (official United States Army photo).

personnel, from enlisted chamber technicians through aerospace medicine specialists, to staff the clinical hyperbaric medicine service. One Army aerospace medicine specialist is periodically selected to attend the Fellowship in Hyperbaric Medicine offered by the United States Air Force at Brooks Air Force Base, Texas.

Plans for further implementation of an Army-wide hospital-based clinical hyperbaric medicine program are being developed. Numerous other nonclinical hyperbaric chambers exist in the Army, primarily in support of hard hat and scuba divers in Special Forces, Ranger Units, and the Corps of Engineers (COE). These chambers, both fixed and portable, are used for emergency treatment of decompression sickness in COE divers who inspect and maintain dams, waterways, underwater pipelines, and other facilities, as well as combat divers in Special Forces and Ranger units.

CIVIL HELICOPTER AEROMEDICAL CONCERNS

Except for the tactical/combat considerations of military aviation, civilian pilots face many of the same problems as their Army counterparts;

however, a significant difference occurs in the degree to which the civilian pilot is protected against adversity. The use of protective helmets, boots, gloves, fire-resistant flight clothing, and crashworthy fuel systems is by no means universal in civil flying due to economic, useful load, attitude, local policy, and performance considerations. Should a crash occur the results may therefore be more devastating to a civil pilot and passengers.

In military aviation, an extensive support system provides a high degree of safety surveillance through multiple systems of inspection, including aviation resource management surveys, operational readiness and safety evaluations, and general inspections. These all monitor aviator selection, training, equipment, maintenance, and unit operations. Each pilot undergoes an annual check ride, takes a written examination and flight physical, and meets flight currency requirements. Equivalent programs are not necessarily conducted in the civil sector because of economic or other constraints. What has proved cost-effective in military helicopter aviation, however, could as well save lives and costly equipment in the civilian sector (22).

HELICOPTER AVIATION MEDICINE AND THE FUTURE

The medical evacuation helicopter had a long adolescence during the close of World War II and the Korean conflict, but came of age in Vietnam. Casualties were saved by rapid transport to hospitals where systematic and definitive care was given by teams of specialists. This same service was later offered to many civilian communities in the proximity of military installations through the Military Assistance to Safety and Traffic (MAST) program authorized by Congress in 1975, and is still permitted to serve communities without civilian air ambulance service. Many civil helicopter ambulance services have offered similar services to rapidly transport patients to medical centers for definitive and highly specialized care.

Present day technology, coupled with the definitive emergency care available at medical centers and larger hospitals, has drastically altered previous mortality and morbidity statistics for many diseases and categories of trauma. This advanced technology must be utilized early in the patient's course to be effective; thus, the helicopter is ideally suited to transport critical patients to medical specialists and their equipment. The ability to land at the accident site or rural hospital parking lot together with the lack of pressure changes at flying altitudes make the helicopter a true ambulance without roads. Recent examples of types of trauma which benefit from rapid transport to trauma centers include: victims of head and other trauma for early computerized axial tomography (CAT) or MRI and definitive surgical treatment; patients with spinal cord injury requiring hyperbaric oxygen therapy available only at a few locations; and those needing emergency coronary artery surgery following the onset of angina (Chapter 20).

These and other important medical advances will be available to many people through helicopter transport systems. The aviation medicine specialist plays a critical role in the planning, design, and operational aspects of the aeromedical rescue and transport of critical patients. The general medical orientation of most aviation medicine specialists proves highly valuable for these needs; however, those with additional clinical specialties will add critical and specific information to a growing body of aeromedical knowledge.

The Army has made a major commitment to rotary wing aircraft to satisfy needs for mobility and firepower over large and diffused battlefields, for logistic support, and for evacuation of casualties. New generation helicopters will be capable of extended ranges, carry large useful loads, and approach or exceed the cost and complexity of many jet fighter aircraft.

The pilots of these and future Army helicopters will find themselves seated in aircraft capable of $> 3-4 + Gz + Gz$ and 0.5 to 1.0 $- Gz$ and equipped with complex armaments for air-to-air and air-to-ground combat. Multiple image intensifiers integrated with weapons and aircraft instrument presentations, highly accurate navigation systems, electronic countermeasure equipment, and devices to counter microwave and laser energies will all be used by the aviator during combat flight to enhance effectiveness and counter the threats. Filtered positive pressure environmental control systems to counter chemical and toxic threats, and an on-board oxygen generating system for night and mountain operations will also be present.

Human engineering with automation of flight control, weapons, communication, countermeasure, and weapons systems will be employed wherever possible to reduce workload and capitalize on the human capability. Higher fidelity simulators and automated training devices will reduce training costs; however, investments in aircraft and the crew will remain substantial. Army aviation will undergo greater specialization resulting in increasing specific requirements for aeromedical support. The unit flight surgeon will continue to apply specific medical and scientific information to support training and specific mission requirements to help the commander achieve optimal combat effectiveness. The aerospace medicine specialist will be vitally important to this process.

As rapid technological growth has outpaced the native ability of man, aviation medicine must concentrate on the development of information systems to correlate performance with measurable physical and psychological guidelines. Flight surgeon involvement in research, development, and acquisition of new aviation systems will assure the optimal human-machine interface. The flight surgeon's close involvement in combat doctrine development will help counter chemical, toxic, biological, and electromagnetic energy threats. Medical expertise critical to research and development of protective equipment, systems, and techniques will protect the aviator and maintain optimal performance. Preventive medicine principles will become ingrained in the aviation force to meet the medical, physiological, and psychological challenges of the worldwide mission. The multifaceted contributions of the Army flight surgeon will maintain aviation safety and combat readiness to meet tomorrow's challenges and help Army aviation live up to its motto: ABOVE THE BEST!

ACKNOWLEDGMENTS

The Authors wish to thank other Army personnel for their contributions to this chapter: Rhonda Cornum, M.D., Ph.D., John Crowley, M.D., M.P.H., Warner Farr, M.D., M.P.H., Dan Fitzpatrick D.O., M.P.H., Joseph Haley, Jr., B.S., Jerry Hope, M.D., M.P.H., Nick Johnson, B.S., MBA, David Lam, M.D., M.P.H., J.D. LaMothe, Ph.D., Keith Martin, M.D., M.P.H., Kevin Mason, M.D., M.P.H., Dennis Shanahan, M.D., M.P.H., David Wehrly, M.D., M.P.H., Robert Weien, M.D., M.P.H., and Roger Wiley, Ph.D.

REFERENCES

1. Politella D. Operation grasshopper. Tyler: Robert R Longo Company Inc, 1958.
2. Tierney RK. Forty years of army aviation, part 3: Combat. US Army Aviation Digest 1982;28:19–32.
3. Link MM, Coleman HA. Medical support of the Army Air Forces in World War II. Washington, DC: Office of the Surgeon General, USAF, 1955.
4. Neel SH, Shamburek RH. History of Army Aviation medicine. US Army Aviation Digest 1963;9:34–9.
5. Wright RH. Night vision system performance criteria. Fort Rucker: US Army Aeromedical Research Laboratory, LR 75-20-4-2, 1974.
6. Rash CE, Verona RW, Crowley JS. Human factors and safety considerations of night vision systems flight using imaging systems. SPIE Proceedings: Optical Engineering and Photonics in Aerospace Sensing. Orlando, 1990.
7. Mitchell GW, Knox FS, et al. Microclimate cooling and the aircrew chemical defense ensemble. Fort Rucker: US Army Aeromedical Laboratory Report 86–12, 1986.
8. Johnson JC, Priser DB. Vibration levels in army helicopters-measurement recommendations and data. Fort Rucker: US Army Aeromedical Research Laboratory, TR 81–5, 1982.
9. North Atlantic Treaty Organization Advisory Group for Aerospace Research and Development. Backache and back discomfort. AGARD-CP-378, 1986.
10. Department of the Army. Crash survival design guide. Fort Eustis: US Army Air Mobility Research and Development Laboratory, TR 71–22, 1971.
11. Department of Defense Military Standard. Light fixed- and rotary-wing crash worthiness. Washington, DC: Department of Defense, MIL-STD-1290 (Av), 1974.
12. Shanahan DF, Shanahan MO. Injury in U.S. Army helicopter crashes October 1979–September 1985. J Trauma 1989;29:415–423.
13. Shanahan DF, Shanahan MO. Kinematics of U.S. Army helicopter crashes 1979–1985. Aviat Space Environ Med 1989;60:112–121.
14. Singley GT III. Army aircraft occupant crash-impact protection. Army RD&A 1981;22:10–12.
15. Springate CS, McMeekin RR, Ruehle CJ. Fire deaths in aircraft without the crashworthy fuel system. Aviat Space Environ Med 1989;60(Suppl):B35–8.
16. Sand LD. Comparative injury patterns in U.S. Army helicopters, U.S. Army Agency for Aviation Safety. In: Operational helicopter aviation medicine. Neuilly-sur-Seine, France: AGARD Conference, 1978. Proceedings No. 255; 54–1 to 54–7.
17. Reading TE, Haley JL, et al. SPH-4 U.S. Army flight helmet performance, 1972–1983. Aviat Space Environ Med 1989;60(Suppl):B110–20.
18. Department of the Army. Army flight surgeons' manual. Fort Rucker: US Army Aeromedical Center 1976;ST-105-8.
19. Department of the Army. Aeromedical training for flight personnel. Washington, DC: Dept of the Army, Jan 1979;TC 1–20.
20. Department of the Army. Standards of medical fitness. Washington, DC: Dept of the Army, Aug 1995;AR 40–501.
21. Edwards RJ, Price DR. Descriptive analysis of medical attrition in U.S. Army Aviation. Aviat Space Environ Med 1989;60(Suppl):A92–7.
22. Rhee KJ, Holmes EM, et al. A Comparison of Emergency Medical Helicopter Accident Rates in the United States and in the Federal Republic of Germany. Aviat Space Environ Med 1990;61:750–2.

Chapter 23

Naval Aerospace Medicine

Captain Ronald Ohslund,

MC, USN-Ret

Naval Aerospace Medicine

Resident Classes 1990 & 1991

The whole principle of naval fighting is to be free to go anywhere with every damned thing the Navy possesses.

Sir John Fisher, 1919

Operating aircraft from ships makes naval aviation unique. The naval aviator is routinely subjected to levels of stress and danger that are not experienced elsewhere, such as jockeying a fighter to an arrested landing on a pitching carrier deck steaming at 30 knots, or landing a helicopter on the stern of a bobbing destroyer at night. The first solo carrier landing requires the highest levels of skill, confidence, and support with no margin for error; each subsequent landing is a matter of refining technique and gaining experience. Aviation training not only demands proficiency and accuracy but also the ability to perform in progressively more difficult environments, such as "Blue Water" operations, where the ship provides the only dry landing area available (Fig. 23.1).

Many similarities exist between naval aviators and those who choose to practice naval aerospace medicine. Naval flight surgeon training is challenging, but the anxiety of being part of a small, isolated medical practice, responsible for the care and safety of thousands of personnel, is overcome by the challenge and excitement of living "on the edge."

HISTORY OF NAVAL AEROSPACE MEDICINE

The destiny of the Navy has been uniquely shaped through the concerted efforts of the naval aviation team. Throughout the last seventy years, flight surgeons have been an integral part of that team, whose efforts achieved victory in World War II and which has since participated in other limited-intensity conflicts in the last two decades.

Technologic advances have made it possible to fly at supersonic speed and at altitudes limited only by the supply of oxidants; they have enabled us to put humans in space, to land them on the Moon, and to envision the exploration of other planets. Many of those responsible for the early work associated with these accomplishments, as well as ongoing efforts toward future goals, have done their research and training through Navy-sponsored programs.

Early Years

Within a decade after the Wright brothers changed history at Kitty Hawk, people of vision

731

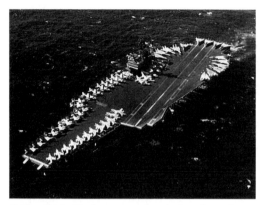

Figure 23.1. Modern operational aircraft carrier underway.

realized the value of aircraft at sea. In 1911, the first launch and recovery of an aircraft from a ship was achieved. Recognizing the unique character of problems associated with aviation, both ashore and afloat, the Navy sent its first five flight surgeons for training at the Army's School of Aviation Medicine at Mitchell Field in New York between 1922 and 1926.

In 1922, the first United States aircraft carrier, USS Langley, was commissioned, and the Bureau of Medicine and Surgery established its Aviation Medicine Division. After the successful launch of naval aviation medicine, the Great Depression sharply curtailed expansion of these programs. Between 1926 and 1934, only 25 naval flight surgeons were trained; many were assigned to general medical duties, often far removed from the aviation community needing their support.

World War II

By the late 1930s, the winds of war were stirring and America was emerging from its depression and geopolitical isolation. Recognizing the revolutionary and far-reaching ability of carrier aircraft to project power at sea and ashore, the Navy developed and procured faster, more powerful aircraft and carriers. These new aircraft could climb to higher altitudes, withstand greater ''G'' loads, carry more avionics, and provide a

broader scope of mission capabilities. They also ultimately subjected their occupants to greater extremes of environmental stress.

This technologic revolution mandated that specially trained physicians, psychologists, and physiologists study, categorize, prevent, and treat those stressors and maladies unique to the naval aviator. Thus, in 1939, the Navy established a School of Aviation Medicine at the Naval Air Station in Pensacola, Florida, and launched its first graduates in 1940. Since its inception, nearly 4500 physicians have been trained and designated as naval flight surgeons.

At the start of World War II, there were approximately 50 naval flight surgeons on active duty. By the end of the war, the Navy had 80 aircraft carriers afloat, and more than 1200 medical officers and flight surgeons directly supporting Navy and Marine Corps aviation units. Others remaining at home established the Navy's first research laboratories to study such problems as G-induced loss of consciousness, aviator selection, physical standards, hypoxia, vertigo, and the early foundations of ergonomics associated with the human-machine interface. Flaws in physiology training, protective equipment, and survival gear were discovered, often through tragic mishaps. Programs were implemented to improve efficiency, performance, and survivability of both humans and machines. Curricula were developed for training technicians in aviation medicine, aerospace physiology, and search and rescue. This expansion of resources and training programs during the latter stages of World War II has never been equalled.

Post-War Years

The solutions to many of the problems identified during World War II remained elusive. Research concentrated on spatial disorientation, visual illusions, motion sickness, emergency egress and life-support equipment, protective clothing, ergonomics, and the psychological disorders associated with flight. The Naval Aviation Physiology program was established in 1951 in recognition of the increasingly complex field of aviation medicine.

The next two decades witnessed significant milestones. In 1956, a Residency in Aerospace Medicine, approved by the American Board of Preventive Medicine, was established at the Naval Aviation Medical Institute, later renamed the Naval Aerospace and Operational Medical Institute (NAMI) in Pensacola, Florida. The forum of the Special Board of Flight Surgeons evolved for disposition of difficult aeromedical cases. The Navy conducted extensive research and development for the National Aeronautics and Space Administration in support of the Mercury, Gemini, and Apollo programs, and naval aviators made significant contributions to the manned space programs. Alan Shepard, the first American in space, John Glenn, the first American in orbit, and Neil Armstrong, the first man on the moon were all naval aviators. The first space shuttle missions were piloted by naval aviators, John Young and Robert Crippen. Vital segments of their training were accomplished through the efforts of NAMI and the Naval Air Development Center's research centrifuge in Warminster, Pennsylvania. A coriolis accelerator platform and vestibular research unit were also established, leading to better understanding of spatial disorientation, "G"-induced loss of consciousness, vertigo, and space sickness syndrome. Flight surgeons and physiologists at NAMI also developed several devices which enhanced water survival training, helping to reduce fatalities associated with ditching at sea.

In 1970, the research wing of NAMI was renamed the Naval Aerospace Medical Research Laboratory (NAMRL) and designated a separate command. The tasking of both commands are described in detail in subsequent sections of this chapter.

Towards the Year 2000

As this century comes to a close, we can anticipate further quantum leaps in aerospace technology. No longer will an aviator be limited to fixed-wing versus rotary-wing aircraft. The Osprey represents both types in one airframe. Vehicles are being developed that will allow suborbital, high-speed intercontinental travel, allowing warfare to extend beyond the atmosphere into space. The High Frontier project heralds the development of powerful new directed-energy weapons. Plans are also underway for permanently manned space stations and interplanetary exploration of several years duration.

Each of these projects presents the Navy's aerospace medicine community with new hazards, stressors, and challenges. No matter where our naval forces sail, whether upon the high seas or among the stars, as Fleet Admiral Nimitz stated, "... the Navy is this nation's strongest instrument of policy in peace and its first line of defense in war." Support of the fleet in the defense of our country remains the mission of the aerospace medicine professionals who are launched from the Naval Aerospace and Operational Medical Institute.

BASIC NAVAL FLIGHT SURGEON TRAINING

Any physician desiring to pursue training as a naval flight surgeon must have earned a medical degree from an approved medical or osteopathic school, and have completed at least one year of graduate medical education. Over the years, many physicians with diverse medical specialties and subspecialties have also trained to be flight surgeons, enhancing the pool of talented physicians in the Navy's aerospace medical community.

Naval flight surgeons are trained to be operational medicine specialists. They practice clinical and preventive medicine away from land-based hospitals and clinics, working closely with their line counterparts "in the field." They must be physically qualified to fly, meeting Class II aviation standards. They must be in good overall health with benign medical histories and must have eyesight correctable to 20/20 in each eye with a refractive error no greater than ±5.50

diopters. Student flight surgeons meeting more exacting vision requirements have the opportunity to solo during the flight training phase of the program.

Once chosen, the student is ordered to NAMI at the Naval Air Station, Pensacola, where all Navy and Marine Corps aviators and aircrew receive their initial training. Here begins the six-month period of training leading to designation as a naval flight surgeon. NAMI has the capability of training one hundred flight surgeons per year, as well as aerospace physiologists, aerospace experimental psychologists, and allied foreign flight surgeon students.

The standard flight surgeon course is divided into two phases. Twelve weeks of didactic and clinical studies at NAMI comprise phase one. Included is special training in the fields particularly important to aviation medicine: ophthalmology, otorhinolaryngology, cardiology, neuropsychiatry, physiology, infectious diseases, dermatology, and toxicology. In addition, the students gain experience in special problem areas created by simulators and disorientation devices. Student flight surgeons also attend, as observers, Special Boards of Flight Surgeons which deliberate on referred complex aeromedical cases. They receive extensive training in aircraft mishap investigations, and learn aviation-related physical standards.

During the final phase of their training, the student flight surgeons report to Naval Air Training Schools Command and Naval Air Station Whiting Field for twelve weeks of ground school and flight training. The students fly the Beechcraft T-34C (Turbo Mentor) or the Bell TH-57C (Jet Ranger), following the same initial syllabus prescribed for all Navy and Marine Corps student aviators. The goal is to complete the familiarization portion of the primary flight syllabus, including solo flight when physically qualified.

Naval flight surgeon Wings of Gold are awarded upon graduation. They signify that physicians will apply well-rounded medical education with initiative, self-confidence, and atten-

tion to detail to support their command in meeting their operational commitments.

NAVAL FLIGHT SURGEON ASSIGNMENTS

After designation, naval flight surgeons are assigned to a variety of aviation units which reflect the diversity of naval aviation. Flight surgeons may be assigned to carrier airwings, Fleet Marine Force aviation units, patrol and helicopter squadrons, or to overseas or continental United States air stations. These assignments are made based on the needs of the service and take into account the desires of the individual flight surgeon.

Carrier Airwings

Perhaps nothing better embodies the unique role of the naval flight surgeon than serving with a carrier airwing. This visible, publicized and even romanticized collection of aircraft, people, and warships is ready to project power and demonstrate military presence in areas far removed from land-based assets. Usually two flight surgeons are assigned to the Commander, Carrier Air Wing (CAG) staff, sharing responsibility for nine squadrons. Locations for air-wing units are displayed in Table 23.1.

Typically, an airwing is composed of the following squadrons: two fighter (F-14A Tomcat), two light attack (F/A-18 Hornet or A-7E Corsair), one medium attack (A-6E Intruder), one electronic counter-measures (EA-6B Prowler), one helicopter antisubmarine warfare/search and rescue (SH-3 Sea King), one fixed-wing antisubmarine warfare (S-3A Viking), and an airborne early warning (E-2C Hawkeye) squadron. Thus, while the airwing commander is the reporting senior officer, flight surgeons also serve the needs of the commanding officers of the various squadrons over which they have cognizance, as well as the senior medical officer of the carrier or shore-based branch clinic or hospital (Fig. 23.2).

The airwing commander and staff are based at various Naval Air Stations when not de-

Table 23.1
Location of Naval Aircraft Squadrons

Aircraft	COMNAVAIRPAC*	COMNAVAIRLANT
A-6E	NAS Whidbey, WA	NAS Oceana, VA
A-7E	NAS Lemoore, CA	NAS Cecil Field, FL
E-2C	NAS Miramar, CA	NAS Norfolk, VA
EA-6B	NAS Whidbey, WA	NAS Oceana, VA
F-14A/A+	NAS Miramar, CA	NAS Oceana, VA
F/A-18A	NAS Lemoore, CA	NAS Cecil Field, FL
H-3	NAS North Island, CA	NAS Jacksonville, FL
S-3A	NAS North Island, CA	NAS Cecil Field, FL

* Carrier Airwing 5 which deploys on-board USS Midway is forward homeported in Naval Air Facility, Atsugi, Japan and is composed of F/A-18, A-6E, EA-6B, and H-3 squadrons.

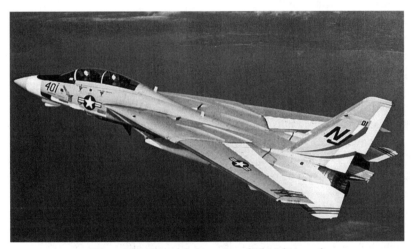

Figure 23.2. Naval fighter aircraft F-14 (Tomcat).

ployed. The squadrons are assigned to Commander, US Naval Air Forces, Pacific (COMNAVAIRPAC) and Commander, US Naval Air Forces, Atlantic (COMNAVAIRLANT). Squadrons flying similar aircraft are grouped into functional wings located at one air station on each coast (Table 23.1). This arrangement helps coordinate training and maintenance by concentrating similar aircraft. The aircraft carriers on which the wings operate are likewise homeported in different locations. The logistics of wedding the various wing squadrons with the ship are complex and challenging.

Aircraft Carrier Medical Department

The modern aircraft carrier has been described as the most dangerous occupational setting in the world. The aviation and industrial activities of a 6000 person ship with 90 aircraft operating day and night in all weather conditions from four acres of flight deck in a maze of passages, ladders, conduits, pipes, cables, and machinery are conducive to a wide range of injuries. This environment of high-mass, high-energy, jet fuel and ordnance carries an ever-present potential for disaster. When considering shipboard operations from the first training cycle to the completion of a combat cruise, every member of the crew and embarked airwing must not only be proficient in their assigned duties but be fully trained to react properly to every potential disaster. Any ship, even when tied to a pier, presents a multitude of potential dangers to the unwary and careless crewmember. Time spent steaming only magnifies the risks.

Fire, collision, person overboard, electrocution, exposure to toxins, novice, falls, burns, or aircraft-related accidents are only a few of the more common causes of injury and death. Every crewmember is trained in self-help and buddy-aid, because the first priority in any disaster is to save the ship. Definitive medical care is only available when the ship is no longer in extreme danger. Medical Department personnel, therefore, must be first-aid instructors, practitioners of preventive medicine, safety inspectors, counselors, and compatriots. Although the tasks are demanding and the deployments long, the airwing billet is one of the most sought after by junior flight surgeons.

Medical Department staff includes the Senior Medical Officer (SMO), the two airwing flight surgeons, a general surgeon, a general medical officer, a physician's assistant, a nurse-anesthetist, a general duty nurse, a medical administrative officer, and 40–45 corpsmen. The Dental Department, with three dentists and an oral surgeon, is a separate entity which joins assets with the medical department during emergencies. Medical Department duties include sick call, physical examinations, ward patient care and departmental or ship-wide training. Additionally, watchstanding and coverage of the ship's ER rotates among the physicians, both at sea and upon reaching liberty or working ports. The carrier Medical Department includes its own laboratory, pharmacy, radiographic suite, operating rooms, physical examination suite with hearing booth, lens fabrication lab, eye examination lanes (including slit lamp and phoropter), and a 70-bed hospital ward.

Senior Medical Officers, usually Commanders or Captains, are frequently graduates of the Navy's Residency in Aerospace Medicine. They are permanent members of the ship's company for their two-year tours. Besides responsibility for the medical care and readiness of the carrier crew, they are also medical advisors for their entire deployed battle group, which may include a dozen smaller ships with 2000–3000 total crewmembers, in addition to the 5000–6000 aboard the carrier. The carrier serves as a floating referral center for the other ships in the battle group, which generally do not have medical officers aboard. The carrier also provides aeromedical support to the aviation detachments (usually helicopters) aboard escort or support ships.

Aircraft Carrier Deployment Cycle

The typical aircraft carrier deployment is based on an 18-month cycle: six months for pre-deployment exercises and "work-ups"; six months deployed, generally to the Western Pacific/Indian Ocean or to the Mediterranean; and six months post-cruise stand down.

Predeployment work-ups reunite the elements of the airwing after six months of independent operations, culminating in a major strike exercise, where the wing flight surgeon has an opportunity to fly in each of the multi-seat aircraft assigned to the wing. The airwing then rejoins the carrier for Carrier Qualifications, Refresher Training, Weapons Training and an Operational Readiness Exercise, each representing about two weeks at sea. During these evolutions, the squadron aircraft, personnel, medical records, and communication centers ferry back and forth between home base and the carrier.

For the flight surgeon, this is also the period when immunizations must be updated for all personnel, squadron records screened, physicals performed for those who will be working the flight deck, and eyeglasses and any non-standard medications ordered.

One recurrent portion of the pre-deployment cycle is the staging of mass casualty and conflagration exercises which test the entire ship in its ability to isolate and minimize fire and damages, respond to the injured, and practice military triage and transport. These large-scale exercises occur throughout the work-up cycle, culminating in a major mass casualty drill during the final Operational Readiness Exam (ORE). This is a key test upon which the skill of the medical department is judged. Well-honed teamwork from a large variety of medical and non-medical personnel positioned throughout the ship is essential to its success. When all these diverse training evolutions have been completed, the carrier and airwing enter a month of final preparations and a relaxed tempo of operations which allow personnel to prepare themselves and their families for deployment.

While deployed, the airwing flight surgeon is assigned to the ship's medical department, working under the direction of the Senior Medical Officer, but retaining the airwing and squadron responsibilities. One flight surgeon is generally given responsibility for the Flight Deck Battle Dressing Station, which is staffed by two corpsmen at all times during flight operations, and which serves as a staging area for flight deck casualties. During actual or drill general-quarters situations (when the ship is fully prepared for combat with all personnel at their battle stations and all weapon, damage control, and other systems activated), the flight surgeon staffs this station, conducting training or providing direct medical support and treatment until casualties can be transported to the main medical spaces.

Usually the two airwing flight surgeons rotate the flight surgeon duty, so that one will always be on board and available for aeromedical problems, such as flight physicals, and mishaps. The other will be flying, delivering briefs to the squadrons, touring workspaces, or generally being available to the aircrews.

At the end of the six-month deployment, the embarked airwing disperses to the various home bases. This transition period also sees replacement personnel joining the squadron, and the training syllabus for all aircrew starts a new cycle. Generally, squadrons train independently during this six-month period, with short detachments for bombing and gunnery practice, tactical exercises, and hosted operations with other Navy, Air Force, or Marine units.

The carrier mission, the crew, and aircraft of the airwing provide exciting and challenging opportunities for flight surgeons to hone their medical skills and judgment, and to operate in an unparalleled environment. Carrier medicine combines the mundane with the state of the art: sanitation, hygiene, radiation, lasers, infrared, biological and chemical hazards, sexually transmitted diseases, sustained operations and the psychological implications of family separation, job stress and crowding. All these—the opportunity to launch in a thundering jet down a screaming catapult, the chance to travel and serve both the nation and some of the finest people in the world—make the job of the airwing flight surgeon one of the most exciting in Navy medicine.

Maritime Patrol

Submarine forces pose a unique threat. To protect freedom of navigation, worldwide surveillance is maintained by Navy maritime-patrol squadrons flying the P-3C Orion aircraft. The P-3C is a multi-engine, multi-piloted, transoceanic aircraft flying from shore air stations. COMNAVAIRLANT has maritime-patrol squadrons at NAS Brunswick, Maine and NAS Jacksonville, Florida, while COMNAVAIRPAC squadrons are at NAS Moffett Field, CA, and NAS Barbers Point, HI. Each base has six squadrons, with two squadrons deployed to forward operational bases. Normally, squadrons deploy for six months alternated with 12 months at home base.

The patrol squadron consists of nine airplanes, 36 aviators, 24 naval flight officers, and 280 enlisted personnel. Squadron medical support is provided by a flight surgeon and three hospital corpsmen. The medical support accompanies the squadron during deployment.

Flight surgeons are responsible to the Commanding Officer for occupational and preventive medicine programs, such as immunization, respirator usage, physical examination program, and health record maintenance. They fly with all aircrews to become familiar with mission and personnel factors.

P-3Cs typically fly long-duration (up to 13 hours), low-level, all-weather, day and night missions. Various sensors include passive and active sonobuoys, magnetic detectors, and optical scanners. Weapons carried on board the P-3C include torpedoes, depth charges, mines, bombs, and Harpoon air-to-surface missiles. Flight crews consist of three aviators, two naval flight officers, and eight enlisted aircrew. Up to 23 total aircrew can be accommodated aboard the aircraft when needed. The potential stresses attending such missions require the active presence of the flight surgeon to monitor aircrew and maintenance personnel.

Helicopter Squadron and Air Station Assignments

The Navy flies helicopters in support of fleet operational requirements in a variety of missions. One Anti-Submarine Warfare (ASW) squadron, flying the SH-3 Sea King or SH-60F Seahawk, is assigned with each carrier airwing and supported by the airwing flight surgeons. Additionally, detachments fly the SH-2F and SH-60B aircraft from frigates, destroyers, and cruisers in the LAMPS (Light Airborne Multipurpose System) mission, including Surface Surveillance, Search and Control (SSSC), ASW, logistic, and medevac. These single-plane detachments consist of four pilots with 10 maintenance personnel and are supported by flight surgeons assigned to the homebase squadron.

Similarly, detachments of CH-46s conduct vertical replenishment (VERTREP) missions to provide logistical support for operational needs, ferrying supplies and material between supply ships and combatants. Squadrons and detachments of the MH-53E provide airborne mine-countermeasures support, as needed, for operations such as mine sweeping. When these units do not have integral flight surgeon support, personnel requiring aviation medical care are referred to the carrier battle group or the nearest Navy shore base with aviation medicine capability (Fig. 23.3).

Naval flight surgeons are also assigned to a number of other aviation units: VXE-6 from Point Mugu, CA (operating C-130 and UH-1N

aircraft to support scientific exploration of the Antarctic continent); the Presidential Helicopter Squadron (HMX-1 at Quantico, Virginia); Naval Air Test Center, Patuxent River, Maryland; Naval Air Warfare Center, Patuxent River, Maryland; Naval Weapons Center, China Lake, California; and the Blue Angels Flight Demonstration Team. A number of flight surgeons are also assigned to overseas squadrons and naval air stations.

Marine Corps Aviation

The United States Marine Corps is a separate uniformed service under the aegis of the Department of the Navy. The Navy Medical Department supports the Marine Corps, and naval flight surgeons support Marine aviation units. Marine Corps aviation units have unique organizational and command relationships during operational utilization.

The Marine Corps operational doctrine emphasizes the air-ground team integrated at relatively low command levels. The smallest such unit is the Marine Expeditionary Unit (MEU). Routinely, one MEU is kept in readiness afloat in both the Mediterranean and the Western Pacific regions. Three components to the MEU exist: composite helicopter squadron, infantry battalion, and additional support/maintenance units. The composite helicopter squadron has medium transport, heavy lift, utility, and attack helicopters, and at least four AV-8B Harrier jet aircraft. One flight surgeon and three Navy corpsmen are assigned to provide aeromedical support. The MEU also has one infantry battalion, with artillery, tanks, amphibious tractors, engineer, medical, and maintenance units. Normally, the entire MEU deploys aboard three to five amphibious ships of which at least one is an amphibious assault ship (Fig. 23.4).

While underway, the flight surgeon integrates into the ship's medical department. When the composite helicopter squadron deploys ashore, the surgeon accompanies the squadron. Support may be provided from a sick call box in a tent, from a small medical facility in a flight line

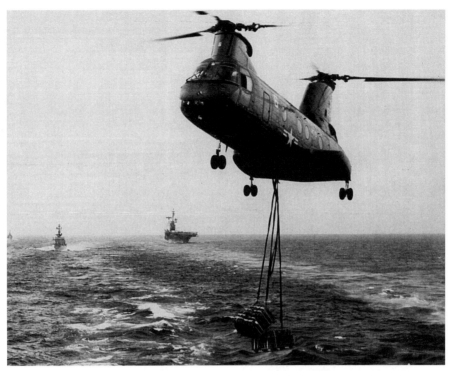

Figure 23.3. CH-46 Conducting vertical replenishment.

shack at an expeditionary air field, or from co-located medical treatment facilities. Prepacked medical supplies sufficient to support 15 days of combat operations are stored aboard the amphibious assault ships used for shore operations. Aboard the larger assault ships, medical facilities are available, including operating rooms, intensive care units, a ward facility, isolation rooms, laboratory, radiography, pharmacy, sick call, and administrative spaces. Often, assault ships deploy with a Mobile Medical Augmentation Readiness Team (MMART) aboard, which have a full operating room team, including general surgeon, orthopedic surgeon, and anesthesiologist.

The next larger operational unit is the Marine Expeditionary Brigade (MEB), which carries 30 days of supplies. There are three components of a MEB: a Marine Air Group (MAG), a Marine infantry regiment, and support/maintenance units. The Marine Air Group will include both fixed-wing and helicopter squadrons. The larg-est Marine operational unit is the Marine Expeditionary Force (MEF) composed of a Marine Aircraft Wing (MAW), a Marine Division (MARDIV), and support/maintenance units. This force of 50,000 Marines and Sailors carries 60 days of supplies. Aeromedical as well as general medical support is integrated into a MEF or MEB.

The Marine Corps emphasizes high standards of readiness under the most adverse circumstances. Marine squadrons (including fixed-wing) may deploy to the field and operate from tents. Air-traffic control and other support units are included in such field operations. Operating under spartan conditions is embraced as a challenge. The Marines are expected to be at maximum operational readiness; they demand no less from their medical support. The flight surgeons may spend half of their operational tour operating from a variety of environments: austere field conditions, mountainous areas, deserts, snow/arctic environments, and

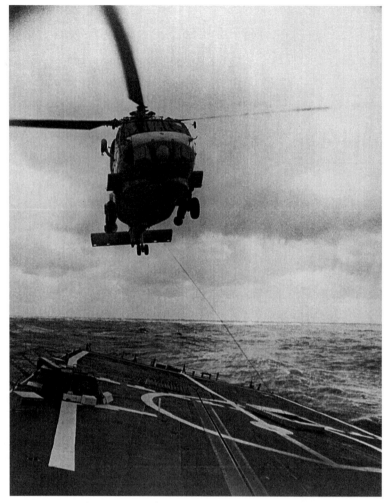

Figure 23.4. Helicopter landing on assault ship.

aboard ships. Marine squadrons have a reputation for integrating their flight surgeon support
into daily operations.

AEROSPACE MEDICINE RESIDENCY

For flight surgeons who desire to pursue a career
path in aviation and aerospace medicine, the
Navy offers a three-year residency program. The
special concern of the Navy program is tied to
the role of the Navy aeromedical specialist in the
deployed environment. The resident completing
this training is prepared to serve in a leadership
capacity, initially as the Senior Medical Officer

aboard an aircraft carrier. Further assignments
may include major staff positions with major
operational and administrative commands
ashore or afloat, and with the Fleet Marine
Forces. The Navy's residency in aerospace medicine encompasses all aspects of the American
Board of Preventive Medicine's requirements,
augmenting those requirements with specific
Navy training.

A strong background in clinical medicine is
required by the Navy, because the medical department of the aircraft carrier is the referral center for all ships in company during periods of
forward deployment. However, the special re-

quirements of preventive medicine, mastered by the resident in aerospace medicine, are also essential to the health of the task group of carrier and ships in company.

The three-year aerospace medicine residency includes Navy sponsorship of an academic year in an accredited School of Public Health, or its equivalent. The remaining two years are spent at NAMI, where the resident is given two or three months advanced training in each of the Institute's specialty clinics: Internal Medicine/Cardiology, Ophthalmology, Otorhinolaryngology, Neuropsychiatry and Aviation Physical Qualifications.

Each resident is also required to attend a variety of meetings and courses given throughout the country, including the Aerospace Medicine Association annual scientific meeting; Navy, Army and Air Force Operational Aeromedical Problems Courses; Advanced Aircraft Crash Survival Investigation School; a space medicine module at the Johnson Space Flight Center in Houston; Navy Undersea Medicine Course, Naval Diving School; a month-long rotation at the Burn Unit, US Army Institute of Surgical Research; Global Medicine at the USAF School of Aerospace Medicine; and a rotation in emergency medicine/trauma at a local civilian hospital center.

Other responsibilities include training of student flight surgeons, student aviation corpsmen, enlisted staff training, visiting lectures to Navy training wings, etc. Residents must maintain currency in annual physical examinations, physiology and water survival, and flight-time participation.

The residents perform a variety of additional duties while assigned to NAMI. They stand as flight surgeon coordinator for the Pensacola area, and may be tasked to provide aeromedical support for aircraft mishaps when other flight surgeons are not available. Physically qualified residents serve as hyperbaric medicine advisors after Navy Undersea Medicine training at Panama City, Florida. As such, they provide medical support for the hyperbaric chamber operations

and treat both aviation and diving decompression sickness cases.

The residents are required to participate in research in an area of personal interest on aviation-related topics. Research projects at NAMI or NAMRL are available. Up to two months of the first practicum may be used exclusively for research activities. One intent of these requirements is to encourage residents to submit articles for publication.

The residency in aerospace medicine provides the Navy with a steady flow of broadly trained aeromedical experts who are capable in general preventive, occupational, and industrial medicine as well as the clinical arena. This breadth of training and experience makes them uniquely qualified to assume roles of leadership and management in the Navy's demanding environments.

AEROMEDICAL SELECTION

The selection of candidates for aviation programs is an art that both line and medical advisors have sought to perfect for decades. The elusive ideal combination of physical attributes, psychomotor skills, and motivation essential to a successful and safe flyer has been a focus of attention since aviation programs began.

Psychological Selection

By World War I, it was recognized that a majority of aviation accidents could be attributed to pilot error, and that human factors were a major concern in aviation safety. The large cost of training and of the aircraft prompted careful selection of aviation candidates. Many aptitude and fitness tests and standards were applied, some of which proved invalid, while others have continued for lack of more precise or reliable tests. No single physical or psychological ideal emerged, although certain characteristics and biographic items have a high correlation with success in training and subsequent performance. By its nature, considerable self-selection among applicants occurs, and they tend to form a rather homogeneous group.

During World War II, the physical standards were relatively strict, and psychological factors received increased attention. An indomitable will to fight and win were considered essential. The effects of anxiety, temperament, and personality were soon as great a concern as physical condition. Stamina, intact senses, and lack of handicap were considered essential to success in aviation. Particularly, visual acuity, normal color vision, adequate depth perception, normal vestibular function, and good hand-eye coordination were considered necessary. Reaction-time, emotional stability, aptitude, and adaptability were some of the psychological characteristics considered important. Training, and the response to training, fatigability, and performance tests came into use as predictors of success.

Since 1947, the United States Navy has relied on the Aviation Qualification Test (AQT) of general ability and the Flight Aptitude Rating (FAR) to select naval aviators. This collection of tests determining mechanical comprehension, spatial aptitude and biographical data have proved useful. Still, the attrition rate among selectees during the past 20 years still remains relatively high (20–25%), although less than previously. A number of automated and computerized tests show promise. NAMRL demonstrated the ability to predict success at flight training, to predict an individual's flight grade and the number of flight hours required to complete primary training, and even to predict air combat performance of fleet pilots. Emphasis on newer personality tests—including the Defense Mechanism Test, the Personality Research Form, the Locus of Control, Work and Family Orientation Questionnaire, and Extended Personality Attributes Questionnaire—promise improved success at selection and improved aviation safety in the coming decade. No test or combination of tests is likely to provide the ultimate answer of motivation, innate ability, training, experience, and determination that has been the ultimate determinate

of success in aviation; however, quantitative methods, with a blend of human and humane inquiry and compassion, are likely to find better ways to determine "the right stuff."

Medical Selection

In the Navy, aircrew candidates are selected by the line community. The Medical Department, as a staff corps, makes recommendations to the line regarding medical fitness for special duty in aviation. Medical selection criteria are specified in Chapter 15 of the Manual of the Medical Department. Prior to assignment to aviation special duty and training leading to enlistment or commissioning, a physical examination is performed for the purpose of identifying physical defects and psychological problems which would jeopardize an aircrew member's ability to perform duties normally assigned. Depending upon the needs of the Navy, the standards cited in the Manual of the Medical Department are subject to change. Such changes are based on years of cumulative experience of naval aviation medicine and the work of individuals dedicated to research in aircrew selection. In general, if a defect were to constitute a menace or endangerment to health, general welfare, or aviation safety, it would be considered disqualifying. Medical standards for candidates, students, or designated aviation groups are detailed. Specific criteria in the specialties of otolaryngology, ophthalmology, medicine, neurology, and psychiatry are enumerated. The standards for special duty, including aviation duty, are determined by the Secretary of the Navy. An aviation medical examination is performed by an authorized aviation medical officer or proper authority designated by the Army or Air Force to perform such examination.

Medical Qualifications and Disposition

Aeromedical qualifications are used to ensure maximal flight safety and operational readiness. They are based on physical qualifications and aeronautical adaptability. Physical qualifications involve compliance with defined standards recommended by the Bureau of Medicine and Surgery (BUMED), Washington, DC, and approved by the Chief of Naval Operations (CNO) or Commandant of Marine Corps (CMC), as appropriate. Physical qualifications are periodically updated to reflect changes in aeromedical considerations. The understanding of Aeronautical Adaptability (AA) is based on certain related concepts regarding personality traits and disorders and the level of defensive functioning. Aeronautically Adaptable is a term reserved for candidates and students in aviation. These individuals have the potential to adapt to the rigors of the aviation environment by possessing the temperament, flexibility, and appropriate defense mechanisms necessary to suppress anxiety, maintain full attention to flight and successfully complete the mission. Aeronautically Adapted is a term reserved for designated aviators and aircrew. These individuals have demonstrated on a long-term basis the ability to utilize appropriate defense mechanisms, display temperament and personality traits necessary to maintain a compatible mood, suppress anxiety and devote full attention to flight safety and mission execution. In this context, mission execution includes not only the ability to successfully complete the mission, but also to participate harmoniously in flight crew coordination. From a psychiatric viewpoint, an Axis I diagnosis from the current Diagnostic and Statistical Manual of Mental Disorders (DSM) warrants treatment and would be considered not physically qualified (NPQ), while an Axis II diagnosis for personality disorders or maladaptive traits is considered not aeronautically adaptable/adapted (NAA). Personality traits which are considered maladaptive are those which negatively impact safety of flight, crew coordination and/or mission execution. An example would be an aviator whose obsessive-compulsive personality traits impair safety of flight when the aviator fixates on minor details in the cockpit and is unable to respond quickly enough in an emergency. Waivers may be considered for personnel who are found not

physically qualified; however, a finding of not aeronautically adaptable/adapted is considered permanent and not subject to waiver.

The physical standards requirements for naval aviation personnel are separated into two classes. Class I personnel are involved in duty involving actual control of the aircraft (DIACA), while Class II personnel are involved in duty involving flight (DIF). Within Class I, designated naval aviators (DNAs) are subdivided into three service groups, and student naval aviators (SNAs) constitute a special group. SNAs have the most stringent physical standards. Service Group I aviators have no medical limitations on aircraft assignment or in-flight duties. Service Group II aviators have medical limitations that preclude them from flying in single-piloted, tactical aircraft from ships, although they may fly as pilots in command of helicopters aboard ships, multi-piloted maritime/patrol/transport airplanes, and shore-based tactical aircraft. Service Group III aviators have medical limitations that prevent them from flying as pilot-in-command in fixed-wing or helicopters, but they may fly as copilots. Class II personnel are not formally subdivided; however, several subgroupings are maintained. Class II personnel include naval flight officers (NFOs), such as radar intercept officers (RIOs), bombardier-navigators (BNs), electronic warfare counter-measures officers (ECMOs), and tactical coordination and control officers (TACCOs). Flight surgeons, aerospace physiologists, and aerospace psychologists are considered Class II personnel, as are enlisted aircrew and air-traffic controllers.

Flight status personnel who are found not physically qualified (NPQ) may apply for a waiver of standards to Chief of Naval Operations or the Commandant of the Marine Corps after recommendation by the Bureau of Medicine and Surgery (BUMED). This process begins with the aviator's flight surgeon completing an aeromedical summary, including physical examination and appropriate consultations. The flight surgeon then formally requests a waiver of standards to CNO or CMC via the aviator's Commanding Officer and BUMED. NAMI serves as the representative for BUMED and acts on most waiver requests by endorsement. BUMED's recommendation is forwarded to CNO/CMC, who actually grant the waiver of physical standards.

When the aviator's flight surgeon has some concern about the disposition, he or she may request that the aviator's Commanding Officer convene a Local Board of Flight Surgeons (LBFS). The LBFS consists of three or more flight surgeons who review the case and make recommendations. In remote locations, one flight surgeon may constitute the LBFS. The LBFS has the authority to return an aviator to flight duties immediately, pending review by NAMI and CNO/CMC if considered appropriate. More difficult cases may be referred to NAMI for review by the Special Board of Flight Surgeons (SBFS). Upon referral, the aviator is examined by all NAMI clinical specialists, as well as other consultants as required. The aviator sits before the SBFS while his or her case is presented to the NAMI flight surgeons and clinical experts. The board reviews the many factors in the human-machine-mission interface and makes recommendations for aeromedical disposition. Occasionally, these recommendations are reviewed by the Senior Board of Flight Surgeons at BUMED, Washington, DC. The recommendations are then considered by CNO/CMC, who may waive standards as appropriate.

The Navy relies on its flight surgeons to operate independently from remote locations in providing quality aeromedical support to operational units. Naval flight surgeons must operate with minimal medical specialist support in dealing with a wide spectrum of disease processes. Well-trained flight surgeons are required who know the aeromedical standards, disposition procedures, and waiver process to expedite the handling of medically relevant issues.

RESEARCH IN NAVAL AVIATION MEDICINE

The Naval Aerospace Medical Research Laboratory (NAMRL), in Pensacola is the research component of naval aviation medicine, which began concomitant with the Naval School of Aviation Medicine in 1939. It performs an important and vital role in conducting research in support of fleet operations, aircrew selection, aircraft design, and mission effectiveness.

NAMRL is subordinate to the Naval Medical Research and Development Command within the Medical Department of the Navy, and has its own extensive physical plant and mission base. The laboratory conducts its research to meet expressed fleet needs. Areas of current research include: acceleration, spatial awareness, spatial disorientation, aircrew selection, sustained operations, aircrew equipment/systems test and evaluation, virtual reality and virtual environments patterns, aided and unaided night vision and instrument scan.

Civilian and military scientists are supported by professional, technical, and support personnel in maintaining a continuing flow of scientific reports describing the work of the laboratory, supporting the education and training missions of NAMI, and providing lecture and laboratory support for special groups involved in advanced aeromedical education.

NAMRL conducts basic and applied research to assess human performance of aircrew in operational tasks and develops a scientific rationale for performance standards used in selection, retention, and classification of aircrew. It also seeks ways to enhance physiologic performance of aircrew, and develops methods and devices to prevent and treat casualties in naval aviation operations.

Examples of problems addressed include sound attenuation data on the SPH-3C flight helmet, kits to train aided as well as unaided night vision, a device to aid accurate NVG focusing, a manual describing a physical fitness program designed to enhance aircrew G-tolerance, and interim guidelines for the use of stimulants to enhance human performance in sustained operations.

Another focus of NAMRL involves the physiologic and psychological response of Navy and

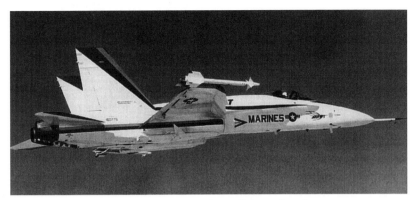

Figure 23.5. Marine Corps fighter aircraft.

Marine Corps personnel to physical and chemical environments associated with Navy equipment, operating procedures, or natural phenomena in deployment areas. In addition, tests and procedures for assessing the ability of individuals to succeed in flight training and as aircrew, secondary assessment decisions regarding operational assignment and classification, automation of measurement devices, identification of aviator skills, and personnel retention and motivation are being investigated.

Examples of findings that have affected the Navy and Marine Corps mission include: radio-frequency current meters developed for shipboard use to quantitate the radio-frequency-induced currents in shipboard personnel who work near high frequency transmitting antennas; tests that reduce the uncertainty of predicting performance during flight training; and specific absorption rate (SAR) measurements in shipboard working conditions to predict safe topside areas when high frequency fields are a consideration.

Research at NAMRL is coordinated with and supplemented by research conducted at the Naval Air Warfare Center in Warminster, Pennsylvania, which conducts research in air vehicle and crew systems, human factors and protective systems, escape systems, and advanced life-support systems. The Center also supports a vision laboratory, thermal chamber, ejection tower, and a multidimensional centrifuge for G-induced

loss of consciousness research and training. Both facilities provide the research, development, testing, and evaluation in aviation medicine and allied sciences that impact the human-machine interface and ensure the health, safety, and readiness of Navy and Marine Corps personnel (Fig. 23.5).

FUTURE DIRECTION

Today's aeromedical specialist is faced with ever-increasing professional demands compounded by the scientific and technologic advances and complexities of an inherently dangerous aviation environment. Tomorrow's specialists will be challenged to provide and render quality aeromedical services through knowledge and experience gained directly from academic and operational training.

The Naval Aerospace and Operational Medical Institute will continue to support the Navy's operational commitments and their extraordinary medical demands by selecting and training residents in aerospace medicine. NAMI will also continue to train flight surgeons, aerospace physiologists, aerospace experimental psychologists, and other aeromedical personnel to meet and effectively deal with the complex physical and psychological problems created by the aviation environment.

Chapter 24

Civil Aviation Medicine

Stanley R. Mohler

The commonplace of the schoolbooks of tomorrow is the adventure of today, and that is what we are engaged in.

Jacob Brownowski

The air transport industry, including the airframe manufacturers, the airlines, general aviation, and a myriad of supporting activities of every variety, has become a major force in the nation's, as well as the world's, economy and industry. The original lead established by the United States with the introduction of the DC-2/DC-3 series aircraft in the 1930s has never been relinquished. Every year, the aviation industry contributes over $50 billion to the gross national product and provides employment for over 1 million individuals. Approximately 50% of the world's civilian transports were manufactured in the United States.

Today in the United States, public air carriers have become a primary long-haul mover of people. It is estimated that 85% of long-haul public carrier transportation is by air and that 95% of international travel is by air. The U.S. scheduled airlines move nearly 400 million persons per year, the equivalent of moving nearly twice the entire U.S. population from one place to another. Of equal significance has been the enormous growth of general aviation—the private, corporate, and business fleet—which now flies 100 million people both domestically and internationally.

Significant aeromedical factors are involved in civil aviation. These factors will be discussed with a particular emphasis on their application to general aviation. These factors represent a combination of specialized aeromedical knowledge, general medical information, and, as importantly, common sense.

The practitioner engaged in civil aviation medicine must be receptive to new concepts and data developed from research, aircraft accident investigations, and direct clinical experience. Professional and ethical concerns must bridge the chasm between obligations to the aviator and obligations to the public safety.

SCOPE OF CIVIL AVIATION MEDICINE

Aeromedical support to civil aviation is complex because of two primary factors. First, aeronautic systems range in complexity from balloons, gliders, and ultralights to large jumbo and sleek supersonic commercial jet transports (Figs. 24.1 and 24.2). Second is the diversity of education, training, experience, sophistication, and health status of the aviator flying these systems.

Airline Operations

Within the United States, 4017 airline turbojet aircraft belong to more than 77 airline carriers and fly over 4164 million miles annually. The long-term trend in the number of passengers

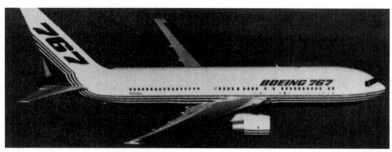

Figure 24.1. The Boeing 767 airliner contains advanced technology design features. It is certified by the Federal Aviation Administration for a flight deck crew of two, a result of diminished crew workload through the extensive use of automation. The supercritical wing airfoils and the two-engine configuration provide fuel-efficient operations. The Boeing 767 can carry 211 passengers and has a maximum range of 5200 km (photo courtesy of the Boeing Company).

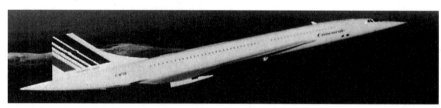

Figure 24.2. The Mach 2 supersonic transport Anglo-French Concorde has halved the flight times from Europe to the Americas (it is also used on Europe to mid-East runs). It carries up to 140 passengers and can cruise at an altitude of 20,000 m. At a weight in the range of 171,000 kg, or 376,000 lb (190,000 lb of this weight is fuel), it can carry a payload of 11,400 kg. Because of the continuous sonic-boom "carpet" produced during supersonic flight, the Concorde confines speeds of Mach 1 and above to over ocean segments when flying between Europe and the Americas (photo courtesy of the British Aerospace Corporation).

carried continues to increase. It has been estimated that in 1990, 4055 airline aircraft carried 460 million passengers within the United States and 40 million to and from outside destinations.

Worldwide, nearly 10,000 airline aircraft are in operation, providing air transport service to over 600 million passengers. These aircraft log over 700,000 million passenger-miles per year.

The captain (pilot-in-command) of these aircraft must have an airline transport pilot certificate and a Class 1 medical certificate. The first-officer (copilot) and flight engineer positions require a commercial pilot and flight engineer certificate, respectively, and a Class 2 medical certificate. On March 15, 1960, the then Federal Aviation Agency imposed a controversial upper age limit of 60 years on the pilot-in-command and copilot aboard airline transports.

The limit was not applied to flight engineers because there is no stated justification for doing so.

Since the promulgation of this rule, it has been the subject of increasing scrutiny and controversy. The Federal Aviation Administration (FAA) has defended the age 60 rule as necessary to protect the public from age-related performance decrements in pilots, contending that such deterioration cannot be measured dependably. On the other side, persons who oppose the rule (and many are physicians) say it is discriminatory because it is based on age alone and does not consider the individual's ability to do his or her job; arbitrary, because there is no scientific basis for choosing age 60; and unnecessary because it is now feasible to measure individual performance and estimate the risk of incapacitation (1).

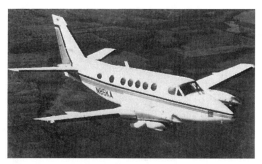

Figure 24.3. The Beechcraft King Air B-100 is a turboprop corporate, freight, air taxi, or commuter aircraft that has a passenger capacity of eight plus a crew of two. It is fully equipped with anti-icing equipment and can operate in virtually any kind of weather (photo courtesy of the Beech Aircraft Company).

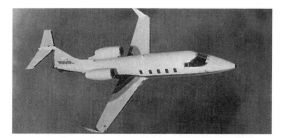

Figure 24.4. The Lear Model 55 represents an efficient sign in corporate jet technology. The aircraft is capable of cruising at 16,000 m with a maximum range of 3600 km. It can carry 10 passengers with a crew of two. The wing incorporates the winglets, developed by the National Aeronautics and Space Administration, to increase aerodynamic efficiency (photo courtesy of the Gates Learjet Company).

Air Taxi and Air Commuter Operations

In 1990, air taxi and air commuter operations carried 35 million people, usually using aircraft at the smaller end of the passenger capacity scale (9 to 60 passengers). The continuing growth of this segment of aviation is forecast by the aviation authorities. Many of the aircraft used in this type of passenger transport are designed for short field operations and include rotary-wing helicopters (Fig. 24.3).

Aircrew members of these aircraft must have at least a commercial pilot certificate and a Class 2 medical certificate. No upper age limit applies to these aircrew members.

Corporate and Business Flying

Businesses of all sizes are finding the use of small and, at times, large aircraft a useful adjunct in meeting their executive travel needs. The aircraft operated may range from single-engine or twin-engine propeller aircraft through turboprop and small turbojet aircraft (Fig. 24.4).

Corporate pilots may be corporate officers or, more often, career pilots. No upper age limit applies to these crewmembers. When flying for hire, the crewmembers must hold a Class 2 medical certificate and a commercial pilot certifi-

cate. Occasionally, a corporation may operate certain of its aircraft as a revenue-generating activity in charter operations.

Aerial Application

Agricultural spray operations include the application of insecticides, weed control chemicals, defoliants, fertilizers, fire control substances, sterile male screwworm fly larvae, and other materials. Many of the chemicals used are highly toxic and most can cause illness and death. Crashes have occurred as a result of impairment caused by exposure to these substances.

Aerial application flying, also referred to as crop dusting, or top dressing in New Zealand and Australia, is governed by FAA regulations. Operators must demonstrate a knowledge of the chemicals they use, including their purposes and toxic characteristics. Many of the aircraft used in these operations are specifically designed for the purpose (Fig. 24.5). The aircraft are more maneuverable, have significantly more powerful engines, and have a crash-resistant cockpit area. Other special design features may include wire cutters on the landing gear struts to sever any power or telephone lines that are inadvertently struck. The pilots must have a commercial pilot certificate and a Class 2 medical certificate when

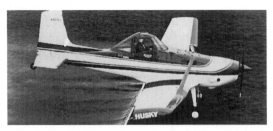

Figure 24.5. The Cessna Husky, an aerial applicator aircraft, can carry 920 L of liquid for dispersal. Rates of dispersal range from less than 1 L/acre to more than 20 L/acre. The cabin has air conditioning, and the aircraft can be equipped with external lights for night spray operations. "Automatic flagmen," little flags dropped at the end of each swath, can be used to improve the precision and efficiency of spraying (photo courtesy of the Cessna Aircraft Company).

flying for hire. No upper age limit applies. Cantor and Booze (2) investigated mortality among pesticide aerial applicators and flight instructors from aircraft crashes and cancer. The cohort mortality study calculated standardized mortality ratios (SMRs) for 9677 applicators and 9727 instructors. Overall excess mortality among applicators resulted from airlane crashes. Deaths from most chronic diseases, including cancer, was less than anticipated.

A few of the major categories of toxic substances used in aerial application are discussed in the following sections to provide a better understanding of their toxic potential.

Organophosphate Insecticides

Insecticidal and mammalian toxic effects in the organophosphate insecticides are derived from the inhibition of acetylcholinesterase enzymes in the nerve cells, as is the case with parathion. Symptoms may include nausea, vomiting, sweating, salivation, visual disturbances, bradycardia, and respiratory cessation. Death may follow. Pilocarpine-like pupillary constriction is ordinarily present, but dilated pupils also may be found.

Washing the contaminated areas with soap and water is the first treatment, followed by atropine for symptomatic relief, if necessary, and

pralidoxime (2-PAM) for cholinesterase enzyme reactivation.

Plasma cholinesterase enzyme measurements are useful as indicators of exposure during the spraying season. Heparin is the desired anticoagulant for freshly drawn blood samples because other anticoagulants may inactivate the enzyme.

Carbamate Insecticides

The symptoms, signs, and course of poisoning by carbamate insecticides are similar to, but do not last as long as, those of the organophosphates. A representative carbamate is tetraethyl pyrophosphate (TEPP). Carbamates also produce motor paralysis. Atropine is used for symptomatic treatment. Pralidoxime is ineffective.

Red blood cell cholinesterase enzyme measurements may be used to assess the degree of exposure. Again, heparin is the desired anticoagulant for the blood samples.

Chlorinated Insecticides

Because of increasing restrictions on their use, chlorinated insecticides (e.g., DDT, dieldrin, aldrin, endrin) are now rarely used by aerial sprayers in the United States. The toxic symptoms derive from central nervous system effects, including convulsions. Intermediate-duration barbiturates such as amobarbital (Amytal) and pentobarbital are used in treatment. The intermediate barbiturates help ensure that the stimulant effect of the pesticide is not exceeded by the depressant effect of the barbiturate.

Chlorinated Herbicides

Broad-leaf plants are especially susceptible to the chlorinated herbicides. These chemicals cause growth stimulation, including the production of bizarre plant configuration and plant death. Toxicity is low in humans. During the Vietnam War, herbicides were often disseminated by aircraft, and these chemicals have served as a focal point for a wide range of medical complaints alleged by veterans of that war.

To investigate the alleged health effects of these compounds, often referred to as Agent

Orange, and the highly toxic compound, dioxin, that contaminated the herbicides, the United States Air Force is conducting an extensive epidemiologic study of the aircrew associated with its aerial application. Although combat troops on the ground may have come in contact with the herbicide, by far the highest level of exposure was experienced by the aircrew flying the spray missions.

Nitrophenols

Nitrophenols produce ovicidal, acaricidal, and insecticidal effects. This group of chemicals also has herbicidal effects. In some cases, these substances are used as defoliants. Signs of poisoning include excessive sweating, thirst, euphoria, and subsequent fatigue. Immediate treatment for contamination consists of washing off the chemicals with soap and water. No antidote exists.

Paraquat

Paraquat is a potent irritant to the skin, although it is not readily absorbed. Oral intake of small amounts causes severe damage to the mouth, throat, and esophagus followed by pulmonary edema, pulmonary hemorrhage, and renal toxicity effects. There is no antidote.

Chemical Logbook

The former Soviet Union made an advance relating to aerial application flight safety: the chemical logbook (3). Each agricultural pilot in that former country maintains a chemical logbook, an entity separate from the flight logbook. The chemical log records the specific chemicals used during aerial application flights plus the times of exposures. This log is especially valuable to the attending physician should symptoms or signs of illness develop.

Private Flying

In the United States, there are more than 190,000 light aircraft and about 700,000 active general aviation pilots. These pilots may own an aircraft, belong to a flying club, or rent aircraft.

The pilots need have only a Class 3 medical certificate, which for student pilots may be the combined student/pilot medical certificate. The certificate is valid for 3 years; the lower age limit is 16 years, with no upper age limit. All general aviation pilots receive instruction about hypoxia, pressure changes, and disorientation, and the written examination for the pilot certificate includes questions on these subjects. Because of the importance of the material, aeromedical practitioners need to review with their pilot populations these physiologic concerns. Periodically, situations arise in which pilots are misinformed regarding their own limitations or those of the equipment they use. For example, a publication circulated among hang-glider enthusiasts advocated flights to 6096 m (20,000 ft) without oxygen. Such advice could lead to fatal mistakes. The physician must assist in providing sound and rational advice to the flyer.

The spectrum of recreational flying continues to expand. The small, fixed-wing, single-engine aircraft is by far the most common aircraft used in civil flying (Figs. 24.6 and 24.7). Gliding remains popular. Efficient, long-wing, powerless aircraft have achieved altitudes requiring supplemental oxygen and may remain airborne for many hours in long-duration flight. Each year, the skies near Albuquerque, New Mexico, become filled as hundreds of hot-air balloons participate in mass ascension. Hang-glider flying and parachuting are both recreational activities with growing numbers of participants. The ultralights do not require a FAA certificate, nor must the pilot be certified. These very small aircraft must weigh less than 70.3 kg and carry 6.8 kg or less of fuel (Fig. 24.8).

Pilot Medical Certification Exceptions

At the minimum, civil pilots require the medical and pilot certificates necessary for the type of flight operations conducted. In the case of United States glider and balloon operations, only self-proclamation of health status is necessary. Public safety is the concept underlying medical

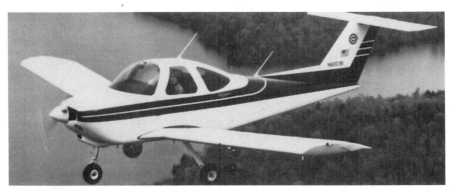

Figure 24.6. The Beechcraft Model 77 Skipper, a two-seat training plane, reflects a typical light plane design of the late 1970s. It has a 115-hp Lycoming engine and cruises at 105 knots. An inertia-reel shoulder harness is provided for each seat (photo courtesy of the Beech Aircraft Company).

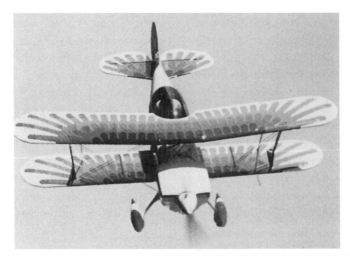

Figure 24.7. The Cristen Eagle II is a top two-seat aerobatic aircraft. Introduced in the 1970s, it is capable of maneuvers in excess of $+9$ G and -6 G. It can perform almost any conceivable aerobatic maneuver, including multiple inverted snap rolls, multiple turning tail slides, prolonged inverted spins, knife-edge flight, and Lomcovaks (photo courtesy of Christen Industries).

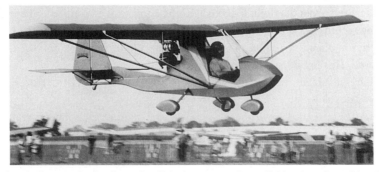

Figure 24.8. The Challenger single-place ultralight is a currently available aircraft. Neither it nor the pilot require Federal Aviation Administration certification. (Photo by Hal Adkins. Courtesy Quad City Ultralight Aircraft Corp., Moline, IL.)

Table 24.1.
Certificates Held in 1987

Type of Certificate	Number
Pilot	699,653
Student	146,016
Private	300,949
Commercial	143,645
Airline transport	91,287
Glider (only)	7,901
Helicopter (only)	8,702
Lighter than air	1,153
Nonpilot	370,602
Engineers	49,328
Navigators	1,445
Air traffic specialists	22,651
Aircraft mechanics	297,178

Table 24.3.
Civil Aircraft Active in the United States, 1989

Aircraft Group	Number
Fixed wing	204,067 (subtotal)
Turbine powered	9,612 (subtotal)
Turbojet	4,338
Turboprop	5,274
Piston-powered	194,455 (subtotal)
Multiengine	23,419
Single-engine	171,035
Rotary wing (includes autogyros)	6,333 (subtotal)
Turbine	3,520
Piston	2,813
Gliders/lighter than air	6,783
Total	217,183

FAA Stat Handbook CY 1989.

Table 24.2.
Civil Airmen Medical Certifications

Medical Certification	Number
Class 1	83,254
Class 2	157,219
Class 3	427,059
Total	667,532

(Total airmen certified as of December 31, 1989)

certification. In 1987, about 700,000 civil airmen held certificates (Table 24.1). Approximately one third of these aviators held instrument flying qualifications. The medical certificate levels are shown in Table 24.2.

Persons who do not meet all of the medical standards subsequently may become certified through the waiver route (the FAA concludes that there are compensatory factors in a pilot's requesting reconsideration that safely allow medical certification), the exception route (the FAA decides that in a specific case, the condition, although disqualifying by regulatory provisions, is no longer a safety hazard), or the judicial route (the National Transportation Safety Board or the courts overturn a prior medical certificate denial based on appeal information supplied by the plaintiff, frequently consisting of expert medical testimony by front-line physicians emphasizing medical advances in diagnosis and treatment).

In issuing a waiver, the FAA may base the decision on a "Statement of Demonstrated Ability." This statement is obtained by the requesting pilot, who may have paraplegia, monocular vision, color vision deficiency, hearing loss, or other impairment, after a satisfactory demonstration of performance to an FAA inspector. The inspectors have protocols for dozens of conditions that arise in this connection from time to time. Pilots with the following conditions have been individually certified on appeal: replacement heart valve, coronary bypass surgery, cerebral fluid shunt, chronic or paroxysmal atrial fibrillation, and cardiac pacemaker.

Aircraft Certification

The design, performance, and operational safety characteristics of an aircraft are determined by the FAA from data supplied by the manufacturer or obtained by flight tests. Table 24.3 provides data illustrating the progressive increase in civil aircraft.

The categories of airworthiness include fixed-wing airline aircraft (5670 kg and over) and general aviation aircraft. Rotary-wing aircraft and lighter-than-air categories also are specified.

A complex body of regulations has evolved regarding civil aircraft certification and operations progressively augmented whenever a new aircraft is developed. An infinite series of profiles showing cabin altitude versus time can be obtained between 2438 m (8000 ft), the upper allowable routine cabin altitude in United States civil airline operations, and the maximum cruising altitudes of civil aircraft. Selected key altitudes for civil aviation certification and operational purposes are as follows (given in feet, as in regulatory documents) (4).

Key Altitudes

8000 feet (2400 m)—Cabin altitude provides a blood oxygen saturation of approximately 93% in the resting individual who does not suffer from advanced cardiovascular or pulmonary disease. After suffering a hypoxic experience, this is the ceiling altitude to which an individual should be returned for physiologic compensatory mechanisms to effectively reoxygenate the body. Operationally, this altitude has been prescribed as the altitude above which passenger oxygen must be available in specified amounts.

10,000 feet (3000 m)—Cabin altitude provides a blood oxygen saturation of approximately 89%. After a period of time at this level, the more complex cerebral functions, such as making mathematical computations, begin to suffer, and night vision is markedly impaired. Crewmembers must use oxygen when the cabin pressure altitudes exceed 3048 m (10,000 ft).

12,000 feet (3600 m)—The blood oxygen saturation falls to approximately 87%. Some mathematical computation becomes difficult, short-term memory begins to be impaired, and errors of omission increase with extended exposure. Oxygen must be used by each crewmember on flight duty and must be provided for each crewmember during the flight when the cabin altitude is above 3600 m in consideration of these physiologic findings.

12,500 feet (3750 m)—The use of oxygen is required by the flight crew of unpressurized aircraft beginning at altitudes above 3750 m (the crew can fly for about 30 minutes without oxygen between 3750 and 4200 m, a compromise zone, for example, in which they can fly the

aircraft over the crest of a mountain). The blood oxygen saturation is 87%.

14,000 feet (4200 m)—The blood oxygen saturation is approximately 83%, and all persons are impaired to a greater or lesser extent with respect to mental functions, including intellectual and emotional alterations. Thus, at a cabin altitude of 4200 m (14,000 ft), oxygen will be provided for at least 10% of the passengers in recognition of the marginal physiologic aspects of this altitude and the decompensations experienced by a variable proportion of the general population.

15,000 feet (4500 m)—At this altitude blood oxygen saturation is approximately 80%, and all persons are impaired, some seriously. The FAA regulations provide that oxygen be available for 30% of the passengers at a cabin altitude between 4200 and 4500 m (15,000 ft). Above a 4650 m cabin altitude, oxygen must be available for all passengers because everyone is seriously impaired above this cabin altitude.

20,000 feet (6000 m)—The blood oxygen saturation is 65%, and all unacclimatized persons become torpid and increasingly stuporous and lose useful consciousness in about 10 minutes. The time of useful consciousness (TUC) is determined generally from the time breathing oxygen is lost from the respiratory tract with reference to an initial safe level to the time when purposeful activity, such as the ability to don an oxygen mask, is lost. Although for most persons the TUC at 6000 m (20,000 ft) is about 10 minutes, for some it may be 20 minutes and for a few, 30 minutes.

25,000 feet (7500 m)—This altitude and above produces a blood oxygen saturation below 60%. A TUC of about 2.5 minutes exists at this altitude. Above 7500 m (25,000 ft) the rate of occurrence of bends (nitrogen bubble evolution and embolism) increases as a threat after decompression. If an airline pilot leaves a duty station at an altitude above 7500 m, the other pilot must have an oxygen mask in place to protect against problems should decompression occur.

37,000 feet (11,100 m)—At this altitude, the

TUC is approximately 18 seconds. Provision of 100% oxygen will produce approximately 80% blood oxygen saturation. As this altitude is exceeded, the oxygen begins to leave the blood unless positive-pressure oxygen is supplied. A draft standard covering this altitude was prepared when the United States was developing its own supersonic transport (SST). With the demise of the United States SST program, the standard was not put into the regulations but has been used as a guide in approving the British-French SST Concorde for operations in the United States.

45,000 feet (13,000 m)—The TUC is approximately 15 seconds, and positive-pressure oxygen decreases in practicality because of the increasing inability to exhale against the oxygen pressure.

Certain executive jet aircraft have been certified to an altitude of 51,000 ft (15,300 m) (Gates Learjet). Specific service histories and rational analyses showing a high degree of pressure vessel integrity (that portion of the aircraft hull designed to hold atmospheric pressure higher than that outside), a low probability of catastrophic or major pressurization failures, and certain in-place emergency procedures in the event of a decompression or pressurization problem form the basis for this certification. The civil airline aircraft with the highest certified cruise altitude is the British-French SST Concorde (range, 60,000 ft, or 18,000 m).

MEDICAL FACTORS IN GENERAL AVIATION ACCIDENTS

The three major factors in fatal general aviation accidents are (1) mixing alcohol with flying (15%); (2) conducting unwarranted, low-level, maneuvers that satisfy some emotional need that overrides logic (30%); and (3) penetrating known adverse weather beyond the pilot or aircraft capabilities (40%)—many such accidents are due to an emotional drive to reach the destination. The remaining 15% of fatal accidents include carbon monoxide poisoning from heater leaks (about 12 cases per year), drug impairment of the pilot (several dozen cases per year), in-flight heart attacks (about four to six per year), and a miscellaneous group, including in-flight incapacitation due to renal colic. General aviation accident rates are presented in Figure 24.9.

Pilot suicides through flying into a bar, church, school, or other structure or geographic area occur several times per year. Strictly speaking, these are not accidents and are not used in accident rate computations by the National Transportation Safety Board.

Two or three hypoxia accidents occur each year, including decompression and loss of consciousness by those on board. Two such hypoxia cases are described here.

On the evening of January 11, 1980, a Cessna 441 departed Shreveport, Louisiana, for Baton Rouge; the pilot and one passenger were on board. The pilot notified air traffic control at about 2130 hours that bad weather had been encountered. He requested an eastern routing, and the flight was cleared to 7010 m (21,000 ft). The controllers, however, subsequently noticed that the aircraft continued climbing beyond the assigned altitude. As the flight proceeded to the east, it continued to climb. It was tracked along its northeast route, and two Air Force planes were dispatched from Seymour-Johnson Air Force Base in Goldsboro, North Carolina. These aircraft picked up the Cessna shortly after midnight, 15 miles west of Raleigh, North Carolina, at 12,000 m (40,000 ft) flying at a speed of 410 kilometers per hour (kph). Fuel exhaustion occurred over the Atlantic Ocean at 12,300 m (41,000 ft). The Cessna began a spiraling turn and struck the water.

Investigators concluded the Cessna was on autopilot and that its occupants had become incapacitated from hypoxia, with hypoxic death occurring several minutes thereafter. The incapacitation was thought to have occurred when the aircraft was climbing near 7010 m (21,000 ft).

Four months earlier, on September 25, 1979, a Beech King Air 200 departed Stansted Airfield,

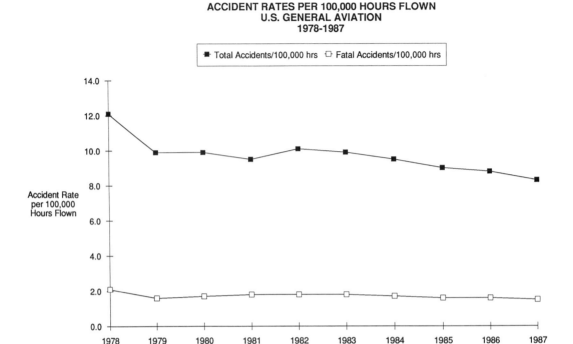

ACCIDENT RATES PER 100,000 HOURS FLOWN
U.S. GENERAL AVIATION
1978-1987

■ Total Accidents/100,000 hrs   □ Fatal Accidents/100,000 hrs

Figure 24.9. General aviation accident rates have slowly improved over the years. More effort is needed to ensure that the aeromedical factors related to fatal and nonfatal accidents can be more adequately addressed within the pilot population. (Federal Aviation Administration Statistical Handbook, 1989).

England, at 1341 hours so that the left seat pilot could receive a checkout. After a few practice landing approaches, the aircraft received clearance to climb to 9144 m (30,000 ft). Nothing further was heard from the aircraft, which flew across the English Channel toward France at an altitude of 9144 m.

A British Nimrod intercepted the King Air and followed it along. No radio contact could be established. In addition, a French Air Force Mirage flew close to the King Air and observed the flashing warning lights in the cockpit indicating that the cabin altitude was above 3810 m (12,500 ft). Fuel exhaustion brought the aircraft down in a crash near Nantes, France, at 2035 hours.

Investigators found that both pilots had been wearing oxygen masks and concluded that a practice decompression had gone wrong in that oxygen had not flowed into the masks. The TUC at 9144 m (30,000 ft) is about 30 seconds, and

the crew apparently did not recognize the early symptoms of hypoxia and thus did not initiate an emergency descent.

It was concluded that both pilots had lost consciousness during a practice decompression followed by subsequent death in situ.

Evidence indicated that an incorrect connection of mask assembly pipes and flight deck bulkhead supply points may have existed. The oxygen supply pipe bayonet may have been incorrectly inserted in its socket, resulting in failure of depression of a valve necessary for oxygen flow. This could have happened because the bayonet can appear to be inserted properly but not actually be so. Further complicating this situation are two oxygen control handles that can be confused in an emergency in that one handle has a manual override for the passenger system that can be selected accidentally when the pilot actually wants the other handle. If this happens, oxygen is not delivered as desired. These are factors for preflight consideration and have aeromedical importance.

SPECIFIC CIVIL AVIATION MEDICINE TOPICS

Alcohol

The euphoria produced by the consumption of alcohol is extremely hazardous for persons who fly while under its influence. Judgment is modified in the intoxicated state, and the pilots may attempt maneuvers that they would not undertake while sober.

In addition to its euphoric effect, alcohol tends to promote a narrowed span of attention, producing visual and concentration fixation effects. The time of concentration may be shortened, leading to a flight of ideas and a false sense of well-being. With increasing levels of intoxication, coordination becomes impaired and drowsiness occurs. All of these changes are incompatible with safe pilot performance.

In-flight studies of pilots with varying blood levels of alcohol have shown that levels as low as 0.04% (40 mg/dl), three standard alcoholic drinks for the average person, result in markedly impaired pilot performance on instrument landing system (ILS) approaches (5). Laboratory studies have revealed performance degradations at levels below the 0.04% level.

FAA Regulation 91.17 provides that no person may act as a crewmember of a civil aircraft: (1) within 8 hours after the consumption of any alcoholic beverage; (2) while under the influence of alcohol; or (3) while using any drug that affects his or her faculties in any way that could be unsafe. A consideration regarding this regulation is that the crewmembers must be alert to the detrimental effects of hangovers; effects that can last 24 to 48 hours after consuming alcohol, especially consumption in amounts exceeding one or two standard drinks.

Drugs

The two main considerations in regard to the adverse effects of a drug on a pilot are whether the drug impairs judgment and whether it impairs alertness. Some drugs may exert these effects directly or may bring them about through emotional, sleep-disturbing, or physiologic actions. In addition, drugs that degrade vision, impair coordination, or interfere with elimination functions are incompatible with safe flight, as are drugs that lower a pilot's tolerance to in-flight G forces.

For purposes of civil aviation, drugs may be categorized as follows:

1. Flight duties are normally permitted when taking the drug (e.g., aspirin, candicidin, ascorbic acid, ethynodiol, and phenacetin).
2. Flight duties are permitted if the flight surgeon (aviation medical examiner) or the FAA gives permission (e.g., ampicillin, chloroquine, metronidazole, oxytetracycline, and pyrimethamine).
3. Flight duties may be approved by the FAA (e.g., allopurinol, benzthiazide, chlorthalidone, propranolol, and thyroid preparations).
4. Flight duties are not permitted until the drug is discontinued and cleared from the body (clearance time of three times the drug's half-life) (e.g., amobarbital, buclizine, codeine, glutethimide, prednisolone, and tripelennamine).
5. The condition for which the drug is taken precludes flight duties (e.g., bishydroxycoumarin, bretylium tosylate, digitoxin, diphenylhydantoin, insulin, nitroglycerine, and tolbutamide).
6. The adverse effect of the drug precludes flight duties (clearance time of five times the drug's half-life) (e.g., amphetamine, carbamazepine, chlorpromazine, diazepam, doxepin, hydralazine, meperidine, and reserpine).
7. The drug either is illicit or is disapproved by the Food and Drug Administration (e.g., cocaine, heroin, LSD, and marijuana). Disapproved drugs include azaribine and triparanol.

A great deal could be said concerning the placement of specific drugs in the scheme

Section IV: Operational Aerospace Medicine

described above. Judgment by competent aeromedical and pharmacologic authorities must be applied, allowing maximum benefit to the pilot with no adverse effect on safety. Research results and accident data are valuable aids in arriving at decisions concerning specific drugs. Of special concern are the potential side effects of the drug.

Aerobatics

Civil sport aerobatic activities can result in pilot G_z axis accelerations in excess of $+7G$ and -5 G. During aerobatic training, pilots are taught methods of countering the adverse effects of G forces.

Some fatalities occur each year that are apparently related to the loss of consciousness during positive G_z maneuvers. On occasion, these accidents are attributed to pilots who undertook aerobatics while ill or anemic. Fatalities have been attributed to the loss-of-consciousness effect of sequentially conducting a powerful negative G_z maneuver ($-3 G_z$) followed by a powerful positive G_z maneuver (6). This latter sequence results in a transient desensitization of the carotid and aortic sinus blood pressure reflexes during the negative G_z maneuver, with a delay in activation of the reflexes during the immediate positive G_z maneuver. Unconsciousness at the 7 to 9 o'clock position is very apt to occur. The solution to avoiding the unconsciousness is to perform the positive G_z maneuver first, and then immediately undertake the negative G_z maneuver (Fig. 24.10).

Civil aerobatic pilots who regularly perform at air shows or in periodic competitions develop amazing tolerances to imposed G forces, illustrating significant increases of physiologic adaptation. This tolerance is rapidly lost after a few months of nonaerobatic flying. Unlike military aircraft, most civilian aerobatic aircraft are not equipped to handle G-suit inflations; hence, no anti-G gear is worn.

The Vertical "8"

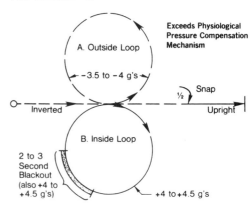

Figure 24.10. This diagram is cast in the Aresti system for portraying aerobic maneuvers. To perform the vertical 8, an aircraft enters inverted horizontal flight (left dashed line). An "outside" loop is performed (the head is to the outside with the blood consequently centrifuged cephalad) followed by a lower "inside" loop (the head is to the inside with the blood centrifuged toward the feet). The loop is completed in the inverted portion, and recovering to upright is achieved by a half-snap roll. Desensitization of the carotid pressure sensors during the outside loop results in a sluggish response during the 7 to 9 o'clock position in the inside loop, resulting in hypotension and the high likelihood of loss of consciousness for several seconds. Conducting the (+)G loop first, followed by a (−)G loop does not result in a blackout.

Fatigue

The circadian oscillator is located in the suprachiasmic area of the brain, and by its cyclic alteration in alertness, it can cause degradation in performance levels if work is attempted during the low phase of the cycle (7). Accumulated sleep deficits can move the work cycle toward the low phase and play a powerful role in decreasing pilot alertness during flight. Pilot education on these phenomena is a cornerstone of air safety. Fatigue is significant to single-pilot operations involving less experienced pilots, as well as multicrew airline operations.

The key scheduling factors contributing to the development of aircrew fatigue are multiple night flights, multiple time-zone displacements, flights departing 24 hours after an evening arrival, and multiple takeoffs and landings. Additional aggravating factors include departure delays of several hours that require pilots to lounge about airports, in-flight malfunctions, emergencies, adverse weather, or other factors that markedly increase workload. In aerial application flying, the required low-level maneuvers, long hours, and chemical exposures promote the onset of fatigue.

The worst aircraft accident in aviation history occurred between two Boeing 747 aircraft on March 27, 1977, at Los Rodeos Airport, Santa Cruz de Tenerife, Tenerife, Canary Islands (583 fatalities) (8). The Spanish investigators, assisted by U.S. and Dutch specialists, found that relatively recent changes in Dutch flight-time regulations removing the captain's flexibility regarding discretionary duty time extensions contributed to the cause of the accident. A number of significant safety lessons can be derived from this accident for flight surgeons and those working in the area of air safety.

The specific incident leading to this catastrophe was a terrorist bomb explosion in the terminal of the Las Palmas Airport, the original destination of the two aircraft. Because of the explosion, incoming aircraft were diverted to Los Rodeos Airport, about 60 statute miles away.

KLM 747 PH-SUF arrived at Los Rodeos Airport at 1338 hours and was parked at the end of the taxiway. Other aircraft arrived, including a Pan Am 747 (N1736) at 1415 hours. This airplane was parked near the KLM 747. Because of the small ramp size and the number of aircraft that landed, the Pan Am aircraft was blocked from taxiing to the runway by those behind it and by the KLM aircraft. The passengers were kept on board both aircraft.

Cockpit voice recorder data from the two aircraft reveal that the captain of the KLM aircraft was very concerned that the diversion and delay would bring about a violation of the Dutch flight-time limitations in effect. These regulations were rigid, did not allow judgmental extensions by the captain, and carried severe penalties

for those who exceeded them (including loss of license). The phrases, "Yes, that would mean imprisonment" and "Yes, then you are hanged from the highest tree," occur during the KLM cockpit discussions. The captain elected to refuel (55,000 L) on Tenerife so that after flying to Las Palmas, the departure for the return flight to Amsterdam could be made with a minimum delay (no refueling). A crewmember states, "I can do without Las Palmas." The discussions also note concern about the airport weather: "Hurry, or else it will close again complete."

The Pan Am crew became upset with the refueling decision by the KLM crew because it delayed the former's departure by an hour, the result of the slow refueling process. This is revealed in the cockpit voice recorder data. Discussions about being "ready for the sack" also took place. Las Palmas was the crew change point for this flight.

At 1650 hours, the KLM crew received engine start-up clearance. Shortly thereafter, the Pan Am crew received clearance. As the aircraft taxied, light rain and fog developed over the runway, with runway visibilities dropping to 300 m. The temperature and dew point held at 14° and 13°C, respectively.

The aircraft taxied down runway 12 in trail, the KLM crew aware that the Pan Am aircraft was behind them. The tower controller could not see the two aircraft because of the fog. He cleared the KLM aircraft to the end of the runway for a 180° turn so that the KLM departure on runway 30 could be expedited. The runway is 3400 m long and 45 m wide. The Pan Am aircraft was directed to turn left from the runway on taxiway C-3, "the third taxiway." The turnoff was tricky for large aircraft because it was a 90° turn. An ambiguity problem occurred, however, in that the third taxiway from the aircraft was actually taxiway C-4, thus the Pan Am aircraft was kept on the runway for a longer time.

At 1705 hours, the KLM crew were given the departure clearance to Las Palmas, which was read back by the crew. The crew reported at 1706 hours that they were in a takeoff position. The

Pan Am crew immediately informed the tower, "We're still taxiing down the runway." The tower requested, "Report the runway clear."

At 1706 hours, one Pan Am crewmember said to another, "He's anxious, isn't he" (referring to the KLM captain). The reply was, "Yeah, after he held us up for an hour and a half, that ***." (*** stands for profanity.) "Now he's in a rush," the other crewmember said. The captain then said, "There he is—look at him—***—that, that *** is coming!" A crewmember said, "Get off! Get off!" The impact then occurred, tearing off the top of the Pan Am 747. The aircraft then began burning as the emergency escape procedures were activated.

The KLM crew could not see the Pan Am aircraft because of the fog. A brief discussion had occurred concerning whether the Pan Am 747 was clear of the runway, and the KLM captain concluded that it must be. The fog was worsening, the runway center-line lights were not working, and the flight-time limits reviewed by high-frequency radio with KLM headquarters would run out if the departure did not occur soon (the crew would not be able to fly the Las Palmas to Amsterdam return flight, disrupting the schedules and passenger and crew plans).

Still within the 1706 time frame, the KLM initiated takeoff (cockpit voices in Dutch, translated to English as follows):

1706:32—KLM crewmember: "Isn't he off then?"

1706:34—KLM captain: "What do you say?"

1706:34—KLM crewmember: "He is not off, that Pan American?"

1706:35—KLM captain: "Yes, well!"

1706:43—KLM copilot: "V One." (This is the go or no-go decision speed.)

1706:47—KLM captain: "Oh god-damn!"

1706:49—sound of impact

The KLM aircraft lifted off the ground and struck the top of the Pan Am aircraft, burst into flames and fell back to earth, and everyone on board was killed (14 crewmembers and 234 passengers). Of the 396 persons on board the burn-

ing Pan Am aircraft, 9 crewmembers and 326 passengers died. The total dead were 583.

The investigators concluded that the KLM captain took off without clearance and did not interrupt takeoff on learning that the Pan Am aircraft was still on the runway. When asked by the flight engineer if the Pan Am aircraft had left the runway, the captain had replied emphatically, "Yes."

The investigators concluded that the major reasons for the accident were as follows:

1. A growing feeling of tension as the KLM captain's problems mounted (strict flight-time limitations)
2. Deteriorating weather conditions
3. Two transmissions occurring simultaneously, blocking for the KLM captain the Pan Am transmission, "We are still taxiing down the runway"
4. Certain language problems, in which the KLM copilot stated, "We are now at takeoff," was misunderstood by the tower controller, who had not granted takeoff clearance
5. The communication confusion between the tower and the Pan Am crew about the third intersection" being the C-3 or C-4 intersection (a minor point because the Pan Am crew twice advised that the aircraft was still on the runway)
6. The unusual traffic congestion leading to shortcuts allowing taxiing down runways

Flight surgeons who work with crewmembers, airline companies, and controllers can actively participate in preventive activities in regard to the above factors. These include a continued assessment of flight-time limitations and how changes can affect future operations. Conducting educational programs for crewmembers concerning emotional factors and the effects of fatigue is important. The comprehensibility of communications, including the tendencies under stress to "hear" or perceive what one wants to hear, should be emphasized. The slogans, "when in doubt, reassess" and "if you are in a hurry, you are in danger,'' apply to the above-mentioned disaster, aviation's worst accident.

The present United States flight-time regulations do not incorporate any circadian component, although physiologic indices exist that can be applied in scoring specific flight schedules for their fatigue potential (9,10). Application of the indices has been slow to evolve, but one can forecast their increasing use as the general knowledge regarding fatigue and circadian rhythms increases.

Flight Attendants

The medical aspects of flight attendant work have emerged relatively recently as a significant added dimension in aerospace medicine. Beginning May 15, 1930, when United Airlines' predecessor, Boeing Air Transport, hired the first eight stewardesses, and into the 1960s, U.S. flight attendants were predominantly young, petite, white females. If the flight attendant became overweight, got married, or became pregnant, she almost always was terminated by the airlines. Sprogis versus United Airlines (1970) and other cases settled the marriage issue. The Civil Rights Act of 1964 and the Age Discrimination in Employment Act of 1967, plus many legal suits brought by flight attendants, have led to the elimination of virtually all of the old restrictions arbitrarily imposed by marketing-oriented airline managers. Today, approximately 50,000 people of diverse sex, race, and age groups (the potential upper-age limit is 70 years) work for the airlines as flight attendants.

Flight attendants are the front line of passenger safety when aircraft disasters occur, serving a critical role in the accomplishment of emergency evacuations. Accidents may happen on land or water, near airports, or in remote locations. Flight attendants are also the primary inflight providers of emergency aid to passengers should illness, injury, or aircraft decompressions occur.

Among the environmental factors that are significant to flight attendants' health and well-being are the need for fresh air flow; absence of gaseous or particulate contaminants (including cigarette smoke and other pollutants); absence of ozone (or quantities below 0.1 ppm by volume); temperature and humidity control; circadian rhythm scheduling; and adequate nutrition, layover facilities, and rest periods. The work environment requires energy expenditures in the range of 3 to 5 mets. Flight attendants with normal, uncomplicated pregnancies can fly on many airlines into the third trimester. Recent concern has been voiced regarding radiation and reproductive factors. Flight attendants also can fly with well-controlled diabetes and a history of epilepsy if the condition is controlled by medication. Turbulence injuries, accident impact, and fire injuries are potential occupational hazards.

The aeromedical practitioner has the opportunity to assist in the assurance that flight attendants are provided adequate support medically, operationally, and environmentally to perform a quality job.

Age

Age, race, and sex traditionally have been limiting factors on the range of work activities available to a given individual. Modern concepts and medical progress in understanding, diagnosis, and treatment (prodded by legal actions) have progressively whittled these limitations to a few rearguard areas.

It is now known that the normal aging process is a developmental continuum, proceeding along a species-specific time line. Graying hair and lost hair are genetically determined changes of no consequence to flying abilities. In similar fashion, wrinkling of the skin and changes due to years of exposure to the elements are inconsequential.

The progressively extending visual near point occurring in most persons in their 40s can be fully refracted and is, therefore, of no significance to aviation activities. Acquired chronic diseases, especially those related to cardiovascular risk factors, may be significant. These diseases occur in individuals who have lived long enough for the chronicity aspect to develop, but the diseases are not a part of the normal aging process, as demonstrated by the many persons who maintain low risk factors, and reach an advanced age of 80 years or more without these diseases appearing. Medical screening and performance tests are available for individual health assessment irrespective of age, race, or sex.

The significant factors in regard to safe pilot performance are (1) ability to perform, (2) freedom from impairing disease, and (3) motivation to fly (11). Age, race, and sex are not indicators of a pilot's competency. Analyses of observed versus expected accidents in commercial and airline transport pilots from 1978 to 1979 reveal that beginning in the 30s age bracket, fewer accidents actually occur per 1000 pilots than is the case with younger pilots. Maturity, experience, and better judgment are key factors in the improving safety record accompanying increasing age. In 1981, the median age of U.S. Boeing 747 captains was 58 years; for the Lockheed 1011, 58; for the McDonnell-Douglas DC-10, 57; for the Air Bus A-300, 56; for the DC-8, 54;, for the B-707, 52; for the B-727, 50; for the DC-9, 48; and for the B-737 47. The wide-body, advanced, jet aircraft are flown by the senior, most experienced captains in their late 50s. The overall safety record of these aircraft reflects the direct correlation between air safety and the improved judgment and experience accompanying normal, healthy aging.

Accidents per 1000 pilots-in-command for civilians having commercial or air transport pilot certificates are shown in Table 24.4. As is the case with automobile accidents, increasing maturity and experience (concomitants of the aging process) are positively correlated with a decreasing accident incidence (more than twofold decrease from the teenage period to the late 50s and older). Some critics have decried the absence of precise exposure data, but this aspect is not critical to pilot safety because each pilot-in-command determines the risk to which he or she

Table 24.4.
Pilot Age and Accidents Composite, 1982–1985

Age	Mean Number of Active Pilots	Accidents Observed	Accidents Expected	Accidents per 1000 Pilots
16–19	227	14	4	15
20–24	10,636	212	158	5
25–29	24,476	372	364	4
30–34	30,257	507	450	4
35–39	40,534	664	602	4
40–44	36,696	514	546	4
45–49	30,240	374	449	3
50–54	23,957	315	356	3
55–59	16,113	237	239	4
60+	22,733	297	338	3
Total	235,869	3506	3506	

Pilots in command with commercial and airline transport certificates.
General aviation accidents.
From: NTSB and FAA Stat Handbook. Washington, D.C.: US Govt Printing Office, 1982–1985.

is exposed; deliberate penetration of thunderstorms, intentional, unwarranted, low-level maneuvers, and flight under the influence of alcohol or drugs are all related to immaturity and impulse control problems. As with automobile accidents, about 90% of aircraft accidents result from operator error.

Improved screening methods for significant diseases in pilots are increasingly available, as is better understanding of the role of cardiovascular risk factors in disease causation. A growing movement is developing to abolish all upper age limits in regard to pilot duties. This movement is impelled further by the remarkable increase in health and longevity in the U.S. population. The average length of an individual's life is currently in the neighborhood of 73 years and is rapidly moving toward a healthy 85 years. The implications for the continued productive employment of aircrew members are clear, as is the role to be played by the aeromedical specialist under these circumstances.

Mental Functions

The main requisites for safe pilot performance are sensory accuracy, cognitive capacity—

including judgment, motor efficiency, and emotional stability—and drive. All of these elements can be evaluated either in the clinic or through flight performance. The two accident reports that follow fall into the realm of mental dysfunction.

A United McDonnell-Douglas DC-8 passenger flight incurred complete fuel exhaustion at night on December 28, 1978, over Portland, Oregon (12). Ten persons on board received fatal injuries in the deadstick landing that followed. Investigators determined that the pilot had not properly monitored the fuel supply because his attention had been diverted by a landing gear malfunction. The investigators also felt that the first officer and the flight engineer did not fully appreciate the development of a critically low fuel state. They concluded that these two crewmembers should have been more alert to the status of the fuel supply and should have been more assertive in communicating the developing problem to the captain.

In the other accident report, the attitude indicators failed on a night flight in a Transamerica Lockheed L-188 near Salt Lake City, Utah, on November 18, 1978 (13). The turn needle and directional heading indicator remained functional, but the captain became spatially disoriented when he attempted to integrate unreliable attitude information and the information from the other instruments. The large turboprop aircraft entered a typical graveyard spiral and broke up in flight, killing the three crewmembers. Insidious failures of critical flight instruments still remain a major hazard in flight activities, as demonstrated by this accident. A mental state of alertness to possible partial failures of flight instruments is necessary if recognition and proper actions are to be taken.

Civil Protective Equipment

The basic protective equipment available in civil aviation relates to the nature of the aircraft, the flight mission, and the minimal standards for this type of equipment.

Gliders, agricultural aircraft, aerobatic aircraft, and most airline aircraft have been equipped with shoulder harnesses since the 1960s. Only since the late 1970s have other newly manufactured general aviation aircraft required shoulder harnesses, and there are even exceptions to this.

It can be forecast that approximately half of the annual general aviation accident fatalities can be prevented by the simple expedient of using a proper shoulder harness seat-belt restraint system.

"Delethalized" instrument panels and controls have helped to prevent fatalities in general aviation, but much more remains to be done, including protection against pyrolysis and heat from fire.

The requirement for protective equipment aboard airline aircraft is extensive and depends, in part, on the routes flown. Water survival equipment is, of course, necessary for prolonged flights over water. For general aviation aircraft, the requirements are not as extensive. Most single-engine private aircraft fly without oxygen equipment. If the owner wishes to fly at altitudes requiring oxygen supplementation, however, inexpensive portable oxygen systems are available. Most aircraft now carry emergency radio beacons that activate when a crash occurs. Many private pilots equip their aircraft with emergency equipment, that is, water, first-aid kit, survival kit, and food. The aeromedical specialist can provide assistance to those pilots wishing to prepare such an emergency kit for carrying aboard their aircraft.

International Civil Aviation Medicine

Civil aviation activities among the world's countries are coordinated by the International Civil Aviation Organization (ICAO), a component of the United Nations (see Chapter 27). Recommended standards and practices are developed, and member nations—virtually all countries—either adhere to these standards or file "exceptions." The United States has more general aviation activities and pilots than all of the rest of the world combined and has perhaps filed more exceptions to the ICAO standards than any other nation. This is felt by many to reflect the progressive actions in the field of general aviation historically taken by the United States.

The Future and Civil Aviation Medicine

The trend in medical certification in the United States is to move away from arbitrarily fixed standards toward a more functional approach. For example, the present standards call for binocular vision, but 5000 one-eyed civil United States pilots have been certified based on individual performance capabilities.

Pilots with missing limbs have received medical certificates based on a Statement of Demonstrated Ability, as demonstrated in the flight environment. Paraplegic pilots have been certified, with limitations requiring the use of a specially equipped aircraft. Airline pilots have been recertified with prosthetic replacements for part of the leg. One pilot returned with bilateral artificial hip joints.

Pilots with hearing loss have been certified, with the requirement that a hearing aid be worn. Aphakic pilots have received certification contingent on wearing proper contact lenses. More than 1088 recovering alcoholic airline pilots have received medical certification by special issuance, a process involving inpatient treatment, cessation of intake of all alcoholic beverages, and the institution of a periodic follow-up program (Table 24.5).

In the United States, pilots also have been returned to commercial flight duties (airline captain, corporate pilot) after coronary bypass surgery on appeal to the National Transportation Safety Board. The same return to duty by airline pilots has been accomplished in Canada. As medical research develops new understanding of disease, new diagnostic techniques, and new treatments, a marked individualization of medical certification for those having various conditions is predicted. It is anticipated that all arbitrary upper age limits will give way to individual

Table 24.5.
Overview of FAA Medical Rejections, Reconsiderations, and Special Issuances at Varying Appeal Levels in FAA, 1989

Initial rejection cause
(note: 99% of applicants achieve certification):

	No.
Medical history	104,115
Vision	54,739
Blood Pressure or Pulse	7,634
Hearing	22,018
Other	171,219
Total	359,725

Reconsiderations and special issuances	
Eye	8
Cardiovascular	750
Neurologic	34
Psychiatric (includes alcoholism)	38
Bone/joint	1
Miscellaneous	36
Total	867

FAA, Federal Aviation Administration.

assessments of functional capability and freedom from disease when the desire to continue flying exists.

A direction taken by the civil medical standards and certification process is the elimination of the mandatory denials based on medical history. This action leaves the individual determination of certification essentials to decisions by the FAA based on the current health and functional status of the applicant (special issuance procedures). Consideration will be given to the probability that no significant change in medical status is likely to occur within 3 years from the date of certification, the longest potential duration of a medical certificate not otherwise time-limited.

Among the key medical issues for the coming decades in civil aviation medicine are the following:

1. The quantification of crew workload levels at specific flight phases (including sensory, cognitive, and motor elements)
2. The management of crew fatigue, including scheduling aspects related to multiple night

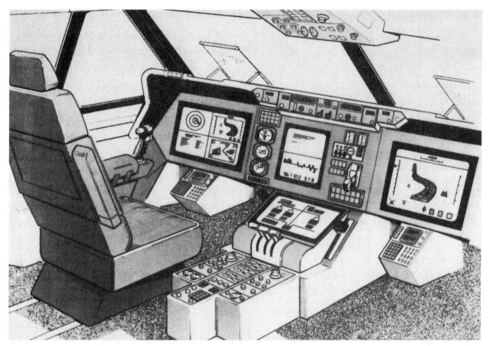

Figure 24.11. This illustration demonstrates how modern technology can simultaneously simplify and improve displays for future airline aircraft. Available to the crew is a head-up windshield and a cathode ray tube (CRT) display that projects a "pathway in the sky," enabling the pilots to easily follow either inertial coordinates or external electronic navigation beams to a specific point. Virtually all necessary operating data can be called up for display on the CRTs. A side control replaces the traditional yoke, giving a superior view of the instrument panel (courtesy of the Lockheed Georgia Company).

flights, transmeridian desynchronization, 24-hour layovers after night arrivals, and multiple takeoffs and landings

3. Biomedical assessments of flight display characteristics, emphasizing the increasing replacement of mechanical instruments by cathode ray tube (CRT) displays and other electronic optical instruments, including flat panel dot-matrix displays (Fig. 24.11)

4. Institution of programs that deal with pilot fitness and behavior, medical standards, and exceptions to these standards

5. Further research and pilot education programs on the acute and long-term effects of alcohol and drugs on crew performance

6. Refinement of the understanding of in-flight environmental factors, including G forces, hypoxia, and spatial disorientation

7. An air traffic control system that will be increasingly automated, further removing the human controllers from the pilot/air traffic controller interactions

8. Improved accident investigation methods, leading to a better understanding of the underlying causes of accidents so that preventive programs can be enhanced

9. Improved aircraft accident survivability, including impact attenuation, crash fire minimization and control, and improved emergency escape systems

New generations of civil aircraft will contain increasing levels of automation and will extend current limits of aerodynamic envelopes. The hypersonic transport, flying several times the speed of sound at altitudes in the 60,000 m (200,000-ft) range, is projected to provide a 3-hour flight from New York to Australia. Civil aerospace medicine physicians must increasingly incorporate in their work new biomedical advances so that these advances can be applied in preventing human failure in flight activities.

REFERENCES

1. Institute of Medicine: Airline Pilot Age, Health, and Performance. Washington, D.C., National Academy Press:, 1981.
2. Cantor KP, Booze CF: Mortality Among Aerial Pesticide Applicators and Flight Instructors. Arch Env Health 1990;45(5):295–302, 1990.
3. Mohler SR: Agricultural aviation medicine in the Soviet Union. Aviat Space Environ Med,1980; 51:515, 1980.
4. Mohler SR: Physiologically Tolerable Decompression Profiles for Supersonic Transport Type Certification. Office of Aviation Medicine Report AM-70–12. U.S. Government Printing Office, Federal Aviation Administration, Washington, D.C. July 1970.
5. Billings CE, Wick RL, Gerke RJ, Chase, RC, et al. Effects of Alcohol on Pilot Performance During Instrument Flight. Office of Aviation Medicine Report AM-72–4. U.S. Government Printing Office, Washington, D.C.:, Federal Aviation Administration, 1972.
6. Mohler SR: G Effects on the Pilot During Aerobatics. Office of Aviation Medicine Report AM-72–28. U.S. Government Printing Office, Federal Aviation Administration, Washington, D.C., 1972.
7. Klein KE: Significance of Circadian Rhythms in Aero-space Activities. Agardograph 247. National Technical Information Services. North Atlantic Treaty Organization, Springfield, Virginia: 1980.
8. Spanish Government: Accident Report, Fatal Collision, KLM Boeing B-747 (PH-SUF) and Pan American Boeing B-747 (N1736), Los Rodeos Airport, Tenerife, Canary Islands, March 27, 1977.
9. Federal Aviation Administration.: Flight-Time Limitations. Subpart Q, Domestic Air Carriers; Subpart R, Flag Air Carriers; Subpart S, Supplemental Air Carriers and Commercial Operators. Federal Aviation Regulations 21, Title 14. Washington, DC: U.S. Government Printing Office, 1982.
10. Wegmann HM: Models to Predict Loads of Flight Schedules on Cockpit Personnel. Twenty-ninth International Congress of Aviation and Space Medicine, Nancy, France, 1981.
11. Mohler SR: Reasons for eliminating the "age 60" regulation for airline pilots. Aviat Space Environ Med, 1981;52:445, 1981.
12. National Transportation Safety Board.: Aircraft Accident Report, United Airlines, Inc., McDonnell-Douglas DC-861, N8082U, Portland, Oregon, December 28, 1978. NTSB-AAR-79–7. Washington, DC: U.S. Government Printing Office, June 7, 1979.
13. National Transportation Safety Board.: Aircraft Accident Report, Transamerica Airlines, Inc. Lockheed L-188, N859U, Salt Lake City, Utah, November 28, 1979. NTSB-AAR-80–11. Washington, DC: U.S. Government Printing Office, August 26, 1980.

Chapter 25

Aeromedical Support to Airline and Civilian Professional Aircrew

Richard L. Masters, Gary M. Kohn

The Divine Hippocrates informs us, that when a physician visits a patient, he ought to inquire into many things, by putting questions to the patient and to bystanders. You must ask, says he, what uneasiness he is under, what was the cause of it, how many days he had been ill, how his belly is affected and what food he eats. To which I presume to add one interrogation more; namely, what trade he is of. But I find it very seldom minded in the common course of practice, or if the physician knows it without asking he takes little notice of it.

Bernardino Ramazzini, 1700

Approximately 55,000 professional airline pilots in the United States are employed by some 45 air carriers. These carriers are classified by the Civil Aeronautics Board according to income as major, national, and regional carriers. The carriers also range in size, as measured by the number of pilots employed, from those employing over 7000 pilots to those with less than 25 pilots. Fewer than 50% of U.S. airline pilots work for companies employing a full-time medical director. Air carrier size generally is unrelated to the employment of a physician because large carriers may have no physician or may employ several physicians. Small carriers usually employ no physician, or they maintain a consulting relationship with a physician in the local community where the carrier is based. Hence, a significant number of professional airline pilots do not receive the services of a formal corporate medical department, making the provision of alternative specialty resources necessary. In terms of aerospace medicine specialty representation in private practice, these other sources have been insufficiently provided. The long-standing lack of aerospace medicine specialist support for many professional airline pilots has necessitated the development of resources through the initiative of the major airline pilots' representative union, the Air Line Pilots Association (ALPA). This chapter outlines the scope of aeromedical problems facing professional airline pilots and the services provided by medical and other professional resources both within and outside of airline medical departments.

AEROMEDICAL SERVICES

Needed and Provided Medical Services

Professional airline pilots constitute one of the few professions in which sustained good health is an absolute prerequisite for productivity and employment. Airline pilots not only must meet Federal Aviation Administration (FAA) periodic certification examinations, but also are expected to maintain their health in a manner consonant with the highest level of air safety. Employers typically do not provide FAA periodic certification examinations but may assist pilots in special follow-up evaluations and referral to specialists in the event disqualifying conditions raise questions as to their continued eligibility for flying duties. Air carrier physicians assist in the referral of pilots to competent treatment resources and in the oversight of rehabilitation, continuing care, and monitoring. Pilots who do not have medical services provided by their airline must seek those services on their own. How, by whom, and at what facilities these services are provided, as well as their quality and quantity, are proper matters for consideration. As with all medical care, quality will vary with the physician and the health facility. Ideally, the aerospace medical specialist provides the major source of quality control. The number of such specialists, unfortunately, is limited.

Federal Aviation Administration Periodic Medical Certification Examinations

The FAA requires periodic medical certification examinations of all pilots who operate aircraft. The details and protocols of such examinations are specified in the applicable portions of the Federal Aviation Regulations (FARs) and in manuals and directives issued by the FAA Office of Aviation Medicine. Detailed information pertaining to medical certification and to the requirements are contained in Chapter 26. The examinations are conducted by designated physician aviation medical examiners (AMEs), who are selected and trained by the FAA and who are located throughout the United States. In addition, some AMEs are located overseas. The examinations are not designed to encourage or require the practice of preventive medicine because they constitute an examination of an individual's physical condition at a static point in

time. The AME is required to determine whether a pilot meets the medical standards, and if so, that physician is empowered to issue the pilot's FAA certificate. The results of the examinations are forwarded to the FAA for review to determine whether the decision made was consonant with the regulations. If the pilot is qualified, the certificate remains in force for a specified period of time, with future required evaluations at established intervals. Airline pilots seek their FAA examinations from senior AMEs, physicians designated to perform First Class FAA airman medical examinations. AMEs assume varying degrees of responsibility for the pilots they examine. For example, some AMEs may feel that acting as an agent of the federal government, they are required strictly to perform the examination and make no basic decisions if any disqualifying condition is discovered. This minimal service often is inadequate, and the pilot may have to seek further evaluation elsewhere. Other AMEs do what is necessary to get thorough specialists' evaluations and follow-up to ensure that the information presented to the FAA is as complete as possible.

FAA Special Follow-Up Evaluations

In the event that the AME or FAA physicians determine that some conditions may not be in accordance with the standards, special follow-up evaluations may be required. For example, a pilot who has borderline hypertension and is receiving treatment with diuretics or other medication may be allowed to fly but be required to have follow-up evaluations specifically directed at blood pressure and cardiovascular health. Such evaluations may be requested by the AME, the pilot's personal physician, or a medical specialist. The determining factor here is the protocol for the follow-up evaluation and which physician would be asked by the FAA to provide the information.

Specialist's Evaluations

When a deviation from normal is detected, the pilot usually is referred to a medical specialist.

The specialist provides information necessary for the AME and the FAA to determine whether the pilot meets the standards and, if not, whether the standards could be set aside in a particular instance without adversely affecting flight safety. Many medical specialties are involved in these evaluations, but the most common are cardiology, ophthalmology, orthopedics, and neuropsychiatry; other specialties are involved to a lesser degree. The airline pilot often cannot identify highly qualified specialists for a particular condition. Hence, the specialists in aerospace medicine should refer pilots to appropriate high-quality specialists. Because the FAA must depend almost entirely on the quality of the medical reports it receives in determining a pilot's continued eligibility for medical certification, a deficient, incomplete, or overly brief report serves neither the pilot nor the interests of aviation safety.

Treatment

The aim of treatment must be to restore pilots to their premorbid condition and to ensure that their recovery returns them to a level of functioning that is fully consistent with the safe and efficient performance of their duties. Overseeing the health and specific medical problems of pilots is the proper responsibility of the specialist in aerospace medicine. He or she acts, in a narrow sense, as the generalist and ensures, through appropriate consultation, that the highest quality medical treatment is focused on complete recovery and/or rehabilitation. Specialists in aerospace medicine can play an important role in the management of a given patient if they choose to be in charge of treatment, using specialists for required areas. Usually, however, they play a somewhat different role, monitoring the treatment of pilots and their progress after having directed them to the highest quality resources. These aerospace physicians can be helpful in explaining to the specialists the requirements for FAA medical certification, the job requirements for return to work, and any special needs in preparing the pilot for reconsideration and recertifi-

cation. Often, they must take special precautions to ensure that the pilot continues after the normal course of treatment into the stages of recovery and rehabilitation necessary for a return to flying duties, which may not be recognized by the treating physician. The treating physician often may have one goal in mind, whereas the goal of professional pilots may be quite different.

Rehabilitation

The aim of rehabilitation of pilots cannot be limited. Rather, rehabilitation must be aimed in every aspect toward returning them to a level of optimal functioning consistent with their ability to return to duty. The importance of rehabilitation cannot be overemphasized because of the necessity, both economic and humane, to preserve and protect the professional capabilities of pilots. The costs of training an airline pilot are estimated to approach $500,000. It thus is not feasible to discard such highly skilled professionals as long as they can be rehabilitated and safely returned to flying duties. In achieving the major aim of the reestablishment of full premorbid functional capacity, the flight surgeon must be guided by the comprehensive knowledge of job requirements, physical capacity, the aviation environment, and the details of operator-machine interactions. Often, professional pilots find themselves in a situation in which guidance by specialists in aerospace medicine is required. Rehabilitation experts should rely on this background knowledge in individualizing the rehabilitation plan for optimal results. An example of this is the situation in which rehabilitation is directed toward the return of functional capacity, say, of an individual with an injured ankle. The orthopedist or the rehabilitation director may be quite satisfied if the person is able to walk, whereas the professional pilot must direct rehabilitation to the point at which ankle function is compatible not only with the use of rudder pedals under normal operating conditions but also under emergency conditions should hydraulic power be lost. Factors such as these may be unknown to the treating physician and can provide delays and misunderstandings in the ultimate attempt of an injured pilot to regain flying duties.

Continuing Care and Monitoring

Certain illnesses may require that the pilot undergo continuing care and that the condition be monitored for extended periods of time. For example, a pilot who has been rehabilitated after a cardiovascular disability should be monitored periodically by specialists' evaluations. Reevaluations necessary to the continuing certification and qualification for flying duties must be timely, complete, and accurate. Certification decisions are affected by the ability of the FAA to ensure continued stability of the pilot's medical condition. This becomes especially critical in the special services area, notably alcoholism and drug rehabilitation, and is addressed later in this chapter.

Recertification Evaluations

After prolonged illnesses or conditions resulting in decertification, the FAA, upon petition from the affected pilot, will consider recertification. Such reconsideration is judged on the pilot's state of health, appropriate treatment, and state of rehabilitation. The FAA requires complete information pertaining to the pilot's medical history and treatment, as well as documented evidence of recovery. Recertification decisions are based on the pilot's ability to return to cockpit duties free of any condition deemed detrimental to the safe performance of duties.

Other Evaluations

The professional pilot's career is punctuated by various evaluations and physical examinations that are required for a number of reasons. For example, professional pilots frequently come to air carrier employment from a background of military service and have undergone a number of physical examinations during their military career. Also, many air carrier pilots maintain their affiliation with Air National Guard or military reserve units after their separation from active duty and incur additional examinations. Preplacement medical examinations are required by a number of air carriers. Some air carriers, however, simply accept a pilot as physically qualified for the job if he or she is able to demonstrate the ability to hold a First Class FAA medical certificate. Some carriers also require periodic physical examinations. Carriers also may require evaluations after long or serious illnesses or when there is reason to believe that the pilot may not meet job performance or safety standards. Examinations to determine eligibility for medical disability pay, as well as for purposes of termination evaluations, inevitably are required. These evaluations are obtained from various resources, either at the direction of the requesting organization or at the selection of the individual pilot. In the case of disputed claims, a neutral physician sometimes is selected to make the final determination. Often, disability determinations rest on the opinion of the pilot's personal physician, who may be unfamiliar with the specific requirements of the airline environment. In some cases, the pilot's physician believes the patient is disabled, but the company physician feels otherwise; and, of course, the converse may apply. In most instances, final disability determination depends on the applicant fulfilling a specified set of procedures that are designed to be fair to the disabled pilot as well as to the providers of the funds that support disability payments.

Factors Affecting Aeromedical Efficiency

Mechanisms for providing health care to professional airline pilots lack uniformity. Standardization may occur within a specific airline medical department, but there is, for all practical purposes, no uniformity among airline medical departments. Carriers without medical departments often lack even a foundation for establishing uniformity. Some air carriers adopt the physical standards of the FAA as their own; other airlines have physical standards that are applied by their medical departments, whereas still others may have physical standards that are unwritten or are interpreted by nonspecialists.

Some carriers provide appropriate disability insurance benefits for pilots who lose their medical certificates. Other airlines have less desirable plans, and still others have no medical disability insurance. Within the medical disability insurance programs, some carriers allow pilots to be retained on the seniority rolls for certain periods of time so that, upon recovery, return to flying status is possible.

A major factor affecting system efficiency is the lack of sufficient numbers of aeromedical specialists throughout the country. There are very few trained aeromedical specialists, and few are entering the field; however, the need for these specialists is not diminishing. The sporadic disappearance of airline medical departments does nothing to diminish the need but shifts the burden to aeromedical specialists in private practice.

For a preventive medicine system to be effective, knowledge of the epidemiologic background of the population is needed. Hidden diseases within the airline pilot population are possible and are a matter of continuing concern. The incidence and prevalence of disease within this population is difficult to determine. The systematic collection of such information is lacking. FAA medical data lack closure information. For example, if a pilot takes an FAA examination one day, the pilot conceivably could become ill the next day and never fly again because of that illness, but the FAA might never know about the illness. The FAA does not have a systematic follow-up program for detecting unreported disease, and the open-ended nature of their information system thus renders their ''epidemiologic'' evaluations incomplete. In a 1981 report, the National Academy of Sciences pointed to this deficiency of systematic data collection and recommended long-term remedies (1). No corrective steps are evident.

DEVELOPMENT OF AIRLINE MEDICINE

The airline industry evolved gradually during the first 50 years of its existence, and then, some would argue, evolved much more rapidly during the past two decades. A review of this history is useful in understanding the variations that exist in today's airline medical organizations. In the early days of the airline industry, the personnel officer was the first to recognize the need for medical support. These medical needs were twofold: medical evaluation for the selection of new employees, especially flight personnel, and on-site first aid for job-related injuries. These needs usually were fulfilled by sending the applicant to a local physician for a physical examination and hiring a nurse to operate a first-aid facility in the maintenance building. As the industry grew, the needs increased in magnitude and complexity. During the transition, the next step frequently was to employ a consulting physician, first part-time and then full-time. The medical responsibilities began to broaden to include job placement examinations, periodic special examinations to monitor personnel in critical jobs, job safety—including human factors and environmental health—aircraft accident investigation, and consultation on group and workmen's compensation insurance. As a result of this beginning, many airlines' medical departments became part of the human resources department. Occasionally, such an organizational structure was found to be less than optimal, and new organizational arrangements were tried.

One of the first airlines to hire private physicians to support the selection and health maintenance of crewmembers was Pan American. In 1928, this airline employed private physicians to examine its flight crew. Early in its history, Eastern Airlines employed physicians on a fee-for-service basis in various cities along its route structure to accomplish preemployment and flight examinations and to care for injuries or illness involving passengers or employees. In 1936, Eastern Airlines appointed Dr. Ralph N. Green, a former Army pilot and the first U.S. physician to attain military flight status, to develop a medical service for its flight crews. In 1931, American Airlines began to provide medical care for its pilots. Qualified physicians and part-time consultants provided this service. In 1940, the airline established its first medical office and selected as its first medical director Dr. Edward C. Greene. In 1937, the commandant of the U.S. Army's School of Aviation Medicine at San Antonio, Texas, Col. A.D. Tuttle, was hired by United Airlines with an appropriation to set up the first airline medical clinic in the company's headquarters across the street from Chicago's Midway Airport. Early grumbling by pilots and profit-minded shareholders alike were dispensed with, citing the inherent logic of "preventative maintenance" for air crewmembers as well as airframes.

As medical departments were developing in the United States, Canadian airlines began establishing medical departments as well. In 1937, Dr. Kenneth Dowd was named airline medical director for Trans Canadian Airlines.

Many leaders in the field of aerospace medicine were actively involved in the development of airline medical departments, for example, Drs. Eric S. Lilenkrantz, Ross McFarland, and John Tamisiea. Other early names associated with the medical support to airlines were Dr. W. Randolph Lovelace and Dr. Jan H. Tillisch.

In 1944, physician members of medical departments for commercial airlines met in St. Louis and formed their own unique professional society—the Airline Medical Directors Association (AMDA). With Dr. Arnold D. Tuttle of the United States as its first president, the association took on as its objective "to improve the practice and standards of aviation and industrial medicine, particularly as pertaining to domestic and international airline operations, and to encourage research and study of medical problems in these fields (2)."

The rapid technical developments during and immediately after World War II brought about the need for more specialized training for the airline physician. Airplanes were becoming more sophisticated as they flew faster and higher, and materials used to make and maintain them became more exotic and hazardous. The cost of operating an airline became increasingly expensive, especially those costs related to flight training, crew salaries, and insurance and retirement programs. At the same time that the value of human resources was escalating and leading to the need for aeromedical specialists, the American Board of Preventive Medicine began certification in the subspecialty of aviation medicine in 1953.

Since the deregulation of domestic airlines in 1978, an additional emphasis on cost containment has permeated support services for all airline management staff. Thus, nonoperational functions such as personnel, medical, legal, and training functions have been reduced or eliminated by many carriers. From the medical vantage point, a few large carriers have maintained or increased their corporate visibility and contributions, while many others, unfortunately, have declined in import or been eliminated outright. At this time, only American and United Airlines have system medical responsibilities with a geographically allocated system of flight surgeons and support staff dedicated to the aeromedical and occupational health needs of airline employees. Most other major carriers are served by a single-site medical function and/or outside consultants.

ORGANIZATION AND STRUCTURE OF AIRLINE AND UNION MEDICAL FUNCTIONS

One of the unique features of medical practice in the airline setting is the considerable concern for the public's safety and the possibility of liability resulting from activities and decisions in connection with practicing aviation medicine. Regardless of the structure through which aviation medicine support is provided, it is imperative that the physician never lose sight of his or her obligations to public safety. Airline medical departments also must be sensitive to the fact that flight crewmembers are regulated by the FAA, which is concerned with medical fitness and safety.

Self-Contained Medical Departments

It is common to find the airline medical department located in the corporation's major headquarters. For the larger airlines, it is standard practice for a considerable portion of the medical resources to be concentrated at the home office. Regional medical offices also may be established and house at least one physician and additional paraprofessional and support personnel. The offices are normally located at one of the major hubs of the airline route structure where aircrew are domiciled. This location provides the crewmember ease of access to medical services. One major airline centralized its medical resources and uses its system to bring the employee to the physician. In acute medical situations, consultants have been identified throughout the United States who can support the medical needs of the crewmember. In determining the medical services structure within a corporation, a cost-benefit analysis is appropriate, and, as developed below, current studies in the general occupational setting tend to favor in-plant over out-of-plant medical care.

Title and organizational level can be significant influencing factors in obtaining or sustaining a program or in making decisions within a company. Some airlines overcome the difficulty by designating the medical department as a separate, high-level department reporting directly to the president of the airline. The chief physician in such a structure carries the title of Corporate Medical Director or Vice President of Medical Services. Employees for other medical functions report to a senior officer in the personnel, human resources, or employee relations division.

Functions traditionally associated with medical concerns, such as industrial hygiene, ground and flight safety, and employee assistance staff, may report directly to the medical office, exist in a matrix management arrangement with other operation or support functions, or report directly to another area of the company.

Contractual Services

Other airlines have elected not to develop a medical department within their own corporate structure rather to rely on a contractual arrangement. In these situations, it is common for the airline to turn to a nationally recognized clinic or specialist for the necessary medical support. Each airline must, in turn, weigh the benefits of this arrangement against those of developing their own medical department. At times using a separate clinic proves to be less convenient to both the employee and the airline. Further, the clinic may be unable to adjust to corporate needs as expeditiously as the airline company might desire. Such an arrangement, however, reduces the potential for conflicts of interest regarding the employee's health status. Another advantage to this arrangement is that senior consultants frequently are readily available as members of the clinic staff.

Contingency and Fee-for-Service Arrangements

Among the smaller airlines, medical support commonly is provided through a contingency arrangement with a private practitioner or simply on a fee-for-service basis. Aerospace medical specialists or physicians knowledgeable in the field of aviation medicine often are available near the nation's major airports. Smaller airlines turn to these physicians for medical support requirements. This procedure is frequently an acceptable alternative in view of the routine nature of the services required. These same physicians may provide en-route medical support to even the major airlines. The availability of their services at or near airports can be particularly attractive.

Union Medical Function

The unavailability and lack of uniformity of medical services for airline pilots caused the board of directors of the Air Line Pilots Association (ALPA) to establish the position of Aero-medical Advisor in 1968.

The ALPA is a union of professional pilots having some 40,000 members and representing pilots from most major U.S. air carriers. In existence for over 60 years, its interests include wages and working conditions, representation services, safety, and health and welfare of the membership.

One of the authors (RLM) was the first Aeromedical Advisor, and opened the office in 1969. The service provides, on request, medical advice and assistance to members whose FAA medical certificates are in question or whose ability to meet medical standards has been challenged. Additionally, the office advises the ALPA president and elected officers on all matters pertaining to the health and welfare of the general membership, matters pertaining to human factors, the aerospace environment, and government regulations. By 1987, several other pilot unions were providing similar services to their members.

ALPA physicians provide case management assistance to members. This involves discussing the case, taking a careful history, reviewing all medical records available, and recommending specialist evaluations. After the records are gathered and analyzed, the pilot is advised of the favorable or unfavorable aspects of the case and the potential impact on air safety related to the condition. If the case warrants appeal to the FAA or air carrier medical department (or both), the Aeromedical Advisor will, with the pilot's signed authorization, present the case for consideration. Should the pilot's condition be deemed unsafe, he or she would be so advised. The pilot still has the right to request direct consideration from the FAA or company, whereupon the case would be forwarded.

In 1991, the results of a review of the most recent 10,500 cases from an active aeromedical consultation group practice were released (3). This paper analyzed the numbers and types of airline pilot cases managed by the practice, and compared the results to a major FAA study of medically disqualified pilots that covered the same relative time period. Overall, the two studies were quite comparable, with the FAA neuropsychiatric category (includes substance abuse and the entire spectrum of psychiatric diagnoses) ranking as the most prevalent cause of disqualification in all 5 year cohorts from age 30 to 49. For age groups 50–54 and 55–59, the cardiovascular disease group rose to number one, by large margins. Overall, because of the weight of the large numbers of cardiovascular cases, 29% of all office cases were cardiovascular, with 19% neuropsychiatric, and the miscellaneous, abdominal, bones/joints, ear, nose and throat, and others accounting for the remainder of 87% of all cases. Because of the nature of the practice, administrative assistance questions accounted for the remaining 13%. While neuropsychiatric case rates were relatively stable with age, cardiovascular rates quintupled between the 30–34 age group and the 55–59 age group. In the FAA data, the denial rates for cardiovascular disease was 0.1/1,000 in age groups 25–29, 30–34, and 35–39; at 45–49, the rate was 2.7/1,000 and reached 11.9/1,000 in the age 55–59 category. These data are indicative of the need for diligent attention to the need for case finding, intervention and prevention oriented programs.

Preventive and Health Maintenance Needs of Pilots

Given the interdependent relationship between maintaining good health and preserving a career in aviation, there is ample motivation for the provision of prevention-oriented medical services. Airlines and unions alike pursue a policy to provide for a broad preventive medicine program and to encourage the pilots to maintain the highest levels of health. Ongoing efforts in these areas may fall short of total success; however, they must be pursued with vigor.

Comprehensive programs involving a sound patient-physician relationship, accomplishing thorough prevention-oriented physical examinations, counseling and directing clients in preventive measures, and formal programs aimed at diminishing or deferring the impact of career-threatening diseases are scarce indeed. Those air carriers with well-supported medical departments perform well in this area. The handful of private physicians who offer such programs around the country are too few. A few centers and practitioners offer a comprehensive type of service to pilots. Some pilots seek out the services only when they have a health problem; others may participate in the hope of preventing disease in the future. Perhaps providers would step forward to assume roles of comprehensive health care for professional pilots if they sensed the demand for such services.

Pilots must be educated about the importance and efficacy of prevention-oriented health maintenance programs. Although the usefulness of health maintenance programs that involve periodic comprehensive physical examinations may indeed be questioned among the general population, their use in specific populations such as airline pilots is undoubtedly cost-effective. Given the high cost of pilot replacement and the impact of good health on air safety, it behooves both employers and employees to encourage participation in the programs. The development of programs is controversial, and the reluctance of pilots to participate in them hangs largely on their fear of adverse FAA certificate action. The FAA may take the position that a finding is indicative of a disqualifying disorder. Because professional pilots have no assurance that adverse findings would not disqualify them, they are reluctant to participate. Hence, regulatory concepts have a negative motivating effect on preventive maintenance programs for professional airline pilots. If positive findings in a health maintenance physical were viewed as risk factors warranting more in-depth study rather than as disqualifying criteria, preventive programs and pilots' health would be better served. A broadened understanding of the importance and necessity of preventive programs may lead to accommodation between carriers, the FAA, and the various providers of medical service to professional pilots, resulting in the encourage-

ment of effective prevention-oriented health maintenance programs.

Cardiovascular Disease in the Pilot Program

The actual incidence and prevalence of cardiovascular disorders in the professional pilot population are uncertain, but one study that used estimates based on medical loss of license claims points to a lower incidence of cardiovascular disease than that of the U.S. white male population (4). It would not be unexpected that the incidence of heart disease in the pilot population would be lower, but it is interesting that the figures show the relentless progression of the disease with age (Table 25.1). In fact, starting from a very low incidence, which can largely be accounted for by selection, the prevalence of the condition has almost approached that of the U.S. white male population by ages 55 to 59 (as represented by the Framingham study results.)

The overall decline in cardiovascular disease in the general U.S. population over the past two decades appears to be real and sustainable. Various explanations have been advanced to account for this change, but most likely a combination of factors, such as improved lifestyle (diet, exercise) and marked improvements in treatment and treatment availability explain this for-

Table 25.1.
Incidence of Coronary Heart Disease, Airline Pilots Association (ALPA) and Framingham Study of White Males (Age-Specific Incidences per 1000 Persons)

Age Group	Framingham Study	ALPA	Framingham/ ALPA Ratio
29–34	2.93	0.151	19.40
35–39	2.44	0.678	3.60
40–44	5.16	2.050	2.52
45–49	7.23	4.460	1.62
50–54	12.70	8.740	1.45
55–59	19.80	15.900	1.25

Adapted from Kulak LL, Wick RL Jr., Billings CE. Epidemiological study of in-flight airline pilot incapacitation. Aerospace Med 1971;42:670–672.

tunate turn of events. Based on unpublished data, the ALPA group demonstrated an approximate decline in cardiovascular disease cases of 27% between 1978 and 1991 (3).

Acquired Immune Deficiency Syndrome

Acquired immune deficiency syndrome (AIDS) has come into public prominence in the last decade. The aeromedical and safety implications of the several forms of this disease have been and will continue to be matters of heated debate. Variables in the manifestations, progression, rate of progression, and complications reduce prediction, at best, to a conundrum unlikely to be solved. The FAA and aeromedical specialists have long favored evaluations for determining eligibility for flight duty on an individual case basis. But, to take just one example, the insidious nature of the dementia that may be seen in HIV-positive individuals, and the discomfort level with neuropsychological test specificity and sensitivity, makes for a tragic dilemma where ruling on the side of safety often is the prudent course (see Chapters 18 and 19).

Drug Abuse and Alcoholism

In the ALPA experience, incidents involving drug abuse in the professional airline population are rare. Except for cases in which polydrug abuse is seen in association with alcoholism, only one isolated case of drug abuse was seen in over 1100 alcohol cases. Some use of marijuana and other drugs might be expected in younger pilots, reflecting sociocultural attitudes, but it is not clinically manifested. The incidence of alcoholism among commercial crewmembers is impossible to state precisely but is believed to be in the same general proportion as that found among white-collar and professional persons in the U.S. population.

Since the initiation of federally mandated random drug testing in late 1989, positive tests have been found to be quite low in the professional airline pilot population. For example, two of the largest U.S. carriers, employing together about 15,000 pilots, found no positive random tests in their first year of testing. While it is arguable whether this bears a close relationship to the actual numbers, there certainly appeared to be a very low rate in the pilot population of abuse of the five DOT-specified drugs for which the tests were given.

The FAA experience with air traffic controllers and pilots has shown a confirmed positive rate of 0.06%, at a cost of about $45,000 per positive result. It might prove far more fruitful if these funds were used to educate the population about drugs and teach supervisors to recognize behavioral changes, performance decrements, and other factors that could lead to early intervention. Too much reliance can be placed on random testing as being "the program," allowing neglect of preventive and case-finding techniques.

Environmental Protection

Aviation Physiology

Adverse physiologic effects resulting from low humidity in aircraft cabin atmospheres, pressurization problems (including rapid decompression), cabin air quality, and hypoxia are the concerns of the airframe manufacturers and air carriers. They are directly involved in providing protection from such adverse conditions. The flight surgeon's concern is to monitor these conditions for any trends and changes in the frequency or severity of incidents and to interact with the proper authorities.

Hazardous Cargo

The safe carriage of hazardous materials, including explosives, flammable substances, and biologic and radioactive materials is a matter of ongoing concern to the FAA, carriers, pilots, and passengers. Pilot committees follow this subject very carefully and encourage the enforcement of regulatory controls to protect both passengers and crew from unwarranted exposure to hazardous substances. Specific FAA regulations involving the protective measures to be taken when such materials are transported are carefully monitored, but that task generally is outside the purview of the aerospace medicine practitioner. To physicians fall the responsibility of providing treatment, analyzing medical effects and providing long-term follow-up and monitoring for those harmed by exposures.

A substance that may constitute hazardous cargo is carbon dioxide. Dry ice frequently is used in the shipment of perishables in the frozen state, and the amount of dry ice on board a commercial airliner may be substantial. Airline rules generally require passengers to declare dry ice that is being checked in baggage and limit the amount of dry ice that may be placed aboard an aircraft. Carbon dioxide, if released in significant amounts, could displace oxygen and enhance hypoxia.

Atmosphere Agents

Ozone has been a cause of concern to both passengers and crewmembers in recent years. Complaints of symptoms by passengers and crew have led to FAA regulations that delineate the maximum allowable levels of ozone in cabin atmospheres. Also specified are certain preventive measures, including the use of onboard equipment to reduce ozone levels.

Communicable Disease

Although flight attendants are more likely to be exposed to communicable diseases carried by passengers, pilots may be similarly exposed. In addition, crewmembers may be billeted in areas of the world where they may be exposed to contagious illnesses and hence must be informed regarding epidemic communicable diseases. Good hygiene and appropriate precautions in the consumption of local foods and liquids are important. Generally, air carriers maintain careful surveillance of appropriate lodging and eating facilities and arrange to billet crewmembers in inspected quarters. Primary preventive measures include proper inoculation and the use of antimalarial agents where indicated, and geographic infectious disease warnings (See Chapter 33).

Ionizing Radiation

With the possible exception of supersonic aircraft, the exposure of pilots to ionizing radiation is within the standards provided for radiation workers. No hard data confirm an increased prevalence or incidence of radiation-induced illnesses such as malignant tumors. Hence, no concrete information is available on which to base standards different from those now in effect. Continued monitoring of the possible occurrence of increased or decreased amounts of ionizing radiation and associated morbidity or mortality continues.

Nonionizing Radiation

Nonionizing radiation exposure in the form of microwave radiation is a known potential cause of cataracts, and an alleged cause of numerous other maladies, none of which have been proven.

Generally, radar is turned off when aircraft are parked on the ground, but occasionally is left on and continues to operate.

In such circumstances, pilots performing their walk-around inspections or persons standing on the ground near the aircraft may be exposed to hazardous levels of microwave radiation. Advances in design may obviate this problem, since radar automatically turns off at touchdown on newer aircraft.

Microwave is not the only nor the most problematic of nonionizing radiation wavelengths. Far more prevalent is ultraviolet light. A 1987 study of cataracts in airline pilots found a prevalence 2.34 times greater than in non-airline pilots.

The study also found that the average age of onset, 47 years, was significantly younger in airline pilots than would be expected in the general population (5).

Crew Scheduling, Desynchronosis, and Fatigue

Few areas are more controversial than scheduling, especially as this may relate to the prevention or alleviation of fatigue and the prevention of the undesirable effects of desynchronosis. The exigencies of the air carrier business require some flights to begin and end at undesirable times for economic or competitive reasons; or aircraft must be stationed at a given airfield so as to be available at a later scheduled use time. Therefore, some crews are scheduled to fly at all hours. In some scheduling situations fatigue can play a potentially serious role in the functional capability of the crewmembers. The complexity of the scheduling system and the varying degree of compliance with the principles of rest and nutrition for the crew, on the part of both carriers and crewmembers, complicate the problem further. Review of Aviation Safety Reporting System (ASRS) data reveals that in a full 20% of reported incidents, crew fatigue is cited as a factor. Desynchronosis and fatigue have been the subject of intense research since the early 1980s, led by the National Aeronautics and Space Administration (NASA) Ames Research Center, with cooperation from several international government and aeromedical organizations.

Commercial passenger operations must and have dealt with the work schedule problems. In many cases, the work rules have been altered by agreements between pilots and management. Joint scheduling committees, composed of flight operations management, crew scheduling professionals and pilots have reorganized flight schedules, provided augmented crews, and installed comfortable crew rest facilities on aircraft. Even the controversial idea of allowing napping inflight ('controlled rest on the flight deck') is likely to be resolved in the near future (6). Boredom is a very important area of concern in the newer highly automated cockpits of today and in the future. Add fatigue to boredom and the result can be disastrous. Controlled napping in cockpits can and will allow heightened alertness for inflight duties, and approach and landing high work loads. However, this expedient must never substitute for good sleep hygiene,

adequate rest before, during and after trips; and it is not an excuse for extended duty periods.

Overnight cargo operations add yet another dimension to the issues under consideration here. NASA studied these operations in 1987 and 1988. Using volunteer crews, NASA investigators studied trip makeup, duty times, onboard inflight observations, psychological test instruments, physiological measurements and crew self-reporting. The report, released in 1995, concludes, among other things, that nighttime flying imposes different physiological challenges that should, wherever possible, be taken into account in trip construction, timing and duration of rest periods, and the number of consecutive nights of flying. Crew members are urged to attempt to improve their alertness and performance through education and training on the physiological causes of fatigue, its potential operational consequences, and personal countermeasure strategies to minimize its effects (7).

Airline pilot and cabin crewmembers (flight attendants) are shift workers. In fact, the nature of their scheduling makes these workers irregularly irregular shift workers. The FAA currently is reviewing public comments solicited by a notice of proposed rule making (NPRM No. 95–18) (8). This announcement proposes to amend existing regulations to establish one set of duty period limitations, flight time limitations and rest requirements for flight crewmembers engaged in air transportation. The FAA states that the proposal stems from public and congressional interest, NTSB safety recommendations, petitions for rule making, and scientific data contained in recent NASA studies. The purpose of this highly detailed proposal is stated to be to ensure that flight crewmembers are provided with the opportunity to obtain sufficient rest to perform their routine and emergency safety duties. The final rule is expected to take several years to produce.

Human Error and Aircraft Accidents

Although no U.S. scheduled commercial air carrier jet accident has been attributed to pilot

Note that medical complications, aberrant behavior patterns, and disturbed social functioning are key elements of these definitions. Not all elements are necessary to the establishment of a diagnosis of alcoholism for a given individual, and their detection may be related to the severity of the illness; accuracy of the history; willingness of significant persons close to the suspected alcoholic to discuss the facts openly; and the comfort, knowledge, and the understanding with which the physician approaches the case.

Impact and Prevalence

Alcoholism is at once a manifest and a hidden disease in our society. Long ignored or deliberately suppressed as a diagnosis, alcoholism has been understated both as a primary condition and as an underlying factor in associated conditions and known complications and concomitants of the disease. Estimates of alcoholism prevalence in the U.S. range from 5–10% of the population. The economic and social costs to the nation are staggering and include billions in costs for lost productivity, health and medical expenses, motor vehicle accidents, violent crimes, and social responses.

Etiology

A number of theories have been advanced regarding the possible cause of alcoholism. Psychodynamic models, pathophysiologic mechanisms, endocrine effects, genetic predisposition, sociologic models, and ethnic differences, to mention but a few, have been investigated. Although many theories are being academically pursued, no method of primary prevention is available. Hence, only secondary and tertiary mechanisms of prevention are applicable.

Pathophysiology

The effect of alcohol on the body is widespread. The gastrointestinal tract; liver; hematopoietic system; nervous system; and cardiovascular, musculoskeletal, and endocrine systems often are adversely affected by alcohol. Cardiomyopathy, coronary artery occlusive disease, and atrial fibrillation, for example, are associated with heavy alcohol consumption. The hallmark effects of alcohol on the liver include alcoholic hepatitis and cirrhosis. Nervous system effects include peripheral neuropathy, a general depressant effect on the central nervous system, and with long-term abuse, organic brain damage, which can be irreversible. Neoplasia of various organ systems is known to be increased in the alcoholic person.

Psychosocial Aspects

The deterioration of psychosocial behavior patterns of the alcoholic person is generally relentless and progressive and has characteristic symptoms and signs that Johnson (11) feels are present in persons addicted to other chemicals. He delineates the progression to the universal alcoholic profile as a series of steps involving the learning behavior of the alcoholic person, increasing use and discomfort, waning feelings of self-worth, and ebbing ego strength through self-destructive and, finally, suicidal emotional attitudes. The well-known psychologic defense mechanisms of projection, rationalization, repression, and denial interact to contribute to a delusional memory system in which alcoholic persons are unable to understand what is happening to them and thus may not be able to seek help on their own.

Alcohol Rules in Aviation

The consumption of alcohol followed by the operation of an aircraft is prohibited by the FAA regulations. FAA rules prohibit aircraft operation under the influence of alcohol and specify an 8-hour period after alcohol consumption during which attempted aircraft operation would constitute a violation (FAR 91.11). In addition, air carriers have internal operating procedures that either parallel the FAA regulations or establish more stringent prohibitions. No alcohol or drug-caused accidents are acceptable, hence rigid prohibitions are fully supportable.

Industry and FAA Attitudes Toward Alcoholism

Early Industry Attitudes

Few conditions in medicine are as socially sensitive as alcoholism. The stigmas attached to alcoholism are so thoroughly ingrained in society that it is easily understood why air carrier executives want to avoid even the suggestion that their pilots might be alcoholic. Given this concern, as well as the persisting public attitude toward alcoholism as an untreatable illness or moral weakness, air carrier leaders formerly felt a sense of hopelessness in dealing with the condition and ignored, hid, or fired alcoholic pilots. Some leaders in air carrier medical departments have worked quietly to change these attitudes, although little effective action has been taken elsewhere. Loss of lives and careers were the inevitable consequences in a majority of cases prior to the 1970s. Most importantly, no uniform approach affected alcoholic pilots across the industry.

Early ALPA Attitudes

Attitudes prevalent in the general public and airline management carried over to the leadership and membership of the ALPA. That is, in addition to the general disdain and feeling of helplessness in dealing with the problem, "sweeping it under the rug" avoided for pilots the abhorrent consequences of public condemnation, as well as the equally abhorrent responsibility for destroying the careers of fellow pilots. Every pilot knew well that disclosure of alcoholism to the FAA meant mandatory and permanent denial of medical certification.

Early Federal Regulatory Attitudes

A 1976 FAS letter on alcoholism and airline flight crewmembers outlines the FAA position on the disease and its management. It points out that: "An individual who has a medical history or clinical diagnosis of alcoholism does not meet the medical standards and may not act as a flight crewmember, unless an exemption to the medi-

cal standards has been granted. Between 1960 and 1971, there were eight petitions from air transport pilots for exemption from the alcohol standard. None were granted. . . ." Thus, all three major elements of the airline industry—the carriers, the pilots, and the regulatory agency—either implied or practiced attitudes that precluded alcoholic pilots from continuing their career even if the condition was treated.

The Underground System

Given the prevalent attitudes outlined above, pilots with a history of alcohol abuse or alcoholism could turn only to covert methods of dealing with the problem. Those persons with knowledge of the problem in others often ignored it and, by so doing, silently condoned the activity or took action that almost certainly led to discharge or permanent medical disqualification. Fear of discovery often prevented alcoholic pilots from seeking help from qualified treatment resources, further decreasing the likelihood of treating the illness. Even those pilots who managed their illness through the effective methods of Alcoholic Anonymous were denied the ability to shed themselves of the cloak of secrecy. The persistence of the underground system was, in fact, locked by societal attitudes and a punitive regulatory atmosphere.

Treatment

Intervention

The alcoholic person's life can be described as being punctuated by crises. As the disease progresses, the person is beset with social problems (e.g., drunk driving arrests, legal entanglements), marital and family problems, and occupational threats. The alcoholic person is unable to cope effectively with the series of crises, and the downhill spiral continues. It is during these repeated crises common to alcoholics that the best opportunity exists for assisting the person and his or her family, concerned friends, and employer. Years of practical experience have led to the development of Johnson's principles of intervention (12). The basic assumption is that the chemically dependent person can accept reality when it is presented to him in a receivable form. The goal of the intervention process, which involves several steps that must be followed carefully, is to have the alcoholic individual see and accept reality enough to admit the need for help. The technique avoids the pitfalls of failure, and it works.

Modern Concepts of Treatment

Ill-conceived approaches to the alcoholic person, including one-on-one confrontations by physicians and construing alcoholism as a mental illness or a deficiency of moral character, are doomed to failure. Physicians who intend to deal with alcoholism in an effective manner must expose themselves to educational efforts to overcome the dearth of information they received through most standard medical school curricula. Careful preparation of family members and significant others in approaching the alcoholic individual is important. The psychoanalytic approaches of insight-oriented or in-depth psychotherapy are considered contraindicated, and alcoholism must be treated as a primary illness. A multidisciplinary approach is most likely to expose the broad symptomatology and dynamics of the illness and includes a team consisting of physicians, nurses, psychologists, social workers, and lay counselors with personal experience with Alcoholics Anonymous and group therapy. They must learn that treatment (recovery) is always ongoing; in fact, the term is not used in the past tense. Family-oriented treatment is a paramount consideration, and individualized aftercare (or continuing care) plans often comprise the essential elements of successful rehabilitation. Both inpatient and extended outpatient modes of treatment are available and, at least in the general population, appear to meet with similar success. In experience with air carrier pilots, however, the preferred mode is inpatient treatment, which provides a structured approach and wider patient access to specialists to deal with any physical and psychosociologic

complications or accompaniments of the illness. In all cases, the goal of treatment must be to reestablish the premorbid state and to take the steps necessary to assist the pilot in attaining long-lasting, total abstinence. A comprehensive program must be capable of meeting and dealing with relapses if they occur.

Model for Industry Alcoholism Programs

Evolution of Program Concepts

The attitude of the public and the medical professions changed gradually from 1965 to 1975. It became recognized practice to use the motivational force of the threat of job loss as a means of encouraging alcoholic persons into self-help programs and into the professional treatment programs that were developing. With this development of so-called occupational alcoholism programs—later more commonly titled employee assistance programs (EAPs)—awareness of their efficacy spread. Some air carriers discreetly developed in-house programs, but for the most part, no formal industry-wide methods evolved, and pilots remained underserved in a vital health care area. In 1974, the ALPA Human Intervention and Motivation Study (HIMS) was begun with the assistance of government demonstration grant funds (13). A continuation program (HIMS-II) has been funded by the FAA. The major aim of the HIMS was to encourage a nonpunitive atmosphere in which the combined forces of union, management, and the FAA could cooperate to bring pilots needed assistance in obtaining careful evaluation, referral to competent treatment resources, recovery with comfortable sobriety, and rehabilitation and return to work. This aim was achieved, but only because of the long-term cooperative efforts of all segments of the tripartite group. All parties conceded that the most important matter was the safe rehabilitation of pilots, and this required both ALPA and management to forego some traditional but counterproductive premises in the disciplinary area. ALPA established peer identification systems because traditional day-to-day supervisory roles are absent in the industry. A new stance and a change of policy was adopted by the FAA. The FAA first developed a 1976 policy letter allowing recertification by exemption from applicable portions of FAR Part 67. In May 1982, the FARs were amended to abolish mandatory denial of recertification for alcoholism and to allow discretionary special issuance of medical certificates to certain recovering, abstinent applicants.

Evolution of Program Concepts

FAA regulations and policies specify rigid conditions under which recertification is granted to recovering alcoholic or drug dependent pilots. Medical certificates are limited to six months validity, and pilots are monitored by their chief pilots, union representatives (peer monitors) and medical sponsors for continued certification recommendations. Although monitoring is required for 24 months, it is only terminated after 24 months with the written approval of the evaluating psychiatrist, medical sponsor and Federal Air Surgeon. Relapse rates over the past twenty years have ranged between 7% and 15%. Under certain circumstances, retreatment is permitted. By January 1996, some 1500 pilots recovering from alcohol abuse received Special Issuance certification (14). The HIMS consists of three concurrent efforts—education, case management, and model program development, refinement and feedback. Educational efforts utilize mailings to all pilots and families, discussions relating to FAA regulations, company and HIMS policies, and the showing of specifically designed films and videos at pilot recurrent training, ground training and safety briefings. Seminars, both initial and recurrent, are offered to all EAP, management and pilots who participate in the program. These seminars, given at both individual locations and centrally, last from one to three days, and are jointly administered by widely known experts. Attendance numbers from 25 to 200 persons. Case management, while varying with each carrier, generally complies with the overall program goals and always

mandatory abstinence from alcohol or mind altering and controlled substances. Program modeling and upgrading are continuously carried out by carrier and HIMS-II functions.

Program Needs

Carriers employing collectively over 95% of U.S. airline pilots with medical officers and/or professional alcohol and drug abuse counselors have the on-property expertise to establish and carry out rehabilitation programs. Experience in intervention, evaluation, treatment referral, follow-up, monitoring of aftercare, and continued observation of pilots returned to flying status are needed. Peer identification by trained pilots and supervisors (chief pilots) bring over 80% of cases to the attention of the program personnel. The remainder are identified through proficiency problems and self-referral (13). Carriers not having medical services available must rely on union medical resources or independent services having expertise with pilots.

Managing Continuing Needs

The requirements for an industry-wide alcoholism rehabilitation program ensures the continued long-term cooperation among ALPA, air carrier managements, and the FAA. Education of pilots and management regarding the disease nature of alcoholism and systems available to deal with the problem continues. Refinement of techniques and ongoing quality control are vital to ensure excellence of the programs. The development of a network of independent medical sponsors capable of handling the exigencies of pilot alcohol cases continues. The developing medical care delivery systems in the U.S. have resulted in disestablishment of many traditional inpatient and outpatient substance abuse treatment programs. It will be a serious challenge to employers and pilots to make appropriate arrangements with health maintenance and managed care organizations to provide vital recovery services.

CLINICAL SERVICES OF AN AIRLINE MEDICAL DEPARTMENT

The functions of airline medical services depend on the size and complexity of the corporations. The focus here is on a major airline's medical department. Many activities, programs, and services can be required and quickly move the scope of the medical services from aviation medicine to occupational medicine to the broad spectrum of preventive medicine. Such services would include those necessary for the selection and health maintenance of flight deck and cabin crews, aircraft maintenance personnel, aircraft servicing personnel, counter and administrative personnel, and executives. Typical services available to the employee advisory personnel are as follows:

Preplacement assessment
Periodic medical examination
On-the-job illness and injury treatment
Counseling services
Health hazards screening
Health and safety educational activities
Employee assistance for substance abuse/drug testing
Work hazard assessment
Consultative services
Benefits review and consultation

Preplacement Assessment

The preplacement assessment (after an offer of employment) is tailored to the specific position the prospective employee will be expected to fill. The degree of sophistication of this assessment is divided into two categories: crewmembers and all other.

Crewmember Preplacement Assessment

The success of the airline is in large measure dependent on adequate flight crews to operate the aircraft. It is to the airline's advantage to select crewmembers who can reasonably be expected to maintain their good health and meet medical and FAA standards throughout their working lives. The medical department must be careful to consider potential legal ramifications of employment decisions. Any handicap, perceived or actual, which does not impinge upon bona fide occupational requirements (BFOQs) cannot be considered disqualifying per se. Similarly, risks for future disability need to be evaluated in the context of a crewmember's ability to perform the job now and for a "reasonable" period in the future.

Historically, the airlines had drawn most of their flight deck personnel from the military; therefore, the candidate would frequently have proven academic credentials, demonstrated leadership skills, and 2000 or more flying hours. He or she would have satisfactorily met the medical standards for commissioning in the armed forces, as well as the more stringent standards required for pilot training. It is not surprising, then, that the majority of airline pilot candidates came to the physical assessment in a state of unusually good health. Because of the excess of applicants for available positions in recent years, it was not necessary for the airlines to consider employment of any but the healthiest individuals. This, however, is not currently the case, and the medical standards for employment required by a particular airline company during any specific year depend primarily on supply and demand. Nevertheless, the aviation medical specialist frequently plays a key role in the employment decision of safety sensitive airline crewmembers.

Nonpilot Preplacement Assessment

In the preemployment assessment of all other employees, the medical examination usually is not as stringent as it is for pilots. However, there are categories of prospective safety sensitive employees, such as flight attendants, crane operators, and motor vehicle operators, who also should be medically evaluated against established health standards. There may be other categories of employees who require a license with medical qualification as a precondition to their employment. One of the features for most flight attendants that should not be overlooked is the need for food handler certification issued by a public health authority. Employees entering the administrative, clerical, or reservations category may require nothing more than a health survey. Special attention should be given to the musculoskeletal system and to establishing an audiologic baseline in individuals seeking placement in heavy industry or maintenance work.

In the late 1950s, flight attendants with U.S. airlines had a job expectancy of approximately 2 years. Nearly all flight attendants were female, young, and unmarried. Since then, major changes have occurred in the social expectations and federal legislation addressing employee discrimination. Flight attendants are now of both sexes, capable of working beyond the age of 70, may be married, and, in fact, may perform cabin duties while pregnant. The flight attendant is the primary cabin safety guarantor during in-flight or ground emergencies. The absolute minimum number of flight attendants for a given flight and their distribution within the cabin of the aircraft during takeoff and landing are specified by regulations. Currently, an estimated 90,000 flight attendants are employed by U.S. air carriers. Preventive medicine and health promotion programs directed toward flight attendants have been outlined by Alter and Mohler (15). Basically, the concerns are the same as those that must be addressed by the aviation medicine specialist when dealing with flight deck crews. Unfortunately, the application of preventive medicine and health promotion programs to the occupation of flight attendant has lagged behind the progress of medical and engineering sciences. The airline medical departments must provide a realistic and needs-specific program directed to the requirements of these cabin personnel.

In a number of corporation settings within the United States, it is becoming standard practice to require a candidate for a high executive position to undergo an extensive medical examination, including cardiac stress testing. The type of evaluation and sophistication of the assessment is frequently established by the medical department, with the approval of corporate management. Thus, the aviation medicine practitioner not only is responsible for conducting such an assessment but, more importantly, may be the individual who establishes its need and scope. With the implementation of the Americans with Disabilities Act, airlines have adjusted their preplacement assessment procedures.

Periodic Medical Examinations

Periodic medical examinations are normally done on pilots and corporate executives. The degree to which other employees are afforded the opportunity for periodic health assessments depends on the airline. The flight crews are normally the only employee group for whom the frequency of the examination is set without consideration for age. For all other categories, examinations are scheduled periodically based on the individual's age at the time of the examination. A schedule that has been found acceptable in some industrial settings begins the periodic assessment at 30 years of age, with subsequent examinations at 35, 40, 43, 46, 49, and 52 years of age and each even-year anniversary thereafter. The components of the periodic assessment depend on the category of the employee. Again, it should be pointed out that the physician generally is not only responsible for conducting such assessments but for establishing their periodicity and scope.

Periodic Medical Assessments of Pilots

The airline medical departments provide a system of preventive health maintenance for their flight deck crews. This system may demonstrate the presence of early disease, and by initiating ameliorative programs, crewmembers who might otherwise have lost their medical license and thereby their livelihood are saved. In addition to the periodic assessment required by the airline and conducted by its medical personnel, the pilot possessing a Class 1 medical certificate must undergo a medical examination by an FAA-designated senior medical examiner every 6 months.

In 1960, the designated AME system was established for the purpose of identifying medical examiners to perform assessments on all civil airmen required by regulation to hold a valid FAA medical certificate. Currently, it is permissible, though infrequent, for the airline aviation medical physician to conduct the FAA-certifying examination, provided the physician is a senior AME. In general, such examinations are most likely to be performed in the context of a "special issuance" medical certificate.

With respect to medical examinations conducted by the AMEs, there are several areas of interest. Because commercial airline pilots may turn outside the company for their periodic medical examination, several considerations are involved in choosing a particular physician to conduct the medical examination. These considerations include such factors as cost, availability, convenience, and the reputation of the examining physician. In this particular circumstance, one must be cautious in judging the elements that establish the physician's reputation. Unlike a patient seeking a physician who may be best able to diagnose and treat a medical condition, it is conceivable that an airline pilot would seek a medical examiner who is less precise and detailed in the examination and more cavalier in the history-taking. The pilot may mistakenly judge it an advantage to have a less thorough medical examination because it lessens the possibility of medical conditions being identified that could compromise his or her medical certificate. This statement is not meant to imply that most pilots would seek a superficial examination but is meant to alert the aviation medical specialist to that possibility and to remind the specialist that the selection of medical examiners is not a chance occurrence.

Within most airlines, those pilots who occupy the copilot and engineer positions are required

by federal regulation to meet only the requirements of a valid Second Class medical certificate. In reality, the majority of these pilots maintain a First Class certificate.

Within the airline corporate structure, the aviation medical practitioner walks a thin line. On one side of the line is the commitment to the operation, public safety, and federal law. On the other side is the ethical obligation to the patient (the employee) and the representative body (the union). This situation, then, calls for a delicate balance between services primarily designed to benefit the flight crewmember and those actions that must be taken in compliance with the regulatory requirements. In the air carrier industry, one specific article is common in contracts between organized crewmembers and the airline: no medical information obtained by the airline medical department will be released to the regulatory agency without the expressed written permission of the involved crewmember. Further, pilots will be deemed to be medically fit as long as they possess a current, valid FAA medical certificate. A potentially explosive situation is created in which the airlines, through their more thorough examinations, may become aware of a medical condition that is not known to the FAA. Actions taken by the medical department or the operations division of the airline to prevent a pilot from flying as a result of a disqualifying defect may be appropriate, but are subject to the established grievance procedures in the contract. The medical practitioner is again reminded that the FAA Class 1 examination is neither sophisticated nor extensive, and it does not require provocative or stress testing or the use of high-technology procedures or facilities. The examination is performed by a senior medical examiner in the privacy of an office, and is dependent on the conscientiousness of both parties with regard to history and physical assessment.

Nonpilot Periodic Health Assessment

The scope and periodicity of nonpilot health assessments are normally determined by the airline medical personnel. Factors involved in making the decision are the age of the employee, employment category, degree of safety risk, and cost benefits of such assessments. It is important that the philosophy of periodic assessment not be confused with the need for periodic biologic monitoring as a result of the work environment. The periodic medical examination is designed to focus on particular organs that are susceptible to disease over time. The goal is to reduce the significance of the effects of impairment from diseases common to the population. Periodic biologic monitoring focuses on body systems that may be susceptible to harm from exposures within the work environment and are unique to the conditions of employment rather than to the population as a whole.

Job-Related Illness and Injury

A corporation has both a legal and moral obligation to ensure emergency care follow-up, and, if necessary, rehabilitation of any employee injured under conditions of employment. Fortunately, the more common injuries are readily cared for within a first-aid setting. Serious injuries could well require immediate evacuation of the employee to a major medical center for stabilization and appropriate care. The medical department arranges for the provision of such care throughout the entire airline system and, where numbers of employees dictate, provides the facilities and personnel to satisfy these requirements. The airline is faced with the full spectrum of occupational hazards, although some hazards are obviously more prevalent than others. One of the major flight-line occupational hazards is noise. Consequently, an airline medical department must ensure that procedures are established to protect employees from noise-induced hearing loss early through appropriate preventive measures. The medical department must work closely with safety, industrial hygiene, and operational personnel to ensure that employees receive and use noise protection devices. Numerous other potential physical hazards, including temperature extremes, radiation, and hypoxia,

are possible constituents of the work environment. Because the airline serves as a common carrier, the potential exists for employees to be exposed to toxic chemicals, zoonoses, imported or transported contagion, plant products, and other hazardous substances.

Occupational illnesses are often subtle and easily can be confused with common medical conditions. A high index of suspicion on the part of the examiner is frequently the key to the diagnosis. Because of the character of airline operations, the kind of insult or hazard that could result in the manifestation of illness is nearly unlimited. In an airline medical department, little purpose is served by subdividing the medical practice into aviation and occupational medicine. In fact, the full spectrum of the components of both are at work. Fortunately, the principles of both aviation and occupational medicine have their foundations in preventive medicine, and a physician trained in the discipline can serve both fields well.

The employee returning to work after an illness usually is not of major concern. It is common practice to restrict employees, when necessary, to limited duty to ensure that recovery is rapid and not complicated by the stresses of the job. For flight crews, this is far more difficult. Because of the potential safety risks in the environment of flight, it may not be appropriate to return an otherwise essentially healthy individual to work. For example, a moderately severe cold that would be only an inconvenience to a mechanic could result in the temporary incapacitation of a crewmember because of the possibility of barotrauma.

Counseling Services

The medical department's counseling service has two focuses. The first involves those services provided to the employees, who derive direct benefit to themselves or to members of their family. This type of counseling is frequently provided to employees seeking reassurance or further explanation of a situation that they don't fully understand and do not feel comfortable in pursuing further with their private physician. An employee may seek advice regarding health maintenance activities such as a dietary regimen for weight control, assistance in understanding his or her recently diagnosed hypertension, advice regarding a fitness regimen, or recommendations on health services available in the community. The same questions may be asked by an employee but with reference to family members. With all the medical attention focused on potential hazards introduced into the home from the workplace, an employee may request reassurance or clarification.

The second major focus of counseling is directed at supervisors and management. The concern here is mainly an employee with a medical problem who needs to be helped to cope with the stresses this problem brings to the workplace. These counseling activities often focus on personality aberrations of or substance abuse by the employee. Aviation medicine specialists do a disservice to management if they fail to encourage employees to avail themselves of counseling expertise in dealing with these sorts of problems. Generally, the medical officer is best trained to advise on the employee whose behavioral change is related to the work environment.

Advice should be offered, whether asked or not, to the supervisor of an employee returning to work after a major health crisis. Employees returning after serious trauma, loss of a loved one, recovery from a myocardial infarction, or a diagnosis of cancer are examples of cases in which assistance to the supervisor may be helpful.

Health Hazard Assessments

A medical department has many reasons for establishing a program of health hazard assessments for the airline employees, including compliance with federal law or regulatory requirements, compensation costs, union demands, insurance considerations, and altruistic motivations of the company. Such a program

that is pervasive among the airline companies is the "hearing conversation" effort. This program is designed to identify methods of reducing noise generation and exposure to workers susceptible to hearing loss in the high-noise environment of aircraft operations. Another program focuses on individuals who may be exposed to toxic chemicals and require periodic biologic monitoring that consists of physical examination and specific blood and urine chemistry analyses. Other periodic assessment programs may be established for those employees who may be exposed to ionizing or nonionizing radiation, hazardous vibration, or a variety of toxins and other physical hazards.

Such assessments fulfill only a part of the obligation of a company to the health and welfare of its employees. Parallel to the biologic monitoring is an entire system of work-site monitoring efforts. Environmental engineers, industrial hygienists, and technicians assess the noise profile and noise hazard areas, measure the adequacy of ventilation in paint shops and fueling stands, monitor both ionizing and nonionizing radiation fields with dosimeters, and assess with other monitors a variety of hazards within the work environment.

It is clear from the foregoing discussion that a close working relationship between medical and industrial hygiene functions are essential. This interaction can be accomplished with the industrial hygiene function reporting directly to the medical department or being associated in some other matrix arrangement. The important point is regular and frequent communication by the professional staffs of the two specialties.

Other aspects of a selective health screening program are those activities periodically conducted for the benefit of the employee. The medical staff may choose to mobilize its resources in parallel with a national drive to focus on a particular medical affliction. For example, screening might be made available to the entire population for conditions such as hypertension, diabetes, pulmonary disease, or glaucoma.

Health Hazard Inspection of the Work Environment

One of the more challenging activities of an airline medical department is understanding and describing the potential hazards of the workplace to the workers. For the aeromedical specialist, the initial step to understanding the environment is an indoctrination tour of the company. Because of the nature of airline operations and the shift work of many employees, it is necessary to visit each shift because different activities are frequently conducted in response to the flight schedule. The flight service ramp is a dynamic environment, with numerous individual operations going on simultaneously but, again, all activities are coordinated with the flight schedule. While aircraft taxi, ground service vehicles move about as service personnel move over, around, and in between the vehicles. Noise is ubiquitous. Weather conditions vary. Oil and fuel are everywhere and at times are mixed with deicing solution. Food service is loading at one end of the aircraft while the sanitary systems are being serviced at the other end. All of this is complicated by the press of time and the competitive environment.

In the maintenance hangars, nearly every industrial process from painting to degreasing and from welding to engine teardown can be found. Eye, ear, and respiratory protection are frequently required.

For the aviation medical specialist, one of the most important working environments to visit is the operational flight deck. A full appreciation for the workload and performance requirements of the crewmember comes only after in-flight observations in a variety of flight conditions. Flying in all types of weather, both day and night, is necessary to make one truly appreciate the professional skill, talent, and coordination of the typical airline flight deck crew.

After being oriented to the workplace, the physician is better able to make sound recommendations regarding environmental health surveys, compliance with the Occupational Safety and Health Administration, etc. Such recommendations normally are made in consultation with an industrial hygienist or technician. Frequently, the physician who sees an occupationally induced illness will recommend an environmental survey of that particular place to determine the appropriate corrective measures. Having visited the workplace, the physician is much more sensitive to the specific categories of occupational illness and their potential significance for a particular employee. Further, the physician can make a more rational recommendation regarding the degree of work restrictions for a convalescing employee returning to work but not yet fully recovered.

Employee Assistance Programs

Most airlines have established or contracted for EAPs for those individuals who have found their lives altered because of substance abuse. Although many forms of drug abuse are dealt with in these programs, ranging from prescription drugs to illicit drugs, the drug of the greatest abuse among airline employees, including flight crews, is alcohol. In developing programs to address this very sensitive issue, it is necessary to gain the support of many different constituencies. The medical department needs the commitment of all levels of management, support from employee organizations, commitment from trade associations outside the airline, and, not infrequently, a working arrangement with a regulatory agency. Once it is agreed to proceed with such a program, an extensive educational effort must be undertaken to advise all employees and to remove any aspects of a witch hunt. In this medical program more than most, it is perception rather than reality that determines the success of case finding. The cooperation of the ALPA, in concert with several commercial airlines, has been gratifying.

Even giving the benefit of the doubt to airline companies, it can be reasonably expected that 5% to 10% of employees have a substance-abuse problem of some magnitude. Unfortunately, many of these employees are among the most effective and productive of the workforce, and their value eventually will be compromised unless effective employee assistance is provided. In the industrial setting, the problem drinker generates excessive costs—three times the company average in terms of absenteeism, accidents, and illness benefits. It is difficult to calculate other costs that may be of greater magnitude, including the loss of the experienced employee, friction in the work group, lowered morale, inefficiency, waste of supervisory time, bad decisions, damage to customer and public relations, and, when dealing with the flight deck crew member, a potential compromise of public safety.

For an effective substance abuse program, the airline should commit to and publicize a number of principles. Recommended corporate policy regarding substance abuse should (1) recognize substance abuse as a health problem affecting the employee's job performance; (2) recognize the need for early identification and treatment of substance abuse to maximize the recovery rate; (3) make the company's health benefits programs, including sick leave and group insurance benefits, available for employees participating in an approved treatment program; (4) ensure that identification of an abuser per se is not cause for termination; (5) avoid the appearance of a moral crusade under the auspices of the substance abuse rehabilitation program; and (6) recognize that the airline does not supervise its employee's social habits, provided substance abuse does not threaten safety.

Once recovery has begun, the employee, with the support of the airline, often turns to a community-based support organization. One of the most effective support organizations is Alcoholics Anonymous. By using such an organization, the recovering individual has a broad-based support system, including the medical department of the airline, the philosophy of the company, coworkers or the union, the home, and the community.

For the recovering alcoholic pilot, provisions are made for a return to the cockpit after evidence of satisfactory progress in a recovery program. In the case of a recovering alcoholic, a return to social drinking is not permitted. It should be noted that a return to drinking occuring soon after discharge from an alcohol rehabilitation facility is not rare and would not necessarily preclude a return to flying status provided the crewmember followed a successful course of recycling treatment. It is reassuring to all associated with airline operations to witness the high recovery rate of pilots entering the alcohol rehabilitation program.

EAPs in the airline industry, as well as in other occupational settings, have evolved into more "broad-brush" efforts than before. Whereas most such programs were known as "alcohol programs" in their infancy, most now offer intake and referral services for other abused substances, family problems, workplace adjustment concerns, and sometimes even legal and financial problems. Paradoxically, this has resulted in increased diagnoses of alcoholism, because alcoholic employees often present with complaints other than substance abuse.

One large carrier reports that 50% of its consultations deal with substance abuse (primarily alcohol), while the other half are concerned with mental health problem issues.

Within the implementation in 1990 of Department of Transportation regulations concerning drug testing of safety-sensitive personnel, EAP efforts have become mandatory pieces of the process by which "positive" patients are processed. It remains critically important for EAP professionals to maintain their compassion, objectivity, and sensitivity.

Mental Health Services

Just as increased emphasis in cardiovascular disease prevention mirrors the prevalence in the pilot population, so must there be a substantial time commitment to mental health services. The services should cover individuals troubled by use and abuse of chemical substances, as well as persons troubled by psychological disorders, interpersonal problems, financial problems, domestic problems, and job-related behavior dysfunction. The general principle that should apply is that regardless of cause, a troubled pilot is prone to errors and misjudgments which can make him or her a performance and safety risk.

A wide variety of psychiatric abnormalities are seen in the professional pilot ranks. Depression is, in our experience, the most common entity, with alcoholism ranking next and anxiety a distant third. Other chemical substance abuse is rare.

Depression should be handled aggressively with appropriate evaluation and use of antidepressant medications to diminish, if possible, the severity and duration of the condition. Pilots often express frustration and unhappiness over the duration of their treatment, during which time they cannot operate aircraft. They must understand that rushing the treatment or stopping drugs prematurely can lead to recurrence; then return to flight status becomes more problematic. We ask the pilot to allow the treating psychiatrist leeway to handle the case so as to avoid recurrence. In severe cases, electroconvulsive treatment may be required but does not necessarily preclude FAA recertification.

The concept of ''fear of flying'' and its management by administrative action stems from military aviation experience. Cadets entering pilot training occasionally exhibit behavior which indicates that they have anxiety about aircraft and the flying milieu. This is termed fear of flying, and the student pilot is relieved of training duties to be placed in a nonflying position or discharged from military service.

Because most professional air carrier pilots were recruited from the military, preselection accounted for very few cases being seen in air carrier practice. A slight increase in frequency of such cases has been noted in the past decade. This may be a result of more pilots coming into air carrier service with civilian training backgrounds and somewhat less rigid criteria for elimination from training.

Airline pilots who exhibit symptoms of anxiety associated with their work are more likely to receive a behavioral evaluation by aviation-oriented mental health professionals. It would be rare to see such a case termed fear of flying; rather, it would be characterized, for example, as anxiety or phobic reaction to a specific element of flight (e.g., phobic reaction to adverse weather conditions). Some pilots have been treated and returned to work; others have not responded to treatment and have been grounded.

Consultation and Advice to Management

The airline medical department has an opportunity to serve management in a far wider role than simply performing its clinical activities. This consultative role may range from international health activities to educational activities.

Health and Sanitation

For those U.S. air carriers operating in the international air carrier system, the medical department must be up to date regarding disease incidence and prevalence in the regions of the world served by the airline. It is necessary to establish and maintain the immunologic status of crewmembers and to ensure appropriate prophylaxis for diseases such as malaria. Crews must be educated in ways of reducing the potential exposure to food-borne diseases and in awareness of the hazards of hepatitis, tuberculosis, and other contagious diseases. It is appropriate that a member of the medical staff visit the various domiciliary sites throughout the international route structure. Necessary health care must be provided in the same way that such care is arranged in the domestic setting. It is the responsibility of the medical department to ensure the competency of the local physician who is to care for the crewmembers and may be called on in passenger emergencies.

Although the subject of international sanitation is covered by various regulatory agencies, the airline medical department should have established methods to validate such standards periodically. Inspection of food service facilities providing local support to the airline is an obvious responsibility. Such inspections should stress sanitation, including food and water sources, refrigerated storage, and insect and rodent control. The source of potable water and the way it is handled should be inspected and tested.

The medical department, in association with industrial hygiene staff, should periodically review the insect control methods employed by the airline. Although disinfection is also a subject of international health regulations, options are available to the airline, and the aviation medical physician should make sure that the most effective methods available are being employed while creating minimal inconvenience to the air traveling public.

Educational Activities

The airline medical department has an obligation both to management and to the employee to publicize the services that are available. In addition, the medical department frequently is required to publicize specific health or safety information throughout the corporation. For example, a recent hearing survey may have indicated the need for a greater emphasis on the use of hearing protection, or an industrial accident may highlight the need for emphasis on the use of eye protection. Appropriate educational programs go hand in hand with the periodic health assessments and special health screening programs and are far more effective when accompanied by appropriate educational media attention. One example of a satisfactory combined health screening and educational program conducted by an airline was related to colon cancer. A significant portion of the EAP effort may entail management education and consultation, as discussed previously.

Cargo Service

The medical department will be expected to establish protective health standards for the carriage of dangerous or toxic cargo. Such cargos that are rather frequently carried in the cargo compartments of aircraft include radioactive materials, live virulent cultures for manufacturers and research laboratories, toxic gases—including carbon dioxide from the sublimation of dry ice—and dangerous or diseased animals. The medical department needs to be available to assist industrial safety staff in making arrangements and to advise on the proper management of personnel and facilities involved in transporting potentially hazardous cargo. In the unlikely event that a misadventure occurs, resulting in spill or leakage, on-site medical support at the airport may be required to ensure the safe and proper cleanup and protection of personnel.

HUMAN FACTORS AND AIRCRAFT INCIDENT INVESTIGATION

Human Factors

Working closely with the engineering department, the airline aeromedical physician can provide expert advice on human factors in aeronautic systems. During the upgrading of aircraft or the purchase of new equipment, the opportunity occurs to ensure that human factors are considered and optimized. Aircraft cockpit instrumentation has been undergoing a revolution and currently is capable of presenting nearly any dynamic information desired in a vast array of formulations via a number of cathode ray tube displays or flat-plate displays. The physician should be prepared to advise on the selection of such instrumentation with regard to alphanumerics, character size, color rendition, brightness, and impact to overall crewmember workload.

The flight deck crew may request consultation regarding the use of sunglasses and visual corrective devices (including contact lenses) and other issues related to the visual environment of the cockpit.

Within the human factors arena, one area is exceptionally sensitive between management and the union. This area relates to optimizing the work-rest cycle with regard to crewmember duties. Management's desires and requirements, as expressed through operations, may have significant counterpoint among the flight crew, including both cabin and flight deck personnel. Although regulatory requirements have been established, and new FAA rules are proposed, considerable leeway for implementation is left with airline management. The medical department and consultants can provide sound scientific advice and assist in selecting the optimal solution for scheduling crew duty.

A specialist in aerospace medicine is expected to provide consultation to management on a variety of human factors related to airline operation. Additional concerns are situations resulting from the environmental flight conditions at altitude. Such issues as the quality, flow rates, and types of oxygen equipment to be provided both in the cabin and on the flight deck are issues on which the medical specialist can provide advice. In dealing with the subject of hypobarics, advice can be provided regarding the pressurization differential, reliability of the system, and planning contingency operations in case of rapid decompression. Other altitude-related factors include the potential for industrial radiation exposure to both cabin and flight deck crews. Generally, the question is one of chronic exposure based on industrial standards for the working life of the crewmember; thus, the energy of radiation received, duration of exposure, methods of dosimetry, and procedures for protection are areas for recommendation and consultation.

Human factors related to ground escape by passengers in an emergency ground egress situation are subject to medical advice. Medical input is often helpful with regard to training for emergency escape, use of onboard oxygen equipment, number, location, and content of onboard emergency first-aid kits, type and number of smoke masks, and other aspects of emergency aircraft operation.

Other factors related to the aviation environment, such as sudden descent in turbulence,

cabin air quality, ozone contamination of the cabin air, onboard crew rest facilities, and the issues of diurnal work-rest cycles related to flying safety, provide a challenge to the aeromedical specialist.

Cockpit Design

Although not of specific concern to the private practitioner of aerospace medicine, cockpit design has long been a matter of serious deliberation by airlines, manufacturers, and pilot groups. Standing committees interact in an attempt to modernize and make more efficient the design of airframes and cockpits. In the past, commercial airline cockpits were designed for either two or three operating crewmembers. In 1981, a presidential commission determined that future aircraft may use two crewmembers without detriment to flight safety. The capability of two pilots to operate highly advanced modern aircraft has been attributed to advances in control instrumentation and cockpit design and to improved computerized systems to assist pilots in their cockpit duties.

Incident Investigation

The initial steps in any accident or incident investigation begin well before the actual event. The airline medical director and the staff must consider the improbable and develop procedures for handling a multitude of challenges that arise when an aircraft is involved in a serious accident. It is important to ensure that emergency equipment, facilities, and personnel are available at airports serviced by the airline. The medical director should be aware of the procedures at these major airports in case of an on-field accident or an off-field catastrophe.

Once the event has occurred, the physician assumes some part of the responsibility in coordination and monitoring the treatment and disposition of survivors. Concern is directed toward both crew and passengers. Once the press of the emergency has subsided, the physician must then turn to the difficult task of informing the family and friends of those aboard the aircraft. It is important that an airline representative be available to answer questions and, when possible, to allay concern. When deaths occur as a result of the accident, the airline is asked to assist in the identification of the deceased. Such activities must be coordinated with the NTSB and the local medical authority (the coroner's office, the sheriff's department, or the local magistrate). Frequently, resources are not available at the accident site to provide the necessary forensic support, and the airline may find it necessary to bring professionals with this experience to the site.

Among the many agencies involved in aircraft accident investigation, the NTSB is charged with the primary investigative responsibilities. Medical personnel from the airline and union may be requested to provide assistance to the investigative effort, but more probably these individuals deal with circumstances and situations peculiar to airline operations. If it becomes evident that human factors are involved in the accident, the aeromedical specialist should work closely with airline operations to reduce the probability of a similar event recurring within the airline. Once the immediate ramifications of the accident have been resolved, the medical director will eventually be asked to assist the airline's legal department in handling the inevitable litigation that will arise from the accident. Scientific and expert medical advice can provide invaluable assistance in developing the airline's legal position. However, such legal advice does not prevent physicians from being requested to participate at the direction of the NTSB in its investigative procedures. It would not be uncommon for the medical records of the crew involved in the accident to be subpoenaed as part of the investigative procedures and for a physician to be asked to appear and testify relative to those records.

PASSENGER SERVICES

The obligation of a common carrier to receive and transport passengers and freight without dis-crimination in the choice of accommodations has come down from the common law of medieval Europe. The travel and transportation of goods in those early days was considerably more hazardous, and the merchant was dependent on the carrier. Thus, it was decided that the carrier was liable for damages if it refused to accept goods for transport. The logical development was to extend this obligation to passengers as well. Consequently, from the beginning of the establishment of our judicial system, it has been recognized as the duty of a common carrier to accept and carry, without discrimination, those who offered themselves as passengers. The carrier also was charged with the responsibility to transport its passengers safely to their destination. This extraordinary responsibility has served society well, despite the revolutionary changes that have occurred in the modes of transportation. It is a long way from the sailing ship to the palatial ocean liner, from ancient caravans to the modern passenger train, from the oxcart to the automobile, and from the stage coach to the airliner of today.

Services provided the typical airline passenger range from adequate to opulent. Passengers are reasonably secure in the belief that they will travel from their point of departure to their destination in a safe and timely fashion. The airline makes a reasonable effort to ensure their comfort and diligently tries to satisfy all reasonable requests. Efforts are made to cater to the needs of the young and the aged and to provide for the physically handicapped. It is considered the law, however, that passengers who are so mentally or physically infirm as to be unable to care for themselves or who may become a burden on their fellow passengers or demand medical assistance may be refused transport. Should infirm passengers be voluntarily accepted, their inability to care for themselves having been made evident to the airline prior to or at the time of their acceptance, a greater duty and responsibility are placed on the carrier. This section does not address those passengers who, in fact, are patients and require aeromedical transportation (see

Chapter 20, The Passenger and the Patient in Flight).

If passengers become ill or helpless after having started their journey, it is considered the duty of the carrier to extend reasonable and necessary help to them until suitable provisions can be made. This duty may require that a passenger be removed from the aircraft and left at a suitable place until he or she is well enough to resume the journey or obtains other appropriate aid. A carrier's duty to other passengers cannot be overlooked, however, in observing the rights of any individual traveler. If a passenger's conduct or condition is such as to render his or her presence dangerous or offensive to fellow passengers or create a serious annoyance or discomfort to those passengers, it is the duty of the airline to remove the offending passenger. These general guidelines have been tested extensively in the courts.

One example of a court's decision is in the case of Casteel versus American Airlines, Inc. This case involved an initial acceptance to carry a passenger who was known to be very ill with tuberculosis and was subsequently removed because his condition worsened en route. The courts concluded that the nature of the business and the machine made it almost necessary that the court sanction a reasonable discretion in these matters on the part of the operator and that their judgment, if exercised in good faith and on reasonable grounds, should be accepted prima facie as justification.

In March 1990, the Department of Transportation (FAA) published final rules concerning nondiscrimination on the basis of handicap in air travel, as well as exit-row seating. As the issue remains subject to probable legal challenges on both sides of the argument, it behooves the airline medical staff to remain current on the status of this and other federal regulations concerning passenger travel.

Transporting the Ill Patient

To accommodate a stretcher patient, several commercial airline carriers have developed unique and convenient stretcher kits that fit essentially all aircraft without the necessity of removing seats. These kits are located strategically at several airports along the flight route and are ready for quick installation. The seat backs are designed to fold down into the arms of the seat, and a stretcher platform is then secured over these folded down seats adjacent to the windows. A foam rubber mattress is placed on top of the platform to make a more comfortable bed. The seats on the aisle are available for the patient's attendant, who must accompany any stretcher passenger. To provide privacy, curtains can be attached to the overhead storage compartment and surround the four seats containing the stretcher. It should be evident, however, that transportation of this type is not without some considerable expense because this requires paying for four first-class seats. Obviously, prior arrangements must be made with the airline.

It is not uncommon for an airline medical director to be consulted regarding the possible transfer of an ill passenger. In the majority of cases, arrangements can be made for the adequate and safe transport of the passenger. Provisions can be made for special diets and for medical oxygen. If it is not possible to load the passenger via the standard ramp or mobile lounge, arrangements can be made for a forklift or an elevating truck bed. Passengers with an orthopedic apparatus who can not board through the normal passenger door frequently can be boarded using the galley entrance.

In-Flight Medical Incidents

One major airline reports having approximately 1500 to 2000 in-flight medical incidents per year. This number represents about one incident per 10 million passenger-miles flown. Despite the potential of serious illness developing during flight, the incidence has proven to be quite low. Nevertheless, airlines do make nonscheduled landings either to obtain emergency medical aid for an ill patient or to seek consultation about and relief of non–life-threatening symptoms.

Table 25.2.
Medical Kit Contents

Sphygmomanometer
Oropharyngeal airways (3)
Needles
Epinephrine 1:1000
Nitroglycerine tablets
Stethoscope
Syringes
50% Dextrose (50 ml)
Diphenhydramine injectable
Instruction book

Experience has shown that these diversions occur once per 2 million passengers carried, or once per approximately 3000 million passenger-miles flown. Advance planning by the potential passenger and, when in doubt, consultation with the airline medical department, can minimize untold developments from occurring in flight. Deaths occurring in flight from natural causes have likewise been infrequent events and can be expected to occur approximately once per 2 to 3 million passengers flown. The same airline reports further that there were a total of 287 injuries in 1 year, in which 5.8 million passengers were carried 5650 million passenger-miles. During the same time frame, the number of illnesses reported in flight totaled 342.

Federal regulations require all U.S. air carriers to maintain and carry an enhanced medical kit (Table 25.2). The most commonly used medical supplies included the stethoscope and sphygmomanometer (80%) and oxygen (60%). Other medications and supplies were used 17% of the time. Provider assessments indicated that the kit was somewhat useful or very useful in over 80% of the incidents. Sixty-nine percent of the medical incidents that led to inflight kit usage can be categorized into one of seven major diagnostic groupings, including syncope/near syncope (29%), cardiac/chest pain (15%), asthma/lung disease/shortness of breath (10%), and allergic reactions (5%). Onboard illness appeared to be random and not associated with aircraft type or flight duration (16).

COST-EFFECTIVENESS OF AN AIRLINE MEDICAL DEPARTMENT

The resources necessary to support an airline medical department must compete with the other areas of expenditure on the airline's cost ledger. Because it is the nature of the airline medical department to provide long-range, tangible cost benefits, it becomes difficult to establish the cost-effectiveness ratio for these departments solely on the basis of short-term gains. Nevertheless, it is essential, if one is to ensure the survivability of such departments, to clearly demonstrate the cost-effectiveness to the airline profit motive. The medical program should not be considered as primarily a fringe benefit or an altruistic expression by the airline toward its employees. A dynamic preventive program conducted by the airline medical department makes smart business sense.

While few airline medical departments have accumulated and maintained records sufficient to establish a sophisticated cost-benefit analysis, several reviewers have published data on cost-effectiveness studies (which evaluate the economic implications of alternative ways of doing the same task), and some simple cost-benefit efforts have been produced. Existing studies generally fall short of the scientific ideal; however, they point out reasonably conclusively the cost benefit of absence surveillance and EAP efforts. They point out, somewhat less conclusively, the cost benefit of periodic and preemployment medical examinations (17).

One major exception is the medical department of Trans World Airlines (TWA), and these data have been reported by Anderson and Gullet (18). In 1971, Kulak and colleagues (4) reported a study on in-flight airline pilot incapacitation. Age-specific incidence rates of fatal and nonfatal causes of career termination for an 11-year period were compiled from members of the ALPA. When the rates of incapacitation were compared with national population norms, the pilots fared far better in all disease categories and in all age groupings, with the exception of

Table 25.3.
**Estimated Probability of Pilot
In-flight Incapacitation**

Age Group	Annual Events
30–34	1/58,000 pilots
35–39	1/36,000 pilots
40–44	1/16,000 pilots
45–49	1/9500 pilots
50–54	1/5500 pilots
55–59	1/3500 pilots

From Kulak LL, Wick RL, Billings CE. Epidemiological study of inflight airline pilot incapacitation. Aerospace Med 1971;42(6): 670–672.

younger pilots dying from aircraft accidents. The "healthy worker effect" was clearly evident in the rates derived from this study. Two other points are evident in the review of this important epidemiologic investigation. First, it was possible to establish an expected incidence rate for potential serious in-flight pilot failure, and second, the data provide a baseline to compare a preventive medicine program under airline medical sponsorship.

Based on these epidemiologic findings, the expected incidence rate for in-flight failure was established for serious disease manifestations such as sudden coronary death or convulsive seizures (Table 25.3). As is evident, annual in-flight pilot incapacitation is estimated to be extremely low, and it would be difficult to justify an airline medical program purely on the premise of reducing these already low figures.

The study conducted by Anderson and Gullet (18) addressed the long-term payback potential of a preventive medicine program for airline pilots. Over time, many airlines changed the emphasis of their traditional cockpit crew safety medical examinations to a more comprehensive program that stressed the principles of preventive medicine. Because of the enormous expenses incurred in pilot training and in disability programs, efforts were geared to ameliorate diseases that could be most effectively addressed by preventive measures. Aviation safety has remained an important consideration, but the em-

phasis clearly has shifted to one of economics. This approach has taken on even greater significance as the flight deck crewmembers have grown older with the stability of the airline industry in the past several decades.

The medical director of TWA retained the authority to determine the eligibility for pilot benefits and whether the individual qualified for disability retirement status should the crewmember inadvertently lose his or her medical certification. Consequently, the medical department has been able to maintain oversight and records on each incident of pilot disability occurring at the airline since 1948.

The study conducted by Kulak and colleagues (4) previously described and a subsequent study that was published as part of the report by the National Institute on Aging, *Panel on the Experienced Pilot Study* (19), served as a comparison base for the TWA program.

The crew disability rate reported for the TWA pilots remained remarkably constant from 1962, averaging 7.9 pilots per 1000 pilot-years. This occurred during a period when the average age of the crew increased from 36 to older than 46 years. The progressive decline in the age-adjusted disability rate at TWA was influenced most significantly by a drop in the rate of disability for pilots in the oldest age group, followed by a lesser drop in the age groups 45 to 49 years and 50 to 54 years. This decline in disability rates in the older age groups suggested a major influence from TWA's preventive medicine program. Undocumented reports from several sources suggest that airlines not providing preventive medicine programs have disability rates significantly higher than those demonstrated by TWA. When the baseline studies were compared with the TWA study, the age-adjusted rate of disability resulting from disease in TWA pilots was significantly better than those from ALPA-represented pilots (7.92/1000 to 10.92/1000, P < 0.0005.)

Comparison with the ALPA disability data supports the thesis that the TWA pilots became disabled at a rate significantly below that of the

Table 25.4.
Estimated Cost Avoidance Associated with TWA Pilot Preventive Medicine Program

Age	Pilot Wastage		Net Gain	Cost Avoidance* (millions of dollars)
	TWA Experience	Expected Experience		
35–44	22	27	5	3.5
45–54	28	53	25	13.0
55–59	49	71	22	9.8
Total	99	151	52	26.3

* Cost based on $200,000 per pilot in training and disability payments. From Anderson R, Gullet CC. Airline pilot disability: Economic impact of an airline preventive medicine program. Aviat Space Environ Med 1982;53(4):398–402.

other airline pilots. An appropriate assumption has been made that this difference is attributable to the comprehensive medical program.

To quantify the economic impact, a detailed analysis of cost benefits to TWA was developed and is summarized in Table 25.4. The preventive medicine program demonstrated the ability to reduce the disability of airline pilots by one third while demonstrating a cost avoidance to the airline exceeding $6 million annually, with a yield-to-investment ratio of 6:1. It is difficult to establish the cost of savings of a nonevent that has been avoided; however, it is an economic reality that within a free enterprise system these economic factors must be determined. Excellent records, sound data, and sophisticated analyses conducted over time are required to establish cost-benefit ratios.

In 1987, Holt, Taylor, and Carter studied the impact of airline medical departments on pilot disability. They compared three different approaches to medical monitoring of pilots and found that airlines with active medical departments had lower pilot disability rates than airlines without such departments (3). They also concluded that preemployment screening and assessment of individual disability claims were more important determinants of long-term disability rates than other medical activities (20).

The 1980s saw numerous studies whose purpose was to evaluate the cost-benefit ratios of EAPs. One of the most rigorous came out of a 4-year study of mental health treatment at McDonnell Douglas Corporation. In 1989, Dr. John Mahoney found the following to be true:

- In general, employers can shrink their bill for mental health care by taking the long view, especially by using effective EAP personnel, even if that means spending more in the early stages of treatment.
- An EAP that screens troubled patients confidentially and refers them for appropriate treatment is much more effective than treatment obtained by employees seeking their own help.
- Forty percent of employees treated outside the EAP for drug or alcohol abuse left the company within 4 years compared with just 7.5% of those who used the EAP.
- McDonnell Douglas estimated $5.1 million in savings over the ensuing 3 years for the 1032 patients who began treatment through the EAP in 1988, as opposed to the costs of outside programs. Of the total, $2 million would come from reduced employee medical claims, $2.3 million from reduced dependent medical claims, and $800,000 from reduced absenteeism.

While the general issue of substitution of in-plant for out-of-plant resources has not been clearly identified as a cost-effectiveness issue, all recent studies have favored in-plant treatment on a cost basis (21).

The medical departments of the U.S. air carriers are expected to meet numerous responsibilities in providing for the physical and mental health of personnel and to contribute to the economic well-being of the airline. A properly trained and managed medical function, administered by the physician trained as a specialist in aerospace medicine, will be likely to satisfy the expectations of the corporation by providing a professional aviation safety service while assisting in conserving the airline's most valuable resource: its employees.

AEROSPACE MEDICINE AND ETHICS

The air carrier medical officer, whether an employee or consultant, may be criticized for trying to represent too many viewpoints at the same time. He or she is subject to allegations of being a "double agent," or, at times, even a triple agent. Take for example the case of a physician who serves as medical director for a carrier and may be required to balance his or her interests between best serving the company, the pilot (or pilot union), and the FAA interests of safety. The judgment of how well the physician performs these functions comes from all sides and varies depending on the viewpoint of each observer.

The relationship between a pilot and the company medical officer may be fraught with mistrust. Here, the pilot more clearly may see the potential conflict of interest caused by the company physician's necessary loyalty to the employer. More conflict may be seen when the company medical department's physician (or physicians) also has FAA AME duties. Here we see the triple-agent effect.

How, then, can the medical officer avoid or minimize the conflicts of interest perceived by others? Mere claims of honesty and integrity go unheard until and unless the practitioner has demonstrated his or her intentions in action. It must be borne in mind that no single case is worth sacrificing ethical principles. Pressured by pilots, management, and the FAA, the practitioner must maintain equanimity and base decisions on fact. The single overview of the physician must be an unanswerable conviction to protect the public safety.

Flight surgeons are encouraged to get to know their pilots, and some are better than others at cultivating close ties. When friendships develop, it is not uncommon for a pilot to expect special treatment. Indeed, the pilot may feel that anything short of total commitment is inadequate. An advocacy role often is sought, and the pilot may feel betrayed if the physician does not prevail on the pilot's behalf.

The physician's responsibility is not to keep every pilot flying, but rather to keep every safe pilot flying safely.

So, too, the role of union physicians must be tempered by their responsibility for safety. They cannot be guided by other than fact, and their presentations to federal authority for certification decisions must be objective and factual. They certainly can express their professional opinion regarding the pilot's ability to do his or her job with no compromise to flight safety. But beyond that they should not tread. Advocacy must be buttressed by thorough documentation.

In dealing with the pilot, the physician should make clear his or her methods and means of case management. The pilot who is examined by the company physician must realize that the physician may be obliged to bring disqualification to the attention of management. So to that extent, the patient-physician privilege of strict privacy may be inoperative. Even in this case, however, communication should be limited to the question of fitness for duty and not the specific diagnosis.

Ethical dilemmas confront the aeromedical specialist in various settings. A pilot may seek advice in private consultation with the physician and may even demand a guarantee of confidentiality before discussing any aspect of the case. Confidentiality thus becomes the key to opening the history to scrutiny. In the course of the history, it may become clear that a disqualifying condition or event is present. It is not incumbent upon the physician to play the role of an enforcer of regulations or law, unless there is a specific law applying to that situation.

In the area of patient-physician confidentiality, medical professionals generally adhere closely to the strict interpretation to keep the rule inviolate. Exceptions would be rare, and usually only when the law makes provisions for exceptions, such as in the reporting of a serious communicable disease or where a court has ordered declaration in the interest of public safety or justice.

This does not mean that the physician should not discuss the disqualification with the pilot;

indeed, it is the physician's duty to do so and to inform the pilot, in clear and understandable terms, the pilot's obligation to remove himself or herself from the flight status and to report the matter to responsible authorities. As long as the pilot does not fly with a known defect, he or she violates no federal rules; hence, a thorough evaluation can be carried out to determine the nature of the problem, the etiology, the prognosis, and an estimate of the likelihood of recurrence.

In our experience, the professional pilot, when confronted with an established diagnosis of a disqualifying condition, will follow the flight surgeon's advice and proceed to remove himself or herself from flight duty while a complete evaluation is presented to the FAA for decision. Should a pilot refuse to report the condition and prohibit the physician from so doing, then the physician should withdraw from the case.

If the physician consulted is an AME for the FAA, then he or she has an obligation to the FAA to so advise the pilot. If a disqualification is established after appropriate specialist consultation, then no ethical requirement to treat the matter confidentially exists. The report to the FAA is proper, since the AME acts as a representative of the FAA.

Some pilots opt to seek personal and/or family care services from their AME, thus potentially enabling a future conflict of interest to develop. When the physician, acting properly, reports disqualifying data to the FAA, the pilot may feel betrayed. The resulting feeling of distrust may render any constructive attempts at assistance by the AME worthless. This is the double-agent problem referred to earlier.

Operating an aircraft, particularly one belonging to an air carrier, is a privilege carefully regulated by law. It is not a right, and the government has an obligation to maintain the public safety. FARs Part 121, governing air carrier operations, further require the carrier to maintain the highest level of air safety achievable. Specifically, the carrier may not use the services of a pilot as a flight crewmember, if they know, or have reason

to know, that the pilot has a disqualifying condition. Hence, both the pilot and the air carrier have obligations to air safety that override the privilege to fly or operate passenger-carrying aircraft in public commerce.

Deliberate failure to declare a disqualifying defect, or history thereof, is punishable as a felony by federal statute. Sanctions include incarceration and substantial monetary fines. Each pilot applicant, in completing the FAA history form at the time of his or her periodic examination, is required to acknowledge that he or she has read and understands the law. (18, U.S. Code Secs. 1001;3571).

Some medical professional organizations or societies have enunciated their codes of ethics by approval of the membership; others have not. The American Medical Association and the American College of Occupational and Environmental Medicine have codes, as do many others. The codes, usually lay out the general parameters of ethical practice for the group and proscribe certain activities and functions as unethical.

ACKNOWLEDGMENTS

The editor acknowledges the contributions made by the chapter authors of the first edition: R.L. DeHart and C.C. Gullet.

REFERENCES

1. Institute of Medicine, National Academy of Sciences. Airline pilot age, health and performance. Washington, DC: National Academy Press, 1981.
2. Airlines medical directors association handbook. Washinton, DC: Airlines Medical Directors Association, 1989.
3. Masters RL, Masters RR. Major disqualifying illnesses among pilots. Airline Pilot October 1991;15–19.
4. Kulak LL, Wick RL Jr. Billings CE. Epidemiological study of in-flight airline pilot incapacitation. Aerospace Med, 1971;42(6):670–672.
5. Masters R.R. Cataracts in airline pilots. University of Colorado, Department of Preventive Medicine and Biomedics; 1987. Thesis.
6. NASA Technical Publication, in press. Principles and guidelines for duty and rest scheduling in commercial aviation. Washington, DC: NASA, 1–10, 1995.

7. NASA Technical Memorandum, in press. Crew factors in flight operations VII: psychophysiological responses to overnight cargo operations. Washington, DC: NASA, 1–49, 1995.

8. Department of Transportation, Federal Aviation Administration. Notice of proposed rulemaking No. 95–18. Washington, DC: U.S. Department of Transportation, 1–46, 1995.

9. Kowalsky NB, et al. An analysis of pilot error related aircraft accidents. NASA CR-2444. Washington, DC: National Aeronautics and Space Administration, 1974.

10. Department of Transportation, Federal Aviation Administration. Revision of airmen medical standards and certification procedures and duration of medical certificates, amendment Nos. 61–99, 67–17. Federal Register 1996;61:11238-11263.

11. Morse RM, Flavin DK. The definition of alcoholism. JAMA 1992;268:1012–1014.

12. Johnson VE. I'll quit tomorrow. 2nd ed. New York: Harper and Row, 1980.

13. Hoover EP, Kowalsky NB, Masters RL. An employee assistance program for professional pilots (an eight year review). Denver, CO: Air Line Pilots Association, International, Human Intervention and Motivation Study,

NIAAA Grant No. 1 R18 AA01484 Report, 1–32, plus appendices, 1982.

14. Pakull B, Chief, Behavioral Sciences, Office of Aviation Medicine, Federal Aviation Administration. Personal communications, 1996.

15. Alter JD, Mohler SR. Preventive medicine aspects and health promotion programs for flight attendants. Aviat Space Environ Med,1980;51(2):168–175.

16. Aerospace facts and figures, 1982/83. Washington, DC: Aerospace Industrial Association of America Inc., 1982.

17. Jacobs P, Choval A. Economic evaluation of corporate medical programs. J Occ Med 1983;25(4):273–278.

18. Anderson R, Gullet CC. Airline pilot disability: economic impact of an airline preventive medicine program. Aviat Space Environ Med 1982;53(4):398–402.

19. Report of the National Institute on Aging. Panel on the experienced pilot study. Bethesda, Maryland. U.S. Department of Health and Human Services. Washington, DC: U.S. Government Printing Office, 1981.

20. Holt GW, Taylor WF, Carter ET. Airline pilot disability: a comparison between three airlines with different approaches to medical monitoring. Aviat Space Environ Med 1987;788–792.

21. Mahoney J. McDonnell Douglas Corporation's EAP produces hard data. The Almacan 1989;19(8):226–231.

Chapter 26

Aviation Medicine in the Federal Aviation Administration

Jon L. Jordan, William H. Hark,

Guillermo J. Salazar

Not within a thousand years would man ever fly.
Wilbur Wright, 1901

The Air Commerce Act of 1926 was signed into law by President Calvin Coolidge on May 20, 1926. The act instructed the Secretary of Commerce to: foster air commerce; designate and establish airways; establish, operate, and maintain aid to air navigation (except airports); institute research and development to improve such aid; issue airworthiness certificates for aircraft and major aircraft components; investigate accidents; and license pilots. Herbert Hoover, then Secretary of Commerce, established the Aeronautics Branch in his department to administer this new responsibility. The Air Regulations Division and the Air Information Division were created within this branch; aeronautical activities were grouped by function within both of these. In addition to organizations with responsibilities in inspection, engineering, licensing, and enforcement, the Medical Section was placed in the Air Regulations Division.

In November, 1926, Louis H. Bauer, MD, was appointed the first director of civil aviation medicine. Dr. Bauer was a former Army flight surgeon who brought a considerable background of training and experience in the relatively new field of aviation medicine. He was a major in the Medical Corps at his appointment and was a veteran of 13 years service in the United States

Army, seven years of which were with the Air Service. Early in his tenure as director of the medical service, Dr. Bauer developed the first civil physical standards and examination frequencies for determining the medical fitness of pilots. In determining these standards, he took into consideration the physical standards of the International Commission for Air Navigation which were instituted by approximately 20 countries. He also considered British, as well as United States, military medical qualification standards. In the development of these standards, Dr. Bauer concluded that strict adherence to military standards was not required for civil aviation because the military requirements related not only to flying but to performing other military duties. He also recognized that military standards were designed to establish a selection process that would assure a long and useful military career for the aviator and that such considerations did not apply to civilian pilots.

In developing the medical standards, Dr. Bauer corresponded with several medical authorities who had been involved with the physical standards for flying during World War I. For the actual drafting of the standards, he called upon a small group of physicians to corroborate his findings concerning the physical requirements for flying. The result of this collaboration was publication of a set of standards contained in the Air Commerce Regulations. These standards became effective December 31, 1926.

To conduct required examinations of pilot applicants and to apply the newly established set of medical standards, Dr. Bauer established a system of physician examiners. This system used private medical practitioners scattered throughout the United States. A list of 57 physicians qualified to direct medical examinations for pilot licenses was published in *Domestic Air News*, the official journal of the Aeronautics Branch. By October 1, 1927, the number of qualified physicians had grown to 188. Besides these civilian medical examiners, all military flight surgeons were qualified ex officio to conduct pilot physical examinations.

A training program for these physicians was developed; on December 9, 1927, the first conference of medical examiners was held in Washington, DC. Thirteen physicians were present to discuss medical problems in civil aviation and to receive training that would permit the appropriate application of the standards. Examiners for the medical certification system issued temporary medical certificates that were subject to ratification by the Washington office within 60 days after examination. Twelve training conferences for aviation medical examiners (AMEs) were conducted in 1929 and 1930.

Prior to his resignation on November 26, 1930, Dr. Bauer reached a number of milestones in the establishment of a medical regulatory system for civil aviation. He proposed a system of federally employed district flight surgeons in 1928, completed studies of the correlation of physical deficiencies with aircraft accident and training success, and established procedures for conducting practical flight tests for granting "waivers" of medical standards.

Such was the evolution of aviation medicine in the federal government: from a service that only determined the qualifications of pilots, to an organization that now provides multiple services to a large number of aviation disciplines and users.

ORGANIZATION AND RESPONSIBILITIES

Federal Aviation Administration

In 1938, a major change occurred in the federal government's regulatory responsibilities concerning civil aviation. As a result of the Civil Aeronautics Act of 1938, the responsibilities were transferred from the Department of Commerce to the independent Civil Aeronautics Authority (CAA). The act created a new kind of federal agency: one designed to keep its functions as an agent of Congress distinct from its functions as an agent of the president. The five-member Authority was given the responsibility for fostering civil aeronautics and commerce, operating civil airways, maintaining air navigation facilities, regulating air traffic, and inquiring into the cause of aircraft accidents. Within the Authority, an Office of Administrator was created for executive and operational functions and an Air Safety Board was created for inquiring into aircraft accidents. This governmental organization remained in place until 1940 when, under President Franklin Roosevelt's reorganization plan, the five-member Authority was transferred back to the Department of Commerce and renamed the Civil Aeronautics Board (CAB). CAB retained technical and operational independence for aviation rule-making, adjudication, and accident investigation, but organizationally reported to Congress and the president through the Secretary of Commerce. The functions of the administrator within the CAA were also transferred to the Department of Commerce. A new organization, the Civil Aeronautics Administration, was established to carry out these responsibilities, which were gradually expanded to include licensing of pilots and other aircrew; research; training; certain delegated aircraft investigation and safety regulation activities; certification of airports; and certification of design, manufacture, and performance of civil aircraft. This organization reported directly to the Secretary of Commerce. The Air Safety Board was abolished and its accident investigation functions were assigned to the new CAB.

The organizational placement of federal responsibilities for regulating and promoting air commerce remained within the Department of Commerce and was essentially unchanged for nearly two decades. In 1958, however, the Federal Aviation Act established a new independent governmental organization, the Federal Aviation Agency. A number of factors contributed to the creation of the agency and the transfer of aviation regulatory responsibilities from the Department of Commerce. The most important was the growing urgency after World War II for a single air-navigation and air-traffic control system, equipped with modern facilities, to serve the vastly increased demands of both civil and military aviation. In the early postwar years, both Congress and the Executive Branch became convinced that, with aircraft increasing rapidly in both number and speed, a modern uniform system was imperative for the safe and efficient use of the nation's airspace. Enactment of legislation creating the agency was also spurred by a midair collision of two airliners over the Grand Canyon in June, 1956 and two midair collisions between military and civil aircraft in the spring of 1958 (1).

Under the Federal Aviation Act, the Federal Aviation Agency inherited the organization and functions of the CAB and most of the authority for safety regulation and enforcement. The CAB, which was freed of its administrative ties to the Department of Commerce and became an independent agency, retained responsibility for economic regulation of the air carriers and for accident investigation and determination of probable cause. In addition to the authority acquired at the expense of the CAB and from the CAA, the Federal Aviation Agency was assigned sole responsibility for managing the nation's airspace.

Eight years later, as a result of the Department of Transportation Act of 1966, the federal government's aviation function again lost its independent status. Under this legislation, the Federal Aviation Agency became the Federal Aviation Administration (FAA), a major component of the new Department of Transportation (DOT). All functions, powers, and duties of the Federal Aviation Agency were transferred to the Secretary of Transportation, but those pertaining to aviation safety were specifically transferred by the statute back to the FAA administrator. The responsibility for establishing probable cause of civil aviation accidents and of exercising appellate jurisdiction over safety rule enforcement involving modification, ratification, or suspension of a certificate or license were transferred from the CAB to the new department. Here, however, they were assigned to the National Transportation Safety Board (NTSB), a departmental component authorized to act independently of the secretary. The NTSB is discussed in more detail later in this chapter.

Currently, the FAA consists of approximately 48,000 persons, half of whom are employed in the operation of the air-traffic control system. Although this system is the most visible and publicly recognized function of the agency, countless other regulatory and operational activities are performed by the FAA. Aviation is a vast enterprise in the United States consisting of over 639,000 active pilots, 170,000 active general aviation aircraft, 18,700 air carrier aircraft, 18,200 airports, and a myriad of people and facilities performing allied activities. In support of this extensive and vital system, the FAA operates 476 air-traffic control towers, 21 air-route-traffic control centers, 106 flight service stations, 52 agency support and inspection aircraft centers, and countless other facilities. With overall responsibility over the national airspace system, the FAA administrator in Washington, DC oversees the function and coordination of the headquarters' organization, 9 regions (Figure 26.1), the Mike Monroney Aeronautical Center in Oklahoma City, Oklahoma, the FAA Technical Center in Atlantic City, New Jersey, and several FAA field offices in foreign countries.

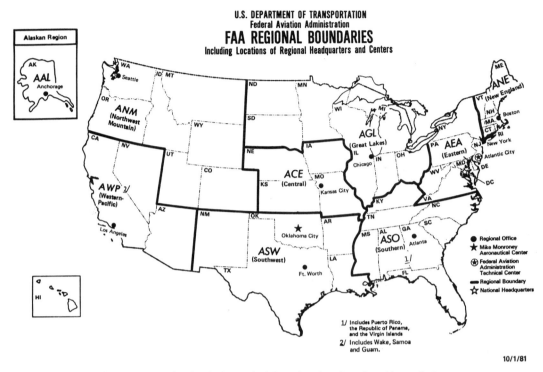

Figure 26.1. Federal Aviation Administration (FAA) regional boundaries.

Office of Aviation Medicine

From its modest beginning in 1926, when its only staff consisted of a director and a secretary, the aviation medical program within the FAA has grown to approximately 380 employees with an annual operations budget of more than $28 million and a research budget of $12 million. The Office of Aviation Medicine (Figure 26.2) is directed by the Federal Air Surgeon, who is located in the Washington headquarters. The Federal Air Surgeon is supported at the Washington level by three divisions; the Program Management Division, the Medical Specialties Division, and the Drug Abatement Division. The divisions report to the Deputy Federal Air Surgeon. The Program Management Division provides general administrative support, including budget planning and personnel management, as well as program evaluation activities. The Medical Specialties Division is comprised of the Psychiatric Staff, the Certification Appeals Branch, the Aeromedical Standards and Substance

Abuse Staff, the Employee Health Branch, and the Research and Special Projects Staff. The Drug Abatement Division oversees the aviation industry drug and alcohol abatement programs and is comprised of the Program Implementation Branch, the Compliance and Enforcement Branch, and the Special Projects Branch. Regional medical divisions located in each of the nine regional FAA offices are directed by regional flight surgeons who report to the Deputy Federal Air Surgeon. The Civil Aeromedical Institute (CAMI), which is located in Oklahoma City, is comprised of the Aeromedical Certification Division, the Aeromedical Education Division, the Human Resources Research Division, the Aeromedical Research Division, and the Occupational Health Division. These divisions report to the Director of CAMI who, in turn, reports to the Federal Air Surgeon. The medical programs directed by the Federal Air Surgeon and developed and administered by various medical divisions include aeromedical standards, airman medical certification, occupational

OFFICE OF AVIATION MEDICINE ORGANIZATIONAL STRUCTURE

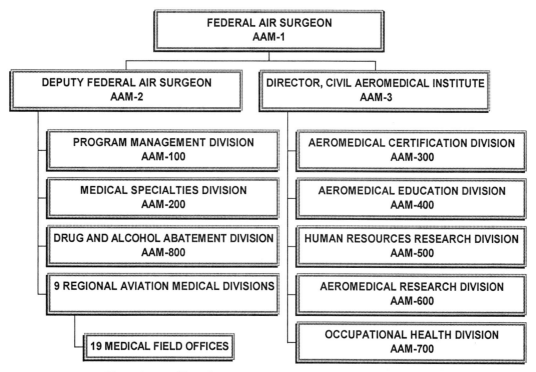

Figure 26.2. Office of Aviation Medicine organizational structure.

and employee health, aeromedical research, aeromedical education, and medical factors in aircraft accident investigation. The mission of the Office of Aviation Medicine is to apply aviation medical knowledge and research technology to the safety and promotion of civil aviation.

Federal Air Surgeon

The Federal Air Surgeon provides medical support to agency management and is responsible for the direction and management of all medical activities within the FAA. Although the Federal Air Surgeon reports directly to the Associate Administrator for Regulation and Certification, medical decisions of the Federal Air Surgeon are subject to review only by the FAA Administrator.

The Federal Air Surgeon is delegated the authority to determine the medical qualifications of applicants for aircrew medical certificates and to issue or deny medical certificates. To assist in performing these responsibilities, the Federal Air Surgeon also has been delegated the authority to designate physicians in a variety of medical practices to perform medical examinations of applicants and to make initial certification decisions. In addition, the Federal Air Surgeon develops procedures for ensuring compliance with medical standards and issues notices of proposed rule-making related to the establishment of medical rules and regulations.

Program Management Division

The Program Management Division is the principal element of the Office of Aviation Medicine with respect to the administrative management of medical operations and the evaluation of medical program activities. It develops policies and procedures in areas of: program planning, budget, and financial management; information management, organization, and staffing; human resource management; and automation. The division administers an evaluation program that reviews the operational adequacy of medical policies, standards, and procedures and determines the effectiveness of medical programs.

Medical Specialties Division

The Medical Specialties Division administers the drug and alcohol abatement program for agency employees. Division staff provide technical expertise and professional advice to the Federal Air Surgeon, other medical divisions, and other agency elements with respect to medical rule-making, research, psychiatry, medical certification, accident investigation, and employee and occupational health.

The division conducts employee health awareness activities, operates a medical treatment facility in the Washington headquarters, coordinates international aviation medical activities, develops medical regulations, coordinates national medical accident investigation activities, and provides advice and staff support to the Federal Air Surgeon for the administration of the FAA's medical research program.

Drug and Alcohol Abatement Division

The Drug and Alcohol Abatement Division develops regulations, policies, and procedures for the conduct of aviation industry drug and alcohol testing programs. Division personnel approve employers' substance abuse programs, and conduct compliance and enforcement assessments to ensure proper program implementation and conduct.

Regional Aviation Medical Divisions

Regional flight surgeons manage regional medical offices and are responsible for the direction of national aviation medical programs at that level. They direct aircrew medical certification, occupational health, and designated AME programs regionally. They also participate in the investigation of civil aircraft accidents and assist in conducting medical education programs for pilots, AME's and agency employees. In exercising these responsibilities, the regional flight surgeons process selected certification cases referred by the Aeromedical Certification Division in Oklahoma City, administer occupational health and health awareness programs for regional employees, assist in the investigation of aircraft accidents, and determine the medical fitness of air-traffic control specialists (ATCS) regionally. Regional management of the FAA's internal substance abuse control program is also a responsibility of the regional flight surgeons, who serve as medical review officers (MROs) for the program. FAA medical personnel, who are stationed at clinics in air-traffic control centers within the region, administer the aviation medical programs in support of the regional medical office and report to the regional flight surgeon.

Regional medical offices are located in Boston, New York, Atlanta, Chicago, Fort Worth, Kansas City, Los Angeles, Seattle, and Anchorage.

Civil Aeromedical Institute

CAMI plays an essential role not only in the design and development of FAA medical programs but also in the field implementation of these programs. Personnel at CAMI conduct medical research projects applicable to the FAA's mission, maintain a system for the medical certification of US civil pilots, administer airman and AME education programs, and provide direction for FAA occupational health and industrial hygiene programs.

Aeromedical Certification Division

The Aeromedical Certification Division is responsible for management of the airman medical certification program. It serves as the repository of airman medical records and is responsible for developing and furnishing statistical data from airman medical certification records for support of agency certification policies, procedures, and regulations. Personnel within the division evaluate the effectiveness of medical certification activities and develop medical qualification requirements for all pilots and non-FAA air-traffic controllers.

Aeromedical Education Division

The Aeromedical Education Division is responsible for the FAA's medical education programs. The division maintains a central repository of information related to the selection, training, and management of AME's. In addition to conducting professional seminars for AME's, the division also trains FAA pilots, inspectors, and medical personnel in aviation physiology, global survival, and medical aspects of aircraft accident investigation. The division also disseminates medical information through reports, booklets, films, and lectures to FAA personnel and the aviation public. It administers a centralized medical education program and supports a national accident prevention program for pilots, including displays of medical exhibits at accident prevention seminars. In addition, it conducts a high-altitude physiology indoctrination program through cooperative agreements with the US Air Force and Navy, and the National Aeronautics and Space Administration (NASA).

Human Resources Research Division

The Human Resources Research Division conducts an integrated program of field and laboratory research in the behavioral, personnel, organizational, and human factors involved in aviation work environments. Research includes agency work force optimization, reliability analyses of human performance, performance effects of advanced automation systems, and psychophysiologic aspects of work proficiency and safety in aviation.

With respect to this research, division personnel assess the psychological dimensions of compatibility of individuals with their work environments and conduct research concerned with human factors influenced by stress, such as workload and work shifts on team and individual performance. Human resources and human factor issues, such as pilot-controller communication, cockpit resource management, and performance errors are also studied, as are selection and training programs for aviation personnel.

Aeromedical Research Division

The Aeromedical Research Division evaluates human performance in aviation and air-traffic controller environments, both simulated and actual, through multidisciplinary medical, physiologic, and biochemical studies. Protection and survival research is conducted in this division, as well as research into the effects of drugs and toxic chemicals on human performance.

Personnel within the division investigate selected general aviation and air carrier accidents in search of biomedical or clinical evidence of disease or chemical abuse as causes of accidents. Data concerning medical and human engineering design aspects of those accidents are maintained within the division.

Occupational Health Division

The Occupational Health Division assists in the management of the agency's health program for FAA Air Traffic Control Specialists and develops and recommends medical qualification criteria for these employees. In coordination with the Medical Specialties Division, it initiates projects designed to identify clinical factors that may impact aviation safety, reviews the results of medical evaluations of applicants for the Office of Workers' Compensation Programs (OWCP) benefits, and provides guidance to regional aviation medical divisions for disposition of OWCP cases. Division personnel also operate a medical clinic at the Mike Monroney Aeronautical Center and provide industrial hygiene expertise for the Office of Aviation Medicine.

MEDICAL STANDARDS

Evolution of Standards

During World War I, Army personnel who had been rejected by the infantry for medical reasons frequently became pilots. The army soon recognized, however, that pilots with physical defects had a much higher accident rate than did those without defects. This recognition led to the first medical standards for pilots and to the development of aviation medicine as a specialty. Because few people had experience in the aeromedical field, the first standards were largely arbitrary and geared to the type of equipment and flying environments of the time, namely goggles and open cockpit aircraft.

The military standards were rigid, and when a pilot was disqualified, no avenue of appeal was available. The first civil standards established in 1926 by the Department of Commerce grew out of military experience. Like military standards, civil standards were also empirical in origin. Moreover, they bore the same rigid characteristics as the military standards, and they retained these characteristics for many years.

Early Standards

The first physical standards for civil pilots became effective on December 31, 1926, and were contained in Chapter 4, Section 66 of the Air Commerce Regulations. Dr. Bauer, with the assistance of other medical experts, identified disqualifying conditions that he concluded could cause sudden incapacitation or death while at the controls of aircraft, or could otherwise compromise the pilot's ability to operate an aircraft in a manner compatible with an acceptable level of safety. Three levels of physical qualification were established, one for each class of pilot created by the new regulations: private pilot, industrial pilot, and transportation pilot (2).

Private Pilots

Absence of organic disease or defect that would interfere with safe handling of an airplane

under the conditions for private flying; visual acuity of at least 20/40 in each eye ($< 20/40$ may be accepted when the pilot wears goggles with appropriate correction and has normal judgment of distance without correction); good judgment of distance; no diplopia in any position; normal visual fields and color vision; and no organic disease of the eye or internal ear.

Industrial Pilots

Absence of organic disease or defect that would interfere with the safe handling of an airplane; visual acuity of not less than 20/30 in each eye, although in certain instances less than 20/30 may be accepted when the applicant wears correction to 20/20 in the goggles and has good judgment of distance without correction; good judgment of distance; no diplopia in any field; normal visual fields and color vision; and absence of organic disease of the eye, ear, nose, and throat.

Transportation Pilots

Unremarkable medical history; sound pulmonary, cardiovascular, gastrointestinal, and central nervous and genitourinary systems; freedom from material structural defects or limitations; freedom from disease of the ductless glands; normal central, peripheral, and color vision; normal judgment of distance; only slight defects of ocular muscle balance; freedom from ocular disease; absence of obstruction or disease conditions of the ear, nose, and throat; no abnormalities of equilibrium that would interfere with flying.

In March, 1927, a fourth class of certificate, "limited commercial," was added to the standards for transportation pilots, and student pilots were included under the private pilot standards. Transport and limited commercial pilots were required to undergo a physical examination every six months, and industrial and private pilots required renewal of medical certificates every 12 months.

These standards were essentially the same as those in use for certifying Army pilots. Dr.

Bauer originally intended that waivers of the standards would not be granted to new student pilot applicants but would be reserved for pilots who had operational experience. Under congressional and industry pressure, however, and in part because of the erroneous issuance of medical certificates by the department's designated medical examiners to applicants who did not meet the standards, waivers were soon granted to both new and experienced pilots.

Dr. Bauer's reluctance to grant waivers to new student pilots put him at odds with the aviation community. His critics pointed out that citizens had a right to assume risks and that the job of the Department of Commerce was to foster the growth of aviation, not stifle it with rules (3).

Except for the establishment of a requirement in 1929 that glider pilots meet the physical standards for private pilots, the regulations remained unchanged until early January, 1931. The decline of new student pilot certificates in 1930 was attributed to "unreasonable medical standards" rather than to the difficult economic times brought on by the Great Depression. Despite studies by Dr. Bauer and Dr. Harold J. Cooper showing poor progress in training and higher accident rates for pilots with physical defects, the visual standards were relaxed for student and private pilots.

The distant visual standard for student and private pilots was decreased from 20/40 in each eye without correction, to 20/50 in each eye without correction. Under the new standard, a pilot was disqualified when uncorrected vision was worse than 20/50. Concurrently, the medical standard for diplopia was also relaxed permitting a private pilot to qualify for medical certification provided the condition did not interfere with central vision.

Further modification was made to the visual standards in 1931. The uncorrected distant visual acuity limitation for student, private, and glider pilots was eliminated. If the visual defect could be corrected to 20/30, the applicant would be certified. The justification for changing the vision standards was based on technical im-

provements in aircraft design. Engineering improvements to aircraft cowlings and the advent of enclosed cockpits decreased the likelihood of "prop blast" knocking off glasses or goggles of the pilot. In 1934, the vision standards were changed for industrial pilots. The change provided for an uncorrected distant visual acuity standard of 20/50 corrected to 20/30 or better. In 1938, the distant visual acuity standard for transport pilots was changed to permit medical certification of individuals with uncorrected visual defects of up to 20/50 who corrected to 20/20.

In addition to the changes in visual standards, the 1930s also saw modification of other aeromedical regulations as a result of the continuing pressure for relaxation of medical certification standards. Examples include the introduction of certifying pilots with static physical defects, such as loss of a limb, and the interval between physical examinations for noncommercial pilots was lengthened from one year to two years.

The most significant change in the regulations was made in 1959 when the FAA identified nine medical conditions with a high risk of sudden incapacitation or altered judgment that required denial for any class of airman medical certificate. An established medical history or clinical diagnosis of myocardial infarction or angina pectoris; epilepsy, a disturbance of consciousness without satisfactory medical explanation of the cause; diabetes mellitus requiring insulin or other hypoglycemic drug for control; psychosis; drug addiction; alcoholism; or a character disorder severe enough to have repeatedly manifested by overt acts were all identified as "mandatorily" disqualifying under the standards. Although the Federal Air Surgeon could not issue "waivers" to these individuals with these conditions, exemptions could be granted by the FAA Administrator. Exemption authority was later delegated to the Federal Air Surgeon.

Further changes in the regulations were not made until 1972, when the standards for mental disorders were clarified by differentiating psychiatric from neurologic disorders. In addition, current psychiatric nomenclature of the time was adopted, and standardized definitions for alcoholism, drug dependence, and personality disorders were introduced. In 1976, vision standards were modified to permit the use of contact lenses in lieu of spectacles.

In May, 1982, medical standards were further amended. This change was prompted by three factors: a lawsuit against the agency regarding the granting of exemptions from the nine ''mandatory'' denial conditions; a Federal court decision finding that the alcoholism standard was in conflict with the Comprehensive Alcohol Abuse and Alcoholism Prevention, Treatment, and Rehabilitation Act of 1970; and FAA concern regarding misinterpretation of the cardiovascular standards by the NTSB. The regulations were amended:

1. To permit the special issuance of medical certificates (i.e., ''waiver'') under established standards rather than through an exemption process for those people with ''mandatorily'' disqualifying conditions;
2. To permit the issuance of a medical certificate under the regulations to an individual with alcoholism who could show evidence, satisfactory to the Federal Air Surgeon, of recovery; including sustained total abstinence from alcohol for not less than the preceding two years;
3. To clearly indicate that significant coronary heart disease, even when treated, is disqualifying; and,
4. To preclude the granting of first-class medical certificates with functional limitations (e.g., limiting a pilot to specified duties, such as those of a second pilot in command or flight engineer).

No further significant activity occurred with the regulations until 1995, when an important amendment was made to Part 67 to provide authority for the denial of medical certification to a pilot based on the use of medication that would be considered contrary to aviation safety. This amendment was issued after a decision by the US Court of Appeals for the 7th Circuit found that the medical standards in force prior to that time did not provide sufficient legal basis for the denial of pilot medical certification based solely on the use of medication (4).

Shortly after issuance of the rule regarding medication, a comprehensive revision of Part 67 was made in early 1996. In addition to the Part 67 revision, an amendment of Part 61 changed the duration of validity of medical certificates for private pilots. Although changes to Part 67 did not substantially alter the application of regulations already in place for medical certification of pilots, the revisions implemented a number of comprehensive medical and administrative recommendations proposed earlier in an extensive review on the subject. Revisions of medical standards were necessary to reflect current medical knowledge, practice, and terminology. In addition, standards were recodified to reflect current federal government numbering. This materially altered the numbering scheme identifying various sections containing the medical standards. Previous Part 67 sections 67.1 through 67.31 were renumbered as 67.1 through 67.415. The changes implemented are reflected in the section that follows.

Current Standards

Federal Aviation Regulations (FAR) are contained in Title 14 of the Code of Federal Regulations (14 CFR). Parts 61, 63, and 65 provide the certification requirements for pilots and flight instructors, flight crewmembers other than pilots, and aircrew other than flight crewmembers. Part 67 contains the medical standards for certification of US civil pilots and foreign pilots operating US-registered aircraft.

Under these parts of the regulations, a pilot must hold a first-class medical certificate to perform duties requiring an airline transport pilot certificate; a second-class medical certificate must be held for performing duties requiring a commercial pilot certificate; and a third-class medical certificate must be held for performing duties that require a recreational, private, or student pilot certificate. Flight engineers are required to hold a second-class medical certificate, as are civil air-traffic-control-tower operators not employed by the FAA, the Department of Defense, or the US Coast Guard. Persons who hold only glider or free balloon ratings are not required to meet any established set of medical standards; however, they must certify that they have no known medical defect that makes them unable to pilot a glider or free balloon. Under section 23 of Part 61 (Part 61.23) of the regulations, a first-class medical certificate is valid for six months after the month of the examination date; a second-class medical certificate is valid for 12 months after the month of the examination date; and a third-class medical certificate is valid for 36 months after the month of the examination date for pilots below the age of 40, and for 24 months for those age 40 or older.

Part 67

The medical standards contained in Part 67 of the FAR are divided into three categories applicable to first-, second-, and third-class medical certificates. With a few exceptions, the standards are identical from class to class.

Under the changes instituted in the 1996 revision of Part 67, the nine conditions that were originally specifically disqualifying were expanded to a total of fifteen. These include an established medical history or clinical diagnosis of:

1. Myocardial infarction;
2. Angina pectoris;
3. Coronary heart disease that has required treatment, or when untreated has been symptomatic or clinically significant;
4. Cardiac valve replacement;
5. Permanent cardiac pacemaker implantation;
6. Heart replacement;
7. Epilepsy;
8. Transient loss of nervous system function

control without satisfactory medical explanation of the cause;
9. Disturbance of consciousness without satisfactory medical explanation of the cause;
10. Personality disorder severe enough to have repeatedly manifested by overt acts;
11. Psychosis;
12. Bipolar disorder;
13. Substance dependence, unless established clinical evidence—satisfactory to the Federal Air Surgeon—indicates recovery including sustained total abstinence for not less than the preceding two years;
14. Substance abuse within the preceding two years; and,
15. Diabetes mellitus that requires insulin or any hypoglycemic drug for control.

Distant vision standards for first- and second-class medical certificates were changed to delete the uncorrected vision standard. Corrected vision in each eye must nevertheless be 20/20. For third-class medical certification, the new standard mandates visual acuity of 20/40 or better in each eye, with or without correction. Near visual acuity standards were changed for first- and second-class medical certificates to 20/40 or better, corrected or uncorrected, in each eye at 16 inches. A new intermediate vision requirement of 20/40 or better, corrected or uncorrected, in each eye at 32 inches, was added for people over the age of 50 desiring first- or second-class medical certificates. For third-class medical certification, a near visual acuity standard of 20/40 or better, corrected or uncorrected, in each eye at 16 inches was added. Color vision standards for all classes of certificate were amended to read: "ability to perceive those colors necessary for the safe performance of airman duties."

Hearing standards were modified, as was the standard referring to disorders of the ear. The latter was modified to specifically include vertigo and, in addition, other conditions that may affect equilibrium. The "whispered voice" test was deleted for all classes and replaced by a requirement that the applicant be able to satisfactorily accomplish one of the following three tests:

1. Conversational voice test of both ears at six feet, with the back turned to the examiner;
2. Acceptable understanding of speech as determined by an audiometric speech discrimination test score of at least 70% obtained in one ear or in a sound field environment; or
3. Acceptable results of pure tone audiometric testing of unaided hearing acuity according to the following table of worst acceptable thresholds:

Frequency (Hz)	500	1000	2000	3000
Better ear (dB)	35	30	30	40
Poorer ear (dB)	35	50	50	60

Significant changes were made to the standards relating to neurologic disorders, mental disease, and use of drugs, including alcohol. The neurologic concept of transient loss of nervous system control was introduced to more effectively identify conditions that were not fully covered with the standard that applies to disturbance of consciousness. The word "seizure" was substituted for "convulsive." The term "psychosis" was better defined to include any condition in which the individual had delusions, hallucinations, or grossly bizarre or disorganized behavior. The diagnosis of "bipolar disorder" was added to the standards to reflect terminology contained in the Diagnostic and Statistical Manual of Mental Disorders, Fourth Edition (DSM IV). The terms "substance dependence" and "substance abuse" were introduced to replace "alcoholism" and "drug dependence." The new terminology was introduced to provide greater authority in dealing with pilots who use drugs and alcohol.

General medical standards remained unchanged to provide a vehicle for the agency to evaluate a variety of conditions not specifically identified by organ system as disqualifying. The terminology for a special issuance ("waiver") was changed to an "authorization for special is-

suance of a medical certificate," or simply "authorization." In order to grant an authorization, the Federal Air Surgeon may require the pilot to undergo a special medical flight test, practical test, or medical evaluation to make this determination. This authorization is time limited and the individual must requalify for renewal. In addition, under section 67.401, the Federal Air Surgeon may issue a Statement of Demonstrated Ability (SODA) instead of an authorization when the condition to be "waivered" is static or nonprogressive (e.g., loss of limb or loss of eye). The individual must be found fit to perform pilot duties without endangering public safety. The SODA is not time limited; it must be renewed only when the medical condition changes.

Certification Policies

To supplement the medical standards contained in Part 67 of the Federal Aviation Regulations, substantial guidance material is provided by the Office of Aviation Medicine specifically for use by designated AMEs. This material, *Guide for Aviation Medical Examiners*, is designed to assist in the interpretation and application of the regulations. This document contains general information outlining the legal responsibilities of designees and sets forth the conditions under which examinations are performed. The guide describes examination techniques and criteria for qualification, as well as instructions for completion of the application form. Through the guide, the Office of Aviation Medicine provides substantial information regarding the many potentially disqualifying medical conditions that are not covered in the medical standards.

In addition to the guide, current information on agency certification policies is disseminated at AME seminars. These seminars are conducted at various locations throughout the United States each year. The seminars provide training with respect to certification policies and practices and cover various medical specialty areas relevant to the aviation environment.

Regulatory and Policy Updating

The federal government's regulatory process is complicated and lengthy. To achieve even a minor change in the regulations, an extensive intra-governmental and public review process is involved. It is not unusual for several years to elapse between the internal establishment of a rules project and actual amendment of the regulations. In developing a regulatory project, an initial determination is made regarding the sufficiency of information to proceed with a proposal. If it appears that a regulatory change may be indicated but that insufficient information is available to clearly formulate a proposal, an Advanced Notice of Proposed Rulemaking (ANPRM) is issued. The purpose of the ANPRM is to gather information and views on the suggested change. When the FAA has sufficient data indicating that rule-making action is warranted, a Notice of Proposed Rule-making (NPRM) is issued setting out the basis for the proposed rule, as well as the proposal itself. After providing an opportunity for public comment and conducting public hearings that may be required, the FAA reassesses the proposal and determines whether to proceed with an amendment of the regulations. If it is decided that a regulatory amendment is indicated, the amendment is issued by the administrator with an effective date that allows pilots and/or other employees of the aviation industry to come into compliance with the requirements of the new rule.

Recommendations for amendment of the regulations and for changes in FAA policies regarding aircrew medical certification originate from a variety of sources. These include, among others, the NTSB, the Comptroller General of the United States, individual members of Congress, special studies supported by the FAA, medical staff within the agency, agency medical consultants, pilots' organizations, treating physicians, and the pilots themselves.

Major studies of the regulations and certification policies by outside medical groups have included the First Bethesda Conference of the American College of Cardiology held in 1965 and the Eighth Bethesda Conference held in 1975 (5,6). A study of the neurologic and neurosurgical conditions associated with aviation safety was made by members of the American Academy of Neurology and the American Association of Neurological Surgeons. The results of the joint study were published in the *Archives of Neurology* in November, 1979 (7). More recently, under the auspices of the American Medical Association (AMA), an extensive review of all elements of Part 67 of the Federal Aviation Regulations and the policies and procedures for the medical certification of civil pilots was conducted by 13 task groups composed of experts in various specialties of medicine that are important to aviation safety (8). The FAA received the AMA's report in the early months of 1986. The AMA report, together with other studies as a background, served as the foundation for the 1996 changes in regulations.

Aviation Medical Examiners

Two months after the first physical standards were established on December 31, 1926, the AME system was implemented with the appointment of 57 physicians located in 46 cities. The first medical examiners specially designated to conduct airline pilot examinations were selected in 1935, and except for a period between 1945 and 1960, when any competent, licensed physician could examine student and private pilots, the medical certification system has relied on physical examinations conducted exclusively by designated AMEs.

As of December 31, 1994, 5,276 designated examiners existed in the United States and 375 in foreign countries. In addition, 138 military flight surgeons were designated to conduct second- and third-class examinations. The majority of physicians who conduct examinations are family practitioners (Figure 26.3). Approximately 50% of the examiners are pilots.

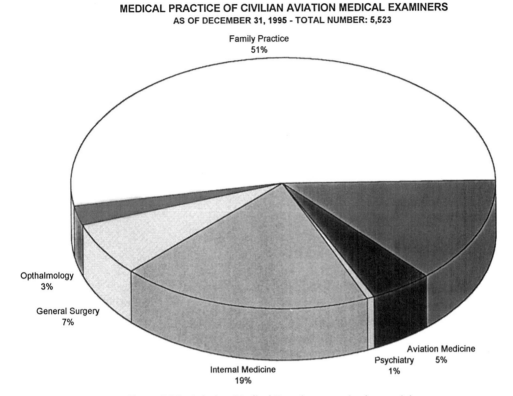

MEDICAL PRACTICE OF CIVILIAN AVIATION MEDICAL EXAMINERS
AS OF DECEMBER 31, 1995 - TOTAL NUMBER: 5,523

Family Practice
51%

Opthalmology
3%

General Surgery
7%

Internal Medicine
19%

Psychiatry
1%

Aviation Medicine
5%

Figure 26.3. Aviation Medical Examiner practice by specialty.

Management of the national civilian AME system has been delegated to regional flight surgeons. Practicing, fully-licensed physicians in good standing are designated on the basis of training and experience, adequacy of facilities for performing prescribed examinations, and the need for examiners in the geographic area. Typically, preference for designation is given to those physicians who have extensive experience or training in aerospace medicine or who have demonstrated familiarity with aviation operations.

Designation as an AME authorizes the physician to perform medical examinations for the issuance of third- and second-class medical certificates and to issue or deny issuance of certificates of those classes. Designation as a senior AME with authority to examine and certify applicants for all classes, including first-class certificates, requires three years of experience as an AME and additional equipment for performing

examinations. All designations are made for one year and renewal is contingent, in part, upon the continuing interest of the AME in FAA programs, accuracy in reporting examination results and making certification decisions, the number of examinations performed, and participation in the FAA's AME seminar and workshop programs. The fee for an examination is paid to the AME by the pilot. Although it is not established by the FAA, the amount of the fee is expected to be comparable to the prevailing rate for a similar medical service in the physician's locality.

Prior to the initial designation, the physician is required to attend a five-day FAA-sponsored seminar on aviation medicine, as well as complete a four-hour computer-based instruction (CBI) course in the accurate processing of the medical application form. This CBI course must also be successfully completed by any member of the AME's office staff involved in processing application forms. Thereafter, as a condition of continued designation, AMEs must receive FAA-provided continuing aeromedical education at least once every three years and a member of their office staff must complete the CBI course at least once every three years.

With authority to designate physicians as AMEs, regional flight surgeons also have been delegated authority to terminate designations. Designations may be terminated for a number of reasons, including: high error rate in reporting examination results; failure to conduct a sufficient number of examinations; disregard of, or failure to demonstrate knowledge of, FAA rules, regulations, policies, and procedures; failure to attend AME seminars; change of practice location; loss, restriction, or limitation of a license to practice medicine; any illness that may affect the physician's sound professional judgment; or personal conduct or public notoriety that may reflect adversely on the FAA.

The authority to designate AMEs in countries other than the United States and at US military medical facilities has been delegated to the manager of the Aeromedical Education Division at CAMI. Designation of physicians in foreign countries is based principally upon the need for an examiner in the physician's locality. Criteria for designation of international examiners are generally the same as those for AMEs in the United States, but some flexibility is permitted with respect to seminar attendance and the requirement to serve as an examiner for at least three years before designation as a senior AME.

A change in internal policies regarding the designation of military medical facilities and NASA clinics now requires that specifically identified military flight surgeons and NASA physicians, rather than the facilities, be designated. This change in policy prevents military physicians other than the designated flight surgeon from conducting examinations and issuing FAA medical certificates. In agreement with the respective Surgeons General of the various military services, military flight surgeons are not authorized to conduct first-class medical examinations or issue first-class medical certificates.

OPERATIONS PROGRAMS

Aircrew Medical Certification

Applications for aircrew medical certification that contain the results of physical examinations conducted by the AMEs are forwarded to the Aeromedical Certification Division of CAMI for data collection and application processing. During 1995, 441,827 applications were received. These included 174,522 applications for first-class medical certificates, 110,456 for second-class certificates, and 156,849 for third-class certificates (9).

Over 2,000 applications for medical certification are received by the Aeromedical Certification Division each working day. Documents are sorted for routine or priority processing according to issuance, denial, or deferral of certification by the AME and are assigned identification numbers that provide subsequent document control. Alphanumeric codes are assigned to medical and administrative data contained in the application, and the coded applications are sent to the Data Conversion Unit, where the data are prepared for computer input. Data are processed through several edit programs to ensure a complete record, and each application is screened for significant deviations from established medical criteria and compared with data on the applicant that are contained in agency files. With the finding of an administrative or medical discrepancy, the computer rejects the application and creates documentation that requires review by division medical records technicians. Technicians initiate corrective action or make appropriate certification decisions. Approximately 10% of rejected cases require review and adjudication by division medical officers. When applications contain inadequate documentation or errors, division personnel are required to contact the applicant or the examining physician for additional information or correction of errors.

In early 1992, the Aeromedical Certification Division implemented an option for the electronic transmittal of aircrew medical certification examination data directly from the AME to the FAA. Titled the Aeromedical Certification Subsystem (AMCS), this option was designed to modernize the certification process, decrease the time required to make certification decisions, and assure that all data transmitted to the FAA are complete and accurate. Beginning in January, 1996, all newly designated AMEs were required to transmit examination results through AMCS. By May, 1996, approximately 23% of all applications received by the Certification Division were being received through AMCS.

Applicants who have been refused issuance of medical certificates by an AME may request reconsideration by the FAA and may be asked to provide additional information to support the request. Depending upon the complexity of the case, division medical officers may review the available medical data and make determinations regarding the applicant's eligibility. When necessary, medical files are referred to consultant medical specialists located throughout the United States for review and recommendations regarding certification. Because many of the cases requiring specialist review involve cardiovascular disease, a group of cardiology consultants meets periodically in Oklahoma City to review cases and make recommendations for certification. For the most part, this element of the review process is reserved for consideration of significant cardiovascular conditions in air carrier pilots or for those cases under review in which a decision would establish a significant precedent or deviation from established certification policies.

Pilot applicants who are denied certification by the manager of the Aeromedical Certification Division may request reconsideration by the Federal Air Surgeon. When necessary, the support staff in the Medical Specialties Division of the Office of Aviation Medicine obtains additional information for the Federal Air Surgeon or obtains additional opinions from consultants. Reversal of decisions made by the manager of the Aeromedical Certification Division is infrequent, however, because extensive file docu-

mentation and consultant review are usually obtained at that level.

Authorization for Special Issuance of Medical Certificate (Authorization)

The authority to grant an authorization (waiver) is contained in section 67.401 of the Federal Aviation Regulations. This authority is delegated not only to the Federal Air Surgeon, but to the manager of the Aeromedical Certification Division and to each regional flight surgeon. At the discretion of these agency officials, a medical certificate may be issued to an applicant who does not meet the medical standards when the applicant shows, to the satisfaction of agency officials, that the duties authorized by the class of medical certificate can be performed without endangering air commerce during the period in which the certificate would be in force. For purposes of determining whether an authorization may be granted, the agency may authorize a special medical flight test, practical test, or medical evaluation. An applicant's operational experience and medical factors are taken into consideration. In determining whether the special issuance of a third-class medical certificate should be granted, consideration is given to the concept that in the exercise of the privileges of a private pilot certificate, the pilot should be free to accept reasonable risks that are not acceptable in the exercise of commercial or airline transport pilot privileges.

In issuing a medical certificate under Section 67.401, limitations may be placed on the duration of the certificate; follow-up special medical tests, examinations, or evaluations may be required; and operational limitations may be imposed (e.g., requiring the applicant to wear lenses, hearing aids, or prosthetic device). Functional limitations (e.g., those that restrict pilot duties that may be performed) may be imposed on second- or third-class medical certificates, but not on first-class certificates.

Consideration for authorization may be given in the case of any disqualifying medical condition. Risk to aviation safety is minimized through requirements that applicants with known significant disease undergo extensive clinical evaluations and, when certified, provide periodic special evaluations to assess disease progression. By placing these requirements or limitations on certification, the agency's intent is to establish a level of safety for those granted an authorization that is equivalent to persons in the general pilot population who have no known disease.

Authorizations have been granted for all classes of medical certificates and for almost all disqualifying conditions as described under the provisions of Part 67. These include authorizations to persons with histories of angina pectoris, myocardial infarction, other significant coronary heart disease, psychosis, significant personality disorders, substance abuse, substance dependence, epilepsy, disturbances of consciousness, diabetes requiring certain medications, and a variety of other conditions. In 1994, the FAA issued 1,209 first-class medical certificates to pilots with one or more of these medical conditions. Approximately 840 of these issuances were to pilots who had successfully undergone recovery programs for alcoholism, and slightly more than 300 were to pilots with histories of significant cardiovascular conditions, including valve replacement, pacemaker implantation, coronary artery bypass surgery, coronary angioplasty, and myocardial infarction.

Although the range of conditions for which authorizations may be granted is quite broad, criteria for proving recovery and stability are stringent. Flexibility in the granting of authorizations increases as the degree of pilot responsibilities diminishes. Therefore, greater flexibility exists in granting third-class certification as opposed to first- or second-class certification, especially when the duties do not involve the transport of passengers for compensation or hire.

Appeal Procedures

Within 60 days after final denial of certification by the FAA, a pilot may petition the NTSB for a review of the denial. This review is limited to a determination of whether the agency has appropriately applied its standards, not whether the standards themselves are appropriate. Upon receipt of a petition for review, the NTSB assigns an Administrative Law Judge (ALJ) to hear the petition. A hearing is scheduled and conducted, usually at a location convenient to the pilot and his or her witnesses. The rules of evidence for these hearings are relaxed. The pilot has the right to be represented by legal counsel, and the FAA is always represented by legal counsel. Medical testimony is received from witnesses on behalf of the pilot and the agency.

On the basis of the information submitted at the hearing, as well as the testimony by experts, a determination is made by the ALJ as to whether the pilot qualifies under the medical standards. Either the pilot or the FAA may appeal an adverse decision to the Full Board. The Full Board relies upon the record established at the hearing and briefs submitted by each of the parties. The Full Board rarely hears oral arguments.

In those circumstances in which an NTSB proceeding results from a pilot's appeal of an FAA action taken within 60 days of the issuance of a medical certificate (either a denial of certification or a request for information followed by a denial), the burden of proving qualification is on the pilot. If the FAA action were taken more than 60 days after the issuance of a certificate, the burden of proof would be on the agency. For this reason, timely receipt and review of applications for which AMEs have issued medical certificates are important objectives of the medical certification program. NTSB rules of practice in air safety proceedings are published in 49 CFR Part 821.

If the Full Board were to find for the agency, the pilot may appeal that decision to a US Court of Appeals in the circuit in which the pilot resides or in the District of Columbia. The FAA may also appeal an adverse NTSB decision to the courts but only in cases where eligibility for medical certification is challenged by the FAA more than 60 days after the issuance of the medical certificate.

Occupational Health

The FAA maintains an active occupational health program for its approximately 50,000 employees. Foremost in this program are medical support and qualification determinations for agency employees who perform safety-related duties. Among others, these include FAA air traffic control specialists, federal air marshals, aviation safety inspectors, and FAA pilots. As a major element of this program, the air-traffic controller health program serves air-traffic personnel working in air-traffic control centers, towers, and flight service stations.

Through the conduct of annual physical examinations and the application of qualification standards developed by the FAA, determinations are made with respect to the continuing eligibility of these employees to perform air-traffic control and flight-service-station duties. Federal air marshals must meet the second-class airman medical standards, modified to meet the specific job requirements for a security specialist. Aviation Safety Inspectors and FAA pilots are required to meet Part 67 medical standards and annually obtain second-class medical certificates.

Occupational health services for agency employees are provided through clinics in regional offices, as well as medical facilities located in some air-traffic control centers. To supplement the relatively small agency medical staff, specially designated AMEs assist in performing the required periodic medical examinations of agency employees.

Although most occupational health resources are directed toward the conduct of periodic medical evaluations on selected FAA employees, increasing emphasis is placed upon providing consultative health services to all FAA employees, especially with respect to preventive medicine concepts and health awareness.

As an important element of the occupational

health program, an industrial hygienist located in the Occupational Health Division of CAMI oversees and provides guidance and technical information related to environmental health issues. As may be expected for any large organization with employees located in different facilities in various geographical areas, resolution of industrial hygiene issues plays a major role in ensuring employee health. Asbestos health hazards, facility air quality, toxicity of chemicals used in agency facilities, and radiation hazards are only a few of the problem areas that confront the industrial hygienist.

Antidrug Programs

The use of alcohol and drugs has been regulated for years for pilots and other aircrew under Part 91.17. Among others, this rule provides that no person may act as a crewmember of a civil aircraft within eight hours after consuming alcohol, while under the influence of alcohol, or while using any drug that affects an individual's facilities. In 1990, the FAA also implemented an amendment to Part 61 of the Code of Federal Regulations to provide the authority to revoke or suspend the aircrew certificate or rating when an individual has two or more alcohol- or drug-related motor vehicle convictions or state motor vehicle administrative actions within a three-year period. For enforcement purposes the rule requires pilots to report all alcohol- and drug-related state motor vehicle convictions or administrative actions. The medical certification rules were amended to include an ''express consent'' provision that authorizes the FAA to obtain information from the National Driver Register. In addition to these rules, the DOT and the FAA issued regulations covering the aviation industry and established a program for agency employees in safety-related positions that mandate drug and alcohol testing.

Intra-agency Drug and Alcohol Testing

On February 15, 1987, the FAA initiated an antidrug program for agency employees in certain safety-related positions. The program included urine testing for prohibited drugs of selected FAA employees, including air-traffic control specialists, federal air marshals, aviation safety inspectors, and agency pilots. Under this program, urine testing was performed in conjunction with preemployment and annual medical examinations. On September 10, 1987, as a concurrent drug abatement initiative, the Department of Transportation implemented random urine drug testing of certain department employees, including those in the FAA. Included in the departmental program are employees in safety-related positions (e.g., railroad safety inspection, aviation security, and vessel-traffic control) and employees who require a "top secret" clearance.

Under the program that now exists, urine specimens are collected from applicants for positions covered under the program, and employees in these positions are subject to random testing, postaccident testing, testing for reasonable suspicion of drug use, and followup testing during a drug rehabilitation program. Urine specimens are collected and sent to a contract laboratory approved by the Department of Health and Human Services where they are tested for cocaine, marijuana, phencyclidine, opiates, and amphetamines. A two-step drug testing process is used. As an initial screen, the specimens are subjected to enzyme immunoassay. When the screening test reveals evidence of drugs in a concentration that exceeds established cutoff levels, a confirmatory test is performed using gas chromatography/mass spectrometry.

A positive test does not automatically identify an applicant or employee as a problem drug user. For FAA employees, agency-employed physicians acting as MROs conduct investigations to determine whether there may be alternative medical explanations for a positive test result. This action includes the conduct of employee medical interviews, review of employee medical histories, and review of any other relevant factors. The MRO reviews all medical records made available by the tested employee when a confirmed positive test may have resulted from legally prescribed medication. Prior to verifying a test as positive for drugs, the FAA MRO consults with the Departmental MRO who reviews all positive urine tests of applicants for covered positions, as well as DOT employees subject to testing.

Although applicants who are found to have a drug problem are denied employment, employees are offered the opportunity for rehabilitation as a condition of continued employment. Those who decline rehabilitation are discharged from the FAA. After counseling, treatment, and rehabilitation, employees are returned to safety-related duties contingent upon receiving medical clearance by the MRO. Once returned to duty, the employee is subject to unannounced testing for at least one year. Employees who do not maintain abstinence from drugs may be discharged from the FAA.

As of December 31, 1995, 97,372 random specimens had been collected from FAA employees. Of these, 286 (approximately 0.29%) were verified as positive for substance abuse. These data make it clear that while drug abuse exists among FAA employees, the prevalence is quite low.

In December, 1994, additional authority was granted to permit the agency to begin testing employees and applicants for employment in safety-sensitive positions for the use of alcohol. As with the drug program, agency employees may be alcohol tested for any of four reasons: random selection, postaccident, reasonable suspicion, or as followup during an alcohol treatment program. The method selected for testing is breath alcohol using evidentiary quality breath testing equipment. An employee with an alcohol concentration of 0.02 or greater is prohibited from functioning in any safety-sensitive capacity. Although no adverse action is taken at levels of 0.02–0.039 an employee who tests positive a second time at those levels may be subject to disciplinary action. At levels of ≥ 0.04, the employee violates agency policy and is subject to a variety of disciplinary actions, including dismissal from the agency. Prior to any disciplinary action, the employee is offered the opportunity to enter a substance abuse rehabilitation program which, when successfully completed, allows the employee to return to safety-sensitive duties. As of the end of fiscal year 1995, of 2,630 employees tested, 6 tested positive for alcohol (i.e., ≥ 0.04) and 3 tested as not ready for duty (i.e., < 0.04).

Industry Drug and Alcohol Testing

Drug testing has been required by the FAA for aviation industry employees since 1989. The rule-making to institute the antidrug program began in 1986 when the FAA issued an Advance Notice of Proposed Rule-making (ANPRM) for public comments. A Notice of Proposed Rule-making (NPRM) was issued in March, 1988, followed by publication of the final rule in November, 1988 (*Anti-Drug Program for Personnel Engaged in Specified Aviation Activities*). Drug testing began in December, 1989, with all Part 121 and large Part 135 certificate holders required to implement programs first. The remaining cited employers were required to implement programs during 1990 and 1991, depending on the size and/or type of employer. Although the antidrug rule has been amended a number of times, the basic elements have remained largely unchanged.

Alcohol testing of aviation industry employees began January 1, 1995, and is being phased in by size and type of employer. The development of alcohol misuse prevention regulations was directed by Congress in the Omnibus Transportation Employee Testing Act of 1991 (the Act), which also effectively codified the FAA's existing antidrug program. The alcohol rule-making was a combined effort involving the Office of the Secretary of Transportation, the FAA, and the four operating administrations that regulate the motor carrier, railroad, transit, and pipeline industries. An NPRM was published in December, 1992, and the final rule issued in February, 1994.

The FAA's drug and alcohol testing rules require domestic and supplemental air carriers, air taxi and commuter operators, noncertified sightseeing operators, and air-traffic control facilities not operated by the FAA or the military to implement substance abuse prevention programs for their safety-sensitive employees. The regulations define safety-sensitive employees as those who perform the following functions: flight crewmember duties, flight attendant duties, flight instruction duties, aircraft dispatcher duties, aircraft maintenance or preventive maintenance duties, aviation screening duties, ground security coordinator duties, and air-traffic control duties. Although many other functions could affect aviation safety, the FAA chose to impose testing programs only on these categories of employees to ensure that the rules did not intrude unduly into constitutionally protected privacy interests.

The rules require testing under the following conditions: random, postaccident, reasonable cause/suspicion, return to duty, and followup. Preemployment drug testing is required; preemployment alcohol testing, although initially required, has been suspended indefinitely. Periodic drug testing is required for airman medical certificate holders during the first year of a new employer's antidrug program.

The minimum annual, random, drug testing rate was reduced from 50% to 25% effective January 1, 1995, under a recent amendment to the antidrug rule. Alcohol testing began at 25%. Each rule provides for an increase in the testing rate to 50% should the rate of positive drug or alcohol random tests reach ≥ 1% in any calendar year.

The antidrug rule prohibits the use of controlled substances except as authorized by law or lawful prescription, but the consequences of the rule primarily attach to positive drug tests. Because alcohol use is generally lawful, specific uses of alcohol are prohibited under the FAA's alcohol misuse prevention rule: use during the performance of safety-sensitive functions, performance of a safety-sensitive function within four to eight hours of using alcohol (depending on the safety-sensitive function), use after an accident, or reporting for duty or remaining on duty requiring the performance of safety-sensitive functions with an alcohol concentration of ≥ 0.04.

Specific consequences occur with rule violations, including removal from safety-sensitive functions, required evaluation by a substance abuse professional, and reporting to the FAA of refusals to submit to required tests by aircrew certificate holders. As required by the act, employees who use drugs or alcohol on-duty, or have two positive tests are permanently barred from the safety-sensitive duties they performed prior to the violation.

Aviation employers must submit antidrug plans/alcohol certification statements to the FAA for approval prior to program implementation.

Based on the statistical summaries submitted by employers from 1990–1995, the prevalence of prohibited drug use has remained at a low level. The positive rate (number of positive random tests divided by total random tests) has been $< 1\%$ in all but one of these years, averaging about 0.5%. Data on alcohol testing are limited, but it appears that the violation rate (i.e., number of random alcohol tests of ≥ 0.04 divided by total random tests) for 1995 will be low.

Aeromedical Education

FAA aeromedical education activities support a broad range of users. The education program promotes aviation safety through the development, dissemination, and presentation of educational materials that use the principles of flight physiology, aviation psychology, and survival skills. Altitude chamber training demonstrates to pilots the effects of hypoxia and the proper use of oxygen equipment. Drugs, alcohol, vision, and physical and emotional problems are other common topics, and emphasis is placed on the preflight assessment of both pilots and their aircraft to determine individual fitness to fly on a day-to-day basis.

Because it is a frequent cause of fatal aviation accidents, the effects of spatial disorientation are demonstrated in exhibits using portable Barany-type chairs. In addition, a more sophisticated and realistic device, the Vertigon, is used to demonstrate physiologic disorientation.

Division personnel conduct courses with special emphasis on accident investigation and global survival training for flight crews and hold seminars for AMEs at various locations across the country. The AME seminars are designed for continuing medical education and for training in current FAA medical certification policies, practices, and procedures. During 1994, 1,531 physicians attended 15 AME seminars held at locations throughout the United States.

Whenever possible, FAA flight surgeons meet with pilots at safety seminars and "hangar flying" sessions. AMEs also participate in these educational sessions and are provided with materials, such as films, slides, and brochures, to assist in medically-oriented presentations.

Research

Historically, the FAA's medical research program has emphasized analysis, assessment, and improvement of the human operator role in the air-traffic control system, the performance and work environment of the pilot, the safety and health of pilots and aircrew, and the safety of passengers and persons on the ground. Aeromedical research in civil aviation began soon after the establishment of the Medical Service in the Department of Commerce. Bauer and Cooper reviewed pilot records of 9,102 student pilots and analyzed physical defects as they related to progress in pilot training and accidents. The results of the review were first published in 1930. Bauer and Cooper concluded that physical defects diminished a student's flying ability, and that although an individual who did not meet the physical standards probably could learn to fly, there was no doubt that the flying hazards were greatly increased (10–12).

Using a more traditional definition, civil aviation medical research in the federal government began in 1935 with Roy E. Whitehead, MD, who was a pioneer in the study of oxygen requirements for flight crewmembers and passengers. In 1935, Dr. Whitehead arranged with the US National Bureau of Standards to use its low-pressure chamber to conduct oxygen deprivation experiments at simulated flight altitudes. In conjunction with scientists from the US National Bureau of Standards, chamber tests were conducted on several subjects at altitudes up to 22,000 feet.

The first FAA medical research facility, the Medical Science Station, was established in Kansas City, Missouri, in April, 1938. It was headed by Dr. Wade H. Miller, one of the original group of AMEs appointed by the Department of Commerce in 1927. Establishment of this facility and Dr. Miller's appointment as the first aviation medical research director resulted from a proposal for a special fatigue study of airline pilots. When the Medical Science Station opened in April, 1938, it was announced that the areas to be studied at the facility included pilot fatigue, creation of new and more applicable physical standards for commercial and noncommercial pilots, and the effects of hypoxia in airline transport operations. Kansas City was selected as the site of the station because of its central geographic location and because of the opportunities for conducting analyses and studies offered by its varied and concentrated flying activities in commercial, military, and airline operations.

Unfortunately, the Medical Science Station did not last long. As a result of CAA organizational problems in the fall of 1938, the medical research function was neglected, and the facility underwent delays in equipment installation and approval of research plans. In addition, enthusiasm for studies of pilot fatigue waned because of CAA sanctioning of an 85-hour flight rule for airline pilots. A third reason for early demise of the Medical Science Station related to a belief that adequate laboratory facilities were already available in universities and research foundations with a strong backing in the scientific community. It was concluded that scarce federal funds for medical research activities should be directed to those organizations; as a result, the Medical Science Station closed in the summer of 1940.

Plans were laid in 1941 for the establishment of a medical research facility at the CAA's Standardization Center in Houston; however, these plans were overshadowed by the need for a rapid buildup of US efforts in World War II. When the Standardization Center was moved to the new Aeronautical Center in Oklahoma City in 1946, however, the Aviation Medical Branch was established there. In 1953, the branch was moved to Columbus, Ohio, where it was renamed the Civil Aeromedical Research Laboratory. It was returned to Oklahoma City in 1958 and later became the Protection and Survival Laboratory of the Civil Aeromedical Research Institute. The work of this branch related to crash injury and survival research that included: assessment of restraint systems; use of padding and deformable materials in aircraft interiors; emergency evacuation procedures; and equipment that provided protection from hypoxia, decompression, ditching, and fire and smoke.

Another significant event in the development of aeromedical research in the federal government occurred with the establishment of the Georgetown Clinical Research Institute (GCRI) at the Georgetown University Medical Center in Washington, DC, in 1960. Establishment of the institute followed implementation of an agency rule that prohibits an individual from serving as a pilot in any aircraft engaged in air carrier operations when that individual has reached 60 years of age. Although this rule, which is commonly referred to as the Age 60 Rule, relied upon an arbitrarily selected chronologic age, the agency recognized the desirability of basing pilot retirement on physiologic age. The GCRI was established for the purpose of conducting aging research. At approximately the same time as the establishment of the GCRI, the Bureau of Aviation Medicine contracted with the Lovelace Foundation for Medical Education and Research in Albuquerque, New Mexico, to identify the criteria for studies that would provide the basis for a physiologic age rating. The Lovelace Foundation subsequently submitted its FAA contract report to the Public Health Service (PHS) as a grant application. After approval of the application, the Foundation began a funded study for PHS to develop a physiologic age rating schedule.

Based upon concerns expressed by Congress and elements of the aviation industry regarding duplication of research efforts and the effective use of limited funds for aeromedical research, the GCRI was closed in 1966, and its functions were transferred to CAMI. None of the scientists employed at the Institute moved to Oklahoma City, and no useful physiologic age indices were developed from the accumulated data.

Almost coincidental with the establishment of the GCRI, the Civil Aeromedical Research Institute (CARI) was established in Oklahoma City in 1960. The Civil Aviation Medical Research Laboratory, which had moved from Columbus to Oklahoma City in 1958, served as the nucleus for the new research institute. Six branches specializing in the areas of biochemistry, biodynamics, environmental physiology, psychology, protection and survival, and neurophysiology were added. Twenty-one positions were authorized, and researchers concentrated on such projects as the human aging process in relationship to chronologic age and pilot proficiency, selection criteria for air-traffic controllers exposed to environmental stress factors, and flight crewmember fatigue. Researchers were housed in facilities owned by the University of Oklahoma until a new facility was built at the Aeronautical Center in October, 1962. In late 1965, CARI became the Research Branch of CAMI, which also included the medical certification and clinical branches and an administrative support group.

Over the years, important research has been conducted at the FAA's facility in Oklahoma City, including research on the following: air-traffic controller selection; studies of color vision requirements and testing; aircraft accident correlation with age, weight, vision disorders, and static defects; effect of spatial disorientation on pilot performance; pesticide poisoning, drugs, and circadian rhythm; effects of ionizing and microwave radiation; crew smoke protection; emergency evacuation; child restraint systems; and ditching survival.

Aeromedical Research

Much of the aeromedical research conducted at CAMI is related to improving the safety of various aviation hardware and systems, such as seats, restraints, and protective breathing and floatation gear. With the objective of identifying required medical research and preventing future accidents, the research staff participates extensively in the investigation of aircraft accidents.

In keeping with the philosophy of concentrating on specific research areas, active expansion occurred in testing of aviation seat and restraint systems (Figure 26.4). This work has

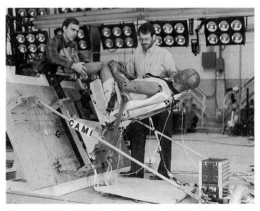

Figure 26.4. Civil Aeromedical Institute (CAMI) researchers inspect pretest conditions of a vertical test configuration. The test of an aircraft seat in this configuration simulates a downward-direction crash. The seat, with a dummy in it, is tested to ensure conformity to standards of spinal compression landing.

contributed significantly to available data concerning seat strength and restraint systems, as well as performance of infant restraint systems. In achieving this, the capabilities of CAMI's dynamic impact test facility have been made available to manufacturers of existing and developmental seat and restraint models.

Researchers have also engaged in the evaluation of passenger protective breathing devices designed to improve passenger survivability in a smoke- and fume-filled environment. As an example, tests have been conducted using a standard passenger mask fitted with a rebreather bag designed to conserve and recycle oxygen-rich air and reduce the inhalation of cabin air. Testing showed that although the device functioned adequately with nominal resting ventilation conditions, specific design deficiencies were documented during actual altitude chamber tests at higher exercise-induced ventilation rates. The accumulated data were made available to the manufacturer for design improvement and to elements of the FAA that have responsibility for regulatory development and implementation. Ongoing efforts in this area include performance tests of various new designs of protective breathing devices for both crew and passengers. As a part of an international study group composed of scientists from Canada, the United Kingdom, and France, devices with self-contained air/gas supplies are being studied.

Researchers continue to work on the development of viable and cost-effective water survival concepts and procedures. Through practical test methods, standards are developed for floatation platforms and cushion buoyancy. The focus of this research activity is on airport water-rescue requirements and rescue equipment compatibility.

In the area of evacuation research, studies of actual and estimated evacuation routes used by passengers are conducted. These investigations support the development of agency regulations pertaining to the number and spacing of emergency exits. Evacuation studies also contribute to the development of FAA exit and escape route lighting requirements for transport aircraft, an important safety initiative for improving passenger survivability in a smoke-filled cabin.

Other important work conducted by scientists of CAMI include study of ionizing and radiofrequency/microwave radiation hazards to crewmembers and passengers. Data accumulated and analyzed suggest increased health risks to some flight crewmembers and passengers as a result of galactic cosmic radiation (13). Characteristics of cosmic radiation have been reviewed and estimates made of the dose equivalents from galactic cosmic radiation received on air carrier flights on a variety of routes to and from, or within the contiguous United States. The annual dose equivalents received on the flights were estimated to range 0.2–9.1 mSv (20–910 mrem), or 0.4–18% of the recommended annual limit for occupational exposure of an adult. This study has provided calculations for estimating radiation-induced risks of malignancies, genetic defects, and harm to an embryo or fetus. It was estimated that the increased risk of dying from cancer because of galactic radiation exposure received during 20 years of flying ranges 0.1–5 in 1,000. For the adult population in the United States, the risk of dying from cancer is approximately 220 in 1,000.

Aeromedical research has also focused on neurophysiologic responses to pesticides and other toxicant exposures in the aviation environment. Cooperative projects with the FAA Technical Center in Atlantic City have involved the testing of aircraft cabin interior materials for flammability and smoke toxicity. Participation by CAMI scientists has included thermodegradation using a combustion tube furnace and a radiant panel furnace.

Research is also conducted to improve techniques for determining accident causation and support is provided to other elements of the FAA and to the NTSB in the evaluation of postmortem blood and tissue samples from victims of general aviation and air carrier accidents. Screening checks are carried out for a broad profile of chemicals, including alcohol, cannabinoids and cocaine metabolites.

Aviation physiology research emphasizes the documentation of human responses to a variety of aviation-associated stressors. Some of these include hypoxia, circadian shifts, and ozone exposure. Studies are also conducted on the effects of alcohol and other chemicals on human tolerance to the aviation environment. This work has contributed significantly to the development of educational material, to the adoption of blood alcohol limits for pilots, and to the regulation of flight crewmember exposure to ozone.

Categorized as "aeromedical program support," some of the research effort is directed to meeting the Federal Air Surgeon's responsibilities for the development and management of occupational health, medical accident investigation, and aeromedical education programs. In addition, research efforts have contributed to the establishment of medical certification guidelines for aphakia, intraocular lens implantation, and glaucoma. Certain antihypertensive and other medications have been assessed regarding their use by pilots and impact on aviation safety. Major studies are being conducted to determine the possible relationship between a pilot's chronologic age and aircraft accidents and to develop an automated test battery for the assessment of cognitive function in pilots.

Human Resources Research

CAMI's human resources research plays an important role in the agency's overall research program through the collection and evaluation of ATCS and flight crewmember performance data.

The objectives of this research are to: improve ATCS selection procedures; evaluate the effectiveness of university-based ATCS training programs; evaluate existing ATCS selection, screening, and training programs (Figure 26.5); validate color-vision requirements for current and future ATCS workstations; and study job

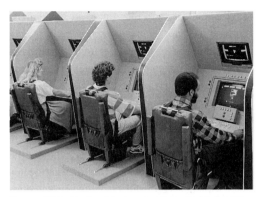

Figure 26.5. Test subjects are given multiple aviation-related performance tasks to evaluate the effects of fatigue and other stressors.

task analysis data to identify those critical tasks associated with operational errors.

Defining and identifying stress in the context of air-traffic personnel and performance have been thorny issues for the FAA for years. Psychological, physiologic, and biochemical test results have not indicated any predilection for controller anxiety, although employees at certain locations have relatively high workloads. Studies done in this area have not identified air-traffic control as a highly stressful occupation. A comprehensive five-year study of air-traffic controller health was completed in 1978 by Rose et al. (14). The most frequent, single, chronic illness identified among air-traffic controllers was hypertension. Although the study indicated that it could not be concluded that air-traffic control work, per se, causes hypertension, it appeared that the work increases the risk, or possibly hastens the rate of development of hypertension in individuals who are predisposed because of genetic and biologic factors. Approximately one-half of the men in the study had at least one psychiatric problem, as defined by study criteria; however, most of them did not receive professional treatment. The most prevalent psychiatric difficulties were impulse control disturbances. Alcohol use was quite high, but alcohol abuse was not considered a significant problem. Anxiety and depression were at levels equal to or less than that found in the general population.

The FAA has emphasized policies for the improvement of its own employee/employer relations. Research personnel have served as principal coordinators and analysts in agency-sanctioned FAA employee surveys. The surveys have solicited feedback on perceived supervisor/employee relationships, as well as on other aspects of the FAA work climate. Data collected have been analyzed and distributed to agency managers for the purpose of improving work climate and enhancing the productivity of employees.

The impact of the introduction of color coding in the modern cockpit, as well as in the air-traffic control system, has also been assessed. A relatively high incidence of color-vision deficiency occurs among applicants for employment as air-traffic controllers and applicants for pilot medical certificates. Accordingly, the requirements for equal employment opportunity and reasonable accommodation of persons with disabilities have heightened the importance of establishing valid, job-related screening tests for color vision.

In response to renewed FAA emphasis on general aviation accident prevention and the initiation of a comprehensive assessment of the relationship between human factors and accident causation, research tasks have been developed to assess factors involved in pilot/controller miscommunication and the analysis of aviation accidents and incidents. An in-depth analysis of human errors is expected to lead to recommendations for improved training and modification of system procedures that will significantly reduce certain accidents and incidents.

Other research tasks cover a wide range of issues related to both air-traffic controller and pilot performance in relationship to accident causation. Efforts to develop and validate a performance test for "readiness to perform" is being assessed as a method of determining fatigue-related declines in performance that may be causal factors in operational incidents and accidents. Extensive studies have added substan-

tially to the body of knowledge concerning the relevance of age to accidents.

AIRCRAFT ACCIDENT INVESTIGATION IN FAA

The NTSB is responsible for civil aircraft investigation in the United States. The NTSB is an independent federal agency whose objective is promoting aviation, railroad, highway, marine, pipeline, and hazardous materials safety. Established in 1967, the Board is mandated to investigate transportation accidents, determine probable cause, issue safety recommendations, study transportation safety issues, and evaluate the safety effectiveness of government agencies involved in transportation.

Although the NTSB has prime responsibility for the investigation of all aviation accidents, a considerable part of general aviation accident investigation has been delegated to the FAA. This includes most nonfatal, general aviation accidents and those fatal accidents involving aerial application and home-built aircraft. Other fatal accidents and selected nonfatal accidents are reserved for Board investigation, although FAA personnel participate in many of the investigations both actively and as observers.

Accident Causation

During 1995, 35 accidents involved major United States scheduled and charter airlines, 12 involved commuter air carrier operations, 76 involved air taxi operations, 2,066 involved general aviation operations, and preliminary figures showed 162 rotorcraft accidents. These accidents represent a combined total of 1,040 fatalities in 1995. Of these, 175 occurred in accidents involving scheduled airlines; however, the majority, 732, involved general aviation accidents.

When considering the high degree of aviation activity in the United States, it becomes apparent that an exceptional safety record has been established. Manufacturers produce aircraft with reliability that far exceeds the reliability of human performance. Although structural or mechanical system failures occur, human factors account for the vast majority of aircraft accidents. In 1994, the NTSB assigned pilot involvement as the broad cause/factor in 76% of all general aviation accidents and for 82% of the accidents that involved fatalities (15). Failure to maintain airspeed, inadvertent stall, improper inflight planning, fuel exhaustion, and failure to maintain a proper altitude were among the most prevalent human-factor causes of serious accidents.

FAA Role

The Office of Aviation Medicine provides medical support for the FAA's accident investigation program. This support is provided by agency physicians located in regional offices, air-traffic control centers, CAMI, and headquarters. AMEs are sometimes called upon to assist in investigations because of the wide geographic distribution of aviation accidents and because of the limited availability of FAA physicians. Medical investigations include autopsies and toxicologic examinations in fatal accidents.

Agency physicians receive notification of fatal aircraft accidents through central FAA communication centers. Based upon logistical considerations, an AME may be contacted to assist in an investigation either by an NTSB investigator or by regional medical personnel. One of the principal duties of the AME is to aid in the collection of blood, urine, and other specimens that are sent to CAMI for toxicologic examination. Because of familiarity with the local medical community, the AME is in a position to facilitate arrangements for autopsies and for the collection of toxicologic specimens.

Medical participation in the investigation of aircraft accidents may reveal information vital to: the validation of the medical standards used in the pilot medical certification program; the effectiveness of the medical examination process, which identifies those who may be a hazard to themselves and others; and the identification of human factors that need further evaluation.

Fatigue, lack of coordination, inattentiveness, failure to adequately communicate, loss of consciousness, and impairment from alcohol and drugs are but a few of the factors that demand an aggressive medical accident investigation program.

Increased emphasis on the FAA's accident investigation program has called for a greater degree of involvement of medical personnel. Since late 1959, there has been concerted effort to ensure the medical investigation of all fatal air carrier accidents. Approximately 90% of general aviation fatal accidents now receive some form of medical investigation. In these accidents, as in the air carrier accidents, the study of injury patterns, evacuation sequence, and the concentration of inhaled combustible products in the bodies of accident victims has led to a fuller understanding of factors that affect escape and survival after an accident. Information obtained from these investigations is used in the design of specific research studies to develop equipment or procedures that will increase the probability of escape and survival.

THE FUTURE

Forecasts indicate expanding growth in aviation. Aviation activity from fiscal year 1996 to fiscal year 2007 is expected to increase by 19% at towered airports, 27% at air-traffic control centers, and 8.4% in flight services performed. Hours flown by general aviation are forecasted to increase 10.5% and revenue passenger miles 58.8%, with scheduled international revenue passenger miles increasing 76.6% and domestic carrier revenue passenger miles increasing 52.3% (16).

The FAA will meet forecasted demands in a way that ensures safe and efficient transportation for all people who use and depend upon the National Airspace System. With the impact of technologic advances in the design of aircraft and air-traffic control systems and instrumentation, new challenges will face the FAA's medical program. To meet these challenges, modifications will be required not only in the programs themselves but also in the manner in which medical support and expertise are provided to users both within and outside the agency. Significant changes are underway to meet these future needs.

The Office of Aviation Medicine will be called upon more frequently to address the concerns of the general public and respond to societal mandates:

Are the skies safe for passengers, or does alcohol or other substance abuse now degrade what has been the safest transportation system in the world?

Will aging transport aircraft remain safely on the line through the skilled efforts of maintenance personnel and engineering staffs, or will tragedies in structural failure follow human failure?

Is the cabin environment safe for crew and passengers, or do contaminants of cabin air and cosmic radiation pose significant present and future danger?

Can occupants survive and escape the inevitable aircraft accidents that will occur?

Are occupational safety and health programs adequate for the thousands of aviation industry employees who keep the system operating?

Does the system ensure that crewmembers and air-traffic controllers are as free from the risk of incapacitation as medical science can provide, yet permit skilled persons with disabilities the opportunity to be gainfully employed in their chosen aviation fields?

Are the established medical standards for every job appropriate, necessary for task completion and safety, and nondiscriminatory?

These questions establish both broad and specific goals for the Office of Aviation Medicine as the 21st century approaches. No longer will the individual medical examination for pilots and the review of the medical certification documents be of overriding importance in the allocation of resources. These operations will be ac-

complished more accurately, faster, and more efficiently as current efforts to automate and to recognize modern medical technology come to fruition. The standards for pilot medical certification have already been reviewed by expert medical specialty groups under the auspices of the AMA, and a new set of standards, the first since 1959, were put in place in 1996. Continuing evolution of organization and operating mechanisms within the medical elements of the FAA matches this progress.

Focused research by CAMI, by other agency medical elements, or through contract with other organizations is accelerating to meet these challenges. Human factors, as they pertain to aging aircraft, are the subjects of new studies that will continue throughout the 1990s and into the next century. The results may also have significance for occupational safety and health among industry workers.

CAMI reported that radiation research in the high-altitude aviation environment has identified potential dangers for air carrier crewmembers and passengers. New efforts are underway to further evaluate this risk, to inform the medical community, and to provide sources of information for the aviation community and general public. The Office of Aviation Medicine, jointly with agency flight standards and operations elements, will pursue means to avoid or minimize radiation exposure. Future research should more clearly delineate the risks to humans, including fetuses, and provide viable solutions.

The future will bring further efforts to allay public concern about the passenger environment. Ozone, carbon dioxide, and other contaminants must be reduced or eliminated and potentially hazardous materials should be identified and removed. Better accident protection and survival mechanisms are needed, and CAMI will lead these efforts of the Office of Aviation Medicine.

With respect to the effects of aging on pilots, the Office of Aviation Medicine increasingly will accomplish or support work to better define and to detect those medical factors or functional changes that may affect flight safety. CAMI will further refine and expand available age-related accident data and continue its research on the causes and implications of cognitive deficit, particularly as related to aging and to the use of alcohol. The public remains divided and concerned about aging pilots and worries about aging aircraft. Should either continue to fly? Both require ongoing attention.

The Office of Aviation Medicine has led the FAA into the forefront of the nation's battle against substance abuse. Among the first federal civilian agencies to develop a comprehensive program to identify and remove from air traffic and other safety and security positions employees who are involved with drugs, the FAA extended a similar program to the aviation industry. To ensure a drug-free transportation industry work force, testing for drugs as a deterrent has become necessary, and the Office of Aviation Medicine accepted the initial responsibility for providing a fair, effective, and efficient program. Only time will tell whether the final goal can be reached, but major educational, regulatory, and enforcement efforts are expected to be necessary for many years.

It is clear that the challenges of the future are substantial. Major medical issues must be resolved, and problems related to an ever-expanding aviation system must be met. Through innovative changes in program administration and judicious use of resources, the Office of Aviation Medicine plans to meet these challenges in a manner that will not only continue to ensure safety in air commerce, but will also promote the growth and expansion of aviation.

REFERENCES

1. Briddon AE, Champie EA. FAA historical fact book—1926–1963. Washington, DC: Federal Aviation Agency, 1966.
2. U. S. Department of Commerce. Air Commerce Regulations. Washington, DC, 1926.
3. Holbrook HA. Civil aviation medicine in the bureaucracy. Bethesda: Banner Publishing Company, 1974.
4. Bullwinkel V. Federal Aviation Administration, 23 F.3d 167, (7th Circuit, rehearing denied).
5. First Bethesda Conference of the American College of Cardiology. Standards of physical fitness for aircrew. Am J Cardiol 1966;18:630.
6. Eighth Bethesda Conference of the American College of Cardiology. Cardiovascular problems associated with aviation safety. Am J Cardiol 1975;36:573.
7. American Medical Association. Neurological and neurosurgical conditions associated with aviation safety. Arch Neurol 1979;36:731.
8. American Medical Association. Review of Part 67 of the Federal Air Regulations and the medical certification of civilian airmen. Contract #DTFA01–83-C-20066. Chicago: American Medical Association, 1986.
9. Civil Aeromedical Institute. Aeromedical certification statistical handbook. AC 8500–1. Federal Aviation Administration. Oklahoma City: Office of Aviation Medicine, 1995.
10. Bauer LH, Cooper HJ. Regulating air commerce, Article V—Medical. Aviation 1929;1:520.
11. Cooper HJ. The relation between physical deficiencies and decreased performance. J Aviat Med 1930;1:4.
12. Cooper HJ. Further studies in the effect of physical defects on flying ability. J Aviat Med 1931;2:162.
13. Friedberg W, Faulkner DN, Snyder J, Darden EB, O'Brien K. Galactic cosmic radiation exposure and associated health risks for air carrier crewmembers. Aviat Space Environ Med 1989;60:1104.
14. Rose RM, Jenkins CD, Hurst MW. Air traffic controller health change study. Federal Aviation Administration, Office of Aviation Medicine Report No. 78–39. Washington, DC, 1978.
15. National Transportation Safety Board. Annual review of aircraft accident data: U.S. general aviation calendar year 1994. Report No. NTSB/ARG-96/01, PB96–138160. Washington, DC, 1996.
16. Federal Aviation Administration. FAA aviation forecasts: fiscal years 1996–2007. Federal Aviation Administration, APO 90–1. Washington, DC, 1996.

Chapter 27

International Aviation Medicine

S. Finkelstein

Physical environmental stresses in international civil aviation are similar in all regions of the world; however, approaches to the interpretation and solution of problems are significantly different. Worldwide cultural differences make international civil aviation medicine a most fascinating and challenging field.

S. Finkelstein

1995 was the ninth consecutive year in which more than one billion passengers were carried on scheduled air services throughout the world. This number is equivalent to about one fifth of the world's population. Over half of all air traffic was international, and this segment has continued to grow faster than domestic air traffic. The safety of air travel has shown continuous improvement; measured in terms of passenger fatalities per 100 million passenger-miles, the 1989 figure of 0.064 represents a 26% reduction in the average rate over the past 6 years.

The magnitude of aviation operations indicates the need for international standardization of all aspects of international civil aviation. The major medical responsibility lies with optimizing the interaction of human beings, machines, and environment.

This chapter will therefore cover the aviation medicine implications of the international specifications permitting air travel to be accomplished in a safe and orderly way. The activities and terms of reference of international organizations of the United Nations system which have direct relevance to aviation medicine will be discussed. Other organizations that substantially

contribute to the aviation medical aspects of flight safety will also be briefly described.

INTERNATIONAL REGULATIONS—ORIGIN AND NEEDS

On December 17, 1903, in North Carolina, a frail structure of metal, wood, and fabric struggled into the air and carried a single passenger 269 m. This was the first recorded flight by a heavier-than-air powered machine, but it was also the culmination of experiments made in many nations during the previous century. For even at the moment of its birth, the airplane was a creation of no one nation or of no one technology. Today, more than three quarters of a century later, the international character of air transport is self-evident. The world is enveloped by a network of air routes. The air has become a highway for world commerce.

This development of the airplane into a major instrument of transport has brought with it international challenges—the coordination of techniques and laws, the dissemination of technical and economic information—far beyond the ability of individual governments to solve. The need for safety and regularity in air transport involves the necessity of building airports, of setting up navigation aids, and of establishing weather reporting systems. Of fundamental importance is the optimum selection of aviation personnel and their adequate training. The standardization of operational practices for international services is of importance, so that there may be no error caused by misunderstanding or inexperience. The establishment of such standards, standards for rules of the air, for air traffic control, for personnel licensing (including medical requirements), for the design of airports, and for so many details of prime importance to air safety, all require more than national action.

The Chicago Convention

World War II had a major effect upon the technical development of the airplane, telescoping a quarter-century of normal peacetime development into 6 years. A vast network of passenger and freight carriage was set up, but there were many problems, both political and technical, to which solutions had to be found to benefit and support a world at peace. There was the question of commercial rights—what arrangements would be made for airlines of one country to fly into and through the territories of another. There were other concerns with regard to the legal and economic conflicts that might come with peacetime flying across national borders, such as how to maintain existing air navigation facilities, many of which were located in sparsely settled areas. For these reasons the U.S. government conducted exploratory discussions with allied nations during the early months of 1944. On the basis of the talks, invitations were sent to 55 allied and neutral states to meet in Chicago in November 1944. Of these 55 states, 52 attended. For 5 weeks, these delegates considered the problems of international civil aviation. The outcome was the Convention on International Civil Aviation Organization. The Provisional International Civil Aviation Organization (PICAO) was established and functioned from June 6, 1945, to

April 4, 1947. By March 5, 1947, the 26th ratification having been received, the International Civil Aviation Organization (ICAO) came into being on April 4, 1947. In October 1947, it became a specialized agency of the United Nations linked to its Economic and Social Council.

INTERGOVERNMENTAL ORGANIZATIONS IN RELATION TO THE UNITED NATIONS

International Civil Aviation Organization

The permanent body charged with the administration of this convention is the ICAO, based in Montreal and with seven Regional Offices in all geographic areas of the world.

ICAO aims at developing the principles and techniques of international air navigation and fostering the planning and development of international air transport so as to ensure safe and orderly growth of international civil aviation throughout the world; encourage aircraft design and operation for peaceful purposes; meet the needs of the peoples of the world for safe, regular, efficient, and economic air transport; prevent economic waste caused by unreasonable competition; ensure that the rights of contracting states are fully respected and that every contracting state has a fair opportunity to operate international airlines.

To achieve such aims, ICAO regularly revises the standards and recommended practices contained in the Annexes to the Chicago Convention and Procedures for Air Navigation Services. ICAO studies current problems, aiming to apply new technology in different fields of civil aviation, such as aviation medicine, air navigation, air transport, and legal matters, and provides technical assistance, in the form of country and intercountry projects, to the developing countries through the United Nations Development Program and other funding sources. Assistance includes the provision of experts for advice and assistance, equipment for operations and training purposes, and training of national personnel by means of awards of fellowships and scholarships.

The sovereign body of ICAO is the Assembly, which meets regularly every 3 years. On occasion, extraordinary sessions of the Assembly have been held to deal with specific matters. For the day-to-day operation of the organization, the Council is the executive body. Elected by the Assembly, it is composed of representatives of 133 contracting states elected for 3 years in three different categories: representatives of states of chief importance to air transport, states which make the largest contribution to the provision of facilities for international air transport, and states ensuring geographic representation.

Several committees report to the Council, such as the Air Transport Committee, the Committee on Joint Support of Air Navigation Services, and the Committee on Unlawful Interference. A separate subordinate body of the Council is the Air Navigation Commission, which is composed of 15 experts nominated by contracting states and appointed by the Council. These experts, according to the Chicago Convention, should possess qualifications in the field of aeronautics and work as individuals not necessarily representing the opinion of the administrations to which they belong. To assist the deliberative bodies of ICAO, there is a permanent Secretariat subdivided into five bureaus: Air Navigation, Air Transport, Technical Cooperation, Legal, and Administration, and Services. Senior officials are recruited on a broad international basis.

In addition to the establishment located at ICAO headquarters in Montreal, seven regional offices are distributed throughout the world. They are located in Bangkok, Cairo, Dakar, Lima, Mexico City, Nairobi, and Paris. They are primarily responsible for the implementation of regional air navigation plans, and their principal function is to assist states to which they are accredited in interpretation and implementation of ICAO's specifications.

World Health Organization

Another agency of the United Nations system based in Geneva with which ICAO is in continuous coordination regarding matters of mutual interest is the World Health Organization (WHO). Its aims are as follows:

The WHO is a specialized agency with primary responsibility for international health matters and public health. The constitution of WHO defines health as "a state of complete physical, mental and social well-being and not merely the absence of disease or infirmity." Article 1 of the constitution states: "The objective of WHO shall be the attainment by all peoples of the highest possible level of health." Consequently, a wide range of functions revolves around WHO, so as to accomplish the following:

1. Act as the directing and coordinating authority on international health work
2. Assist governments, upon request, in strengthening health services
3. Furnish appropriate technical assistance and, in emergencies, necessary aid upon the request or acceptance of governments
4. Stimulate and advance work to eradicate or control epidemics and other disease
5. Promote, in cooperation with other specialized agencies when necessary, improvement of nutrition, housing, sanitation, recreation, economic or working conditions, and other aspects of environmental hygiene
6. Promote cooperation among scientific and professional groups that contribute to advancement of health
7. Promote maternal and child health and welfare and foster the ability to live harmoniously in a changing total environment
8. Foster activities in the field of mental health, especially those that affect the harmony of human relations
9. Promote and conduct research in the field of health
10. Promote improved standards of teaching and training in the health, medical, and related professions
11. Study and report on, in cooperation with other specialized agencies when necessary, administrative and social techniques affect-

ing public health and medical care from preventive and curative points of view, including hospital services and social security
12. Assist in developing an informed public opinion among all peoples on matters of health

Of direct relevance to international aviation medicine are three publications developed by WHO. The first, titled *Guide to Hygiene and Sanitation in Aviation*, contains, in addition to general considerations, recommendations related to the following topics:

1. Food
2. Water
3. Toilet sanitation and liquid wastes disposal
4. Solid wastes
5. Aircraft interior cleaning
6. Vector control

Another WHO publication of relevance to aviation, titled *International Health Regulations*, contains specifications recommended by the agency concerning international travel. Finally, the *Weekly Epidemiological Record* periodically provides updated reports of the epidemiologic situation of the world. The latter publication serves as a guideline for aviation medical practitioners, enabling them to provide timely advice and recommendations for flight crews and passengers.

ICAO's Aviation Medicine Section is in continuous coordination with relevant units of WHO on matters of mutual interest. In 1991 liaison was maintained with the Director of the Global Programme on AIDS and with the Division on Mental Health and later on with the Director of the Programme of Substance Abuse on this subject. Very recently (1995), the aviation medicine section of ICAO, with the assistance of our international study group, developed a manual covering the matter of prevention of problematic substance use in the aviation environment. Since 1992 continuous coordination was held with the director of the Tobacco and

Health Programme. The significant work accomplished in this area led both organizations to adopt, at assembly level, resolutions related to smoking restrictions in international flight.

International Labor Organization

The International Labor Organization (ILO) was established in Versailles, France, in June 1919, and became associated with the United Nations in 1946. It is linked to the Economic and Social Council. Its major responsibility consists of monitoring working and living standards throughout the world. In connection with aviation medical activities, the most important considerations are those related to the development of policies and recommendations with reference to working conditions.

Two publications specifically related to aviation medicine, although dated, are worthy of mention: *Occupational Health and Safety in Civil Aviation*, published by the Tripartite Meeting for Civil Aviation, and the *Encyclopedia of Occupational Health and Safety*.

Technical Annexes to the ICAO Convention

Since ICAO came into being in 1947, a main feature of its technical work has been the achievement of agreement of the contracting states on the necessary level of standardization for the operation of safe, regular, and efficient air services. In turn, this has resulted in high levels of reliability being achieved in all the many areas which collectively make up international civil aviation. This has particularly been so with respect to aircraft, the crews that operate them, and ground-based facilities and services. The necessary standardization has been achieved by ICAO primarily through the creation, adoption, and amendment by the Council Annexes to the Convention on International Civil Aviation that are specifications known as International Standards and Recommended Practices (SARPs). The Standard is a specification, the uniform application of which is necessary for the safety or regularity of international civil air navigation, while the Recommended Practice is one considered desirable but not essential. At present there are 18 sets of international Standards and Recommended Practices; 17 of these are in the technical field. The Annexes contain specifications as follows:

Annex 1: Personnel Licensing

Annex 2: Rules of the Air

Annex 3: Meteorological Service for International Air Navigation

Annex 4: Aeronautical Charts

Annex 5: Units of Measurement to Be Used in Air & Ground Operations

Annex 6: Operation of Aircraft

Annex 7: Aircraft Nationality and Registration Marks

Annex 8: Airworthiness of Aircraft

Annex 9: Facilitation

Annex 10: Aeronautical Telecommunications

Annex 11: Air Traffic Services

Annex 12: Search and Rescue

Annex 13: Aircraft Accident Investigation

Annex 14: Aerodromes

Annex 15: Aeronautical Information Services

Annex 16: Environmental Protection

Annex 17: Security—Safeguarding International Civil Aviation Against Acts of Unlawful Interference

Annex 18: The Safe Transport of Dangerous Goods by Air Provisions of a medical nature are found primarily in Annexes 1,2,6,9, and 13.

Need for International Standardization

To better understand the need for international standardization, it should be recalled that during flight, the crew of an aircraft frequently communicates with stations on the ground. They may seek authorization for flight maneuvers, obtain information necessary to avoid collision, receive an update of weather conditions ahead, or question the operational status of navigational aids en route or at destination. There is a continuous invisible link between the aircraft and the ground stations, and among the ground stations themselves. Many ground facilities and supporting services are needed for the safe and efficient operation of aircraft. To achieve harmonious functioning of all these ground facilities and services, international standardization is necessary.

To ensure safety, regularity, and efficiency of international and civil aviation operations, international standardization is essential in all matters affecting them—in the licensing (including medical requirements) and training of aviation personnel; in the operation of aircraft; and aircraft airworthiness and the numerous facilities and services required in their support, such as airports, telecommunications, navigational aids, meteorology, air traffic services, search and rescue, aeronautical information services, and aeronautical charts. A common understanding among the countries of the world on these matters is absolutely necessary.

ICAO'S AVIATION MEDICINE ACTIVITIES

From its beginning, the ICAO considered aviation medicine a vital element in flight safety. Since its inception, an aviation medicine section has been included within the Air Navigation Bureau of the permanent Secretariat. This section is responsible for undertaking studies and providing specialized aeromedical advice on medical problems associated with flight and flight crew performance, air traffic control, licensing standards and conditions of work, biological and psychologic problems relating to passengers and crews, first aid and survival equipment, medical aspects of accident investigation, and prevention.

In fulfilling its constitutional responsibilities, the Section works on projects and tasks belonging to one of these three categories:

1. Maintenance of current and valid specifications of a medical nature found in ICAO's regulatory documents and related guidance material

2. Projects leading to the standardization and greater effectiveness of training for designated medical examiners, with the objective of achieving a worldwide uniform interpretation and implementation of medical SARPs

3. Projects related to the continuous monitoring and surveillance of all the medical aspects of flight safety.

Standards and recommended practices with a medical component are contained mostly in Annex 1 (Personnel Licensing). Medical standards of an administrative nature are found in Chapter 1 of the Annex. A few selected definitions and general rules concerning licenses are presented in Appendix A. These definitions have international judicial strength and are in force throughout the world.

Specific medical standards are contained in Chapter 6 (Medical Provisions for Licensing). These current standards have been adopted by ICAO's Council to be implemented worldwide by all contracting states (currently 183 member states in 1995). Medical specifications which included physical, mental, visual, color perception, and hearing requirements are adopted to complement specifications related to age, skill, experience, and knowledge necessary for licensing aviation personnel. As in all the regulatory annexes, ICAO's standards are the minimum standards to be implemented by contracting states to ensure the safety of civil aviation operations. In exercising their sovereignty, contracting states may adopt stricter standards. If for any reason a contracting state is unable to incorporate into its national legislation the minimum standards adopted by ICAO, that state is under the obligation, in accordance with Article 38 of the Chicago Convention, to give immediate notification to ICAO of the differences between its own practice and that established by the international standards. ICAO periodically publishes supplements to the annexes describing the differences filed by states.

In order to permit proper uniform interpretation and implementation of international standards, the Aviation Medicine Section is actively involved in an ongoing educational program. This program encompasses several aspects, as follows:

1. Production of guidance material: *A Manual of Civil Aviation Medicine* was first issued in 1974. Several amendments to the first edition have been published; the second edition was published in 1985. This manual is available in English, French, Spanish, and Russian. Its purpose is to assist medical examiners and licensing authorities in their interpretation of the international standards.

2. Convening of Regional Civil Aviation Medicine Seminars. This program has proven to be very successful; it started in 1974 with one or two seminars held every year depending upon the desires of contracting states and the availability of human and financial resources. Matters covered in these seminars are described in Appendix B.

3. Publication of guidelines and circular letters. These contain aviation medicine information of an international nature which are periodically sent from the ICAO Aviation Medicine Section to chief medical officers of civil aviation administrations and medical directors of international carriers.

At the present time (1995), the Section continues to work on several projects of international significance such as prevention of drug abuse in the workplace by aviation personnel; the implications of AIDS in the civil aviation environment; medical aspects of flight crew fatigue, including considerations related to duty time and rest periods; medical supplies to be carried on board international flights; smoking in aircraft from a flight safety point of view; assessment of upper age limits for pilots; medical aspects of human factors in civil aviation; and the continuous provision of specialized aeromedical advice to contracting states.

NONGOVERNMENTAL ORGANIZATIONS

International Air Transport Association

The International Air Transport Association (IATA) acts as the agency through which airlines seek to solve jointly those problems they cannot surmount alone. Its work begins only after governments have promulgated a formal exchange of traffic and other rights (bilateral air transport agreements) and have licensed the airlines selected to perform the service. From that point on, the activity of the Association spreads through every phase of air transport operations. IATA's operational task is to ensure that the aircraft used to carry the world's passengers and goods are able to proceed with maximum safety and efficiency, under clearly defined and universally understood regulations. Its commercial objective is to ensure that people, cargo, and mail can move everywhere on the vast global network that constitutes the various airlines worldwide as though they were on a single line within a single country. These two activities are closely related in their connection with the cost of airline operation, the carrier's charges to the public, and the desire to keep both of these as low as possible, commensurate with safety.

Cooperation of the airlines in operational and technical matters is channeled through the Technical Committee and its various global and regional working groups. IATA's technical activity is founded upon full exchange of information and experience among all the airlines. Out of these data the airlines select common requirements and observations which guide the standardization and unification of their own activities, determine their practical advice and assistance to governments, and act as guides to future development in transport technology. IATA has played, and continues to play, an important part in the drafting of the ICAO Standards and Recommended Practices which form the accepted international pattern for the technical regulation of civil aviation, and the Association cooperates closely with ICAO to encourage governments to implement them fully and keep them up to date. In addition, IATA provides means for member airlines to enter into consultation with ICAO, with individual states, or with the countries composing a particular region on the planning and implementation of air navigation facilities and services (this work is generally carried out, under the control of the Technical Committee, by global and regional working groups which deal with new and developing problems in all technical fields of air transport operations). The Technical Department of IATA coordinates the airlines' involvement in the fields of medicine, which includes the physiologic and psychologic factors that might affect the safety and well-being of flight crews and passengers. IATA has permanent observer status in ICAO's Air Navigation Commission.

International Federation of Air Line Pilots' Associations

The International Federation of Air Line Pilots' Associations (IFALPA) was founded on April 7, 1948, in London, as the World Federation of Air Line Pilots. Its aims are to coordinate activities of airline pilots' associations and provide a vehicle for expression of the considered opinion of pilots in relation to technical and professional matters; assist and advise in development of a safe and orderly system of air transportation; promote the interests of the airline piloting profession and safeguard the rights, individually and collectively, of members; foster support and sponsor the passage of legislation and increase the safety of pilots' working conditions. In the aviation medical field, ICAO maintains liaison with IFALPA through the latter's Human Performance Committee.

International Academy of Aviation and Space Medicine

The International Academy of Aviation and Space Medicine (IAASM) was founded on April 27, 1959, in Los Angeles, as the successor body to the International Board of Aviation Medicine. Its aims are to promote development and research in the realm of aviation and space biology and medicine, improve and extend exchange of information and ideas in these fields, contribute to the search for new knowledge and its applications, and improve teaching and training. A general assembly and an executive council usually meet twice a year. The Academy sponsors international congresses on aerospace medicine, which are usually attended by ICAO's aviation medical officers.

APPENDIX A
Relevant Definitions and General Rules Concerning Licenses—Extracted From Chapter 1 of Annex 1

1.1   Definitions

Accredited medical conclusion. The conclusion reached by one or more medical experts acceptable to the Licensing Authority for the purposes of the case concerned, in consultation with flight operations or other experts as necessary.

Flight Crew Member. A licensed crew member charged with duties essential to the operation of an aircraft during flight time.

Flight Time. The total time from the moment the aircraft first moves under its own power for the purpose of taking off until the moment it comes to rest at the end of the flight.

Licensing Authority. The authority designated by a Contracting State as responsible for the licensing of personnel.

Medical Assessment. The evidence issued by a Contracting State that the license holder meets specific requirements of medical fitness. It is issued following an evaluation by the Licensing Authority of the report submitted by the designated medical examiner who conducted the examination of the applicant for the license.

Pilot-in-Command. The pilot responsible for the operation and safety of the aircraft during flight time.

1.2   General rules concerning licenses.

1.2.4.   Medical fitness 1.2.4.1. An appli-

cant for a license shall, when applicable, hold a Medical Assessment issued in accordance with the provisions of Chapter 6.

1.2.4.4.   Contracting States shall designate medical examiners, qualified and licensed in the practice of medicine, to conduct medical examinations of fitness of applications for the issue or renewal of the licenses or ratings specified in Chapters 2 and 3, and of the appropriate licenses specified in Chapter 4.

1.2.4.4.1. Medical examiners shall have had, or shall receive, training in aviation medicine.

1.2.4.4.2. Recommendation. Medical examiners should acquire practical knowledge and experience of the conditions in which the holders of licenses and ratings carry out their duties.

1.2.4.7.   Contracting States shall use the services of physicians experienced in the practice of aviation medicine when it is necessary to evaluate reports submitted to the Licensing Authority by medical examiners.

1.2.4.8.   If the medical Standards prescribed in Chapter 6 for a particular license are not met, the appropriate Medical Assessment shall not be issued or renewed unless the following conditions are fulfilled:

a)   Accredited medical conclusion indicates that in special circumstances the applicant's failure to meet any requirement, whether numerical or otherwise, is such that exercise of the privileges of the license applied for is not likely to jeopardize flight safety;

b)   Relevant ability, skill and experience of the applicant and operational conditions have been given due consideration; and

c) The license is endorsed with any special limitation or limitations when the safe performance of the license holder's duties is dependent on compliance with such limitation or limitations.

1.2.6.   Decrease in medical fitness.

1.2.6.1.   License holders shall not exercise the privileges of their licenses and related ratings at any time when they are aware of any decrease in their medical fitness which might render them unable to safely exercise these privileges.

1.2.6.1.1.   Recommendation. Each Contracting State should, as far as practicable, ensure that license holders do not exercise the privileges of their licenses and related ratings during any period in which their medical fitness has, from any cause, decreased to an extent that would have prevented the issue or renewal of their Medical Assessment.

APPENDIX B
Standardized International Curriculum for Training Aviation Medical Examiners

Programs of Lectures, Clinical Presentations and Round-Table Discussions

Introduction: This curriculum has been used in ICAO-sponsored Regional Civil Aviation Medicine Seminars. As a complement to academic activities, familiarization visits are carried out to aviation facilities and different specialty clinics. The latter enable participants to observe and practice recent evaluation techniques. In relation to the above curriculum, the following reference material is utilized:

ICAO Annex 1
ICAO Annex 13

ICAO Manual of Civil Aviation Medicine (Doc 8984-AN/895)

ICAO Manual of Aircraft Accident Investigation (Doc 6920)

A standard textbook in aviation medicine

The following program could be conducted in one week at a very intensive pace. On several occasions, it has been used as a two-week training program.

Lecture Units:

1. a) Introduction—Course organization and curriculum
   b) Human factors in the aviation system Responsibility of the designated medical examiner in air safety
   c) Aviation medicine: history and evolution
   d) International and national regulations—Chicago Convention—Annex 1
   e) ICAO Manual of Civil Aviation Medicine: origin, objectives, contents

2. a) Medical requirements—Basic principles in the assessment of fitness for aviation duties
   b) General medical requirements for licenses
   c) Physical and mental requirements for licenses
   d) Visual requirements for license
   e) Color perception requirements for licenses
   f) Hearing requirements for licenses
   g) Aviation physiology—Basic principles
   h) Operational and environmental conditions
   i) Barometric pressure—Hypoxia—Decompression—Pressurization
   j) Accelerations—Basic principles—Effects on human beings
   k) Respiratory system—Annex 1 requirements

Assessment of applicants with respiratory problems

Lung infections—Tuberculosis

Post-surgical conditions

Asthma and its treatment

3. a) Cardiovascular system—Basic principles of cardiovascular physiology
   b) Relation to aviation duties—Risk of sudden incapacitation
   c) Examination procedures—Laboratory and special examinations
   d) Specific cardiovascular conditions—Hypertension and its treatment
   e) Ischemic heart disease—ECG findings
   f) Angina pectoris
   g) Assessment of satisfactory recovery from myocardial infarction
   h) Cardiomyopathies—Pericarditis—Rheumatic heart disease
   i) Arrhythmias—Conduction defects
   j) Congenital heart disease—Post-surgical conditions

4. a) Digestive System—Basic principles
   b) Abdominal Pain—Gastrointestinal and biliary post-surgical conditions
   c) Gastritis—Uncomplicated peptic ulcer and its treatment—Complications: recurrence, bleeding and perforations
   d) Biliary tract disorders
   e) Pancreatitis
   f) Irritable colon
   g) Hernias

5. a) Diabetes mellitus—Basic principles, definitions, etiology, symptomatology
   b) Diagnostic criteria
   c) Glucose tolerance tests
   d) Classification
   e) Anti diabetic therapy
   f) Operational aspects in aviation
   g) Licensing considerations
   h) Satisfactory control criteria for aviation duties

6. a) Hematology—Anemias—Leukemias
   b) Platelet disorders
   c) Hemoglobinopathies, geographical distribution, classification, sickling conditions
   d) Assessment of medical fitness for aviation duties

7. a) Urinary system. Basic principles. Risk of sudden incapacitation. Urine findings: Hematuria, Albuminuria, Nephritis, Pyelonephritis, Obstructive uropathies, Tuberculosis. Lithiasis: single episode, recurrence, post-surgical conditions

8. a) Gynecology-obstetrics. Basic principles. Performance of aviation duties
   b) Risk of sudden incapacitation
   c) Menstrual disorders
   d) Pregnancy and aviation duties
   e) Abortion

9. a) Mental fitness and Neurological disorders
   b) Assessment of mental fitness for aviation duties
   c) Normal mental development. Psychological testing of intelligence and personality
   d) Psychiatric disorders in aviation personnel: Neurosis, personality disorders, psychosis, organic mental illness
   e) Diseases of the nervous system, inflammation, intoxication, vascular diseases, tumors, head trauma, post-traumatic states, disturbance of consciousness, epilepsy
   f) Electroencephalography in aviation medicine

10. Tropical Diseases: Basic principles. General sanitation, diseases transmitted by vectors, food and water borne diseases, parasitic disease. Hygiene and sanitation in relation with aviation. Prevention and spread diseases. Disinfection of aircraft. Vaccination. General health principles. Food poisoning. Incapacitation. Catering services, food, water.

11. Otorhinolaryngology: The external ear. The tympanic membrane. The middle ear. Post-surgical conditions. The vestibular system, hearing assessment, audiometry, nose and para-nasal sinuses, pathological conditions, special testing on the ENT system.

12. Ophthalmology. Examination techniques, visual acuity assessment, visual aids, visual fields, ocular muscle balance, assessment of

pathological eye conditions, glaucoma, color vision.

13. Flight crew fatigue. Flight duty time. Flight time limitation. Circadian rhythms. General health status. Basic principles, operational and environmental conditions.

14. On-duty incapacitation. Sudden, subtle, complete, partial, medical aspects, operational aspects.

15. Flexibility, waivers. Consideration of knowledge, skill and experience. Trained versus untrained crews. Medical flight test.

16. Accident investigation and prevention, the human factors aspect, the role of the medical examiner, identification of the victim, determination of the causes; circumstances and events.

17. Hazards of medication and drugs in aviation medicine.

18. General course revision. Appraisal and evaluation.

RECOMMENDED READINGS

Convention on international civil aviation (Doc 7300) 6th ed. Montreal: International Civil Aviation Organization, 1980.

International standards and recommended practices. Personnel licensing annex 1 to the convention on international civil aviation, 8th ed. July 1988, applicable on 16 November, 1989. Montreal: International Civil Aviation Organization, 1988.

Manual of civil aviation medicine (Doc 8984) 2nd ed. Montreal: International Civil Aviation Organization, 1985.

Occupational health and safety in civil aviation tripartite technical meeting for civil aviation. Geneva: International Labor Organization, 1977.

Occupational health and safety. Geneva: International Labor Organization, 1971.

Guide to hygiene and sanitation in aviation. Geneva: World Health Organization, 1978.

Yearbook of international organizations. 25th ed. New York: Saur, 1988–1989.

Work program (program budget) of the organization, 1990–1991–1992 (Doc 9532). Montreal: International Civil Aviation Organization, 1989.

Manual on prevention of problematic use of substances in the aviation workplace (Doc 9654). Montreal: International Civil Aviation Organization, 1995.

Chapter 28

Aircraft Accident Investigation

Robert R. McMeekin

Aviation itself is not inherently dangerous. But to an even greater degree than the sea, it is terribly unforgiving of any carelessness, incapacity or neglect.

Unknown

Aircraft accidents are not new occurrences. An accident badly damaged the front rudder frame of the Wright Flyer, cutting short the early flights of Wilbur and Orville Wright in the first successfully controlled, powered, and manned heavier-than-air machine near Kitty Hawk, North Carolina, on Thursday, December 17, 1903.

The first reported aircraft fatality in the United States occurred when the Wright brothers were demonstrating their standard Wright Type A Flyer to the U.S. Army Signal Corps at Fort Myer, Virginia, on September 17, 1908. When a crack developed in the starboard propeller of the Flyer, causing violent vibrations, Orville, who was at the controls of the aircraft, was unable to prevent the nosedive and resulting crash (Fig. 28.1). First Lieutenant Thomas E. Selfridge, who was aboard as an observer, died as a result of a compound, comminuted fracture of the base of the skull suffered during the crash. An autopsy was performed, and Captain H.H. Bailey (Medical Corps, U.S. Army) determined the cause of death. An aeronautical board investigated to determine the cause of the crash.

Most people considered flying to be particularly dangerous in the early days of flight, and fatal aircraft crashes were not surprising. Tran-

scontinental and Western Air flight no. 6, en route from Los Angeles to New York with intermediate stops in Albuquerque, New Mexico; Kansas City, Missouri; Columbus, Ohio; and Pittsburgh, Pennsylvania; crashed in dense fog near Millard, Missouri, on May 6, 1935. Few people would have taken notice of this crash, which killed five persons, except that Senator Bronson M. Cutting (R-New Mexico) was among those who died.

As a result of this crash, an outraged Senate quickly authorized the Committee on Commerce:

> to investigate . . . [the Cutting crash] . . . and any other accidents or wrecks of airplanes engaged in interstate commerce in which lives have been lost; and to investigate . . . interstate air commerce, the precautions and safeguards provided therein, both by those engaged in such interstate air transportation and by officials or departments of the United States Government; and to investigate . . . the activities of those entrusted by the Government with the protection of property and life by [sic] air transportation, and the degree, adequacy, and efficiency of supervision by any agency of Government including inspection and frequency thereof . . . (1)

This action established federal interest in aircraft accident investigations.

Although investigation into the mechanical causes of crashes progressed, it was not until the 1950s that the value of medical investigation of aircraft crashes became apparent. Several mysterious crashes of jet-powered British Comets, a new generation of pressurized aircraft, led to medical investigations that marked the beginning of modern aerospace pathology. One Comet crashed on January 10, 1954, with 35 persons on board approximately 25 minutes after taking off from Rome, Italy, en route to London, England. Another Comet crashed en route to Cairo, Egypt, from Rome on April 8, 1954, with 21 persons on board. Both planes crashed at sea, and there were no indications as to the cause. Postmortem examination of the remains of the passengers and crew who floated to the surface allowed pathologists to determine that an explosive decompression had occurred. This structural failure resulted from insufficient hull strength to withstand the pressure differential between the cabin and the outside atmosphere at altitude (2).

Until the development of jumbo airliners led to the potential for numerous fatalities associated with crashes, "mass disaster" meant up to 50 or perhaps 100 fatalities. Nevertheless, few people were prepared to comprehend the collision of two Boeing 747 jumbo airliners at Tenerife in the Canary islands on March 27, 1977, nor could they understand the problems that more than 580 fatalities presented (Fig. 28.2). This accident focused attention on the problems that aircraft accidents and other mass disasters can present (see Chapters 24 and 32).

There are a number of reasons to investigate aircraft accidents and incidents. The general public has a morbid curiosity about death. Certainly, a sudden occurrence such as an aircraft accident arouses public concern, and individuals have a pressing interest in the results of an aircraft accident investigation. Survivors of those who die in the crash are interested in obtaining adequate documentation to substantiate their claims for damages when they sue in the courts. The local government has an interest in ensuring

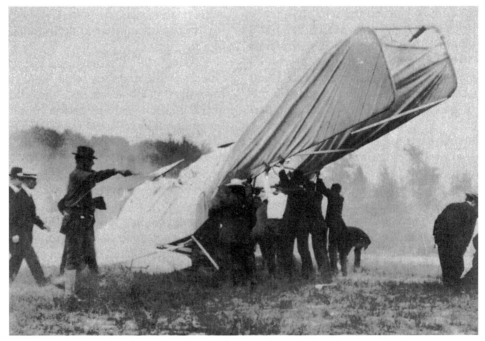

Figure 28.1. Crash of the Wright Flyer at Fort Myer, Virginia, on September 17, 1908 (Armed Forces Institute of Pathology photo).

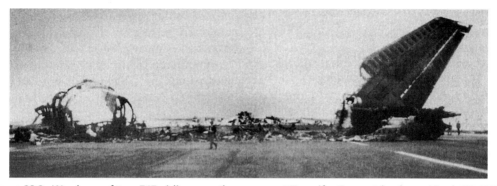

Figure 28.2. Wreckage of two 747 airliners on the runway at Tenerife, Canary Islands, on March 27, 1977 (Armed Forces Institute of Pathology photo).

the public health, safety, and welfare. It wants to be sure that no crime against the state or individuals has been committed and that there is no risk of infectious diseases. The federal government has many of the same interests as the local government. In addition, it has other interests, such as the safe and efficient operation of interstate commerce.

Investigators feel the pressure of all these interests, but they must not forget that the primary purpose of aircraft accident investigation is to prevent future accidents, injuries, and fatalities. To achieve this goal, they must thoroughly investigate all injuries and circumstances of a mishap.

Although this chapter uses aircraft accidents to illustrate the techniques for the investigation of accidents, identification of the victims, and evaluation of injuries, the methods are in most cases directly applicable to accidents involving other modes of transportation.

ORGANIZATION OF THE INVESTIGATION

The development of a multidisciplinary team approach to accident investigation leads to coordinated efforts in the following general areas of interest:

1. Operations
2. Structures
3. Power plants
4. Human factors
5. Aircraft systems
6. Witnesses
7. Air traffic control
8. Weather
9. Flight data recorder
10. Maintenance records
11. Evacuation, search, rescue, and firefighting

One or more team members are often assigned to each of these areas, but the actual composition of the accident investigation team always depends on the circumstances of the accident and the number of persons involved. For example, human factors teams generally consider the crashworthiness aspects of the investigation, with particular emphasis on organization, identification, injury tolerance, and analysis of injury patterns. The human factors investigation evaluates the cause of injuries received by the occupants and the psychologic or physiologic factors that may have contributed to the accident. These observations are the basis of recommendations for changes in standards for the physical examination of aircrew and pilot selection. They also lead to improvements in cockpit or passenger compartment layout and the design of seats, restraints, protective equipment, and escape mechanisms and pathways.

Phases of the Investigation

The immediate post-accident period may seem chaotic, and experienced investigators recognize the importance of the early development of an organizational plan that considers the following five general phases:

1. Preliminary evaluation
2. Data collection
3. Data analysis
4. Conclusions
5. Recommendations

The Joint Committee on Aviation Pathology (JCAP) prepared an outline of six steps for the pathologist to take when investigating fatal aircraft accidents. These steps are an adaptation of the five investigation steps listed above, and they are useful guidelines for any investigating physician. Although no rigid protocol can describe in detail how to investigate all accident types that a pathologist may encounter, JCAP recommends the following steps for the investigation of injuries sustained by the victims of a crash:

The first step in the investigation is for the pathologist to familiarize himself thoroughly with the type of aircraft—its internal structure, seating arrangement, ejection mechanism, and general layout and, if possible, to examine an intact plane of the type in question. An exact knowledge of the size, contour, and color of the objects that the pilot's body may have hit is extremely helpful in evaluating the injuries observed in and on the body. The pathologist should confer with pilots, engineers, and other experts who are familiar with the aircraft, parachute, ejection mechanism, and other equipment, to gain first-hand knowledge.

The second step in the investigation is for the pathologist to acquaint himself with all available information relative to the flight: the nature of the accident, severity of damage at the crash site, known factors about the weather, airfield, the health record and past performance of the pilot and his condition prior to and during flight, information regarding the passengers, the nature of any radio contact, and other pertinent information.

The third step in the pathologist's investiga-

tion consists of careful observation and written and photographic records of the position of the body and its relation to the total wreckage (or the parachute and other escape mechanism) and the conditions under which the body was found. The pathologist should examine carefully the pilot's protective helmet, clothing, shoes, and any other attachments. In the absence of the pathologist on the crash scene, these items should be left on the body as recovered. No article of clothing, harness, and so on should be cut or removed prior to inspection by the pathologist. The protective helmet and articles of clothing, shoes, gloves, and so forth, may reveal important information about the crash and may suggest defects in the design of the plane. Cytologic and ultraviolet light studies may offer helpful data.

The fourth step performed by the pathologist and his assistants will consist of meticulous examination of the exterior of the body and the viscera, with necessary close-up photographs and radiographs, and removal of properly selected tissue for chemical, toxicologic, and histopathologic examination. Special attention must be given to the detailed examination of all abrasions, lacerations, superficial and deep wounds. For example, a single small wound on the lateral or posterior portion of the lower legs may be strong evidence that ejection occurred but that the individual's feet were not positioned properly at the time. Photographing such wounds will be of great assistance in later correlation of the findings. Specimens of urine, blood, liver, kidney, and brain (unfixed) are best suited for the identification of poisons. For histopathologic examination, tissue sections from all organs, including the skin, bone, middle and inner ears, entire brain, spinal cord, entire heart and aorta, and organs showing significant lesions, should be preserved in 10% neutral formalin. These sections should include not only the diseased or traumatized area but also its margin and the adjacent normal area. In cases where a less than complete body is recovered, the examination of the remains should be carried out as conditions permit. It is essential to find as much of the body and internal organs as possible. The condition of the heart, brain, spinal cord, larynx, liver, skeletal muscle, and bone may well explain the cause of the crash.

The fifth stage in the investigation consists of microscopic study of the sections and chemical analysis for poisons. The pathologist must take special notice of the occurrence of vital processes such as vascular dilatation and the cellular exudation of early inflammation in the proximity of burns, contusions, etc.

The final step in the investigation is completed by summarizing the report of the accident and correlating it with the findings of the autopsy. The pathologist may participate in the proceedings of the Investigating Board (3).

Preliminary Evaluation

Preliminary evaluation of the crash site, nature of the casualties, available resources, and the chain of events that immediately preceded the crash will save time in the long run and will allow the investigator to determine the most efficient course to follow. This early phase, which is easily underemphasized, is certainly the most important.

The investigator must become familiar with the type of aircraft, seating arrangement, restraint systems, structural arrangement, and personal equipment. He or she should examine an intact aircraft of the same type. If possible, this aircraft should be available for comparisons during examination of the wreckage.

Examining the cockpit of a similar aircraft may provide important clues. Comparison of details of the paint scheme of the crashed aircraft with the location of paint fragments found at the crash site may help in determining the kinematics of the occupant in the crash. Review of manuals for the operation of the aircraft and its systems and for information about the injury patterns and accident circumstances associated with previous crashes of the same or similar types of aircraft may also be helpful.

Data Collection

The initial phases of accident investigation involve gathering information about the circumstance of the accident and the casualties. The investigator begins collecting data to evaluate many factors; background information about the general health, emotional attitude, experience level, and training of the crew is particularly important. The investigator should look for behavior patterns that might have led to errors of judgment or errors of action or reaction on the part of crewmembers, as well as for the presence of adverse physiologic conditions that might have impaired the crew. The investigator should seek clues regarding the speed, direction, and attitude of impact, which will be helpful later in analyzing injury patterns.

The investigator must be particularly alert in obtaining all available information about the circumstances of the accident and must coordinate this information with other groups involved in the investigation. The investigator should interview any witnesses because their observations may give clues about what occurred immediately prior to the crash. Even seemingly insignificant factors can be valuable to the human factors investigator in understanding the kinematics of the crash and in evaluating the causes of any unusual injuries. For example, severe turbulence associated with thunderstorms may explain the wreckage distribution after in-flight breakup.

Security at the crash site is important to ensure that no one alters the wreckage and its valuable clues as to the cause of the crash. Taking photographs and making diagrams is essential before anyone disturbs the wreckage. Well-meaning investigators often create problems by unintentionally altering crash sites. Nothing should be disturbed until someone photographs or otherwise documents the site. This, of course, assumes that survivors already have been evacuated from the site.

Adequate investigation requires careful documentation of the scene, and all participants in the investigation need to consider the final

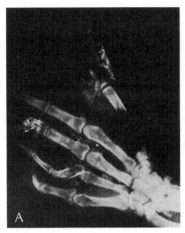 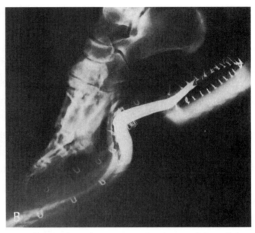

Figure 28.3. Radiograph of hand (A) and foot (B) indicate that these were the extremities of the pilot, who was at the controls when this accident occurred (Armed Forces Institute of Pathology photo).

location of the debris. The investigator should note the exact location of various parts of the wreckage, the location and configuration of ground impact, the stopping distance of the aircraft, and the exact amount of crush of the aircraft structure and should record this information on a scaled diagram. The diagram should also note the location of the bodies. These notes will be helpful in the identification of bodies, estimation of crash forces, and determination of the sequence of events.

A thorough description of the nature and extent of each injury will also be helpful, and photographs, radiographs, and diagrams will be useful in documenting injuries. Careful examination to document pre-existing disease and toxicologic studies to evaluate possible toxic substances or self-medication are also important.

Radiologic examination of the entire body, particularly the hands, feet, and vertebrae, is important. Radiographs often enable the investigator to determine who was operating the vehicle controls at the time of the crash or estimate the magnitude and direction of impact (Fig. 28.3).

A complete autopsy examination of all fatalities is essential. Autopsies of fatally injured crewmembers may uncover preexisting disease, incapacitation, or the presence of toxic substances in aircraft. Autopsies of the passengers may speed their identification and allow correlation of the design features of the aircraft or peculiarities of the accident that are responsible for the deaths of some passengers and the survival of others.

Data Analysis

The investigator must diligently collect and evaluate the data. Having collected the facts, he or she must then carefully analyze the questions to be answered. Given properly posed questions and adequate investigation, most answers follow surprisingly easily. Although initial impressions as to the cause of an accident may be tempting conclusions, the investigator must not summarily dismiss any observation as insignificant. The investigator must remain unbiased while conducting the investigation and be continually aware of possible new areas in which to pursue the investigation before forming conclusions. Each piece of factual information must be weighed as to its validity. The investigator must even suspect the witnesses' observations if they cannot be substantiated with factual information. Proper evaluation of the factual data that have been collected involves ruling out all other possible explanations.

Conclusions

After determining and evaluating the facts, the investigator must reach conclusions as to the cause both of the accident and of the injuries received by the passengers and crew. Three of five important questions that Fryer proposed must be answered in the conclusion and recommendation phases:

Why did the fatally injured lose their lives?
To what feature of the accident or of the aircraft can be attributed the escape of the survivors?
Is there any indication that the main or any subsidiary causes of the accident might have been of a medical nature (4)?

The conclusions should reflect the investigator's best opinions based on the available factual information. The cause of the accident or of specific injuries need to be proven beyond any shadow of doubt because the questions that require this degree of certainty are matters for the courts and collateral boards of investigation to determine. After defining substantiating facts, reasonable speculation is of definite value in deriving conclusions. A determination of ''cause: undetermined'' does nothing to advance the prevention of accidents and injuries.

Recommendations

The investigation is not complete until the investigator makes recommendations for changes that will prevent similar injuries and fatalities and, if possible, prevent the recurrence of the factors that caused the accident. The recommendations should address at least Fryer's (4) last two questions:

1. Would any modification of the aircraft or of its equipment have improved the chances of survival of those killed or reduced the severity of injury of the survivors?
2. Would the incorporation of such modifica-

tions have a detrimental effect on the chances of any of the survivors?

JURISDICTION

The jurisdiction to conduct investigations of deaths usually rests with the government of the territory in which the death occurs. Nevertheless, disputes occur at the state, national, and international levels over jurisdiction to conduct postmortem investigations, including autopsies of aircraft accident fatalities.

Jurisdiction for postmortem investigation at the international level is usually clear, if not entirely satisfactory, to the parties. According to customary international law, in the absence of a contrary agreement, a sovereign nation may establish whatever laws it chooses with respect to matters that are essentially within its domestic jurisdiction. One country cannot enforce its laws within the territory of another country, and the law of the country where an act is done wholly determines the character of the act. Treaties, conventions, and executive agreements resolve many of the problems that result from differences in laws among countries. The 1944 Chicago Convention provides for international participation by the state of registry in investigations of civil aviation accidents, as follows:

In the event of an accident to an aircraft of a contracting State occurring in the territory of another contracting State, and involving death or serious injury, or indicating serious technical defect in the aircraft or air navigation facilities, the State in which the accident occurs will institute an inquiry into the circumstances of the accident, in accordance, so far as its laws permit, with the procedure which may be recommended by the International Civil Aviation Organization. The State in which the aircraft is registered shall be given the opportunity to appoint observers to be present at the inquiry and the State holding the inquiry shall communicate the report and findings in the matter to that State (5).

Effective international cooperation resulted when a major air disaster involving two Boeing

747s occurred in Tenerife in the Canary islands in 1977. U.S. representatives participated in the investigation, and the Spanish government permitted the removal of the fatally injured U.S. passengers from Tenerife to Dover (Delaware) Air Force Base for identification.

Jurisdiction disputes also occur at the functional level between government agencies. The National Transportation Safety Board (NTSB), the Federal Bureau of Investigation (FBI), and the Department of Defense (DOD) are only a few of the U.S. agencies with interest in accident investigation. Although their interests may occasionally be diverse, personnel from the agencies are able to work together harmoniously. Statutes, regulations, and letters of agreement covering most situations clearly define the relationships between the various federal agencies.

Serious conflicts over postmortem jurisdiction occur most frequently between federal and state interests. In the United States, by virtue of the 10th amendment to the Constitution, the individual states retain jurisdiction over matters that federal legislation has not preempted. State laws regarding postmortem investigations differ considerably, and the official who authorizes postmortem examinations varies from state to state. Autopsy is available in some states only when this official suspects that a death resulted from unlawful means. Strong arguments maintain that this authority does not extend to fatalities resulting from aircraft accidents.

The U.S. military services, as well as armed forces from many other countries, recognize the importance of the pathologic investigation of fatal aircraft accidents, and they have published regulations requiring the postmortem examination of all fatally injured crewmembers. Civil jurisdictions, on the other hand, do not universally recognize this role of pathology, and the investigators encounter major problems when fatal military aircraft accidents occur outside exclusively federal jurisdiction. Even when they acknowledge the federal interest, these civil jurisdictions consider it secondary to their own authority. The result is that many postmortem investigations of military aircraft accident fatalities are inadequate.

Adequacy of Investigations

Investigations of aircraft accident fatalities are inadequate or unavailable in certain circumstances because appropriate legislative authority is lacking. Approximately 90% of U.S. military aircraft accident fatalities occur in areas where the federal government has no authority to obtain postmortem information that may be essential to aviation safety and accident prevention and where many local officials refuse to fully cooperate with the military investigations.

The primary interest of coroners and medical examiners is in determining the cause and manner of death and seldom in collecting information concerning aircraft accident and injury prevention. The authorizing official or examining pathologist may have no interest in aircraft accidents and may have no knowledge, experience, or training in the techniques involved. These officials often conduct only an external description of the body, frequently omitting the microscopic and toxicologic examinations necessary to determine the presence of toxic substances in the aircraft and preexisting disease in the aircrew. Even when local officials have the authority to conduct complete autopsy examinations, they may elect not to perform them. In one instance, in answering a request for information about his investigation after a fatal aircraft accident, a coroner's pathologist responded that ''according to local interpretation of state law, a coroner's autopsy precedes to [sic] the cause of death and is not an academic endeavor. When the cause of death is obvious in the gross autopsy, as is usually the case in aircraft accidents, microscopic examinations are not performed.'' In such cases, the military must depend on local civilian officials to conduct whatever examinations they deem advisable.

Even the presence of trained forensic pathologists with experience in investigating aircraft accidents does not ensure adequate examinations.

Statutory authority often limits even these trained investigators in the scope of postmortem examinations. Most coroners and medical examiners do not have sufficient funds or staffs to permit the more than 2 workdays often needed for a thorough investigation. Situations in which it is not clear who, if anyone, has jurisdiction, are especially disconcerting because nothing is accomplished, even though everyone agrees that postmortem examinations are needed. In the above-mentioned major air disaster involving two Boeing 747s at Tenerife, there were more than 580 fatalities, of which more than half were U.S. citizens. Of the 396 persons aboard the Pan American aircraft, 334 died. The jurisdiction of Spain to investigate the accident and of the United States to participate was clear under the provisions of the Chicago Convention. Logistics, however, necessitated the removal of the U.S. fatalities to Dover Air Force Base, where easier access to communications facilities aided the identification process. Detailed postmortem examination could have determined the exact cause of death and why so few survived this ground collision, but no one established the jurisdiction to conduct complete autopsy examinations. Without these examinations, the investigation was incomplete. The state of Delaware could not give adequate authorization for postmortem examinations because the deaths did not occur in Delaware. The NTSB did not have jurisdiction because Spain was in charge of the investigation. Everyone agreed that the investigations were necessary, but no one could cite a proper authority. The result was that the investigators used only those methods necessary to establish the identity of the bodies. Valuable information was lost that could have contributed to the furtherance of air safety.

Other cases of particular concern involve deaths of (1) personnel on board foreign military aircraft, (2) contractor and Department of Defense civilians who fly military aircraft, and (3) manufacturers' maintenance and test personnel who fly aircraft being constructed under contract for sale to the military and other federal agen-

cies. If a fatal accident involving one or more of these persons as crewmembers occurs outside exclusively federal jurisdiction, the federal government must depend on the scope of local civil laws regarding autopsies. Even if local officials agree that postmortem investigations should be done, they cannot be conducted if the state laws provide for autopsies only in cases where it is suspected that death occurred by unlawful means.

Federal Interest in Aircraft Accident Investigation

Congress has expressed an interest in the investigation of aircraft accident fatalities. Congress determined that the federal government has an overriding interest in aviation safety and enacted legislation to ensure thorough investigations, including autopsies, of all civil aircraft accidents. The NTSB may conduct these autopsies regardless of provisions of local law unless the local laws pertaining to autopsies are based on the protection of religious beliefs, as follows:

. . . In the case of any fatal accident, the Board is authorized to examine the remains of any deceased person aboard the aircraft at the time of the accident, who dies as a result of the accident, and to conduct autopsies or such other tests thereof as may be necessary to the investigation of the accident: Provided, That to the extent consistent with the needs of the accident investigation, provisions of local law protecting religious beliefs with respect to autopsies shall be observed (6).

A similar federal interest exists in military aircraft accidents in which the economic effects and the impact on national defense are critical, but the authority of the NTSB does not extend to the investigation of accidents involving military aircraft only. Statutes authorize the U.S. Army and Air Force to conduct autopsies of persons fatally injured on board military aircraft when a fatal accident occurs on a military reservation where there is sole U.S. military jurisdiction. The military services recognize the importance of postmortem investigations of all fatally injured military crewmembers, and their regulations require autopsy examination regardless of where death occurred. Regulations give military commanders power, similar to that of coroners, to direct the performance of autopsies of aircraft accident fatalities involving military personnel.

The Office of the Armed Forces Medical Examiner (OAME), located at the Armed Forces Institute of Pathology (AFIP) and staffed by fully trained forensic pathologists, investigates all fatal U.S. military aircraft accidents. The AFIP also provides consultation and pathology support to the NTSB and other government agencies. Active aviation pathology departments also exist in Germany, the United Kingdom, and other countries.

Preemptive Federal Authority

Federal, state, and local jurisdictions have legitimate interests in the investigation of aircraft accident fatalities. The difficult question is which interest prevails when more than one jurisdiction asserts its interest.

Exclusive Jurisdiction

The federal government has exclusive jurisdiction in the case of enumerated powers and when legislation expresses congressional intent to preempt the field.

The federal government also has exclusive jurisdiction over property of the United States, except to the extent that a state, when ceding land to the federal government, reserves jurisdiction or to the extent that Congress enacts legislation granting jurisdiction to the state. This means that an accident does not necessarily come under federal jurisdiction simply because it occurred on federal land.

Concurrent Jurisdiction

When federal and state laws conflict, federal law, under the supremacy clause and the preemption doctrine, supersedes state law. Even if federal and state laws do not conflict, federal law will prevail when Congress intends to provide complete federal regulation on the subject matter. Courts look to the classification of the subject matter in determining congressional intent, and state laws designed to protect the public health or safety of local citizens traditionally are subject to local regulation. Extensive federal legislation in the field is evidence of intent to preempt any state regulation. When the subject matter is of inherent national interest or when state regulation would be inconsistent with federal objectives, federal law prevails. The most consistently controlling factor, however, is the federal interest in uniform, national regulation of the subject matter. A court will balance the nature and extent of the burden against the purposes and merits of the state regulation. Because state coroner and medical examiner statutes protect public health and safety, courts probably will uphold those laws unless there is specific federal legislation such as the statute empowering the NTSB to investigate fatal U.S. civil aircraft accidents.

Conflicting Interpretations of the Law

Major problems occur when fatal accidents involving other than civil-registry aircraft occur outside exclusively federal jurisdiction. The NTSB does not have jurisdiction over these accidents. The NTSB may conduct autopsies on the remains of aircraft accident victims, but the NTSB authority applies only to accidents involving civil aircraft. The NTSB authority does not extend to military, prototype, or manufacturer's aircraft.

Military regulations permit commanders to authorize autopsies on the remains of military personnel who die in military service while serving on active duty or during training, whether these personnel died on or off a military installation. The legal authority for this comes from Title 10 of the U.S. code and from the constitutional powers of the service secretaries, acting as the alter ego of the President, to prescribe rules and regulations having the force and effect of law on the administration of the service.

The extent to which these regulations apply to civilians or to military personnel where there are conflicting state laws is arguable. State law clearly governs investigations of sudden, violent, or unexpected death—except in situations in which Congress has found an overriding federal interest and granted preemptory power, as in the Federal Aviation Act of 1958. The federal government's authority to investigate sudden, violent, or unexpected deaths of military personnel when they occur in areas of exclusively federal jurisdiction is also clear.

It is only arguable whether the federal government has the authority to conduct postmortem investigations in cases of civilian deaths that occur as a result of accidents involving military aircraft or involving experimental, prototype, or manufacturer's aircraft that are not of civil registry and are operating under an approved-type certificate or postmortem investigations of military personnel who die as a result of aircraft accidents occurring outside exclusively federal jurisdiction. Even if military regulations having the force and effect of law apply to postmortem examinations of military personnel on board the aircraft, these regulations apply to civilian crewmembers only if one may consider them part of "the land and naval forces." The authority of the NTSB does not apply because such an accident would not involve an aircraft of civil registry. If an aircraft manufacturer's employee dies in an aircraft that is still in test or production phases and before actual delivery to the military or assignment of civil registration number, a similar situation arises and autopsies may not be performed.

The possible concurrent authority of state officials is an issue, even if the military services have legal authority to conduct the autopsy investigations. Few state officials recognize claims of federal jurisdiction based merely on military regulations. Even if regulations grant commanders power to authorize autopsies of air-

crew who die while serving on board military aircraft, other regulations require the approval of civil authorities before removal of the remains when death occurs at a place other than a military installation. The civil authorities usually require compliance with state laws regarding autopsies before granting approval. The extent of state examinations is generally sufficient to satisfy military requirements because of factors such as limited scope of civil law governing postmortem examinations, limited personnel, financial support, and equipment of local medical examiner and coroner systems, and political conflict. The nature of an autopsy is such that the first examination inevitably distorts or destroys the information that may be obtained during a subsequent investigation.

MASS DISASTERS

Identification of Victims

Investigating a mass disaster is a very complex task, and identifying the casualties is one aspect that can be particularly difficult if it is not approached in a systematic manner. Regardless of the nature of the disaster, be it a natural calamity or transportation-related or other human-induced chaos, investigators participate as members of multidisciplinary teams to determine the cause, assign liability, and establish preventive measures for the future. Unfortunately, the other phases of the investigative process have received disproportionately more attention than has organization of the process of identifying casualties.

Many investigators know about identification techniques, but they have considered them as an isolated process and have not integrated them into the overall investigation. Typically, physicians, dentists, and other medical personnel are assigned tasks based on a preconceived disaster plan that they had no role in developing. The practical aspects of the identification process then usually develop on an ad hoc basis.

The seemingly simplistic nature of identification procedures is deceptive and perhaps explains why systematic organization of the entire process is seldom adequately addressed. The ensuing inefficiency produces conflicts among personnel and increases expenses, delays, and errors of identification.

The identification process is an essential element of an adequate investigation. Accurate identification of all fatalities incurred in an aircraft accident or other mass disaster is often the first step in determining where each person was located at the time of the disaster and what role they may have played in its cause.

Another obvious reason for identification is to allow families to recover the correct body. After some disasters, inexperienced people determined identity solely on the basis of the visual inspection of physical features, clothing, and items of personal effects such as jewelry and dog tags. They allowed families to claim portions of bodies even when no identifying characteristics were present, and when religious beliefs required prompt burial, families were often quick to claim any body. Grieving during the emotional period after the death of a family member sometimes produced denial reactions, and families refused to accept definitive identification of their relative. Although visual inspection is usually more than adequate, possible litigation or insurance claims may hinge on documenting that the victim was, in fact, correctly identified.

The task of identifying disaster victims is not difficult if it is approached in a logical, meticulous manner. Separated into basic elements, the identification process involves (1) the collection of identifying information about the missing persons, (2) the observation of identifying features of the victims, and (3) the comparison of the two groups of information. Identification is impossible if any one of these three elements is inadequate.

Planning for the Unknown

The following discussion of the planning process is largely theoretical, rather than a step-by-step description of a plan. Each community must individualize its disaster plan after full consideration of the types of disasters that may occur.

The most serious drawback of any disaster plan is that no one can determine exactly where a disaster will occur. Although many high-risk areas can be identified, even with today's modern transportation technology, the possibility cannot be eliminated that an accident will occur in dense population areas. For this reason, planners often cannot properly select the necessary facilities until after the disaster has occurred and the investigators know the nature and number of casualties and the location, type, and severity of the disaster.

Regardless of these difficulties, predisaster planning can and, in fact, must take place. Although successful investigation of disaster and identification of the victims may be possible without a plan, the job is much easier when all involved know what their role is and what they must do. But unless the planners have already considered the theoretical aspects by planning, the necessary decisions usually cannot be made rapidly and correctly. Expedition of the identification process after the occurrence of a disaster will more than compensate for all the time spent on predisaster planning.

Planners may be able to follow certain guidelines when developing a preaccident plan, but direct incorporation of someone else's plan usually is not possible without at least some modification to accommodate specific circumstances. The plan must reflect the risks, resources, and decision-making process unique to the community in question. A plan that could be used successfully in New York, for example, may not be suitable for a small town of 3000 to 4000 individuals. The larger cities have more extensive resources with which to purchase equipment and hire full-time staffs, allowing them to respond more efficiently to a wider range of disasters. On the other hand, the larger cities have more bureaucratic channels that often make even the simplest decisions complicated. Even in the most carefully thought-out plans, some unique circumstance may arise that the planners did not anticipate.

Nevertheless, a facility that is prepared for the eventuality of a mass disaster will be able to cope on a larger scale than will the facility that has no organization or plan. The unprepared facility must organize rapidly after a disaster occurs and is likely to make mistakes that would not have been made had more time been available for preparation.

Initiating the Planning Process

The disaster investigation organizer or committee can benefit from reviewing the plans and experiences of other communities, even though the plans may not appear directly applicable. The next step is a brainstorming session to see how many different possible disaster scenarios the planners can develop. The important questions concern (1) what types of disasters might occur (2) where might they occur, (3) the magnitude of the risk of occurrence, (4) how many casualties might occur and (5) what resources will be available.

Type of Disaster

The initial consideration should be to determine what types of disasters might possibly occur in the geographic area encompassed by the plan. Reviewing past disasters may provide useful indicators of possible future events, considering that each city, county, state, or other area has its own unique industries, topography, geography, and people. Denver, Colorado, has little reason to be concerned with hurricanes, and Miami, Florida, has little reason to fear blizzards and driving snow. Cities in the midwestern and southern parts of the United States must be prepared for tornados, and Pacific coastal cities recall their disasters resulting from earthquakes. Cities along rivers need to consider flooding and watercraft disasters.

Location of Disaster

Almost all cities, but especially those located near airports, must be concerned about aircraft crashes. Industrial explosions and other accidents must be anticipated near factories. Highways are an ever-present source of disasters.

Risk

A recurring feature of disasters is that they produce casualties. Having determined the type or types of disaster that the plan must anticipate, the next step is to estimate the likelihood of an occurrence with significant numbers of casualties. If an airport is nearby, how large are the aircraft that land there, how many people do they carry, and what is the safety record?

Casualties

Categories of casualties consist of persons who are killed, injured, or displaced from homes. The nature and severity of the disaster influences the number of persons to be found in each of these categories. Generalizations are difficult, but Lane and Brown (7) studied this problem in relation to 1086 aircraft accidents involving 34,369 occupants. They reported that no occupants were seriously injured in 82% of the accidents, that more than 50% of the occupants were seriously injured in less than 1% of the crashes, and that in most accidents (95%), not more than 25% of the occupants were seriously injured.

Resources

What a community will consider as constituting a disaster will be largely determined by the resources available to cope with it. Some communities would consider an automobile accident resulting in three or four fatalities a mass disaster, but some other cities could easily process 20 or more fatalities. Much depends on the exact circumstances of the accident. A city that would have no difficulty processing 20 fatalities from an aircraft accident that occurred at an airport might be totally incapacitated if the same accident and same number of fatalities occurred on a main street or involved a major administrative building such as that of the police or fire department.

Testing the Plan

Although no amount of planning can totally prepare a community, disaster drills are an effective way to test the plan before an actual disaster occurs (8). The drill may point out weaknesses in the plan; seemingly insignificant details often turn out to be critically important when the actual disaster occurs.

Organizational Concept

Approaching identification of the victims of a mass disaster in a logical manner greatly simplifies the process and increases the efficiency and accuracy of identification. Recognizing the concept of the "3 Cs"—command, communication, cooperation"—is fundamental.

Although the literature contains many accounts of specific disaster investigations, the organizational concept described here was developed as a result of participation by personnel from the AFIP in the investigation of many aircraft crashes and other disasters. These disasters have involved casualties varying in number from a single fatality to nearly 1000 deaths.

The organizational concept developed by the AFIP for identifying disaster victims involves another application of the five distinctive phases of investigation: preliminary evaluation, data collection, data analysis, conclusion, and recommendation.

These five phases apply equally to the identification process and to the investigation in general, and all investigators need to know the importance of this flow in the identification process, complementing and not clashing with other working groups who are participating in the overall investigation.

The AFIP investigators retain flexibility within each of the investigative phases to allow general applicability. This flexibility of the process lends it to general application, and, in fact, recognition of this flexibility factor is the key to understanding the concept of mass disaster casualty identification.

The major emphasis of the AFIP mass casualty identification scheme is on quality control. This control consists of multiple checks during the phases of data collection and analysis, and the AFIP personnel attempt to confirm each identification by all available methods. The AFIP personnel also make an intensive effort to obtain complete antemortem records and descriptions as soon as possible, because they know that no identification will be possible without these data for comparison.

Preliminary Evaluation

The process begins with preliminary evaluation of the location and nature of the disaster, number of casualties, and availability of resources. Careful evaluations of these factors at the outset will allow effective structuring if the individual efforts and the most effective use of available resources.

Security

Security procedures to protect the disaster site are important. Looters can quickly strip all identifying evidence from the scene, and bodies and baggage are inviting targets. Some disruption of the site may be inevitable in the course of rescuing survivors, but beyond this initial stage, strict security measures should allow only trained investigators or other specially instructed personnel to enter the site. Disruption of the disaster site compounds an already difficult identification task, and uncontrolled access to the disaster site or to the investigation facilities can have disastrous effects on the outcome of the investigation.

Likewise, appropriate security measures must be taken at the investigative facility to prevent unauthorized entry. Suitable isolation may be necessary for family, news media, and other persons who have a legitimate interest in the investigation but whose presence may distract investigators and result in errors of identification. This consideration usually dictates selection of a site for the identification facility somewhere other than a centrally located public place.

Jurisdiction

The investigator should determine the legal aspects of jurisdiction to proceed with the investigation because many people have legitimate interests in actively participating in the investigation. Rescue teams are concerned with saving the lives of those who have been injured, and these efforts necessarily take precedence over other investigations. The fire department responds to extinguish the fire and investigate its cause. The police investigate possible wrongdoing, provide security, and control spectators. Many police, fire, and rescue teams may respond, and the question of who has primary jurisdiction may not be clear.

Medical examiners and coroners examine the bodies to document the cause of death, detect possible infectious disease, and assist the police in detecting evidence of foul play. Representatives of the news media have an important role in reporting the circumstances of the event and communicating the extent of any continuing hazards to the community. Undertakers want to prepare the bodies as quickly as possible. The operator of the vehicle or industry involved in the disaster is interested in determining the cause, and relatives want to ascertain the status of missing family members. Attorneys help the potential plaintiffs and defendants determine their possible claims and liabilities. In the case of transportation disasters, representatives of various agencies such as the NTSB and the Federal Aviation Administration (FAA) also participate. The international nature of many disasters poses special problems for international relations.

These are only a few of the individuals and organizations that may have an active interest in the investigation, and the process must provide a framework for all interested parties to work together. Fortunately, even in another's jurisdiction, bona fide offers of assistance are seldom refused.

Leadership

Lack of consensus among the early arrivals as to who should be in charge is one of the greatest problems at the scene of a mass disaster, especially when not all of the investigators were participants in a preconceived plan. Many interdependent decisions are made, and too many people attempting to assert command and give orders only increases the state of mass confusion.

Although each of the activities will have a leader, the various parties with interests must determine who will have primary control of the overall investigation. Selection of this "commander" is particularly important. The commander's most important job is to deal with outsiders and, from a practical standpoint, the greater that person's standing in the community, the more effective he or she will be. This person should have experience in identification techniques, but his or her direct involvement in the identification process is less desirable in larger disaster investigations. Rather than dealing with the technical aspects of the identification process, this individual must see that the needs of the identification personnel are promptly filled and that interruptions are prevented. He or she handles all inquiries from the press, families, undertakers, lawyers, and others and arranges for any support that the identification team needs.

Headquarters Site

The investigator must establish a central headquarters to control and monitor progress in the investigation and to maintain necessary liaison. This headquarters must be easily accessible to transportation and communication, although it need not actually be within the identification facility. In many respects, investigators find it advantageous if the headquarters is separate from the identification facility when it comes to dealing with the press, families, and others whose presence may disrupt the identification process. Accommodations for eating and sleeping may be necessary.

The Identification Facility

As the investigators begin the process of finding a site to set up an identification facility, a number of considerations should come to mind. The facility should be convenient to the disaster site, and the problem of removing casualties should not be complicated by moves of great distances. The investigators will need to make repeated trips from the facility to the disaster site, and these trips may waste time unnecessarily if distances are too great or the terrain is too difficult.

The facility must have adequate equipment or at least be located such that needed equipment can be installed quickly. Commercial power lines or portable or mobile electrical generators can provide adequate electricity to power lights and electrical equipment. Refrigeration may be needed to protect temperature-sensitive reagents and foods, and large refrigerated storage vans may be required to store the bodies prior to identification and release to next of kin. Work gloves, rubber gloves, pencils, clipboards, waterproof tags, plastic bags, sawhorses, and plywood to construct examination tables, and heavy-duty plastic sheets to cover floors may be needed.

Although there are many reasons for conducting the identification process as near the disaster site as possible, other factors may be overriding. For example, the availability of refrigeration, communication systems, and other facilities are important factors the investigator must consider. The problem of working in a hostile environment also must be taken into account.

Given a choice, most investigators opt to set up operations in a well-equipped headquarters that is selected, operated, and equipped exclusively for disaster investigations. Unfortunately, the location of disasters often cannot be foretold. Most communities cannot afford the luxury of a specially designated disaster headquarters and necessary associated facilities, and the number of fatalities in a disaster may far exceed the capacity of established morgue facilities. Fre-

quently, the disaster investigation facility has to be created after the disaster has occurred.

Communications

The establishment of an effective communications system should have high priority. The investigator must seek information from outside sources to correlate with identifying characteristics, and obtaining antemortem records and other information for use in identification may be impossible without adequate means of communication. The coordination of operations at the disaster site, hospitals, mortuary, headquarters, and other facilities also requires communications. Telephones are usually the most needed means, but radio communications may be needed, especially to the disaster site.

The investigator must consider public relations. Often, the success of disaster investigation depends on public support. In many instances, the local community can be of valuable assistance, particularly by providing lodging and mess accommodations, canteen facilities at the disaster site and headquarters, transportation, communications (radio, telephone, and runners), secretarial and clerical help, and general construction help and labor. The dissemination of adequate information requires attention to ensure that the public is aware of the continuing activities and of any needs for local participation. On the other hand, aside from problems of security, continuous and uncontrolled access to the facility by sightseers is not desirable.

To provide reasonable access for press representatives, who invariably have an interest in the causes and effects of the disaster, as well as the conduct of the investigation, the investigator should establish a special press area where the public relations group can provide regular scheduled briefings and other press releases can be made available.

Transportation

The investigator must consider transportation requirements. Injured persons need transportation to medical treatment facilities; bodies must be removed to a mortuary; personnel must be transported to and from the disaster site, mess facilities, and sleeping accommodations; equipment must be brought to the facility for installation; mail and other documents to aid in identification and treatment must be transported; and special requirements may exist for transportation of materials to specialized laboratories for analysis.

Personnel

Typically, communities are entirely unprepared for a disaster. Implementation of a previously designed plan can be the most important step taken when a disaster occurs. But even if the community has elaborate predisaster plans, people will not be sitting in well-organized disaster centers with all of the necessary equipment, poised and ready to go. Therefore, a critical element of any predisaster plan is notifying participants and giving them instructions as to what they must do.

The investigator must determine what personnel will be needed to cope with the emergency and often must select appropriate personnel, equipment, and a work site on short notice and without direct knowledge of the nature and scope of the disaster. Extra attention at this point invariably simplifies subsequent tasks.

Fortunately, finding people who are willing to assist in the investigation is seldom a problem. Most people in a community will respond in any way they can. The more serious problem is finding sufficient professional staff in large-scale disasters.

Care and Feeding

Logistic problems must be solved if food is to be brought into the facility; likewise, transportation requirements are involved if the workers must leave the facility to find mess and sleeping accommodations. The facility should be selected with consideration for the comfort of the workers who will be using the facility. One cannot expect workers to function effectively under extremes of temperature or humidity. Adequate

heat and ventilation must be provided, and mess and sleeping facilities may be required. The conditions under which the investigators must work often influence the speed with which the problems can be resolved. The establishment of work schedules is necessary, especially in adverse climatic conditions. Errors made as a result of fatigue, hypoglycemia, or cold can delay the investigation far more than any possible time-saving from extended hours of work under adverse conditions. AFIP investigators have found that they cannot reasonably expect more than 18 hours' effort from the workers on the first day and 10 hours on subsequent days without unacceptable errors being induced.

Viewing large numbers of casualties imposes tremendous psychologic stress upon all members of the team. Nightmares and altered personal behavior patterns, such as drinking and engaging in hazardous activities, represent potential individual responses that carefully organized psychologic support can often prevent. In practice, most disaster workers consider religious leaders, such as priests, rabbis, and ministers, less threatening than psychologists and psychiatrists. A major key to successful psychologic support in these situations is allowing the workers to express their anxiety and reassuring them that their feelings are normal.

Inventory Control

A key factor in disaster victim identification is inventory control. An inventory system will greatly facilitate keeping track of each fatality and survivor. This control must begin with the first rescuer on the scene.

The problem of inventory may be attacked in a number of ways. One method is to establish an inventory control group. The most effective method involves locating this group at the disaster site, triage area, morgue, hospitals, holding area, and central command post. The duties of the inventory control group are to see that all casualties were properly and securely tagged and not commingled. Further, they should keep a running inventory of exactly where each survivor is located, as well as in what stage of the identification process each fatality may be found.

Rescuers should remove only survivors unless immediate danger threatens further destruction and loss of the identifying features of the fatalities. When survivors are removed, they should be questioned to determine their names and other identifying information in anticipation of the possibility that their conditions may suddenly deteriorate en route to the treatment or holding facility. This questioning is particularly important to avert the situation that occurs in large-scale disasters in which a complete list of missing persons is frequently unavailable, thus rendering the identification of fatalities more difficult.

All survivors are taken to the initial triage area, usually a medical facility, so they can be queried more completely as to their identity. After referral to a holding area, uninjured survivors can be questioned by investigators as to the cause of the disaster. Persons who are displaced from their homes must be accommodated in this area until other arrangements can be made, whereas others may be returned to their homes. Injured survivors may be transferred to the holding area from the hospital after they have been treated.

Injured survivors, depending on the severity of injuries, should be transferred rapidly to a medical treatment facility. Care must be taken to ensure that haste does not interfere with inventory control. When more than one medical treatment facility is being used, it is not difficult to ''lose'' casualties. Investigators must know who is where. Casualties who die en route to or at the medical treatment facility must be transferred to the mortuary facility.

Much more care is necessary in the recovery of fatalities to preserve identification information. Valuable information that would be helpful in identification is often lost when recovery is unplanned and hastily performed. The exact location where the fatality was found must be recorded. In the case of mass disasters such as

aircraft accidents, this record can conveniently take the form of a wreckage diagram indicating the recovery location of each of the bodies. This chart may provide helpful clues in the identification of family members. In the identification of crewmembers in an aircraft accident, knowing which bodies were found in the cockpit wreckage and, if possible, the description of the seats in which each body was found is helpful. Photographs should be taken of each body in place at the scene prior to disturbing the position of the bodies. Although these photographs are primarily of interest to those who are investigating the cause of the accident or the survivability aspects, they may also be useful in identification to detect any errors that may occur in the numbering of bodies. Obviously, for this to be valuable, the body number must be conspicuous in the photographs.

The investigator must consider how and where to store the bodies. Particularly important are the containers for the bodies, the means to preserve the bodies, and a system to allow organized retrieval of specific bodies. Body bags are not always readily available, especially in large quantities. In these cases, sheets, temporary coffins, or even shipping containers may be used.

Although the preservation of the bodies is important, the investigator needs to collect any tissues needed for chemical studies before chemical preservation is used. Refrigeration is perhaps the best method of preserving the bodies until the investigation is completed, although charred bodies do not have the urgent need for refrigeration. Refrigeration is particularly important in warm climates, and the investigators may need to rent refrigerated truck-trailers. Although the design of a typical truck-trailer will accommodate approximately 50 bodies, the inventory and retrieval process is easier if fewer numbers are stored in each vehicle.

Keeping track of more than about 20 bodies at a time is often difficult, and assigning one person to keep track of each body whenever it is out of the storage area is one very effective quality control procedure. This person follows the assigned body as it proceeds through each stage of the identification process and keeps the labels and other paperwork in order.

In an effort to safeguard jewelry from looters, rescue workers often remove personal effects from bodies and place them in bags. Although this procedure may seem reasonable if the personal effects are placed in individual bags and labeled with the number of the corresponding body, the possibility still exists for errors in numbering. The situation in which two bodies have the same number readily illustrates the nature of problems that may be encountered. In any case, the identification investigator can only hope that the personal effects he or she did not personally observe to be attached or associated with a body were properly marked.

Collection of Identification Data

The second phase in the investigative process focuses on data collection. This is a particularly intensive period for personnel, and the effective direction of efforts results in an uneventful and thoroughly successful investigation. Overcoming the initial inertia is one of the hurdles. People often seem to stand around waiting for something to happen, frequently not realizing that they are the ones who must take the first step.

Figure 28.4 shows the organizational flow of

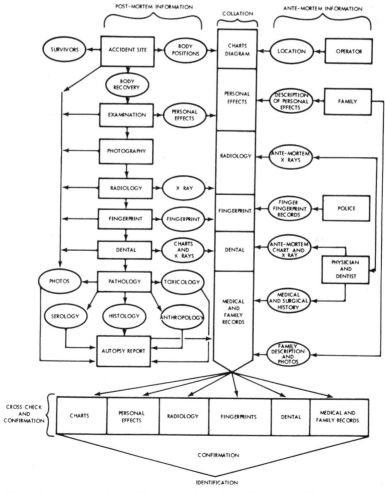

Figure 28.4. Organizational workflow concept for identifying casualties of a mass disaster.

work that AFIP investigators usually follow in collecting and evaluating data. This protocol is not rigid, and I cannot overemphasize the importance of flexibility in applying any organizational scheme to specific situations. Frequent deviations may be necessary to accommodate specific conditions as operational or other requirements necessitate. Nevertheless, this order does allow logical progression in the typical case.

Who Is Missing?

The investigator must accurately determine the answer to this question as early as possible. He or she must take immediate steps to obtain a list of persons believed to be missing and their last reported position. The identification methods to use, the types of additional assistance that may be needed, and the duration of the investigation depend on this list. Finding this information may be extremely difficult, especially in the case of natural disasters; in the case of aircraft accidents, however, this information should be available from the owner or operator in the form of crewmember assignments, flight manifests, passenger lists, and seating assignment charts.

Manifest lists of affinity groups usually are the easiest to determine accurately. For example, when a military aircraft crashes, a manifest, or list of persons on board the aircraft, will almost certainly be available. Unless a last-minute crew change occurred or passengers boarded the aircraft at the last moment without proper documentation, accurate information should be readily available from the flight operations department that dispatched the aircraft. Problems can occur, however; for example, after the crash of an aircraft presumed to have only eight persons on board, investigators recovered 17 feet from the wreckage.

Without a preexisting list of persons suspected of being missing, the problem of identifying the disaster victims may be impossible. Disasters at airport, bus, or train terminals; hotels; and sports stadiums, circuses, and other entertainment sites are only a few examples of situa-

tions in which determination of who is missing is difficult. Almost every large medical examiner's office has had a body that remained unidentified until someone finally noticed that the person was missing and filed a missing-person report.

The problems are even more difficult when people use names other than their own when traveling. This immediately raises questions of illegal activity and foul play. These activities seem particularly prevalent in international travel, but they also occur in domestic travel.

Less sinister reasons are usually the case, such as when a large corporation makes travel reservations for one employee but at the last minute sends a different employee instead. Even such simple errors as misspelled names on a manifest can pose serious problems in discovering the identity of the missing person.

Antemortem Information

After establishing a tentative missing-persons list, knowledge of the general condition of the bodies gained during cursory inspections in the preliminary evaluation phase will allow investigators to pursue the antemortem information needed for comparison with postmortem observations. They may seek some types of information more vigorously than other types, although still recognizing that even the secondary information is important. Medical and dental records may be more helpful than fingerprint records and information about clothing and personal effects in the case of severely burned and charred bodies. On the other hand, in the case of children, medical and dental records may have less importance. This underscores again the importance of the preliminary evaluation phase.

Positive identification can be made only by comparison of observed features with those previously observed and/or recorded. Someone must find records of uniquely identifying characteristics for each of the missing persons if they are to be identified positively. If the investigators cannot obtain this information, positive identification will not be possible. Investigators can ask various sources, such as the missing person's family, friends, employer, physician, and dentist, as well as law enforcement agencies, for information and records. They should make every effort to obtain as much identification information as possible as rapidly as possible.

An effective organization is essential to actively seek and to maintain appropriate chain-of-custody of the required antemortem records. Numerous checklists of desirable identification information are available. Although many of the commercial air carrier operators have detailed questionnaires that can serve as useful checklists, the investigators should inform the interviewers of the specific types of information required for that particular investigation and remind them that the people they interview seldom appreciate the urgency of the request for information and the necessary detail. The immediate acquisition of complete antemortem data is essential if the identification process is to proceed with dispatch and, in fact, if it is to succeed at all.

Postmortem Information

The collecting of postmortem information actually begins with the first person at the disaster site. Although the bodies must, at some point, be recovered from the disaster site and transported to the mortuary facility where identification is to take place, under the best of circumstances the rescuers will leave the bodies in situ until the investigators arrive. Impressing the importance of this on rescue organizations should be part of any disaster plan.

Knowledge of the exact location of each body, its injuries, and its position relative to various parts of the wreckage and to other bodies can be helpful. Prior to removal of any body, the investigator should have someone photograph it, chart its location on a diagram of the disaster site, and apply an identifying tag. The investigator may be able to correlate the body locations with the duty positions of crewmembers or with passenger seat assignments as a preliminary identification procedure. It should be noted that identification by seat or duty assignment is

merely a preliminary step and does not result in positive identification.

Fragmented bodies require special care in collecting, tagging, and identifying each fragment. Investigators must search the disaster site carefully to ensure that they have not overlooked any body fragments. Even small fragments of tissue may aid in identification; small fragments of dentition or printable skin may be the evidence needed to identify some of the casualties. In the example cited earlier, only eight people were missing after one crash, but investigators found body fragments that included 17 feet. Since no one knew of a ninth missing person, the entire process of identification was much more difficult and time-consuming than if some clue to the identity of the ninth missing person had been known.

Rescuers may not be able to recover all of the bodies in some instances, such as in disasters at sea. Investigators must then decide when to terminate further search efforts; they may have to resolve through other aspects of the investigation whether there may have been more victims than the persons reported missing and consider the possibility of foul play.

The information required for the documentation of identity can be provided in most cases by the following:

1. Color photographs of the body (clothed and unclothed);
2. Total-body radiographs (including all extremities);
3. Documentation of all scars, tattoos, deformities, operations;
4. Documentation of body characteristics (hair and eye color, and so on);
5. Documentation of all clothing, jewelry, and personal effects;
6. Dental chart;
7. Fingerprints and footprints;
8. Blood type;
9. Anthropologic measurements and estimates of height, weight, body build, age, race, and sex.

Initial Examination

Even though the initial screening examination of each body does not require much time, it frequently provides immediate clues to identity. The investigator should take particular care at this stage to correlate any associated injuries when removing photographs, labels, and describing clothing and personal effects. Although the personal-effects group will investigate these items further, the information about them should be noted and made available to the investigators at each successive work station. Dentures and other dental material are best left for subsequent examination and removal by the dental investigators.

Complete photographic coverage of this initial examination is important. Photographs of all aspects of the body, particularly specific identifying features of the face, ears, hands, feet, and tattoos, are especially helpful documentation, and the investigator should obtain them before and after removing clothing and personal effects. Additional photographic coverage should be available to document any noteworthy observations made at subsequent work stations.

Radiologic Examination

Radiologic examination has become an increasingly important identification tool. Lichtenstein and colleagues (9) demonstrated its value in screening for foreign materials and identifiable structures, in comparing antemortem radiographic examinations, and in evaluating injury patterns. Obtaining comprehensive radiographs of the entire body frequently pays unexpected dividends. Occasionally, metal fragments from old traumatic injuries or war wounds are demonstrated. In many cases, investigators can obtain further information concerning the circumstances of death and the nature of the forces involved from the interpretation of these radiographs.

The identification value of radiologic examination is greatest in instances in which the deceased is younger than 25 years. In this age group, the interpretation of ossification centers

and closure of the epiphyses can give a close approximation of the age of the individual. For these interpretations, the often overlooked radiographs of the hands and feet are essential.

Investigators can take advantage of travel time when they must travel long distances to the disaster site. When they will not arrive at the disaster site until after the bodies have been removed to mortuary facilities, they can save time by requesting that initial radiologic studies be obtained before their arrival. Dental and fingerprint consultation may also be requested during this travel period. The radiographs, dental charts, and fingerprint records will then be available for immediate review when the team arrives. Additional or complementary radiographs may then be obtained if necessary.

Fingerprints and Footprints

The next step in identification consists of examining hands and feet for the presence of printable surfaces. Fingerprint identification is the first method of choice because it is one of the most accurate and reliable methods for the identification of unknown remains. Experienced investigators can examine fingerprints obtained from disaster victims and, using various coding methods, search the massive files that are kept at organizations such as the FBI in the United States. If records are immediately available, even the physician can make a preliminary comparison. Most countries accept fingerprints and footprints as positive proof of identification.

The use of fingerprints or footprints as means of identification depends on the availability of previous known prints for comparison. Employers, police, and other government agencies can often provide antemortem fingerprints for comparison. Hospitals may have fingerprints of mothers and hand or footprints of children appearing on birth records. Inquiry during the preliminary evaluation phase should reveal whether any of these antemortem records are available. Some countries keep no fingerprint records. In other countries, these records are available only for convicted criminals. In the United States, fingerprint records of many adults are available for comparison, but even the FBI's large file of records contains fingerprints of less than 25% of the population.

Even when no antemortem records are available, the investigator may still be able to obtain latent fingerprints from the missing person's home, office, or vehicle. Good latent prints are often found on objects such as drinking glasses, mirrors, windows, and doorknobs. Satisfactory prints from only the palm of the hand may be on a drinking glass; the investigator must take prints of the entire hand for comparison in this case. The FBI Disaster Squad identified one or more victims through latent fingerprint impressions in the majority of disasters in which they assisted. These techniques are not for the unskilled, but knowing that the techniques are available may greatly shorten the process of identification.

The forensic pathologist or other identification personnel may be able to accomplish many simple screening procedures because comparison of good quality antemortem fingerprint records with sharply defined postmortem impressions is not difficult. In most circumstances, however, the professional assistance of trained fingerprint experts from a local enforcement agency or military police is advisable in obtaining both prints and records.

Even in badly burned or decomposed bodies, satisfactory fingerprints for comparison can often be obtained by special techniques. Badly wrinkled or macerated fingers (''washerwoman skin'') can often be restored to printable condition by the injection of a fluid such as saline. When burn charring involves only the epidermis, scraping away the charred tissue may enable prints or photographs to be made of the underlying dermis. If the facilities to obtain prints are not available, the investigator may remove and retain the finger pads, fingers, or even the entire hand until prints can be made.

In the case of a badly fragmented body, the investigator must make a diligent search for fragments of printable tissue. In one severe crash, after which the investigators could find only minute fragments of tissue, a one-fourth-inch square portion of skin from the thumb of the pilot was found inside the control stick. This not only served to identify the pilot but also indicated that he was probably attempting to control the aircraft at impact.

Dental Examination

Dental identification is probably the most widely used method other than visual recognition for the identification of unknown remains. Dental techniques for the identification of disaster victims have become increasingly important. More people worldwide have dental records than have fingerprint records.

Hill (10) described the dental techniques used by forensic odontologists in the United Kingdom for identifying aircraft accident victims. Morlang (11) described the organizational structure, technical procedures, and methods of documenting dental findings used in the United States. The potential for computer-assisted comparison of the antemortem and postmortem records is particularly interesting. Computer programs allow comparison of other identification information such as age, race, sex, height, weight, hair and eye color, scars, blood type, and surgical implants.

The assistance of a dentist, particularly a forensic odontologist, will greatly facilitate dental charting and identification. The postmortem dental charting should show, as a minimum, the presence or absence of each tooth, the presence and exact location on the tooth of any restorations (fillings), the shape of the restorations, and the presence of cavities. In cases of extensive traumatic injuries, radiographs of the whole body that were obtained at an earlier station in the identification process may aid in the location of dental material that traumatic forces translocated elsewhere in the body.

The dentist can remove any dentures at this time for possible correlation with antemortem dental materials. Dentists often inscribe the person's name or other identifying information on artificial dentures. In many cases, they recognize dental work that they performed and may recognize other characteristics of the person's mouth.

Severe head trauma often dislodges the maxilla, enabling it to be removed with only a scalpel. The dentist may need to remove the mandible and maxilla in some other cases for adequate exposure or further inspection, and if a body still remains unidentified at the completion of the investigation, the dentist should remove and retain the teeth for possible subsequent identification. The technique for removing the teeth intact is simple. With a Stryker saw, the mandible and maxilla can be removed easily, leaving the teeth undisturbed.

The widespread use of radiographic documentation of dental prophylaxis and the decline in the scope of fingerprint identification files are responsible for the great progress in dental identification techniques. Radiographs of teeth may be made to compare the shape of restorations, the location and extent of cavities, the shape of individual teeth and their root structure, or any preexisting abnormalities with antemortem radiographs. Comparison of the root structure of the teeth in antemortem and postmortem radiographs may establish identification even if no restorative dental work has been performed.

The introduction of dental radiographs into the identification process has eliminated the confusion that can follow when the dental chart does not accurately show the actual dental characteristics. In many cases, the dentist verbally transmits his observations to a technician, who records it on the dental chart. Many possible sources for errors exist in this system; it is not unusual to find "left" recorded when "right" was intended or "buccal" recorded when the actual location was lingual. The forensic odontologist can readily verify the correct positions by inspecting the radiographs.

Dental identification depends on the availability of antemortem dental records for comparison. As with fingerprint records, the dental records may not be immediately available. The investigator can save time by taking the radio-graphs and doing the dental charting of the victim while waiting for the antemortem radiographs and charts. Because dental records are not maintained in central, coded repositories as are fingerprint files, finding dental records depends on a reasonably accurate missing persons list. Using this list, the investigator should obtain all available previous records, including dental charts, radiographs, casts, and impressions. Even when the actual dental record is not available, the missing person's dentist can provide the necessary information by telephone.

Victims who had dental work performed subsequent to the last known dental record present a difficult problem of identification. If a victim's dental record indicates that he or she has 32 teeth and no restorations, a victim whose third molars are absent would not seem to be a likely possible match without knowledge that the teeth were extracted subsequent to the date of the record available for comparison. The investigators must take great care to avoid eliminating possible identity matches by errors such as this, and comparison of more detailed anatomic observations of radiographs is usually helpful in avoiding these problems.

Postmortem Examinations

Pathologists discuss the radiographs with radiologists, review the antemortem records, and then perform thorough postmortem pathologic examinations at the next station. The radiographs may show surgical materials, contraceptive devices, or other items of personal effects that were overlooked previously, particularly in the case of burned bodies, and allow the pathologist to recover them for further examination. The postmortem examination should be thorough, and the pathologist should record all weights, measurements, and possible identifying features carefully and collect appropriate tissue specimens for possible toxicologic and serologic studies. The toxicologic examination of tissues or body fluids may reveal the presence of medications that the investigator can correlate with medical records to confirm identification.

Anthropologic and histologic procedures may also be necessary for identification, but this requirement will depend on the availability of antemortem data for comparison. Because the pathologist frequently will not know until some later time whether antemortem data will be available, he or she should consider collecting appropriate measurements and specimens of bone and tissue.

Documentation of body characteristics may serve to further narrow the possibilities of the identity of the deceased. The value of separating tall from short persons is obvious, but investigators often overlook the possibilities for comparing hat size, sleeve length, neck size, waist and inseam length, and shoe size. Measurements that may be affected by postmortem effects on soft tissue must be interpreted with great caution, but they are nevertheless of value in the subjective evaluation of the victims.

Many people have unique identifying body characteristics as a result of exposure to the environment. Other body characteristics may not necessarily be identifying, but they may facilitate further categorization. Categorizing characteristics include surgical scars (such as from an appendectomy), circumcision, and pierced ears, and many tattoos and scars are unique.

The investigator may compare hair obtained from a pillow or comb in a person's home to head hair on an unidentified body. The characteristics of an ear may be compared with those in an antemortem photograph or fingernail clippings found in the home with fingernails on the body. The use of these techniques is less common, and they tend to be last-ditch efforts.

Anthropologic Observations

The direct observation of findings in skeletonized remains (i.e., without resort to the techniques of radiology) may be possible. The investigator can determine age, race, sex, and stature from the interpretation of skeletal remains. Even in intact bodies, the pathologist may excise the pubic symphysis by using a saw and examine the opposing faces of the pubic bones for the presence of parturition pits, indicating a past pregnancy, or to determine age.

DNA

Recent advances in application of laboratory comparison testing of antemortem and postmortem specimens for DNA are encouraging. This new technique is especially important since fewer people have fingerprint records on file, and water flouridation and improved dental care result in fewer readily identifiable dental characteristics. One of the principle advantages of DNA identification techniques is that they can be used with very small tissue samples. Until very recently, DNA analysis was used only to reassociate body parts. However, the U.S. military has been collecting blood and oral swab samples from military personnel into a data repository since 1992, making DNA identification one of the most promising techniques for the future. The theoretical accuracy of DNA identification is much more reliable than any other method. Although some of the laboratory procedures still require particular care, the examinations yield very reliable results for identification when conducted carefully by trained personnel.

Personal Effects

Personal effects can provide clues to identity. These helpful materials may vary from specific information such as identification cards containing photographs and fingerprints to less specific items such as jewelry, clothing labels, and watches. Careful chain-of-custody throughout the identification process is important. Photographs are helpful for documenting each item, and the investigator can circulate the photographs among the identification groups or show them to relatives without having to handle the actual material excessively.

Laboratory Examination of Tissue

The investigator first examines the tissue grossly to determine its general appearance, texture, consistency, and the presence of any odor. This may allow him to determine whether the

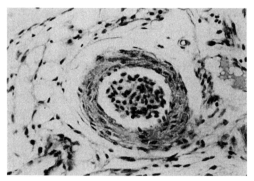

Figure 28.5. Nucleated erythrocytes from bird-strike accident (Armed Forces Institute of Pathology photo).

material is tissue and, if so, whether it is human and what part of the body it is from (12). The pathologist may be able to determine whether materials found at the crash site are mammalian by examining them under the microscope. The erythrocytes of all species other than mammals have nuclei. Figure 28.5 illustrates the nucleated erythrocytes from tissue found at the site of an accident caused by a bird strike. Serologic studies may be helpful (some of these are described later in the chapter).

The intensive effort during this data-collection phase is critical. With tissue, observations must be documented as quickly as possible before postmortem changes obscure them. The lack of suitable antemortem data for comparison will make much of the postmortem information useless, but the investigators risk incorrect identification of some of the casualties if they fail to document all possible identifying features.

Application of Identification Techniques

Certain techniques, such as the comparison of fingerprint, dental, and DNA records, are more reliable and provide definitive identifications directly. On the other end of the reliability scale are such characteristics as height, weight, skin color, and hair color that may be subjective, difficult to measure, and are subject to change; however, even combinations of these subjective characteristics may provide reliable and, in some

cases, the only identification. The "odd-man-out" method (described in the Techniques section) is a practical screening technique that can lead to identification in carefully selected instances even in the absence of identifying features. The careful application of these techniques and avoidance of the pitfalls will enable even the inexperienced investigator to collect valuable information to simplify and shorten the identification process.

A method of identification can be successful only if it adequately meets each of the following three requirements: The body feature must be unique, it must be attached to the body, and a suitable antemortem record must exist. Uniqueness, attachment, and what constitutes a record can vary. While fingerprints are singularly unique, the presence of pierced ears is not. Teeth are attached to the body, but personal effects such as jewelry can be removed. Antemortem records can vary from vague personal recollections to records prepared specifically for the purpose of casualty identification.

Certainty of Identification

One issue in the course of the mass disaster identification process is how certain the identification of each victim must be. How positive are the investigators that they have made correct identifications? As a practical matter, in some disasters, in which bodies are severely fragmented and burned or little antemortem information is available for comparison, identification of all of the casualties may not be possible.

Hardly a person has not at some time seen an apparent acquaintance at a distance only to find on closer observation that the identification was incorrect. Perhaps this occurred because the physical resemblance between the suspected and actual persons was great or because the observer based his or her determination on limited information. An observer can seldom be certain about identification when he or she observes only a part of the whole. For example, the identification of a known person from the posterior aspects of the head is possible, but this identification is not usually as reliable as when the observer makes the identification after seeing the person's face. Hair length is no longer a reliable basis for distinguishing males from females.

The reasons for the certainty in identification are more than academic. Of course, social and moral reasons pressure the investigator to identify casualties and return them to their families. In different societies, pressure may be expressed in a variety of ways. Some cultures are meticulous in the desire to identify all casualties with certainty; in other cultures, the pressure is more to release a body to the family before some religious deadline. In the latter circumstance, it often seems that the desire is for the determination of certainty of death rather than for the certainty of identity of each individual body. Some governments have issued individual death certificates on the basis of the aircraft manifests and held mass burials when they presumed that all persons on board were dead.

Careless identification techniques can initiate a parade of horrors. The problems usually begin with insurance claims, survivors benefits, and other disposition of personal property. In one case, the haste in providing early identification and release of the body of a prominent political figure was for naught. Investigators had to have the body exhumed when it was discovered that they had incorrectly identified it. Cases of borrowed clothing and dog tags have also occurred. The importance of clearly understanding the distinction between definitive and supportive evidence of identity is readily apparent.

An important question that the investigator must answer at the onset of the investigation is, "How, with all of the various methods of identification that are available, can I most efficiently achieve certainty of identification of these casualties?" Four general categories of procedures are available: definitive, secondary, cumulative, and confirmatory. Obviously, any one procedure may fall into more than one of these categories, depending on the circumstances in which it is used.

Definitive Methods

The methods of identification that stand alone as means of identification are definitive methods. Theoretically, these methods assume that only one person can have a particular set of characteristics. As a practical matter, investigators can seldom, if ever, achieve this degree of certainty. As a result, they tend to settle for a degree of certainty of identification on the basis that the probability of any other person having those particular characteristics is low. Labels in dental restorations that contain the deceased's name and identifying number are examples of "absolutely" definitive methods of identification. Of course, even this evidence is not 100% reliable, unless the investigator is certain that the deceased or the preparer had no motive to falsify the identity, that no mistakes occurred in the antemortem preparation of the labels or in the postmortem examination process, and that the antemortem records are correct.

All methods of identification involve the comparison of observed characteristics of the bodies with known or reported characteristics of persons missing or presumed to be dead, and definitive identification of a person occurs when investigators identify a sufficient number of objective features that belong to the missing person and only to that person. Theoretically, two people may have certain characteristics that are similar enough to be identical for all practical purposes. For this reason, the investigator must assign a degree of probability to each method of identification. The greater the number of identical characteristics found, the more certain the probability that the identification is correct. For example, the probability is much greater if 25 matching fingerprint or dental characteristics are present than if the only comparable feature is blood type A.

How many presumptive correlations are necessary to approximate a definitive identification? No set number applies unequivocally to all circumstances. Correlation of three characteristics such as height, weight, and hair color usually are not as corroborative as the correlation of the evidence of surgery and other scars, congenital defects, and dental restorations. On the other hand, if only one of the missing persons weighed over 150 pounds, and if he or she happened to weigh 250 pounds, this might be a very significant identifying characteristic indeed.

A high degree of negative correlation may also be of great value in limiting the number of persons under consideration. For example, if investigators determine that 20% of the victims have blood type A, the missing persons known to have blood types AB, B or O are not likely to provide a match.

Secondary Methods

Secondary methods of identification are those methods which use characteristics that could belong to more than one person and which, therefore, do not by themselves give a high degree of probability of certainty of identification. On the other hand, in many instances, secondary methods that are considered by themselves to have a low probability may, in fact, provide almost certain identification. Secondary methods are most useful when they are used in combination with the cumulative methods described in the following section. Examples of secondary materials and characteristics are age, sex, hair color, and color and type of clothing. Secondary methods can give highly reliable results, but the positivity seldom approaches that of the definitive methods. The limited value of determining that the sex of an unidentified body is male when all of the missing persons are male is easy to appreciate; likewise, a similar determination is of little assistance when half of a large group of missing persons are male. On the other hand, the finding of a male body is highly significant when only one male is missing.

Cumulative Methods

Especially when using secondary methods of identification, the investigator needs to somehow increase the probability that identifications are correct. Using the cumulative methods to analyze several secondary characteristics, the com-

Table 28.1.
Example of the Cumulative Identification Method

Victim	Sex	Dental Data
Person A	M	Edentulous
Person B	M	Present
Person C	F	Edentulous

bined probability of certainty of identification increases. In the hypothetic example in Table 28.1, finding a male body cannot result in definitive identification; similarly, finding an edentulous body cannot result in definitive identification. A male body could be either person A or person B, and an edentulous body could be either person A or person C. But by cumulating these findings, assuming that these three bodies do, in fact, represent three missing persons, an edentulous male body can be only person A. Thus, methods that have an inherently low probability of definitive identification can be combined using cumulative techniques to provide certain identification.

Fingerprint identification is a widely used method of definitive identification, but this technique is actually an example of the cumulative identification methods. The theoretical possibility of any two persons having identical sets of fingerprints depends on the degree of cumulation used. Dental examination, another of the commonly used means of ''positive'' identification, also could be considered a cumulative method, and one could likewise calculate degrees of certainty of this identification method.

Confirmatory Methods

The use of confirmatory methods is another variation of the cumulative technique. For example, using the hypothetic situation described in Table 28.1, having identified body A using the cumulative methods, the investigator may find it possible to obtain definitive identification. Fingerprint or dental records may be available for comparison, or, in unusual cases, investigators may obtain latent fingerprints from the missing person's home for comparison.

Selecting the Identification Techniques

How are investigators to select which of these methods to use in particular situations? The practical answer is that they must use every method that they reasonably can in every case. Even in the situation where definitive methods are readily available, investigators must always be on guard against the possibility that there may be an error in the records or the observations.

Missing persons lists are frequently incorrect in at least some aspect. When commercial modes of transportation are involved, these errors are almost a routine occurrence.

Errors may occur because of fraud or mistake; even criminal misconduct may occur. Certain errors may occur as a normal course of business and may not be detected without knowledge of the business practices. When using prenumbered forms for recording observations of the unidentified bodies, an observer can very easily record findings on an incorrect form. When many bodies are involved, especially when identifying features are not readily apparent (as in severely burned bodies), observations may be correctly charted but may be from a different body. Clerks may file records in an incorrect folder or, when using wall charts, may place an "X" in an incorrect column.

How are investigators to avoid the pitfalls that these errors can induce? They cannot entirely. They must always be alert to the possibility that errors may exist, and they must continually take steps to minimize the effect these errors will have on the overall investigation; they should take whatever steps are possible to detect the existence of errors. Investigators should be especially wary of methods that tend to remove a missing person from consideration too early.

From a practical standpoint, three general rules are helpful. First, do the best you can with what is available. Second, do the easiest things first. Finally, don't release a body before making definitive identification.

Data Analysis

Data analysis occurs in the third phase of the investigation, as working groups continue to evaluate the data they collected in the data-collection phase. The investigators who observed the postmortem findings are best suited to analyze the data, but substantially fewer people are necessary. Reducing the total number of personnel by 50% or more is usually possible at this stage.

Analyzing the data consists of integrating the information from the antemortem records and the postmortem observations. Of particular importance is organization of the techniques for recording, charting, and storing antemortem and postmortem data so that investigators can easily find the necessary information. The early installation of appropriate quality control procedures and careful consideration of which identification techniques, such as spotting, mix-and-match, exclusion, or odd-man-out, will be most productive and will increase the efficiency of the data analysis process.

Quality Control

The antemortem records almost invariably contain some inaccuracies, and other errors will probably occur in the observing and recording of postmortem findings. Transposition of left and right occurs frequently in medical records, and estimating the height, weight, sex, or age of fragmented or severely burned bodies can be extremely difficult. Recognizing the probability of these errors caused by human frailty allows the investigator to plan to avoid the most serious pitfall, misidentification as a result of an irreversible error.

Early adoption and strict adherence to quality control procedures will minimize these errors. More than one observer should confirm each postmortem finding, and each of the working groups should reexamine observation notes from the preliminary examination and from other working groups. Each member of the working group should verify all of the postmortem evidence from a matching antemortem record before making an identification, and making this evidence available to all of the other working groups provides an additional measure of control. Rigid adherence to these seemingly tedious and often redundant procedures will save valuable time in the long run.

Morlang (11) described a computer program used to assist in the identification of victims of the 1977 Tenerife disaster, and computers are now becoming as essential as paper and pencils for data collection and analysis. Converting the antemortem and postmortem data to an acceptable format for the computer requires substantial effort. Opportunities to test these computer applications under actual disaster conditions are infrequent, and investigators have been unable to agree on a standard terminology to describe identifying characteristics that the computer will accept. Nevertheless, small, portable, yet powerful computer systems are receiving increasing acceptance, and the logical nature of the procedures in the data analysis phase is ideally suited for their application in facilitating the scientific identification of disaster victims.

Techniques

The methods of analyzing identification data fall into four general categories. Spotting depends on investigators remembering characteristics observed at the postmortem examination when they encounter similar features as they review the antemortem records. The initial review of the records frequently reveals several obvious identities, and investigators may even correctly identify some victims whose postmortem characteristics were recorded incompletely, inaccurately, or perhaps not at all.

Mix-and-match consists of the logical manipulation of the records into groups that have characteristics in common. Selecting all of the casualties that have a particular characteristic in common, such as age, sex, or race; that have dental or fingerprint information available; or that have unique items or personal effects such as rings or watches will allow the investigators

to focus their attention on more likely identification matches. They should prepare lists grouping these possible matches and make their lists available to all of the other working groups for possible confirmation. As this "mixing" occurs, identity "matches" may become apparent, but this preliminary match must not be the sole basis for positive identification.

Identification by exclusion is another data analysis technique, but investigators should apply it with great caution. When two crewmembers are missing and investigators have positively identified one, the temptation is great to conclude that the second body found within the wreckage is the other missing crewmember. This conclusion may be correct in many instances, but it becomes infamously wrong when the missing persons list turns out to be incorrect. Investigators should avoid the temptation to regress to identification by exclusion when the identification process progresses more slowly than expected. They may need to reexamine the bodies or resort to other methods of identification.

Investigators may be able to identify some victims by a process of elimination if they are certain that all of the bodies have been recovered. If they are reasonably certain that the missing persons list corresponds to the identities of the recovered bodies, the problems of identification are much simpler. In this situation, the degree of certainty necessary for identification need not be as great. Identification by exclusion cannot occur, however, unless all of the bodies have been recovered and the list of missing persons is complete.

The exclusion techniques are also useful in other ways. Tables of exclusion are often helpful for the early categorization of identifying features by the mix-and-match method. Determination of sex is usually easy, and this may exclude a large number of possible missing persons from further consideration. The investigators can exclude person C on the basis of sex and person B by the presence of teeth, and the cumulation of these observations greatly increases the probability that the victim in the example in Table 28.1 is person A.

After first applying the best and most positive methods in attempting to identify victims, a few bodies without definite identifiable features may still remain. In these cases, methods that would not otherwise establish identification may be useful when investigators apply them to a large number of bodies using the odd-man-out technique to produce good evidence of identification. Mason (13) proposed the odd-man-out technique for the evaluation of distinctive injury patterns in reconstructing the cause and sequence of events in an aircraft accident. The logic process of Mason's injury analysis technique applies equally to the preliminary identification of fatalities, in which it relies on the cumulation of observations or, in some instances, the absence of certain observations, and in some applications is an extension of the exclusion method of identification.

Initial screening examination of the bodies usually reveals that some of the bodies have characteristics for which the investigators will almost certainly discover comparison data. Pregnancy and the presence of a glass eye or an artificial limb are identifying data that identification questionnaires seldom seek, but finding this information can be extremely valuable. The presence of any one body with features different from all other bodies found in the wreckage sets the odd-man-out process in motion.

Simplification of the identification process by the odd-man-out method does not require that the characteristics be totally unique. If all of the passengers and crew were male except for one female flight attendant, the investigators could presumptively identify the only female body found as the female flight attendant. Investigators occasionally find an identifying feature that almost certainly must be unique—a feature that only one person in the whole world could possibly have—but, unfortunately, will find nothing in any antemortem record of the missing persons to substantiate the characteristic.

Investigators must exercise great care to avoid eliminating a particular body or missing person from consideration prematurely on the basis of a characteristic that was not unique or that was described improperly. This caution applies especially to the application of the exclusion and odd-man-out methods.

Conclusion Phase

The conclusion phase begins when a working group makes a presumptive identification. Other members of the working group check the observations to confirm the presumptive match first and then refer the presumptive match to other working groups, where confirmation will lead to preliminary identification.

The working group may be unable to reach a presumptive identity determination, but their list of possible matches may be helpful to another group. When a second group reviews the list, their observations may provide additional clues to focus on the identities. This aspect of the conclusion phase overlaps somewhat with the data-analysis phase.

Each working group examines all of the data. If they find no inconsistencies, the responsible senior investigator then reviews the observations that support the match before confirming the positive identification. The senior investigator should release no body before each working group reviews the identification data and he or she confirms their determination. Adequate records should reflect this observation and review process.

Recommendation Phase

The recommendation phase involves more than just identification. Usually, investigators must prepare to make other recommendations as well. They must decide when to abandon search efforts for additional bodies or body fragments, especially in circumstances such as disasters at sea, in which rescuers may be unable to recover all of the bodies; they must determine whether, particularly in the case of fragmented bodies, there may have been more victims than persons reported missing and whether continued searches for additional information will be productive. They also must provide other investigators with recommendations about whether to pursue any possibility of foul play as a cause of any of the casualties.

Investigators finally must determine what to do about any unidentified bodies or body parts that remain. They must thoroughly reexamine each of the fragments to ensure that they have not overlooked any clues to identity, and they may be able to match some of these fragments with previously identified bodies by means of blood type, injury patterns, or hair and fingernail characteristics. This problem is another reason for investigators to take special care to document findings and maintain records throughout the identification process.

Investigators should thoroughly document the remaining body fragments using photographs, radiographs, diagrams, and written descriptions. Retaining mandibles, maxillas, and fingers will make subsequent dental and fingerprint comparison possible. The remaining body fragments should be retained for a reasonable period of time, the length of which will depend on the location and condition of the fragments and the likelihood of finding suitable antemortem information for comparison.

Whether to dispose of the remaining fragments or to bury them depends on the bulk of the tissue, whether identifying characteristics are present, and whether the investigation accounted for all of the missing persons. Burial of each unidentified body, or of all associated body parts in the case of fragments, in individual, numbered sites, will facilitate subsequent exhumation should the investigators discover additional identifying information.

INJURY PATTERN ANALYSIS

Determining the sequence of events in an aircraft crash is essential to any crashworthiness investigation, and injury pattern analysis focuses on

that determination. Various combinations of injuries form certain characteristic patterns that relate to the sequence of events in the accident, and careful analysis of these patterns often explains otherwise obscure circumstances of an accident. Trauma, the environment, and preexisting diseases are the significant factors the investigator must consider.

Tolerance and Injury

The tolerance of each part of the body to injury varies considerably. The force may have no residual effect, may result in minor injury, or may produce irreversible or even lethal injuries. The ultimate consequences of force that amputates an arm are quite different from those of force that, when applied to the neck, results in decapitation.

Although humans have a definable tolerance to injury, much confusion exists in the literature as to what constitutes an acceptable degree of injury. One controversy concerns whether greater effort should be spent on preventing fatal injuries rather than less serious ones. The number of fatalities from crashes is relatively small compared with the number of injuries, and the total cost of treating the injuries is much greater than the cost of dealing with the fatalities. Accepting some fatalities may be the price paid to reduce more frequent and costly injuries.

The better approach gives equal consideration to the prevention of injuries and fatalities. Although evaluation of the injury tolerance issues may appear difficult, the investigator must avoid any first impulse, when confronted with fragmented bodies and wreckage, to conclude that survival would have been impossible.

Injury Pattern

An injury pattern is simply the enumeration of injuries that a victim sustained during or as a result of a crash. After investigators determine the specific event that caused each injury pattern, they can prepare charts to use in comparing the pattern of injuries observed in one person with those seen in others. They can compare the injury patterns of casualties in the same aircraft accident or compare the injury patterns in one accident with injuries observed in another crash. Finding many burned bodies near an exit in an aircraft destroyed by fire suggests malfunction of the exit, and bodies or parts of the aircraft located far from the main wreckage suggests breakup of the aircraft in flight.

Investigators must document each injury pattern carefully and correlate it with the circumstances of the accident. This information is essential to making any modifications that will prevent similar injuries in the future. Because few injuries are specific for aircraft accidents, accident investigators may apply general forensic pathology techniques in interpreting the injuries.

A number of factors directly influence the specific injuries and patterns of injury. Decelerative forces, environmental factors, and the structural configuration of the aircraft produce injuries. Incisions, lacerations, fractures, thermal injuries, and interference with respiration are specific types of injuries, but the severity of each injury may range from minimal to fatal.

The most difficult problems facing investigators are the determinations of (1) exactly when an injury occurred, (2) the nature of the force that produced the injury, and (3) whether the observed injuries are the result of the impact forces or an artificial change induced by the postcrash environment. Did the injury occur before or after death, or did it perhaps even exist before the crash occurred? How much force was required to produce the injury, and how was the force applied? Is the injury pattern misleading, being in fact something other than what it appears to be?

Injuries have misled investigators because they erroneously appeared to be classic, diagnostic accident injury patterns when they were actually caused by entirely different factors or were artifactual. These preexisting injuries and artifacts are probably the most frequent cause of erroneous interpretations of injury patterns and the sequence of events in the crash.

Injury patterns and specific injuries are directly related to the following:

1. The magnitude, duration, direction, and pulse shape of the acceleration forces;
2. The cockpit or passenger compartment configuration;
3. The nature of the accident and subsequent occurrences;
4. The occupant kinematics in the accident, particularly those relating to the restraint systems.

Acceleration Forces

The magnitude, duration, direction, and pulse shape of acceleration forces affect the pattern of injuries and are major factors in determining injury tolerance. Certain levels of force produce minimal injury, whereas greater force may produce transient injuries. Still greater force may produce irreversible injury or even death.

Eiband (14) suggested that the magnitude of tolerable acceleration is inversely related to the duration of its application. Human volunteers tolerated acceleration forces of great magnitude for short periods of time. Colonel John P. Stapp experienced more than $45 - G_x$ on a rocket sled. Early ejection system experiments exposed human subjects to more than $25 + G_z$, with vertebral fractures as the only resulting injuries.

Many people have survived apparently impossible circumstances of high G deceleration such as falls of more than 300 m. The factors that contributed to survival in these cases are poorly defined, but perhaps the high velocity resulted in reduced pulse duration and increased tolerance. By contrast, only 1 G in the $- G_z$ acceleration field may be fatal within a period of several hours. These two examples, representing the extremes of the acceleration scale, illustrate the complexity of the problems associated with tolerance to acceleration.

Cockpit or Passenger Compartment Configuration

The configuration of the compartment may restrict expeditious exit after the crash. The occupant may strike some part of the cockpit or passenger compartment and sustain fatal injuries in what would have otherwise been a survivable accident. Loose objects set in motion by the crash forces may strike the occupant, or he or she may strike the fuselage or be crushed by it or by other objects in the immediate vicinity. The likelihood of injuries increases significantly if external objects penetrate the occupant space or if the space is crushed by the crash forces. Engine, transmission, and still-turning rotor blades may penetrate the occupant space and cause fatal injuries during helicopter crashes.

Nature of the Accident

The nature of the accident and subsequent events will explain many injury patterns. In general, the types of injuries seen in helicopter accidents are different from those that result from crashes of fighter or large transport aircraft. This is due in large part to the differences in operational activities of each of these aircraft.

The nature of the accident and the sequence of events influence the character and severity of crewmember injuries after ejection from an aircraft. Bird strikes, in-flight explosion, striking part of the aircraft or ejection seat after exiting the aircraft, parachute-opening deceleration, or impacts during or after landing may produce similar injury patterns. Investigators must seek trace evidence such as paint scrapings or tissue fragments from suspected contact points to reconstruct the sequence of events.

Mason (12) suggested the odd-man-out technique for the evaluation of injuries. He compared injuries received by multiple fatalities in a single crash with those received by fatalities in separate crashes and looked for similarities in injury patterns. If investigators find dissimilar injury patterns, they must determine what the individuals with each injury pattern were doing that was different. Finding cabin crewmember injury patterns that are similar to passenger injury patterns suggests that the cabin was prepared for the crash, but dissimilar injury patterns would indicate that the occupants may not have anticipated the crash. The finding of leg fractures may explain why many occupants did not exit the aircraft, even though fire may not have developed until many minutes after the crash.

Occupant Kinematics

Many factors influence the trajectory an occupant follows during a crash. The magnitude and direction of the acceleration vector, the shape of the acceleration pulse, the amount of crushable material in the aircraft, and the nature of the seat and restraint systems can vary the trajectory considerably and greatly influence the force applied to the occupant. Investigators must evaluate all of these factors carefully before reconstructing the occupant kinematics during the crash. Special techniques, such as computer simulation, may be helpful.

Various types of protective devices and equipment, such as specially designed seats and other restraint systems, helmets, and protective clothing, frequently modify injury patterns. Most protective systems have many components, and the failure or inadequate design of almost any of these system elements can exponentially increase the force applied to the occupant and lead to injury or death. If an attachment point of a seat to the basic structure fails, the occupant will feel an acceleration force of shorter duration but of much greater magnitude. Force magnification also occurs when the restraint system fails or, because of elasticity or plasticity, allows the occupant's motion to extend to lethal areas outside the protective envelope.

Traumatic Injuries

Head Injuries

Head injuries are the most frequent cause of death in aircraft accident victims. These injuries often result when the head, neck, and upper torso flex over a lap belt because they are unrestrained by a shoulder harness system. This allows the unprotected head, chest, and extremities to strike exposed structures, resulting in serious or fatal injuries.

The skull provides reasonable protection to the cranial contents, but an impact that damages the integrity of the cranial system or transmits the impact force to particularly sensitive areas is often fatal. Concentrations of impact force are particularly lethal, and designs that distribute the force greatly increase the magnitude of the impact the head can withstand.

Certain preventive measures can reduce, if not entirely prevent, these head injuries. Helmets can provide energy absorption and distribute the impact force, and shoulder restraint systems can reduce the range within which the head could strike cockpit objects. Aircraft designers can avoid introducing possible injurious impact surfaces into the cockpit during the development phase.

Linear fractures of the skull tend to occur in the plane in which the force was applied. This has sometimes led investigators to believe erroneously that transverse fractures of the base of the skull, extending from ear to ear and across the sella turcica, could result only from a blow to the side of the head (Fig. 28.6). At least as

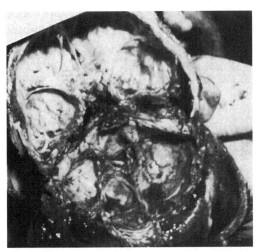

Figure 28.6. Transverse fracture of the base of the skull (Armed Forces Institute of Pathology photo).

frequent a cause of the transverse fractures, however, are blows to the bottom of the skull, transmitted via the mandibular rami when the face impacts with an instrument panel.

Ring fractures, fractures around the circumference of the foramen magnum, may result from force transmitted up the spine in $+G_z$ impacts. Although this fracture pattern can occur from force transmitted from a blow to the top of the head, this possibility is rare. Because the center of gravity of the skull is forward of the spine, a blow to the top of the head tends to produce flexion, resulting in asymmetric application of force to the foramen magnum. This results in anterior cervical fracture and Jefferson's fracture (see Spinal Injuries section) rather than ring fractures.

Skull fractures tend to be subtle, and investigators may not be able to see them without careful observation. They must meticulously remove the dura before concluding that no skull fractures are present. Blunt trauma of greater magnitude may produce eggshell fractures of the skull. Even more severe impact, especially when the upper torso is not restrained or when the upper-torso restraint system fails, results in partial or complete decapitation.

Head injuries sometimes mislead investigators if they rely on examination of the strike envelope alone in considering the possible causes of the injuries. They should consider the possibility that collapse of the aircraft structure or impact with loose objects produced the injury. Figure 28.7 illustrates such a case. The pilot of a small, single-engine plane received fatal head injuries during the crash. Brain tissue was on the instrument panel, and investigators found imprints of the knobs and instrument dials on the pilot's face. The investigators believed that the pilot did not have an upper-torso restraint system available, and they suspected that this deficiency allowed his upper torso to flex forward and his head to strike the instrument panel, which resulted in the fatal head injuries. Examination of the cockpit of the wrecked aircraft, however, clearly indicated that the injuries resulted from

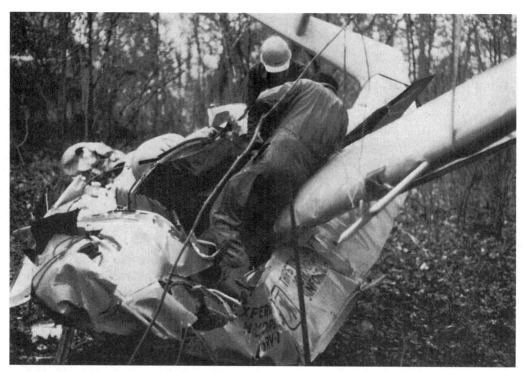

Figure 28.7. Buckling of fuselage at impact was the primary cause of injuries in this accident (Armed Forces Institute of Pathology photo).

the pilot's head being crushed between the instrument panel and the aft overhead cockpit bulkhead despite use of shoulder harness restraint. This occurred when the aircraft fuselage buckled at impact.

Unusual head injuries may lead to erroneous conclusions, especially when the investigator is not fully cognizant of the circumstances of the accident. Figure 28.8 is a photograph of a crewman who walked into the tail rotor of a helicopter. Figure 28.9 illustrates a blowout fracture of the skull from increased intracranial pressure that resulted from steam production as the postcrash fire heated the skull.

Internal Injuries

Crash forces can damage the internal organs of the chest and abdomen by any of several mechanisms, and this damage may result in death if prompt medical and surgical assistance is not available. Because the internal organs are relatively unrestrained and are suspended only by attachments within the chest and abdomen, they move during the impact sequence in a manner that may be quite different from the deceleration of the body as a whole. This frequently means that decelerative forces acting on these organs are much greater than those acting on other, more restrained body parts. Internal tears may be caused by shearing forces applied as a result of differences in the mass of various tissues, and organ asymmetry may introduce torsional forces.

The direct application of force to internal organs as a result of penetration of the body cavities by external objects or as a result of impact with cockpit structures or seat belts can cause serious injuries. Overlying bony structures, such as the ribs and pelvis, provide a measure of protection to many of the internal organs, but other organs are more vulnerable.

The ribs, sternum, scapulae, and thoracic vertebrae, being bony structures, protect the organs of the chest. Application of about 2250 kg of

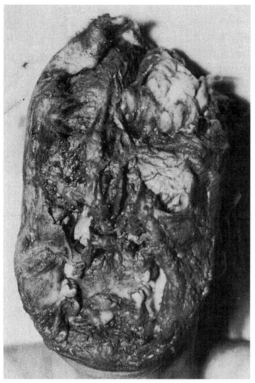

Figure 28.8. Head injury as a result of walking into the tail rotor of a helicopter (Armed Forces Institute of Pathology photo).

force by a restraint belt may produce rib fractures. The jagged ends of a broken rib may lacerate the heart and lungs and even some of the abdominal organs such as the spleen, kidneys, and liver.

Approximately 13% of aircraft accident fatal-

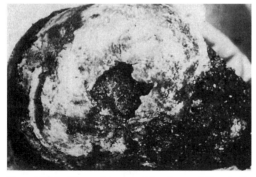

Figure 28.9. Steam blow-out fracture of the skull (Armed Forces Institute of Pathology photo).

ities involve significant cardiovascular injury. Missiles, broken ribs, or portions of the aircraft cockpit or controls may penetrate the chest and puncture the heart or major blood vessels. The heart or great blood vessels may burst as a result of being compressed between the sternum and vertebrae or from force transmitted from compression of the chest and abdomen. Once adequately designed cockpit enclosures, torso restraints, and head protection systems are in use, the tolerance of the cardiovascular system will determine the magnitude of the decelerative force that humans can survive.

Tears of the aorta are frequent findings in air-crash fatalities who have little external evidence of injury, and the pathologist must carefully examine the heart and the aorta in situ and avoid introducing artifactual lacerations. Aortic rupture as an isolated finding is more common just distal to the left subclavian artery, but in cases of cardiac injury, 65% of the tears are in the ascending aorta just above the aortic valve. The origins of the subclavian and carotid blood vessels at the aortic arch provide relatively fixed attachment points for the heart and descending aorta, and even if a restraint system prevents significant movement of the upper torso, decelerative force may cause the heart and descending aorta to swing forward, like pendulums, during a crash. Because the heart is asymmetric (because the left ventricle is more muscular than the right ventricle), the deceleration may concentrate torsional forces and produce tears in the ascending aorta. Concentration of the shearing forces that result from the different deceleration rates of the heart and descending aorta from deceleration of the aortic arch produces tears of the ascending and descending aorta near the insertions of the ligamentum arteriosum.

Blunt force applied to the abdomen can produce lacerations, tears, or rupture of the abdominal organs, and blunt trauma to the thorax or abdomen may rupture the diaphragm. Although both liver and spleen receive some protection from the rib cage, the liver is the more vulnerable of the two organs to impact injury. An improperly positioned or loosely fitted seat belt or a soft seat cushion may allow a seat occupant to slide under, or "submarine" beneath, the restraint system. This increases the frequency of spinal fractures and rupture of abdominal viscera.

Spinal Injuries

Examination of the spine provides the investigator with especially valuable information, particularly the evidence needed to determine the direction and magnitude of impact.

Vertebral fracture occurs frequently with vertical forces ($+g_z$) greater than about 20 g. Compression fractures of vertebrae occur from the imposition of high $+g_z$ forces, especially in ejections from fighter aircraft or hard landings in helicopters. Two thirds of subjects sustain vertebral fracture at g levels greater than $+26$ g_z, but vertebral fracture can occur at forces as low as 10 to 12 g, especially when the positioning of the spine is not entirely vertical. Multiple compression fractures in one individual are unusual and seldom occur at levels less than $+35$ g_z.

g_y or g_x forces in excess of 250 to 400 g may produce shearing fractures of the vertebrae, especially in high-speed crashes (Fig. 28.10). The mass of the more dense vertebral end-plate, which is greater than the mass of the vertebra, may contribute to this injury pattern. When crash force is applied, this inertia creates much the same situation as can be shown by the elementary demonstration of inertia in which a book is placed on a piece of paper to illustrate that the paper can be removed without dislodging the book.

Pure compression fractures ($+g_z$), shearing fractures ($+/-g_x$ or $+/-g_y$), or Chance fractures ($-g_z$) are rarely seen. Most vertebral fractures result from combined x, y, and z force vectors but especially from the x-axis and z-axis. This causes a fracture pattern much like that which would be produced by a crowbar—with compression of the anterior portion of the vertebra and pulling apart of the posterior bony or

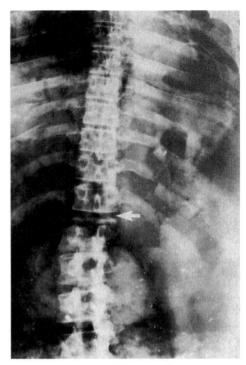

Figure 28.10. Shearing fracture of vertebra (Armed Forces Institute of Pathology photo).

ligamentous portions in tension (Fig. 28.11). This results because the force vector effectively places the fulcrum in the anterior portion of a vertebra.

Various crash circumstances may apply force to the neck and cervical vertebrae, causing

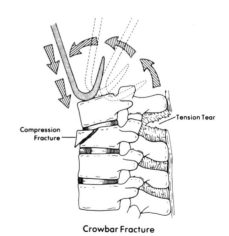

Crowbar Fracture

Figure 28.11. Mechanism producing crowbar fracture of vertebra.

fractures and dislocations. Windblast during ejection from an aircraft may cause the aviator's protective helmet to rotate and the edge of the helmet to strike the neck, much like a guillotine, causing fracture or dislocation of cervical vertebrae. Aircraft wiring and parachute lines entangling the neck are examples of mechanisms that result in "hangman's" fractures of the pedicles of the C-2 vertebra (Fig. 28.12). Impact to the top of the head may cause Jefferson's fracture, which consists of vertical splitting of the ring or lateral masses of the C-1 vertebra and lateral displacement of fragments of the vertebral body. Dissection of the anterior and posterior neck, followed by careful examination, is often helpful in these cases.

Injuries of the Extremities

Injuries to the extremities result from the flailing of unrestrained extremities and from impact with structures; these injuries are seldom fatal unless complicated by other factors. Excessive loss of blood may result from multiple injuries, and injuries of the extremities may prevent or impair escape from a hazardous postcrash environment.

Flailing of arms and legs during ejection from an aircraft may generate sufficient force to cause fractures. The flailing motion, much like that of cracking a whip, concentrates the force more distally, producing fractures of the tibia, fibula, radius, and ulna more frequently than of the femur and humerus. Femoral fractures may result from force applied by the anterior edge of the ejection seat.

Unrestrained extremities may contact aircraft structures within the strike envelope with sufficient force to produce injuries. The legs and arms may strike the instrument panel or a seat in front. "Dashboard femoral fracture" may result from the knee impacting with the instrument panel. Although extremity injuries are of little help in estimating the impact velocity and the parameters of the crash pulse, they may produce patterns that will indicate to the investigator exactly what structure the occupant struck.

Injury patterns of the hands and feet may provide good evidence of who was controlling the aircraft at the time of the crash, especially if other data, such as trace evidence, correlate with the patterns of injury. The best evidence of control is fracture of carpal, metacarpal, tarsal, and metatarsal bones, with associated patterned lacerations of the palms and soles of the hands and feet. Coltart (15) described "aviator's astragalus," fractures of the talar neck in pilots of aircraft with toebrakes. Fractures of the phalanges may be helpful indicators of control, but they are less reliable. Dummit and Reid (16) described unique tibial shaft fractures in helicopter pilots. Similar tibial fractures also occur in pilots of other aircraft.

Environmental Factors

Environmental factors can contribute to the cause of an accident, can cause injuries, and can modify the appearance of injuries. Bird strikes, adverse weather conditions, hypoxia, fire, and water are some of the most significant hazards.

Bird Strikes

Each year, many aircraft collide with birds in flight. These collisions are significant, especially when they involve larger birds, supersonic aircraft, or the ingestion of birds into an engine.

Determination of a bird strike as an event is seldom difficult if investigators examine the wreckage carefully. Even in the most severe cases, they can find remnants of the bird. An ornithologist, on examining the feathers, bone, or other fragments of a bird, can often determine the species and sex and estimate its age and weight. Laboratory personnel can examine fragments of tissue microscopically for nucleated erythrocytes and can perform other serologic tests.

Weather

Turbulence, thunderstorms, and temperature extremes are examples of weather conditions that can influence the course of events in an

Figure 28.12. Cervical fracture resulting from entanglement with helmet microphone cord. (A) Anterior dissection; (B) Posterior dissection (Armed Forces Institute of Pathology photos).

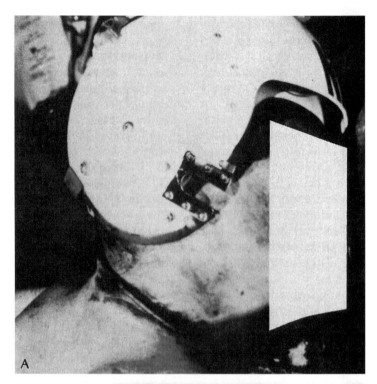

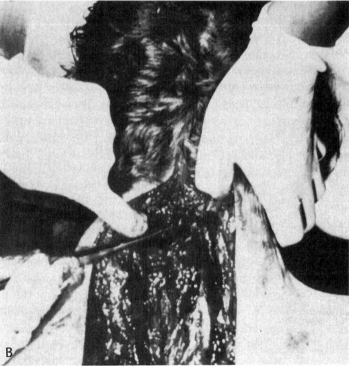

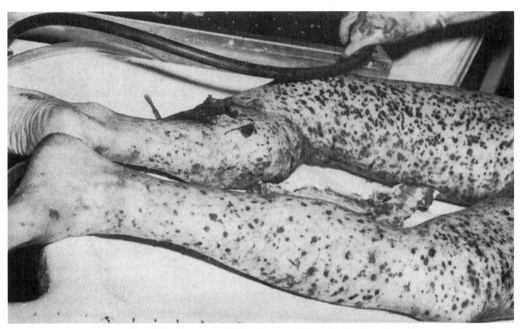

Figure 28.13. Injuries resulting from impact with hailstones after ejection in a thunderstorm (Armed Forces Institute of Pathology photo).

accident. Turbulent weather conditions can produce in-flight breakup of the aircraft. If some of the occupants are thrown from the aircraft as a result, as in the case of the Comet disasters, they will have different injury patterns, due to falling from altitude, than those who remained inside the aircraft.

Thunderstorms are a source of extreme turbulence, hail, and electrical activity. The cold temperatures at altitude and the lifting energy and moisture of thunderstorms combine to create hailstones up to several inches in diameter. These hailstones can damage lifting surfaces, cause engines to fail, and break windscreens. They also may be responsible for some abrasions and contusions in crewmembers after ejection in or near a thunderstorm. The effects of striking these hailstones is not as serious as the injuries inflicted on the crewmembers by the same extreme turbulent force that hurls hailstones thousands of feet in the air (Fig. 28.13) (13).

Many persons on the ground have died after being struck by lightning, but few similar deaths have occurred in occupants of aircraft. The electrical discharge passes primarily along the surface rather than through the center of a conductor. This "skin effect" diverts the electrical charge over the surface of the aircraft and protects the occupants except in a very few cases. Deaths have occurred in occupants of small planes and gliders, especially fabric-covered craft, that have passed directly in the path of a lightning discharge. Pinpoint burns of entry and exit, an arborization pattern of cutaneous erythema, and deposits from the arcing of electrical discharge along zippers and other metal objects among personal effects are evidence of a lightning strike.

Hypoxia

Hypoxia may occur suddenly, as in cases of rapid decompression at high altitude, or may be more insidious, as in prolonged flight at intermediate altitudes of 3000 to 4500 m (10,000 to 15,000 ft). Information such as flight-planned altitude and radio transmissions provide key clues to suggest the incapacitation of crewmembers by hypoxia, and the laboratory determination of lactic acid in the brain will provide confirmation.

Fire

In-flight fires, impact "flash" fires, and post-crash fires produce characteristic patterns. In-flight fires produce streaming patterns of soot deposition, usually seen best on aircraft surfaces rather than in the bodies of the victims. Flash fires, as from the fireball of ignited fuel at impact, produce first- and second-degree burns of unprotected skin surfaces. The interpretation of injury patterns in the case of a postcrash fire is much more difficult.

Burn fatalities occur when occupants have insufficient time to escape because of the rapid onset and propagation of fire, when incapacitating injuries prevent them from exiting the aircraft, when exits are jammed or obstructed, when personal protective equipment is inadequate, or when rescue and fire-suppression efforts are ineffective. The investigator must answer the following key questions:

1. Was the victim alive at the time of impact?
2. Was the victim incapacitated by preexisting disease, medications, toxic gases, or fire injury before impact?
3. Were the burns received post mortem; that is, were fatal injuries sustained at impact, with the burns occurring after death?
4. Did death occur because the victim was unable to exit the aircraft because of injury, toxic gas, smoke, or problems with emergency egress systems before being overcome by smoke and fire?

The most difficult determination is whether burn injuries occurred after death, yet the answer to this question is often the most important. Whether the burns resulting from the postcrash fire or the injuries inflicted by the impact were more responsible for the victim's death influences whether the investigator recommends improvements of egress systems and fire preven-

tion or of seats, restraint systems, and structural design.

The occurrence of burn injuries in U.S. Air Force aircraft accident victims increased from 27.4 to 40.2% from 1953 to 1967, and injuries from fire as the primary cause of death increased from 6.7 to 17.0% (17). Burns as the primary cause of death in U.S. Army aircraft victims also increased, from about 25% in 1957 to more than 40% in 1969, but the installation of a crashworthy fuel system on board Army UH-1 helicopters has virtually eliminated burn injuries as a cause of death in crashes of these helicopters. This is a dramatic illustration of the importance of the correct interpretation of whether burns occurred before or after death.

Laboratory determination of lactic acid levels in the brain and of blood carboxyhemoglobin saturation may be of value in determining whether a crash victim was alive during the postcrash fire. The pathologist may also examine the respiratory system grossly for soot deposits and microscopically for a conclusive histologic response to combustion products of the fire.

Inexperienced investigators often conclude that fire-related postmortem artifactual changes were antemortem injuries. Heat-induced muscle contraction causes the body to assume a pugilistic attitude, as if the victim were protecting himself from the fire. The strongest muscle groups prevail, resulting in flexion of the hips, knees, and elbows but hyperextension of the neck. These heat contractions of muscles are frequently strong enough to produce bone fractures at the muscle attachment points. Rectangular bone fragments are characteristic in heat fractures of long bones.

Increased intracranial steam pressure that results from heating of the skull in a fire may produce blow-out fractures that appear similar to an impact injury. Finding bone fragments within the cranial cavity may help distinguish these fractures. Heating of the skull may also force blood into the extradural space, creating the appearance of extradural hemorrhage. Exposure of the skin to gasoline or other aviation fuels produces epidermolysis, skin bullae, erythema, and the artifactual appearance of burn injury.

The investigator can usually relate the cutaneous burn pattern to protective equipment or to specific agents. Location of flare guns and oxygen bottles may provide clues to the cause of localized, severe burns. Extra thickness of clothing, such as pockets, belts, and waistbands, provide extra protection from burns.

Water

Postcrash survival in water is difficult. Drowning is a frequent cause of death after an aircraft crashes into water, but the exact frequency is difficult to estimate. No one autopsy finding or laboratory test is diagnostic of drowning; the investigator must consider many factors before reaching this diagnosis, largely by excluding other diagnoses. Nevertheless, the correct determination of whether death occurred from drowning or from impact injuries is important.

A few of the external autopsy findings associated with drowning are a mushroom of froth in the nose and mouth and, occasionally, petechial hemorrhages beneath the conjunctiva. Prolonged exposure produces wrinkling of skin, so-called washerwoman's skin, but this finding may occur after death and is not an indicator of drowning. Internal findings include dilated blood vessels engorged with dark-red blood that does not clot, congested lungs with petechial hemorrhages, and hemorrhage into the temporal bones. Microscopic examination may detect diatoms in blood or tissues, but this finding is of little value without comparison with samples of the water from the crash site. Laboratory tests to compare the concentrations of various electrolytes in the blood from the left and right sides of the heart and to determine lactic acid concentration in the brain may be helpful (these tests are discussed in the Blood Electrolytes and Brain Lactic Acid sections).

PREEXISTING DISEASES

Pilots are not immune to the wide variety of diseases that affect the general population. The literature contains reports of almost every imaginable disease process, including a congenital anomaly, cardiovascular disease, neoplasm, and infection, causing a crash; however, the selection criteria, physical standards, and frequent medical supervision of flight crews probably detect most preexisting disease before an acute catastrophic health condition occurs in flight. The accident investigator is more likely to encounter what most people consider minor disease processes.

Did the disease cause the accident? The investigator will want to answer this question. Minor diseases play a much greater role in causing accidents than most investigators have been willing to accept, and diseases that remain undisclosed at autopsy, such as epilepsy and cardiac arrhythmias, are of particular concern.

Detection of Preexisting Disease

After an accident, the first suspicion that preexisting disease may be present often comes from examining the medical records of the crew. Examination of their medical records early in the course of the accident investigation, certainly prior to the autopsy examination, can be a valuable time-saving step. In fact, the documentation of some preexisting conditions may require special techniques that the pathologist would not usually employ, and if the medical records are not available until after the autopsy has been completed, the pathologist may be unable to identify a suspected preexisting disease.

A careful, complete autopsy usually will disclose any preexisting injury or disease that is present, but even when the cause of death appears obvious, the investigator must be alert for underlying preexisting conditions. Although the pathologist can easily detect most preexisting diseases by gross examination of the tissues, the discovery or confirmation of some conditions will require toxicologic or microscopic examination. Histologic examination may be the only way to determine whether a contusion occurred days or weeks prior to the crash, during the crash, or after death. Pilot incapacitation has resulted from acute appendicitis, acute glaucoma, and Meniere's disease, but the investigator may not detect these conditions until he or she examines the histologic sections.

Significance of Preexisting Disease

The presence of preexisting injuries or disease can be a source of confusion. Distinguishing acute from chronic disease processes is not always easy, and even a preexisting, long-standing disease process can precipitate an acute catastrophic event. Distinguishing between those disease processes that might have contributed to the accident and those that were entirely unrelated to the cause of the crash is especially important but often very difficult. The mere presence of preexisting disease does not mean that it was a factor in causing the accident. Investigators may have a difficult time proving that it was a cause, but the preexisting disease may have been a contributing factor in causing a "pilot error" or "cause-undetermined" mishap.

The most significant disease is one that goes undetected in the screening process, contributes to the cause of an accident, and remains undetected during the investigation process. Careful scientific analysis is necessary to find any previous disease and to distinguish merely incidental pathologic findings from disease entities causing disability of crewmembers.

Neurologic Disease

Review of aircraft accident investigation data has disclosed few cases attributed to neurologic disease. The AFIP files contain a few aircraft accident cases involving crewmembers with neurologic disorders such as Parkinson's disease, Meniere's disease, and space-occupying intracranial lesions, including pituitary adenomas and colloid cyst of the third ventricle.

Well-documented cases in which investigators have shown epilepsy to be the cause of an aircraft accident are conspicuously absent, but incapaci-

tation of professional pilots due to epilepsy have occurred in flight. The U.S. Air Force reported that 33% of 30 asymptomatic crewmembers who had abnormal electroencephalographic findings were involved in accidents or incidents or had a neurologically related clinical event. It also reported that 13% died in accidents.

Cardiovascular Disease

Cardiovascular disease in crewmembers is part of the normal aging process and is of major concern as a cause of fatal incapacitation and accidents. It is quite prevalent, even in the relatively young military population. Pettyjohn and McMeekin (18) reported the AFIP's experience in reviewing autopsies of 6500 aircraft accident victims. Of these fatalities, 816 (13%) had preexisting, nontraumatic heart disease.

The literature contains numerous reports of pilots having heart attacks at the controls, but few crashes have occurred. The U.S. Air Force concluded that in-flight myocardial infarction is a rare event after it found only two cases of confirmed and five cases of suspected in-flight myocardial infarction between 1962 and 1972. One international airline reported that only 17 of its pilots experienced health-related incidents between 1948 and 1972. Of the 13 incidents related to the cardiovascular system, only 11 were coronary infarcts, and no crashes occurred.

This low incidence is consistent with the experience of other airlines, and the statistics may be quite accurate, considering the fact that most airlines have cockpit voice and flight data recorders. Nevertheless, the general flying public worries about the health of airline pilots who literally hold the passengers' lives in their hands. Most investigators reflect this concern.

Histologic examination of the heart is particularly helpful. The shearing forces of trauma (Fig. 28.14) and the coagulating effect of heat from fire may create lesions that appear grossly like coronary thrombosis. Careful microscopic examination of multiple sections may reveal the foci of myocarditis. Because these foci also occur in

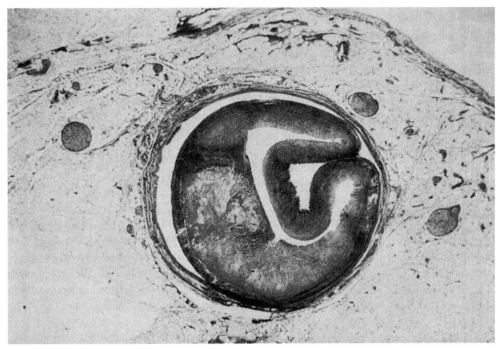

Figure 28.14. Traumatic force separated the intima and media from the less dense adventitia, creating the artifactual appearance of coronary occlusion (Armed Forces Institute of Pathology photo).

healthy people who die, they may be simply minor injury patterns representing the normal wear and tear of repetitive cardiac contractions. The investigator should evaluate the finding of myocarditis carefully, with full consideration of all the facts associated with the accident.

The pathologist may occasionally encounter myocardial infarction associated with an aircraft accident, but trying to find evidence to prove early myocardial infarction, especially in the absence of coronary thrombosis, is especially frustrating. Although histologic examination may be helpful in estimating when the infarction occurred in relation to the time of death, the most optimistic histochemical tests purport to detect myocardial ischemia only as early as 30 minutes after onset, and this is of no value when a crash precipitously follows the acute myocardial event.

Sarcoidosis

Sarcoidosis is a relatively common disease that may cause sudden incapacitation and even death,

but the incidence of clinical manifestations is low. Balfour (19) reported 16 cases of "sarcoid-like granulomas" in autopsies of 852 crewmembers, although the reported incidence of clinical sarcoidosis in the United Kingdom is only about 3 per 100,000 individuals per year. Only one of his subjects had cardiac involvement. Pettyjohn and colleagues (20) reported on 36 U.S. militarycrewmembers with clinical sarcoidosis. Thirty-three percent had evidence of cardiac involvement; four of the 36 had significant cardiac abnormalities, and eight had electrocardiographic abnormalities. These findings are higher than the reported incidence of 13 to 20% in the general population.

Although no evidence clearly establishes that sarcoidosis causes aircraft accidents or that aviation duties make crewmembers more susceptible than others to the lesions of sarcoid, investigators may be underestimating the importance of sarcoidosis as a significant etiologic factor in aircraft accidents. Figure 28.15 illustrates the case of a pilot with severe sarcoidosis with

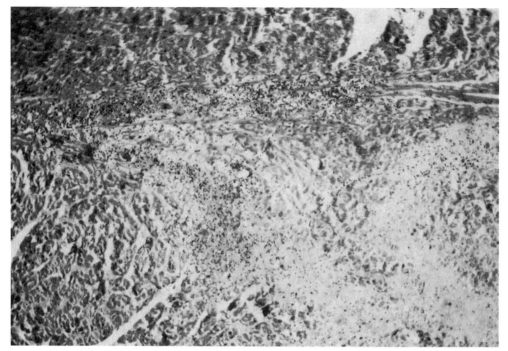

Figure 28.15. Sarcoid granulomas in the heart (Armed Forces Institute of Pathology photo).

multiple organ involvement, including the heart. Investigators concluded that the cardiac involvement probably resulted in incapacitation of the pilot. The injury pattern observed in the passenger of this small aircraft suggested that the passenger and not the pilot was operating the controls at the time of the crash.

Infections

Infections in the upper respiratory tract, especially those involving the sinuses, occur frequently in crewmembers as a result of repeated barotrauma from ascending and descending during flight. These infections may lead to ear involvement, disturbances of equilibrium, and a subsequent accident. The frequency of "nonspecific but definitely abnormal" respiratory tracts in pilots of unexplained, single-seat, high-performance aircraft that crashed impressed Mason (21), and he suggested that these infections may cause more crashes than investigators have been willing to acknowledge.

Tumors

The AFIP reported reviewing 6405 aircraft accident fatalities and finding 90 unsuspected tumors (Fig. 28.16). This number is impressive considering the following factors:

1. The tumors occurred in crewmembers who were required to have a physical examination at least once each year.
2. The pathologists were able to obtain tissue for microscopic examination in less than 50% of the cases.
3. Microscopic examination was present in less than 30% of the cases.
4. The microscopic examination in other cases was superficial.

Alcohol, Self-Medication, and Substance Abuse

The ingestion of alcohol, prescribed or illicit drugs, self-medication with over-the-counter

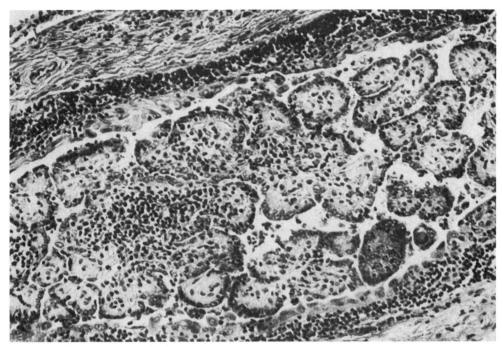

Figure 28.16. Carcinoma of the thyroid (Armed Forces Institute of Pathology photo).

drugs, or even the excessive consumption of various food products can lead to impaired function of crewmembers.

Aircraft accident toxicology laboratories find that crewmembers ingest ethyl alcohol more than any other toxic substance. Of the unusually large number of aircraft accident victims found "positive" for alcohol before about 1965, many were probably positive as a result of postmortem putrefaction or inadequate laboratory methods; however, even after the introduction of better collection and preservation techniques and gas chromatography, the incidence is still greater than 10%. Many positive results are still caused by postmortem decomposition with the resultant bacterial production of alcohol.

The U.S. Air Force reported that the ingestion of ethyl alcohol was associated with 28 of approximately 4200 aircraft accidents from 1962 through 1974 (22). The FAA reported that alcohol levels in 28 (13.9%) of 202 general aviation accidents were greater than 50 mg/100 g (23). General aviation accidents in the United Kingdom during a similar period of a study, 1964

through 1973, resulted in positive alcohol determinations in 34 of 102 pilots; however, only 12 accidents (11.6%) involved alcohol ingestion before flight.

The AFIP toxicology laboratory found the substances listed in Table 28.2 when they examined 2326 occupants involved in aircraft mishaps in 1983. Some of these substances (e.g., lidocaine) may have been used in resuscitation efforts by rescue personnel; other agents, such as the cannabinoids, would certainly be associated with drug abuse. The presence of drugs such as chloroquine probably represent cases of approved usage. Although the use of drugs such as salicylates or acetaminophen may have been approved in some instances, most cases involved the self-medication of an underlying condition that would have been disqualifying for flight duties.

LABORATORY TESTS AND INTERPRETATION OF RESULTS

Many laboratory tests are available to assist the investigator, but the correct choice of the

Table 28.2.
Drugs Found on Examination of 2326 Occupants of Aircraft Mishaps in 1983

Substance	Number of Occupants
Salicylates	109
Acetaminophen	61
Cannabinoids	54
Ethanol	51
Opiates	18
Chloroquine	6
Barbiturates	5
Amphetamines	2
Benzodiazepines	1
Chlorpheniramine	1
Cocaine	1
Diphenhydramine	1
Furosemide	1
Hydrochlorothiazide	1
Lidocaine	1
Phencyclidine	1
Total	314

methods and careful interpretation of the results are important.

Serologic Studies

Serologic studies, such as the determination of blood type, are often useful in narrowing the possible identities of an unknown body. The investigator must exercise caution in the performance and interpretation of serologic studies, because numerous possibilities exist for error and for the introduction of artifacts.

Perhaps the simplest serologic test is the use of antihuman globulin (Coombs' serum) to determine whether a tissue is human or nonhuman. Using proper techniques, this distinction can be made even on dried bones that are more than 100 years old. This test is of particular value in cases in which a long time has lapsed from the occurrence of the disaster to the time of discovery and in which the possibility exists of commingling with animal remains. The technique is also useful in the investigation of aircraft accidents in which a bird strike is suspected.

The detection of A and B blood group substances in blood, tissue, or fluids is helpful in determining the blood type of the deceased. Dried blood in these tests produce the best results, which is advantageous because the investigator cannot always draw blood immediately after death and separate serum and cells. Of the blood group substances, A and B seem more stable than others after death. Many other blood group substances deteriorate rapidly, and even A and B substances may give erratic results to the laboratory tests.

Positive benzidine, orthotoluidine, or phenolphthalein tests may indicate the presence of blood, but interference by many plant, chemical, and other animal sources of peroxidase activity may result in false-positive results. The determination of hemochromogen crystals by procedures such as the Takayama test or of hemin crystals by the Teichmann test also indicates that blood is present.

If blood is present, the investigator may use the absorption-inhibition, absorption-elution, Lattes crust test, or Howard-Martin cellulose acetate sheet test to determine the blood type. The absorption-elution tests are sensitive and accurate, and only small amounts of dried material are needed. Direct agglutination techniques using known antisera give erroneous results because the blood cells are damaged in dried stains, and postmortem changes introduce numerous artifacts.

Several techniques allow the determination of the species of origin of a bloodstain or tissue. The interfacial ring-precipitin test, the Ouchterlony gel double-diffusion test, and the antiglobulin-inhibition technique are three common methods using species-specific antisera.

Toxicologic Studies

Toxicologists have methods to detect many drugs and to determine the levels of substances that occur normally in human tissues. They are especially capable of performing these analyses on postmortem tissues and fluids that would be very difficult for one to perform reliably in the usual hospital laboratory.

Drugs and Volatile Substances

Many toxicology laboratories use solvent-solvent extraction followed by gas chromatographic and mass spectrographic examinations for drugs in the nonvolatile organic acid, basic, and neutral groups. Volatile substances (e.g., alcohol) can be detected by headspace gas chromatography. The investigator should remember that these procedures screen only for classes of compounds; many substances can be detected only by procedures that test for them specifically.

Blood Glucose

Hypoglycemia may be a factor in the cause of aircraft accidents, but the accurate determination of the glucose level in the blood of a fatally injured crewmember at the time of the crash is difficult. The cells continue metabolism for a short time after death, causing blood glucose to fall to very low levels. Then, as tissue breakdown occurs, the blood glucose level becomes very elevated. Depending on where the blood is collected from, but especially if it is collected from the inferior vena cava, the glucose level may be greater than 1000 mg/dl. Glucose levels in the vitreous of the eye do not change as rapidly, making the vitreous a good source of fluid for estimating the postmortem glucose level. Rapid chilling further inhibits the postmortem fall in concentrations of vitreous humor glucose.

Brain Lactic Acid

Dominguez and colleagues (24) reported an association of brain lactic acid concentrations greater than 200 mg/100 g with asphyxial deaths. The determination of the lactic concentration in the brain by ultraviolet spectroscopy requires approximately 500 mg of gray matter. The myelinated white matter and peripheral nerves give unreliable results.

Finding elevated concentrations of lactic acid in the brain is helpful in cases of drowning, death occurring in fires, and altitude hypoxia, but the mechanism that produces this elevation is not clear. The reason is probably not that of simply shutting down the aerobic respiratory pathways. Perhaps it results from adrenal hyperactivity causing increased mobilization of lactate precursors during an agonal period of stress. Certainly, the most frequent cause of an elevated postmortem lactic acid level in the brain is resuscitation efforts with intravenous fluids.

Carbon Monoxide, Cyanide, and Other Combustion Products

Blood carboxyhemoglobin saturation gives an indication of the magnitude of antemortem exposure to carbon monoxide. More reliable laboratory methods and equipment, such as differential colorimetric spectroscopy and gas chromatography, now allow the accurate determination of carboxyhemoglobin saturations less than 1%, rather than the 10% level generally considered significant; however, a wise investigator will seek an explanation of even the lowest carboxyhemoglobin saturations.

The ambient concentration of carbon monoxide in the breathed air and the length and exposure determine the level of carboxyhemoglobin saturation. Smokers seldom have carboxyhemoglobin saturations greater than 10%, although higher levels may occur in cigar smokers. One crewmember who smoked more than two packages of cigarettes in less than 30 minutes en route to the hospital after a crash had a carboxyhemoglobin saturation of 17%. Victims may breathe the products of a postcrash fire for more than 1 minute without reaching 20% carboxyhemoglobin saturation and for more than 5 minutes without reaching 50% saturation. In rapid conflagration situations, victims who survived the impact forces may be found to have died in the postcrash fire before the carboxyhemoglobin saturation reached even 10%. Thus, the investigator should seek an explanation for even low carboxyhemoglobin saturations.

Carbon monoxide has a great affinity for hemoglobin and competes for its oxygen-carrying capacity. The reduced oxygen-carrying capacity of hemoglobin generally was considered to produce sufficient hypoxia to cause death in fire victims. This may still be the reason for these deaths, but it has been suggested that the true mechanism by which carbon monoxide causes deaths in fires is its effect on cellular respiration by binding of intracellular cytochrome a^3 in competition with oxygen. Thus, the carbon monoxide dissolved in plasma, entering the cells, and binding cytochrome a^3 may be more significant than the limitation of the oxygen-carrying capacity of hemoglobin by carboxyhemoglobin. This would explain why some unburned victims die with relatively low carboxyhemoglobin concentrations and some survivors recover even after reaching carboxyhemoglobin saturations greater than 50%.

Many other products result from combustion, depending on the fuels and the composition of the atmosphere in which they burn. Many plastics, when burned, produce cyanide gas. Cyanide is a potent enzyme poison but may not be more toxic than carbon monoxide in this regard. Other materials, such as electrical wiring, may produce halogenated hydrocarbon products, and laboratory measurements of chloride and fluoride may be helpful.

Blood Electrolytes

The comparison of electrolyte concentrations in blood from the left and right heart chambers as a diagnostic test for drowning is controversial. Theoretically, freshwater drowning dilutes the electrolytes in the left heart chambers, and saltwater drowning concentrates some of the electrolytes in the left heart chambers; postmortem changes increase the complexity of these interpretations.

The Gettler test relied on finding a difference in chloride concentration of 25 mg/dl between the left and right heart chambers. The interpretation of results is even more complicated when drowning occurs in brackish water, because the chloride concentration of the water may not be very different from the chloride concentration in the blood. The measurement of other electrolytes, such as magnesium, may be helpful in these cases. Collecting a sample of the water at the drowning site will allow the laboratory to select the electrolytes that might be useful in the comparison.

Artifact and Error

Many factors influence the reliability of various laboratory tests. Investigators should carefully consider the reliability of the test methods used by a particular laboratory, the technical ability of the technicians, and the quality control procedures in use when they select a laboratory to perform toxicology analysis. They must also collect the specimens carefully to avoid contaminating the containers. The indelible ink markers used to label containers may be a source of contamination with organic solvents.

Soil, vegetation, and fuel may contaminate the specimens at the crash site, and immersion may dilute the concentrations of the substances being measured. Fire, burning, and putrefaction may change the composition of the tissues or may produce substances that interfere with the test. The duration and temperature of postcrash exposure have significant effects on the rate of the decomposition process.

The postmortem production of alcohol by bacteria frequently causes difficulty in determining whether the ingestion of alcohol may have impaired a crewmember's judgment. The bacterial production of alcohol usually amounts to less than 50 mg/100 g of tissue, but in rare instances, the production of more than 100 mg/100 g has occurred.

Aircraft accidents are not new, but few persons obtain much experience in aircraft accident investigation. As a result, when called on to participate in an accident investigation, investigators make many mistakes of omission and commission. They can avoid the most serious mistakes by careful planning and by following logical steps, such as the six steps recommended by the JCAP. Determining the role of the participants and the jurisdiction to conduct the investigation is important.

Identifying the victims is an unpleasant but

relatively simple matter. Planning and organization are essential. Someone must obtain sufficient antemortem records before identification can be possible. Once these data are obtained, examination of the bodies and application of various identification techniques, such as fingerprint, dental, radiologic, and DNA methods, can proceed rapidly.

Injury patterns are determined by the acceleration forces, cockpit configuration, nature of the accident, and occupant kinematics. Investigators can conveniently classify injury patterns by cause: traumatic, environmental, and preexisting disease factors.

The procedures are not difficult, but investigators must collect and assimilate much information in a short period of time. They must not draw conclusions too quickly lest they make irreparable mistakes.

ACKNOWLEDGMENTS

The author gratefully acknowledges the valuable assistance of Colonel Charles Ruehle, USAF, MC, retired former Chief of the Armed Forces Institute of Pathology Division of Aerospace Pathology, and his staff, especially Charles Springate, MC, USA, who located and shepherded many of the photographic negatives, illustrations, and references.

REFERENCES

1. United States Congress, Senate Committee on Commerce: Safety in air hearings (3 parts), before a subcommittee, pursuant to Senate Resolution 146, Seventy-fourth Congress, Second Session, and Seventy-fifth Congress, First Session, 1936–1937. Part 1, Page 1, February 10, 1936 (Copeland Hearings).
2. Armstrong JA, Fryer DI, Stewart WK, et al. Interpretation of injuries in the Comet aircraft disasters. Lancet 1955;1:1135.
3. Joint Committee on Aviation Pathology. Memorandum No. 1: An autopsy guide for aircraft accident fatalities. Washington, DC: Joint Committee on Aviation Pathology, 1957.
4. Fryer DI. The medical investigation of accidents. In: Gillies JA, ed. Textbook of aviation physiology. Oxford: Pergamon Press, 1965:1200.
5. Chicago Convention on International Civil Aviation. Article 26, 61 Statute 1180, T.I.A.S. no. 1591, December 7, 1944.
6. Federal Aviation Act of 1958. Section 701, 72 Statute 781, as amended by 76 Statute 921. Forty-ninth Congress. §1441.
7. Lan, JC, Brown TC. Probability of casualties in an airport disaster. Aviat Space Environ Med 1975;46:958.
8. Hays MB, Stefanki JX, Cheu DH. Planning an airport disaster drill. Aviat Space Environ Med 1976;47:556.
9. Lichtenstein JD, et al. Role of radiology in aviation accident investigation. Aviat Space Environ Med 1980;51:1004.
10. Hill IR. Dental identification in fatal aircraft accidents. Aviat Space Environ Med 1980;51:1021.
11. Morlang WM. Forensic dentistry. Aviat Space Environ Med 1982;53:27.
12. Petty AE, McMeekin RR. Laboratory examination of unidentified tissue fragments found at aircraft sites. Aviat Space Environ Med 1977;48:937.
13. Mason JK. Passenger tie-down failure: injuries and accident reconstruction. Aerospace Med 1970;41:781.
14. Eiband AM. Human tolerance to rapidly applied accelerations. NASA Memo 5–19–59E. Washington, DC: National Aeronautics and Space Administration, June, 1959.
15. Coltart WD. Aviators astragalus. J. Bone Joint Surg 1952;34–B:545.
16. Dummit ES, Reid RL. Unique tibial shaft fractures resulting from helicopter crashes. Clin Orthoped 1969;66:155.
17. Smelsey SO. Diagnostic patterns of injury and death in USAF aviation accidents. Aerospace Med 1970;41:790.
18. Pettyjohn FS, McMeekin RR. Coronary artery disease and preventive cardiology in aviation medicine. Aviat Space Environ Med 1975;46:1299.
19. Balfour AJC. Sarcoidosis in aircrew. Aviat Space Environ Med 1982;53:269.
20. Pettyjohn FS, Spoor DH, Buckendorf WA. Sarcoid and the heart—an aeromedical risk. Aviat Space Environ Med 1977;48:955.
21. Mason JK. Previous disease in aircrew killed in flying accidents. Aviat Space Environ Med 1975;46:1271.
22. Zeller AF. Alcohol and other drugs in aircraft accidents. Aviat Space Environ Med 1974;46:1271.
23. Smith PW, Lacefield DJ, Crance CR. Toxicological findings in aircraft accident investigation. Aviat Space Environ Med 1970;41:760.
24. Dominguez AM, et al. Significance of elevated lactic acid in the postmortem brain. Aerospace Med, 1960;31:897.

Chapter 29

Human Factors in Aerospace Medicine

Thomas B. Sheridan,

Laurence R. Young

Know then thyself, presume not God to scan, The proper study of mankind is man.

Alexander Pope

Human factors, sometimes called human factors engineering, is the science and art of interfacing people with the machines they operate. One important interface is with the physical hardware, such as displays, controls, and settings. A second interface is soft, in the sense of procedures for doing the task or training, and the computer software that the operator may have to use directly. The third interface is with the operational environment, such as temperature, vibration, acceleration, radiation, chemical properties, and ambient pressure. The fourth interface of interest is social interaction with other people.

The subject of human factors is primarily identified with the hardware interface, and this chapter will emphasize that interaction. This is certainly the emphasis of the various human factors data books and standards available (1–5). The software interface always has been critical in relation to hardware, and the importance of software is certainly evident as computers become more important in mediating the operator's relationship to the machine. Problems regarding environmental stressors are dealt with in several other chapters of this text. Social interaction, although too often neglected in the design of complex human-machine systems, is a subject both too large and not sufficiently well

codified to treat here. In the chapter that follows, Parker and Shepherd address the management of human resources.

In contrast to medicine, which is concerned primarily with the health of the individual, human factors engineering is concerned with the performance of the overall system: human performance is of interest as it enhances system performance, and safety is intrinsic to system performance.

The human-machine system is depicted in Figure 29.1. The human operator is subdivided into sensory, control processing/memory, and motor functions. On the machine side of the interface are displays that convert electrical, mechanical, and other signals from the vehicle or system into a form understandable to the human senses of vision, hearing, and touch. Correspondingly, conventional control devices, such as joysticks, push-buttons, or pedals, transduce the operator's voluntary motor responses back to electrical and mechanical signals capable of driving the system. Advanced control devices actuated, for example, by voice, eye position, or brain waves, are beyond the scope of this chapter. As shown in Figure 29.2, the information travels in a closed loop. This closed-loop system is essential for the operator to achieve real-time control.

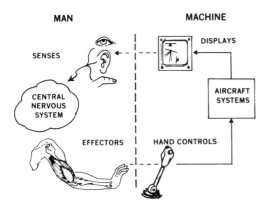

Figure 29.1. The human-machine system.

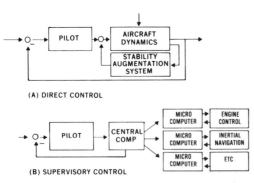

Figure 29.2. Block diagrams of direct and supervisory control.

Increasingly, the human operator is removed from the simple task of closing a feedback loop or driving the vehicle and is placed in a supervisory or monitoring role. When the operator's interactions with the vehicle or controlled process are mediated by a computer, the simply closed loop of Figure 29.2A is modified, as shown in Figure 29.2B. The computer now serves as a direct controller, and the human operator's new role becomes that of supervisor of an otherwise automatic control loop. As a supervisor, the pilot selects autopilot modes, sets altitude or waypoints, etc.

HUMAN FACTORS IN AIRCREW TASKS

Human factors considerations are involved intimately with almost every aspect of manned flight, from the initial selection of pilot candidates through test pilot evaluation of vehicle handling qualities to pilot workload evaluation of changes in crew complement. Although a complete discussion of human factors in aviation is not possible in one chapter, a few examples of relevance to aviation can be presented.

When selecting individuals for pilot training by the military or for initial employment by the commercial airlines, it is commonplace to use both psychologic and physiologic assessment measures. Although no unanimity exists on the validity of these measurement techniques, the typical characteristics of the traditional pilot have been identified over the years. Continuing study has concerned the desirability of a two-track selection in which the psychologic and physical characteristics of transport pilots are separated from those characteristics appropriate for fighter pilots.

Once a candidate is selected for pilot training, he or she will be exposed to a variety of training devices, including various types of aircraft systems trainers. The increased reliance on interactive, computer-driven teaching programs will take training beyond the level of the tape-slide or videotape presentation. When properly programmed and appropriately combined with face-to-face instruction, such programs have proven their effectiveness in aircrew training and can provide the motivation, reinforcement, and effectiveness of self-paced study. Cockpit procedures and flying skills may be taught on any of four different devices: a part-task trainer, a cockpit procedures trainer, a flight simulator, or the aircraft itself. These devices are progressively more expensive and of higher fidelity. Although a pilot's first reaction may be to want to do as much training as possible in the air, the quest for fidelity often is misplaced. For teaching a sequence of procedures, as in the case of an engine fire, it is neither necessary nor desirable to provide the full fidelity of the aircraft or flight simulator. Furthermore, for the crew coordination practice, a part-task trainer in which switches and controls are active but aircraft dynamics are not simulated may be as effective as the aircraft.

For teaching special flying skills, such as engine-out landings or reaction to an engine-out takeoff, repeated practice in a high-fidelity flight simulator with added visual scenery is much more effective, hour for hour, than training in the air. On the other hand, given the current limitations on computer-generated or model-board visual scenes in a simulator, certain skills, such as low-level navigation or treetop flying in a helicopter, are difficult to teach adequately in a simulator. The important human factors considerations in training involve identifying the training goals and providing a device that is capable of meeting these goals rather than one that mimics the aircraft in all respects.

Once the pilot enters the cockpit, the human factors of aviation become readily apparent, particularly as they create problems. Seat adjustments must accommodate the entire range of aircrew anthropometrics, both male and female. Aircraft seat comfort may be limited by the hardness required for the safe use of the ejection seat. Layout of the flight instruments should be in keeping with human factors design rules, grouping the commonly used instruments in the central visual field and placing associated instruments together. All of the important instrument information to be scanned must be readily visible from the pilot's position without interference with the view outside the cockpit. Cockpit noise levels should be kept acceptably low to facilitate communication and reduce aircrew fatigue.

The design of the cockpit instruments themselves must take human factors principles into account, presenting information in a manner that is easily recognizable and interpretable, with a precision commensurate with their use and in an orientation consistent with the required control action. A devastating example of the results of nonconformity with human factors principles is seen in altimeter displays. The older, three-pointer altimeter was easily misinterpreted and blamed for numerous fatalities. The newer, drum-type altimeter and particularly the easy-to-

read and precise vertical-tape altimeter greatly reduce the likelihood of errors in altitude readings under conditions of stress, poor lighting, or turbulence.

The move from mechanical to electromechanical to electronic displays permits the designer to create almost any form of information display desired for the pilot. Although the earlier electronic displays tended to mimic their electromechanical predecessors, human factors considerations are moving the field toward the increased use of ''integrated'' displays. In a well-designed integrated display, aircraft information about many related variables is presented in a single, easily interpreted computer-graphic display. Any required dynamic compensation or quickening easily can be introduced into the command display or flight director. Information not previously displayed to the pilot, such as malfunction checklists, can now be presented on a cockpit display unit driven by an airborne computer and associated mass storage elements.

Human factors considerations of the appropriate computer-aided checklists and procedures remain to be established. The limitations of the pilot in aircraft or spacecraft control become particularly apparent under stressful conditions, either because of increased workload, fatigue, or environmental disturbances. Communication and display design should leave a sufficient margin so that the additional work required does not lead to an inability to attend to the primary flying objectives. A thorough understanding of pilot workload is necessary, although its measurement remains difficult. Despite significant attempts to develop physiologic measures of workload, subjective rating scales, or side task measurements, the final decision on acceptable workload usually depends on the assessment of pilot performance under stress. Pilots must be made aware of their individual limitations, both psychologic and physical. Aircraft control cannot be expected to be as precise when a pilot is simultaneously loaded with communication, navigation, and checklist tasks. Pilots and designers alike should be made aware of the phenomenon of perceptual narrowing, in which objects in the peripheral visual field are literally not seen while attention is focused on either a visual or nonvisual central task.

The functioning of a pilot or astronaut as a member of a continuous control loop introduces the human factors specialty of manual control. Although the ideal and easiest control task is one in which the vehicle or controlled element is compensated so that the pilot commands its velocity, this situation is not always possible under normal or emergency conditions. Predictable situations leading to pilot-induced oscillations result from excessive delays in human or machine response within a control loop, more than two integrations in a control loop, the absence of easily discernible error-rate information, or the need to perform separate parallel tracking tasks. Although one of the major reasons for retaining manual control as opposed to fully automatic piloting is to take advantage of human adaptability, rapidly changing vehicle dynamics can stress the pilot severely. Aerial refueling, for example, involves significant changes in the relationship between control effort and aircraft movement. Similarly, approaching the runway under instrument landing conditions can easily lead to pilot-induced oscillation.

DISPLAYS

Display Function Classification

Displays, that is, any means for communicating information to a pilot or crewmember, can be categorized as follows:

Primary flight displays
  Attitude indicator/flight director
  Radar/pressure altimeter
  Rate of climb
  Airspeed
  Compass/heading
Navigation displays
  Course
  Waypoint

Radar
Wind direction
Moving map, including weather and traffic
Engineer instruments
  Revolutions per minute (rpm)
  Temperature
  Fuel and flow
  Oil and pressure
Autopilot display
  Settable indicators and autopilot mode
  Altitude clearance
  Command heading
  Takeoff/landing ''speed bugs''
  Decision height
Alarms
  Stall
  Fire
Radio/communications
Status of stores
Other aircraft systems
View out of windscreen
Maps, reports, procedures, other texts and
  graphics
Auditory information from other crewmembers
  and miscellaneous sounds or aircraft systems
  operating

Note that in modern aircraft many of these displays are combined and integrated into computer-graphic presentations. In newer commercial aircraft the multifunction flight management system incorporates many of them. The last six categories listed are not usually thought of as displays, but they are extremely important in complementing the panel instruments.

It is sometimes useful to classify displays by whether they are (1) alarms, that is, discrete attention-getting stimuli; (2) check-reading or status monitoring displays, indicating whether conditions are normal and in some cases a qualitative degree of abnormality; (3) quantitative displays, which provide numeric information in digital or analog form; and (4) tracking displays, to be used in conjunction with controls for nulling differences.

Alarms such as stall and fire may be auditory,

visual, or other. (The "stick shaker" stall warning is an effective way of getting the pilot's attention.) The obvious advantage of an auditory alarm is that the pilot does not have to be looking in any particular place. Traditionally, auditory alarms have been Klaxon horns and buzzers, loud enough to be heard clearly but not loud enough to damage the pilot's hearing or interfere with control of the aircraft.

Computer-generated speech is now inexpensive and reliable and offers many possibilities for providing alarm and warning signals. Such displays not only can alert the pilot but also can tell her what the condition is, with qualitative or quantitative modifiers, if necessary, to suit the momentary circumstances. Such displays can be presented at a loudness befitting the occasion and are especially valuable when a pilot's eyes must be fixed on a display or out the window, as in the glide-slope voice warning of deviation from an instrument landing system (ILS) during landing. Voice displays sometimes are combined with other sounds, as in the "whoop, whoop, pull-up, pull-up" terrain-avoidance warning.

The discriminability of alarms, whether light or sound, is an important consideration. Pilots frequently complain that they cannot keep track of what the multiple warning lights and sounds mean, especially under stress. Therefore, the use of synthetic speech is appropriate to tell the pilot the meaning of an alarm after getting her attention, possibly by conventional means. In any case, tonal qualities, location, colors, or other features of alarms should be different from each other and, insofar as possible, should connote their meaning. Flashing lights are useful for attracting the pilot's attention and for discriminating the newly lit alarm or important alarm from status lights. Red lights should be used for emergencies requiring immediate attention; orange or yellow lights for warning or change status; and green, light blue, or white lights for normal operations. Beyond the few most critical alarms, common practice has been to use master alarms that can tell the pilot that something is wrong

within a whole set of functions. The pilot must then visually or manually access some lower-level visual display to find out specifically what is wrong.

Check-reading displays, those to be scanned regularly to check whether the pertinent variable is as expected, conventionally take the form of lights, flags (windows that change color), and linear tapes. Lights are used for discrete on-off information. Flags can indicate several discrete states (e.g., red, green, yellow). Linear or ribbon tapes are used when only qualitative information is necessary and when a quick verification scan is sufficient. The linear tape, depending on its size, can convey quantitative information for a closer second look if that is desired. It can also easily show a variable's rate of change and whether it is above or below some reference. Stacking linear tapes side by side (e.g., for engine variables) is useful for making comparisons and checking against normal operating ranges.

True quantitative displays, in which numeric information is meaningful, may be analog (long linear tapes or circular dials) or digital. The quick, qualitative impression sometimes may be important too (e.g., looking only at the first digit of the numeric display). Thus, the qualitative versus quantitative distinction is seldom a clean one. The altimeter, rpm, compass, and radiofrequency indicators are examples of quantitative displays.

Finally, the tracking or nulling display (for example, the altitude indicator with or without flight director command bars) is necessarily analog. Nulling a digital display is an awkward task; therefore, digital displays are not recommended for this function. Occasionally, displays combine the analog and digital elements, as in a conventional drum altimeter. Figure 29.3 provides some samples.

Cathode Ray Tube Displays

The preceding discussion has not emphasized the cathode ray tube (CRT) as a display, although it may serve all four of the functions

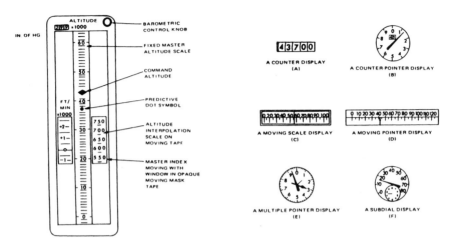

Figure 29.3. Conventional displays formats. (Bioastronautics data book, NASA SP-3006, 2nd ed., 1973.)

described and is extremely flexible. Information is limited only by the physical constraints of the CRT and display generation electronics (number of separable picture elements or pixels) in length, width and speed for generating a new picture. The CRT display has drawbacks such as its depth (roughly equal to its width), high voltage and power requirements, fragility, and problems with legibility in direct sunlight.

A good-quality aircraft CRT is from 512 × 512 to 2000 × 2000 pixels, depending on size. If a raster display generator (left-to-right sweeps successively from top to bottom, like an ordinary television) is used, arbitrary colors and shapes can be rendered. White on color line drawings and small objects can be generated quickly, although regeneration of a larger complex map, for example, rotating to keep heading up, may take up to several seconds. To avoid flicker, displays should be refreshed approximately 30 times each second, depending on brightness.

From a human factors viewpoint, perhaps the most important capability of the CRT is permitting the integration of displays. For example, the computer-generated electronic altitude director instrument (EADI) provides the primary flight director display. It can combine pitch and roll, altitude and ground speed, and glide slope and localizer deviations. Figure 29.4A shows an example.

The CRT can provide a current list of all variables that are either abnormal or about to become so. It can provide maps, diagrams, checklists, reminders, and procedural information. Various displays now in use or being developed combine map and waypoint information, weather radar, and position of all aircraft within a slice of airspace, with range adjustment in both altitude and map scale. Figure 29.4B shows the electronic horizontal situation indicator in the Boeing 767, which embodies many of these features. Figure 29.5 shows multiple CRTs in use in a prototype experimental cockpit.

CRT displays also can be used to provide different information formats at different times, depending on what the pilot or other operator requests. To have some standardization, it has become common practice to use a hierarchy or tree of pages, where a top-level page may represent the whole aircraft and the principal variables concerning its main subsystems. If more detailed information is wanted about some aspect of the top-level page, one could use the "page down" command and thereby call up a full page concerning a single engine and its variables. This page, in turn, could have lower-level pages associated with it. More than three levels of paging usually is not recommended. Recommended practice for formatting a single page follow the same rules as for designing in general.

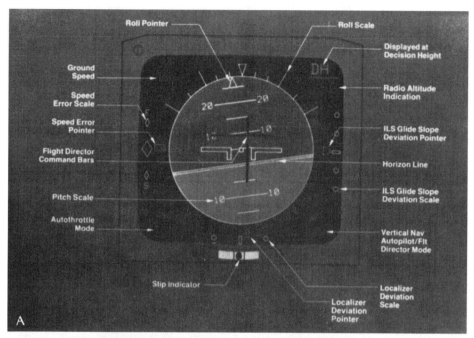

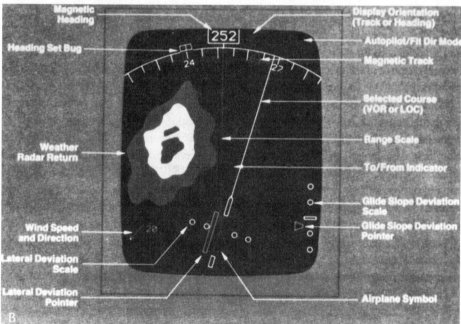

Figure 29.4. A. Electronic attitude director indicator; B. Electronic horizontal situation indicator VOR/ILS mode (Courtesy of the Boeing Company).

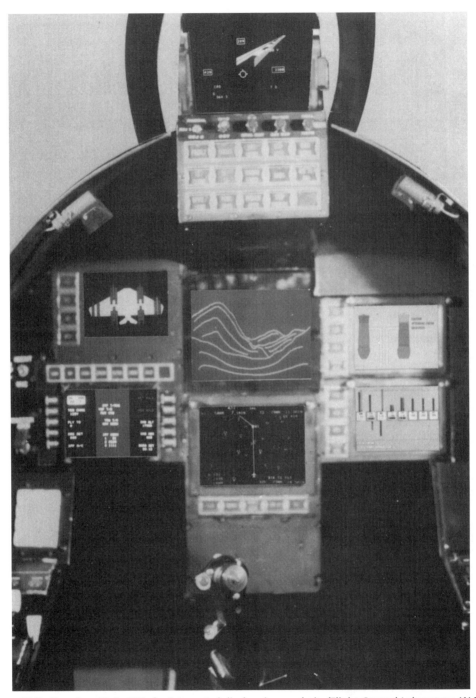

Figure 29.5. Use of multiple CRTs for integrated displays in a cockpit. (Flight Control Laboratory, W-PAFB, Ohio-USAF photo.)

One generalization is that not more than 20% of the total page area should be taken up with symbols or figures. Further, because lines and edges cannot be drawn as sharply on a CRT display as they can be printed on paper or instrument scales, the designer should be conservative in crowding scales, symbols, and text together.

The same CRT display also can be used to call up different types of variables at the same level in the paging tree. For example, one page could be hydraulics, another page electrical power, a third page weapons, and so on. The CRT display can be useful for presenting branching programs for abnormal procedures, troubleshooting, or checklists.

The CRT display can provide trend information on a multitude of variables, scaled on whatever basis is convenient to the user, provided the necessary information has been stored in the computer. History, trends, and anticipated values can be compared. Thus, for failure detection and diagnosis, the CRT display is invaluable.

Other technologies are competing to replace the CRT display, but thus far none has its overall capability. New techniques include gas plasma and light-emitting diode (LED) displays (now in multicolors), and liquid crystal display (LCD) and active matrix arrays. The latter, because they are popular for portable computers, are undergoing rapid improvement in both resolution and color. All of these displays have the advantage of flatness, but cost, power (plasma), resolution (LED), or the need for adequate incident light (LCD) pose problems.

The head-up display (HUD) commonly is used in conjunction with weapons aiming, landing aids, or the altitude-flight director CRT displays. This display is a combining mirror and lens arrangement that superimposes the CRT display image directly on the pilot's front view through the windscreen at optical infinity. Use of the HUD saves the time involved in changing gaze and the time needed to reaccommodate in changing between out-the-window viewing and instrument viewing.

Criteria for Display Location and Design

The location of visual displays or of elements within an integrated computer-graphic display is necessarily a trade-off among many criteria, such as the following:

1. Function or casual order, that is, mimicking left-to-right or top-to-bottom the cause-and-effect chains
2. Left-to-right or top-to-bottom position in terms of normal procedural sequences
3. Same for emergency procedures
4. General direction of where the corresponding physical system is located (e.g., engines, landing gear)
5. Front and center position for most important displays for normal use
6. Same as for emergency use
7. Subsystem grouping
8. Optimum use of panel space
9. Position where the pilots say they want them and are used to having them

A second set of criteria, not necessarily in conflict with the first, considers the succession of responses the operator must make. Operators first must find the proper display or determine that a display has something to tell them, either because they are looking for it or because it is, in a sense, looking for them. A stereotyped scan pattern combined with easy-to-remember locations, as well as brightness, contrast, and size, help with location and detectability. Next, the pilot must read the details of the display. This reading includes recognizing numbers or symbols, knowing where the pointers are pointing, or knowing what the color represents. Finally, the pilot must know what action to take in response to what he or she has read. The display should suggest the direction to move a control or the numbers to set into a keyboard. By convention, aircraft tracking displays are of the inside-looking-out or fly-to design, in which an error is negated by flying the aircraft toward the deviation indicator. Raising the gear handle to raise the landing gear is an unambiguous situation. Similarly, throttle forward means more thrust. Moving the control level forward to command the wing forward in a swing-wing fighter was rejected by pilots, however, because it had the effect of slowing the aircraft, thus being inconsistent with the throttle direction.

Conditions for Good Vision

Good vision is a function of a number of interrelated variables. These empiric relations are well established in the literature of visual psychophysiology (2,6–9). This chapter will examine only the first-order relationships.

The three variables most easily related to visual acuity in terms of ability to resolve two separate points or lines are spatial separation (or size), figure-ground contrast (in percentage of difference in magnitude of illumination relative to the background illumination), and back-

ground illumination level. Larger, brighter, higher-contrast displays generally can be seen better. The interrelation among the variables has well been established (Fig. 29.6). Long parallel lines are easier by an order of magnitude to resolve than dots, other factors remaining the same. One minute of arc is taken visually as a reasonable two-point separation measure of visual acuity for a normal healthy person under good light and contrast.

The retina seems to integrate light intensity over time up to roughly 100 ms (the Bunsen-Roscoe law), so that a very short but very bright electronic strobe is just as discriminable and even looks the same as a much longer and less bright incandescent flashbulb. Obviously, acuity is much better at the fovea than at the periphery, provided that vision is photoptic, that is, the light is bright enough to stimulate the cones. Night

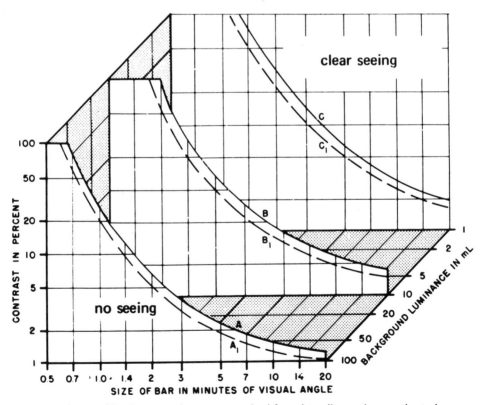

Figure 29.6. Background luminance and contrast required for subtending various angles to be seen under daylight conditions. (From Chapanis A, et al. Applied experimental psychology: human factors in engineering design. New York, John Wiley and Sons, Inc., 1955.)

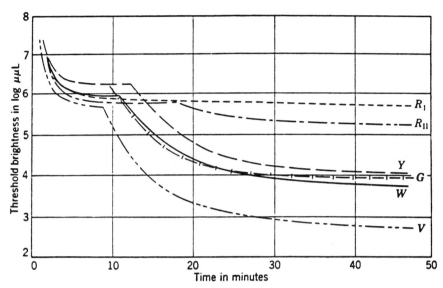

Figure 29.7. Dark adaptation. Curves show the dominant visible light of different colors seen after various periods of darkness (after Chapanis). These curves show the dimmest light one can see at various times after going into the dark. It takes about 30 minutes for the eye to reach full sensitivity. Notice that one finally becomes most sensitive to violet (V) and that one is least sensitive to deep red (R_1) and reddish-orange (R_{11}) light. (From Chapanis A, et al. Applied experimental psychology: human factors in engineering design. New York: John Wiley and Sons, Inc., 1955.)

vision is best about 20° off the optic axis, where rod density is greatest. Other factors, such as vibration of the display or the subject and color of the image, also affect visual acuity.

When exposed to bright light, the visual threshold increases significantly, then falls back slowly when the impact is removed. The impact of flash blindness on display discriminability is significant. Figure 29.7 shows a curve for adaptation to darkness after exposure to bright sunlight. The discontinuity in the curve is the transition from cone to rod vision. Note that only after 30 minutes does the eye reach full sensitivity, becoming most sensitive to violet and least sensitive to dark red and reddish-orange.

Because rod sensitivity or night vision washout depends on sufficient luminant energy within those shorter wavelength colors to which the rods are sensitive, it had been customary in night missions for pilots to wear red glasses and/or to have red filters on cockpit light sources. The light is then kept in a spectral region in which cone vision functions but rod vision is

minimally affected. After removing the red glasses, rod vision is well adapted to low light levels in the higher-frequency, shorter-wavelength range. Current practice is to dim white light for most transport instrument lights.

Design of Instrument Scales and Letters

Based on considerable experimental research, it is clear that some scales are better than others in terms of reading speed and error. Principal number subdivisions of tens or twos (or their multiples) are both fast and accurate, whereas other number subdivisions are not. In the tens case, secondary subdivision by five is appropriate. Fine scale marks at unit intervals are appropriate in both cases if there is room, although a cleaner-looking scale is preferred if the fine marks would lie too close together.

Various studies have been conducted on the effects of letter shape and font (1,7). A letter height-to-letter-width ratio of 1.4:1.7 has been found to be the best, with the letter height-to-stroke (line) width ratio of 6:8. Sans serif fonts are not only cleaner but easier to read than fonts with serifs. Mixing capital and lowercase letters is quite acceptable and preferred to using all capital letters.

For visibility, the military standard 1472 recommends black letters on white background rather than white letters on black background or black letters on yellow background (or other combinations). In most situations with good light, the difference is not critical to reading speed or accuracy.

Color often is used for coding displays. Military standard 1472 recommends that red be used for abnormal situations, yellow for warning, green for normal, and blue for background or nonessential lines or for status advisory signals of a neutral quality, all in combination with white and black and observing the requirements for sufficient contrast, size, and illumination. These recommendations also apply to CRTs.

Commonsense Factors in Visual Displays

Certain human factors of critical importance are not so amenable to scientific research but must be dealt with using common sense. One such factor is text and abbreviations on labels and warnings. Candidate text should be reviewed by a fair sample of the user-operator community to make sure the text is understandable, unambiguous, and not overly complex. Abbreviations should be consistent.

Auditory Signaling and Speech Communication

The first and most important aspect of a sound signal is that it be heard. In Figure 29.8, the standard threshold curve (for no ambient noise) is the 0 decibel line. The other curves show equivalent perceived loudness relative to a reference tone at 1000 Hz at various decibel levels. When masking noise (unwanted ambient background sound) is present, however, the desired sound must be at a higher energy level to be heard, depending on its frequency. Typically, ambient noise is broad band (energy spread over

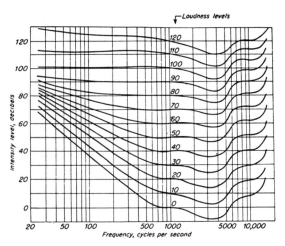

Figure 29.8. Equivalent perceived loudness relative to a reference tone. (Bioastronautics data book, NASA 88–3006, 1964.)

many frequencies, for example, engine noise, air conditioner noise, or speech). The masking effect on a narrow-band signal is defined as the decibel increase in the signal over the unmasked or no-noise threshold in order to be heard. This increase is roughly proportional to the decibel level of the noise in a ''critical band'' of frequencies 50 to 100 Hz wide centered on the signal frequency. For noise outside this critical band, the masking effect drops off sharply and becomes negligible as the noise is at a wholly different frequency range than the signal. Military standard 1472 recommends a 20-decibel margin for signaling above noise within a one-octave band between 200 and 500 Hz.

The same general masking rule is operative with speech signal masking by ambient speech or other broad-band noise, where in this case the result is a combined effect of speech or noise components in each critical band. Figure 29.9 shows how speech is masked by white noise. Obviously, the line for detectability (knowing that the speaker is present) is at a lower decibel level than that for intelligibility. The extra bandwidth required for intelligible speech transmission is one of the factors supporting communication of coded data instead of speech.

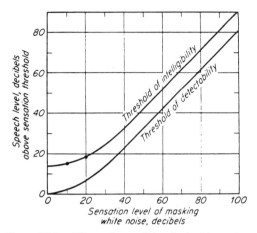

Figure 29.9. Effect of overall level of white noise on the thresholds of intelligibility and of detectability of speech. (From Hawkins J, Stevens S. The masking of pure tones and of speed by white noise. J Acoust Soc Am, 22:6–13, 1964.)

CONTROLS

Human Control Function Classification

Pilot control tasks are categorized as follows:

Primary flight control
    Attitude
    Speed
    Altitude
    Heading
Autopilot controls
    Autopilot mode
    Flight director
    Turn and climb rate
    Heading/inertial navigation
    Altitude
Engine Controls
    Alarm responses
Communications
Operations of stores
Control of other systems
Interpersonal interaction

Primary flight control may be accomplished by pure manual control or by several levels of autopilot use. Autopilot control levels involve increasing equipment sophistication, in which each higher level more or less subsumes the previous or lower level.

Controls may be analogic, meaning that their spatial movement or force bears some continuous geometric isomorphism with the control effect. Joysticks, levers, and pedals are examples of analogic controls. Symbolic (normally discrete) controls, on the other hand, are keys or switches with a label or coding scheme that is read or learned. An alphanumeric keypad or individual buttons or switches are symbolic controls in this sense.

Analogic and symbolic controls may be combined; for example, the joystick with discrete thumb and finger buttons attached, shown in the lower part of Figure 29.5, is an example of a design problem that has received considerable human factors attention. Finger movements are used to arm and fire weapons as well as to adjust trim tabs or other control parameters of the aircraft during time-critical periods when the pilot's eyes are busy. At such times, reaching forward to a particular location on the control panel would be difficult because of high G forces. To further preclude inadvertent actuation of the joystick during high-G maneuvers, a side arm controller may be used, as on the F-16 or the Airbus 330–340. Such a device senses force with only a very small displacement. The arm is supported on a shelf, and the wrist is used to provide pitch and roll displacements.

A newer form of analogic control involves the use of the head or the eyes to drive aiming signals, especially when the pilot's hands are occupied or the pilot is under the stress of high-G turns (10).

Control may be either direct or supervisory. Supervisory control means the pilot or other human operator supervises a computer while the computer itself is the in-the-loop controller (Fig. 29.2). Once the supervisor has programmed and selected the mode for the computer, unless and until the program runs it to the end or some contingency occurs that stops it short, the computer will not need further action by the human supervisor. It may, however, need monitoring by him to check that things are going as expected or to take action if they are not. In the supervisory mode, the human operator performs the following functions:

1. Planning what subgoals the aircraft should achieve over the next time interval in view of given criteria (e.g., nominal schedule) and constraints (e.g., speed, fuel, weather)
2. Programming the computer(s) to control the aircraft or its systems to achieve the subgoal, with the suitable contingency plans built into the program
3. Monitoring the (semi) automatic control of the aircraft or other systems by the computer
4. Intervening to stop or modify the program if necessary or to assume direct manual control or to do repairs
5. Learning from experience

Aerospace vehicles, both government and commercial, are increasingly being controlled in supervisory fashion through autopilots and flight management systems. In newer commercial aircraft the pilot's right hand rests on a computer keypad.

Control by CRT Displays and Computer Recognition

It is common to think of CRTs as display devices but less usual to consider them as control devices. When augmented by various types of touch-sensitive overlay devices, however, they can become virtual control panels (e.g., the display becomes an arrangement of push buttons). When the screen or touch device is pushed with sufficient force at a given button or location, an auditory or visual signal (click or color change) may acknowledge that the computer has received the push information, and the CRT display may then change to provide further feedback or to prepare the operator for the next step in a procedure. This inexpensive and flexible generation of control panels is particularly use-

ful for interactive training programs, such as flight control procedures training.

With especially critical actions, it is useful to require a two-step action in which the first button press results in an "enabled to do X" state, giving the operator a chance to confirm that X is indeed what he intends. Pressing the second button then initiates the X action.

Computer speech recognition offers many possibilities for the pilot or other crewmember to input signals into the computer, especially when the hands are busy or the body is not likely to be positioned conveniently for a manual response. Computer speech recognition systems depend both on training by a given speaker's voice and on the size of the vocabulary of words or utterances. For a single speaker and limited set of commands, available systems are relatively reliable and inexpensive. Voice changes within a speaker, however (e.g., as he or she becomes stressed or fatigued), and recognition of connected words pose difficult problems. Active research and development will lead to more extensive application of this technology.

Criteria for Control

Verification of the accomplishment of the appropriate control requires some feedback. For any discrete response element, the feedback might have one of the following forms:

1. Having the right thoughts about which control to look for
2. Moving the head, eyes, body, and arms in the right direction
3. Grasping the correct control
4. Moving the control in the correct direction
5. Stopping the control at the correct point
6. Achieving the desired response from the aircraft or system

At each stage, it is important to provide feedback cues that are appropriate to correct any error or discrepancy. At the first stage, it might involve a mental model of what the task is or of what procedures and criteria are appropriate, against which the pilot can compare her thoughts. At the second stage, the feedback must be based on familiarity with the aircraft and knowing where to look for needed controls and displays. At the third stage, feedback involves seeing and feeling the control or reading its associated label. At the fourth stage, feedback is essentially tactile and kinesthetic, and the same is true at the fifth stage, although the final position of a critical control often is visually evident as well, as in the case of flap angle in large aircraft.

Closely associated with the factors listed is the criterion of display-control compatibility. Controls should be located adjacent to or below the corresponding displays. If multiple displays of the same type are lined up in left-to-right order, the corresponding controls should be lined up in the same order. Even more important, the direction of movement of the display pointer or indicator should be geometrically the same as the direction of movement of the control that causes that movement.

Earlier, the dilemma of display-control compatibility in aircraft was referred to as the issue of outside-in versus inside-out control display relationships, as illustrated in Figure 29.10, which uses the example of roll control. Figure 29.10A shows the outside-in display, providing the perspective of roll as viewed by an observer fixed relative to earth. A leftward displacement of the joystick rolls the aircraft symbol counterclockwise with the horizon line fixed. Figure 29.10B shows the inside-out display, providing the perspective of the pilot fixed relative to the aircraft. A leftward displacement of the joystick rolls the horizon line clockwise, with the aircraft symbol fixed. The latter display corresponds to what the pilot sees the actual horizon and is used commonly in aircraft.

For discrete control-setting, the pilot reaction and movement time varies upward from 0.25 second, depending on several factors:

1. Accuracy and distance—the effect on reaction and movement time is given by Fitts' law, which states that this time increases with the distance the hand must move and with the required accuracy of the movement (11).
2. Selection from among alternatives—Hick's law states that the reaction and movement time is proportional to the logarithm of the number of (equally probable) alternative selections (12).
3. Anticipation—this factor can effectively reduce the apparent reaction time to zero as an operator predicts the stimulus.
4. Dynamics—the mass-elasticity-viscosity characteristics of the control affect movement time. Starting from a resting position, all three characteristics, if present at a significant level, tend to increase movement time.
5. Display-control compatibility—controls that are not compatible with displays take longer to find and use.

Continuous Manual Control

Mathematical models have been developed that are capable of predicting pilot tracking response in aircraft and helicopter flying. The models are functions of the statistical properties of disturbances (wind gusts), the dynamic properties of the controlled process (aircraft), display characteristics, training, and other factors.

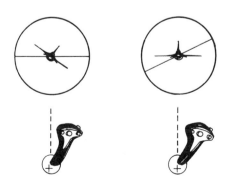

(A) OUTSIDE-IN DISPLAY   (B) INSIDE-OUT DISPLAY

Figure 29.10. Outside-in and inside-out altitude displays in response to stick deflection.

The pilot is treated as a control element (servomechanism) in a closed loop, as shown in Figure 29.2A. A large body of experimental literature derived mostly from simulator experiments has shown that when the input-output differential equation of the pilot is combined with that of the aircraft, the combined open-loop transfer function from tracking error [e(t)] to aircraft response [y(t)] is quite invariant over task and operator conditions and has the form:

$$y(t) = K \int e(t - T_e)dt \qquad (1)$$

K is called loop gain and indicates the sensitivity of pilot response to error, and T_e is the effective time delay in operator response due to neural processing, central processing, and muscle response time (13).

Empirically, parameters K and T_e have been shown to vary systematically, but only slightly, as a function of both the bandwidth or spectrum of energies in the disturbance signal and the dynamic characteristics of the controlled element, in this case the aircraft and its control system, excluding the pilot. This crossover model, as it is known in the aircraft industry, says in effect that the pilot tends to shape his or her own transfer characteristic to compensate for the dynamics of the remainder of the control loop. In doing so, he or she produces combination open-loop characteristics which approximate that of a simple integrator, with an output rate proportional to the error to be neglected. This process, it turns out, is exactly the way a good servomechanism is designed, except for the time delay T_e inherent in the pilot.

To characterize and compare their experimental results and models, manual control researchers tend to use the frequency domain, that is, plots of input-output gain and phase as a function of frequency. The frequency response of the pilot is often characterized in terms of the crossover model, so named because it matches a simple integrator quite well in the region where the forward loop gain line crosses unity. Similar results are obtained with a more general method using a state-space approach to derive the optimal control model of the human operator (14).

It is common to extract statistically that fraction of the total human response energy which is not determined (perfectly correlated with) the model and call that noise. The noise power can be shown to decrease with training and increase with disturbance and other task difficulty parameters.

Within a disturbance frequency range of up to 1 to 2 Hz for controlled-element dynamics varying from a pure gain to a double integrator, the human operator can follow reasonably well, and the crossover model fits. When the controlled element increases to third order (a triple integrator), the human operator can no longer follow; the loop goes unstable. Aircraft are designed with electronic compensation devices to make the net controlled element, from the joystick or control wheel to the observed aircraft response, behave well within the stable and easy-to-control range. This includes force aiding or power steering, making modern aircraft very different from early predecessors that required the pilot to exert considerable stick forces. It is good practice, however, to retain enough force feedback in the control stick to provide tactile feedback cues of the control forces being applied to the aircraft.

The ideal controlled element has dynamics of pure integration, or simply rate control, that permits the operator to merely command a control proportional to observed error and results in an easy task for most tracking.

Figure 29.11 shows that pilot ratings of aircraft handling qualities vary systematically with aircraft dynamics. In assessing the handling qualities of aircraft, test pilots customarily use the Cooper-Harper subjective rating scale (Fig. 29.12). Interestingly, this scale correlates rather well with certain gross parameters of the physical control system, such that ideal systems are not too sluggish, are not close to instability, are not overly sensitive, and do not require excessive control motion.

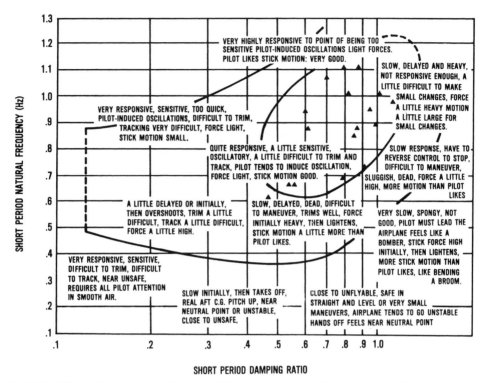

Figure 29.11. Pilot opinion as a function of vehicle second-order system dynamics. (Bioastronautics data book, NASA 88-3006, 1964.)

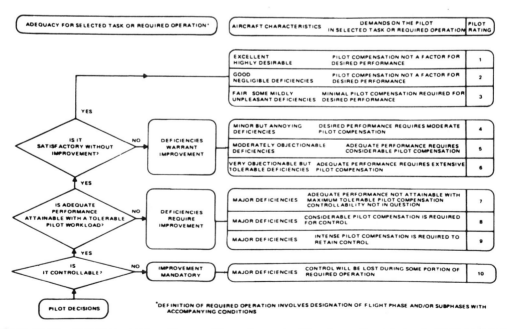

Figure 29.12. Cooper-Harper handling qualities rating scale. (Bioastronautics data book, NASA 88–3006, 1964.)

ANTHROPOMETRY AND GENERAL COCKPIT/WORKPLACE LAYOUT

One aspect of human factors engineering not emphasized thus far in the discussion of displays and controls is whether pilots and operators can see and reach the displays and controls. This criterion must be viewed in terms of the entire population of expected users, a few of whom may be either very large or very small, unless, of course, these individuals are not allowed to operate the equipment. Most operators are near average. Thus, it is important to use statistics in the specification of cockpit or equipment panels, workplaces, and seating.

Anthropometric data are available for various military subpopulations, both men and women, and are further specified for pilots and, in some cases, maintenance personnel (1). Certain key dimensions have been measured for those populations, such as overall height, knee height, and reach. From these data, statistical distributions may be estimated and statistical properties, such as means and confidence limits, determined. The 5% and 95% confidence limits are considered reasonable bounds, meaning that it is reasonable not to have to accommodate those who fall outside this range but to accommodate everyone within it. Actually, the range from the 5% confidence limit for females to the 95% confidence limit for males is the operative range if both males and females are being considered and are present in equal numbers. This approach can pose difficulties, however, because if the seat and knee-space arrangements are large enough for the largest man, other dimensions may then be too great for adequate reach for the smallest woman.

By making certain assumptions, for example, that a seated operator can conveniently see any display within a 30° cone of vision from a horizontal straight-ahead center line, the range of good vision may then be determined between the 5% confidence limit for females and the 95% confidence limit for males. Figure 29.13 is an example of the kinds of reach and vision anthropometric diagrams available in the literature.

Another popular fallacy is that the person who falls at 5% on the distribution for one dimension (e.g., overall height) will fall at the same place on the distribution for another dimension (e.g., reach). Although correlation exists between such measures within individuals, it is far from perfect. Thus, by staying between 5% and 95% confidence limits for one or a few different dimensions, far more than 10% of the population may be excluded on other dimensions.

One must be cautious about using some of the available anthropometric data because they were collected in the late 1940s and 1950s. Since then, the general population of both males and females—has steadily increased in height, by an average of 2.5 cm.

Besides operator body size characteristics, other factors are the forces that can be exerted and the accuracies achieved with controls located in various positions. Large force considerations usually are not critical for pilots and equipment operators in modern aircraft, although they may be for maintenance personnel. Controls should be located where they can be positioned easily and accurately without the inadvertent actuation of other controls.

MENTAL WORKLOAD

During the last two decades, interest in mental workload has been increasing (15,16). The subject is controversial, not because of disagreement over whether it is important, but because of disagreement over how to define and measure it. Nevertheless, military specifications for mental workload are being prepared, based on the assumption that mental workload measures will predict, either at the design stage or during a flight or other operation, whether the operation can succeed. In other words, it is believed that measurements of mental workload will be more sensitive in anticipating when pilot or operator performance will break down than are

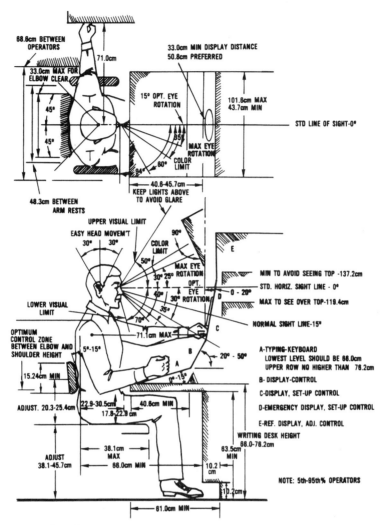

Figure 29.13. Range of reach and vision for the seated operator. (From Van Cott H, Kinkade R. Human engineering guide to equipment design. Washington, DC: U.S. Government Printing Office, 1959.)

conventional measures of performance of the human-machine system.

Currently, mental workload is a construct similar to intelligence. It must be inferred; it cannot be observed directly, as human control response or system performance can, although it might be defined operationally in terms of one or several tests. One clear distinction is between mental and physical workload; the latter is the rate of doing mechanical work and expending calories.

Concern is for situations having long-duration, sustained, mental workload. Many aircraft missions continue to require such efforts by the crew. On the other hand, the introduction of computers and automation in many systems has come to mean that for long periods of time the crew has nothing to do; the workload may be so low as to result in boredom, complacency, and serious decrement in alertness. Then, suddenly the operator may be expected to observe events on a display and make some critical judgments, indeed, even to detect an abnormality, diagnose what failed, and take over control from the automatic system. One concern is that the operator, not being in the control loop, will not have kept up with the situation, and valuable time will be lost as he or she reacquires the knowledge and orientation needed to make the proper diagnosis or take over control. Of additional concern is that at the beginning of the transient, the computer-based information will be opaque to the pilot, and it will take some time even to figure out how to access and retrieve the information needed from the system.

Four approaches have been used to measure mental workload. One approach, which has been used by aircraft manufacturers, avoids coping directly with measurements of the operator per se by basing workload on a task time-line analysis: the more tasks the operator has to do per unit of time, the greater the workload. This approach may provide a relative index of workload, other factors being equal, but it does not address the mental workload of any individual relative to his or her capability, training, or behavior during overload.

The second approach is perhaps the simplest: to use the operator's own subjective judgment rating of his perceived mental workload either during or after the events judged. One form of this approach is a single-category scale similar to the Cooper-Harper scale for rating the handling quality of an aircraft. Perhaps more interesting is a three-attribute scale. There is some agreement that the fraction of total time the crewmember is busy, cognitive complexity, and emotional stress are rather different characteristics of mental workload. These scales have been used by the military services and aircraft manufacturers, with the criticism that people are not always good judges of what their own ability to perform will be in the future. Some pilots may judge themselves to be quite capable of further effort at a high level when, in fact, they are not.

The third approach is the so-called secondary task or reserve capacity technique. Here, the pilot being tested is asked to allocate whatever attention is left from performing the primary task to some unrelated secondary task, such as doing arithmetic problems or tracking a dot on a CRT display with a small joystick. Theoretically, the better performance on the secondary task, the less time required and, therefore, the less the mental workload associated with the primary task. The criticism of this technique is that it is intrusive; it may itself reduce the attention allocated to the primary task and, therefore, be a self-contaminating measure.

The fourth and final technique is a category of only partially explored possibilities—the use of physiologic measures. Many have been proposed, including changes in the electroencephalogram (ongoing or steady state), evoked response potential (the best candidate is the attenuation and latency of the so-called P_{300}, occurring on average 300 ms after the onset of a challenging stimulus), heart rate variability, galvanic skin response, eye scan pattern, pupillary diameter, integrated muscular activity, and frequency spectrum of the voice. No single physiologic measure, however, has been accepted as a valid measure of mental workload.

If mental workload appears to be excessive, several avenues are open for reducing or compensating for it. First, one should examine the situation to see if workload causality can be established and if the casual factors can be redesigned to be quicker, easier, or less anxiety-producing. If this approach is not possible, perhaps parts of the task can be reassigned to other individuals who are less loaded, or the procedure can be altered so as to stretch out in time the succession of events loading the operator. Finally, one may consider giving all or part of the task to a computer or automatic system.

TELEOPERATORS AND VIRTUAL ENVIRONMENTS

Teleoperation and Telepresence

Teleoperation means the extension of a person's sensing, manipulation, or vehicle movement capability to a remote location by communicating through a manual control to a robotic sensor, arm/hand, or vehicle (called teleoperator), which in turn executes the commanded actions and sends visual or position-force feedback to the human operator. Teleoperators can be master-slave devices which mimic the human's arm and hand positions. Or, they can be joystick-rate controlled, which is the most popular mode for current space teleoperators, such as that on the space shuttles. In the latter a three-axis joystick in the astronaut's left hand drives the position of the robotic hand, while a three-axis joystick in the astronaut's right hand drives the orientation of the robotic hand (17).

Teleoperators can also be controlled in supervisory fashion rather than direct manual control, in which the human's instructions specify higher-level goals, constraints, or procedures to be followed rather than instant-by-instant commands. An intermediary computer then must translate these commands into action, much as does an aircraft's autopilot. Supervisory-controlled teleoperators are called telerobots. Remotely piloted aircraft or rotocraft, planetary roving vehicles, or spacecraft operated by humans from earth or other locations in space are examples of telerobots in this sense. Many teleoperators make allowance for either manual or supervisory control.

When the human operator of a teleoperator wears an instrument head-mounted display (e.g., a miniature CRT attached to a helmet) which, when the head is moved to any new position or orientation, drives the remote video camera to a corresponding position and orientation, the operator can look around as he or she would normally and tend to have a sense of being at the remote site. This sensation is called telepresence. If, in addition, he or she feels on the hand an accurate force or touch representation of forces imposed on the teleoperator hand, the sense of telepresence is enhanced, and performance in many telemanipulation tasks can be improved significantly (17).

Virtual Environments for Training and Operations

A virtual environment, called "virtual reality" in the popular media, is a presentation to one's visual, auditory, or haptic (muscle and skin) senses that makes one perceive oneself to be in another environment, one which, unlike that for telepresence, is totally synthetic. One can achieve this virtual presence by wearing a head-mounted display, the position and orientation of which commands the computer to generate a scene which corresponds to the head's position and orientation. In a way, one can look around and walk within an artificial world which exists only in software. By generating a slightly different scene for each eye and using a miniature CRT for each eye, synthetic stereoscopy can be achieved.

Armstrong Aeromedical Research Laboratory, Wright-Patterson Air Force Base (Ohio), and the National Aeronautics and Space Administration (NASA) Ames Research Center, Moffett Field (California), have pioneered in virtual environment technology. It is being used for training and experimentation on systems and missions which are computer prototyped but not yet built in hardware. Since computer-generated images can be superposed easily into normal video images (as with the head-up display), virtual environments can also be added to real ones during actual flight operations, for example, to allow the pilot to see through weather to other aircraft, or to see radar or missile sites which are known in location to a computer database but not normally visible to the naked eye.

Whereas binaural sound presentation (in a horizontal plane) can be synthesized by presenting sounds of different loudness and time difference to the two ears, three-dimensional sound presentation is synthesized by filtering each ear's sound patterns through a "head-related transfer function," a mathematical transformation which mimics what the outer ears (pinnae) achieve for hearing in free three-dimensional space. This new capability achieves an auditory virtual environment.

Virtual environment technology is not complete without synthetic haptic sensations, forces applied to the muscles, tendon, joints and skin which, when reaching out and grasping or touching objects in the synthesized world, correspond to their real world counterparts. "Data gloves" and articulated devices which measure the location and pose of the hands and fingers are available, but generation of realistic tactile sensation still eludes technologists (17).

TASK AND DECISION ANALYSIS

Several types of graphic tools are helpful in analyzing aircrew tasks and decisions for purposes of designing equipment and procedures. Figure 29.14 shows a critical path diagram of tasks that must be done during a nominal mission. The arrows indicate necessary temporal order: A must be done before D, both B and C before E, and D, E, and F before G. Otherwise, these tasks may be done at any time; thus, the precedence of A, B, C, and F is not specified relative to one another. In planning whole missions or detailed procedures for using equipment such as computers, it is important to do this analysis so that design errors will not result from a lack of awareness of priorities.

This approach presupposes that a critical path analysis has been done so that the activities are correctly ordered. The purpose of this analysis is to establish coordination, fully realizing that in many missions, circumstances will cause one individual to assume an activity normally done by another or force the activities to be done in a somewhat different order. Nevertheless, this

has been found to be a useful analysis, especially in a time-critical, high-workload mission.

Figure 29.15 is an event-decision tree. The order of events is from left to right. After each event, several alternative, mutually exclusive events are usually indicated by lines emanating from the preceding event, with the conditional probability indicated. For example, given that event A occurs, there is a 0.7 probability that event C will then occur and a 0.3 probability that event D will occur. After C, three events may occur. The probabilities leaving a block must total 1. In some cases, the succession of events is certain, that is, $p = 1$. Note that some events may be the result of more than one preceding event. Note also in this case that the sum of probabilities entering a block can be anything; the contingent probabilities need not total 1. At the right, consequences (dollars, damage) based on the final column of events are shown. By multiplying through the probabilities for each chain of events that can result in any one consequence and then adding the results for each consequence, one can determine the probability of that consequence occurring. The product of that consequence and its probabilities is the expected consequence, and the sum of these products is the net expected consequence for the whole situation.

The discussion above takes the viewpoint that the succession of events is determined by nature; that is, it occurs without intervention by a person or machine to manipulate which paths are taken. The other viewpoint may be taken, which assumes that each alternative column is a decision manipulated by a person or machine, and the next column is a result (i.e., a decision by nature). In this case, the person or machine is unconstrained in choosing from the alternatives that follow each result; the probabilities in brackets no longer apply. Now one can work back from the consequences and decide exactly which of the alternative responses maximizes the expected value. After C, one can choose the greatest of $(.6C_J + .4C_K)$ for F, $(.4C_L + .6C_M)$ for G, and C_M for H. This value then becomes

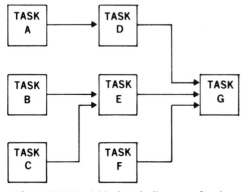

Figure 29.14. Critical path diagram of tasks.

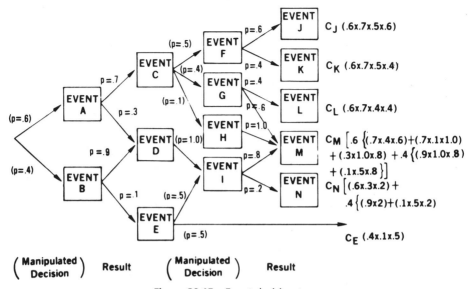

Figure 29.15. Event-decision tree.

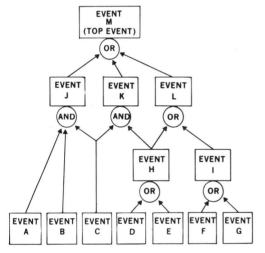

Figure 29.16. Fault tree with logical causality of failures.

the expected consequence of C, assuming one chooses F, G, or H to maximize the expected consequence. Similarly, the expected consequence of D and E can be determined. Finally, a similar analysis can be performed in choosing alternatives A and B, doing whichever has the greatest expected consequence and expecting that consequence, on the average.

Figure 29.16 shows a fault tree. The purpose

of this diagram is to show the logical causality of failures. Cause and effect goes from bottom to top, as does time. In this example all the events are defined as failures. (They could just as easily have been defined as successes, which means the ANDs become ORs and vice-versa.) For example, the AND connecting A, B, and C to J means that all three of the lower failures must occur before the J failure occurs. Either D or E can cause the H failure, but it then takes C and H to cause the K failure. Because there are ORs all the way up the right side, either F or G can make I fail, which is sure to make L fail, which is sure to cause the top event, presumably the failure to which the whole analysis was directed. The same is true for D and E. If probabilities are known for the events along the bottom row, and if events are independent, expected failure or success paths can be traced. The AND means the probabilities must be multiplied for the set of lines coming to the next higher event to determine the probability of that event. In the OR case, the probability of an event is the sum of the two probabilities minus their product. If the convergent events are not independent, more sophisticated statistical analysis is required. This type of analysis can be applied to a combination of human and machine error; that is, the blocks can represent people or machine events (failures or success).

It is common, for example, in the nuclear power industry, to use the fault trees and event-decision trees in combination to perform reliability analysis of complex human-machine systems. To do this, failure probabilities must be estimated for both machine and human components. Conservative estimates for machine components are determined from bench-life tests under severe environmental conditions and from operating records. Failure probabilities for the human components are more difficult to obtain. The following considerations enter into such estimates:

1. People tend to make common mode errors. If they learn two responses together or the procedures call for doing them together, if they err on one of the pair, they are likely to err on the other of the pair.
2. If there is a well-learned sequence of steps, say A B C, and if a different procedure calls for X B Y, people tend to go off on the wrong track (i.e., to do X B C).
3. Both stress and the rate of mental processing demanded increase the tendency to err.
4. People tend to persevere and continue to err long after contrary evidence accumulates. On the other hand, people tend to discover their own errors and correct them before serious consequences result.

No science of human error is well codified, and these considerations are only a few of the acceptable generalities. The best error prevention is good design and good training. Errors may be prevented by not exposing people, that is, not giving them the opportunity to err. This can be done by isolating controls or displays that have particularly critical functions from those with which they might otherwise be confused, by using guards, by recessing push buttons, or by requiring two-step (enable, activate) operation sequences. A final technique is the use of warn-

ing labels, but this technique should be used sparingly if at all; more than a few warning labels on a panel can result in clutter and distraction (18).

The majority of aviation accidents are attributed to operator error. Close examination may reveal that the root cause goes back to a system design in failing to account for human capacity or limitations. For example, the operator errors associated with misreading a poor altimeter display, mishearing a communication in a high-noise environment, or missing a procedure step during a high-workload crisis can be reduced by proper attention to human factors considerations. The time to apply human factors is in the design stage rather than as a remedy after an aircraft accident investigation.

REFERENCES

1. Parker JF, West VR, eds. Bioastronautics data book. 2nd ed. Washington,DC: National Aeronautics and Space Administration, 1973.
2. Boff K, Kaufman L, Thomas JP, eds. Handbook of perception and human performance. New York: Wiley, 1986.
3. Military standard: human engineering design criteria for military systems, equipment and facilities. MIL-STD-1472C. Washington, DC: U.S. Government Printing Office, 1981.
4. Salvendy G, ed. Handbook of human factors. New York: Wiley, 1987.
5. Helander M, ed. Handbook of human-computer interaction. New York: Elsevier North Holland, 1988.
6. Stevens SS, ed. Handbook of experimental psychology. New York: Wiley, 1951.
7. Sanders MS, McCormick EJ. Human factors in engineering and design. 7th ed. New York: McGraw Hill, 1993.
8. Banks WW, Gertman DI, Peterson RJ. Human engineering design considerations for cathode ray tube-generated displays. Nuclear Regulatory Commission. NUREG/CR-2496. Washington DC: U.S. Government Printing Office, 1982.
9. Kantowitz BH, Sorkin RD. Human factors. New York: Wiley, 1983.
10. Young LR, Sheena D. Eye movement measurement techniques. Am Psychol 1975;30(3):315–330.
11. Fitts PM. The information capacity of the human motor system in controlling the amplitude of movement. J Exp Psychol 1954;47:381–391.
12. Hic, WE. On the rate of gain of information. Q J Exp Psychol 1952;4:11–26.
13. McRuer D, Graham D, Krendel E, et al. Human pilot

dynamics in compensatory systems: theory models and experiments with controlled element and forcing function variations. AFFDL-TR-65-15. Wright-Patterson Air Force Base, Ohio, 1965.

14. Kleinman DL, Baron S, Levison W. A control theoretic approach to manual vehicle systems analysis. New York: Institute of Electrical and Electronics Transactions, 1971:824–832.

15. Moray N. Mental workload. New York: Plenum Press, 1979.

16. Wickins CD. Engineering psychology and human performance. Columbus, OH: Merrill, 1984.

17. Sheridan TB. Telerobotics, automation, and human supervisory control, Cambridge, MA: MIT Press, 1992.

18. Senders JW, Moray NP. Human error: cause, prediction and reduction. Hillsdale, NJ: Erlbaum, 1991.

Chapter 30

Management of Human Resources in Air Transport Operations

James F. Parker, Jr.,

William T. Shepherd

People are the common denominator of progress.

John Kenneth Galbraith, 1964

The growth of the air transport industry in the United States represents a notable success by any standard. Air travel is readily accessible; it is affordable; and it is remarkably safe. While the industry has grown steadily since World War II, the rate of growth increased after the Airline Deregulation Act of 1978. In addition to stimulating growth, this Act changed the economics of airline operations. Increased competition resulted in a growing demand for aircraft and brought new financial pressures. In this, there was a message. Successful airline management would require that airline resources, whether they be equipment, finances, or personnel, be used in a manner designed for optimum benefit and productivity.

Personnel employed within the air transport industry, particularly flight crewmembers and maintenance technicians, represent one of the industry's most valuable resources, a resource which must be given proper management and support if the safety and efficiency goals of the industry are to be achieved. Scheduled U.S. airlines now employ over 500,000 men and women compared to 329,000 at the time of deregulation in 1978. This growth has changed the character of the industry and presents significant challenges for health professionals and behavioral scientists working to ensure the health and productivity of this workforce.

Airlines must remain competitive and, at the same time, comply with an array of regulatory requirements. To accomplish this, careful management of operating resources is essential. Direct operating resources of commercial airlines are shown in Table 30.1 (1,2). From an airline point of view, the aircraft itself is high priority. The more revenue-hours the aircraft flies, the more likely the airline is to survive. There is continual pressure to keep an airplane flying productively for as many hours a day as possible. For some aircraft, those that fly nonstop for longer distances, daily schedules having 12 or even 13 flight hours are not uncommon.

The extent to which aircraft can and are being used directly relates to the management of other airline resources. Flight crews must operate the aircraft productively and safely. Maintenance personnel must ensure that aircraft are mechanically sound and safe for flight as the schedule calls. Any break-down in the performance of either of these groups directly affects aircraft use, airline revenue, and flight safety. It is most

Table 30.1.
Commercial Airline Direct Operating Resources (1994)

Resources	Number
Large jet aircraft	4,485
Flight personnel (pilots and copilots)	53,203
Maintenance personnel (mechanics)	56,124
Flight attendants	87,085

Source: Federal Aviation Administration (1), Air Transport Association of America (2).

important for an airline to manage all resources wisely.

Many features of the workday can affect the performance of flight and maintenance crews. Issues of work scheduling and workload, the working environment, management relations, communications, and use of equipment illustrate variables of consequence in determining worker effectiveness. The importance of a number of these variables has been recognized for some time. For example, one of the first matters addressed by the Air Line Pilots Association (ALPA), organized in 1931, was that of pilot fatigue (3). Some of the early airlines were requiring that pilots fly up to 150 hours a month. ALPA claimed that long hours of exposure to vibration, noise, and flying conditions were doing pilots irreparable harm and increasing the likelihood of accidents. After continual pressure from ALPA, which enlisted the support of the Aeromedical Association in its cause, the National Labor Board in 1934 ruled that 85 hours per month would be the flight-time limitation for pilots of the five airlines which had become involved in the labor dispute. Subsequently, the Federal Aviation Administration (FAA) set limits for domestic carrier crews at 1000 hours in a calendar year, 100 hours in a calendar month, and 30 hours in 7 consecutive days. Generally, union contracts set these flight times at lesser values. However, although the issue of flight time has been given considerable attention, fatigue remains even today an example of biomedical and behavioral variables that can affect performance both of flight crews and maintenance crews.

ROLE AND CONTRIBUTION OF BIOMEDICAL AND BEHAVIORAL SCIENTISTS

Biomedical and behavioral specialists have been prominent in aviation since its infancy. As with many other aspects of aviation, their contributions usually followed accidents or mishaps. Physicians, early players in the World War I era, were called upon to examine the alarming noncombat accidents that were decimating airmen and airplanes. Through their work, medical selection criteria and tests for such factors as vision and motor coordination were developed. Behavioral scientists did little at this time because they were few in number and because it was not readily apparent that some of the problems were in fact attributable to nonphysiologic factors. These specialists rose to prominence at the time of World War II, particularly through their development of selection tests and methods. These tests were used, with reasonable reliability, to predict success in military aviation career fields, including piloting and maintenance. The years after World War II saw an expansion of the roles of physicians and psychologists in studies of human performance and in the investigation of such factors as stress and fatigue.

The body of knowledge concerning human performance in aviation has grown exponentially in the last 40 years. We have moved from relatively simple selection batteries to complex models of human performance that account for a wide array of physiologic and behavioral characteristics. We know a great deal about task performance of individuals and teams in aviation and we can confidently specify conditions which result in improved performance, primarily for pilots and air traffic controllers.

In spite of progress over the last few decades, much remains to be done. Further theoretical development is needed, and application of existing knowledge is just beginning to bear fruit. For example, cockpit resource management (CRM) concepts (discussed later in the chapter), developed in the last 15 years, are now employed in many air carrier training and evaluation programs. These essential concepts are now being studied for their application in the aircraft maintenance field. For years our attention in the study of human performance has been almost exclusively on pilots and air traffic controllers. Only recently have we been reminded that the performance of aviation maintenance and inspection technicians can be just as vital to aviation safety.

Studies of maintenance performance require that biomedical and behavioral scientists determine the influence of such variables as training, vigilance, boredom, environmental stressors, and physiologic factors on performance. The FAA currently is conducting research on maintenance performance. The importance of this research is realized when one looks into the future and sees an accelerating retirement rate for the existing maintenance workforce and a smaller pool of available applicants to take its place. These demographic facts of life, coupled with dramatic increases in the level of technology employed in new generation transport aircraft, mean that action must be taken now to ensure that the performance of the incoming workforce is optimal. The demands on this workforce will be greater than now because not only must technicians work with new state-of-the-art technology but old technology as well, since a certain segment of the fleet will always be "aging." Economic factors mean that air carriers will retain aircraft in service for longer periods of time, hence the required knowledge and performance span for technicians will necessarily be broader than today. It will be up to the scientific community to develop the supporting technology and procedures necessary for the inevitable "people" changes in the air carrier industry. These changes will affect pilots, maintenance technicians, and others with crucial roles in the safety of air carrier operations. Research and planning for these changes are underway now in a partnership of government, industry, and academia.

THE AIR TRANSPORT INDUSTRY

The air transport industry is an indispensable force sustaining the quality of life of American citizens and the robustness of the national economy. Airlines offer the public an opportunity to

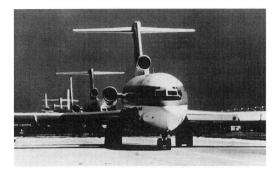

Figure 30.1. Airplanes lined up for takeoff at Chicago's O'Hare Airport. (Photo courtesy of Federal Aviation Administration.)

travel readily to all parts of the country. Businesses operate in the competitive environment of national and international commerce through the rapid movement of goods by air. Both the public and business have come to rely on a growing air transport industry as a necessary feature of day-to-day life. Evidence of growth to date is seen in Figure 30.1, which shows a typical queue of aircraft awaiting takeoff at O'Hare Airport in Chicago. Such sights are common at this airport, which is used by more than 60 million passengers each year.

What we think of as a national air transport industry is by no means monolithic. Commercial air carriers fall into four broad categories, based largely on the service provided, the aircraft operated, and the size of the operation. These categories are as follows:

Majors—These are carriers having annual operating revenues in excess of $1 billion. They fly the longer intercity routes in the United States, including coast-to-coast flights. They also are the principal international operators. In this group, two-engine aircraft (A-300, A-310, and B-767) are the fastest growing segment, expected to increase by about 11% annually through the 1990s (1).

Nationals—Operating revenues for these carriers exceed $75 million annually. Generally, routes flown here center on one part of the country, such as Hawaii or Alaska. Aircraft flown are those best suited for short-haul operations, such as the MD-80, DC-9, D-727, and B-737.

Large/Medium Regionals—Carriers here have

annual operating revenues less than $75 million. These carriers provide localized service, frequently operating as feeder airlines for the majors. Regional fleets are composed predominantly of aircraft having 60 seats or fewer. Most of the aircraft in this fleet are of foreign manufacture.

Commuters—These are small certificated carriers operating aircraft frequently having fewer than 20 passenger seats. The average load is roughly 10 passengers. Operations include intercity routes and feeder service for the majors. Most aircraft flown, again, are of foreign manufacture.

The groupings shown above for the air transport industry illustrate two features of interest for biomedical and behavioral specialists. First, the experience levels and performance requirements for flight crews in regional/commuter operations are different from those for the major carriers. Second, and here the differences are even more pronounced, aircraft maintenance facilities and procedures for regional/commuter carriers may bear only a nominal resemblance to those of the majors. These differences can affect workforce productivity.

Industry Directions

The air transport industry has had a pattern of regular growth during recent years, which is expected to continue. In the decade from 1990 to 2000, passenger enplanements for combined domestic and international operations are forecast to increase from 471 million to well over 700 million, an increase of over 50% (1). The growth for regional/commuter operations will be even greater. Forecasts call for more than 70 million passengers to be carried by regionals/commuters in the year 2001, more than double the 1989 number.

The forecast increase in passenger load necessarily means an increase in the size of the air carrier fleet. Taking into account the anticipated retirement of some aircraft, the U.S. commercial air carrier fleet is projected to increase from an inventory of 3870 large jet aircraft in 1989 to 4949 aircraft by the year 2001. The largest increase, in terms of number of aircraft, is projected to occur in the two-engine, narrow-body aircraft category.

National Airspace System Plan

The present growth in air travel is placing serious demands on supporting services and structures, and these demands will only increase. Airports, surrounding roadway systems, and aircraft manufacturers are all affected by the growth in air travel, but probably none more than the air traffic control system. Recognizing this growth pattern, and realizing that much of its equipment was becoming obsolescent, the FAA in 1981 adopted a comprehensive National Airspace System (NAS) Plan for modernizing and improving air traffic control and airway facilities services through the year 2000. Each year the plan is updated as situations and opportunities change.

The NAS Plan envisions a modern, automated network of facilities and equipment in which the latest levels of available technology are integrated into a coordinated system for air traffic control and air navigation (4). The theme of the plan relies on greater use of automation, consolidation of major facilities, and application of new technological solutions. Some features of the plan include the following:

Major en route and terminal systems will be consolidated from more than 200 facilities today to fewer than 30 by the year 2000.

Common modular computers, software, and controller workstations will be used to increase system capacity and airspace availability. The new workstations, called sector suites, consist of displays presenting a plan view of the current situation including (1) position of the aircraft and real-time weather, (2) electronic display of flight data (eliminating the need for manual flight strips), and (3) display of planning information and automated control functions.

Higher levels of automation will be used to improve safety, fuel efficiency, and productivity. One will be the Automated En route Air Traffic Control System (AERA), in which computer systems will offer fuel-efficient instrument flight plans, predict flight paths to detect possible conflicts, and assist with many flight control functions, thereby increasing controller productivity.

Advanced Aircraft

New aircraft now being designed and developed will aid in meeting future needs of the air transport industry. The aircraft will have improved characteristics and capabilities and will present a new environment for flight crews and maintenance teams. Each aircraft will bring with it higher levels of automation. This in turn will mean new roles and procedures for flight crews. For maintenance personnel, automation will bring additional training requirements as well as a new generation of sophisticated diagnostic and repair equipment.

The Boeing 757/767 and the Airbus Industries series of aircraft are representative of a new generation now employed in airline service. These aircraft use advanced avionics and increased automation for flight control and navigation. They also, in a sense, serve as test beds for evaluations of flight deck procedures and maintenance bay requirements for the coming decade.

An example of a different type of aircraft being considered as an answer to heavier demand for short-haul, intercity travel is the Bell-Boeing tilt-rotor airplane, a preview of which is shown in Figure 30.2. This airplane uses turboprop engines which rotate to the vertical for takeoff and landing, allowing operation much like a helicopter at such times. This, of course, greatly reduces the space necessary for landing and opens the possibility of operating from sites well within city limits.

For travel in the distant future, manufacturers are beginning to consider a high-speed civil transport (HSCT) aircraft. Since such a plane necessarily will operate supersonically at times,

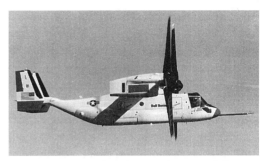

Figure 30.2. V-22 aircraft, a predecessor of the civil tilt-rotor aircraft. (Photo courtesy of Bell Helicopter Textron, Inc.)

a host of environmental and noise issues must be addressed before the aircraft can be built. However, there is every reason to believe that supersonic travel, with all of its implications for flight and maintenance crews, will grow in the future.

Airline Personnel Systems

Flight Personnel

Currently there are over 50,000 pilots flying for U.S. airlines. Of this number about 15% fly for regional or commuter carriers, and the rest fly for the majors. Less than 2% of these pilots are women, but the number of female air carrier pilots has been steadily growing (1). Approximately 85% of major airline pilots are unionized. Most regional airline pilots are nonunion, but organized labor has been increasing its efforts to unionize these pilot groups.

The regional airline pilot personnel system is thought of by many as a "farm club" for major airlines. Most pilots flying for regional carriers are working to obtain sufficient flight time and experience to qualify for a job with one of the major airlines. This poses a problem for the regionals, where 50 to 100% turnover rates for pilot personnel in a year are not unusual. The regionals are constantly faced with recruitment and training of new pilot personnel. This can be very expensive. Since few regional airlines own simulators or operate extensive training departments, they must perform a good deal of their training in their own airplanes or use commercial organizations such as Flight Safety International. These organizations have large investments in training facilities and own simulators and aircraft of the types used by regional airlines.

Turnover of pilots employed by major airlines is relatively low. Salaries and benefits are typically much better in majors than in regional carriers. Also, job progression in major airlines is heavily dependent on seniority. If a pilot leaves one airline to work for another, he or she usually is relegated to the bottom of the seniority list at the new carrier. This tends to stem circulation of pilot personnel among the majors.

Many regional carriers are now affiliated with or even owned outright by major airlines. The majors provide various kinds of support to their regional affiliates, including financial and management aid and, in some cases, regional pilots with seniority numbers at the major carrier. This allows a pilot to build seniority while employed by a regional airline and tends to keep regional pilots flying longer for their employer before making the transition to the majors. This helps to increase the stability of regionals.

Maintenance Personnel

The people who inspect and maintain civil air carrier aircraft are growing in importance. As noted previously, demographic projections suggest a shrinking pool of available, talented people able to assume the responsible role of aviation maintenance technician (AMT). Competition from other industries offering higher salaries, better working conditions, and day-shift operations will further reduce the potential group of AMTs. Also, the number of persons with military experience (a significant present-day source of personnel) is expected to decline substantially in the years ahead.

Currently, airlines are able to attract only 25 to 30% of graduates of airframe and powerplant (A&P) schools. The rest go to manufacturers, fixed-base operators, air taxi operators and other industries. This disparity will almost certainly

increase unless the air carrier industry initiates action to head off this trend.

The FAA currently shows a total of more than 325,000 mechanic certificates in force. However, this number is not very revealing because it only tells the total number of certificates issued since the FAA began accumulating this statistic. There is no way of telling how many of these certificate holders are active or where they may be working since the FAA does not currently seek this information. Many of these certificate holders work for general aviation operations. Almost certainly, many of these certificate holders are retired, deceased, or otherwise no longer functional in the aircraft maintenance industry.

A recent survey of member operators by the Air Transport Association (ATA) found 4000 mechanic jobs currently vacant out of 69,000 available or currently filled positions, and the demand for AMTs is expected to grow at the rate of about 10% a year. An estimate by the Future Aviation Professionals of America (FAPA) suggests that the airlines will need 46,000 new AMTs by 1999. However, the yearly number of newly licensed mechanics has been declining in the last few years.

The projected need for people is partly due to recent FAA requirements for modifications to older aircraft, but it is also due to the record pace of new aircraft acquisition by the airline industry. The fleet will be much larger in future years due to an anticipated growth in air travel. The fleet will be made up of a mix of new and old technology aircraft as carriers retain older aircraft in service for longer periods of time. This of course contributes to the complexity of the AMT task.

FLIGHT OPERATIONS

Crew Structure and Responsibilities

The typical air carrier cockpit crew complement is getting smaller. In years past, prior to the advent of automated cockpit systems, cockpits were crowded with people, particularly in long-range or overwater operations. It was not uncommon to find several pilots, a navigator, radio operator, and flight engineer. With improvements in radio and system automation, the required cockpit team has been reduced to two people in many cases and three at most. Three-person crews are found in older aircraft, but new-generation aircraft, even large aircraft such as the Boeing 747-400, operate with just two pilots. Some people even talk about the days when a single pilot will operate air carrier flights, but at least for now, this is a distant and unlikely possibility.

Airline cockpit crews have traditionally followed a system of military-like command structure. The captain has unquestioned authority to direct all phases of flight and other crewmembers are subordinate to his or her authority. (Coupled with this authority is the rarely disputed responsibility for everything that happens on the flight deck; when someone does something wrong, the captain usually is charged with failing to prevent the action). The captain's role is as much that of a manager as that of control manipulator to direct the flight of the airplane. System automation has further underscored this role identification. The captain decides what the flight operating parameters will be and in many cases directs other cockpit personnel or commands cockpit systems to execute these wishes. In a sense this resembles the role of the sea captain who rarely touches the ship's wheel or other bridge systems, but has ultimate authority and responsibility for safe operation of the ship.

In most air carrier operations, first and second officers are, like the captain, also pilots. The flight engineer's position, formerly held by non-pilot specialists in many cases, is now the responsibility of the second officer, usually a pilot with a flight engineer's certificate. However, as noted previously, the flight engineer's position no longer exists in most newer air transports, and eventually all air carrier aircraft likely will be operated by two-person cockpit crews—a captain and first officer.

Almost always, the cockpit crew consists of

people who are working their way up from junior positions, such as second officer, to more senior jobs, with the captain's assignment being the ultimate to which most crewmembers aspire. Union contracts typically mandate a strict seniority approach to advancement, and this policy is also observed in most nonunion environments.

Flight attendants complete the typical air transport crew. These crewmembers are responsible for the safety of passengers in the cabin. They are trained to deal with emergencies such as in-flight fires and particularly situations that require emergency evacuation of the cabin. Flight attendants, like the junior members of the cockpit crew, are subordinate to the command of the captain, although most air carrier operations with more than one flight attendant usually consist of one senior or lead flight attendant to manage the activities of the others. In practice, the senior flight attendant has primary responsibility for cabin safety, and the wise captain defers to his or her knowledge and skill in this area.

Not all air carrier operations require flight attendants. Commuter or regional operators with aircraft having fewer than 19 seats do not require flight attendants. These operations are usually accomplished under Part 135 of the Federal Aviation Regulations (FARs). This part of the FARs is aimed at what are sometimes referred to as air taxi operations, although certain types of scheduled air carrier operations are included.

Flight Crew Requirements

Most major airline activity is governed by Part 121 of the FARs. Slightly different standards apply in the two cases regarding crew training, qualification, and performance. However, Parts 121 and 135 are more similar than different as far as flight crew requirements are concerned. In both cases (with only rare exceptions) the captain or pilot-in-command must possess an Airline Transport Pilot (ATP) certificate, the highest level pilot certificate granted by the FAA. There currently are some differences in regulatory requirements for pilot flight and duty time limits between Parts 121 and 135. For example, Part 121 states a maximum of 100 flying hours per month, whereas Part 135 permits 120 flying hours per month. There are other small differences between the two sets of regulations, such as required rest periods between flights and training and testing requirements. In practice, most Part 121 operations do not schedule pilots to fly 100 hours per month, nor do Part 135 pilots routinely fly 120 hours per month since the annual regulatory flying limits are 1000 and 1200 hours, respectively. As this publication goes to press, the FAA is considering harmonization of regulations contained in FAR Parts 121 and 135. In these revisions, most Part 121 requirements supersede existing Part 135 requirements. These rulemaking changes are expected to take place in 1996.

Flight crews spend considerably more time at their jobs than just the time spent at the controls. They are required to report well in advance of each flight for briefings on factors such as weather, fuel and passenger loads, aircraft condition, and destination airport status. Sometimes, flight crews have to "dead-head," or fly from their domicile to another location, to join their flight and may also have to dead-head home from the last stop of their flight. These additional activities add considerably to the amount of time flight crews spend "on the job."

Performance Measurement

The FAA requires regular evaluation of pilot skills and performance through a system of tests and checks. These consist of written and oral tests, proficiency checks, and flight checks. These are given usually at intervals of 6 and 12 months, with more stringent requirements for captains and pilots-in-command. Tests evaluate knowledge of such factors as FARs, meteorology, weight and balance, air traffic control procedures, and aircraft systems. Flight checks can be instrument proficiency checks, line checks, and flying proficiency checks. Instrument proficiency checks evaluate a pilot's ability to per-

form various types of approaches, execute emergency procedures, and navigate by instruments. These checks include oral or written tests as well as flight demonstrations. A line check is typically a demonstration by a pilot-in-command of ability to fly proficiently over a typical part of the air carrier's route. Flying proficiency checks involve demonstration of specific procedures and maneuvers, such as steep turns, crosswind landings, and emergency procedures. A considerable amount of the testing and checking can be accomplished in flight simulators. Simulators have become so sophisticated and have such fidelity to actual flight that they readily mimic the performance of the real airplane without leaving the ground. They are extremely useful in evaluating pilot performance in potentially hazardous operations such as wind shear avoidance and engine-out maneuvers.

Factors Affecting Flight Crew Performance

Training
In addition to all the assessment procedures discussed above, operators are required to conduct training programs for their crews, including flight attendants. They must provide initial training, recurrent training, differences training, transition training, upgrade training, and other training which may be appropriate for given circumstances. Training can be ground or flight training; ground training is usually classroom oriented; flight training can be accomplished in an actual airplane or a simulator. In recent years air carrier simulator training has shifted from intensive attention to specific procedures, such as engine failure after takeoff, to a process called Line-Oriented Flight Training (LOFT). LOFT simulates a typical entire air carrier flight segment during which abnormal conditions may be introduced. These could range from dealing with difficult air traffic control instructions during a simulated weather diversion, to dealing with a passenger with a heart attack in the cabin. LOFT provides opportunities to observe and train

entire crews on coordination and interaction as well as procedures for dealing with system malfunctions. LOFT blends training and performance assessment in that a crew's performance during training often is critiqued. LOFT scenarios frequently are videotaped to allow later review and discussion of the crew's actions during the "flight."

Crew Scheduling

Commercial air crews follow flight schedules dictated by operational and economic factors, regulatory constraints, and union contractual rules. For short-haul operations, a workday may consist of a number of short legs and a flight duty day of possibly 12 to 14 hours (5). By contrast, long-haul flights may last for many hours and cross many time zones before reaching their destination. Indeed, the length of long-haul stages certainly will increase, as reflected by the ranges of the Boeing 747–400 and the McDonnell-Douglas MD-11, each of which can extend beyond 14 hours.

The schedules followed by flight crews can create problems. Most important are fatigue and circadian desynchronization (see Chapter 14). While flight crews certainly are able to cope with the flight fatigue and disruption of daily rhythms, the issues nonetheless exist and can increase the likelihood of errors in performance. As Green noted in a study of the relationship between stress and aviation accidents, subtle errors in pilot performance can have large consequences (6).

Green examined reports maintained in a confidential database describing in-flight incidents and found many referring to sleep and fatigue problems. In a number of the incidents, crewmembers actually fell asleep during flight. In some cases a single pilot was flying alone at night, with little contact with Air Traffic Control. One report, however, describes how the entire crew of a trans-Atlantic aircraft fell asleep, only to be awakened by an audio warning. Green also discusses research conducted by the Royal Air Force Institute of Aviation Medicine, which

found that pilots fatigued by sleep deprivation committed more and larger procedural errors during in-flight instrument operations than did rested pilots. He concludes that fatigue and sleep deprivation are ongoing problems in aviation and may be underestimated as causes of in-flight incidents and accidents.

An extensive program of research dealing with flight crew fatigue and problems of desynchronization has been conducted at the National Aeronautics and Space Administration (NASA) Ames Research Center. Much of the research has been cooperative, involving members of international laboratories, U.S. researchers, and volunteer crews from different airlines. The research has examined both the fatigue effects of short-haul flying and desynchronosis problems in long-haul international flights (7). The work of the NASA team provides considerable information for those concerned with crew scheduling and its possible impact on crew performance. In the NASA studies, sleepiness is generally equated with fatigue, since sleepiness is viewed by most aviation professionals as the most operationally significant aspect of fatigue.

In the short-haul research program, schedules of two U.S. carriers were identified that included some combination of early morning or late evening departures, long duty days, many segments, long en route layovers, and/or minimal overnight rest. Crews operating with this type of scheduling served as study participants. Some of the principal findings regarding these flight crews include the following:

1. Short-haul crews experience sleep loss despite overnight rest schedules that meet the regulatory and contractual requirements for time off duty and for quality of accommodations. As Graeber notes (7), these findings might be expected for crews who fly mostly at night but are somewhat surprising for crews who operate primarily during daylight.
2. The development of fatigue is more a function of the timing of trips than the length of the duty day or the number of segments

flown. Pilots have difficulty adjusting their sleep habits to get as much sleep as they get at home. Pilots did not go to sleep early enough to compensate for early morning departures; they simply stay up later on trips than they do at home.

3. One surprising finding is the positive relationship between the intensity of a day's duty and the length and quality of sleep that night. This supports the preference of most crews to keep flying with brief stopovers. This also supports the finding that crews may be able to pace themselves or somehow anticipate at the beginning of a trip the fatigue level they will experience over the length of the trip. This pacing obviously is aided through the use of napping when opportunities arise. Findings show the frequency of napping began to increase on the second day of the trip and reached a sharp peak during the first day home.

4. Flying more segments led to increased sleep duration and more restful sleep that night. Quality of sleep was measured by lower heart rates and activity during sleep and by higher sleep-quality ratings after wake-up. These findings were valid for increases up to six or seven flights per day. Findings also showed that it was the number of daily flight hours, not daily duty hours, that was associated with longer sleep duration.

Graeber considered the significance of fatigue and sleep loss in short-haul crews and whether this might affect safety and operational efficiency. Based on reports received at the NASA Aviation Safety Reporting System, he concluded that such fatigue does operate detrimentally. However, in a simulator study run in concert with the field study, results supported the view that increased crew coordination resulting from several consecutive days of flying can substantially counterbalance the detrimental effects of fatigue.

Results of studies of long-haul operational flights also lead to certain conclusions regarding the scheduling of crews flying across many time zones. The findings were as follows:

1. While circadian desynchronization affects many physiologic and behavioral functions, flight crews complain most about fatigue and sleep loss.

2. Sleep quality decreased more after eastward flights than westward flights. Sleep was more variable and fragmented after eastward night flights. The fact that sleep patterns, as well as other behavioral and physiologic variables, are more disrupted by eastward than westward flights illustrates that humans have difficulty in shortening their day.

3. Average sleep patterns for all groups used in the study, as well as those reported for nonpilot groups, were similar. These curves show a gradual increase in sleepiness through the day, reaching a maximum in late afternoon, and followed by a gradual decline into the evening. These sleepiness rhythms persisted on home base time after flights transiting many time zones. Graeber suggests that the apparent stability of the sleepiness curve might allow crews to predict when they could fall asleep most readily and thereby develop better strategies for sleeping or napping while on travel.

4. Physiologic measures of sleepiness, such as electroencephalographic recordings, do not match subjective estimates of sleepiness. This implies that crewmembers on duty are not able to reliably assess their own state of fatigue and thus may not be aware of when they are most at risk for reduced vigilance because of sleepiness.

5. Based on project findings, researchers recommended that crews limit their sleep immediately after arrival in new time zones and prolong the subsequent wakeful period to end at about the normal local time for sleep. Proper sleep scheduling during the first 24 hours of a layover is critical, and crewmembers therefore should develop a discipline to terminate their initial sleep even though they

could sleep longer. This will considerably improve subsequent sleep periods.

6. Research findings suggest that, under acceptable operational circumstances, limited-duration naps can be of benefit in improving alertness for a useful period. If feasible, controlled napping on the flight deck could be of benefit. Graeber concludes that it is more important to have an alert, well-performing crewmember available upon descent than to have a tired, error-prone individual who has the dubious distinction of having fought off sleep during several boring hours of cruising over the ocean.

Cockpit Resource Management

Cockpit resource management (CRM) is a training activity that is becoming more widespread in the airline industry. CRM evolved from recognition that many airline accidents result from failure of flight crews to interact properly in emergency or deteriorating conditions. Air carrier accidents are filled with examples in which aircrews allowed manageable situations to deteriorate to a point at which accidents were unavoidable.

Fuel exhaustion accidents are an example of situations that should never occur, yet still do. One of the classic accidents cited to buttress the need for CRM training is one that occurred several years ago, in which a DC-8 crew flew around aimlessly for a lengthy period, attempting to deal with an apparent landing gear malfunction (8). The combination of poor team management by an autocratic captain and a submissive junior crew led to eventual fuel exhaustion and subsequent crash with loss of life. It was clear from analysis of the cockpit voice recorder tape that not only did the captain mismanage the situation, but that the crew had failed to take many opportunities to forcefully point out the critical fuel state of the airplane. As it turned out, the landing gear malfunction became the least of the crew's difficulties.

Other accidents demonstrate similar lack of productive interaction on the part of the crew.

Postaccident investigations usually reveal several common threads. Deficient crew coordination and decision making, ineffective communication, and poor management and leadership on the part of the captain are frequently cited as contributing to the accident.

For a long time, experts in the behavioral and social sciences were absent from most accident investigations. Events that were not attributable to equipment or system failure were lumped under the rubric "pilot error." Unfortunately, this did little to identify the real causes of accidents. In the 1960s, use of cockpit voice recorders and more thorough accident investigations revealed that poor crew interaction and lack of communication were major accident causes. Questions arose as to how to deal with these and other issues related to team management and "cockpit sociology."

Scientists at the NASA-Ames Research Center were instrumental in developing an understanding of underlying problems and in formulating approaches to solutions. They coined the term cockpit resource management in recognition of the many resources available in the cockpit (including human resources) for safe flight operation (9,10). NASA scientists developed prototype training methods and tested them in their extensive simulator facilities. They found that application of CRM training improved crew interaction and communication and reduced errors that can lead to accidents. CRM training programs have since been widely implemented in the worldwide air carrier industry.

The Dutch national carrier KLM developed the first CRM course, perhaps in recognition of the poor crew coordination that led to the disastrous Tenerife accident (11) (see Chapter 28). United Airlines was also an early leader in the development and implementation of a CRM program for its aircrews. Since then most major airlines instituted such training. In fact, FAA rules now require CRM-type training in Part 121 air carrier operations.

The NASA research team recommends that several key features be a part of CRM training programs. First, CRM training should emphasize functioning of the crew as a team, not a group of individuals. Individual "lone-wolf" operation in the cockpit has been the cause of many accidents. The training should provide opportunities for crews to practice together; this is why LOFT is frequently used to reinforce CRM classroom training. Also, it is recommended that CRM include at least three distinct phases:

1. An awareness phase in which CRM principles are presented and discussed.
2. A practice and feedback phase in which flight crews are given opportunities to interact in cockpit scenarios using the principles learned in the first phase. Role playing and feedback to team members on their attitudes and interpersonal styles are common in this phase.
3. A reinforcement phase which is actually a continuous phase, recognizing that one-shot training sessions are unlikely to produce desired, lasting changes in attitudes and behavior that have developed over a lifetime.

CRM reinforcement should be incorporated as a permanent part of the recurrent training required for all flight crews. Six major topics are recommended in CRM programs (12).

1. Communications/interpersonal skills, including listening, feedback and participation.
2. Situation awareness; focusing on maintaining current and forecast knowledge of what is going on inside the cockpit and outside the aircraft.
3. Problem solving/decision-making; emphasizing "head-work" to analyze situations and make rational decisions.
4. Leadership/followership, including discussion of professionalism, the need for assertiveness, and managerial and supervisory skills.
5. Stress management; teaching crewmembers to recognize the effects of fatigue, emotional problems, and other personal problems and

to develop methods for coping with the resultant stress.
6. Critique, involving development of the ability to analyze a plan of action.

All major carriers now have some form of CRM training for flight crews, and at least one airline brings flight attendants into this training in recognition of the fact that these people also play a vital role in the safe execution of flight operations. The hope now is that CRM will also find its way into training for regional and commuter carriers. These airlines typically do not have the training resources that the majors have, such as simulation capability and training departments staffed with several full-time professionals. However, as more regional carriers become affiliated with major airlines, opportunities for CRM training will inevitably increase. Further, a number of independent training companies that offer flight training under contract to regional carriers are now including CRM in their curricula.

As pilot shortages grow, a trend has developed to provide ab initio pilot training for people who wish to pursue an airline flying career. These aspirants often enter training programs with no prior pilot time. They are trained from the first day in the concepts of CRM. The emphasis in these programs is on team performance rather than on single pilot operations. The University of North Dakota pioneered one of these programs, and others are in various stages of development. In some cases, airlines have teamed with training institutions such as junior colleges to provide pilot training with an airline emphasis. These airlines typically provide support to these programs through use of simulators and training personnel and through curricula development. The benefit to the airline comes through access to a group of new pilots who have an airline flying perspective as well as thorough exposure to CRM principles.

The growth of CRM training in the air carrier industry is an acknowledgment of its strong potential for improving safety. Team coordination, communication, leadership, and decision making are all vital for safe flight operations. Many feel that these same concepts can be profitably applied elsewhere, such as within the ranks of the airline management and maintenance workforces.

Automation

The progress of cockpit automation in airline aircraft has been steady since the introduction of the first autopilot systems in U.S. operations in 1931 (13). Notable strides were made, however, over the last two decades, based in large measure on revolutionary changes in microprocessor and display technology. An important application of these technologies has been in the development of the ''glass cockpit.'' The term glass cockpit has come to refer to the full array of new automation systems and information displays which make the flight deck of the 1990s truly different from that of 20 years ago. The 747–400 flight deck, shown in Figure 30.3, is a glass cockpit which incorporates advanced digital technology to reduce workload and allow two-pilot operation. The display system minimizes clutter in the instrument panel while pro-

viding the crew with the flexibility to call up additional information when necessary. Airplane systems and flight status are displayed on six cathode ray tubes (CRTs). Two of the CRTs are used for primary flight display (PFD), two for navigation display (ND), and two for the engine indicating and crew alerting system (EICAS). System simplification and automation have reduced the number of lights, gauges, and switches to the level found on a two-engine commercial jet airplane.

There are many definitions of automation as applied to aircraft operation. In Wiener's definition (14), automation means that some tasks or portions of tasks performed by the human crew can be assigned, by the choice of the crew, to machinery. Wiener also notes that automation may refer to cockpit warning and alerting systems, which may be thought of as the machine monitoring the human. Under either definition, automated systems directly replace a crewmember in task performance or assist the crewmember in that performance. The extent to which automation now can perform relatively complex functions previously considered the responsibility of the flight crew is shown in the

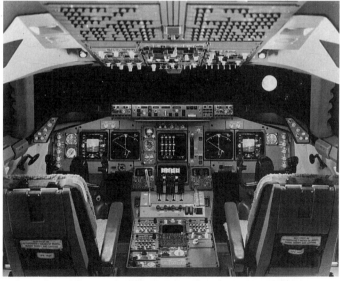

Figure 30.3. Flight deck of the Boeing 747–400 airplane. (Photo courtesy of Boeing Commercial Airplane Group.)

automation achievements of the original Airbus A-300 aircraft, as follows (15).

Automatic throttle from brakes-off to touchdown

Automatic angle-of-attack protection and speed reference system, both being instrumental against windshear incidents

Automatic two- and one-engine go-around

Thrust computer linked to autothrottle, allowing derated engine operation/increased engine life

The purposes and advantages of automating flight tasks such as those listed above include (1) safety, (2) flight precision, (3) economy, and (4) reduction of workload for the flight crew. Automation, applied appropriately, obviously can produce the first three advantages. Automated warning systems improve safety. Modern autopilots maintain flight paths with great precision. Automated engine controls result in fuel economy. The hoped-for advantage in workload reduction, however, remains a matter for discussion.

Crewmember workload has been a concern for aircraft designers, airline operators, regulatory agencies, and behavioral scientists for many years. The demands of aircraft operation, communications, navigation, and systems management can result in heavy workload, particularly during instrument flight when expected routings may change suddenly. Sustained periods of high workload can overtax the crew and increase the likelihood of control or communications errors, with a corresponding decrease in the desired margin of safety. Sharing the workload with automated systems is the obvious solution to the greater demands of new and more sophisticated aircraft as well as those caused by the growing complexity of the airspace environment.

Studies attempting to describe the extent to which automation reduces cockpit workload encounter two immediate problems. First, workload is difficult to define. There is no generally agreed-upon definition in the technical literature, although everyone agrees that cockpit workload involves primarily subjective mental workload. Physical workload is of a lesser order. Second, there is no best way to measure workload. Although many physiologic and performance measurement techniques have been tried, most research depends on subjective rating methods of workload. Subjective ratings appear to give useful results and have the additional advantages of simplicity of administration and analysis.

In one study of workload in the Boeing 757 aircraft, Wiener, along with associates at the NASA Ames Research Center, interviewed a number of pilots, with interesting results (16). While most of the pilots reported favorable impressions of the glass cockpit environment, at least one half felt that automation increases rather than reduces workload. They felt that workload becomes excessive with revisions of a flight plan, such as route changes and speed changes, because of new data entry requirements for the flight management computer. This problem generally occurs below 10,000 feet while maneuvering during an airport approach. Data entry into a flight computer can be demanding, since it must be accurate, and requires the undivided attention of one pilot. If the other pilot is observing to see that the operation is done correctly, the result is a head-down operation in which no one is looking outside. This is not desirable when in the vicinity of an airport.

Pilots in Wiener's study also expressed some concern over their ability to maintain flying skills after working in an automated aircraft. To prevent this, almost all pilots fly the aircraft by hand during part of every trip. Maintaining flying skills can be very important if a pilot transfers at some point to another aircraft not having the same level of automation.

Another issue Wiener encountered is that of flight deck organizational structure. The normal division of roles between crewmembers tends to become less clear-cut as the computer assumes the role of a third crewmember. Also, the usual standardized assignment of duties may be disrupted when one pilot attempts to "help" the other pilot with computer programming duties. Wiener feels that the CRM training now being offered by many airlines may resolve these organizational issues, particularly if the training is tailored to advanced technology aircraft.

In considering the issues identified to date with highly automated aircraft, certain conclusions can be drawn. The first is that pilots generally approve of the automated cockpit and are receptive to continuing automation. However, it is by no means clear that automation necessarily reduces crew workload. During periods of high demand, workload may actually increase. In other phases of flight, such as long periods of cruise, workload may decrease to the point where boredom and/or inattention may be of consequence. There also is the problem of maintaining flying skills as cockpit tasks move more and more to those required by computer operation. Finally, unique issues of cockpit organization and task assignments in a glass-cockpit aircraft must be addressed or at least given proper attention during crew training.

MAINTENANCE OPERATIONS

Commercial aircraft are exceedingly complex vehicles that operate under a wide range of environmental conditions and follow demanding schedules. These aircraft represent significant investments and must be in the best possible condition if safety and economic objectives of airlines are to be met. High quality maintenance is critical. The maintenance department is an essential component in an airline organization.

As the commercial aircraft fleet in the United States grows in size, and as the average age of the fleet increases, the burden on maintenance becomes heavier. The maintenance industry today is large and continues to grow in parallel with the expansion of airline operations. Almost 60,000 mechanics are employed today by the commercial airline fleet, with a total cost for maintenance operations exceeding $9 billion per year (2).

Most maintenance work is done by the airline itself. However, major carriers consistently contract about 11% of their maintenance work, while smaller national carriers may contract about 40% (17). Even when work is contracted, however, airlines must provide their own inspectors to monitor the maintenance. The contracting activity has given rise to another industry, i.e., repair stations, which have become an important part of the maintenance picture.

Repair stations are rapidly growing, with some stations showing a growth rate in the order of 30% a year (18). These stations provide a useful service for airlines and other air carriers since they offer a quality maintenance program without the carrier having to build or expand its own facilities. For the carrier, one disadvantage is that the maintenance staff at the repair station is not under direct control. Therefore, issues of workforce management and workforce productivity cannot be addressed. From the repair station point of view, one disadvantage is that there are many customers to be served. One repair station may deal with major carriers, freight and package carriers, federal aircraft, and foreign governments. Even when the aircraft are the same, each customer may want the work done in a particular way. Another issue is that a repair station must maintain a staff qualified to work on a number of different aircraft. This produces serious problems in staffing and training.

Aging Aircraft

The Airline Deregulation Act of 1978 initiated a general period of growth for the U.S. air transport industry. Since 1983, this growth has been sustained, and the size of the fleet increases each year. While new aircraft are being added, however, older aircraft are not being retired at a corresponding rate. Thus, the commercial carrier fleet is growing older just as it is growing larger. The aging characteristics of the U.S. fleet are shown in Table 30.2 (19).

The FAA has been aware of the aging of the civil fleet for years, particularly as a number of aircraft began to exceed their economic design

Table 30.2.
Average Age of U.S. Commercial Airline Fleet (1990)

Age	No. of Aircraft	% of Fleet
Under 5 years	707	19.2
5–10 years	747	20.3
10–15 years	515	14.0
15–20 years	742	20.3
20 years and older	960	26.2
Average age, 12.7 years		

Adapted from Kizer (19).

life objective. This objective is established during the design of the airplane and is not set as a limitation on its service life. The prevailing philosophy was that aircraft could continue flying for years providing proper inspections were conducted and proper repairs were made.

On April 28, 1988, a Boeing 737 airplane operated by Aloha Airlines had a dramatic in-flight incident in which approximately 18 feet of the cabin skin and roof structure aft of the cabin entrance door and above the passenger floor line separated from the airplane. Miraculously, the flight crew was able to control the aircraft during an emergency descent and successful landing, with only one fatality. Within hours, the FAA issued a telegraphic airworthiness directive limiting cabin pressure differentials on Boeing 737s to a lower level. Within a few days another airworthiness directive was issued requiring special inspections of lap splices on the 737.

The larger result of the Aloha incident was that fundamental questions about aging aircraft were raised, particularly concerning the design, inspection, and maintenance of airplanes in general, and especially as they approach and exceed their economic design goal (20). The degree of damage suffered by the Aloha airplane caused the FAA to rethink the issue of aging aircraft. The result has been a change from the old philosophy of inspect and repair to a new approach toward replacement of items at specific intervals. More important, increased attention was immediately given to maintenance procedures

for the U.S. carrier fleet and overall use of maintenance resources.

Factors Affecting Maintenance Performance

Communications

At a conference to review human factors issues in aircraft maintenance and inspection, recommendations for improvement made by attendees noted "communications" more frequently than any other issue (21). There are many ways in which information must be transmitted through the maintenance industry, and each transmission system has its own set of problems.

At an organizational level, aircraft manufacturers, airlines, and government regulatory agencies, principally the FAA, form a three-legged stool to maintain the industry. The communication network among these three principal members is the basis on which the system works. Each member of the three-legged stool has a responsibility, yet each must understand the responsibilities of the others. Manufacturers depend on airlines to provide data supporting the design and performance characteristics of aircraft. Airlines depend on manufacturers to provide product support information such as fleet and systems reliability data. The FAA depends on the airlines and the manufacturer for data concerning in-service difficulties and product reliability in order to provide industry oversight and to ensure appropriate safety levels. In all of this, the ATA serves a coordinating function. The existing organizational communications system works, but in many respects it does not work rapidly enough. For instance, the use of service difficulty reports to provide information concerning specific aircraft problems may require as long as 6 months for the information to reach all interested parties (19).

Prior to airline deregulation, there existed an effective communication network among airline operators, which also included manufacturers. Useful information concerning common problems was passed through this network. This network is no longer as effective, and efforts are being made to replace it with a more formal system.

Communication problems also exist at the maintenance technician level. In a large maintenance base, which might have as many as 12,000 employees, each technician will be involved in many information transactions every day (22). Maintenance documentation to support these transactions takes many forms, ranging from aircraft maintenance manuals to work cards. The sheer amount of this documentation can be overwhelming. As of 1996, Boeing maintains 1,980 active maintenance manuals for 6,846 airplanes and 594 operators. In these manuals, over 56 million different pages must be maintained and revised as necessary (23).

To keep information in maintenance documentation as error free as possible, manufacturers and airlines have worked to develop a simplified English. For example, Boeing created a limited vocabulary for use by technical writers and engineers in the preparation of maintenance documentation (23). In this vocabulary, an access area in an aircraft must be referred to as a hatch. It cannot be called a door, a panel, a limited-access area, or any of many other similar terms. It always is a hatch. The advantage is that if a technician wishes to retrieve all items having to do with "hatch," he need ask only one question and not 20.

Communications around an airplane while work is underway also are important. These communications serve both to coordinate the work effort and to support personal safety. Two problems affect these communications. The first is the noise level that exists at times. For example, in a riveting operation, one mechanic is on the inside and one on the outside of the aircraft. They must coordinate this effort by voice since they are not able to see each other. Yet the noise of the operation requires hearing protection equipment. This presents an obvious communication problem.

Another problem exists at times when mainte- nance personnel come from different national groups. The natural language of two mechanics working together may be Spanish. If they use this language, English-speaking personnel near- by will not be aware of their intentions, and safety problems can arise. For this reason, airlines require English to be used during actual maintenance. However, this requirement is not always observed.

Small portable radios have been used by airlines to assist in communications around an airplane during maintenance. Although expensive radios have been purchased, problems still exist. One is that mechanics occasionally use the radio for a hammer or may drop it. Neither action is good for service life. Another problem is with the steel structure interference encountered in maintenance bays. In all, portable radios help but have not been the ultimate solution.

Training

Training for airline maintenance personnel, just as training for flight crews, has been experiencing change. Federal Aviation Regulations (Part 147) that specify the curricula to be followed by maintenance training schools have been revised for the first time in a number of years. While the new training procedures are more appropriate for the needs of air carriers, additional training and experience is necessary before technicians can become proficient in maintaining sophisticated airline equipment.

Training requirements for inspectors also are becoming more demanding. According to a maintenance manager at a major airline, "It takes an inspector at an airline such as ours two years to become effective; six years to become efficient." (24)

Because of forecast shortages in personnel and possible reductions in quality of available people, training will become a much more important tool in ensuring effective personnel performance. New training technologies are developing which can be profitably applied in the airline industry. These technologies, based heavily on use of artificial intelligence and computer-based instruction (CBI) were, in large measure, developed by NASA and the Department of Defense for training astronauts and technicians. One of the latest developments is the Intelligent Tutoring System (ITS).

The ITS goes several steps beyond the capability of CBI, in which students receive rudimentary instruction and then key in answers to screen-presented questions. A typical old-style CBI system response to an incorrect student input might be "wrong answer-try again." This provides little real interaction with the student and does not give much help to the student in reasoning through to the correct answer. The ideal system would function much like a classroom led by an expert instructor who knows the individual capabilities of his or her students and can adapt the instruction and explanations to the students' abilities and knowledge. ITS attempts to simulate this type of instructional environment.

ITSs are usually described with some version of the diagram shown in Figure 30.4. The center of the diagram depicts the instructional environ-

ment which, along with the student interface, comprises what is usually found in traditional CBI systems. The software that differentiates ITSs from CBIs are the models of the expert, instructor, and student. The expert model provides a detailed understanding of the topic or system being studied. The instructor model sequences instruction based on the level of apparent student competence and also provides detailed feedback which goes considerably beyond the "wrong answer-try again" responses of CBI systems. The instructor model is an expert system which does not need to know anything about the technical details of the instructed topic. The student model is a dynamic record of individual student performance vis-a-vis the topic under study.

The challenge facing the air carrier, manufacturing, and training industries is to develop ITSs which can successfully supplement the traditional on-the-job training and classroom lecture methods. Most training experts feel this capability will go a long way toward improving training effectiveness and efficiency in the airline industry.

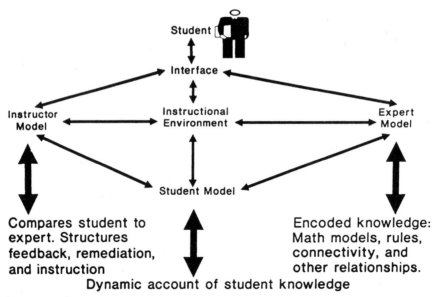

Figure 30.4. Components of an intelligent tutoring system (ITS).

Personnel Health and Well-Being

The health and productivity of maintenance workers are important issues in airline operations, just as for flight crews. Maintenance technicians must be in good health and able to work shift schedules as well as overtime when necessary. Physical demands also can be heavy as workers carry equipment and parts to different areas of an airplane.

Each airline establishes its own health requirements for maintenance personnel, with most relying on a routine physical examination administered by qualified medical personnel. These examinations usually include audiometric testing to establish a hearing baseline in view of the noise environment in which a maintenance technician may work.

While maintenance activities require good health, especially good vision and good hearing, the physical requirements of the maintenance workplace are not excessive. Normal strength and physical condition generally are adequate. The need for establishing physical standards unique to maintenance operations has not been established. Consideration has been given to the establishment of visual standards for maintenance inspectors, but the requirement has not yet been validated. For those with visual deficiencies, use of proper eyeglasses appears adequate.

Environmental Monitoring

A number of maintenance operations use chemicals or substances with potentially toxic qualities. While protective equipment is used to control such hazards, continuous or periodic monitoring is required to ensure that the equipment is used properly and exposures are controlled.

Paint stripping and repainting of aircraft occur frequently and use chemicals with toxic qualities. Paint stripping is done within the confines of the maintenance hangar bay and requires careful attention to proper ventilation and to use of protective equipment. The chemical of greatest concern is methylene chloride (CH_2CL_2). This chemical can be used in paint stripping operations during two shifts per month, with each shift employing four individuals for 8 hours. Methylene chloride produces adverse health effects if inhaled and can cause drunken-like behavior which would impair maintenance performance. Skin contact can result in burns and dermatitis. Maintenance personnel doing paint stripping wear a jumpsuit with gloves, rubber boots taped at the cuffs, a hard hat with a face shield, and a powered air purifying respirator (PAPR).

During winter months, airlines use ethylene glycol ($C_2H_4(NO_3)_2$) as a deicing agent. Concern here is mostly over contact dermatitis through skin exposure. Inhalation is usually not a problem due to low vapor pressure, but there have been occasional incidents of headache, nausea, and similar symptoms after long exposures. This is generally not a problem for maintenance technicians but rather one for aircraft servicing personnel, who wear full jumpsuits with gloves, hard hat, and respirator.

Two other substances requiring some monitoring are aircraft hydraulic fluid and jet fuel. Hydraulic fluid is used throughout the aircraft in aircraft systems, including wing flaps and engines. Hydraulic fluid is a very strong eye irritant and occasionally causes problems as it drips into a technician's eyes during aircraft inspection. For this reason, goggles generally are worn during inspections of these systems.

Jet fuel (Jet A or Jet B) is a skin and eye irritant. Exposure may occur due to overflow of fuel tanks. Technicians usually use rubber gloves and goggles when working with these tanks.

Radioactive materials may be used in some maintenance work. For instance, radioisotopes may be inserted into the central shaft of a jet engine to obtain radiographic pictures of the interior. While this is an excellent means of inspection, it does introduce a hazardous material into the operation. Use of radioisotopes is restricted only to those inspectors with special training who use appropriate protective equipment. The testing area is closely monitored while inspections are underway.

Task Performance

Aircraft maintenance, including both inspection and repair, is an operation which must strive to be error free. As the commercial carrier fleet ages, error-free task performance by maintenance personnel becomes increasingly important. Yet, behavioral scientists recognize that the human is never an error-free component in any large system. While humans can do almost anything reasonably well, the error rate in human performance can be high. An individual asked to perform some critical task repeatedly and do it exactly right every time generally will be unable to do so. In human factors design terms, this means it is a mistake to design a system in which 100% reliability is required of the human operator (25).

The objective of human factors design is to understand the capabilities and limits of the human and then to adjust task demands and other features of the job so that reliability of performance is maximized. Human and machine components must be matched so that overall system reliability is higher than that of either component acting independently.

Vigilance

Visual inspection is the primary method of aircraft examination, possibly 95% of an aircraft is inspected in this manner (26). The philosophy in using visual inspection is to establish a maintenance interval of sufficient time so that a defect too small to be detected on one inspection will have grown sufficiently that it will be detected on the next. This, of course, places great reliance on the second inspection being error free.

Visual inspections are a matter of vigilance, and considerable research has demonstrated that vigilance performance is not error free. However, by understanding those features of tasks which contribute to vigilance errors, one can structure an inspection process to reduce inspection errors. Reports by Wiener (14) and Drury (25) describe certain features of vigilance tasks which affect performance, as follows:

1. Vigilance performance shows a decrement through time. Wiener (14) reports one study involving a 48-minute vigil in which probability of detection dropped from just below 80% in the initial stages to approximately 60% at the conclusion.
2. If the rate of appearance of a signal is low, the probability of detecting it is lowered. In aviation this means that the higher the quality of the product, the lower the signal event rate, and therefore the lower the probability of detection of any given fault.
3. There is a steady decrease in search effectiveness as a flaw is moved away from direct vision. Drury (25) reports a study in which subjects could identify a defect with a 10-minute visual angle size at 20° off central visual axis. At 40° off axis, the detectable size increased to 20 minutes.
4. When inspectors are very rapidly provided feedback concerning performance, inspection performance improves. In one instance, performance was essentially doubled by providing more rapid feedback.
5. Feed-forward information, i.e., telling an inspector precisely the characteristics of the flaw for which he or she is searching, will improve performance. Ambiguity in inspection contributes to errors.

Fatigue

Maintenance personnel frequently are called upon to work overtime. Overtime demands can be high in the inspection department because there may not be enough inspectors for heavy activity periods. Generally overtime involves an additional 4 hours. On occasion it can be for 8 additional hours, but this is avoided if possible because of the increased overtime expense. Overtime operations bring subjective reports of increased fatigue. However, there is little evidence that inspection performance or aircraft repair noticeably suffers. If errors are made by a mechanic, they are likely to be caught at the check at the end of the shift or during the next inspection.

The research literature shows that performance decreases in vigilance tasks as the period of sustained vigilance increases. However, there is little if any information as to the effect on performance if a vigilance task is started when an inspector already has been on the job for 12 hours.

Job Pressures

The goals of aircraft inspectors are not identical with those of aircraft mechanics and their supervisors. Inspectors have the pressure of making certain an aircraft is airworthy before it leaves maintenance for revenue service. Maintenance crews have the pressure of getting the aircraft to the gate at its scheduled time. While each group is fully committed to safety, differences do arise as to what is airworthy and what is not.

Conflicting pressures of quality versus time cause some job stress. This appears to be truer for regional or commuter operations, where virtually all maintenance is conducted at night in anticipation of early morning departures, than for the major carriers. For commuters, it is not unusual for an aircraft to arrive at midnight for maintenance with a run-up time of 5:00 A.M. to meet a departure at 6:00 A.M. This puts pressure on both maintenance and inspection groups and can cause friction between the two groups (27).

Cognitive and Perceptual Demands

Aviation maintenance places certain cognitive and perceptual demands on maintenance technicians and inspectors. While these demands are not severe, they are important as they affect safety and job efficiency. An understanding of these cognitive and perceptual requirements can aid in establishing a work environment that minimizes maintenance error.

Decision Making

Maintenance personnel, and inspectors in particular, face a variety of situations requiring decisions. An inspector searching for aircraft flaws, whether relying on visual search or use of a nondestructive test (NDT) system such as the eddy-current device, makes a series of decisions. These decisions will be more or less accurate depending on how the task is structured.

An inspector making a decision concerning an aircraft flaw is, in effect, comparing what he or she sees with a standard. It has long been known that comparative judgment (against an available standard) is more accurate than absolute judgment (against a remembered standard) (25). Standards maintained at the working point, which allow a comparative judgment to be made, can be extremely effective. In one instance noted by Drury (25), introduction of such work point standards reduced the average error of a trained inspector to 64% of its magnitude before such standards were used.

An inspector working with an NDT system, such as in eddy-current testing (Fig. 30.5), evaluates the response of the NDT probe as a meter deflection or as a pattern on an oscilloscope. For the most part, no standard is used at the work site. Thus the inspector is making an absolute rather than a comparative judgment.

A repetitive decision-making task is improved if appropriate performance feedback is provided. For maintenance inspectors, performance feedback frequently is not rapid or obvious (25). If an inspector marks a defect, it will be repaired at a later time and then reinspected, likely by a different inspector. Unless the original inspector deliberately seeks feedback concerning the validity of his initial decision, he or she may not know whether his or her decision was correct or not. Appropriate feedback is not being provided. Also, as Drury notes, some repairs destroy an identified ''defect'' without confirming it. An indication of a small crack in the aircraft skin may be corrected simply by drilling an oversized hole and using a larger rivet. The initial decision is neither confirmed nor rejected. Use of a confirmation system would improve the reliability of inspector performance.

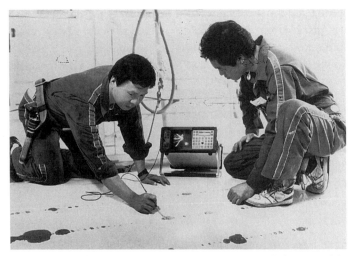

Figure 30.5. Eddy-current testing for stress cracks around rivets in aircraft fuselage. (Photo courtesy of United Airlines.)

Visual Acuity

Maintenance inspection and repair tasks require good vision. However, no standards for visual acuity have been established that take into account any unique visual demands of maintenance. Inspectors, who perform the most visually demanding tasks, use a variety of visual aids. Figure 30.6 shows an inspector using a borescope for inspection of the combustion chamber of a jet engine.

Each airline can set its own rules for testing vision. Such testing usually is included in the routine physical examination. Even here, however, there is no prescribed interval for physical examinations, and such examinations may be given only at the time of hiring. The responsibility for maintaining good visual acuity rests with the inspector. Inspectors certainly are aware of the need for good vision and meet this responsibility through use of proper eyeglasses plus aids such as magnifying glasses.

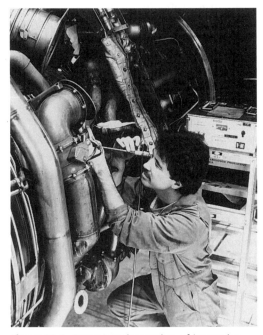

Figure 30.6. Borescope inspection of jet engine. (Photo courtesy of United Airlines.)

Auditory Acuity

Auditory acuity is important for communications and for safety. The ability to hear properly is most important when maintenance personnel are working in a high noise environment, such as areas where metal repairs are being made or

engine tests conducted. As with vision, there are no standards for auditory acuity based on specific maintenance tasks. However, hearing generally is tested more frequently than is vision, in part because of an airline's hearing conservation program. Either personal injury suffered from failure to hear a warning command, or hearing loss occurring after extended work in a high noise area, are of concern to management and employees. To assess employee hearing and control liability claims for hearing loss, portable booths frequently are used to obtain audiograms and establish a permanent record of hearing capability for each employee.

Environmental Factors

The environment in which work is conducted can be a major source of human error. Optimum human performance requires attention to a number of environmental factors. Physical features of the environment, such as lighting and temperature, are important. Attention also must be given to functional characteristics so that work can flow smoothly, and to social features so that workers are comfortable.

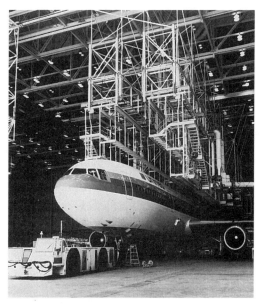

Figure 30.7. Boeing DC-10 aircraft being towed from dock facility scaffolding. (Photo courtesy of United Airlines.)

Workplace Structure

The nature of aircraft maintenance means that certain features of the workplace environment will be less than optimal. Maintenance facilities are large because they must hold aircraft, test stands, and maintenance equipment. Since the structure must be open to accommodate aircraft movements from time to time, environmental control can never be perfect. Accessibility of different parts of the aircraft also presents problems. Major airlines, however, are working to control these problems in newer maintenance facilities. For instance, massive test structures, which can enclose a large airplane, now are being used to increase accessibility of the aircraft and to improve safety. Figure 30.7 shows a DC-10 aircraft being moved from an enclosing test structure. Structures such as this are expensive and may be beyond the reach of smaller airlines, particularly those in regional and commuter operations. However, the value of the structures is apparent in Figure 30.8, which shows ready access to difficult aircraft parts, such as the vertical stabilizer.

A review of maintenance operations by the FAA found that most operators continue to use a

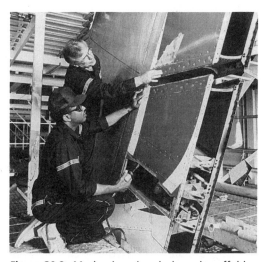

Figure 30.8. Mechanics using dock-work scaffolding for easy access to vertical stabilizer on Boeing 737 aircraft. (Photo courtesy of United Airlines.)

variety of scaffolds, ladders, stools, and "cherry pickers" for maintenance (28). While the work accomplished was satisfactory, the potential for these work platforms to produce increased fatigue was noted, particularly if the work stand requires working in an awkward position. Use of cherry pickers is of particular concern because of their inherent instability. This increases the difficulty of detailed visual inspection and/or maintenance, especially if torsional forces are required.

Climate Conditions

Climate control, involving temperature, humidity, and air movement, is satisfactory in the maintenance facilities of major carriers. Temperatures generally range between 21° and 26.6°C, with only a few instances noted of temperatures exceeding 26.6°C. Measured humidities are within the range of 10 to 60%. When maintenance is performed on the flight line, temperature and humidity conditions obviously will be whatever prevails at that time. For regional and commuter operators, temperature and humidity control is more of a problem since considerable maintenance is performed at the flight line, and the maintenance facilities are not as elaborate as those for the major carriers.

Hancock (29) reviewed the literature on the effect of thermal extremes on vigilance performance and concluded that such performance is impaired by exposure to temperatures greater than 32°C. Hancock also noted that there is a rather complex relationship between heat stress and performance. In general, conditions which act to increase body temperature degrade performance, while a stable hyperthermic body state may prove beneficial. In a heat environment which does not produce changes in body temperature, immediate entry into a hotter environment can aid performance efficiency. Only a few studies have examined the effect of cold on vigilance. In general, the best conclusion is that cold per se impairs vigilance performance.

Lighting

Proper lighting is essential for the various tasks in aircraft maintenance. While inspection and repair can be conducted under less than optimal lighting conditions, any effort toward error-free maintenance must provide proper task illumination. Attention should be given to the inten-

Table 30.3.
Measured Illumination Levels at Major Air Carriers Compared With Recommended Levels

	Measured (footcandles)	
	Day	Night
Hangar area	66	51
Below wings, fuselage and in cargo areas	26	15
Within fuselage	23	18
Visual inspection (2 D-cell flashlight)	100–500	

	Recommended (footcandles)
	Min. Level
Aircraft repair, general	75
Aircraft visual inspection	
Ordinary area	50
Difficult	100
Highly difficult	200

Source: Thackray (28).

sity of lighting, to location of lights, to the ability of technicians to adjust and relocate lights as necessary, and to control of glare sources.

An FAA audit of major air carriers included a survey of lighting conditions (28). Various lighting systems were found, including mercury vapor, metal halide, and high-pressure sodium lights. While these lights differ in color rendition, the differences were not deemed of real importance. The principal problem was with level of illumination. Table 30.3 shows average illumination levels measured at different maintenance work areas, both for day shifts and night shifts. For work performed on upper and lateral surfaces of the aircraft, illumination levels were deemed adequate. Problems arise for work conducted below wings, the fuselage, and within cargo and engine areas. Because these areas are shielded from overhead light, supplemental light sources are employed. These usually are quartz halogen stand lights, dual 40-watt fluorescent stand fixtures, single hand-held fluorescent lamps, and flashlights. Figure 30.9 shows an inspector using a Burton-jet light to provide intensified local lighting during inspection of jet engine fan blades.

The problem with most supplemental lighting systems, with the exception of hand-held flashlights, is that usually they are placed too far from

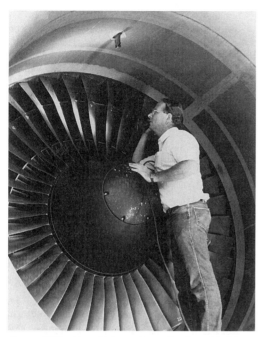

Figure 30.9. Aircraft inspector using hand-held light source for engine inspection. (Photo courtesy of United Airlines.)

the work being performed and are too few in number. The result is that, on occasion, illumination levels ranging from 1 to about 10 to 14 foot-candles (ft-c) were obtained in shielded regions. For work within fuselage areas, comparable illumination levels were measured, ranging from 23 ft-c during the day and 18 ft-c at night. However, some readings as low as 1 ft-c were obtained. Aircraft inspectors generally use standard two D-cell flashlights as light sources. These provide illumination ranging from 100 to 500 ft-c and are completely acceptable for visual inspection.

Table 30.3 also shows recommended minimum illumination levels for aircraft repair and inspection tasks, as determined by the Illuminating Engineering Society. A minimum level of 75 ft-c is recommended for virtually all repair tasks. Many aircraft repair sites, as shown in Table 30.3, fall considerably below this recommended level. Improper lighting, considering both location of light sources and general level of illumination, could represent one source of error in aircraft maintenance operations.

Noise

In any industrial operation where mechanical repairs are made, noise exposure is a matter of concern. Noise measurements made in maintenance bays of major air carriers range generally between 70 and 75 dBA. This is an acceptable level for an industrial environment and requires no hearing protection. At certain times during maintenance, when riveting or other pneumatic tools were being used, levels above 90 dBA were recorded. Since these high noise level periods were infrequent and discontinuous, hearing protective devices would be required only for the workers using the tools and for those working close by (see Chapter 10).

Hearing protectors are of value only if used when needed and if used properly. Workers in areas adjacent to riveting operations were observed not wearing any form of hearing protection. When earplugs were used, they were not always inserted properly. The first line of responsibility for ensuring proper use of such devices is with the crew supervisor. If lapses in proper use are observed, the crew supervisor should be reminded of this responsibility by medical and safety personnel.

Physical Demands

Both maintenance and inspection activities can place a variety of physical demands on technicians. One such demand is having to leave the work location frequently to get materials or instructions. Every effort is made to control these demands. Both supervisors and mechanics plan maintenance so that mechanics will never leave the job once they are there. Mechanics should get their work item card and all called-for materials before leaving for the job. Additionally, racks of frequently used stock (standard screws, nuts, bolts) often are placed directly at the work site. However, materials accessibility remains an ongoing issue.

Access to aircraft inspection and repair areas is a larger problem. In a study conducted at the Douglas Aircraft Company (30), maintenance personnel listed "access and weight" as the most important problems they faced. Certain sites in an aircraft, such as the interior of a vertical stabilizer, are virtually inaccessible. Components that mechanics or inspectors must move during their work can weigh in the order of 50 lb. Majoros (30) describes research in which workload demands for various aircraft sites and for different maintenance tasks are computed. The objective is to define required working envelopes for aircraft components that might be specified, and adjusted as necessary, during initial design of an airplane.

Maintenance Resource Management

Over the past decade CRM has been introduced as part of the flight training program for major air carriers. One definition of CRM is "the effective utilization of all available resources—hardware, software, and liveware—to achieve safe, efficient flight operations" (31). CRM, described earlier for flight crews, addresses many features of intracockpit dynamics in order to make best use of total resources available, especially the skills and expertise of crewmembers.

The apparent benefits achieved through use of CRM with flight crews led to consideration of its applicability in aviation maintenance. To explore this, Pan American World Airways began development of a CRM-type training program, similar to that used for flight crews, that might be appropriate for maintenance managers, ranging from crew supervisors to the vice president of maintenance and engineering. The program was called MELD, for maintenance, engineering, and logistics development, and was intended to develop resource management skills for personnel in those departments.

The first session of the Pan Am program was held in 1988. The purpose of the first test session was to determine the acceptability of this type of training effort for maintenance and engineering personnel. A questionnaire administered at the completion of the MELD training showed that a high percentage of attendees found the training

to be personally useful (32). No one judged it as being a waste of time or only slightly useful.

The maintenance resource management training program was delivered through use of eight training modules, which are listed below in descending order of usefulness as judged by attendees.

Training in interpersonal communications and skills
Assertion and conflict management
Managing stress and recognizing its influence
Development of critiquing skills
Understanding the value of briefings
Developing situation awareness
Understanding leadership behavior
Review of case studies in flight operations

The acceptance given the first three modules, "training in interpersonal communications and skills," "managing assertion and conflict and using assertion properly," and "dealing with stress and recognizing the influence of stress on the job and how it can affect the day-to-day problem-solving process" is directly in line with the purposes of the resource management program. In addition to personal acceptance of this training, attendees unanimously agreed that this type of training effort would help to improve overall safety and effectiveness on the job.

The program at Pan Am is continuing and ultimately will be given to all maintenance managers and crew supervisors. Follow-up training will be given at regular intervals. Those conducting the program will attempt to track attitude changes and actual behavior changes as the program progresses. Ultimately, use of this resource management program will be related, to the extent feasible, to direct measures of safety and productivity in the maintenance and engineering workforce.

Directions in Maintenance and Inspection

New Technologies

New technologies are regularly being introduced into the maintenance and inspection of aircraft. Many of these are devoted to improving information flow at maintenance sites. It is critical that correct information be provided to the AMT on a timely basis so that proper servicing and repairs can be quickly accomplished.

Most air carrier aircraft are scheduled for service throughout the day. Daily utilization rates of 12 to 13 hours or more are not uncommon. These rates reflect customer needs to travel mostly during the day, otherwise utilization rates might be even higher. Unscheduled maintenance or maintenance delays cause disruption that can have a ripple effect throughout an airline's system. Most carriers do not have extra planes and crews poised to take up the slack caused by maintenance problems because of the obvious cost and logistical problems. There is strong pressure to ensure that airplanes scheduled for certain flights are ready at the appointed time. Problems that occur during a schedule must be dealt with during stops. This makes it all the more important for service personnel to be able to quickly pinpoint problems and perform correct repairs.

Many of the new technologies that are developing to assist this process are, as might be expected, computer based. These range from aircraft onboard diagnostic systems to ground-based hypermedia systems that allow technicians to quickly access several sources of information to diagnose and repair malfunctions. Currently, technicians may have to go to several different sources, such as manuals, microfiche readers, and job cards, to get all the information needed to make a repair. Lengthy verbal consultations with other technicians may be needed to not only discuss a diagnosis or repair, but to find out where to get the needed information. Often, the information sources are found in different locations, requiring the AMT to spend time traveling about to get the needed information.

Boeing is using computer technology to improve work task cards, frequently called job cards, to provide maintenance information (33). Use of work task cards by mechanics is a time-honored procedure. The card tells a mechanic what to do and when to do it. He or she then consults the maintenance manual for specific details on the task. Information from the maintenance manual may be provided in the form of printouts from a microfilm reader/printer. The Boeing Automated Customized Task Card method computerizes the preparation of task cards. With the new cards, a mechanic now has everything he or she needs to properly conduct a maintenance task. The automated system reduces time spent in preparing and revising work cards, eliminates use of microfilm and the microfilm reader, and reduces errors due to manually transferring and retyping the manufacturer's maintenance data. The Boeing program is but one in a number of industry efforts to aid technician performance through use of computer-based systems.

Hypertext, in which users interactively take control of a set of dynamic links among units of information, is being considered as one system for managing maintenance (34). Hypertext not only can bring all the information to a single point, but can take the technician through the diagnostic and repair sequence in a much more efficient manner. The savings in technician time can be dramatic, but the real payoff will come in the added safety brought by correct repairs and through avoidance of ''fixing'' systems that are not broken.

The U.S. Air Force is developing a system called the Integrated Maintenance Information System (IMIS) which allows a technician to take a portable computerized system to the flight line (35). The technician, through keyboard input and electronic-display output, can diagnose system faults and see such information as repair sequences, repair part numbers, and exploded views of systems and can even determine the technician specialties and estimated manhours needed to make the repairs. It would seem that there is a clear application of this technology to the civil sector, particularly for maintenance at the gate, where mechanics and aircraft are distant from the hangar containing specialized test equipment and information sources.

A common issue associated with emerging technologies for maintenance is the need for facility with computer systems, particularly keyboard skills to interact with these systems. Many high schools now include some sort of computer training in their curricula. This training can be an important primer for the future AMT who in all likelihood will be using computer-based systems on the job.

Airplane manufacturers are developing onboard systems that will continuously monitor several components such as engines or hydraulic systems. Some of these onboard systems will be capable of telemetering information, possibly via satellite, to the carriers' maintenance bases. Ground-based maintenance managers will be able to diagnose problems on aircraft in flight and arrange for repairs at appropriate places and times. When the aircraft arrives at the desired place, prepared technicians will be able to quickly attack the repair, forearmed with all needed information and parts. Detection of potentially urgent problems will permit the safe diversion of a flight before a problem becomes severe enough to cause an emergency condition.

New technologies will have a dramatic impact on maintenance and inspection of the future air carrier fleet. New systems are constantly being developed that will improve the performance of tomorrow's maintenance workforce. The benefits to safety and efficiency are eagerly awaited by industry and the traveling public.

REFERENCES

1. Federal Aviation Administration: FAA aviation forecasts—fiscal years 1990–2001 (FAA-APO 90–1). Springfield, VA: National Technical Information Service, March 1990.
2. Air Transport Association of America: Air transport 1990—the annual report of the U.S. scheduled airline industry. Washington, DC: Air Transport Association of America, June 1990.
3. Holbrook HA. Civil aviation medicine in the bureaucracy. Bethesda, MD: Banner Publishing Company, 1974.
4. Department of Transportation/Federal Aviation Administration: National airspace system plan. Washington, DC: Federal Aviation Administration, September 1989.
5. Stone RR, Babcock GL. Airline pilots' perspective. In: Wiener EL, Nagel DC, eds. Human factors in aviation. San Diego: Academic Press, 1988;529–560.
6. Green RG. Stress and accidents. Aviat Space Environ Med 1985;58:638–641.
7. Graeber RC. Aircrew fatigue and circadian rhythmicity. In:. Wiener EL, Nagel DC, eds. Human factors in aviation. San Diego: Academic Press, 1988;305–344.
8. National Transportation Safety Board: Accident investigation report: United Airlines (McDonnell-Douglas DC-8-61, No. N8082U) accident in Portland, Oregon on December 28, 1978. Washington, DC: National Transportation Safety Board, 1979.
9. Lauber JK. Resource management in the cockpit. Air Line Pilot, September 1984.
10. Foushe HC, Helmreich RL. Group interaction and flight crew performance. In:. Wiener EL, Nagel DC, eds. Human factors in aviation. San Diego: Academic Press, 1988.
11. International Civil Aviation Organization: KLM and Pan Am Collision at Tenerife Airport, Spain on 27 March 1977 (ICAO Circular 153-AN/56), pp 22–24 and 54–55, Montreal: ICAO, 1977.
12. International Civil Aviation Organization: Flight crew training: cockpit resource management (CRM) and line oriented flight training (LOFT) (ICAO Circular 217-AN/132). Human Factors Digest No. 2. Montreal: ICAO, 1989.
13. McFarland RA. Human factors in air transportation. 1st ed. New York: McGraw-Hill Book Company, 1953.
14. Wiener EL. Cockpit automation. In: Wiener EL, Nagel DC, eds. Human factors in aviation. San Diego: Academic Press, 1988;433–461.
15. Speyer JJ, Bloomberg RD. Workload and automation. In: Human error avoidance techniques: proceedings of the second conference (P-229). Warrendale, PA: Society of Automotive Engineers, Inc., December 1989.
16. Wiener EL. Human factors of advanced technology ('glass cockpit') transport aircraft (NASA CR-177528). Moffett Field, CA: NASA Ames Research Center, June 1989.
17. Office of Technology Assessment: Safe skies for tomorrow: aviation safety in a competitive environment (OTA-SET-381). Washington, DC: U.S. Government Printing Office, 1988.
18. Rose M. Training at the repair station. In: Third federal aviation administration meeting on human factors in aircraft maintenance and inspection: 'training issues.' Falls Church, VA: BioTechnology, Inc., November 1990.
19. Kizer CR. Major Air Carrier Perspective. In: Second federal aviation administration meeting on human factors issues in aircraft maintenance and inspection: information exchange and communications. ParkerJF Jr., ed. Washington, DC: Office of Aviation Medicine, Federal Aviation Administration, May 1990.
20. Keith LA. Transport aircraft certification. In: Proceedings of FAA/DOT second annual international conference on aging aircraft (DOT/FAA/CT-89-35). Springfield, VA: National Technical Information Service, February 1990.

21. Shepherd WT, Parker JF Jr, eds. Human factors issues in aircraft maintenance and inspection (DOT/FAA/AAM-89/9). Springfield, VA: National Technical Information Service, October 1989.

22. Doll R. Maintenance and inspection issues in air carrier operations. In: Shepherd WT, Parker JF Jr., eds. Human factors issues in aircraft maintenance and inspection (DOT/FAA/AAM-89/9). Springfield, VA: National Technical Information Service, October 1989.

23. Higgins RG. Better utilization of aircraft maintenance manuals. In: Parker JF Jr., ed. Second federal aviation administration meeting on human factors issues in aircraft maintenance and inspection: information exchange and communications. Washington, DC: Office of Aviation Medicine, Federal Aviation Administration, May 1990.

24. Lutzinger RT. Day-to-day problems in air carrier maintenance and inspection operations. In: Shepherd WT, Parker JF Jr., eds. Human factors issues in aircraft maintenance and inspection (DOT/FAA/AAM-89/9). Springfield, VA: National Technical Information Service, October 1989.

25. Drury CG. The human operator as an inspector: aided and unaided. In: Proceedings of FAA/DOT second annual international conference on aging aircraft (DOT/FAA/CT-89–35). Springfield, VA: National Technical Information Service, October 1989.

26. Ansley G. Nondestructive inspection equipment and procedures. In: Shepherd WT, Parker JF Jr., eds. Human factors issues in aircraft maintenance and inspection (DOT/FAA/AAM-89/9). Springfield, VA: National Technical Information Service, October 1989.

27. Grubb NS. Commuter air carrier maintenance and inspection. In: Shepherd WT, Parker JF Jr., eds. Human factors issues in aircraft maintenance and inspection (DOT/FAA/AAM-89/9). Springfield, VA: National Technical Information Service, October 1989.

28. Thackray RI. Aging fleet evaluation summary report: human factors. Washington, DC: Office of Aviation Medicine, Federal Aviation Administration Aging Fleet Inspection Team, 1990.

29. Hancock PA. Environmental stressors. In: Warm JS, ed. Sustained attention in human performance. New York: Wiley, 1984.

30. Majoros AE. Human performance in aircraft maintenance: the role of aircraft design. In: Shepherd WT, Parker JF Jr., eds. Human factors issues in aircraft maintenance and inspection (DOT/FAA/AAM-89/9). Springfield, VA: National Technical Information Service, October 1989.

31. National Aeronautics and Space Administration: Spinoff 1989. Washington, DC: Technology Utilization Division, NASA Headquarters, 1989.

32. Taggart WR. Introducing CRM into maintenance training. In: Third federal aviation administration meeting on human factors in aircraft maintenance and inspection: 'training issues.' Falls Church, VA: BioTechnology, November 1990.

33. Oldani RL. Maintenance and inspection from the manufacturer's point of view. In: Shepherd WT, Parker JF Jr., eds. Human factors issues in aircraft maintenance and inspection (DOT/FAA/AAM-89/9). Springfield, VA: National Technical Information Service, October 1989.

34. Nielsen J. Hypertext and hypermedia. San Diego: Academic Press, 1990.

35. Johnson RC. Improved information for maintenance personnel. In: Shepherd WT, Parker JF Jr., eds. Human factors issues in aircraft maintenance and inspection (DOT/FAA/AAM-89/9). Springfield, VA: National Technical Information Service, October 1989.

Chapter 31

Biomedical Challenges of Spaceflight

Arnold E. Nicogossian,

Karen Gaiser

Life is short; the art long; opportunity fleeting: Judgment difficult, experience fallacious.

Hippocrates

In the past two decades, significant progress has been made in characterizing the biomedical effects of weightlessness on living organisms. Most of this information was derived from actual spaceflight and ground-based simulation studies. These research efforts were justified, considering the novel nature of the space environment and the requirements generated by the technologic achievements necessary to explore the universe beyond the confines of Earth. Until 1971, when the Soviet Union launched the first manned space station (Salyut 1), opportunities for in-flight experimentation were quite limited due to spacecraft size and operational constraints. Thus, prior to 1970, most biomedical studies were conducted before and after flight to determine the net changes undergone during flight and the rate and time-course of the re-adaptation process to a 1-g environment.

With the advent of Skylab (1973 to 1974), with subsequent Soviet Salyut missions of up to 6 months' duration (1977 to 1986), and the Soviet Mir flights of up to 1 year (1987 to present), the time-course of acclimatization to the weightlessness environment itself could be repeatedly studied through carefully designed in-flight biomedical experiments.

These studies, although mostly observational and often designed to evaluate biomedical changes observed in previous missions, nevertheless have contributed to our general understanding of the gross physiologic changes associated mostly with single exposures to spaceflights of varied duration. As the number of missions increased, as more biomedical data was accrued, as individuals flew repeated missions, and as space endurance records were extended further, a clustering of events began to occur that has allowed scientists to approximate physiologic trends and formulate newer hypotheses.

Despite significant limitations, such as operational constraints, concomitant use of countermeasures, and large intersubject variabilities in a highly select population, the data obtained so far point to the fact that humans do adapt to and can function usefully in the space environment if adequate medical support is provided. Much remains to be learned, however, concerning the true nature of the changes observed to date and the best procedures for providing medical support. It may be instructive to examine these aspects of spaceflight and the support of space missions, beginning with a review of the current knowledge regarding the effects of the space-flight environment on several key physiologic systems.

953

PHYSIOLOGIC EFFECTS OF SPACEFLIGHT

Neurovestibular Reactions

One of the primary functions of the neurovestibular system is to provide information about gravity. Previous space missions have shown that when the pull of gravity is neutralized, significant alterations occur in the components of this sensory system and in vestibular interactions with other sensory systems, resulting in numerous side effects.

Clinically, the most important vestibular disturbance associated with spaceflight is space motion sickness. Immediately on entry into the weightless environment, most individuals experience the sensation of bodily inversion. This illusion soon passes but may recur with rapid movement or when moving from a small area to a larger volume within the space vehicle. More susceptible individuals, however, develop symptoms of space motion sickness. Affecting some 40% of all space travelers, it occurs early in the mission, typically within the first 3 days, and usually lasts for 2 to 4 days. Symptoms range from minimal discomfort (stomach awareness) to nausea and vomiting, in rare cases accompanied by pallor and sweating. Head and body movements tend to worsen the discomfort. When the symptoms are severe, crew performance can be affected and mission efficiency severely compromised. During the Apollo IX mission, for example, certain crew activities were delayed by 24 hours due to space motion sickness. Some work time was lost in the first 3 days of the Skylab 3 flight for the same reason.

The classic model for the onset of space motion sickness is found in a description provided by the Soviet cosmonaut Titov (1). For a brief period after transition into orbit, Titov felt that he was flying upside down. This was followed by dizziness associated with head movements. Some time between the fourth and seventh orbits, or 6 or more hours into the flight, he became nauseated and ill. This was the first recorded instance of space motion sickness.

The medical basis for space motion sickness is not well understood, partly because the phenomenon can be studied effectively only during spaceflight. Dietlein and Johnston (2) noted that direct pressure measurements in animal models and human studies using z-axis recumbent rotation largely discounted the etiologic role of cephalad fluid shifts as a basis for space motion sickness. They concluded that the most plausible explanation was the "sensory conflict" hypothesis, according to which the usual afferent visual and somatosensory inputs to the vestibular receptors and/or the central nervous system were no longer appropriate in the weightless environment of space, resulting in aberrant reflexes and/or effector responses. During the adaptation period of several days, new sensory thresholds are established that allow the afferent sensory inputs to once again be correctly interpreted.

In the general population, a number of variables appear to be related to an individual's susceptibility to motion sickness. For example, children younger than 2 years of age are usually immune to motion sickness; susceptibility increases during childhood and reaches its highest level between the ages of 2 and 12 years. Thereafter, susceptibility declines with age (3). Reason and Brand (4) found that women report a significantly greater incidence of motion sickness, suggesting that gender may play some role in susceptibility. Personality variables that are positively correlated with increased susceptibility to motion sickness include introversion, neuroticism, and fear, especially fear of flying. Barrett and Thorton (5) reported a relatively strong relationship between measures of discomfort in a car simulator and scores on a test designed to measure a perceptual style called "field of independence." Presumably, subjects who score higher on tests of field of independence rely more on vestibular and proprioceptive cues for head and body orientation than on external visual cues; they may, therefore, be more susceptible to the conflicting sensory cues associated with motion sickness. In addition, limited postflight data obtained on space shuttle crewmembers confirm that motion sickness susceptibility thresholds remain elevated for some time post-flight (6).

A variety of tests and questionnaires have been devised in an attempt to predict motion sickness susceptibility. Some of these methods measure aspects of vestibular function, and others provide actual exposure to provocative motion stimulation. Although vestibular function tests, particularly the ones that involve actual exposure to Coriolis stimulation, predict susceptibility in 1-g motional environments, they have not successfully predicted space motion sickness susceptibility. Of the potential reasons for the failure of these tests to predict motion sickness susceptibility in space is the variables in individual susceptibility to different motional environments in 1-g.

One approach to reducing susceptibility to space motion sickness has been to subject astronauts to a variety of vestibular loads just prior to flight in an attempt to shorten the required inflight adaptation period. Astronauts have reported that this vestibular conditioning is at least partially effective in reducing the severity and duration of space motion sickness. But time constraints in the immediate preflight period limit the amount of emphasis that can be placed on such conditioning activities.

Initially, the accepted method for preventing or treating the symptoms of space motion sickness was the use of medications, usually scopolamine-dextroamphetamine sulfate (Dexedrine) or promethazine-ephedrine combinations. Such drugs, however, have strong central nervous system activity. Currently, the space shuttle program is using an intramuscular injection of Phenergan. Additional approaches, such as the use of biofeedback, mechanical devices to restrain head and neck movements, and adaptation-training techniques, remain under laboratory investigation.

Cardiovascular Deconditioning

To date, all space travelers have evidenced cardiovascular deconditioning upon returning to Earth. The cardiovascular system exhibits a decreased ability to function effectively against gravitational stress after exposure to weightlessness. Symptoms of orthostatic intolerance have ranged from an elevated heart rate and inappropriate blood pressure responses to a tendency toward spontaneous syncope during orthostatic stress. In flight, reduced orthostatic tolerance has been demonstrated by means of the lower-body negative-pressure (LBNP) stress test. This condition is primarily attributed to the contraction of effective circulating blood volume resulting from the loss of body fluids and electrolytes during the early period of adaptation to weightlessness (7).

The deconditioning of the cardiovascular system occurs early in weightlessness but tends to stabilize after about the fifth week of flight. Response to orthostatic stress in flight was measured for the first time during the Skylab program. Figure 31.1 shows the mean heart rates for a Skylab crewmember before, during, and after the 56-day mission. Note that there is both an increase and variation in heart rate under the -50 mm Hg stress of the LBNP test immediately upon entry into weightlessness. There appears to be a gradual stabilizing of heart rate to a new level of functional efficiency. In even longer Soviet spaceflights (3 months to 1 year), a slight increase in heart rate has been noted, particularly toward the end of the mission (8). Nevertheless, cardiovascular deconditioning appears to be a self-limiting phenomenon that does not continue to worsen with increased flight duration. It represents an adjustment of the cardiovascular system to a new environment in which the load placed on the heart is considerably less than it is on Earth.

Cardiovascular deconditioning becomes a medical problem only after a space traveler is subjected to acceleration forces encountered during reentry or upon return to the constant 1-g stress on Earth. Depending on the duration of the spaceflight and the amount of exercise performed in flight, the return of cardiovascular function to preflight values might take as long

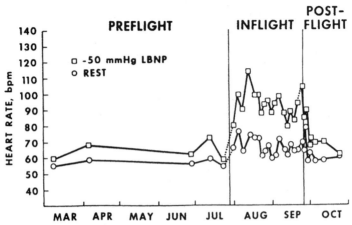

Figure 31.1. Mean heart rate of Skylab 3 pilot under 50 mm Hg of negative pressure during the lower-body negative-pressure stress test.

as 1 month. As spaceflight becomes available to a wider population, the problem of adjusting to reentry forces might be of greater consequence. This would be true in the case of a scientist who might be older and not in the same peak physical condition as astronauts traditionally have been in. In such a case, it would be necessary to conduct a careful assessment of the individual's cardiovascular fitness prior to returning to Earth and the use of appropriate countermeasures. Cardiovascular deconditioning might present a potentially more serious problem in the space shuttle era because the magnitude of accelerative reentry forces is quite different from that of the earlier missions. For example, the first orbital flight of the space shuttle presented a maximum G reentry profile during descent of approximately 1.6 G (Fig. 31.2).

There are at least two methods for dealing with the problem of cardiovascular deconditioning. The first is through use of antigravity suits. When inflated, an anti-G suit provides a restrictive pressure over the lower half of the body, thus preventing the blood from pooling in the lower extremities during the period of reentry stress. A second approach is through the use of rehydration prior to returning to Earth. Dietlein and Johnston (3) referred to simulation studies

that have shown that after 7 and 28 days of bed rest, 1 L of ingested saline solution (156 mEq of sodium) coupled with LBNP (-30 mm Hg pressure for 4 hours) will prevent or greatly lessen the symptoms of cardiovascular deconditioning. The benefits of this relatively simple procedure continue for some 18 to 20 hours and, if used just prior to the end of a mission, should offer protection against the reentry forces. Recent Soviet flights have demonstrated that intensive in-flight physical exercise and an optimal work-rest cycle can have additional prophylactic effects against deconditioning, particularly in long-term missions (8).

Although all observations to date are optimistic with respect to the ability of the cardiovascular system to acclimate to the space environment, several questions remain unanswered. In particular, it is important to further delineate the effects (and time-course) of the early and substantial inflight cephalad fluid shifts (up to 1.5 L from the lower extremities to the upper part of the body) and the resulting reduction in total blood volume on central venous pressure, stroke volume, and cardiac output. Complete information can be gained only by critical, long-term observations in space.

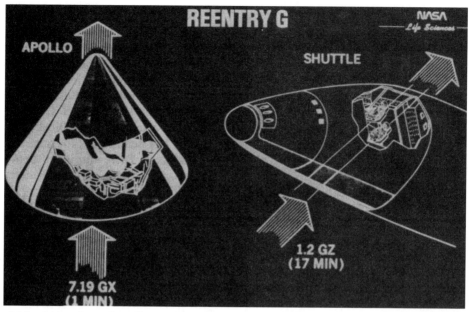

Figure 31.2. Comparison of Apollo and space shuttle reentry profiles. (Courtesy of the National Aeronautics and Space Administration.)

Motor System Disturbances

Among the most dramatic effects of spaceflight are changes in the musculature of the body and disturbances of the motor regulation system. The former changes are ordinarily indicated in flight by a progressive decrease in total body mass, leg volume, and muscular strength. Substantial muscle atrophy also is believed to occur, particularly in antigravity muscles, which is usually considered to be responsible for the postflight motor system changes that are observed. Disturbances in postural and motor coordination, locomotion function, and equilibrium and alterations in proprioceptor activity and spinal reflex mechanisms occur. Although all of these changes appear to be dependent, at least to some extent, on flight duration, they nevertheless have been reversible, and no sequelae have been reported so far.

Body Mass

In-flight weight losses of 3 to 4% were seen in association with early, short-duration spaceflights. With the advent of longer missions, it became apparent that most of weight loss took place during the first 3 to 5 flight days, with a much more gradual decline thereafter. This finding suggested that most of the initial change in body mass was due to the loss of fluids either through diuresis or decreased thirst and fluid intake and that subsequent losses were due to metabolic imbalances and/or muscle atrophy. The changes appear to be self-limiting, with the largest weight losses recorded (6 to 7 kg) being independent of mission duration.

In long-duration space missions, where adequate caloric intake and physical exercise were maintained by some of the crewmembers, actual weight gains have been reported. Such weight gains probably reflect an overall increase in adipose tissue, which was more than sufficient to offset losses of muscle tissue.

In any event, body mass lost in flight is rapidly regained in the postflight period.

Muscle Atrophy

Weightlessness and the loss of accustomed gravitational loads produce a number of structural and functional changes in skeletal muscles.

These changes are most pronounced in the postural, or antigravity, muscles such as the gastrocnemius and the muscles of the back and the neck. There is a gradual atrophy of these muscles along with a decrease in muscle tone. The process is progressive and can be controlled only with a high caloric intake and intensive exercise, especially strength exercises.

Evidence for the deterioration of muscle during spaceflight comes from several sources. In-flight measurements of leg volume show a rapid initial decrease attributed to the headward fluid shift, followed by a gradual recovery. Postflight biostereometric measurements of Skylab astronauts demonstrate more general losses of volume from the abdomen downward, although losses in the abdomen and buttocks are attributed to the loss of fat (9). Postflight urinary analyses reveal in-flight increases in the excretion of a number of metabolites associated with muscle breakdown such as nitrogen, potassium, creatinine, and amino acids. Metabolic balance studies and electromyographic analyses of muscular activity further substantiate the deteriorative effects of zero gravity on muscle function.

Bone and Mineral Changes

It has long been known that removal of muscle forces and weight from bones, as occurs in bed rest or having a limb in a cast, causes a loss of mineral, which is known as disuse osteoporosis. Residence in the weightless environment of space, which represents a form of musculoskeletal disuse, also has been found to cause a loss of bone mineral. Early studies of bone mineral changes using x-ray densitometry suggest that large amounts of bone may be lost during relatively brief periods of spaceflight. The 12 crewmembers who participated in the Gemini 4, 5, and 7 and Apollo 7 and 8 missions averaged postflight losses of bone density from the os calcis of 3.2% compared with preflight baseline values. Some losses also were observed from the radius and ulna after these early flights.

For later Apollo missions and Skylab, a more

accurate method of photon absorptiometry was developed to assess preflight and postflight bone mineral mass changes. Data from the 84-day Skylab mission showed moderate losses of calcium from the os calcis. In contrast to the earlier flights, increased bone mineral losses were not evident in the radius. These losses are believed to be comparable to those seen in subjects after bed rest. There is no evidence that the in-flight bone losses are self-limiting, and it is the current assumption that calcium losses occur progressively throughout the flight. Significant loss of os calcis mass was seen in one Soviet mission which involved substantial exercise, although the Soviets have indicated that extensive exercise programs in later missions decreased skeletal loss (10).

The precise mechanisms underlying the loss of bone mineral during spaceflight are still not known. Studies of animals with immobilized limbs indicate that disuse produces a number of time-dependent changes in bone formation and resorption. It may be that a proportionately larger increase in resorption over formation is responsible for the loss of bone mineral mass, at least in immobilized subjects. Whether the skeletal losses in space are due to relatively larger increases in bone resorption over formation is also still conjectural, but autopsies of three Soviet cosmonauts who died after a 21-day Soyuz spaceflight revealed a number of unusually wide osteocytic lacunae, which may have been due to increased bone resorption. Also not known are the underlying physiologic processes—whether hormonal, neural, electrical, or mechanical—that initiate these changes.

In evaluating the loss of bone mineral during spaceflight, investigators have drawn on bed rest studies as a model. Recently, however, it has been shown that bed-rest results are at variance with the composite calcium balance data for all Skylab missions. In bed rest, urinary calcium excretion peaks at about 5 weeks and then gradually decreases almost to its initial level. Fecal calcium excretion increases over a period of 10 to 12 weeks and plateaus at a level of about 120 mg/day. This is far less than the level of 300 mg/day reached on the 84th day of the Skylab 4 flight. The flight data show a monthly calcium loss for the average Skylab crewman of about 8 g, or about 25 g for the 84-day flight. This would mean a total calcium loss in 1 year of over 300 g, or approximately 25% of the total body supply. Such a loss is much higher than the rate of 6% per year estimated from bed-rest research. The difference appears to lie in the fact that the loss of fecal calcium does not plateau during spaceflight. Dietlein and Johnston (2) speculated that these results might be attributed to a deficiency in 1,25 dihydroxycholecalciferol, key regulator of calcium absorption in the gastrointestinal tract. Loss of bone mineral, if allowed to proceed unchecked, could represent a limiting variable for long-duration space missions. At least two countermeasures, however, are considered to be potentially beneficial. The first countermeasure is exercise. An ideal exercise countermeasure program represents the best possible compromise among efficacy, equipment size, ease of performance, and operational time requirements (11). Thornton (12) stated that although passive forces may modify the rate of calcium loss, the large forces produced by the activity of large muscle masses appear necessary to prevent or reverse the loss of bone mineral. He considered that 1 to 1.5 hours per day of walking or jogging under a 1-g force applied by elastic straps should be adequate to prevent disuse osteoporosis.

A pharmacologic countermeasure also has been considered. Ground-based studies have shown that drugs such as diphosphonate can control the loss of calcium in subjects undergoing bed rest over a period of many weeks. This approach has not been tried during a space mission but may offer a useful means of reducing bone demineralization during the weightless environment of an extended spaceflight. Other possible measures, such as rotation of spacecrafts to produce artificial gravity, might become a necessity if calcium loss cannot be controlled by any other means. Preliminary data

from Soviet missions of 6 months' duration have shown, however, that the mineral loss from weight-bearing bones remains constant and does not exceed 7%. Although these data are encouraging, in view of current hypotheses they do not shed any further light on calcium losses, especially losses from other portions of the skeleton, such as vertebral bodies.

Changes in Blood, Fluid, and Electrolytes

The cephalad shift of fluids in weightlessness, with the resulting contraction of circulating blood volume, is responsible for many of the physiologic changes that occur during adaptation to spaceflight conditions. As has been discussed, it directly affects the functioning of the cardiovascular system. It also has a number of effects on the composition of body fluids, especially blood. The most significant hematologic changes involve a reduction in plasma volume, alterations in red blood cell (RBC) mass, and changes in the distribution of RBC shapes.

Hematologic Changes

From the time of the early Gemini and Vostok missions, a postflight decrease in total RBC mass has been observed in nearly all United States and Soviet astronauts. There is a gradual decrease, with losses averaging about 9% of the total RBC pool over the first 30 to 60 days in flight and values ranging from 2 to 21%. Cosmonauts participating in missions of 18 days to 6 months have shown postflight decrease in erythrocyte counts which returned to baseline values within 6 weeks (13).

The magnitude of the RBC loss does not appear to be related to mission length, except possibly in missions of 30 days or less. Measurements of hemoglobin concentration taken in Skylab astronauts suggested that although RBC mass had declined to the same extent on longer flights as on shorter ones, it had begun to recover before return to Earth in the longer flights. The delay in the RBC mass recovery is apparently independent of spaceflight factors because RBC mass in the crew of Skylab 2 did not begin to recover until several weeks after the crew returned; however, recovery followed roughly the same time-course as in longer missions. A corresponding pattern is seen in the reticulocyte count, which declines initially (26 to 50%) and begins to recover after 30 to 60 days in space.

Accompanying the changes in mass are changes in shapes of RBCs. Normally, discocytes predominate by a wide margin. During spaceflight, the proportion of discocytes decreases sharply, whereas the number of echinocytes, apherocytes, and other atypically shaped cells rises. So far, these alterations in erythrocytes' shape do not affect crew health or function in flight and are rapidly reversed postflight.

There is still some uncertainty as to the primary mechanism responsible for the reduction in RBC mass. Toward the end of the Apollo program, it was believed that the observed RBC loss was due to mild oxygen toxicity produced by the hyperbaric 100% oxygen atmospheres in use in Gemini and some Apollo spacecraft. Results of missions using different atmospheres, however, did not bear out this hypothesis. A later proposal focused on the increased destruction and removal of cells, but experiments conducted on the Apollo-Soyuz flight demonstrated that this was not the case.

The weight of evidence now suggests that the loss of RBC mass is due, instead, to a suppression in RBC production by the bone marrow. The relatively rapid 4 to 16% decline in plasma volume in flight masks a drop in RBC mass by allowing the ratio of cells to plasma to remain roughly normal. Later, as the level of serum phosphorus rises, the RBCs increase their release of oxygen. The oxygen-sensitive kidney then counters the increased release of oxygen by further decreasing RBC production. Eventually, additional biochemical changes probably initiate a resumption of normal RBC production. In lengthy missions, this also may be related to the aging of existing cells as their 120-day life span is reached.

Electrolyte Alterations

The weightlessness-induced fluid shift produces at least a transient increase in central blood volume. From ground-based bed-rest studies, it has been suggested that the stretch receptors in the left atrium interpret this as an increase in total circulating blood volume, triggering a compensatory loss of water, sodium, and potassium from the renal tubules. This is the first event in a series of fluid and electrolyte shifts that occur during the adaptation to weightlessness.

So far, the early diuresis has been observed only in bed-rest studies. It has been difficult to demonstrate during spaceflight because of the problems involved in accurately documenting urine volumes early in flight, and because water intake is usually reduced during the early stages of flight. Nevertheless, data obtained from Skylab indicate that the nine crewmen decreased their water intake by approximately 700 ml/day during the same period, indicating a net loss of water.

Additional supporting observations include the observed in-flight increases in the urinary output of sodium, potassium, and chloride, an in-flight decrease in antidiuretic hormone, and a reduced postflight excretion of sodium (14). Fluid retention has also been a consistent finding in cosmonauts after Soyut flights, but excretion of potassium and calcium was found to increase (13).

Countermeasures that may prove useful against the effects of spaceflight on fluid and electrolytes include water and electrolyte replenishment and increased exercise. Such measures may partly alleviate the problem of contracting plasma volume and diminish the observed incidence of cardiac arrhythmias in flight, which may be partly due to aberrations in electrolyte balance. Increased exercise appears to have multiple benefits as a countermeasure. Perhaps most importantly, it may diminish the loss of electrolytes and metabolites associated with changes in muscle and bone and in mineral metabolism.

Additional changes observed in conjunction with short- and long-duration space missions are summarized in Table 31.1.

Table 31.1.
Physiologic Changes Associated With Short-Term and Long-Term Spaceflight

Physiologic Parameter	Short-Term Spaceflights (1–14 days)[a]	Long-Term Spaceflights (more than 2 weeks)[b]	
		Preflight vs In-flight	Preflight vs Postflight
Cardiopulmonary system			
Heart rate (resting)	Increased postflight; peaks during launch and reentry, normal or decreased during mission; RPB:[c] up to 2 days	Normal or slightly increased	Increased; RPB: 4–5 days
Blood pressure (resting)	Normal or decreased postflight	Diastolic blood pressure reduced	No change
Orthostatic tolerance	Decreased after flights longer than 5 hours. Exaggerated cardiovascular responses to tilt test, stand test, and LBNP postflight; RPB: 3–14 days	Highly exaggerated cardiovascular responses to in-flight LBNP (especially during first 2 weeks), sometimes resulting in presyncope. Last in-flight test comparable to R[d] + 0 (recovery day) test	Exaggerated cardiovascular responses to LBNP; RPB: up to 3 weeks
Cardiac size	Normal or slightly decreased postflight cardiac/thoracic ratio		Decreased postflight cardiac/thoracic ratio
Stroke volume and cardiac output	Decreased postflight; gradual recovery after 5 days postflight	Variable, usually increased during first month (impedance measurements)	Decreased postflight. Gradual recovery 5–21 days, depending on the level of exercise in flight
Electrocardiogram/vectorcardiogram	Moderate rightward shift in QRS and T postflight	Increased PR interval, QT interval, and QRS vector magnitude	Slight increase in QRS duration and magnitude; increase in PR interval duration
Systolic time intervals			Increase in resting and LBNP-stressed PEP/ET ratio/RPB: 2 weeks
Echocardiography			Decreased stroke volume and left end-diastolic volume. Ventricular function plots indicate no postflight myocardial dysfunction
Arrhythmias	Usually premature atrial and ventricular beats (PABs, PVBs). Isolated cases of nodal tachycardia, ectopic beats, and supraventricular bigeminy in–flight	PBVs and occasional PABs; sinus or nodal arrhythmia at release of LBNP in–flight	
Exercise capacity	No change or decreased postflight; increased heart rate for same oxygen consumption; no change in efficiency; RPB: 3–8 days	High exercise capacity in–flight	Decreased postflight; recovery time inversely related to amount of in-flight exercise rather than mission duration

continued

Table 31.1.—*continued*

Physiologic Parameter	Short-Term Spaceflights (1–14 days)[a]	Long-Term Spaceflights (more than 2 weeks)[b]	
		Preflight vs In-flight	Preflight vs Postflight
Lung volume		Vital capacity decreased 10%	No change
Leg volume	Decreased up to 3% postflight. In–flight, leg volume decreases exponentially during first 24 hours and plateaus within 3 to 5 days	Same as short missions	Same as short missions
Leg blood flow		Marked increase	Normal or slightly increased
Venous compliance in legs		Increased; continues to increase for 10 days or more; slow decrease later in–flight	Normal or slightly decreased
Body fluids			
Total body water	Decreased postflight		Decreased postflight
Plasma volume	Decreased postflight (except Gemini 7 and 8)		Markedly decreased postflight; RPB: 2 weeks
Hematocrit	Normal or slightly decreased postflight		Normal R + 0; decreased R + 2 (hydration effect)
Hemoglobin	Normal or slightly increased postflight	Increased first in-flight sample; slowly declines later in flight	Decreased postflight; RPB: 1–2 months
Red blood cell (RBC) mass	Decreased postflight; RPB: at least 2 weeks	Decreased ~15% during first 2–3 weeks in–flight; begins to recover after about 60 days; recovery of RBC mass is independent of the presence or absence of gravity	Decreased postflight; RPB: 2 weeks to 2 months after landing
Red blood cell half-life (^{51}Cr)	No change		No change
Iron turnover			No change
Mean corpuscular volume (MCV)	Increased postflight; RPB: at least 2 weeks		Variable, but within normal limits
Mean corpuscular hemoglobin (MCH)	Increased postflight; RPB: 2 weeks		Variable, but within normal limits
Mean corpuscular hemoglobin concentration (MCHC)	Increased postflight; RPB: at least 2 weeks		Variable, but within normal limits
Reticulocytes	Decreased postflight; RPB: 1 week		Decreased postflight. In Skylab, RPB: 2–3 weeks for 28-day mission, 1 week for 59-day mission, and 1 day for 84-day mission

Table 31.1.—*continued*

Physiologic Parameter	Short-Term Spaceflights (1–14 days)[a]	Long-Term Spaceflights (more than 2 weeks)[b]	
		Preflight vs In-flight	Preflight vs Postflight
White blood cells	Increased postflight, especially neutrophils; lymphocytes decreased; RPB: 1–2 days		Increased, especially neutrophils; postflight reduction in number of T cells and reduced T-cell function as measured by PHA[e] responsiveness; RPB: 3–7 days; transient postflight elevation in T-cells; RPB: 3 days
Red blood cell morphology	No significant changes observed postflight	Increase in percentage of echinocytes; decrease in discocytes	Rapid reversal of in-flight changes in distribution of red blood cell shapes; significantly increased potassium influx; RPB: 3 days
Plasma proteins	Occasional postflight elevations in α_2-globulin due to increases of haptoglobin, ceruloplasmin, and α_2-macroglobulin; elevated IgA and C_3 factor		
Red blood cell enzymes	No consistent postflight changes	Decrease in phosphofructokinase; no evidence of lipid peroxidation and red blood cell damage	No consistent postflight changes
Serum/plasma electrolytes	Decreased potassium and magnesium postflight	Decreased sodium, chloride, and osmolality; slight increase in potassium and phosphate	Postflight decreases in sodium, potassium chloride, and magnesium; increase in phosphate and osmolality
Serum/plasma hormones	Postflight increases in human growth hormone, thyroxine, insulin, angiotensin I, sometimes aldosterone	Increases in cortisol; decreases in adrenocorticotropic hormone and insulin	Postflight increases in angiotensin aldosterone thyroxine, thyroid-stimulating hormone, and growth hormone; decrease in adrenocorticotropic hormone
Serum/plasma metabolites and enzymes	Postflight increases in blood urea nitrogen, creatinine, and glucose; decreases in lactic acid dehydrogenase, creatinine phosphokinase, albumin, triglycerides, cholesterol, and uric acid		Postflight decrease in cholesterol and uric acid
Urine volume	Decreased postflight	Decreased early in–flight	Normal or slightly increased

continued

Table 31.1.—*continued*

Physiologic Parameter	Short-Term Spaceflights (1–14 days)[a]	Long-Term Spaceflights (more than 2 weeks)[b]	
		Preflight vs In-flight	Preflight vs Postflight
Urine electrolytes	Postflight increases in calcium, creatinine, phosphate, and osmolality; decreases in sodium, potassium, chloride, and magnesium	Increased osmolality, sodium, potassium, chloride, magnesium, calcium, and phosphate; decrease in uric acid excretion	Increase in calcium excretion; initial postflight decreases in sodium, potassium, chloride, magnesium, phosphate, and uric acid; sodium and chloride excretion increased in second and third week postflight
Urinary hormones	In-flight decreases in 17-hydroxycorticosteroids increase in aldosterone; postflight increases in cortisol, aldosterone, antidiuretic hormone, and pregnanediol; decreases in epinephrine, 17-hydroxycorticosteroids, androsterone, and etiocholanolone	In-flight increases in cortisol, aldosterone, and total 17-ketosteroids; decrease in antidiuretic hormone	Increase in cortisol, aldosterone, norepinephrine; decrease in total 17-hydroxycorticosteroids and antidiuretic hormone
Urinary amino acids	Postflight increases in taurine and β-alanine; decreases in glycine, alanine, and tyrosine	Increased in–flight	Increased postflight
Sensory systems			
Audition	No change in auditory thresholds postflight		No change in auditory thresholds postflight
Gustation and olfaction	Subjective and varied human experience. No impairments noted	Same as shorter missions	Same as shorter missions
Somatosensory	Subjective and varied human experience. No impairments noted	Subjective experiences (e.g., tingling of feet)	
Vision	Transitory postflight decrease in intraocular tension; postflight decreases in visual field; constriction of blood vessels in retina observed postflight; dark-adapted crews reported light flashes with eyes open or closed; possible postflight changes in color vision. Decrease in visual motor task performance and contrast discrimination	Light flashes reported by dark-adapted subject; frequency related to latitude (highest in South Atlantic anomaly, lowest over poles)	No significant changes except for transient decreases in intraocular pressures

Table 31.1.—*continued*

Physiologic Parameter	Short-Term Spaceflights (1–14 days)[a]	Long-Term Spaceflights (more than 2 weeks)[b]	
		Preflight vs In-flight	Preflight vs Postflight
Vestibular System	Forty to fifty percent of astronauts/cosmonauts exhibit in-flight neurovestibular effects, including immediate reflex motor responses (postural illusions, sensations of tumbling or rotation, nystagmus, dizziness, vertigo) and space motion sickness (pallor, cold sweating, nausea, vomiting). Motion sickness symptoms appear early in–flight and subside or disappear in 2–7 days. Postflight difficulties in postural equilibrium with eyes closed or other vestibular disturbances	In-flight vestibular disturbances are same as for shorter missions; markedly decreased susceptibility to provocative motion stimuli (cross-coupled angular acceleration) after 2–7 days adaptation period. Cosmonauts have reported occasional reappearance of illusions during long-duration missions	Immunity to provocative motion continues for several days postflight. Marked postflight disturbances in postural equilibrium with eyes closed. Some cosmonauts exhibited additional vestibular disturbances postflight, including dizziness, nausea, and vomiting
Musculoskeletal system and anthropometry			
Height	Slight increase during first week in–flight (~1.3 cm); RPB: 1 day	Increased during first 2 weeks in–flight (maximum 3–6 cm); stabilizes thereafter	Height returns to normal on R + 0
Mass	Postflight weight losses average about 3.4%; about two thirds of the loss is due to water loss; the remainder is due to loss of lean body mass and fat	In-flight weight losses average 3–4% during first 5 days; thereafter, weight gradually declines for the remainder of the mission. Early in-flight losses are probably mainly due to loss of fluids; later losses are metabolic	Rapid weight gain during first 5 days postflight, mainly due to replenishment of fluids. Slower weight gain from R + 5[f] to R + 2 or 3 weeks. Amount of postflight weight loss is inversely related to in-flight caloric intake
Body composition		Large losses of water, protein, and fat during first month in flight. Fat is probably regained. Muscle mass, depending on exercise regimens, is partially preserved	
Total body volume	Decreased postflight		Decreased postflight. Center of mass has shifted toward head

continued

Table 31.1.—*continued*

Physiologic Parameter	Short-Term Spaceflights (1–14 days)[a]	Long-Term Spaceflights (more than 2 weeks)[b]	
		Preflight vs In-flight	Preflight vs Postflight
Limb volume	In–flight leg volume decreases exponentially during first mission day; thereafter, rate of decrease declines until reaching a plateau within 3–5 days. Postflight decrements in leg volume up to 3%; rapid increase immediately postflight, followed by slower RPB	Early in-flight period same as short missions. Leg volume may continue to decrease slightly throughout mission. Arm volume decreases slightly	Rapid increase in leg volume immediately postflight, followed by slower RPB
Muscle strength	Decreased in–flight and postflight; RPB: 1–2 weeks		Postflight decrease in leg muscle strength, particularly extensors. Increased use of in-flight exercise appears to reduce postflight strength losses, regardless of mission duration. Arm strength is normal or slightly decreased postflight
Electromyographic analysis	Postflight electromyograms from gastrocnemius suggest increased susceptibility to fatigue and reduced muscular efficiency. Electromyograms, from arm muscles show no change		Postflight electromyograms from gastrocnemius showed shift to higher frequencies, suggesting deterioration of muscle tissue; electromyograms indicated increased susceptibility to fatigue; RPB: about 4 days
Reflexes (Achilles tendon)	Reflex duration decreased postflight		Reflex duration decreased postflight (by 30% or more); reflex magnitude increased; compensatory increase in reflex duration about 2 weeks postflight; RPB: about 1 month
Nitrogen and phosphorus balance		Negative balances early in flight; less negative or slightly positive balances later in flight	Rapid return to markedly positive balances postflight
Bone density	Os calcis density decreased postflight; radius and ulna show variable changes, depending on method used to measure density		Os calcis density decreased postflight; amount of loss is correlated with mission duration; little or no loss from non–weight-bearing bones; RPB is gradual; recovery time is about the same as mission duration

Table 31.1.—*continued*

Physiologic Parameter	Short-Term Spaceflights (1–14 days)[a]	Long-Term Spaceflights (more than 2 weeks)[b]	
		Preflight vs In-flight	Preflight vs Postflight
Calcium balance	Increasing negative calcium balance in flight	Excretion of calcium in urine increases during first month in flight, then plateaus; fecal calcium excretion declines until day 10, then increases continually throughout the flight. Calcium balance is positive before flight, becoming increasingly more negative throughout the flight	Urine calcium content drops below preflight baselines by day 10; fecal calcium content declines but does not reach preflight baseline by day 20. Markedly negative calcium balance postflight, becoming much less negative by day 10. Calcium balance still slightly negative on day 20; RPB: at least several weeks

[a] Compiled from biomedical data collected during the following space programs: Mercury, Gemini, Apollo, Apollo-Soyuz Test Project, Vostok, Voskhod, and Soyuz.
[b] Compiled from biomedical data collected during Skylab and Salyut missions.
[c] RPB: return to preflight baseline.
[d] R: return from flight.
[e] Phytohemagglutination.
[f] Recovery day plus postflight days.

SPACECRAFT ONBOARD LIFE SUPPORT

Most of the physiologic shifts discussed in the preceding sections are either direct or indirect consequences of weightlessness. The space environment, however, includes conditions that are, in themselves, far more hazardous and inhospitable for humans than weightlessness. Prominent among these are temperature extremes and the lack of an atmosphere and atmospheric pressure. Space vehicles provide these environmental conditions at levels that are not only survivable but comfortable. In addition, they provide systems for regenerating air and water, handling wastes, generating necessary power, and even preparing cooked food.

Recent Soviet missions aboard space stations have included experiments directed at the eventual development of a closed ecologic life-support system. Such a system would permit the continuous recycling of organic matter aboard the station, generating food for the crew in the process. It would probably be a prerequisite for very long-term space missions in which resupply was not possible, such as crew supported planetary explorations. For short-term missions in near-Earth orbit, the current state of onboard life support is entirely adequate. It is instructive to examine the progressive development of spacecraft environmental control systems that have culminated in the nearly Earth-normal environment of a vehicle such as the space shuttle.

Requirements

Pressure Control
For all practical purposes, and particularly in the context of spacecraft, acceptable environmental pressures are determined primarily by the required partial pressures of the component gases and by the necessity for change in pressure in the course of a mission. The important criteria are breathability and the avoidance of physiologic injury from decompression. Too great a rate of decompression can cause the explosive decompression syndrome. Slower rates of

decompression may produce decompression sickness if the pressure of dissolved gases in the tissues, particularly nitrogen, exceeds the ambient pressure.

Gas Concentrations

The most important gaseous component of an atmosphere is oxygen. At sea level, the partial pressure of oxygen (P_{O_2}) is 158 mm Hg. Because of the pressure of carbon dioxide and water vapor, the P_{O_2} at the alveoli of the lung averages 100 mm Hg. Without acclimation, human performance begins to show the debilitating effects of hypoxia at an alveolar P_{O_2} of about 85 mm Hg. Hyperoxia results when the P_{O_2} is too high, but a 5-psi (260 mm Hg) 100% oxygen atmosphere has been employed on spacecraft with no adverse effects.

The second gaseous component of concern is carbon dioxide. Normally present on Earth at a concentration of 0.04%, carbon dioxide becomes a serious problem at about 20 mm Hg, when hypercapnia can develop. Air regeneration systems include the means for removing carbon dioxide.

Water vapor, or humidity, is a third atmospheric component of physiologic consequence. Low humidity causes drying of mucous membranes, eyes, and skin. Inactivation of protective cilia in the respiratory tract leads to an increased risk of infection. Extremes of humidity also affect heat exchange. To avoid these problems, a water vapor pressure between 6 and 14 mm Hg is desirable.

Temperature Control

As a hemeothermic organism, humans are able to survive in a range of thermal extremes from subfreezing to tropical—particularly if they are clothed. But in the spacecraft environment, comfort is the primary objective. Thermal discomfort initiates thermoregulatory control responses and subjective sensations that detract from performance. A practical approach is to provide thermostatic control around an optimum point (usually 22°C) and to permit the modification of individual heat balance through clothing selection or air motion control.

Evolution of Control Systems

Mercury Spacecraft

The Mercury spacecraft had a 5-psi oxygen atmosphere supplied from a store of pressurized oxygen. Carbon dioxide was controlled by a lithium hydroxide absorber in the environmental control loop. Temperature control was accomplished through cooling provided by a sublimator heat exchanger. The sublimator vented water vapor overboard, and cooling resulted from the change of state. The crew stayed in their pressure suits, and the onboard environmental control system (ECS) supplied both the pressure suit and the cabin.

Gemini Spacecraft

The Gemini spacecraft retained the 5-psi oxygen atmosphere used in Mercury; however, the primary source of oxygen was now a liquid oxygen tank, with secondary oxygen supplies stored as high pressure oxygen. Carbon dioxide again was controlled by the use of lithium hydroxide absorber. The primary means of heat rejection in the Gemini vehicle was a spacecraft radiator that radiated the heat to space. Heat loss was controlled by the flow of coolant to the radiator and the ECS heat exchangers. In the later Gemini flights, extensive periods were spent outside the pressure suit.

Apollo Spacecraft

The Apollo spacecraft atmosphere control systems were similar to those of the Gemini systems but were improved and more elaborate. The overall ECS included two subsystems: a command module ECS and the lunar landing module ECS. A third module, the service module, carried consumables to support the command module ECS. The atmosphere was 5-psi oxygen, supplied by a cryogenic oxygen supply in the service module. Lithium hydroxide was used to absorb carbon dioxide. Cabin temperature was maintained at 24°C ± 2.8°, with relative humidity limited to the range of 40 to 70%. The primary system for heat rejection was again a space radiator. An evaporator was installed to provide cooling, but it was not used after Apollo 1 except for launch, Earth orbit, and reentry.

Skylab

The Skylab atmosphere control system incorporated some significant changes. Cabin pressure was 5 psi, but to avoid the minor chronic effects of hyperoxia over a long mission and the possible interference of such effects with medical experiments, a two-gas environment was used. The atmospheric composition was 70% oxygen and 30% nitrogen to provide a p_{O_2} just slightly higher than Earth-normal. The two gases could be controlled automatically, but in practice much of the control was accomplished manually to provide constant oxygen pressure during certain medical experiments. Carbon dioxide absorption was accomplished with a regenerable molecular sieve system. A characteristic of this system was that it operated at a nominal carbon dioxide level of about 5 mm Hg, so that although it met the same 7.6 mm Hg carbon dioxide limit as earlier lithium hydroxide systems, the average carbon dioxide level was higher than on earlier spacecraft. The earlier systems had kept carbon dioxide near 1 mm Hg most of the time. The thermal control system for Skylab was primarily a passive one. The vehicle was carefully painted with paints of varying emissivity in specific patterns so that very little active control with radiators or evaporators was necessary.

Space Shuttle

The space shuttle is the first American spacecraft to use a 760 mm Hg (14.6-psi) atmospheric pressure. Gas composition is 80% nitrogen and 20% oxygen, as on Earth. Carbon dioxide absorption is accomplished with disposable lithium hydroxide cartridges, as in pre-Skylab flights, and thermal control is accomplished using radiators on the insides of the cargo bay doors.

The space shuttle ECS provides for temperature control within a range of 18° to 27°C. Under conditions in which a comfortable heat balance is maintained, variations in humidity do not have a strong effect on comfort. When this heat balance can be maintained only at the upper limit of a comfort band or outside a comfort band, however, the humidity becomes very significant. To preserve a strong and effective thermoregulation response to overheating, particularly during the short, transient changes that may be encountered during exercise, an upper value of 0.27 psi P_{H_2O} is a component of the space shuttle orbiter specification.

Space Station Freedom

The Space Station Freedom will provide two different atmospheric pressures during the crew-member-tended capability phase of operations. For mission build (MB) flights, intensive extravehicular activities (EVAs) are expected, thus the atmospheric pressure in the pressurized volume will be maintained at 10.2 per square inch absolute (psia) normoxic. This lower atmosphere reduces the risk of decompression sickness that could be caused by EVAs. For utilization flights (UFs), no EVAs are planned, therefore the atmosphere will be maintained at 14.7 psia dependent on scientific requirements for payloads that are operating during this period. At permanent manned capability (PMC), the station will be continuously maintained at 14.7 psia.

Carbon dioxide absorption will be accomplished using a molecular sieve system. Carbon dioxide levels will not be allowed to exceed a partial pressure of 3.0 mm Hg under normal operating conditions.

The Space Station Environment Control and Life Support System (ECLSS) will maintain internal temperature in the cabin between 65° to 80°F. Relative humidity in the pressurized volume will not exceed 70% in the operational mode.

BIOMEDICAL SUPPORT OF SPACE MISSIONS

Medical Selection Standards

Astronaut Selection

Because of all the unknowns associated with spaceflight when the space program began, early astronaut candidates were subjected to some of the most rigorous selection standards ever employed. To begin with, all candidates were drawn from a highly select pool that consisted of military pilots and test pilots. The selection process involved a detailed review of the individual's biographical and career data, a large array of physical and physiologic tests and examinations, and an extensive physiologic evaluation.

Table 31.2 presents the flight status and age ranges of astronauts who have been selected during the course of the space program. Table 31.3 describes a number of physiologic parameters for astronauts selected before and after 1970; for

male and female astronauts selected after 1970; for male astronauts selected between 1959 and 1990; and finally, for astronauts selected between 1959 and 1990.

The physical and physiologic qualifying criteria remained essentially unchanged from the Mercury program through the Apollo program. The range and stringency of these standards have been modified for space shuttle astronauts and the screening of civilian scientists and technicians as nonpilot payload specialists in the Spacelab program. The mental health standards for the selection of pilots, likewise, have undergone an evolution since the early days of spaceflight.

During the Mercury program, psychologic testing and evaluation took 30 hours and resulted in a specific ranking of candidates according to a number of parameters of mental status.

After the initial experiences in space demonstrated that the psychologic stresses of spaceflight were not extreme, the selection criteria for Gemini and Apollo missions shifted away from a research-oriented approach to proficiency and

Table 31.2.
Description and Status^a of United States Astronaut Selections

| Selection Year | Selection Group | Number of People Selected | Age (yr)^b | | | Current Status | | | |
			Mean	Standard Deviation	Range	Deceased	Resigned (Never Flown)	Active	Inactive (Flown)
1959	1	7	34.6	1.7	32–37	1	0	0	6
1962	2	9	32.3	1.4	31–34	2	0	1	6
1963	3	14	30.8	2.0	27–33	5	0	0	9
1965	4	6	31.5	2.6	28–34	0	2	0	4
1966	5	19	33.0	2.3	29–36	4	1	2	12
1967	6	11	31.2	4.6	25–40	0	4	2	5
1969	7	7	32.4	1.8	31–35	0	0	0	7
1977	8	35 (6 f)	32.1	3.3	26–39	5	0	16	14
1980	9	19 (2 f)	33.2	2.6	28–38	1	0	10	8
1984	10	17 (3 f)	34.1	3.7	28–41	1	0	15	1
1985	11	13 (2 f)	31.8	2.9	26–36	1	0	12	0
1987	12	15 (2 f)	33.3	2.8	30–38	0	0	15	0
1990	13	23 (5 f)	34.1	2.8	29–40	0	0	23	0
Total		195 (20 f)	32.7	3.0	25–41	20	7	96	72

^{a} Status is current as of February 1992.
^{b} Age is in years as of the last birthday prior to July 1 of the year of selection.
f, female.

Table 31.3.
Physiological Parameters for Astronauts Selected Before and After 1970

Selection			Weight (lb)		Blood Pressure[a] (mm Hg)				Cholesterol (mg/dl)		Triglycerides (mg/dl)		Fasting Glucose (mg/dl)		Oxygen (max) (ml/kg)	
					Systolic		Diastolic									
Grp	cYr	N	Mean	SD	Mean	SD	Mean	SD	Mean	SD	Mean	SD	Mean	SD	Mean	SD
						Selection Results for Astronauts Selected Before 1970										
1	1959	7	167	16.0	113	8.0	71	7.2	209	18.5	NA		102	5.5	NA	
2	1962	9	162	12.3	125	7.6	75	7.9	184	34.9	NA		94	6.5	44.2	8.9
3	1963	14	163	13.5	122	11.0	76	7.4	179	19.0	121	56.3	103	10.7	42.0	4.9
4	1965	6	163	11.1	125	11.2	72	7.2	164	74.5	116	35.5	92	15.0	43.0	4.3
5	1966	19	166	14.7	125	11.3	76	7.1	204	39.4	101	20.6	106	9.5	44.2	4.4
6	1967	11	164	21.7	126	10.4	74	6.9	193	56.8	71	33.8	99	10.0	49.4	3.4
7	1969	7	165	14.0	115	8.1	70	6.9	175	11.1	86	38.6	95	6.4	52.0	6.0
1959–69		73	164	14.8	123	10.6	74	7.3	190	40.9	100	40.7	100	10.5	45.3	5.7
						Selection Results for All Astronauts Selected After 1970										
8	1977	35	161	23.0	120	11.8	77	6.7	197	43.3	87	44.8	94	9.6	44.1	8.8
9	1980	19	153	20.6	117	8.9	77	5.6	170	29.6	72	23.9	93	5.4	47.8	6.8
10	1984	17	159	28.3	119	12.9	74	8.7	203	43.0	63	30.3	88	7.0	47.7	7.5
11	1985	13	164	21.8	110	11.6	68	7.0	177	23.3	61	13.2	91	4.8	48.4	6.1
12	1987	15	164	20.5	117	7.8	79	5.9	184	50.8	73	29.7	88	8.6	45.5	5.9
13	1989	23	153	22.2	119	11.6	76	8.8	180	33.7	65	31.6	92	14.1	50.2	11.1
1977–89		122	159	22.8	118	11.2	76	7.8	186	39.8	72	33.9	92	9.5	47.0	8.4
						Selection Results for Male Astronauts Selected After 1970										
8	1977	29	166	19.2	122	11.7	77	7.2	198	42.4	90	47.7	96	9.4	46.1	7.8
9	1980	17	159	14.3	118	9.2	77	5.8	170	31.4	75	23.3	94	4.9	48.7	6.7
10	1984	14	167	22.9	124	6.0	76	7.0	200	45.1	57	27.0	90	6.1	49.6	6.2
11	1985	11	170	18.7	112	9.4	69	6.6	181	23.8	60	13.2	92	5.3	50.2	4.8
12	1987	13	169	16.7	118	8.1	79	6.4	188	51.7	75	31.2	91	4.9	47.0	5.3
13	1989	18	161	15.5	123	9.2	78	8.7	186	33.8	68	35.3	94	15.0	54.2	9.7
1959–89		102	165	18.0	120	9.9	77	7.4	188	39.9	73	35.7	93	9.1	49.0	7.6
						Selection Results for Female Astronauts Selected After 1970										
8	1977	6	134	24.2	111	8.3	77	2.7	192	52.7	73	23.0	84	3.6	34.1	6.1
9	1980	2	111	9.9	114	5.7	79	4.2	169	9.2	46	9.9	86	0.7	40.9	2.6
10	1984	3	121	20.0	94	4.2	62	7.2	214	36.9	91	33.1	80	5.3	38.9	7.4
11	1985	2	134	6.0	97	18.4	60	0.0	158	1.4	65	17.7	90	0.7	39.3	1.9
12	1987	2	134	21.4	115	7.1	79	1.4	162	53.0	58	11.3	72	6.4	38.9	3.3
13	1989	5	123	15.4	106	9.5	70	7.4	156	23.0	53	2.6	85	7.6	38.2	4.2
1959–89		20	126	18.0	106	10.7	72	8.5	177	39.1	65	22.1	83	6.7	37.7	5.0

continued

Table 31.3.—*continued*

Selection			Weight (lb)		Blood Pressure[a] (mm Hg)				Cholesterol (mg/dl)		Triglycerides (mg/dl)		Fasting Glucose (mg/dl)		Oxygen (max) (ml/kg)	
					Systolic		Diastolic									
Grp	Yr	N	Mean	SD	Mean	SD	Mean	SD	Mean	SD	Mean	SD	Mean	SD	Mean	SD
	Selection Results for All Male Astronauts Selected Between 1959 and 1990
1	1959	7	167	16.0	113	8.0	71	7.2	209	18.5	NA		102	5.5	NA	
2	1962	9	162	12.3	125	7.6	75	7.9	184	34.9	NA		94	6.5	44.2	8.9
3	1963	14	163	13.5	122	11.0	76	7.4	179	19.0	121	56.3	103	10.7	42.0	4.9
4	1965	6	163	11.1	125	11.2	72	7.2	164	74.5	116	35.5	92	15.0	43.0	4.3
5	1966	19	166	14.7	125	11.3	76	7.1	204	39.4	101	20.6	106	9.5	44.2	4.4
6	1967	11	164	21.7	126	10.4	74	6.9	193	56.8	71	33.8	99	10.0	49.4	3.4
7	1969	7	165	14.0	115	8.1	70	6.9	175	11.1	86	38.6	95	6.4	52.0	6.0
8	1977	29	166	19.2	122	11.7	77	7.2	198	42.4	90	47.7	96	9.4	46.1	7.8
9	1980	17	159	14.3	118	9.2	77	5.8	170	31.4	75	23.3	94	4.9	48.7	6.7
10	1984	14	167	22.9	124	6.0	76	7.0	200	45.1	57	27.0	90	6.1	49.6	6.2
11	1985	11	170	18.7	112	9.4	69	6.6	181	23.8	60	13.2	92	5.3	50.2	4.8
12	1987	13	169	16.7	118	8.1	79	6.4	188	51.7	75	31.2	91	4.9	47.0	5.3
13	1989	18	161	15.5	123	9.2	78	8.7	186	33.8	68	35.3	94	15.0	54.2	9.7
1959–89		175	165	16.6	121	9.9	75	7.4	189	39.8	83	35.7	96	9.1	47.6	7.6
	Selection Results for All Astronauts Selected Between 1959 and 1990
1	1959	7	167	16.0	113	8.0	71	7.2	209	18.5	NA		102	5.5	NA	
2	1962	9	162	12.3	125	7.6	75	7.9	184	34.9	NA		94	6.5	44.2	8.9
3	1963	14	163	13.5	122	11.0	76	7.4	179	19.0	121	56.3	103	10.7	42.0	4.9
4	1965	6	163	11.1	125	11.2	72	7.2	164	74.5	116	35.5	92	15.0	43.0	4.3
5	1966	19	166	14.7	125	11.3	76	7.1	204	39.4	101	20.6	106	9.5	44.2	4.4
6	1967	11	164	21.7	126	10.4	74	6.9	193	56.8	71	33.8	99	10.0	49.4	3.4
7	1969	7	165	14.0	115	8.1	70	6.9	175	11.1	86	38.6	95	6.4	52.0	6.0
8	1977	35	161	23.0	120	11.8	77	6.7	197	43.3	87	44.8	94	9.6	44.1	8.8
9	1980	19	153	20.6	117	8.9	77	5.6	170	29.6	72	23.9	93	5.4	47.8	6.8
10	1984	17	159	28.3	119	12.9	74	8.7	203	43.0	63	30.3	88	7.0	47.7	7.5
11	1985	13	164	21.8	110	11.6	68	7.0	177	23.3	61	13.2	91	4.8	48.4	6.1
12	1987	15	164	20.5	117	7.8	79	5.9	184	50.8	73	29.7	88	8.6	45.5	5.9
13	1989	23	153	22.2	119	11.6	76	8.8	180	33.7	65	31.6	92	14.1	50.2	11.1
1959–89		195	161	20.3	120	11.2	75	7.6	188	40.2	81	38.3	95	10.7	46.5	7.6

SD, standard deviation.
[a] Sitting blood pressure.

reliability and toward a determination of adaptability to known spaceflight factors.

After the Apollo program, mental health screenings became even more subjective and were based primarily on unstructured interviews with psychiatrists. Currently, no psychologic testing is done; only interviews are employed. The only requirement is that a candidate be free of psychosis, neurosis, and personality disorders. The objective of the screening is no longer to select the best candidate from a psychologic point of view but simply to ensure that each candidate is fully qualified to fly space missions.

Preflight Health Stabilization

The possibility of illness during a space mission—particularly if it involved an infectious disease—was a concern from the beginning of the manned space program. A preflight illness could cost valuable training time and possibly entail the postponement of a mission. In flight, the transient occurrence of space motion sickness was already troublesome; the appearance of infectious diseases could seriously jeopardize crew safety and mission success. For this reason, efforts were made to minimize the risk of such illnesses.

Early Mission Experience

Project Mercury flights were brief, and the risk of developing disease in flight was judged to be low. Even so, efforts were made to restrict the nonessential contact of crewmembers with others during the preflight period. Although some symptoms of upper respiratory tract infection and influenza were manifested postflight, no in-flight illness occurred during Project Mercury.

During the Gemini program, the increase in mission duration also meant an increase in the risk of infectious disease in flight. Medical personnel were able to implement a partial quarantine of crewmembers, screening the personnel with whom the crew came in contact. In particular, access to the crewmembers was closely controlled during the prelaunch period. Again, there were no in-flight illnesses, although there were a number of preflight cases of upper respiratory tract infections and influenza, along with one case of streptococcal pharyngitis and exposure to mumps.

The Apollo program was not so fortunate. During the first mission, Apollo 7, all three crew members were ill with an upper respiratory tract infection throughout most of the flight. After this experience, a medical plan was developed to minimize preflight exposure to infectious diseases in future missions. Conflict with the already-established training schedule reduced the effectiveness of the program, however. During the Apollo 8 preflight period, all crew members contracted viral gastroenteritis. Although treatment seemed to be successful, the commander experienced a recurrence of the disease 18 hours into the flight. In the Apollo 9 preflight period,

all three crewmembers came down with the common cold. For the first time, a manned launch was postponed (3 days) for medical reasons.

During this time, stricter health stabilization measures came into use. Crews were restricted to their quarters at the launch site, access to them was controlled, and personnel with whom they came in contact were carefully screened. Nevertheless, a member of the Apollo 13 primary crew was exposed to rubella before flight, necessitating replacement of the command module pilot by a backup crewmember. This episode finally led to the development of a detailed and strictly enforced program for minimizing the exposure of flight crews to infectious diseases before launch.

Flight Crew Health Stabilization Program

First implemented for the Apollo 14 mission, the Flight Crew Health Stabilization Program (FCHSP), a comprehensive program, involved a 3-week preflight isolation of crewmembers and a careful epidemiologic surveillance of hundreds of primary and secondary contacts during the 3 months prior to launch. The program provided for the rapid diagnosis and prompt treatment of any disease event in the crewmembers or their families. An immunization program was carried out, and strict procedures for preventing the exposure of crewmembers to potential disease-carrying persons were enforced.

The success of the FCHSP is evident in that throughout the remainder of the Apollo program (Apollo missions 14 through 17), during the three missions of the Skylab program, during the Apollo-Soyuz Test Project, and in the flights of the space shuttle, no infectious diseases have occurred in crewmembers in flight or after flight while the FCHSP has been in effect.

In-Flight Monitoring of Physiologic Status

The spaceflight environment produces a number of changes in the human body, many of which are of considerable physiologic significance. The first brief manned flights simply confirmed the nature of some of the more dramatic and immediate of these changes, such as cephalad shift of body fluids and the vestibular effects. Subsequent biomedical studies have confronted the arduous task of identifying all the physiologic effects of spaceflight. The objective of this research has been to answer the following questions:

1. How long can humans stay in space before incurring significant difficulties in performance or long-term health?
2. What are the basic mechanisms of the physiologic changes that occur?
3. What are the most effective preventive countermeasures?

In-flight monitoring of physiologic status provides essential data to support these efforts. It also allows ground control staff to monitor crew status in real time for purposes of decision making and ensuring crew safety. As technology has improved, as mission length has increased, and especially as the size and comfort of space cabins have increased, instrumentation has been added to provide a wider range of functions monitored under a greater variety of conditions. In addition, in-flight biomedical experiments conducted by the crew have added a new dimen-sion to biomedical knowledge derived from spaceflight. Table 31.4 summarizes the illness events observed among U.S. space crews.

Preflight and Postflight Evaluation

Prior to Skylab, the only source of objective data regarding most of the physiologic changes that occurred in spaceflight was the comparison of measurements taken before launch and after return to Earth. Although the inflight medical experiments on Skylab provided a major addition to knowledge in this area, preflight and postflight observations continued to be of great importance.

Mercury flights served primarily to identify some of the changes that occurred in weightlessness. Studies conducted during the Gemini program identified other effects and began to evaluate the extent of these flight-related changes.

Attention was focused to a greater extent on the cardiovascular system. Preflight and postflight studies, however, remained qualitative and were primarily intended to detect gross functional alterations.

Studies were made of blood volume and red blood cell mass, response to lower-body negative pressure, exercise capacity, biochemical changes, bone x-ray densitometry, and microbiologic counts. The results were sufficiently

Table 31.4.
Illness Occurrence in Space Crews[a]

Illness	Number Involved	Phase	Illness	Number Involved	Phase
Bends	2	In flight	Laceration	1	Preflight
Upper respiratory disease	8	Preflight	Serous otitis	1	In flight
Viral gastrointestinal infection	3	Preflight	Eyes and finger injury	1	In flight
Eye-skin irritation (fiberglass)	3	In flight	Sty	1	In flight
Skin infection	2	In flight	Boil	1	In flight
Trauma	1	Landing	Back strain	1	Postflight
Urinary tract infection	1	In flight	Rash	1	In flight
Contact dermatitis	2	In flight	Fatigue work-rest cycles	3	In flight
Arrhythmia	2	In flight	Toxic pneumonia	3	Reentry
Arrhythmia	2	Postflight			

[a] Does not include isolated premature ventricular beats, premature atrial beats, or motion sickness.

Table 31.5.
Ten-Year Trends for Astronauts Selected Before 1970 (N = 57)

Year	Weight		Systolic Blood Pressure		Diastolic Blood Pressure		Cholesterol		Triglycerides		Glucose		Oxygen (max)	
	Mean	Standard Deviation	Mean	Standard Deviation	Mean	Standard Deviation	Mean	Standard Deviation	Mean	Standard Deviation	Mean	Standard Deviation	Mean	Standard Deviation
1969	166	16	120	7.4	75	6.5	184	40.6	102	36.3	94	8.3		ND
1970	167	16	121	10.2	75	6.7	187	29.7	110	35.5	95	8.2		ND
1971	168	15	119	9.5	73	7.8	204	36.7	98	32.0	99	6.9		ND
1972	168	16	116	7.8	74	7.0	202	38.2	103	52.6	99	6.8		ND
1973	166	16	117	8.6	75	7.9	208	32.5	95	40.8	95	7.1		ND
1974	167	15	116	9.4	75	7.5	217	32.5	107	47.0	96	8.6		ND
1975	164	23	119	9.2	71	7.7	220	34.6	103	45.5	97	7.6		ND
1976	163	25	116	8.7	74	7.5	199	38.9	97	38.4	95	8.5		ND
1977	168	16	119	10.4	77	9.7	219	40.2	109	51.0	96	7.3		ND
1978	169	17	117	9.5	77	7.9	224	45.4	108	45.2	96	7.8	43	7.9
1979	165	24	119	9.4	72	7.5	211	39.3	108	46.9	91	7.4	43	7.9

ND, not done; N for 1978, 12; N for 1979, 29.

positive to provide reassurance that the long missions of the Apollo series were feasible.

By the time of the Apollo program, the pattern of preflight and postflight examinations was well established and remains essentially the same. Comprehensive examinations are conducted 30, 15, and 5 days before flight. They include full examinations of internal history and vital signs; ear, nose, and throat; eyes and visual function; skin; lymph nodes; and teeth. In addition, a number of special studies are carried out in the areas of microbiology, hematology and immunology, biochemical analysis of fluids, and cardiopulmonary function. These latter studies in particular form the baseline for comparison with postflight results of the same tests, which are conducted immediately after return to Earth and daily thereafter.

Table 31.5 summarizes the major points of the longitudinal health indices obtained from a cohort of 57 individuals after results over a 10-year period. No significant deviations in these data have been noted over this period.

Longitudinal Surveillance

Thus far, the physiologic changes seen to occur in spaceflight have not been debilitating and have been rapidly reversible upon return to Earth. Primarily, they consist of a degree of car-

diovascular deconditioning and some musculoskeletal deterioration. In flight, space motion sickness is the only remaining medical problem in short-duration missions. But from a strictly epidemiologic point of view, these results are not highly significant. For one thing, the population of space travelers represents a small sample of approximately 200 individuals. In addition, selection standards and preflight, in-flight, and postflight medical procedures have not been consistent over the data collection period.

Two developments now afford the opportunity to bring space biomedical research into accord with standard public health practices and to give its conclusions the validity of more structured and formalized studies. One factor is the development of formal medical standards by the National Aeronautics and Space Administration; the other factor is the advent of the space shuttle program, which is expected to expose relatively large numbers of people to spaceflight conditions (400 individuals by 2000). Indeed, a highly efficient system of biomedical record keeping will be required as part of the biomedical system needed to support the high launch and landing rate and rapid turnaround time of the Space Transportation System.

A major strength of such longitudinal studies would be their specificity for the establishment of a direct or relative measure of risk associated with long-term or repeated exposures to weight-lessness.

Space medicine is still in its evolutionary phase; as the number of flights and the length of stay in space increase, and as a greater number of individuals are exposed to weightlessness, new problems, both medical and physiologic, will be identified. These problems might require unique solutions, and the practice of space medicine will mature when it is practiced in orbit.

REFERENCES

1. Graybiel A, Miller EF II, Homick JL. Equipment M131. Human vestibular function. In: Johnston RS, Dietlein LF, eds. Biomedical Results From Skylab. NASA SP-377. Washington, DC: Government Printing Office, 1977.
2. Dietlein LF, Johnston RS. U.S. manned space flight: the first twenty years. a biomedical status report. Acta Astronautica 1981;8(9–10):893–906.
3. Money, K.E.: Motion sickness. Physiol Rev 1970;50: 1–39.
4. Reason JT, Brand JJ. Motion sickness. New York: Academic Press, 1975.
5. Barrett SV, Thornton CL. Relationship between perceptual style and simulator sickness. J Appl Psychol,1968; 52:304–308.
6. Oman CM, Lichtenberg BR, Money KE. Space motion sickness monitoring experiment: Spacelab 1. In:
7. Nicogossian A, Parker J. Space Physiology and Medicine. NASA SP-447. Washington, DC: Government Printing Office, 1983.
8. Gazenko OG, Genin AM, Yerorov AD. Summary of medical investigations in the U.S.S.R. manned space missions. Acta Astronautica 1981;8(9–10):907–917.
9. Whittle MW, Herron R, Cuzzi J. Biostereometric analysis of body form. In: Johnston RS, Dietlein LF, eds. Biomedical Results From Skylab. NASA SP-377. Washington, DC: Government Printing Office, 1977.
10. Gazenko OG, Genin AM, Yegorov AD. Major medical results of the Salyut-6/Soyuz 185-day space flight. NASA NDB 2747. Proceedings of the XXXII congress of the international astronautical federation. Rome, Italy, 6–12, 1981.
11. Nicogossian A, Sulzman F, Radtke M, et al. Assessment of the efficacy of medical countermeasures in space flight. Acta Astronautica 1988;17(2):195–198.
12. Thornton W. Rationale for excercise in space flight. In: Parker JF Jr, Lewis CS, Christensen DG, eds. Conference proceedings: spaceflight deconditioning and physical fitness. Prepared under National Aeronautics and Space Administration Contract NASW-3469 by Bio-Technology, Inc., Falls Church, VA. Washington, DC: U.S. Government Printing Office, 1981.
13. Vorobyov EI, Gazenko OG, Genin AM, et al. Medical results of Salyut-6 manned space flights. Aviat Space Environ Med 1983;54(Suppl 1):S31–S40.
14. Leach CS. An overview of the endocrine and metabolic changes in manned space flight. Acta Astronautica 1981;8:977–986.

AGARD conference proceedings (CP-372) on motion sickness: mechanisms, prediction, prevention and treatment. Williamsburg, VA, 1984.

Chapter 32

Aircraft Accidents: Prevention, Survival, and Rescue

Harry L. Gibbons,

Richard G. Snyder

Those who will not learn from history are condemned to repeat it.

George Santayana

When one of the first balloon flights occurred in France in the 1700's, someone questioned, "What good is it?" An observer, Benjamin Franklin, answered, "What good is a baby?" Although the "baby" of manned flight was to become extremely useful, not to mention popular, romantic, a major economic factor, and probably the greatest single instrument of war in the history of the world, it has also unfortunately been associated with accidents.

The National Transportation Safety Board (NTSB) defines an accident as "an occurrence associated with the operation of an aircraft which takes place between the time any person boards the aircraft with the intention of flight until such time as all such persons have disembarked, in which any person suffers death or serious injury as a result of being in or upon the aircraft or by direct contact with the aircraft or anything attached thereto, or the aircraft receives substantial damage (1)."

In the tenth edition of *Merriam Webster's Collegiate Dictionary*, an "accident" is defined as an unforseen and unplanned event. Although "accident" is a commonly accepted term, many of the occurrences that are called accidents are not unforseen, and some, to the aviation safety expert, are predictable. The occurrence of the

intent incident, that is, suicide or sabotage, is no longer included in accident rates by the NTSB. Therefore, accidents resulting from suicide and sabotage will not be covered in this chapter. U.S. military forces use the term "mishap" rather that accident. Accidents involving public use aircraft are not usually investigated or reported by the Federal Aviation Adminstration (FAA) or NTSB, and are not included.

To understand aircraft accidents in relation to the overall transportation safety record and with accidents in general, it is appropriate to point out that passenger transportation accidents account for about one fourth of all accidental deaths. Of all types of transportation, only transit buses have a lower death rate than scheduled airlines. General aviation passenger-miles are estimated to exceed that of scheduled airlines. (Table 32.1)

Although numbers are demonstrably impressive, they are included for information purposes only because comparison is not possible without exposure data and rates. Rates are available for only a few years and for only part of the transportation system. Recent data are preliminary and usually subject to change. This accounts for some of the variation in data from different sources (Tables 32.2–32.4, Fig. 32.1).

977

AIR CARRIER ACCIDENTS AND SAFETY

In 1987, *Aviation Week and Space Technology* stated, as part of a commercial state-of-the-art presentation, that the areas of primary concern in air safety are weather, human performance, and sabotage. In the 1980s, airline safety proponents placed a significantly increased emphasis on human performance, specifically human factors and cockpit resource management. This increased intensity was the result of incidents and accidents associated with major changes in the air carrier industry. Although the worldwide record of the air carrier industry is excellent in carrying about one billion passengers a year, or the equivalent of a fifth of the world's population, an NTSB member reminds us that "Even if accident rates are brought down, we may well see an increase in the absolute numbers of accidents."

Without attempting to compare with exposure or the at-risk population, a Boeing safety expert has stated that the total number of fatalities in commercial aviation is far exceeded by the 24,000 people killed annually in the United States in auto accidents in which alcohol is a factor. In the 30-year-period of 1959 through 1988, 16,000 air carrier fatalities occurred, or an average of 546 per year. That same expert related that if a person were born aboard a commercial jet in the United States in the 1980s and remained on board for 24 hours each day, that person would be 2,300 years old before being involved in an aviation accident. The individual would also have a 29% chance of surviving that accident. On the other hand, there were 10 fatal crashes in 1989 that claimed 257 lives. Although attributed by some to deregulation, the NTSB, supported by independent safety experts, found no common thread. There is concern, however, that some of these "operational accidents" might have been prevented by more experience in the cockpit after it was discovered that rapid growth led to coincidental assignment of crewmembers with little experience on the same flight.

Table 32.1.
Transportation Fatalities by Year

Type	Year 1987	1988*	1989*
Aviation			
Air carrier	232	285	277
Air commuter	—	21	32
(combined in 1987)	123		
Air taxi	—	58	86
General aviation	813	796	763
Highway			
Passenger cars	25,132	25,808	24,929
Pedestrians	6,745	6,870	6,525
Pickup and vans	8,058	8,306	8,513
Large trucks	852	911	852
Motorized cycles	3,836	3,662	3,137
Pedal cycles	948	911	830
Other highway	819	619	668
Total	46,390	47,087	45,454
Rail, intercity	616	563	601
Grade crossing	624	689	791
Marine			
Commercial	118	128	95
Recreational	1,036	946	896

* Except for aviation, all fatality data are from the Department of Transportation. Data from 1989 and 1990 are preliminary and subject to change. Aviation data is from the National Transportation Safety Board.
Administrator's Fact Book, U.S. Department of Transportation, Federal Aviation Administration, Washington D.C., Government Printing Office, April, 1991.

Table 32.2.
Report of Numbers of Accidents by Type of Operation and Year

Type	Year 1987	1988	1989*	1990*
Air carrier	36	33	30	26
Commuter	32	19	17	17
Air taxi	98	97	114	103
General aviation	2464	2354	2201	2145

* Preliminary, subject to change.
Administrator's Fact Book, U.S. Department of Transportation, Federal Aviation Administration, Washington D.C., Government Printing Office, April, 1991.

Table 32.3.
Transportation Passenger Accident Death Rate 1986–88

Type	1988 Deaths	1988 Per Billion Miles	1988 Fatalities Per 100 Million Passenger Miles	1986–88 Fatalities Rate Per 100 Million Passenger Miles
Automobiles	25,614	2,143.9	1.19	1.23
Buses	44	127.9	0.03	0.03
School	34	83.2	0.04	0.02
Transit	1	21.6	0.005	0.01
Intercity	6	23.1	0.03	0.03
Railroad trains	2	12.8	0.02	0.06
*Scheduled airlines	273	334.2	0.01	0.03

* Includes large airlines and scheduled commuter airlines; rates exclude suicide/sabotage deaths.
National Safety Council, Accidents Facts, Chicago, 1990.

Table 32.4.
Airlines: Scheduled and Nonscheduled Service Accidents, Fatalities, and Rates 1980–1989

	1980	1981	1982	1983	1984	1985	1986	1987	1988	1989
Accidents										
Total	19	26	20	24	17	22	23	36	32	28
Fatal	1	4	5	4	1	7	2	5	3	11
Total fatalities	1	4	235	15	4	526	4	232	285	274
Aircraft hours flown (thousands)	7380	7126	7040	7299	8165	8710	9918	10534	10998	11050
Aircraft miles flown (hundred thousands)	3044	2921	2939	3069	3428	3631	4054	4335	4500	4567
Departures (thousands)	5729	5575	5351	5444	5899	6307	7247	7504	7590	7625
Accident rate per 100,000 hours flown										
Total	0.26	0.36	0.27	0.33	0.21	0.25	0.22	0.33	0.28	0.25
Fatal	0.01	0.06	0.06	0.06	0.01	0.08	0.01	0.04	0.02	0.1
Accident rate per million miles flown										
Total	0.01	0.01	0.01	0.01	0.01	0.01	0.01	0.01	0.01	0.01
Fatal	0	0	0	0	0	0	0	0	0	0
Accident rate per 100,000 departures										
Total	0.33	0.47	0.36	0.44	0.28	0.35	0.3	0.47	0.41	0.37
Fatal	0.02	0.07	0.08	0.07	0.02	0.11	0.01	0.05	0.03	0.14

(U.S. Air Carriers Operating Under 14 CFR 121)
From the Department of Transportation, Federal Aviation Administration. FAA Statistical Handbook of Aviation, Washington D.C., Government Printing Office, 1989.

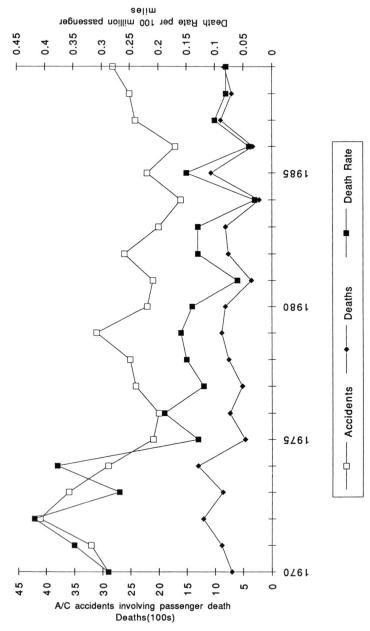

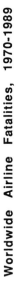

Figure 32.1. Worldwide airline fatalities for 1970 through 1989 illustrating the number of aircraft accidents, deaths, and death rate per 100 million passenger-miles. (National Safety Council, Accident Facts, 1991).

After an air carrier accident in 1987 that killed 156, litigation procedures, (which do not always agree with probable cause findings) placed responsibility on the airline, finding that the airline was negligent in training and supervision and that the negligence of the airline and crew contributed to the accident. The manufacturer of the aircraft was not required to pay damages. Prior to this litigation decision, the NTSB recommended to the FAA that all airlines (operators under the Code of Federal Regulations [CFRs], Parts 121 and 135) and operations inspectors emphasize the importance of disciplined application of standard operating procedures and, in particular, emphasize rigorous adherence to prescribed checklist procedures. In two accidents following an airline merger, human error and cockpit procedures were suspected as contributing to both accidents.

Suggested improvements in airline safety for the 1990s include establishing safety departments for airlines, a renewed drive for both airlines and unions to permit monitoring of pilot performance by routine review of the digital flight recorder, an FAA review of pilot training programs to determine if they meet the needs of a changing work force, and regulations on pilot pairing requiring additional precautions before two inexperienced pilots are assigned to the same flight. Regarding the organization of a safety section or department within airlines, the NTSB believes that the FAA should initiate a joint airline industry program to develop guidelines and regulatory provisions for airline safety programs, applying the same rationale that requires the separation of maintenance and maintenance inspection departments. That is, an independent safety officer who reports to the top manager of the airline.

The director of aviation safety programs for Transport Canada strongly urges airlines in Canada to adopt an independent safety officer program. Transport Canada sponsors a program that includes training for airline chief executives to demonstrate the need and cost benefit for such programs (2). They also provide training seminars for airline safety officers, a service not provided in the United States.

In 1991 the deaths of a U.S. senator and a prominent former senator in two separate commuter accidents drew a great deal of attention and concern to commuter airline safety; however, Table 32.2 does not indicate any major adverse trends over the period of 1987–1990.

AIR CARRIER ACCIDENT PREVENTION

Case Histories

The prevention of problems, incidents, and accidents usually requires identifying questionable or faulty procedures that have developed over a period of time yet suddenly become apparent as a result of an incident or accident. That these problems can be corrected is clearly indicated by the success of one airline. Their experience shows what may be accomplished to change a pattern of problems through cockpit resource management. In 1987 this major U.S. airline experienced six operational incidents attributed to pilot error, including near mid-air collisions, landing at the wrong airport, landing on the wrong runway, and inadvertent in-flight engine shutdown (2). In 1988 this carrier was criticized by both NTSB and FAA for being slow and timid in resolving cockpit procedure problems after a takeoff accident resulted in 14 deaths and 26 serious injuries of 108 persons on board. Reported as a contributing factor was slow implementation of needed changes in operating procedures, manuals, checklists, training, and crew checking programs required as a result of rapid growth and merger. NTSB also faulted FAA for lack of sufficiently aggressive action pertaining to this airline. Specifically, the investigation revealed that the airline did not insist on a standardized approach towards cockpit management (2,3).

The FAA instituted a National Inspection

Team safety audit for this airline in the summer of 1987 after the ''unprecedented series of incidents'' mentioned above. Among other things, the team was charged to review the line check program, evaluate cockpit crew procedures, and audit the overall training program, including an evaluation to determine need of additional instruction in crew coordination and discipline.

The audit reported lack of crew coordination, lapses of discipline, and breakdown in cockpit communications. Crewmembers acting as individuals rather than members of a team were described as the greatest problem. The airline recognized that with the increasingly complex and stressful environment of airline growth, it was necessary to change from a policy of delegating responsibility and discretion to crewmembers, which had been an informal if not casual procedure in the past, to clear-cut, definitive guidance through standardized cockpit procedures (2,3). Review of operating procedures with many changes; extensive rewriting of manuals, checklists, and handbooks; and restructuring of the airline flight standards section with eventual plans for a flight safety section resulted in significant and dramatic lowering of the frequency of even minor incidents. The airline established what has now been described as an excellent standards, flight training, and safety program. As indicated in Table 32.5, although data are not available for every quarter of the years during which the changes occurred, the percent of en

route inspections and cabin safety inspections with deviations from Federal Air Regulations (FARs) or established airline procedures decreased from the range of 7 to 9% down to an acceptable range of 1 to 2%.

DRUG TESTING AND ACCIDENT PREVENTION

November 21, 1988, the FAA published its final drug testing rules, Anti-Drug Program for Personnel Engaged in Specific Activities. These rules require operators under the CFRs, Parts 121 and 135 to establish antidrug programs for employees (including pilots) who perform safety related functions. Over 500,000 aviation employees are affected by this program, which requires testing for five commonly abused drugs: marijuana, cocaine, opiates, amphetamines, and phencyclidine.

Case History

In January, 1988, a commuter airline crashed, killing the two crewmembers and seven of the 15 passengers. The NTSB found that the captain was medically unqualified to serve as a crewmember on the flight due to his use of cocaine before the accident, and that his performance was degraded due to the adverse effects of his use of cocaine before the accident. This degradation was listed as contributing to the accident (4).

Table 32.5.
Safety Audit Results of a Selected Airline

Year/Quarter	En Route Inspections	Cabin Safety Inspections	Total	% Deviations
1987/third	499	49	548	7.0
1987/fourth	532	83	615	9.0
1988/first	626	98	724	6.0
1988/second	475	85	560	6.0
1988/third	482	71	553	5.0
1989/third	NA	NA	400	1.8
1990/second	NA	NA	NA	2.5
1990/third	381	94	475	2.3

Personal Data, HLG, 1991.

In spite of this case, the random drug testing of flight crew employees has clearly indicated that flight crews have a very low incidence of positive tests, and the Air Line Pilots Association (ALPA) has appealed to the administrator of the FAA to eliminate the random testing of flight crews. There appears to be some justification for this request since other drug testing programs, such as the military program, reported a decrease over time in positive findings after the initial results. In the above-cited flight crew random testing, only two positive tests were found (one of those possibly being a false-positive) out of 30,732 tests—a positive test rate of 0.007%. This has led ALPA to point out the questionable cost-effectiveness of the program. However, the value of such testing as a deterrent has not yet been defined.

AIRCRAFT MAINTENANCE, ACCIDENT PREVENTION, AND HUMAN FACTORS

In 1988, after an interisland flight experienced an explosive decompression at 7315 m (24,000 ft), resulting in one presumed fatality (swept overboard in the decompression) and eight seriously injured of the 95 persons on board, the human factors of air carrier maintenance and inspection became an issue. There was concern about the inspection procedures, especially with pressure to have the aircraft ready to fly the next morning.

Regarding discovery of fatigue cracks, the NTSB noted that a person can be motivated to perform a critical task very well, but when that task is performed repeatedly, expectation of results, boredom, task length, isolation during the inspection task, and environmental conditions all tend to reduce performance reliability. These factors were coupled with probable circadian dysrhythmia complications in that airline maintenance is most often performed at night and during the early morning hours. It has been documented that work in those early hours is often associated with decrements in human performance (5). The possible adverse effects of sleep loss, irregular work and rest schedules, and circadian factors on the performance of both mechanics and inspectors must be considered in order to achieve adequate performance and acceptable safety support. The physical, physiologic, and psychologic limitations of performing the inspection of rivets to detect the type of cracks that apparently led to this explosive decompression were emphasized by experts involved in the NTSB hearing of this case (5).

U.S. AIR FORCE, ARMY, AND NAVY

The past decade has been one of significant improvement by all branches of the service in achieving unprecedented safety records. All branches of service use the same mishap classification criteria. This chapter covers only class A mishaps and does not detail classes B, C, D, or E or foreign-object-damage (FOD) incidents. A Class A flight mishap is an accident or incident that results in loss of life, permanent total disability, destruction of an aircraft, or more than $1 million in property damage.

Since the U.S. Air Force fiscal year is from October 1, through September 30, less than 2 months of Operation Desert Shield is included in the 1990 report. Operation Desert Shield began shortly after Iraq invaded Kuwait on August 2, 1990. In the first 28 days the Military Airlift Command (MAC) flew more than 2000 missions, delivering to the Persian Gulf more than 63,000 armed forces personnel and 81,000 tons of cargo. From August 7 through September 30, 1990, MAC flew an additional 100,000 hours in support of Desert Shield. Of even greater significance, in fiscal year 1990 the air force logged the fewest major flying accidents and the lowest rate of fatalities from flying accidents since it began keeping records in 1921 (Table 32.6) (6).

U.S. Army aviation mishaps and fatalities have steadily decreased since 1956, with the exception of the Vietnam era. The army data are broken down into fixed wing and rotary aircraft

Table 32.6.
U.S. Air Force Class A Mishaps

Fiscal Year	Mishaps	Flying Hours (Million)	Rate/100,000 Flying Hours	Deaths
1985	61	3.48	1.76	89
1986	53	3.46	1.53	47
1987	57	3.46	1.65	61
1988	55	3.34	1.64	48
1989	57	3.41	1.56	76
1990	51	3.46	1.49	43

Air Force Magazine, Air Force Mishap Rates 74(4):98, 1991.

Table 32.7.
U.S. Army Class A Mishaps

Fiscal Year	Flying Hours (Millions)	Fixed Wing No.	Fixed Wing Rate*	Rotary No.	Rotary Rate*	Total No.	Total Rate*
1984	1.54	4	2.23	35	2.57	39	2.53
1985	1.53	5	2.83	40	2.95	45	2.94
1986	1.63	3	1.55	29	2.02	32	1.97
1987	1.70	2	1.04	35	2.31	37	2.17
1988	1.74	1	0.51	31	2.00	32	1.84
1989	1.69	1	0.52	31	2.08	32	1.90
1990	1.70	1	0.53	30	1.99	31	1.83

* Rates are per 100,000 flying hours.
U.S. Army Aviation Safety Center, Ft. Rucker, Alabama, July 1991.

mishaps. The U.S. Army has experienced concern over crew coordination, as mentioned earlier regarding the airline industry. A rotary wing crew coordination study was performed, and six types of crew coordination mishaps were documented. Appropriate steps were and are being taken, including widespread distribution of the study results; rewriting of manuals, training, and planning guides; and development of a video demonstrating crew coordination procedures (Table 32.7) (7).

Thermal injuries in U.S. Army survivable mishaps has almost been eliminated. Prior to installation of Crash Worthy Fuel Systems (CWFS) in helicopters in the 1970s, 13% of survivable mishaps resulted in postcrash fire, with up to 40% of the fatalities resulting from thermal injury. From October 1979 to September 1985 there was only one such mishap. In contrast, the NTSB found in a 14-year general aviation study

that postcrash fire occurred in approximately 8% of the general aviation accidents, with fatalities in 59% of the accidents with postcrash fire (see Chapter 22).

The U.S. Navy has also experienced a consistent and significant trend toward decreasing rates of major mishaps, number of destroyed aircraft, fatal mishaps, and fatalities (8). Only class A mishap data are included in this chapter (Table 32.8).

GENERAL AVIATION ACCIDENTS

General aviation experiences an average of six accidents each day, or about 2000 each year. However, the number of general aviation accidents has decreased dramatically over the past two decades. The peak was reached in 1967, when 6115 accidents were recorded. The 2138 accidents in 1990 were the fewest since general aviation records were initiated in the 1960s (9).

Table 32.8.
U.S. Navy Class A Flight Mishaps

Year	Flying Hours Million	Total Mishaps	Rate*	Fatal Mishaps	Rate*	Fatalities	Rate*
1977	1.98	107	5.40	41	2.07	119	6.01
1978	1.95	108	5.54	50	2.57	128	6.57
1979	1.91	99	5.18	39	2.04	77	4.03
1980	1.92	115	5.97	43	2.23	91	4.72
1981	1.96	92	4.68	38	1.93	81	1.12
1982	2.01	89	4.41	39	1.93	73	3.62
1983	2.00	86	4.29	38	1.90	99	4.94
1984	2.09	69	3.30	32	1.53	79	3.78
1985	2.14	73	3.42	28	1.31	82	3.84
1986	2.15	68	3.16	27	1.26	58	2.70
1987	2.28	74	3.25	27	1.19	66	2.90
1988	2.22	48	2.16	23	1.04	66	2.98
1989	2.23	55	2.46	23	1.03	78	3.48
1990†	2.15	63	2.94	20	0.93	42	1.96

* All rates are per 100,000 flying hours.
† Preliminary, subject to change.
Department of the Navy, Naval Safety Center, Naval Air Station, Norfolk, Virginia, 1991.

Table 32.9.
Accidents, Fatalities, and Rates: U.S. General Aviation 1980–1990

Year	Accidents		Fatalities		Aircraft Hours Flown Million	Accident Rates* per 100,000 Aircraft Hours	
	Total	Fatal	Total	Aboard		Total	Fatal
1980	3590	618	1239	1230	36.4	9.86	1.69
1981	3500	654	1282	1261	36.8	9.51	1.78
1982	3233	591	1187	1171	32.1	10.10	1.84
1983	3075	555	1064	1057	31.0	9.90	1.78
1984	3011	543	1039	1018	31.5	9.55	1.72
1985	2737	497	951	940	30.6	8.94	1.62
1986	2576	473	965	876	29.3	8.79	1.61
1987	2464	431	807	791	29.2	8.43	1.47
1988	2354	447	777	771	29.6	7.94	1.51
1989†	2201	423	757	NA	30.3	7.24	1.38
1990†	2138	424	736	NA	30.5	7.01	1.39

* Accident rates are per 100,000 flying hours; Suicide and sabotage accidents are excluded from rates.
† Preliminary, subject to change.
NA, Not available.
National Transportation Safety Board, Public Affairs, Washington, DC, 1991.

There has been, as indicated in Table 32.9, approximately a 2% increase in the number of fatal accidents that involved fatalities from 1980 to 1990 but a 40% reduction (from 1249 to 736) in total fatalities. Also, the total and fatal accident rates per 100,000 aircraft hours have decreased approximately 20 and 15%, respectively. The Aircraft Owners and Pilots Association attributed the decline of the number of accidents to greater numbers of pilots participating in more professional initial training and more frequent upgrading of skills.

General Aviation Accident Prevention

The efforts of an FAA Flight Surgeon to initiate an extensive education program for general aviation pilots regarding medical factors of accident prevention almost three decades ago resulted in clearly positive and measurable results. This educational program included significant safety enhancement through a nationwide effort. In this program, general aviation pilots were made aware of the effects of hypoxia as well as other safety information usually taught to military pilots by the use of military hypobaric chambers and crews. Many thousands of private and commercial pilots have participated in this training. As FAA Flight Standards and Air Traffic Control accident prevention procedures were added to the curriculum, the interest increased, and this regional recipe for accident prevention through education was provided nationwide. Currently, every FAA General Aviation District Office or Flight Standards District Office has an accident prevention specialist (APS). The practitioner of aviation medicine can obtain valuable assistance through the services of the APS, who has excellent teaching aids, including a Barany chair to demonstrate the greatest single cause of fatal general aviation accidents: spatial disorientation. Excellent aeromedical teaching materials for the FAA Aviation Medical Examiner are also available from the FAA's Civil Aeromedical Institute at Oklahoma City.

Ultralights

It is estimated that there are between 15,000 and 40,000 ultralight vehicles in the United States. Since 1982 the FAA has regulated ultralight aircraft under the CFRs. Because of increasing reports of ultralights being operated in regulated airspace and for nonrecreational purposes, the NTSB found it necessary to evaluate the FAA's regulatory approach. Because of data inadequacies, the NTSB initiated an investigation of all fatal accidents of powered ultralight aircraft involving obvious safety issues (10).

Between March 1983 and September 1984, the NTSB investigated 177 accidents. Of these, 88 involved a total of 93 fatalities. Only 42% of the pilots held an FAA pilot certificate, which is not required. Non–home-built ultralight accidents involving airframe failure constituted 23% of total accidents in contrast to only 2% of comparable general aviation aircraft. Ultralight accidents caused by loss of control constituted 42%, whereas general aviation airplane accidents constituted only 28%.

Lack of experience in flying a specific make and model of ultralight aircraft is a common factor in many of the accidents caused by loss of control. In several instances the operator had significant amounts of flying time in conventional aircraft or other ultralight vehicles. Some of these accidents occurred because loss of control was followed by collision before recovery could be made, or structural failure followed loss of control because the vehicle exceeded the design speed limitations of the vehicle (10).

Alcohol or drug impairment was cited as an underlying factor in six ultralight accidents. The NTSB study also revealed that some ultralight owners and operators are not receiving important safety information. However, in 98% of fatal accidents, available seat belts were used compared to 77% in general aviation accidents. Also, in 98% of ultralight accidents available shoulder harnesses had been used compared to 57% in general aviation accidents. This suggests that the pilots are generally responsible in the use of safety equipment (10).

To improve the safety record of ultralights, it is necessary to improve the skills and knowledge of ultralight pilots; improve the vehicle design, construction, and maintenance; and provide proper notification regarding safety defects. Ballistic parachutes installed in ultralight aircraft have been successfully employed, and one insurance carrier announced a reduced rate for aircraft with such a system installed. Some safety experts state that there is a need for more extensive rules governing the operation of ultralight vehicles. A number of organizations are assisting owners and operators to improve ultralight safety, including the Aircraft Owners and Pilots Association, the Experimental Aircraft Association, and the Powered Ultralight Manufacturers Association.

ROTORCRAFT

Medical Evacuation Aircraft Accidents

The first commercial emergency medical system (EMS) helicopter program began in the United States in 1972. The industry experienced significant growth during the 1980s. By 1984, the NTSB observed a significant rise in the number of accidents when seven major EMS helicopter crashes were investigated that year. In 1985 this had increased to 11. In 1986, 14 major EMS helicopter accidents destroyed or substantially damaged 9% of the total commercial EMS helicopter fleet operating that year. At that time the NTSB undertook a safety study of commercial EMS helicopter operations. A detailed discussion of the air ambulance and its advantages is covered in Chapter 20, but it is not inappropriate to point out in this discussion of accidents that in spite of the serious safety record mentioned here, medical evacuation by air is the only form of air transportation that has saved more lives than it has cost. The data from the Korea and Vietnam conflicts are remarkable.

In the NTSB safety study, 59 commercial EMS helicopter accidents were reviewed. This constituted all accidents that occurred between May 11, 1978, and December 3, 1986. There is not complete agreement on the database due to different parameters of definition and mission description used by different organizations providing data to the NTSB. Only 47 of the 59 accidents were included in determining the accident rate data—accidents in which the helicopter was involved in patient transport at the time of the accident. From 1980 through 1985, the commercial EMS helicopter industry had an estimated accident rate of 12.34 accidents per 100,000 hours flown. This rate is almost double the esti-

mated accident rate of 6.69 per 100,000 hours flown by nonscheduled helicopter air taxi operations and more than one and a half times the rate of 7.35 for all turbine-powered helicopters during the same period. The rate of fatal accidents (those in which one or more occupants are fatally injured) for EMS operations was 5.4—more than triple the 1.6 rate for nonscheduled air taxi operations (11).

This significantly higher rate appears to be the result of EMS helicopters routinely operating in poor weather and at night, serving unimproved areas, and participating in flight without advanced notice. Although the injury accident rate was not remarkably different from that of air taxis, the much higher fatal accident rate is consistent with weather and night accidents. Because EMS helicopters operate 24 hours a day, 365 days a year, poor weather conditions pose the greatest single hazard. The single most common factor in fatal EMS helicopter accidents was unplanned entry into instrument meteorologic conditions, and most of those accidents occurred at night. Spatial disorientation (see Chapter 11) has been reported to be the greatest single cause of fatal aircraft accidents in two reports issued in 1974 and 1981 covering a total of 13 years. Even if a pilot is instrument rated, current, and proficient, success is not guaranteed. Most helicopters require some form of autopilot system in addition to appropriate navigation equipment and instrumentation in order to be approved and certificated for single-pilot flight into instrument conditions. Even then, helicopters are unstable in flight and require constant input from the pilot to remain under control.

ROLE OF THE PHYSICIAN IN AIRCRAFT ACCIDENT PREVENTION

The flight surgeon, the aviation medical officer, and the FAA aviation medical examiner have a role in preventing aircraft accidents. The private practitioner has a role in caring for his or her patient. In some cases, when that patient is a pilot, problems are avoided when physicians not only provide medical care but also take appropriate administrative action regarding the pilot's medical condition and flight duty status. However, accidents have occurred because some physicians participate in misdirected actions under the guise of protecting or assisting the patient. Through the failure of these physicians to (paraphrasing Hippocrates) noise abroad what ought to be noised abroad, not only the patient who was a pilot but also others have been endangered or lost their lives.

Case Histories

A psychiatrist was informed by his patient, an airline pilot, that he was considering flying his airliner with all passengers on board into the ocean. To prevent a potential mishap, the psychiatrist contacted the pilot's wife and indicated that if she did not take appropriate steps, he would have to take action. The wife contacted the airline and the pilot was taken off flying status.

The staff of an emergency room treated an airline pilot for a nearly fatal dose of cocaine. After recovering some degree of alertness, the pilot-patient removed all intravenous and other attachments and left the hospital. The hospital staff was concerned but was not willing to contact the airline because of fear of suit. This and other problem cases, such as flight crewmembers being treated for drug addiction, were emphasized by a major U.S. newspaper and undoubtedly played a role in leading to the FAA drug testing program.

A commuter airline was notified by two of its pilots that a fellow pilot was behaving erratically and had been under psychiatric care for many years. The FAA was requested to investigate and found that the pilot had indeed been under psychiatric care for many years but cleared the pilot to return to flying with an admonishment that the history should have been reported. The airline refused to return the pilot to flight duty until they received the information and all medical records obtained in the investigation. The pilot

filed a lawsuit against the airline, and in the course of the trial it came to light that the pilot had experienced many conflicts with law enforcement and had been treated by numerous physicians who had prescribed over 12 medications, many of which were contraindicated for a pilot. It was the opinion of the expert witness for the airline that the psychiatrist had played down the severity of the illness for which he had treated the pilot for many years and had not mentioned the numerous conflicts with law enforcement. It was also apparent that some of the prescribing physicians were not aware that the patient was a pilot. It is unfortunate if some of the prescribing physicians did not know the occupation of their patient. The great physician-teacher-diagnosticians of the past century felt it necessary to know the occupation of the patient, both for diagnostic assistance and for therapeutic regimen choice; how much more important that is today.

A urologist, treating a pilot for hematuria, noted slurred speech. On questioning, the patient admitted that he was using a number of mind-altering medications for, among other things, panic attacks. The physician immediately called the pilot's employing airline. The pilot was terminated, or he resigned, and the physician was sued. The medical malpractice arbitrators awarded the pilot $11,000. Approximately $0.5 million had been requested. The physician did not agree with the arbitrators' recommendation, and the case was referred to court. Expert aerospace medical testimony emphasized that the pilot should not have been flying, that he had falsified his application for medical certificate, and that had the FAA known of his medical problems and the use of medication, he would have not been medically certified to fly. It was also pointed out that the action taken by the urologist may well have saved the pilot's life as well as his passengers' lives. The court decided for the urologist, who did not let the matter rest with success in court but went to the State Legislature. The State of Ohio now has a law which provides physicians with qualified immunity from lawsuit for breach of patient confidentiality when reporting transportation workers who are medically impaired.

Some years ago, a chartered airline crashed during approach to landing, killing 83 of the 98 persons on board. The investigation revealed that the pilot had apparently died during the approach, and there was not sufficient time for the copilot to recover the aircraft and prevent the crash. The pilot's physician revealed that the pilot had been under treatment for coronary artery disease and diabetes for many years. He was aware that his patient was a pilot. The Civil Aeronautics Board, the agency responsible for the investigation at the time of the accident, reported as follows: "The Board, in conjunction with the FAA, is exploring ways to improve the quality of medical information received from pilots, is attempting to improve the state of the art of medical diagnosis of pilots (the pilot in this case had a normal resting cardiogram in spite of severe disease), and is exploring the possibility of removing legal restraint which prevents physicians from reporting information of importance to the maintenance of aviation safety." The Ardmore accident report cited was released April 4, 1967, but since that time no rules have been made at the federal level although at least two states have taken action. An American Medical Association spokesperson, speaking of ethical and judicial matters, has stated, "The obligation to safeguard patient confidences is subject to certain exceptions which are legally and ethically justified because of overriding social considerations . . . Court is aware of the fact that if an airline pilot is not alert and capable of handling the flight, the lives of many people are at risk." The practitioner needs more concrete guidelines and permission, if not a requirement, to report information necessary for public safety. It appears that by working with state legislatures, state medical associations are the best source of an impetus for appropriate legislation. Unfortunately, it may require more accidents for legislative action to occur.

CRASHWORTHINESS AND SURVIVAL

Child/Infant Restraint

The protection of child and infant aircraft passengers in crash landings, in-flight turbulence, decompression, ditching, or emergency egress had received limited attention until recently. Although all 50 states, all 10 Canadian provinces, and 40 other nations now require restraints in automobiles, similar protection for children in aircraft is not yet mandated.

Case Histories

An airline crash in November 1987 involved five crewmembers and 77 passengers. The forward flight attendant, both pilots, and 25 passengers were killed. Of the three children and two unticketed lap-infants aboard, one child and one infant were fatally injured. The only child to escape injury was a 6-month-old infant held in his father's lap in the middle seat in the very last row, where survival is much more likely to occur.

A wide-body aircraft crashed during an emergency landing in July 1989. Of the 296 persons on board, 110 passengers and 1 flight attendant were killed. Three infants and one small child were being held by adults. One of these four received fatal trauma; the other three were located in an area where 91% of the survivors received only minor injuries. A 2-year-old child was placed on the floor between the mother's legs; during the impact the child was propelled down the aisle toward the front of the cabin and died of asphyxia after smoke inhalation.

A January 1990 crash which occurred on approach involved seven infants under 2 years of age. A 4-month-old was killed, and the other six infants were seriously injured.

In-flight turbulence may also pose a hazard to unrestrained children. In January 1990, a DC-10 encountered turbulence and a 7-week-old infant sustained a fractured occipital bone, subdural hemorrhage, and intracranial bleeding.

In many accidents there are insufficient data

to determine survivability. Neither the FAA nor the NTSB have significant data on most air carrier child and infant injuries. General aviation injury and fatality data for infants and children are essentially nonexistent. A recent study of members of the Ninety-Nines, the international organization of female pilots, found that 39% of 250 pilots carry infants in aircraft using commercially available automotive child restraints or infant seats, but 33% reported using no restraint other than ''held in arms.''

Regulations and Child/Infant Restraint

Current FAR operation rules require a seat belt to be used during takeoff and landing, except for sport parachutists, who can sit on the floor, and children under 2 years of age, who may be held by a seated adult. That is the case for both general aviation and air carrier operations. The rule that a safety belt provided for the occupant of a seat may not be used during takeoff and landing by more than one person who has reached his or her second birthday allows an adult to put an infant under his or her seat belt, a very dangerous practice (12).

In scheduled air carrier helicopter operations a person who has not reached his or her second birthday may be held by a seated adult. In the case of children who have reached their second birthday but not their 12th birthday, a safety belt may be used for two in a single seat if the strength requirements of the seat and safety belt are not exceeded. This is also a dangerous practice, according to many safety researchers.

There is confusion among the agencies regarding the definition of an infant or child. The FAA addresses a ''person'' under 2 years of age. The CFR addresses child restraint systems ''. . . as any device except seat belts Type I (lap belt only) or Type II (combination lap-shoulder belt) designed for use in a motor vehicle or aircraft to restrain, seat, or position children who weigh 50 pounds or less.'' The National Highway Traffic Safety Administration (NHTSA) defines infants as younger than 1 year of age, while the Society of Automotive Engineers aero-

nautical recommended practice refers to infants as weighing less than 20 pounds and/or being too young to sit up and refers to children as weighing between 20 and 40 pounds. Although there is an obvious dearth of safety regulations regarding child and infant restraint, the subject has been extensively discussed since the 1950s. ''Cradle board'' restraints on the bulkhead, under the seat, and on the back of the seat in front of the occupant, and the use of netting have all been considered and have continued to surface as new ideas over the past 30 years but still lack sufficient protective merit. Since 1985 NHTSA is the sole agency responsible for both automotive and aircraft child/infant restraint certification, and the applicable Federal Motor Vehicle Safety Standard 213 applies to both automobiles and aircraft.

The majority of child restraint models that have been approved for aircraft use are rated by size rather than age. Generally, these restraint systems are designed for infants weighing 20 pounds or less, children in the range of 20 to 40 pounds, and some children weighing 50 pounds. There are four general classes of restraints designed for slightly different populations, as follows:

- Infant seats are intended for infants up to 20 pounds who are not able to sit up by themselves. The best protection for infants is with rearward installation to allow the widest distribution over the body of any impact loading. Usually the infant seat is designed to place the occupant in a semireclined position within a padded shell of molded plastic which can also be used as a carrier.
- Convertible seats are designed for infants and toddlers up to 40 pounds, and as the child grows, the seat can be converted from a rearward-facing, semireclined device to a forward-facing, upright position. These systems have three to five belt attach points and often feature a full or partial shield.
- Toddler seats do not recline and are rated for children who weigh up to about 40 pounds.

- Booster seats provide a means to boost or raise the older child who weighs up to about 60 pounds, to provide a better view. Some models make use of the adult lap belt restraint (12).

Several airlines use a device approved in England, Australia, Germany, and other countries that is known as the "belly belt." It consists of an extension lap belt attached to the adult's lap belt and is an attractive way for the operator to resolve the dilemma of the extra seat cost. However, it is considered by most medical researchers to be potentially dangerous and is not approved by the FAA. Tests of this device conducted by the Civil Aeromedical Institute of the FAA in cooperation with Transport Canada demonstrated that it did not offer adequate protection. The infant's unprotected soft abdomen takes all the loading, or the infant may be thrown out or crushed when the adult's upper torso jackknifes over the infant.

Infant/Child Tolerances

A child's body dimensions, proportions, and biomechanical properties are markedly different from those of the adult, and the child cannot be considered a miniature adult. Compared to the adult, very little is known about biomechanical tolerances of the child. However, some data have been derived from free-fall impacts of children who appear to be more fragile, yet resilient, and who can apparently absorb head impacts greater than those an adult can absorb. Based on studies by one of the authors (RGS), conservative injury tolerance limits for impacts to a child's head lie in the range of 150 to 200 g for 3 ms on average, with peak accelerations of 200 to 250 g. Children are unlikely to sustain serious head injuries when impact accelerations are less than this, although the long-term effects are unknown. Of importance, the comparatively large head mass perched on the fragile neck structure of the infant is significantly different from that of the adult. Head impact followed by thoracic injuries

is the major cause of impact injuries and fatalities in infants and children (12).

The Unborn Child

Since pregnant passengers and flight attendants now routinely travel by air—sometimes well into the last trimester—the effect of impact and restraint has been the subject of several studies. It is important that these women wear the lap belt low and snug on takeoff, landing, and especially in turbulence. However, they often place the belt high on the abdomen for comfort, which can be extremely hazardous on impact or in turbulence. Both authors were involved in FAA tests using pregnant baboons on a decelerator. The investigators concluded that the fetus is in a well-protected environment and that the critical factor is the survivability of the mother. When a lap belt is the only restraint, it should be worn low so the load is distributed under the bony pelvis rather than the unprotected soft abdomen. The rearward facing flight attendant with shoulder restraint is not subjected to the lap belt hazards of the passenger.

Presently there is no FAA requirement for use of child restraint. Proposed legislation would mandate restraint use. The FAA recommends their use, but this is voluntary, presumably with parents bringing their own approved restraint device on board. In March 1990 the FAA introduced proposed rule making pertaining to child restraint, but its policy has been to oppose mandated child safety seats based on cost-effectiveness studies indicating that more parents will elect to drive rather than fly, leading to even greater risks. The Aerospace Medical Association has formally passed a resolution strongly supporting the required use of approved child restraints since a lap-held infant or child remains virtually unprotected and at much greater risk. Currently, adults are instructed by airlines to hold a child younger than 2 years of age on their lap, although research has shown that under such conditions the child often becomes a free-flying missile. The inertial force of a 7.9-kg infant at a peak deceleration of 35 g is about 2800N (625 pounds) or four times greater than the strength of the average female and more than twice average male strength. At only 10 g, a 7.99-kg child may have an inertial force in excess of 1000N (225 pounds). Impact studies have shown that with a low-velocity impact of 25 km/h (15 mph), decelerations can exceed 15 g. Even if the adult can successfully hold the infant, flexing forward can cause crushing injuries to the child.

AIR CARRIER SURVIVAL

Every air traveler has seen or heard the demonstrations, either live or on video, relating to seat belt, oxygen mask, flotation device usage, and location of emergency exits. The FAA has instituted new requirements to increase accident and particularly postcrash fire survivability, as follows:

- As of November 1986, floor lighting is mandated which is designed to help passengers find emergency exits under smoky conditions. (Simulation tests indicated a 20% reduction in evacuation times.)
- After a November 1987 requirement, more than 600,000 airline aircraft seat cushions in the U.S. fleet were equipped with fire-blocking materials. This may provide 40 to 60 seconds of additional escape time after postcrash fire. In a previously mentioned 1988 accident involving fire, the fire-blocking material was reported to have played a significant role in saving lives (3).
- In August 1988, the FAA directed more stringent burn tests related to cabin interior, which were designed to drive the technology of cabin materials to improve safety. Maximum allowable peak heat released from burning cabin material was reduced by 35%.
- In February 1989, more stringent tests were required to improve fire containment in Class C (detection and suppression systems) and Class D (containment by oxygen starvation) cargo areas. This requirement of aircraft certification became effective March 1991 for in-

service aircraft. These efforts should decrease death resulting from intense heat and toxic gasses, such as carbon monoxide and hydrogen cyanide, and increase postcrash fire survivability.

Case Histories

When an air carrier jet ran off the runway and into water off an eastern seaboard airport, the city police stated that the rescue was well executed and well coordinated. However, coordination with the U.S. Coast Guard was not adequate. Airport rescue units were at the end of the runway within 90 seconds. Within 10 minutes city emergency units were involved. Use of airport water vehicles was delayed due to inadequate tow for launching, or not available when they were immobilized due to damage during or after launching. Two deaths occurred when the aircraft split apart as it went off the runway. Disaster may have been avoided because the aircraft collapsed a 6-foot-wide pier at the end of the runway. The collapsed pier prevented the fuselage from sinking in 20 to 40 feet of water.

A wide-body jet had overwater engine failure of all three engines and descended from 3962 m (13,000 ft) to 1219 m (4000 ft) before one of the engines was started and a landing was completed. Flight attendants reported that, as usual, many passengers had not watched the predeparture safety briefing with the demonstration of life preserver donning. They also reported that the cabin was particularly noisy during the safety briefing and demonstrations. In preparation for ditching, passengers were briefed and instructed on donning of life preservers. The flight attendants were told by the flight crew only that a ditching was imminent and the passengers were ordered to assume the brace position, where they remained for about 10 minutes until a flight attendant looked out and saw the landing destination, went to the cockpit, and was told that a normal landing would be made. Investigation revealed that the flight crew failed to tell the flight attendant how much time was available from the onset of the emergency to the order to prepare the passengers for a ditching. Consequently, the flight attendants rushed or cut short the preparations before the signal to ditch was made because they thought that they were almost out of time. Some passengers panicked and screamed throughout the preparations, and a few were unable to respond to the flight attendant's instructions. Some nonswimmers panicked and had problems donning life preservers. Some passengers had problems finding the preservers under their seats. Some could not open the plastic protective pouches, and many passengers found it difficult to don their preservers while they were seated with their seat belts fastened and had to stand to don their vests. Parents had problems putting life preservers on their children. Some male passengers refused to assist, and others were not asked to assist because they had consumed too much alcohol.

A wide-body jet with 212 passengers and crew of 13 lost pressurization while descending from 8839 m (29,000 ft). The cabin altitude rose to 6096 m (20,000 ft). Most oxygen masks automatically deployed, and passengers donned their masks immediately, but some of them placed the mask over their mouths only. The flight attendants reported that it was difficult to instruct passengers while also using oxygen equipment.

A wide-body aircraft with 182 passengers and a crew of 12 had decreasing cabin pressure, and at 10,058 m (33,000 ft) the cabin altitude was 4572 m (15,000 ft) and increasing. The oxygen masks deployed. The cabin altitude reached 5486 m (18,000 ft). Only 2 of the 182 passengers properly activated their oxygen systems and donned their oxygen masks.

A wide-body aircraft, after a rejected takeoff, ran off the end of the runway. Of the 393 persons aboard, 50 were killed and 42 seriously injured. All of the fatalities were found in the aft cabin (which seated 167 passengers), near the only exit which was open (the left overwing exit) and used during the evacuation in that section. All of these fatalities, who survived the crash but died from the effects of the fire, failed to use the right side

aisle, which was clear and could have been used to move forward to other available exits. Many of the survivors indicated that their evacuation was not influenced by the passengers' safety information which had been presented. Numerous passengers admitted that they had not read the emergency briefing card, but most did recall the oral briefing which was given in Spanish and English. They said the briefing was hard to hear and difficult to understand (13).

Passenger Briefing

The NTSB has had a long-standing concern that some passengers, in spite of safety efforts, contribute to their own injuries or deaths and that past and present means of conveying information on the use of safety equipment are not entirely effective. A study by the NTSB of the problems of passenger preparation for emergencies by oral briefings and demonstration before takeoff, use of briefing cards, video briefing, and other instructions, sometimes given under the duress of an emergency, reported that passengers do not listen to the oral announcements. However, passengers tend to watch a flight attendant who physically points out the area of exits and retain therefore a general idea of the location of such exits, particulary those nearest to them. Also, there is a need for a properly functioning public address system to ensure that safety messages by the crew are understandable in all parts of the cabin, both on the ground and in flight. Because of these and other findings, the NTSB recommended that the FAA, as priority action, do the following:

• Provide guidelines covering briefings and demonstrations of adults donning oxygen masks before placing masks on accompanying children, fastening an adult-size life preserver or personal flotation device on a child, and brace positions for children.

   The NTSB recommended that the FAA, as an interim measure, do the following:

- Issue an Air Carrier Operations Bulletin to assist FAA inspectors in providing better guidance to airlines.
- Require prelanding safety announcements to reinforce the pretakeoff briefings on release of seat belts, the location of exits, the location and operation of life preservers (in the case of overwater landings) and urge passengers to refer to safety cards prior to landing.
- Require, on airplanes which are equipped with life preservers, that the safety briefings include demonstrations of how to open the life preserver's sealed protective pouch.
- Require that automatically activated safety messages be used for explaining the operation of the supplemental oxygen system after loss of cabin pressurization in all newly manufactured air carrier airplanes and after a specified date in all other air carrier airplanes which operate under CFR Part 121.
- Require that recurrent flight attendant training programs contain instructions on the use of the public address system and techniques for maintaining effective safety briefings and demonstrations, which will improve the motivation of passengers to pay attention to the oral briefings and to the demonstrations.
- Require airlines to include, during initial and recurrent flight attendant training programs, information on how personality and behavior of passengers can be manifested in nonroutine and emergency situations, and to provide instruction on how flight attendants can compensate for these interpersonal dynamics when they must assign duties to passengers in emergencies (13).

The NTSB recommended, as longer term action, that the FAA do the following:

- Develop programs and testing of safety briefings and passenger motivation to listen to briefings.

The NTSB also recommended, as priority actions, that the airline industry do the following:

- Encourage all employees and their families, when flying as passengers for personal or business reasons, to set an example of attentiveness to oral briefings and demonstrations, videos, and safety cards.
- Include articles in in-flight magazines which provide additional and more detailed safety information for passengers.
- Establish a standing committee within appropriate airline organizations to review passenger safety briefing methods and to work closely with the FAA in improving the content and presentation of passenger safety information (13).

AIR CARRIER CABIN SAFETY AND SURVIVAL

A 10-year study (1970–1980) by the NTSB showed that in 58.4% of the 77 survivable or partially survivable aircraft accidents or incidents involving passenger carrying aircraft, there were failures of cabin furnishings. From 1970 to 1980 there were 4800 passengers and crew involved in these accidents, and over 1,850 were injured or killed. Because of these cabin furnishing failures, death and injury occurred as a result of direct trauma. Not uncommon was failure of the seat or the restraint system, allowing the occupant to become a missile traveling at the same velocity as the aircraft just before impact. Death and injury also occurred as a result of occupants being trapped or having evacuation difficulties because of obstacles to egress as a result of failure of cabin furnishings. Regulations dealing with occupant protection in crashes were last updated in the 1950s and do not adequately reflect needs of the aircraft of today, nor do they adequately reflect the existing technology for design and testing to provide updated regulations.

If a crash occurs and the occupant is restrained by lap belt, and the aircraft and occupants experience a rate of onset and duration of forces typical of those experienced in survivable crashes, the human body can withstand whole-body forces at least two to three times greater than those cited in the CFR (9.0 g forward, 4.5 g downward, 1.5 g sideward, and 2.0 g upward) without irreversible injury. Aircraft accident investigation, research, and experimentation, including full-scale crash tests of aircraft, showed the tolerable forces to be as follows:

Direction	g's
Forward	20–25
Downward	15–20
Sideward	10–15
Upward	20

(Duration from 0.1 to 0.2 seconds and rate of onset of 50 gs/second.)

Tests have also shown that the limits in the forward direction can be more than doubled by the use of an upper-torso restraint (shoulder harness).

GENERAL AVIATION CRASHWORTHINESS

Studies indicate that there is a substantial likelihood (60 to 73%, based on four studies) that a general aviation aircraft will be involved in an accident during a 20-year service life. In those accidents in one decade alone, more than 100,000 occupants were injured in approximately 40,000 accidents. Of these accidents, 17.7% involved at least one fatality. NTSB accident investigators report that few changes have been made in cabin interior design or restraint systems which might have eliminated or reduced these injuries. Sharply contrasting with this is the progress in improving automobile crashworthiness. Without comparing impact speeds, general aviation aircraft accidents produce two fatalities for every three serious injuries, whereas automobile accidents have only one fatality for every 10 serious injuries.

The NTSB recognizes that automobile and aircraft accidents statistics are not directly comparable because of different crash loads and ve-

hicle design objectives. However, there should be little disagreement with the NTSB definition of crashworthiness that when crash forces transmitted to occupants through properly designed seats and restraint systems do not exceed the limits of human tolerance to abrupt deceleration, and when the cabin structure remains sufficiently intact to provide a liveable space immediately around the occupants, they should survive the accident without serious injury (14–16).

A study ending in 1952 reported that of 913 accidents involving 1,596 occupants and 15 aircraft models, there were 389 fatalities and that "roughly $\frac{1}{3}$ of the 389 people that were killed ... died unnecessarily." A 1970 report by Bruce and Draper of an aviation consumer project addressing crash safety on general aviation aircraft stated the following, among other things:

- The human body, restrained by seat belt and shoulder harnesses, can tolerate, without injury, forces sufficient to collapse today's general aviation aircraft.
- The general aviation manufacturers have not approached crash injury protection (crashworthiness) with engineering methods which have been applied successfully to the performance aspects (airworthiness) of the aircraft.

The most common deficiencies in general aviation aircraft are the following:

1. Lack of adequate upper torso restraint. Head injuries remain the most frequent injury as well as the major cause of death and serious trauma. This usually occurs when the occupant jackknifes over the seatbelt and contacts hard, sharp, unyielding, or rigid structures.
2. Inability of seats to adequately attenuate vertical compressive forces. Recent attention has been given to improved design of the front seats, but the rear seats do not appear to provide equivalent protection.
3. Lack of adquate seat support and attachment. Even with upper torso restraint and attenu-

ated vertical compressive forces, an inadequately supported and attached seat will reduce injury tolerance.

4. Cabin interiors that contain many lethal surfaces, structures, and objects which cause death or serious trauma upon crash impact. Flailing appendages, even when upper-torso restraints are worn, can contact controls and non-yielding structures.

An FAA report states ''. . . Severe but nonfatal injuries were common in 3 to 5 g accidents. Fatalities and very severe injuries occurred in crash decelerations of 6 to 10 g. At 10 g and above, most present general aviation aircraft disintegrate to the extent that the value of restraint equipment for crash survival is doubtful.'' In contrast, a new-generation agricultural aircraft was manufactured, patterned after a prototype aircraft with a 50-g seat, an integral double upper-torso restraint with inertial reel, a 40-g cockpit box, the storage hopper placed between the engine and the pilot to provide energy absorption, and an overturn structure (rollbar). In a 10-year period these aircraft were in 368 accidents with only 3% fatalities, whereas for the same period the fatality rate in all U.S. general aviation aircraft averaged 12.8% fatalities. If all occupants wear shoulder harnesses, fatalities are expected to be reduced by 20%. Of seriously injured persons in survivable crashes, 88% are expected to experience significantly fewer life-threatening injuries if shoulder harnesses are worn. Thirty-four percent of the seriously injured occupants of survivable accidents are expected to be less seriously injured if energy-absorbing seats are available (14–16).

SEARCH AND RESCUE

Search and rescue (SAR) is defined as the employment of available personnel, equipment, and facilities to render aid to persons and property in distress. Today's SAR had its beginning early in World War II when the German Luftwaffe

established a well-organized air/sea rescue when they were also the first to provide their pilots with life rafts. During the Korean War, U.S. air/sea rescue units evacuated approximately 10,000 wounded from battle areas. During the Vietnam War, U.S. air/sea rescue units rescued downed flyers from friendly and hostile territories. Although aircraft in the U.S. civil fleet are required to have an emergency locator transmitter (ELT) on board, it may not function as intended, its signal may not be received, and it may be regarded as false.

The U.S. Air Force Rescue Coordination Center (AFRCC) at Scott Air Force Base, Illinois, reports aircraft search and rescue activity for the inland United States (Table 32.10). The center director points out that most incidents are resolved by state, local, and volunteer organizations whose role in the national SAR is extremely important. For improvement of SAR to prevent loss of life, the critical time between SAR notification and recovery must be shortened. This can be accomplished by ensuring that ELTs are operational and reliable by increased monitoring of distress frequencies, by increased filing of flight plans, and, as reported by AFRCC, by ''using common sense (17)!''

GENERAL AVIATION SURVIVAL

Case History

A nationally recognized pilot with 20,000 hours of flight time, president of one of the nation's largest pilot organizations, experienced as an FAA pilot examiner, the winner of a U.S. National Unlimited Air Race, recipient of a Three Million Miles Safe Pilot Award, and survivor of several crash landings during racing competition, experienced engine failure due to contaminated fuel. His reputation as a perfectionist, if swashbuckling, but very skilled pilot was justified by his being able to crash-land his aircraft on a frozen lake at an altitude of 11,200 feet. His skill apparently ended at that point since he and his companions died of exposure within 8

Table 32.10.
Annual Air Force Rescue Coordination Center Activity

	1985	1986	1987	1988	1989	1990
Missions	2749	2791	2689	2686	2820	2805
Incidents	9169	7581	8584	7915	8041	7939
ELT event*	6159	5268	6319	5768	6134	5983
Saves	664	650	442	484	315	388

* ELT, emergency locator transmitter.
Department of the Air Force, Air Force Rescue Coordination Center, Annual Report, Scott Air Force Base, Illinois, 1990.

hours of the crash in spite of the availability of fuel, matches, ski clothing, and food. The clothing was partially used, but not wisely. Perhaps the traces of amphetamines and cocaine in the urine of the pilot were indicators of previous central nervous system excitation blocking the sensory perception of cold, but there was no evidence of these substances in the other two passengers, who also had minimal evidence of injury. Perhaps it was their reliance upon the ELT to bring help within hours. Had they acted as if no help would arrive soon, and used all survival material available, there would have been a much greater chance of survival. Even after the ELT was reported, it was some hours before it was considered to be authentic since there was no flight plan and the signal was some distance from any airway.

Water Survival

It is paradoxical that one of the most hostile environments of the earth, water, may offer the greatest chances of surviving an unplanned descent. However, after a controlled impact, the comparatively receptive surface significantly reduces chances of further survival. In 306 cases of water-ditching involving general aviation aircraft, 50% of reported fatalities survived the ditching only to die of drowning or exposure, probably hypothermia. Of those cases for which data are available, 90 to 95% of the aircraft stayed afloat long enough for safe egress (18). With so many cities, and therefore airports, lo-

cated near large bodies of water, general aviation aircraft operators should consider some type of water flotation equipment (as do air carriers) as part of their survival gear. It cannot be stored in the luggage area with the usual survival gear but needs to be immediately available in the aircraft cabin.

Regarding search, there are unfortunate cases in which the search is not for survivors, but for victims. The practitioner of aerospace medicine, particulary those who might have the tragic responsibility of locating those who did not survive, are usually aware of the effective use of dogs in the search procedure. However, not widely known, and not widely accepted in the past, is the knowledge that dogs are also able to locate bodies under water. The American Rescue Dog Association has shown that dogs can find bodies that are totally submerged and that bodies can be precisely located in water as deep as 90 feet. Not as extensively researched but evident is that dogs can find bodies submerged in turbulent water (19).

AIRPORT DISASTER MEDICAL MANAGEMENT

With the increasing number of medical facilities at major airports, the potential for significantly improved medical services exists. However, unless the airport has a well-developed disaster and emergency plan, with coordination and communications arranged with numerous off-airport medical services and full-scale rehearsals on a regular basis, when an actual emergency occurs, the greatest accomplishment may be learning the weaknesses of the emergency plan. Although the development of plans for coping with a mass disaster is a prerequisite to full-airport certification by the FAA, exercising the plans through disaster drills is only a recommendation (20).

Case History

The investigation of a previously mentioned air carrier takeoff accident which resulted in 14 deaths of the 108 persons on board, with 26 serious injuries, also uncovered problems with the disaster plan of this major airport, one of the largest and busiest in the United States. Specifically, there were problems in communications and coordination with off-airport medical units, and the NTSB recommended that the airport do the following:

1. Revise its disaster response notification procedures to provide for timely and effective notification of mutual-aid agencies whose assistance is needed.
2. Revise its procedures for coordinating with area hospitals during mass casualty disasters to provide the hospitals with timely information regarding estimated numbers of victims, injury categories, destinations, and arrival times.
3. Conduct full-scale demonstrations of the airport emergency plan and procedures every 2 years. (The airport involved was in the process of planning a disaster drill when the accident occurred (3).)

The NTSB also recommended that the FAA amend the appropriate CFR to require a full-scale demonstration of certified airport emergency plans and procedure at least once every 2 years (3,20).

Flying as either a passenger or crewmember is associated with a finite degree of risk. This risk has continued to decrease as accident pre-

vention, protection, and survival are improved. If government, manufacturers, airport personnel, crews, and passengers fulfill their responsibility to use the knowledge, equipment, training and information available, the opportunity to survive is excellent should an accident occur.

REFERENCES

1. National Transportation Safety Board: Annual review of aircraft accident data. Washington, DC: Government Printing Office, 1980.
2. FAA urged to increase oversight of airline flight safety programs. Aviation Week and Space Technology 1990; April 16:73–77.
3. Probe finds fault with captain's approach to cockpit discipline. Aviation Week and Space Technology 1990; April 2:62–65.
4. National Transportation Safety Board, Aircraft Accident Report: Trans-Colorado Airlines, Flight 2286, Fairchild Metro III, SA227 AC, N69TC, January 19, 1988. Washington, DC: Government Printing Office, 1989.
5. National Transportation Safety Board, Aircraft Accident Report: Aloha Airlines, Flight 243 Boeing 737–200 N73711, April 28, 1988. Washington, DC: Government Printing Office, 1988.
6. Griswold AD. The safer skies of 1990. Air Force Magazine 1991;74(4):98.
7. U.S. Army Aviation Safety Center. Annual report. Fort Rucker, AL, July, 1991.
8. Department of the Navy, Naval Safety Center. Annual report. Naval Air Station, Norfolk, VA May, 1991.
9. National Transportation Safety Board, Public Affairs, Washington, DC, 1991.
10. National Transportation Safety Board. Safety study: ultralight vehicle accidents. Washington, DC: Government Printing Office, 1981.
11. National Transportation Safety Board. Safety study: commercial emergency medical service helicopter operations. Washington, DC: Government Printing Office, 1988.
12. Snyder RG. The status of infant/child restraint protection in aircraft crash impact. DOT/FAA/AV-89–2 August, 1989. Washington, DC: Government Printing Office, 1989.
13. National Transportation Safety Board. Safety study: airline passenger safety education: a review of methods used to present safety information. Washington, DC: Government Printing Office, 1985.
14. National Transportation Safety Board. Safety report: The status of general aviation aircraft crashworthiness. Washington, DC: Government Printing Office, 1980.
15. National Transportation Safety Board. Safety report: The status of general aviation crashworthiness project: phase two. Washington, DC: Government Printing Office, 1985.

16. National Transportation Safety Board. Safety report: The status of general aviation crashworthiness project: phase III. Washington, DC: Government Printing Office, 1985.

17. Department of the Air Force, Air Force Rescue Coordination Center. Annual report. Scott Air Force Base, Illinois, February, 1991.

18. Snyder RG, Gibbons HL. Aircraft crashworthiness. Charlottesville, VA: University Press of Virginia, 1975: 121–139.

19. Stanley AJ. Water searching with dogs. Journal of Search, Rescue, and Emergency Response 1990;4: 89–94.

20. Barbash GI, et al. Airport preparedness for mass disaster: a proposed plan. Aviat Space Environ Med 1986; 57:77–81.

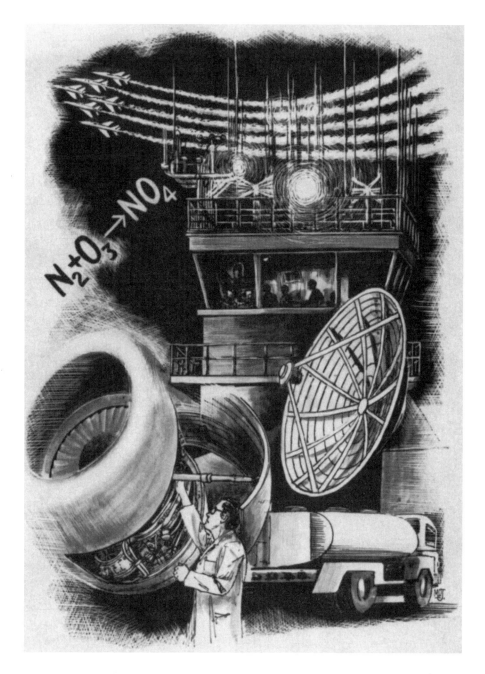

SECTION V

Impact of the Aerospace
Industry on Community
Health

With the establishment of the quarantine by the city-state of Venice, Italy, governments began to formalize procedures to protect the public health from the external influences of commerce. The airplane provides an excellent potential vector for the spread of disease worldwide. Disease has been introduced through aircraft operations by passengers who have not had time to develop clinical symptoms from the time of infection, by insects able to survive the short trip in the relative comfort of the aircraft cabins and by fomites contaminating cargo carried aboard aircraft. Procedures exist to reduce the effectiveness of the aircraft as a disease vector.

Aircraft operations introduce other concerns to the public health. Flight operations generate noise, which is hazardous to those nearby and perhaps injurious to the community health. Air pollution is a concern that has been somewhat alleviated by new jet-engine technology. High altitude flight has been implicated in ozone depletion in the stratosphere. Ground support to flight operations requires an extensive industrial base and thus introduces the practice of occupational medicine and industrial health.

Recommended Readings

Brooks SM, Gochfeld M, Hevzstein J. Environmental medicine. St. Louis: Mosby-Year Book, 1995.

McCunney RJ. A practical approach to occupational and environmental medicine. 2nd ed. Boston, MA: Little, Brown and Co., 1991.

Moser MR, et al. An outbreak of influenza aboard a commercial airliner. Am J Epidemiol, 1979:110(1);1–6.

Moser R Jr. Effective management of occupational and environmental health and safety programs. Boston: OEM Press, 1992.

Naugle DF, Fox DL. Aircraft and air pollution. Environ Sci Technol,1981:15;342.

Potter AE. Environmental effects of the space shuttle. Environ Sci Technol, 1978:8;173.

Randle CJM, et al. Cholera possible infection from aircraft effluent. J Hyg (London), 1978:81(3);361–371.

Rom WWN, ed. Environmental and occupational medicine. 2nd ed. Boston: Little, Brown, and Co., 1992.

Tracor, Inc. Community reaction to airport noise. NASA CR-1761. Washington, DC: National Aeronautics and Space Administration, 1977.

Wald PH, Stave GM, eds. Physical and biological hazards of the workplace. New York: Van Nostrand Reinhold, 1994.

Chapter 33

Role of Aviation in the Transmission of Disease

Mark A. Roberts

When you hear hoof beats think of horses not zebras.

Anonymous

The advice in the quotation above is often used to encourage interns and residents to consider the probabilities of an etiologic agent and diagnosis. Air travel has contributed and probably will continue to contribute the exception to this advice. Air transportation has made it possible for a person to be at the headwaters of the Amazon River today and on Wall Street tomorrow.

HISTORICAL PERSPECTIVE

The concept that disease can be spread by people or their goods in transportation vessels is ancient. Throughout recorded history, movement of populations has been intimately associated with disease. The aggregation of large numbers of disease-susceptible individuals in military units fostered the spread of disease among the armies, but these same troops, in turn, were often responsible for transmitting diseases to civilian populations after the outcome of the conflicts had been determined. An axiom in warfare has been that battle casualties are far fewer than casualties caused by pathogens. "Modern" warfare has reduced the percentage of casualties due to infectious diseases, but morbidity from other causes, such as weather and vehicular injuries, must still be contended with. Likewise, as individuals moved from one area of the world to another, the endemic diseases of one locale were introduced to the susceptible inhabitants of other areas.

One of the earliest documented events of transmission of diseases by an aerial route occurred in Kaffa, in the Crimea, in the 14th century, when invading Tartars catapulted bubonic plague victims over the city walls. It is unlikely that plague was actually transmitted by this route, however (1).

In 630 AD, the concept of a sanitary zone was established by the diocese of Cahors, by Gallus. Armed guards were placed at all points of entry to prohibit movement. The knight Hospitallers of the order of St. John of Jerusalem were the first to adopt the 40-day quarantine because it was the amount of time Christ was in the wilderness. In Venice, Italy, in 1348 AD, vessels, crews, and passengers were detained for 40 days primarily to guard against plague. The idea caught on throughout Europe in the 16th and 17th centuries, and the word "quarantine" entered our vocabulary from the Italian word "quarta," which means 40.

The development of methods of moving larger groups of people in a more economical method modified the patterns of disease transmission. Diseases began to be transmitted by a few individuals to susceptible populations. This was a definite reversal of earlier patterns on diseases after the migration of "hordes," be it pilgrims, armies, or emigrants.

Major outbreaks of cholera followed the rapid increase in travel brought about by the new technologies of steamships and railroads. The forerunner to our major international health organizations was brought about by the need of governments to cooperate to control cholera. Quarantine was attempted but was largely unsuccessful. This failure led to the First International Sanitary Conference in Paris in 1851, which was attended by one physician and one diplomat from each of the two Sicilies, Spain, the Papal States, France, Great Britain, Greece, Portugal, Russia, Sardinia, Tuscany, and Turkey. It agreed on rules of international hygiene and sanitation in international commerce and travel. Over the next 56 years, nine more conferences were held, culminating in the formation of the International Office of Public Health at Paris in 1907. This office was the forerunner to the League of Nations Health Office, which later developed into the World Health Organization (WHO). The first application of international conventions to aircraft was the Pan American Sanitary Code, ratified in 1924 in Havana, Cuba, by 21 countries in the Americas. In 1926, 65 countries were represented at the Thirteenth International Sanitary Conference. The treaty signed that year is the basis for our modern international health laws.

Because of the growing importance of aviation, the first sanitary convention for aerial navigation was held in 1933. It used the existing international maritime laws as a model but modified them to suit the 1933 flying environment. The convention addressed such problems as disinfection, medical inspection, and infectious disease control. It formulated a detailed code to prevent the spread of yellow fever, including methods to eliminate the vector, *Aedes aegypti*. This convention was the forerunner of the WHO Committee on Hygiene and Sanitation in aviation, which now is responsible for the formulation of guidelines protecting the international community from the importation of disease by

military or civilian aircraft. Social and technologic developments have increased the number of people moving from place to place and reduced travel times from weeks to hours, but the population dynamics of disease transmission have remained substantially unchanged.

For the most part, infectious diseases are opportunistic occurrences. Their occurences are new in the sense that they have not been recognized by our medical process. In fact, they may not be so new. Movement of groups of individuals "expose" them to new environments, cultures, food sources, and medical systems. They bring their normal intestinal flora as well. This intermixing results in new selection forces, new subsets of the microbiologic gene pool and new antibiotic pressures that can give rise to "new" outbreaks of disease, all because of transport of people.

IMPACT OF AIR TRAVEL

Prior to the age of air travel, incubation periods for many diseases were shorter than transit times; thus, epidemic diseases usually were evident during transport or upon arrival at the port of entry, where quarantine measures could be imposed. Unfortunately, with modern high-speed, large-volume air travel, illnesses often develop after rather than during travel, decreasing the probability of a diagnosis being made and of recognizing the epidemic potential. Also, the shorter travel times have reduced the significance of geographic separation as an effective barrier to disease transmission.

These factors, combined with the large number of international travelers, make the control of communicable disease a difficult and complex task. Available information for 1995 indicates that world tourist arrivals reached approximately 567 million, 3.8% over 1994. In 1995, the Middle East was the fastest growing region followed by South Asia, East Asia, and the Pacific.

Air travel has been implicated in the transmission of diseases of nearly every etiology. The potential for the transmission of vector-borne diseases is significant because receptive vectors and susceptible populations for many of these diseases are found throughout the temperate zones. Diseases such as malaria, dengue, and yellow fever have been eliminated in many areas, but the reintroduction of these diseases by infected patients or vectors could easily occur. Dengue fever surveillance by the Centers for Disease Control and Prevention (CDC) for the period 1986–1992 serologically confirmed 157 cases of suspected dengue fever (157/788 or 20%) in the United States; a majority of these cases were in travellers to Latin America, the Caribbean, Africa, Asia, or the Pacific Islands. During this time period one indigenous case was identified in Texas (2). The importation of these cases underscores the need for dengue fever's inclusion in the differential diagnosis of individuals presenting with sudden onset of fever, headache, myalgia, rash, nausea, and vomiting with a history of travel to tropical climates which support the mosquito vectors (Americas and Africa) and Asia. Such cases provide the virus necessary to complete the disease cycle since the mosquito vector is present in the southern United States, as indicated by the case in Texas in 1980 (3).

The reintroduction of diseases that had been endemic in an area could be devastating. Each year that the population is shielded from an infectious disease increases the size of the susceptible segment of that population. Vigilance in surveillance and control and effective methods of control need to be available.

Diseases transmitted from person to person are as great a threat now as ever, despite state-of-the-art prevention and treatment efforts. Epidemics of cholera and other highly infectious diseases can be spread far beyond their traditional endemic areas with ease. The movement of refugee populations from southeast Asia, Central America, the Caribbean, and southwestern Asia poses a major disease threat to populations in resettlement areas. The arrival of thousands of Cuban refugees in the United States in the summer of 1980 held the potential for

significant disease problems. The refugees were monitored very closely after arrival to identify any significant health problems that might be transmissible. Fortunately, these refugees were in reasonably good health, unlike many of the southeast Asian refugees. If the influx of refugees from Cuba had taken place during 1981, extensive transmissions of dengue fever might have occurred in the southeastern United States because a large outbreak of this disease swept Cuba that year.

The possibility of foodstuff contamination is often centered on bacterial toxins, but other chemicals should be considered. The offending agent may be unfamiliar and possibly unlicensed in the community where the symptoms are observed. Even efforts to control insects can result in the exposure of aircraft passengers and cargo. Likewise, insect-infested cargo easily could introduce economically significant pests to new areas, thereby severely reducing agricultural productivity and contributing to malnutrition and subsequent disease. Examples of this transport include the Japanese beetle, Dutch elm disease, and chestnut tree fungus.

Hidden travelers are potential sources of imported illness whether it be human stowaways or insects on clothing or in baggage. A random search of 67 airplanes in London in 1987 identified mosquitoes in 12 of the aircraft. In this same report the authors documented the survival of mosquitoes, house flies, and beetles after flights of 6 to 9 hours and temperatures to −42°.

The role of aircraft in disease transmission can be reduced by focusing on three primary factors: people, cargo, and vectors. These elements are addressed in the International Health Regulations adopted by the WHO and are frequently updated to reflect the changing character of endemic and epidemic diseases.

DISEASES SPREAD FROM PERSON TO PERSON

In the discussion of disease of international importance, one often thinks of cholera, yellow fever, malaria, Ebola virus, Lassa fever, or mad cow disease, but by sheer numbers the opportunistic infections of *Shigella*, *Salmonella*, and other enteric bacteria are responsible for more morbidity and mortality (4). Recent new and re-emerging infectious diseases such as waterborne Cryptosporidium, hemorrhagic colitis and renal failure from foodborne *E. coli* 0157:H7, rodent-associated Hantavirus, tuberculosis, pertussis, diphtheria, and plague underscore the fact that the major causes of morbidity and mortality are not always exotic disease.

Cholera

Historically, the spread of cholera has followed passenger traffic routes, and major advances in transportation technology have contributed to pandemics. Prior to 1860, transportation over the old land caravan routes was slow enough to allow most epidemics to die out during the trip. The pandemic of the 1860s, however, was due in large part to the advent of the steamship, which allowed an increased number of pilgrims to travel to and from Mecca far more quickly. Similarly, the spread of cholera within the United States in 1866 and later was rapid and geographically followed the newly built railways.

Pandemic cholera continued in the late 1890s with a pattern of spread along the old land routes leading out of India. An outbreak associated with a pilgrimage to Mecca in 1902 devastated Egypt, with 34,000 deaths in 3 months. The pandemic then spread into most of Europe, following sea lanes. From 1904 to 1923, Europe experienced recurrent waves of cholera. Due to rapid diagnosis, isolation of cases at ports of entry, and improved sanitation, this pandemic failed to spread to Great Britain or the United States.

The next cholera pandemic was the El Tor biotype, which began in Indonesia in 1961. El Tor had been endemic in the Celebes Islands of Indonesia since 1937, but from 1961 to 1962, this strain spread into neighboring island groups along traditional sea routes. It became clear that El Tor cholera was being transported by air as

well as by sea routes when clusters of cases developed around both airports and seaports throughout much of the western Pacific Ocean. By early 1963, the transportation of cholera by air had clearly occurred in Thailand, Vietnam, Cambodia, Japan, and Korea. Air travel also was suspected as a contributing factor in outbreaks of cholera in India, Pakistan, and the Philippines. By 1965, the WHO was concerned enough about the air importation of cholera to publish the numbers of cases occurring in Asian cities serviced by international airlines. In May 1970, El Tor cholera was reported in Guinea, West Africa. Although the index case was never identified, it was believed that the disease had been translocated by aircraft. This was quite likely given that El Tor cholera is more likely to produce asymptomatic cases than symptomatic case (100/1) (5). Guinea was subsequently the focal point for the spread of cholera throughout most of sub-Saharan Africa. Within several months of the Guinea outbreak, the disease spread to Ivory Coast, either by air or sea route, and inland throughout West Africa. By 1971, 22 countries were infected, with 69,000 cases of cholera reported.

Cholera has continued to be a worldwide threat and an opportunist observed in epidemic proportions in areas involved in social unrest. The WHO reported 44,083 cases in 1988 from 30 countries and 48,403 from 35 countries in 1989. Sub-Saharan Africa reported nearly three quarters of the world's cholera cases in 1989 (6).

Not only has the airplane been implicated in the transport of passengers who have become the index cases for major outbreaks, but aircraft effluent also has been implicated as the possible source of sporadic outbreaks of cholera throughout central and western Europe between 1970 and 1975. When outbreaks were mapped, the areas corresponded to the major air routes from Calcutta to Europe (7). Although it has never been proven conclusively that this was the cause of the European outbreaks, this hypothesis has received widespread support and is assumed by some authorities to be the cause of the outbreaks.

In 1992, the largest cholera outbreak of the 20th century in the United States was reported among passengers on a flight from Buenos Aires, Argentina, that stopped in Lima, Peru, and arrived at Los Angeles, California. In all, 75 of the 336 passengers developed diarrhea and had had laboratory evidence of *V. cholera* 01; another 25 cases are suspected to have occurred. The source of their infection was thought to be cold seafood salad prepared by a caterer in Peru (8).

Generally, outbreaks of cholera caused by air transportation have occurred involving movement of people from areas with poor sanitary conditions. We often forget that most of the world has inadequate sanitation and areas of social disruption and destruction often provide the source of new outbreaks. There are indigenous sources of cholera in the United States as evidenced by the presence of *V. cholera* 01 on the Gulf Coast of Louisiana and Texas. More cholera has been attributed to Latin America than to the Gulf Coast but the threat of indigenous cholera cannot be overlooked (9).

Influenza

Epidemiologic mapping of recent influenza epidemics points toward the aircraft as being a major factor in the rapid global spread of new viral strains. Although the aircraft is known to be an efficient ''vector'' of influenza, on rare occasions it has been demonstrated to be the focal environment of a disease outbreak. In 1977, 38 of 53 (72%) interviewed passengers and crewmembers of an Alaskan flight subsequently became ill with influenza A/Texas (H3N2) (10). The index case was identified as a young woman who developed acute respiratory symptoms 15 minutes after boarding the aircraft. The flight aborted because of mechanical difficulty, and most passengers remained on board for more than 3 hours. A nonfunctioning ventilation system, close proximity of the passengers, and low ambient humidity were felt to be contributing factors to the high attack rate. Within

1 week after the incident, a 20% secondary attack rate was discovered along the household contacts of the passengers.

The intensity of transmission of influenza in this outbreak would not have been recognized had it not been for the fact that most of the passengers were seen by one physician who recognized their commonalities and reported the event to health officials.

The influenza A/USSR (H1N1) pandemic of 1978 underscored the transmission speed of influenza in contemporary times. In December 1977, the Soviet Minister of Health notified the WHO that widespread influenza outbreaks had occurred in the Soviet Union. By mid-December 1977, additional reports of influenza A/USSR activity came from Hong Kong, Taiwan, and Finland. A later report from the People's Republic of China to the WHO suggested that the strain had originated from northern China and had been circulating since May 1977. In early January 1978, influenza A/USSR was confirmed in U.S. Air Force personnel stationed at Royal Air Force Base, Upper Heyford, Great Britain. An air force epidemiologic investigation of the Upper Heyford outbreak revealed that all patients were younger than age 25 (consistent with the fact that H1N1 had last circulated from 1947 to 1957) and that the clinical morbidity was sufficient to compromise flying operations. Peculiarly, the outbreak appeared to be initially isolated to the base at Upper Heyford and surrounding communities. Strongly suspected, and later confirmed, was the transmission of the virus from the Soviet Union to Upper Heyford by means of popular tourist flights by air force personnel from Gatwick International Airport to Moscow and Leningrad.

Within 2 weeks of the Upper Heyford outbreak, influenza A/USSR was detected in the United States. A sharp outbreak in a Cheyenne, Wyoming, high school reaffirmed the age distribution and morbidity of the H1N1 strain. Almost simultaneous to the Cheyenne episode was an outbreak at F.E. Warren Air Force Base, Wyoming, adjacent to Cheyenne. It is interesting to note that Royal Air Force Base, Upper Heyford, Great Britain, and F.E. Warren Air Force Base, Wyoming, both contain personnel with common skills and backgrounds and share staff elements that possibly could have been responsible for seeding the HlNl strain so rapidly into a relatively remote section of the United States. By early February 1978, influenza A/USSR had spread to other schools and universities in Wyoming and Colorado. At the U.S. Air Force Academy in Colorado Springs, Colorado, influenza A/USSR caused a particularly severe epidemic that afflicted 76% of the 4300 cadets within 12 days. By March 1978, 16 other U.S. Air Force bases had reported substantial influenza activity, and by the end of the influenza season, influenza A/USSR activity had been confirmed in 19 areas of the United States and in at least 13 countries in Asia and eastern Europe.

Thus, in less than 12 months, a new antigenic variant of influenza had been distributed throughout the population bulk of the world. Had an HlNl or an influenza A/USSR-like strain not previously circulated in the 1950s and conferred demonstrable immunity to the now middle-aged and elderly population, the mortality consequences could have been devastating.

The repetitive propagation of influenza A virus in a population rests with its ability to periodically alter its hemagglutinin (H) and neuraminidase (N) genes. These genetic changes, or antigenic "drifts," are largely the result of forced selective pressures exerted by an immune population. Only when the viral antigenicity has changed sufficiently to avert the cancellation effect of conferred immunity will a "new" strain emerge and become clinically and epidemiologically significant. Perhaps a related mechanism for the production of influenza variants is the process of dual infection with a resulting hybrid or recombinant strain. The 1978 influenza season was remarkable in this regard because three distinct influenza strains (A/Victoria,H3N2; A/Texas,H3N2, and A/USSR,HlNl, were circulating simultaneously, causing substantial morbidity in the same regions of the United States, and

documented dual infections occurred with probable hybridization (H3Nl) (11). If this process is important in the mutation and survival of influenza, it is clear that the frequency of genetic change may be dependent on the number of active cocirculating strains. Thus, the role of strain translocation by aircraft, coupled with the dynamic changes in world politics that has resulted in the mass movement of populations, has the potential to greatly alter the epidemiology of influenza.

Tuberculosis

From January 1993 through February 1995, the CDC completed investigations of six incidents in which passengers or flight crew traveled on commercial aircraft while infectious with tuberculosis (TB). These investigations involved symptomatic TB patients with acid-fast bacillus (AFB) smear-positive, cavitary, pulmonary TB, who were highly infectious at the time of the flight. In none of the six incidents were the airlines aware of the TB-infected passengers. The investigations were undertaken to determine whether exposure to persons with infectious pulmonary TB was associated with transmission of the organism to others traveling on the same aircraft. Two of the investigations indicated that transmission, in fact, occurred from flight attendant to other flight crew and from passenger to passenger. All persons with tuberculin skin test conversions were seated in the same section of the aircraft as the indexed passenger, suggesting that transmission was associated with seating proximity.

To prevent exposure to TB aboard aircraft, when travel is necessary, persons known to have infectious TB should travel by private conveyance and not a commercial carrier. Further, patients with infectious TB should be sputum smear-negative before being placed in indoor environments that could lead to disease transmission. Each decision regarding a patient's TB infectiousness and the ability to travel in public transportation should be made on an individual basis (12).

Human Immunodeficiency Virus

Infection with human immunodeficiency virus (HIV) can realistically be considered a global problem affecting subsets of the population of modern as well as developing nations. Each year the estimates of the number of cases grow. Part of this increase has been the result of definitional changes. Undoubtedly, air transportation is influential in the spread of TB. Popular press articles and books allude to the sexual practices and lifestyles that increase individual risk of developing the disease. Air travel contributes through the mobility that it provides. The very early spread of acquired immunodeficiency syndrome (AIDS) in the United States is attributed by some authors of lay and scientific publications to the sexual exploits of a flight attendant (13). There is no evidence of or scientific plausibility that AIDS can be transmitted through the usual associations of passengers and crew during air travel.

FOODBORNE DISEASE

Foodborne outbreaks are caused by opportunistic organisms that can quite easily find their way into the food we eat. Anytime groups of people are fed at the same time, e.g., banquets, picnics, or transoceanic flights, the possibility for food-related illness is possible. Unfortunately, airline passengers do not share the commonalities of the banquet and picnic attendees; that is, they are less likely to know each other. This lack of readily recognized commonality decreases the likelihood of outbreak recognition.

An epidemic of foodborne illness on board an in-transit aircraft presents logistic and diagnostic challenges not encountered elsewhere. An etiologic diagnosis is often required to rule out the presence of an exotic or quarantinable disease; however, adequate personnel, supplies, and facilities are rarely available to diagnose and treat large numbers of patients. Epidemiologic investigations are complicated by inadequate passenger manifests and the rapid dispersion of passengers after landing. In actuality, once a major quarantinable disease such as cholera is excluded, extensive follow-up investigations are uncommon.

Although most food preparation practices of airline caterers provide bacteriologically safe foods, improper refrigeration or keeping foods warm has contributed to outbreaks of foodborne disease (14). *Clostridium perfringens* was implicated in an outbreak affecting eight separate flights leaving from a southeastern U.S. air terminal. Although 394 persons were at risk, only 18 passengers and 62 crewmembers could be contacted for follow-up investigation, highlighting the difficulty of identifying the true incidence of food-related disease associated with air transportation. Twenty-two of the 62 crewmembers contacted reported illness characterized by diarrhea, nausea, and abdominal cramps. Turkey dinners prepared earlier from whole turkeys that were precooked, frozen, thawed at room temperature, sliced, and then kept at 54°C on board were shown epidemiologically to be the source of the illness.

Food was implicated as the vehicle of a *Vibrio cholerae* outbreak among aircraft passengers in 1972. The apparent lack of enforcement of accepted international standards for the control and surveillance of foodborne diseases aboard aircraft contributed to the outbreak. In 1973, an outbreak of food-borne staphylococcal intoxication on three separate civilian flights was traced to meals prepared by a single caterer. Illness developed in 28 to 84% of the passengers on these flights. First-class passengers and crewmembers had received different meals without the suspected food (custard dessert), and none of them became ill. In 1975, 197 of 344 passengers (57%) aboard a chartered commercial flight and one of 20 crewmembers (5%) experienced symptoms consistent with staphylococcal food poisoning. This outbreak, the largest reported aboard a single aircraft, was traced to ham contaminated by *Staphylococcus aureus* from a cook's inflamed finger lesion. Documented mishandling of the food product over a prolonged period permitted growth of the organism and production of enterotoxin (15). A flight from Rio de Janeiro, Brazil, to New York in 1976 was diverted to San Juan, Puerto Rico, because 16 passengers experienced gastrointestinal illness shown to be caused by chocolate eclairs contaminated with high levels of *S. aureus*.

Aircraft-related foodborne disease can be classified by the type (and length) of flight it will most likely be associated with: in-flight domestic (1 to 4 hours), in-flight international (6 to 20 hours), and postflight outbreaks. Two factors usually determine the classification of an etiologic agent: the elapsed time between food preparation and consumption and the incubation period between ingestion and the onset of clinical illness. Chemical and preformed toxin-related illness, such as staphylotoxicosis, usually occur shortly after consumption of the contaminated meal and thus could be observed on short flights. *S. aureus*, usually linked to ham, meat salads, and custards, has a clinical incubation period of 2 to 4 hours, with a range of 30 minutes to 8 hours. These short incubation outbreaks must be differentiated from motion-induced and psychosomatic-related nausea and vomiting. The communicability of vomiting, particularly in enclosed quarters, is well recognized. Longer flights may be associated with both short and intermediate incubation agents, best exemplified by *C. perfringens* and *Bacillus cereus*. These intoxication illnesses have incubation ranges of 9 to 16 hours and 2 to 16 hours, respectively. *B. cereus* is a contaminant of vegetables and grains and is usually associated with boiled or fried rice. *C. perfringens* intoxication is associated with meat, poultry, or gravy and presents clinically as a complex of abdominal cramps and diarrhea. For extended flights, it is likely that foodborne infections with *V. parahaemolyticus*, *Shigella* species, and *Salmonella* species manifest themselves during a flight or after arrival.

The involvement of crewmembers in an outbreak affecting passengers is confounded by several factors. Civilian pilots of domestic flights are paid per diem and usually eat before the flight or bring a bag lunch; however, meals are available to them on board. Crewmembers on longer international flights are more likely to eat the same meals as passengers, but because of limits on flight time, crews may be changed at intermediate stops and are not as likely to share the extended flight times and multiple meals of the Manila-to-Brussels passenger. U.S. military aircrews and passengers commonly share meals from the same source—inflight kitchens—but the adherence to safe food preparation and storage sanitary standards is considered to be better in this restricted and controlled environment. The prevention of enteric disease transmission among passengers and crew is best achieved by the strict application of hygiene standards and procedures. Basic principles of food preparation and serving must be followed to ensure that contamination of food does not occur. Similarly, the integrity of the potable water sources and onboard storage and distribution system must be maintained. Proper handling and disposal of human wastes from aircraft also must be ensured, including adequate facilities and supplies for the maintenance of personal hygiene. Although outbreaks on aircraft can dramatically affect large numbers of passengers and could conceivably incapacitate the crew, there are no statutory or policy requirements for the pilot and copilot to consume different meals or the same meals at different times.

The contamination of bulk quantities of food products during air transportation is a real probability as well. The movement of manufactured food products by aircraft can provide the mode for the widespread dispersal of contaminated food. In 1973, raw cocoa beans, most likely imported from Ghana, arrived in Canada contaminated with *Salmonella* eastbourne. While the beans were being sorted and cleaned at a Canadian chocolate factory, bean dust cross-contaminated the final product. Christmas chocolate balls from this factory were identified as the source of a major international foodborne outbreak, with cases identified in 23 states in the United States and seven Canadian provinces over a 4-month period. In addition to inadvertent food contamination, misuse of agricultural products, such as chemically treated seed grains not intended for human consumption, has been documented (16). It is conceivable that aircraft support of disaster relief operations could contribute to the widespread distribution of inedible products that, owing to misunderstanding, are consumed as food.

The cultural aspects of foodborne illnesses are equally important. Air travel has brought millions of individuals into new cultures with inherently new and different food items. Their customary methods of food preparation may not be appropriate for the new foods they encounter. In addition, travel may expose the individual to unfamiliar plants that, while appearing similar to more customary plants, may produce significant morbidity and occasionally mortality.

CABIN AIR QUALITY

A growing volume of information is being accumulated about the health complaints attributed to poor indoor air quality in office buildings and residences. The label of "sick building syndrome" is being applied to growing segments of the population without a clear etiology. Air quality in airplanes is susceptible to all the problems associated with a sick building. Most airplanes are better equipped to provide fresh air than most buildings. Modern aircraft are able to provide 5 to 29 air exchanges per hour as compared to the usual office building's rate of 5 to 12 per hour and a typical home's rate of 5 times per hour. This does not take into consideration "dead spaces" within the cabin where decreased air exchange may be more common in fore and aft sections. The source of the air in modern turboprop and jet engines is compressor bleed air and the air is extremely hot as it comes off the engine, typically at temperatures of 250° C or more. This air flow is dependent on the engine's RPMs and thus is routinely decreased

during ground operations. Specific alternative air handling procedures using auxiliary power units or preconditioned air from ground support operations are often overtaxed by environmental conditions and lack of conditioned air.

Air quality in flight is dependent on air recirculation and on the filtration system. Depending on flight conditions and the aircraft, air exchanges can range from 0 to 66%. Air filtration systems include high efficiency filters that should filter out respirable bacteria and fungus. Viral particles are less likely to be filtered out but air exchanges increase the dilutional effect and thus limit the likelihood of transmission when the air system is operating effectively. Suboptimal operation of these systems can lead to indoor conditions conducive to the person-to-person transmission of respiratory infections.

VECTOR-BORNE DISEASE

The control of insect-infested cargo and aircraft also is accomplished through international regulation and cooperation. There are numerous documented instances in which insect pests or vectors of disease have been introduced by humans into new areas. Airport malaria is an excellent example of this occurrence. Airport malaria is the occurrence of a case of human malaria in a person whose history precludes exposure to a possible vector in its natural habitat. Isaacson (17) provided summary data on 29 cases of airport malaria that occurred in Europe from 1969 to 1988. These cases indicate the possibility of vector transportation but also illustrate the difficulty in correctly diagnosing malaria in individuals without a history of travel to a malarious area.

Although malaria is normally considered an insect-borne illness, there have been person-to-person transmissions in the United States and Western Europe. In 1978, a malaria death was reported to the CDC in Atlanta, Georgia. The individual had received a blood transfusion from a donor who had recently traveled abroad. In the 1960s, a minor outbreak of malaria was reported in Fresno, California, among drug abusers. The index case involved a soldier who had recently returned from Southeast Asia. In an earlier instance in northern California in 1952, a Korean War veteran suffered a relapse of vivax malaria while on a weekend camping trip at a popular outdoor recreation area. He was subsequently responsible for at least 35 cases of malaria among a group of Campfire Girls who camped in the same area some weeks later (18). This episode serves as a reminder to all medical care providers that a high index of suspicion must be maintained when dealing with individuals who have recently traveled or have been in contact with other travelers.

A sevenfold increase in the varieties of mosquito species was noted on Guam from 1936 to 1972. Air traffic and seagoing vessels were implicated as the reason for this increase. The history of explosive, nonrepetitive outbreaks of dengue, Japanese B encephalitis, and malaria on Guam may be due to a population of infected individuals or arthropod vectors arriving on the island (19). Air travel can facilitate the rapid and widespread distribution of vectors and pests. During the 1970s, termite-infested cargo from the Philippines and Thailand frequently was intercepted at McClellan and Travis Air Force bases in California. The continuing threat to U.S. agricultural crops posed by the introduction of land snails from Europe and the Far East underscores the necessity to inspect all returning motor vehicles, other cargo, and household goods shipments. Infestations of the devastating stored grain pest, the khapra beetle, were discovered in at least 19 U.S. warehouses and burlap bag establishments in 1981. The beetles were traced to commodities imported from the Middle East.

Human plague is endemic and occasionally epidemic in South America, Africa, and Asia, providing the necessary foci for continued transmission to other parts of the world. In 1989, 770 human cases of plague were reported from 11 countries, including 374 cases from Vietnam and 180 from Madagascar. La Paz, Bolivia, is reported as an endemic area by the CDC and proved to be the source of imported cases of human plague in June 1990. Imported cases are not necessary for the transmission of plague in the United States. An average of 18 cases of plague were reported annually in persons exposed in enzootic areas of the southwestern United States (20).

The detection and elimination of exotic pests on or in cargo is paramount in preventing the transfer of pests and disease vectors between geographically separated land masses. A program that includes the maintenance of clean cargo holding areas, preclearance, inspection, and treatment of cargo prior to shipment is necessary. The surveillance and control of mosquitoes and other vectors around cargo-marshalling areas and flight lines and the proper isolation, treatment, and disposal of galley and other wastes are also important aspects of this program.

The application of insecticide aerosols or micronized dusts inside aircraft to kill mosquitoes and other insects of public health or economic significance is also a vital aspect of quarantine operations. WHO guidelines specify procedures for the disinsection of passenger and cargo compartments in affected areas, in flight, and upon arrival in unaffected areas. Individual countries and agencies selectively apply these recommendations, however. The U.S. Public Health Service requires disinsection only for international flights arriving from areas where there is active vector-borne transmission in the vicinity of the port of embarkation. The point of disinsection is dictated by the country of arrival and often poses problems for airline companies, airport operators, passengers, and government health officials. Four techniques of disinsection have been described and evaluated. Current WHO recommendations for aircraft disinsection include descriptions of methods 1, 2, and 3, as follows (21).

1. Blocks-away disinsection: Aerosol sprays are applied after the cabin is closed and the air-

craft is moved away from the terminal but has not taken off.

2. On-arrival disinsection: Aerosol sprays are applied to the craft upon arrival but before passengers and cargo are removed.
3. Residual disinsection: Longer lasting insecticides are used on the aircraft.
4. Top-of-descent disinsection: Insecticide is applied during the approach for landing.

Methods of insecticide application must take into consideration passenger and crew health. Acute reaction to the insecticide is an emergency that must be considered as must the long-term health effects of repeated crew exposures.

A complete insect inspection and quarantine program should include trained inspectors with knowledge of agricultural and public health pests of international significance; the conscientious inspection of all freight, baggage, cabins, and holds; appropriate insecticidal or other treatment of infested materials and areas; and proper coordination with national and international regulatory authorities.

The movement of exotic and domestic animals among nations, both developed and developing, is extensive. The introduction of foreign zoonotic diseases compounds the diagnostic and logistic challenges facing public health officials. Since November 1989, seven shipments of cynomolgus monkeys imported from three suppliers in the Philippines have been actively infected with filovirus, which is antigenically similar to the African members of the Filoviridae group to which the *Ebola* viruses belong. Transmission among monkeys in quarantine facilities has occurred. Five animal handlers have seroconverted, as detected by immunofluorescence and Western blot tests, using a strain of Filovirus isolated from the infected monkeys. No discernible illness was identified, and no febrile illnesses were reported among the handlers. The infectivity and pathogenicity of laboratory-acquired infection remain unclear.

In April 1996 an outbreak of *Ebola* virus was detected in an animal colony in Alice, Texas in a shipment of monkeys from the Philippines. This occurrence received a large amount of attention from the news media for two reasons. The first is the fact that the Reston, Virginia outbreak among monkeys (of *Outbreak* fame) was linked to the Philippines. Secondly, the public was reassured that this monkey strain was different from the one identified in the outbreak in Zaire. Lost was the fact that at least two strains of the deadly virus were documented in different areas of the world.

Based on the experience in one laboratory, this documentation of laboratory transmission underscores the need for vigilance in adherence to quarantine measures for the importation of animal species (22).

Quarantine restrictions of varying lengths are imposed on animals moving from enzootic rabies areas to rabies-free areas, particularly the island nations and states, such as Great Britain, Australia, Japan, and Hawaii. Another emerging problem is the transportation of diseased livestock from developed nations to both developed and developing nations. In 1980 and 1981, shipment of U.S. cattle and sheep to the European Common Market was halted because the U.S. cattle were infected with blue tongue, an arthropod-borne virus enzootic to North America. The continued expansion of trade between nations and the use of air transport will extend the spectrum of disease entities of concern to agricultural, health, and trade officials.

INFORMATION SOURCES

Various nations have established immunization requirements against specific diseases. Although many of these restrictions are generated by medical and public health concerns, political and cultural motives often come into play. The CDC Traveler's Health Information publishes a "Summary of Health Information for International Travel" (also known as the "Blue Sheet") which provides updates regarding disease of travel importance. The "Blue Sheet" can be obtained by calling the fax number

(404)332–4565 and requesting #220022. A quicker method is available through the Internet via the CDC Travel Information home page. Other sources include medical centers, state health departments, and larger local health departments.

There is a growing volume of information regarding international travel available on the Internet but there are at least two important considerations when accessing these sources. Reliability of information is quite variable and often hard to confirm once you leave the Web pages of the established governmental agencies and medical institutions. In addition, these recommendations are general in nature and may need to be altered depending on an individual's health status and travel itineraries.

FUTURE DEVELOPMENTS

Diseases are oppurtunists and the threat of infectious disease transmission will continue as long as there are segments of the population that are mobile. Mobility brings together diverse cultures, social interactions, behaviors, and gene pools (human, animal, and microbe) which can lead to new occurrences of both new and old diseases. Epidemic diseases are stemmed in one area only to arise in another due to disorganization, destruction, and destitution. Moving people, be it on foot, in ships or aircraft, is conducive to the propagation of disease. Changes in exposure history of populations and lapses in medical attention to the possibility of recurring of ''old'' diseases combined with the current volume, speed, and reach of travel are conducive to the continued occurrence of significant morbidity and mortality associated with air travel.

New diseases and variants of old diseases also are being recognized. The transmission of influenza, dengue, cholera, and other diseases can be enhanced by modern air travel. Continued improvements in the technology of air travel are forecast. The speed of travel and the volume of people and cargo will only increase the risk of disease transmission. Tourism to formerly re-

mote and isolated regions will expose greater numbers of susceptible individuals to disease, as will the increasing number of political and economic refugees. As cargo management shifts from the sea lanes to the air lanes, more ports of entry will be available for the worldwide movement of goods. Thus, the potential for the intermingling of susceptible hosts and agents of disease in a favorable environment will continue to expand.

The effects of space travel and exploration of disease patterns also must be considered. Although the risk of encountering hazardous life forms during foreseeable space explorations may be remote, the effect of the physiologic stresses of prolonged space flight on incubating infectious diseases, latent infections, and commensal saprophytic microflora merit particular attention. The long-term effects of prolonged space flight on the immunologic system and the response of the human organism to the challenge of even common diseases are not yet fully understood. Just as diseases were transported between the old world and the new by 15th and 16th century explorers, we must be aware of the potential risk of transporting disease-producing organisms through interplanetary exploration.

Throughout history, the movement of humans has been associated with the occurrence of disease. We must remain vigilant to the possibilities of exotic diseases manifesting themselves far from their source and share the information with those responsible for tracking diseases. In addition, we must work to remove the social, political, and economic biases that reveal themselves when these diseases are encountered.

Acknowledgments

The author wishes to recognize the contributions to this chapter by George D. Lathrop, M.D., and William H. Wolfe, M.D., authors of this chapter in the first edition of this text.

REFERENCES

1. Doyle RJ, Lee NC. Microbes, warfare, religion, and human institutions. Can J Microbiol 1986;32:193–200.

2. Rigau-Perez JG, Gubler DJ, Vorndam AV, et al. MMWR CDC surveillance summaries 1994;43:7–19.
3. Centers for Disease Control: Imported dengue-United States, 1989. MMWR 1990;39:741–742.
4. Royal L, McCoubrey I. International spread of disease by air travel. Am Fam Physician 1989;40(5):129–36.
5. Glass RI, et al. Cholera in Africa: lessons on transmission and control for Latin America. Lancet 1991;338: 791–795.
6. Centers for Disease Control: Cholera-worldwide, 1989. MMWR 1990;39:365–367.
7. Randle CJM, et al. Cholera: possible infection from aircraft effluent. J Hygiene (London) 1978;81(3):361–371.
8. Driver CR, et al. Cholera among aircraft passengers. JAMA 1994;272:1031–1035.
9. Blake PA. Epidemiology of cholera in the Americas. Gastroenterol Clin North Am 1993;22:639–660.
10. Moser MR, et al. An outbreak of influenza aboard a commercial airliner. Am J Epidemiol 1979;110:1–6.
11. Kendal AP, et al. Laboratory-based surveillance of influenza viruses in the United States during the winter of 1977–1978. Am J Epidemiol 1979;110:462–468.
12. Centers for Disease Control: Exposure of passengers and flight crew to *Mycobacterium tuberculosis* on commercial aircraft, 1992–1995. MMWR 1995;44: 137–140.
13. Shilts, R. And the band played on: politics, people, and the AIDS epidemic. New York: St. Martin's Press, 1988.
14. Bryan FL, et al. Time-temperature observations of food and equipment in airline catering operations. J Food Protect 1978;41:80–92.
15. Eisenberg MS. Staphylococcal food poisoning aboard commercial aircraft. Lancet 1975;II:595–599.
16. Derban LKA. Outbreak of food poisoning due to alkyl-mercury fungicide. Arch Environ Health 1974;28: 49–52.
17. Isaacson M. Airport malaria: a review. Bulletin of the WHO 1989;67:737–743.
18. Brunetti R, Fritz RF, Hollister AC Jr. An outbreak of malaria in California, 1952–1953. Am J Trop Med Hyg 1954;3:779–788.
19. Nowell WR. International quarantine for control of mosquito-borne diseases on Guam. Aviat Space Environ Med 1977;48:53–60.
20. Centers for Disease Control: Imported bubonic plague-District of Columbia. MMWR 1990;39:895–901.
21. Russell RC, Paton R. In-flight disinsection as an efficacious procedure for preventing international transport of insects of public health importance. Bulletin of the WHO 1989;67:543–547.
22. Centers for Disease Control: Update: Filovirus infection in animal handlers. MMWR 1990;39:221.

Chapter 34

Occupational and Environmental Medical Support to the Aviation Industry

Roy L. DeHart

For so runs the oracle of our inspired teacher: ''When you come to a patient's house, you should ask him what sort of pains he has, what caused them, how many days he has been ill, whether the bowels are working and what sort of foods he eats.'' So says Hippocrates in his work AFFLICTIONS. I may venture to add one more question: what occupation does he follow?

Bernardino Ramazzini
1713

INTRODUCTION

In the United States, in 1995, airlines employed approximately 616,200 workers. The majority of these employees were in occupations unrelated to flight crew duties; they were involved in aircraft maintenance, operations, servicing, ramp and baggage handling, ticketing, and counter activities. These employees were subject to most of the workplace hazards found in modern American industry. Added to this worker population are the 444,000 employees of the aircraft manufacturing industry.

Potential workplace hazards are listed in Table 34.1. Although all items in the list are not present in every workplace situation, the common hazards are identified in bold type (1). The type of injuries and illnesses common in American industry by frequency of occurrence are illustrated in Figure 34.1.

Occupational Health

The World Health Organization in 1950 undertook to define Occupational Health as follows:

Occupational Health should aim at the promotion and maintenance of the highest degree of physical, mental, and social well-being of workers in all occupations; the prevention among workers of departures from health caused by their working conditions; the protection of workers in their employment from risks resulting from factors adverse to health; the placing and maintenance of the worker in an occupational environment adapted to his physiological and psychological equipment; and to summarize, the adaptation of work to man and of each man to his job.

It was within the context of this definition that the specialty of Occupational Medicine became

1017

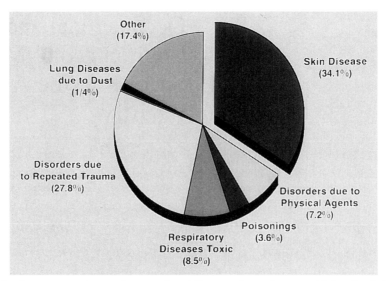

Figure 34.1. The frequency and type of occupational illnesses. From: Bureau of Labor Statistics. Occupational Injuries and Illnesses in 1994. U.S. Department of Labor, 1995.

Table 34.1.
Common Work-Related Medical
Problems of Airline Employees

1. **Neurosensory Hearing Loss**
2. Repetitive Trauma
   - Carpal tunnel syndrome
   - Tenosynovitis
   - Raynaud's syndrome
3. **Strains and Sprains**
   - Low back
   - Cervical
   - Shoulder
4. **Dermatitis**
5. **Cuts and Lacerations**
6. Foreign Body in Eye
7. Respiratory Tract Reaction

formalized. In 1955, a certification program in Occupational Medicine was established by the American Board of Preventive Medicine. As of 1995, over 2,160 physicians have been certified in this specialty. Although the definition above addresses the masculine gender, within the United States, the representation of women in the work force has continually risen to the point that it is approaching 50%.

A key element of Occupational Medicine is its focus on prevention. Not only does the specialty reside within the Board of Preventive Medicine,

but more importantly, many of the tools of the profession are focused on injury and illness prevention, rather than simply limited to treatment and management of affliction, impairment, and disability.

The responsibility of industry is not limited to addressing potential health hazards within the work place, but industry must also address issues beyond the plant boundary as these may impact upon the environment. Release of chemicals, generation of noise, and production of hazardous waste necessitating disposal are examples of environmental issues and concerns that may extend beyond the fence into the neighborhood.

Environmental Medicine

A working definition for Environmental Medicine is:

That branch of medical science which addresses through evaluation, treatment and control, the impact of primarily chemical and physical stressors on the individual or group in a community or dwelling.

Many of the same skills and educational and training experiences are applicable for dealing with both occupational and environmental health concerns. However, there are significant differences in the circumstances of their application. In Occupational Medicine, service is provided to a work force with a demographic characteristic that remains predominantly male in the age group between 18 and 65. Because of the requirements of employment, the majority of the workers are in better health than the general population and enjoy a middle-class living standard (healthy worker effect). Beyond the plant fence, exposure may affect the population including: infants and the elderly, the ill and the well, both genders, and an exposure dose lower than in the factory but chronic and continuous.

The workplace in the aviation industry incorporates many of the materials, processes, and operations common to manufacturing in general: airplane repair and maintenance that includes drilling, riveting, screw fastening, welding, painting, aluminum layout, template work, sub-assembly, fuselage fabrication, manipulating other large units, the placing of motors, engines, propellers, turbines, wing sections, electronic and avionic equipment, and the inspection of the plane, equipment, and machine tool repair. In addition, it is often the aviation industry that introduces new manufacturing processes, such as the fabrication of titanium structures and the build up of metal and carbon fiber composites.

Specialists in Aerospace Medicine should develop and maintain sufficient orientation and motivation in the fields of Environmental and Occupational Medicine to assist management in obtaining and using the consultation necessary to prevent and solve problems involving potential toxic hazards arising out of planned operations, products, and waste. In this way, Aerospace Medicine will better be able to encompass the total program of preventive medicine support to this national economically critical industry.

HISTORY

The relationship of types of work and illness was first addressed by Hippocrates. Centuries later, Ramazzini in his treatise, "Diseases of Work-

ers" described a constellation of afflictions that befall workers in over 50 occupational settings (2). As the book was published in the early 18th century, it would be surprising, indeed, if it mentioned anything regarding the aviation industry. Early in this century, Alice Hamilton, a Professor at Harvard's College of Public Health, began to visit American industries in the Eastern United States, documenting her observations and making recommendations to improve the lot of the worker. Her autobiography "Exploring the Dangerous Trades" details some of her experiences with American industry (3).

More recently, Dhenin, a leader in Aviation Medicine in the United Kingdom, observed that Aviation Medicine is a branch of Occupational Medicine developed from the need to adapt man to the hostile environment of the air (4). Although within the United States, this observation may be considered controversial by some, it does have its advocates. This recognizes the close relationship between Aviation Medicine and Occupational Medicine, particularly when considering commercial airline operations. The author observed in 1990 that among the major airlines in the United States, only 25% of employees were flight deck personnel and flight attendants, while 75% were classified as ground personnel (1). Further, although flight personnel are potentially exposed to many of the hazards of flight as detailed in several chapters of this text, they remain as well susceptible to occupational illnesses and injuries similar to their ground personnel cohorts.

ESTABLISHING AN OCCUPATIONAL AND ENVIRONMENTAL MEDICAL PROGRAM

First and foremost, Occupational and Environmental Medicine (OEM) is a specialty of medicine that is a discipline of Preventive Medicine. The major goal is to prevent injury and disease and should this not be entirely effective, to prevent death and disability, returning the impaired employee to work as soon as is feasible. Providing OEM services is far more complex than

Table 34.2.
Occupational and Environmental Health Services

Clinical Services	Consultative Services
Emergency Response Service	Americans with Disabilities Act
Initial Treatment of Acute Non-Occupationally Related Illness	Community Health
Periodic Health Assessments	Disability Evaluations
Preplacement Examinations	Employee Assistance Program
Return-to-Work Evaluations	Environmental Hazard Evaluation
Substances of Abuse Testing	Epidemiological Studies
Termination Examinations	Expert Testimony
Treatment of Work-Related Injury and Illness	Health Physics
	Human Engineering (Ergonomics)
Special Assessments	Industrial Hazard Evaluation
Audiometric Testing	Industrial Hygiene
Biological Monitoring	Medical Review Officer
Foreign Travel	Research Protocol Development
Functional Capacity Evaluations	Safety Engineering
Prophylactic Immunizations	Toxic Hazard Information Service
Respiratory Clearance	Work-Relatedness of Disease (Causation)
Spirometry	
Visual Screening	*Health Promotion Activities*
X-ray (B-reading)	Fitness
	Health Screening
Educational Services	Smoking Cessation
Back to School	Stress Management
Cardiopulmonary Resuscitation Training	Weight Reduction and Nutrition
First Aid Training	
Hazard Communications: "Right to Know"	*Administrative Services*
Hearing Conservation Program	Evaluation of Health-Related Costs
Vision Conservation	Interaction with Community Physicians
Community Education	Management of Workers' Compensation
	Professional Supervision of On-Site Clinics
	Program Development

The scope of available services will, in large measure, depend on the clinical setting of the practitioner. Such settings range from the limited services of a family physician serving as the plant doctor in his/her community to the major multidisciplinary full services and research program of an international corporation. In all settings, the focus of OEM is on early identification, evaluation, treatment, and prevention.

simply suturing a laceration or performing a preplacement physical examination. The complexities of this practice are complicated by the strong regulatory and legislative influences potentially involved with the practice. Physicians practicing OEM have responsibilities that extend beyond the usual clinical situation. A comprehensive program will provide many of the services listed in Table 34.2.

There are many settings and situations in which OEM services are provided. These range from the office of a family physician to acute care clinics, including multispecialty group practices, hospital-based services, occupational medicine clinics, corporate medical services,

and consulting practitioners. The full list of services cited in Table 34.2 will typically be available only in the larger, more comprehensive programs.

The OEM consultant provides a focused service to the aviation industry. Frequently the consultant has a particular field of expertise, such as toxicology, ergonomics, wellness, or managerial skills, which is available to the industry on a time-limited, but intense, basis. The services of the consultant are usually focused around problem-solving issues and recommendations may include both short term corrections and long term solutions.

In 1993, the American College of

Occupational and Environmental Medicine (ADOEM) outlined its view of the mission of OEM:

The goal of Occupational and Environmental Medicine is to foster the health, safety, productivity, and wellness of workers, their families and the community, and the protection of the environment. This mission is accomplished by the following activities:

- identification, evaluation, prevention, and management of occupational, environmental and personal health risks;
- promotion of the maximum recovery and re-integration of the individual into a fully productive life by the management and treatment of illness and injury;
- assurance of quality care, conservation of resources and reduction on unnecessary costs by efficient management of health care;
- creation of healthy work cultures/promotion of healthy lifestyles;
- expansion and application of the knowledge of toxicology, epidemiology, ergonomics, biostatistics, and related disciplines of occupational and environmental medicine;
- promotion of continuous quality improvement by use of outcome assessments, practice guidelines, integrated health data systems and other methods;
- provision of expert counsel to employees, families, employers, labor organizations, other health professions, government, and the community; and
- development and implementation of a pattern of environmental responsibility.

Approved 7/24/93 by the ACOEM Board of Directors; revised 8/3/93 by the ACOEM Executive Committee.

The Work Place Environment

Centuries ago, Ramazzini reminded physicians that in order to know the employment circumstances of a worker, one must go to the work site. In aviation manufacturing or flight control operations, the complexities of the work environment can only be understood through direct observation. Recognition, evaluation, and control of hazards posed by chemical, biological, and physical agents, ergonomic stresses and safety risks, require occasional on-site visits. Areas for consideration when providing OEM services are listed below (5).

Process Descriptions

Process descriptions are necessary for routine repetitive functions and for special projects, including identification of raw materials, description of processing equipment and conditions, such as temperature and pressure, description of work activities involved, and a description of feed-stock, product and intermediaries, by-products, and waste.

Chemical Inventory

A chemical inventory is required by the Occupational Safety and Health Administration (OSHA) as detailed in the Hazard Communications Standard. The inventory must be comprehensive and include components of mixtures, identification of chemical constituents of trade name products, and remain current.

Toxicology Information

For each chemical in use, information must include chemical and physical properties, toxicity features of animal and human exposure at levels thought to be safe for occasional and daily exposure.

Material Safety Data Sheets (MSDS)

Material Safety Data Sheets (MSDS) are required for each chemical that is used at the industrial site. In addition to toxicological information as described above, there is additional information and other precautions to be observed in handling, storing, and emergency control measures in case of spills. Names and phone numbers of individuals to contact for additional information or assistance are listed.

Listing of Employees

A list of each employee with consecutive job titles and work assignments as well as some method for identifying potential chemical exposures should be available.

Record for Monitoring

Personnel or environmental monitoring of levels of chemical or physical agents indicating sampling strategies, procedures, and dates are commonly required. Ideally, there should be a cross-indexing of workers, job titles, work areas, and projects to allow for comprehensive review of potential past exposures. This is frequently needed for comprehensive medical surveillance of employee exposure.

Reports of Occupational Injury and Illness

Reports of Occupational Injury and Illness are frequently identified in the OSHA 200 Log and identify the injured worker, the circumstances of the injury, and the degree of medical intervention. This record is helpful in identifying work place problems so that solutions can be identified and implemented.

Control Measures

For controls to be effective requires interdisciplinary cooperation between medicine, engineering, industrial hygiene, and management. The implementation of control technologies are most effective and economical if they become a part of the original design and installation. Removing the hazard through control procedures is by far the best preventive medicine action.

Employee Treatment, Evaluation, and Education

Employee treatment, evaluation, and education are Occupational Medicine services that at one time were commonly provided by the employer on site, have become a part of the "Right-Sizing" of American industry and have frequently been out-placed. These types of services, whether in-house or not, have both medical and nonmedical components. Providing

treatment for occupational injury or illness is the obligation of the employer. Such treatment should be handled either by on-site medical personnel or by referral. Complicating health care management is the insurance system existing in all states and in federal agencies known as Worker Compensation which will be discussed in more detail later.

Work Placement

Work placement may depend on the nature and extent of limitations of function caused by medical conditions. Evaluation of such limitations when performing pre-placement medical examinations may influence the proper placement of the potential employee. The OEM physician needs to become familiar with the Americans with Disabilities Act (ADA).

Medical Surveillance

The program of medical surveillance provides information on "target organs" that may be affected by a particular hazard or on all body systems where exposure to multiple or unknown agents may require general documentation of health. Surveillance programs help to assess the adequacy of protective measures. Medical surveillance includes the development of a baseline health inventory followed by periodic re-evaluation.

Epidemiologic Surveillance

Epidemiologic surveillance can help detect possible work-related adverse health effects. Prudence dictates epidemiological evaluation of health indicators for those worker populations having potential exposures to possible health hazards.

Education

Employee and supervisor education concerning work place health factors is vital in preventing illness and injury. There are also significant ethical, legal, regulatory, and employee relations reasons for educating the work force.

Training

Employee and supervisor training in work practices and in the use of personal protective equipment may be required or appropriate. Special training is frequently necessary for employees to meet the emergency, first aid, and cardiopulmonary resuscitation needs of the facility. In certain situations, the OSHA hazard communication standard requires employee training and education.

Employee Assistance Programs (EAP)

Employee Assistance Programs (EAP) provide vitally important services for troubled employees and their families. The comprehensive approach, which may include counseling on marital, financial, and interpersonal issues, is generally more effective than simply limiting such intervention to the traditional alcohol and drug abuse problem. Opportunities for self-referral and confidentiality are important program considerations.

Health Promotion

Wellness programs dealing with non-occupational health situations such as smoking cessation, nutrition, fitness, and other lifestyle issues are increasingly important, and their value to both the worker and industry are now well documented.

Program Administration

Close interaction with company management and employee representative personnel is essential to providing a properly tailored, workable program of occupational health services.

Policies and Procedures

Policies and procedures are management tools that are appropriate to the work site that should be developed by the Occupational Medicine physician with the concurrence and endorsement of management and the union.

Workers' Compensation

The management and administration of Workers' Compensation should assure fairness, encourage appropriate medical management, early recovery, and minimize financial loss to both the worker and the employer. An alternative duty (light duty) policy is a critical element for success in effectively returning the worker to the work place. Laws and procedures vary significantly from state to state and can be a major source of frustration to all. For example, a major airline will have employees stationed in nearly every state in the union, yet each state has its own peculiar regulations with regard to Workers' Compensation. Company policies must address unusual situations such as a flight attendant who is injured due to turbulence while airborne, i.e. which state has jurisdiction of this Workers' Compensation case.

General Liability

General liability considerations are important to prevent claims of willful negligence against the practitioner or the company. Meticulous attention to ethics, medical management, communications, and record keeping are the main stays of defense. Malpractice liability applies to the private practitioner and the corporate physician alike, although the circumstances and degree of liability may vary.

Agency Requirements

Agency requirements must be appropriately addressed by whoever is providing OEM services. Some of the federal agencies with health and safety requirements include:

a. DOT—Department of Transportation
b. EEOC—Equal Employment Opportunity Commission
c. EPA—Environmental Protection Agency
d. FAA—Federal Aviation Administration
e. FDA—Food and Drug Administration
f. NIOSH—National Institute for Occupational Safety and Health
g. NLRB—National Labor Relations Board
h. NRC—Nuclear Regulatory Agency

i. OSHA—Occupational Safety and Health Administration

Communications and Coordination

Communications and coordination are required with workers, technical experts, supervisors, management, and other appropriate people.

Information Management

Information management is a tool providing the basic information necessary for a successful OEM program. Federal requirements concerning retention of medical data must be understood and observed. For example, radiographs obtained as part of an asbestos surveillance program must be retained and available for 30 years past the termination of the employee.

Quality Assurance

Quality assurance provides a management tool that can be used to validate a program's effective, timely, and appropriate use of medical resources in an OEM program. Such assurance may have legal benefit.

Benefits of an Occupational and Environmental Medicine Program

From the viewpoint of the manager, the most valuable asset in industry (and this is particularly true in the aviation industry) is its trained work force. Maintaining and protecting the health of the worker thus becomes a sound industrial investment. Other benefits include:

1. demonstrating management's concern for the health and welfare of the work force, thus enhancing the corporate image;
2. contributing to the productivity and retention of the work force;
3. reducing the cost, both in human and financial terms of Workers' Compensation;
4. lowering the cost of health and disability;
5. eliminating environmentally related problems, thus improving both labor and community relations;
6. producing state-of-the-art spin-off benefits

related to improved instrumentation, computerization, and automation of data on environmental control and the health of the work force;
7. providing internal intelligence on company operations and products, allowing self-initiated correction of faulty planning and design;
8. assuring a necessary bridge between the medical and safety personnel and operating departments, thus helping protect the company from spurious legal attack;
9. serving as the vital link between management and government agencies, competitors, associations, media, and public relations people involved in environmental matters;
10. using preventive health and safety for the work force to expand programs of health protection and conservation to benefit the industrial community and the public at large.

Workers' Compensation

As earlier implied, a common concern for OEM services provided to the airline industry, whether it be in manufacturing or airline operations, is the management of the Workers' Compensation system. For the airlines, as a transportation industry, operating in multiple states and across international borders, the management of various components of Workers' Compensation is frequently involved, complex, and complicated by an enormous governmental bureaucratic system. Airframe manufacturers may have similar concerns as they frequently have multistate operations. In review, Workers' Compensation is a no-fault insurance program with "first dollar pay" for medical expenses that provides protection for both the worker and the employer. In both the state and the federal systems, the worker's only legal remedy for most job-related accidents or injuries is through this system. There is reasonable assurance that the worker will receive medical care at no cost, will receive partial reimbursement for lost wages after a minimum qualifying period, and, should there be permanent impairment or disability resulting from the job-related injury or illness, will receive proportional compensation. At the same time, the employer is spared the inconvenience and expense of law suits for injuries occurring on the plant property. It is intended to assure that the employee receives prompt, free medical care. Coverage is for all employees, including flight crew and ground personnel. Within the United States, each state retains its own regulatory structure which may be a court, a board, or a hearing officer process. A solution achieved by several airlines through labor negotiations involves identifying a single state that will always have jurisdiction of the Workers' Compensation case, regardless of the geographic location of the incident.

WORKPLACE HAZARDS

The aviation industry has the potential of exposing the work force to numerous hazards that may result in adverse health effects. To assist in the systematic review of the major hazards of concern, they are categorized as chemical, physical, or biological.

Chemical Hazards

In many respects, to define a substance as a toxic chemical is redundant. Essentially all chemicals are toxic, given a specific route of exposure or an excessive dose. A gallon of water becomes toxic when inhaled; oxygen can induce convulsions when breathed under hyperbaric conditions; 500 grams of table salt taken orally at one setting will have serious adverse effects on metabolism. The topic of toxicology is complex and still evolving.

Threshold Limit Values

The intent of threshold limit values (TLV) set by consensus within the American Conference of Governmental Industrial Hygienist (ACGIH)

Threshold Limit Value Committee is to provide reliable benchmarks to aid plant engineers, both in designing new facilities and in renovating old ones, so that the possibility of toxicity occurring in the work force would be minimized (6). In this way, other protective measures such as personal protection, limiting exposure time, and special-purpose occupational medical examinations and tests either could be minimized or better still, documented as being totally unnecessary. The basic premise involved in industrial hygiene controls below a permissible (safe) exposure level is that repeated exposures over an eight hour day, five days a week for a working lifetime of approximately 40 years could be allowed for the majority of unprotected employees without harm. Although a few susceptible individuals in the work force might develop evidence of harm, these persons would be detected by close occupational medical surveillance and removed or protected from further exposure prior to sustaining irreversible impairment or disability. The individuals who are sensitive or allergic to the chemical in question would fall outside the proposed permissible limit. According to Hatch, this TLV concept, as illustrated in Figure 34.2, introduces fundamental information to the field of industrial hygiene and the time and effort should be taken to confirm and strengthen these standards with reliable, reproducible data bases on human experience whenever possible (7).

Understanding the Hatch curve is a first step in being able to apply toxicological data to the factory floor or the environment. A healthy individual functioning at point A may respond to environmental stress with a relatively minor and temporary disturbance and will return to point A when the stress is removed. An already impaired individual at point B may find the same kind and degree of stress intolerable and consequently move rapidly up the curve to a position of serious disability and even death. Industrial hygiene engineering controls below a certain level allow the great majority of workers to be exposed safely for up to eight hours per day, five days per week, for up to 40 years. This level

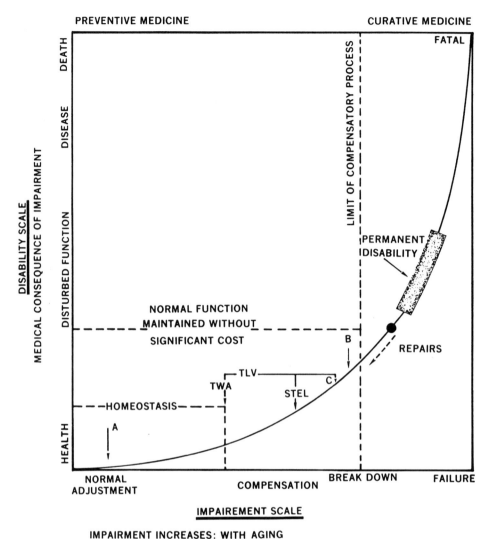

Figure 34.2. Modified Hatch curve. From Hatch TF. Changing objectives in occupational health. Am Indust Hygiene Association J 23(1), 1962.

is known as the threshold limit value-time weighted average (TLV-TWA). The TLV-STEL is defined as the short-term exposure limit, averaged over a period of 15 minutes, which should not be exceeded at any time during a work day (even if the eight hours TWA is within the TLV). Exposures at the STEL should not be for longer than 15 minutes and should not be repeated more than four times per day. Also, there should be at least 60 minutes between successive expo-

sures at the STEL. The TLV-C is a ceiling concentration that should not be exceeded. If any one of these three TLVs is exceeded, a potential hazard from this substance is presumed to exist.

Unfortunately, the facts that would help place matters of environmental and occupational health into proper perspective are not being communicated adequately to many of our citizens. As a result, a climate exists today in which the adverse effects on productivity and the economy are disregarded while sensationalistic, science-fiction-type coverage in the media of environmentally induced illness claims are encouraged and even rewarded. The concept of absolute assurance appears to be the rule that it is reasonable to expect absolutely no risk to the individual, the community, or to the environment from activities of commerce. This tendency toward zero exposure levels for many chemicals is cost prohibitive and may be without scientific merit. The attitude of some that industries must prove the non-event, that is that a chemical is absolutely safe, violates the established and well-recognized limitations of epidemiology. There needs to be greater assurance that appropriate instruction in environmental and occupational health occurs at all levels within the biomedical community.

Toxicology Concepts

Perhaps the most fundamental concept in toxicology is the relationship between the dose of a chemical and the response that occurs in the biological system. Animal models, typically rodents, are used to study the adverse health affects of these chemicals. When the dose is sufficiently high to cause death in the animals, a statistical analysis of the data permits the calculation of the LD_{50} or the dose expected to be lethal in 50% of the animals. If a number of doses of the chemical are delivered by inhalation, then the calculation resulting in 50% mortality is the LC_{50} (2). The LD_{50} or LC_{50} for a chemical, provides the first index of comparative toxicity. The dose response can be expressed as a curve whose slope can define the LD_{50}. In Figure 34.3, substances A and B both have the same LD_{50}, but substance B has a wider margin of safety than substance A as illustrated by the magnitude of the range between a no-effect level and the lethal dose (9).

The toxicity of a chemical is defined as the ability to cause injury to the biological system. The hazard associated with the chemical defines the likelihood it will cause injury in a given environment or situation. As all chemicals are poten-

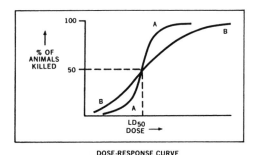

DOSE-RESPONSE CURVE

Figure 34.3. Dose-response curve. (Reproduced with permission from Proctor NH. Setting health standards: Toxicologic concepts. In: Proctor NH, Hughes JP, Fischman ML, eds. Chemical Hazards of the Workplace, 2nd edition. Philadelphia: J. B. Lippincott Company, 1988.)

tially toxic, it is helpful to have a classification for grading the degree of toxicity of a chemical. Table 34.3 provides such a classification system (9).

Regulatory Agencies

The enactment of the Occupational Safety and Health Act (also commonly abbreviated OSHA which is the same as the administration it created in 1970) translated public concern about chemical exposures into law. Subsequently, regulatory strategies were developed, assigning responsibility and accountability for the control of occupational hazards. The regulatory activities of the Act are the responsibility of OSHA, an agency of the Department of Labor.

Created by the same Act was the National Institute for Occupational Safety and Health (NIOSH), an agency charged with research, investigation, and education directed toward workplace safety and health. Also in 1970, the Environmental Protection Agency (EPA) was established. This agency is responsible for the implementation of legislation designed to protect the environment. Standards that relate to air and water are increasingly being based on health effects rather than engineering technology. The Toxic Substance Control Act (TSCA) administered by the EPA requires manufacturers and users to keep records of their chemical inventory. Reports must be submitted if there are any

Table 34.3.
Toxicity Classes

Toxicity Rate	Descriptive Term	LD$_{50}$—weight/kilogram Single Oral Dose Rats	LC$_{50}$—ppm 4-Hour Inhalation Rats
1	Extremely toxic	less than 1 mg	<10
2	Highly toxic	1–50 mg	10–100
3	Moderately toxic	50–500 mg	100–1000
4	Slightly toxic	0.5–5 g	1000–10,000
5	Practically nontoxic	5–15 g	10,000–100,000
6	Relatively harmless	15 g or more	>100,000

From Hodge HC, Sterner JH. Tabulation of toxicity classes. Am Ind Hyg Q 1949;10:93.

allegations of heretofore unknown adverse health effects resulting from chemical exposure. The EPA is also charged with the regulation of toxic waste dumps, and this has clear health implications, not only to the work force, but to the immediate environment.

Another governmental agency, the Agency for Toxic Substances and Disease Registry (ATSDR) is a public health service agency created in 1980 under the superfund legislation. The agency's mission is to conduct activities to protect the public from the adverse health consequences of toxic chemical exposures. It is mandated to establish a disease and exposure registry forming an information base of health effects of toxic substances. The continuing education program which the Agency provides is important to physicians.

Biological Monitoring

Where environmental surveys cannot document adequacy of hazard control below a limiting federal standard (usually ½ the TLV), special purpose occupational medical examinations and biological monitoring may be required, even if proper protection is worn. Biological monitoring, for example, is required when there is asbestos or benzene exposure beyond the regulated levels. Conversely, where environmental data confirm the adequacy of hazard containment, only a preplacement baseline value may need to be established. To accomplish biological monitoring on a routine basis in the absence of poten-

tial hazardous exposures is unjustified due to the administrative burden, the cost of the tests, and the deviation of the worker away from his or her task.

Physical Hazards

Physical hazards are defined by Wald as hazards that result from energy and matter, and the relationship between the two (10). Operationally, these hazards as they exist in the workplace can be organized into worker-material interfaces, the physical environment, and energy and electromagnetic radiation. Each of these is present in the aviation industry. Physical agents are formless and essentially weightless, but may produce hazards to exposed workers by the transfer of energy of various types, resulting in rather specific bioeffects when permissible occupational standards are exceeded. Among the most important potentially harmful physical agents where there is a transfer of energy are (1) oscillatory motions, including noise and vibration; (2) extreme occupational temperature variations in the ambient environment; and (3) ionizing and nonunionizing electromagnetic radiation. Figure 34.4 introduces other forms of physical hazards on the job which are typically defined as ergonomic or biomechanical, but also have important consequences to worker health, safety, and productivity (11).

Noise

In 1979, the ACGIH redefined the TLV from previous considerations at 500, 1000, and 2000

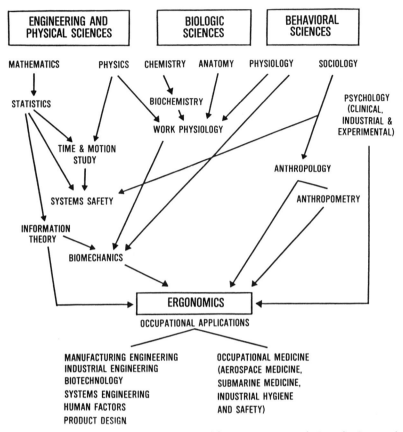

Figure 34.4. Disciplines in Ergonomics. From: Zenz C, Dickerson OB, Horvath EP, eds. Occupational Medicine. 3rd ed. St. Louis, MO: Mosby-Yearbook, Inc., 1994.

Hz, to include as well 3000 and 4000 Hz. However, because of the individual's susceptibility to noise, these figures should not be regarded as fine lines between safe and damaging levels. It is estimated that the TLV should protect the average population against a noise-induced hearing loss that would exceed 2 dB after 40 years of continuous occupational exposure. Table 34.4 lists the TLVs considering the noise level in dBA versus the duration of exposure allowed per day (6).

Accrued liability from noise-induced hearing loss in industry is estimated to be in the billions of dollars. Attempts to implement hearing conservation programs in the past have inadvertently precipitated early retirement and compensation claims solely because of high-frequency losses (above speech frequencies). Effective

Table 34.4.
Threshold Limit Values For Noise

	Duration Per Day	Sound Level dBA
Hours	24	80
	16	82
	8	85
	4	88
	2	91
	1	94
Minutes	30	97
	15	100

From: American Conference of Governmental Industrial Hygienists. Threshold limit values for chemical substance and physical agents. ACGIH, Cincinnati, OH, 1995.

hearing conservation programs are based on proper initial placement, with the establishment of an accurate baseline (or reference) audiogram, as well as follow-up testing in 90 to 120 days, and at least annually thereafter to help insure against unprotected hazardous exposure and temporary hearing loss. If such temporary losses can be prevented, it has been shown that permanent noise-induced changes are unlikely, except in continuous noise such as constant exposure to a rolling mill or waterfall. Even brief removal from continuous hazardous noise exposure tends to limit the progressive loss of hearing; therefore, rotation out of noise and ear-defender protection are components of an effective preventive program. This is especially important in situations where hazardous noise cannot be controlled by engineering means alone such as on the flight line. It should be mentioned that even though 90 dBA is the standard of hazardous noise exposure, the United States Department of Defense and OSHA use the level of greater than 84 dBA-TWA to require inclusion of its workers in a hearing conservation/audiometric testing program. It provides an example of biologic monitoring within a program of occupational health surveillance designed to protect the health of all employees.

The Occupational Safety and Health Act, which has subsequently been modified by the OSHA Hearing Conservation Amendment, established extensive regulations for industries in the United States in order to reduce the incidents of noise-induced hearing loss. After much legal delay, the final rule was published, delineating a specific hearing conservation program in 1983 (12). The guidelines contained in the rule are intended to protect almost all covered workers from substantial occupationally-related noise-induced hearing loss. Further information on noise and communication is available in Chapter 10.

Vibration

Oscillatory motions or vibrations are not currently addressed by federal regulations. Adverse

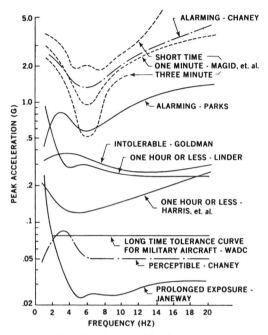

Figure 34.5. Vibration classification and tolerance; acceleration versus frequency versus exposure time. (Reproduced with permission from Ramsey JD. Occupational vibration. In: Zenz C, ed. Occupational medicine: principles and practical applications. Chicago: Yearbook Medical Publishers, 1975.

effects, however, may result from excessive vibratory exposure to the whole body or its parts. Tolerance levels to different degrees of peak acceleration are a function of the frequency and duration of exposure as shown in Figure 34.5 (11).

Research has established that man's sensitivity to external vibration is highest between 0.5 and 20 Hz because the human body absorbs most of the vibratory energy applied within this range, with maximal amplification between 5 and 11 Hz. Posture can greatly affect tolerance in test subjects. There is also wide variability between and within individuals, depending on such other factors as fatigue, physical conditioning, and perceived risk. Standards for human experimentation and aerospace exploration involve the same careful attention to physical and mental fitness and absence of diseases of all types that characterize the selection of individuals for pilot training. Whole-body vibrational stresses of significance are not commonly encountered outside of such military and space environments. A single whole body vibration standard is currently in use in the United States: International Standards Organization (ISO) 2631, ''Evaluation of Human Exposure to Whole Body Vibration.'' A similar standard is that issued by the American National Standards Institute (ANSI), S3.18, ''Guide for the Evaluation of Human Exposure to Whole Body Vibration.'' Standards are also available for segmental or hand-arm vibration. Of particular value is NIOSH #89–106, Criteria for Recommended Standard, ''Occupational Exposure to Hand-Arm Vibration'' released in 1989.

Localized or segmental vibration produces bioeffects from the use of oscillatory and rotary tools in the 25 to 150 Hz range when amplitude is at least 100 μm. For hammer-type tools, the common frequencies for undesirable localized vibration effects are 30 to 50 Hz. In addition to Raynaud's phenomenon, which progressively affects palmar arch and digital arteries, neurologic effects are being recognized that involve tingling and numbness. Adverse effects tend to vary inversely with the weight of the tool. Reduced exposure time appears to be an important controllable factor in protecting against such adverse bioeffects.

Heat Stress

Hot environments are hazardous to life and health because they raise the body's core temperature. Resting deep body temperature is normally about 37.2°C. Variations become intolerable above and below rather narrow physiologic limits, ranging from 35 to 41°C. The TLVs discussed below are based on the assumption that nearly all acclimatized, fully clothed workers with adequate water and salt intake should be able to function effectively under the given working conditions without exceeding a core body temperature of 38°C.

Higher heat exposures than those shown here are permissible under close occupational health surveillance with documentation of workers' tolerance. Workers should not be permitted to continue hot work when their deep body temperature exceeds 38°C (100.4°F).

Physicians responsible for the health of workers in hot climates must understand that any prolonged physical activity results in a higher metabolic rate and, hence, an increase in body temperature. Walking in shorts at 80 m/min for 30 to 40 minutes on a cool day may result in a body temperature of 38.3°C for a 70 kg man, whereas a run of 1500 m in less than 8 minutes under similar conditions may boost the body temperature to 39.5°C, based on maximum oxygen uptake. In the general population, anaerobic metabolism sets in when 40 to 50% of the maximum oxygen uptake is reached and results in decreased efficiency and increased heat production, heart rate, and body temperature without plateauing. Intensive physical conditioning improves heat tolerance, as shown in Figure 34.6, but withholding water eliminates the advantage (11). Heat acclimatization is easily lost after 1 to 3 weeks away from heat stress and must be renewed.

Metabolic body heat and the environmental heat together determine the total body heat load. In order to estimate the metabolic heat generation, it is necessary to categorize the job to establish heat production. In order to determine the thermal TLV, the ACGME has established three categories of work (6):

- Light work which is sitting or standing to control machines, or when performing light hand or arm work rated at 200 kcal/hr;
- Moderate work which is defined as walking about with moderate lifting and pushing producing between 200 and 350 kcal/hr;
- Heavy work such as in performing pick and shovel activities generating 350 to 500 kcal/ hr.

Knowing the category of work, it is possible to estimate the permissible heat exposure TLV

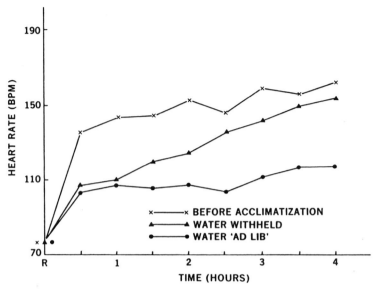

Figure 34.6. The influence of heat acclimatization and water restriction on heart rate response during 4 hours of heat stress. Water restriction entirely eliminates the beneficial influence of heat acclimatization. (Reproduced with permission from Strydom NB. Physical work and heat stress. In: Zenz C, ed. Occupational medicine: principles and practical applications. Chicago: Yearbook Medical Publishers, 1975.

Table 34.5.
Examples of Permissible Heat Exposure Threshold Limit Values In °C And (°F) Wbgt

Work-Rest Pattern	Work Load		
	Light	Moderate	Heavy
Continuous Work	30.0 (86)	26.7 (80)	25.0 (77)
75% Work—25% Rest, each hour	30.6 (87)	28.0 (82)	25.9 (78)
50% Work—50% Rest, each hour	31.4 (89)	29.4 (85)	27.9 (82)
25% Work—75% Rest, each hour	32.2 (90)	31.1 (88)	30.0 (86)

From: American Conference of Governmental Industrial Hygienists. Threshold limit values for chemical substance and physical agents. ACGIH, Cincinnati, OH, 1995.

using Table 34.5. For each work load category, the heat exposure threshold, in both Celsius and Fahrenheit, is given in relationship to the work-rest cycle pattern.

On hot jobs, reasonably cool drinking water (10 to 15°C) should be readily available and consumed by workers at a rate of about 150 ml every 15 to 20 minutes. Where workers are unacclimatized and unable to add sufficient salt to their food to replace that lost in sweat, salt should be added to the drinking water at the rate of 1 g of sodium chloride per liter of water, which produces the desired 0.1% concentration. The use

of salt tablets are not recommended as they generally are poorly absorbed and not well tolerated by the work force. Salt replacement by normal dietary means is preferred.

Permissible heat exposure TLVs are valid only for light-weight, summer-type work clothing. Where insulated or sweat-impervious clothing is required (e.g., firefighters' suits, missile propellant handlers' protective clothing), special attention must be given in arriving at safe limits of exposure. It must be emphasized that the TLVs are valid only for heat-acclimatized workers who are fit physically. Extra caution must

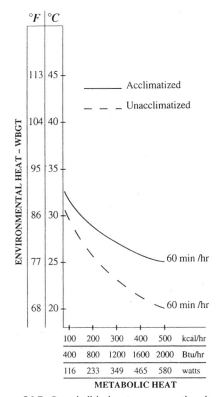

Figure 34.7. Permissible heat exposure threshold limit values for heat acclimatized and unacclimatized workers. (From: American Conference of Governmental Industrial Hygienists, Inc., 1995–1996 Threshold Limit Values™ and Biological Exposure Indices™. Reprinted with permission.)

be used until it can be established both that any unfit workers have been identified and placed in sheltered work situations and that remaining workers are properly acclimatized and instructed in the avoidance of hazardous heat stress.

The TLV specified in Table 34.5 and Figure 34.7 are determined on the assumption that WGBT value of the resting place is the same or very close to that of the workplace (6). Figure 34.7 provides a pictorial representation of the permissible heart exposure threshold limit value for continuous work for both acclimatized and unacclimatized workers.

Heart rates can exceed 170 beats/min the first day of acclimatization but should stabilize within 3 to 4 days to less than 140 beats/min. Daily hot work periods during the process of full

8-hour acclimatization must last a 4 hr/day for 5 to 9 consecutive days. There is no advantage to more than 4 hours, but 2 hours is inadequate. Symptoms of thirst and cramps do not give adequate warning of the hazard of heat stress. Attention of all workers should be directed to the following conditions, which have been associated with increased susceptibility to serious complications of hazardous heat exposure:

1. Lack of acclimatization
2. Obesity
3. Subpar physical fitness
4. Fatigue
5. Lack of sleep
6. Dehydration
7. Febrile illness
8. Acute and convalescent infections
9. Reactions to immunizations
10. Conditions affecting sweating
11. Skin disorders (e.g., heat rash, sunburn)
12. Drug use (e.g., alcohol, barbiturates)
13. Past history of heat injury
14. Previously living in cooler climate
15. Existing chronic diseases (i.e., diabetes, cardiovascular disease)
16. Central nervous system lesions (e.g., of the hypothalamus, brain stem, and cervical part of the spinal cord)
17. Convalescence from certain surgical operations
18. Recent intake of food
19. Sustained muscular exercise
20. Known intolerance to heat

Cold Stress

The cold stress TLVs have been developed to protect workers from the severest effects of hypothermia and cold injury. The objectives are to prevent deep body cooling with the core temperature falling below 36°C (96.8°F) and to prevent cold injury to body parts. For a single occasional exposure to cold, a drop in core temperature to 35°C (95°F) may be tolerated.

Local injury from exposure to excessive cold occurs seasonally among the indigent and infirm

Table 34.6.
Cooling Power of the Wind on Exposed Flesh Expressed as an Equivalent Temperature

Estimated Wind Speed (in kph)	Actual Thermometer Reading (°C)											
	10	4	−1	−7	−12	−18	−23	−29	−34	−40	−46	−51
	Equivalent Temperature (°C)											
calm	10	4	−1	−7	−12	−18	−23	−29	−34	−40	−46	−51
8	9	3	−2	−9	−14	−20	−25	−32	−37	−43	−50	−55
16	5	−2	−6	−15	−22	−30	−35	−42	−48	−55	−63	−69
24	2	−7	−12	−21	−28	−34	−43	−51	−57	−63	−71	−81
32	0	−9	−15	−24	−32	−37	−47	−56	−62	−69	−76	−88
40	−1	−10	−18	−26	−34	−40	−51	−60	−65	−73	−85	−93
48	−2	−11	−19	−28	−36	−42	−53	−63	−68	−76	−89	−97
56	−3	−12	−20	−29	−37	−44	−55	−65	−70	−78	−91	−99
64	−4	−13	−21	−30	−38	−46	−56	−67	−71	−80	−92	−101

(wind speeds greater than 64 kph have little additional effect)	Little danger (for properly clothed person)—maximum danger is false sense of security	Increasing danger—danger from freezing of exposed flesh	Great danger

Trenchfoot and immersion foot may occur at any point on this chart

in northern climates and is also a primary concern of military personnel in the field. It also may occur among civilian workers wherever the predisposing conditions are met such as those outlined in Table 34.6, where exposed flesh is shown to suffer cold injury in the form of freezing (and consequent frostbite) at or below −18°C even at wind velocities as low as 25 kph. The equivalent or wind chill temperature reflects the effective heat loss of an unclothed body exposed to a temperature without wind or at a higher temperature when the wind is blowing. Thus heat loss is the same whether the exposure occurs at −18°C without wind or at −1°C with a wind speed of 24 kph. If the actual temperature is above freezing, water will not freeze regardless of the equivalent wind chill temperature. Special problems obviously exist in arctic regions, where temperatures fall below −40°C and wind speed may reach and maintain hurricane velocities for hours to days at a time. The reader is referred to Chapter 12 for more information on thermal stress.

Electromagnetic Radiation Hazards

The electromagnetic radiation hazards (EMR) spectrum encompasses an unbroken series of ethereal waves, moving with the velocity of light which vary widely in wavelength (Fig. 34.8) from cosmic rays as short as 4×10^{-12} cm to hertzian waves (used in radio and power transmission), which extend several miles in length. For purposes of hazard evaluation and control, EMR falls into two distinct categories based on the ability or inability to dissociate a substance in solution into its constituents, or ions. These categories are universally identified as ionizing and non-ionizing radiation.

Ionizing Radiation (IR)

The degree of IR hazard to living tissues is indicated by the average energy imparted in traversing a specified distance. High linear energy transfer (LET) is characteristic of the particulate emissions of certain elements such as radium. Besides heat and light, radium salts emit three other distinct forms of radiation (alpha, beta, and gamma rays), as well as radon, a radioactive gas. Penetrating power and the range of travel are inversely proportional to LET; hence, high LET radiation (high-energy beta rays or particles, neutrons, and deuterons) would transfer more energy in a specified volume than gamma rays or x-rays of equivalent energy, causing greater

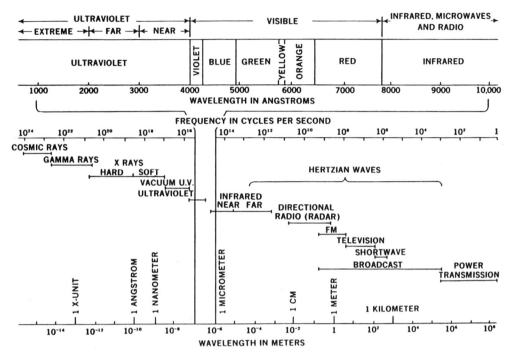

Figure 34.8. The electromagnetic spectrum. (Modified from Zenz C, ed.: Occupational medicine: principles and practical applications. Chicago: Yearbook Medical Publishers, 1975.

damage as a result of secondary ionization induction. Although alpha particles are high LET, their range is so short that a hazard would result only if they were placed in close proximity to a radiosensitive target organ (e.g., cataracts from the use of unshielded thoriated glass in night vision devices or lung cancer from the deposition of radioactive dust in the depths of the lungs, in association with epithelial cells lining the bronchioles). Alpha exposure interacting with skin from outside sources is termed external alpha, whereas alpha particles inhaled, ingested, or absorbed and deposited in or near extremely radiosensitive target organs are termed internal alpha. Chronic exposure to radon releases internal alpha particles which can produce bone sarcoma.

Low LET radiation includes not only external alpha and beta rays or particles but also cosmic, gamma, and x-rays, all of which possess sufficient energy to cause ionization and which share the ability to pass through many substances that are opaque to light. Exposure to a large, single short-term, whole-body dose of ionizing radiation produces a complex of clinical symptoms, signs, and laboratory changes that correlate well with physical measurements of exposure in a predictable way. An algorithm (Fig. 34.9) explicates a step-wise diagnostic process to help determine the presence and extent of acute radiation syndrome following sufficient exposure, as well as therapeutic requirements and ultimate prognosis in such cases (11).

Guidelines have been developed that provide permissible dose limits for exposures in occupational settings and separate limits for the general public. These guidelines have been established by the Department of Energy based on the recommendation of a number of scientific advisory panels. The dose limit guidelines are given in both Radiation Equivalent Man (Rems) and Sieverts in Table 34.7. Although every effort should be made to limit exposure to ionizing radiation to a level that is as low as reasonably achievable, further guidelines exist for emergency occupational exposures. Only actions

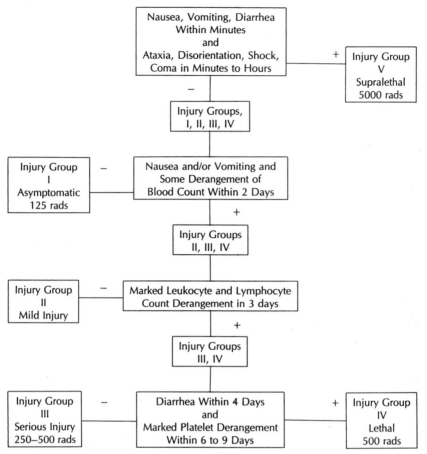

Figure 34.9. Preliminary evaluation of clinical radiation injury following overexposure. Zenz C, Dickerson OB, Horvath EP, eds. Occupational Medicine. 3rd ed. St. Louis, MO: Mosby-Yearbook, 1994.

Table 34.7.
Ionizing Radiation Exposure Guidelines

Category	Dose Limit Guidance	
	Rems	Millisieverts (mSv)
Annual occupational exposure	5.0	50
Lens of eye	15.0	150
Other organs	50.0	500
Unborn child of worker	0.5	5
Annual public exposure	0.1	1
Lifetime cumulative dose	Age × 1	Age × 10

involving life saving response should justify exposures greater than 10 rad (100 mGy) and in truly heroic efforts a dosage should not exceed 100 rad (1 Gy).

Nonionizing Radiation

The major portion of the electromagnetic spectrum is occupied by Nonionizing Radiation (NIR). This ranges from near-ultraviolet through visible light, infrared, radiofrequency, and microwaves to extremely low-frequently radiation. For purposes of regulating hazard prevention, nonionizing radiation is categorized under several broad headings: (1) laser and high-intensity optical sources; (2) ultraviolet (UV); (3) radiofrequency (RF) and microwave (MW);

(4) extremely low-frequency (ELF) radiation; and (5) magnetic fields.

Laser and High-Intensity Optical Sources. Laser and high-intensity optical radiation are considered separately from ionizing radiation, although high irradiances have been known to produce ionization in air and other materials, their principal adverse biologic effects (i.e., those requiring preventive measures) are not related to ionization. Depending on the frequencies involved, lasers produce effects of visible, ultraviolet, or infrared radiation but at levels of intensity previously approached only by the sun, nuclear weapons, burning magnesium, or arclights. Like light, laser beams are reflected, transmitted, and/or absorbed depending on the nature of the surface encountered. Darker materials such as pigment (melanin) absorb more energy than pale or clear tissues; hence, the eye is particularly susceptible to injury due to the pigmented retina.

The threshold for biological injury from a laser beam varies with the wave length of radiation and the operational conditions of the laser as to whether it is pulsed or a continuous wave. Lasers have now been classified using a system described in ANSI Z 136.1. A simplified outline of this classification system follows:

- Class 1 laser—Will not produce injury even if the direct beam is looked at for the maximum possible duration inherent in the design of the laser. For many lasers, this essentially amounts to an unlimited viewing time.
- Class 2 laser—Will not produce injury if the direct beam is viewed for (4) 0.25 sec, the time period necessary for an aversion response. Class 2 lasers are limited to lasers emitting visible light on a continuous basis.
- Class 2A laser—Applies to lasers emitting visible light when the output is not intended to be viewed. The accessible radiation must not exceed that allowed for a class 1 laser for an exposure duration (5) 1000 sec.
- Class 3 laser—Can produce eye damage if the direct beam is viewed. Certain wavelengths

may also damage the skin. This classification is subdivided into classes 3a and 3b. Class 3a, which is limited to the lower accessible outputs of this class, is believed to present less risk of actual injury from a practical standpoint. Class 3b represents those class 3 lasers with higher outputs where the risk of real ocular injury from even momentary viewing of the direct beam is high.
- Class 4 laser—Even the diffuse reflection of lasers with this level of power output can produce biological damage to the eye. The direct laser beam can injure the skin or pose a fire hazard.

For the purpose of establishing TLVs, the optical spectrum has been divided into regions by the ACGIH. These regions are defined in Table 34.8 (6).

Absorption of short UV (200 to 315 nm) and far infrared (1400 to 10^6 nm) radiation occurs principally at the cornea, whereas the near UV radiation (315 to 400 nm) is absorbed primarily in the lens of the eye. Light (400 to 700 nm) and near IR (700 to 1400 nm) are transmitted and refracted by the cornea and lens and absorbed at the retina. The TLVs for viewing a diffuse reflection of a laser beam or an extended source laser and for skin exposure from a laser beam have been published by the ACGIH. Where preventive engineering design criteria are met,

Table 34.8.
Regions Of The Optical Radiation Spectrum

Region	Wavelength Range
Ultraviolet (UV)	100–400 nm
UV-C	100–280 nm
UV-B	280–320 nm
UV-A	320–400 nm
Visible (Light)	380–400 to 760–780 nm
Infrared (IR)	760 nm–1 mm
IR-A	760 nm–1.4 (μm)
IR-B	1.4–3.0 (μm)
IR-C	3.0 (μm − 1 mm)

From: American Conference of Governmental Industrial Hygienists. Threshold limit values for chemical substance and physical agents. ACGIH, Cincinnati, OH, 1995.

special-purpose occupational medical examinations are not ordinarily required as part of routine occupational health surveillance.

In one case, a 65-year-old United States Air Force civil service technician had been tracking magnesium-type flares (dropped from aircraft) with a 24-power telescope using one eye for several hours when he noted he was unable to read with that eye. He was seen by a private ophthalmologist, who agreed that the problem might be related etiologically to exposure at work, stating that the amount of energy required to produce macular degeneration was unknown and thus the possibility that it was due to occupational exposure could not be excluded. A difference in brightness perception also was noted between the left and right eyes.

This claim was discussed with an ophthalmologist experienced in the aviation and military environment who had done considerable experimental research on retinal burns. He demonstrated that the use of a telescope or binoculars spreads light energy focused on the retina rather than concentrating it. Thus, the use of a telescope would actually reduce the chances of macular damage from a high-intensity light source. The amount of energy needed to produce macular degeneration had been extensively studied, and that involved in flare tracking was far lower than would be required to produce injury. A question of aggravation of an existing problem was considered, but in such a case there would have been some evidence of acute local edema in the macular area with subsequent improvement. No such transient effect was observed. The sudden onset of unilateral visual impairment due to macular degeneration is commonly the result of vascular (arteriosclerotic) disease, especially in individuals over the age of 55 to 60 years. There was no reason to suspect that the alleged relationship to an occupational exposure in this case was other than coincidental.

Ultraviolet (UV). For near UV radiation (320 to 400 nm) total irradiance should not exceed 1 mW/cm^2 for periods greater than 16 minutes or 1 J/cm^2 for shorter exposures. Ultraviolet radia-

tion in the UV-C and UV-B bands produce erythema of the skin. If the exposure is more severe, edema and blistering can be expected. Although UV radiation above the 300 nm range is less efficient at producing erythema, there is sufficient energy in the UV-A band from sunlight to cause serious sunburn. Excessive exposure to UV radiation has been causally associated with basal cell carcinoma, squamous cell carcinoma, and mesothelioma. When applying the TLVs, the physician must appreciate that they do not apply to photosensitized individuals or to those exposed concomitantly to photosensitizing agents. These agents may include sulfonamides, chlorothiazides, tetracyclines, and coal tar products.

Radiofrequency (RF) and Microwave (MW) and Electromagnetic Fields (EMF). These forms of radiation produce biologic effects at varying tissue depths depending on the wavelength/frequency relationship, the higher frequencies/shorter wavelengths having less ability to penetrate, similar to IR exposures from heat lamps. Lower frequency/longer wavelengths reach deeper levels, as with therapeutic microwave devices. The lowest/longest type of RF and MW pass completely through tissues without interacting. This explains the varying TLVs shown in Figure 34.10. The results of extensive bioeffects research performed on RF and MW in recent years have indicated the principal bioeffect to be hyperthermia. Extensive medical studies conducted at the USAFSAM of individuals accidentally exposed above permissible occupational limits have failed to document the cataract formation produced experimentally in animals with acute, high MW radiation exposure or any other adverse bioeffects.

In recent years, there has been public concern and numerous epidemiological investigations studying worker populations and community settings in an attempt to define the relative risk for adverse health effects from EMF. The majority of these studies have focused on workers in electrical power generation industries, electrical distribution systems, and individuals living near

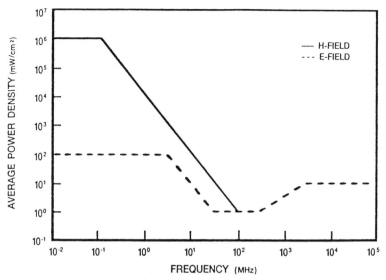

Figure 34.10. Threshold Limit Values (TLV) for Radiofrequency/Microwave Radiation in the workplace (whole-body SAR > than 0.4W/kg). (From: American Conference of Governmental Industrial Hygienists, Inc., 1995–1996 Threshold Limit Values™ and Biological Exposure Indices™. Reprinted with permission.)

transformers or high-voltage power distribution systems. Public concern has focused on reports of increased cancer incidents among children living in the vicinity of power distribution lines and in workers in electrical occupations. There is general agreement among researchers that if the magnetic fields are carcinogenic, they promote, but do not initiate, cancer and that the increased risk is small (13). It is sometimes not appreciated that the earth itself is a magnet and therefore generates a natural magnetic field. This natural magnetic field is approximately 450 mG or .045 mT, and the earth generated electrical field is 120 V/M. Guidelines published by the International Radiation Protection Association (IRPA) for 60 Hertz magnetic fields is limited to 0.5 mT (Tesla) for a complete work day and 5 mT for short term (two hours) exposure. Exposure to electric fields is limited to 10 and 30 kV/m, respectively. The 24 hours exposure for the public is limited to 5 kV/m and 0.1 mT, respectively (14).

BIOLOGICAL HAZARDS

Biological hazards may cause illness as a consequence of their infectious or toxic properties or because they may act as antigens and produce an adverse immune response. Such hazards are uncommon in airframe manufacturing, but of major concern in flight line operations. A noted exception in manufacturing is biological agent contamination of machine cutting fluids which are used to disperse heat and assist in removing metal cuttings.

In 1960, the first Report and Guide to Hygiene and Sanitation in Aviation was published. This addressed many of the flight line operational issues related to biological hazards. Disposal of passenger-generated waste presents a potential infection hazard to ground personnel. Animal transport by air introduces the possibility of spread of zoonoses to airline and ground personnel. The aircraft as a vector for disease transmission is addressed elsewhere (Chapter 35).

ERGONOMIC HAZARDS

Ergonomics has been defined by Chaffin as the science of fitting the job to the worker (15). In both flight line operations and aircraft manufacturing, this interaction of workers with machines focuses on the one hand with compatibility of the worker's capabilities and limitations and the job requirements and machine interface on the other. Ergonomic design is well appreciated in the cockpit, but may receive little consideration in engineering the job of a millwright in a cutting machine operation or the biomechanics of baggage handling for ground personnel. Ergonomic hazards can be defined as physical stressors and environmental conditions that pose a potential risk of injury or illness to a worker. These physical stressors are described as repetition, force, posture, and vibration. To these stressors must be added the issues of poor job design, inadequate work station layout, negative work organizational factors such as work rates, shift work, work-rest cycles, and managerial insensitivity.

Disregarding ergonomic factors can lead to work related injury and disability. Assembly-line work requiring a repetitive cycle of less than 30 seconds has been associated with upper extremity musculoskeletal injury. The application of poor body mechanics to lifting, pulling, or pushing are major contributors to low back pain and disability. The significant increase in carpal tunnel syndrome over the past 20 years has been attributed in part to repetitive injury and biomechanical strain. In 1985, NIOSH released its Proposed National Strategy for the Prevention of Work-Related Musculoskeletal Injury (16). This documented the need to control work related low back injuries as a national goal. One of the resulting strategies was the development of new lifting guidelines. This effort led to the development of the revised 1961 Lifting Equation for Material Handling (17).

To determine ergonomic risk, it is helpful to perform a job analysis which evaluates job requirements and psychophysiological variables, as well as environmental factors. This is the hallmark of prevention: anticipating risks, validating the degree of risk, and then modifying or reducing the risk to avoid biomechanical injury.

ETHICS

For whom do you work? This is a question that each physician must not only ask but answer when entering the field of Occupational Medicine. It must be realized that the simple answer "the patient" may not always be appropriate. Is recommending halting a manufacturing process, because it may have high risk to a worker, even at the cost of the job, serving "the patient?" Is the job applicant upon whom you perform a preplacement examination "a patient?" Is making a recommendation regarding fitness-to-work best serving "the patient" when you have no idea what the duties of the job entail? Do you have a professional, ethical, or moral obligation to the employer who may be paying your salary or the bill?

Ethical issues frequently arise in OEM practice, because of competing interests, economic issues, regulatory requirements, and organizational power structures.

In defining ethics, Rest describes what it is not before indicating what it is. Ethics is neither law nor social custom; it is not personal preference or consensus. Rather she holds that ethics are guides for action that are consistent to held values, principles, or rules that are able to withstand close moral scrutiny.

In 1993, the American College of Occupational and Environmental Medicine, (ACOEM) revised its code of ethical conduct. These standards are intended to guide OEM physicians in their relationship with: the individuals they serve, employers and workers' representatives, colleagues in the health profession, the public, and all levels of government including the judiciary.

Physicians should:

1. accord the highest priority to the health and safety of individuals in both the workplace and the environment;
2. practice on a scientific basis with integrity and strive to acquire and maintain adequate knowledge and expertise upon which to render professional service;
3. relate honestly and ethically in all professional relationships;
4. strive to expand and disseminate medical

knowledge and participate in ethical research efforts as appropriate;

5. keep confidential all individual medical information, releasing such information only when required by law or overriding public health considerations, or to other physicians according to accepted medical practice, or to others at the request of the individual;

6. recognize that employers may be entitled to counsel about an individual's medical work fitness, but not to diagnoses or specific details, except in compliance with laws and regulations;

7. communicate to individuals and/or groups any significant observations and recommendations concerning their health or safety; and

8. recognize those medical impairments in oneself and others, including chemical dependency and abusive personal practices, which interfere with one's ability to follow the above principles, and take appropriate measures.

Professionals of good conscience may differ in the interpretation of such guidelines. The long term focus should not be on the differences but rather on the continuing dialogue which helps to craft refined definitions which meet the expectations of a widening circle of professional colleagues, workers, and employers.

ACKNOWLEDGMENT

Material appearing in a similar chapter of the 1st edition, contributed by Robert T. P. deTreville, appears in this chapter.

REFERENCES

1. DeHart RL. Occupational medicine support for international air carriers. Aviat Space Environ Med 1990; 61: 67–70.
2. Ramazzini B. Diseases of workers. The Classics of Medicine Library, Special Edition. Chicago: University of Chicago Press, 1983.
3. Hamilton A. Exploring the dangerous trades. Boston: Little, Brown, and Company, 1943.
4. Dhenin G, ed. Aviation medicine. London: Tri-Med Books, Ltd., 1978.
5. DeHart RL. Guidelines for establishing an occupational medical program. Am Occup Med Association, 1987.
6. American Conference of Governmental Industrial Hygienists. Threshold limit values for chemical substance and physical agents. ACGIH, Cincinnati, OH, 1995.
7. Hatch TF. Changing objectives in occupational health. Am Indust Hygiene Association J 1962;23:(1),.
8. Proctor NH, Hughes JP, Fischman ML, 2nd ed. Chemical hazards of the workplace. Philadelphia: J.B. Lippincott Co., 1988.
9. Hodge HC, Sterner JH. Tabulation of toxicity classes. Am Indust Hygiene Q 10:93, 1949.
10. Wald PH and Stave GM, ed. Physical and biological hazards of the workplace. New York: Van Nostrand Reinhold, 1994.
11. Zenz C, Dickerson OB, Horvath EP, eds, 3rd ed. Occupational medicine. St. Louis, MO: Mosby—YearBook, Inc., 1994.
12. OSHA. Occupational Noise Exposure: hearing conservation amendment; final rule. Federal Register. 1983; 48:9738–84.
13. Oak Ridge Associated Universities. Health effects of low-frequency electric and magnetic fields. ORAU, 1992.
14. Interventional Radiation Protection Association. Protection of workers against radio-frequency and microwave radiation. Occupational Health and Safety Series #57. International Labor Office, Geneva, 1987.
15. Chaffin DB, Anderson GBJ. Occupational biomechanics. New York: Wiley, 1984.
16. National Institute for Occupational Safety and Health. Proposed national strategy for the prevention of work-related musculoskeletal injury. NIOSH Publication No. 89–129, Cincinnati, 1985.
17. National Institute for Occupational Safety and Health. Guide to manual lifting. NIOSH, Cincinnati, 1993.
18. Rest KM. Ethics and occupational health. In: Levy BS, Wegmon DW, eds. Occupational Health, 2nd ed. Boston: Little, Brown and Co., 1988

Chapter 35

Aviation and the Environment

A. J. Parmet

We see our Earth as a whole planet. We observe the oceans, forests, mountains, cities and roads, and we absolutely do not see the borders between nations.

Cosmonaut Yuri Romankenko

After almost a century of unparalleled and unrestrained technological advances in aviation, there is growing concern that aerospace operations contribute to environmental pollution. Perhaps more important are the air- and space-based observations that contribute to our understanding of the earth's ecology. This chapter will discuss some of the more popular notions and assess the impact of aviation upon understanding our environment.

The effect of aircraft-associated contaminants on crewmembers, passengers, and maintenance personnel has been discussed (see Chapter 34), as have the basics of toxicology and physics. This chapter will focus on the effect of the industry on the general community and how remote sensing has served to change the way we view ourselves and our planet.

ENVIRONMENTAL ASSESSMENT

National Environmental Policy Act

On January 1, 1970, the National Environmental Policy Act (NEPA) of 1969 was signed into law. In part, this law was the result of public awareness brought about by photographs taken from space. Much more than environmental catastro-

phes, such as the contamination of Minimata Bay or Love Canal, the impact of these pictures raised the public consciousness. Within the decade that followed, ecology became a household word and a potent force in contemporary society, influencing everything from international politics to individual lifestyles (1). As stated in the law, the purposes of NEPA are fourfold:

1. To declare a national policy that will encourage productive and enjoyable harmony between humans and their environment.
2. To promote efforts that will prevent or eliminate damage to the environment and biosphere and stimulate the health and welfare of people.
3. To enrich the understanding of the ecologic systems and natural resources important to the nation.
4. To establish a Council of Environment quality.

Federal agencies are directed to use an integrated, interdisciplinary, approach using both the natural and social sciences to evaluate environmental problems. Then they will develop relevant techniques and methods to ensure that unquantifiable amenities receive the same attention

given to the more tangible economic and technological considerations. This dual approach directive evolved into the environmental assessment
process leading to the preparation of detailed environmental consequences of proposed actions
and programs.

Environmental Impact Statements

Every federal agency is now required to include
a detailed environmental impact statement (EIS)
in each recommendation or report on proposals
for legislation and other major federal actions
significantly affecting the quality of the environment. This statement must include the following:

1. Environmental impact of the proposed action
2. Adverse environmental effect that cannot be
   avoided should the action take place
3. Possible alternatives
4. Discussion of short-term versus long-term
   advantages of the proposal
5. Irreversible and irretrievable commitment of
   resources that would be involved if the proposed action were implemented

The concept is simple, but the process of collecting data, writing, reviewing, debating, and
acting on the statement is complex and time-
consuming. Most state and local governments
have legislation similar to NEPA to assist in
making environmentally related decisions.
State, local, and even private-sector actions that
require federal funds require the preparations of
EISs under NEPA.

AIRPORT-COMMUNITY NOISE
PROBLEMS

As a result of advances in aviation technology
and increased air travel, aircraft noise has become increasingly prevalent in communities
during the last decade or so. Along with the
increase in airport noise has been a public
awareness of, and irritation with, the noise.

Sometimes, this irritation has culminated in
complaints and even vigorous opposition to airport operations.

In 1952, Harry Truman convened a President's Airport Commission, the Doolittle Commission, to evaluate the growing airport system.
The Commission concluded the following,
among other things:

*Some excuse may be found for failure to have
foreseen the rapid rate of aeronautical progress
in designing airports in the past, but it is to be
regretted that more consideration was not given
to the comfort and welfare of people living on
the ground in the vicinity of airports. To be sure,
many settled near an airport after it was in operation, with little realization of the potential
nuisance and hazard. The public cannot be expected, however, to anticipate technical developments and it should be informed and protected
by the responsible authorities (2).*

Human Effects of Noise

According to the Department of Transportation,
some 3% of our population, over 7 million persons, have been exposed to an excessive level
of aircraft noise. Older aircraft, such as the
Boeing 707, are still in use and produce about
twice the noise that the Federal Aviation Administration (FAA) rules allow for new airplanes.
Present exposures are generally unacceptable
and create considerable annoyance in most communities.

Temporary or Permanent Hearing Loss

The research basis for the Walsh-Healey Act
Hearing Conservation Standards involved industrial situations with a fairly constant noise
level during an 8-hour workday and an assumed
quiet residential environment for rest and recovery of the auditory system during the other 16
hours of the day. The act now limits an exposure of 106 dBA for a maximum of 1 hr/day
or 100 dBA for a maximum of 2 hr/day. This
maximum approximates the noise level to which

communities closer than 5 to 6 km from airport runways are intermittently exposed. Thus an individual living in a noisy residential environment could be exposed to noise in excess of the cumulative occupational standard.

Physiologic Responses

Noise also can trigger changes in cardiovascular, endocrine, and neurologic functions and is correlated with feelings of distress. Sound levels above 120 dB significantly affect these functions (3).

Speech Interference

The most disruptive and widespread effect of noise is masking, or interference with the reception of speech. This interference is a major factor in aircraft noise annoyance. Surveys conducted in airport neighborhoods indicate that aircraft noise interference with speech, whether in face-to-face conversations, telephone use, or radio and television listening, is more annoying than any other type of noise disturbance except interference with sleep.

Interference with Rest, Privacy, and Sleep

Complaints received by airport authorities indicate that interference with sleep causes relatively more intense annoyance and hostility toward aircraft noise than do daytime interruptions of communications and social functions. Thus, all composite noise indexes place a significance on a nighttime noise exposure equal to 10 daytime exposures. A further concern is that repeated arousal from sleep could generally lead to degradation of health because rest and sleep provide conditions for the recovery from fatigue.

Psychologic Annoyance and Irritability

The interruption of speech and sleep and the nonauditory effects of aircraft noise are undesirable, but these interferences do not necessarily produce equal annoyance or hostility among differently predisposed people. Studies such as the one conducted by Tracor, Inc., reported that when noise exposure was the sole predictor, esti-

mation of community annoyance was poor (4). When other psychologic and social variables were included, the prediction equation was improved. Twenty variables were investigated, including individual susceptibility to noise, distance from the airport, noise adaptability, city of residence, belief in malfeasance on the part of those able to do something about the noise problem, and the extent to which the airport and air transportation were viewed as important by the respondent. Only the fear of aircraft crashing in the neighborhood contributed more to annoyance and irritability than all the other variables.

Complex Noise Measurement

The methods of measuring single noise exposures have proliferated, each method attempting to integrate the different spectral characteristics of different sounds into simple units of equal noisiness or unpleasantness. These units of noise measurement, however, cannot accurately describe units of environmental annoyance. By definition, noise is unwanted sound, and its unwantedness cannot be measured realistically without considering the meaning and emotional content of the noise, as well as its effect in interfering with various desired activities.

Since 1952, techniques have been used to determine how people in natural settings perceived noise and what psychosocial variables influenced their reactions to these noise exposures. The major disadvantages of the survey technique are that data collections are costly and time consuming, and only gross averages of the complex stimulus situations are possible. Engineers and noise abatement officials need to know the independent and interacting contributions of the components of a noise experience to assess the cost benefits of specific proposals for noise reduction.

More recent research at Columbia University placed human subjects in an acoustic laboratory that was furnished as a typical living room in a middle-class home. In this home a quadraphonic sound system was employed to produce a realistic aircraft noise experience in which the plane appeared to fly overhead across the room. This technique controlled the eight basic variables: type of plane, operations, slant distance, time of exposure (and by season), rate per hour, position of the subject, ambient noise, and activities. The subjects rated each randomly allocated experimental noise in terms of the degree of interference with activity, such as watching television, and the degree of annoyance resulting from the interference (5).

Research from the past three decades has produced much useful information on noise propagation and the human response to it. Much more, however, still needs to be learned to answer the practical questions posed by noise abatement officials.

Noise has become regulated, as have all other forms of environmental residue. Environmental Protection Agency (EPA) noise control activities are authorized by the Noise Pollution and Abatement Act of 1970 (Title IV of the Clean Air Act) and the Noise Control Act of 1972 (Public Law 92–574). The Federal Aviation Administration (FAA) also is assigned certain responsibilities in the control and abatement of aircraft noise in Section 7 of the latter act.

The EPA Office of Noise Abatement and Control is responsible for identifying and classifying causes and sources of noise, determining their effects on public health and welfare, and proposing any national standards and regulations necessary to protect the public health and welfare. Noise-monitoring activities are authorized in the Noise Control Act under Section 14, which deals with research, technical assistance to state and local governments, and public information.

The FAA's responsibilities under the Noise Control Act of 1972 are to provide current and future relief from aircraft noise through appropriate noise control and abatement regulations.These goals are accomplished through the Federal Aviation Regulations (FARs). Of particular interest is FAR Part 36, which prescribes noise standards for aircraft type and airworthiness certification. Part 36 was amended, effective April 3, 1978, and prescribes amended noise limits for new airplane designs, limits the noise level increase of certain older airplanes if their designs are changed, and amends noise-measuring points and noise test conditions. This amendment brings U.S. aircraft noise standards into greater conformity with the international standards recently adopted by the International Civil Aviation Organization (ICAO).

ICAO noise standards, found in the ICAO Annex 16, currently divide transport planes into Chapter 2 aircraft (older planes such as the Boeing 727 and 737, Douglas DC-9, and all Soviet-built transports) and Chapter 3 aircraft (all newer planes such as Boeing 757, 767 and 777, McDonnell MD-80 and MD-11 and the Airbus A-300 and A-320) with others being classed as Non-Noise Certificated. In 1987, 4922 Chapter 2 aircraft in operation made up 62% of all commercial passenger-carrying aircraft worldwide. Another 5% were Non-Noise Certificated. By 2005, attrition due to aging or retrofitting should reduce the numbers of Chapter 2 aircraft in operation worldwide to 1650 (6).

FAR Part 150 regulates noise compatibility programs for airports. These programs, along with local rules, restrict certain aircraft types and times of operations. The implementation of these restrictions has not gone unchallenged. A series of legal battles have upheld the community's right to restrict airport traffic. One controversy local authorities have won is to consider peak sound levels instead of average levels. Consider the following: a single event of 110 dB at 2:00 AM may average out to only 65 dB over the entire day, but the annoyance factor is quite high. Possibly the most restrictive community airport in the world is John Wayne Airport, Orange County, California. Operating times are restricted, and noise limits ban many aircraft types. At least six other airports in the United States are in the process of validating their restrictions (7).

Other applicable laws include the Quiet Communities Act (Public Law 95–609), which amends certain portions of the Noise Control Act of 1972, promotes the development of effective state and local noise control programs, and provides for an adequate federal noise control research program. Section 14 of this act also provides for the administrations of a nationwide Quiet Communities Program.

The Aviation Safety and Noise Abatement Act of 1979 (Public Law 96–193) specified noise emission standards and provided for "exemptions from applicable noise standards to permit operation of any non-complying three engine aircraft, but not beyond January 1, 1983 for delivery by January 1, 1985." Similarly, two-engine aircraft were exempted until January 1, 1986, permitting a phased entry for manufacturers to meet deliveries. This act requires that airport operators submit a Noise Compatibility Program to the Secretary of the Department of Transportation. The program addresses, but is not limited to, the following:

1. Implementation of any preferential runway system
2. Restriction of airport use by any type or class of aircraft based on noise characteristics
3. Construction of barriers and acoustic shielding, including sound proofing of public buildings
4. The use of flight procedures to control operations of aircraft to reduce exposure of individuals to noise in areas around the airport
5. Acquisition of land, air rights, easements, and so on to ensure the use of property for purposes that are compatible with airport operations

Section 103 of this act provided for the preparation and submission of noise exposure maps for developmental and planning purposes. The objective is to reduce existing incompatible use.

Final noise rules issued by the FAA in September 1991 implemented the Airport Noise and Capacity Act of 1990 and mandated the elimination of Stage 2 aircraft by the year 2000. Postponement of full compliance until 2003 would be permitted only for those carriers experiencing

financial difficulties. Local airports wishing to impose Stage 2 standards in advance of the Act must allow 180 days notice and permit any interested party to file objections and initiate legal delay. Stage 3 operations can only be implemented voluntarily by all parties (8).

The rule of Stage 2 phaseout requires any given airline to reduce its Stage 2 fleet from the 1991 level by 25% in 1994, 50% by 1996, and 75% by 1998 and to effect Stage 3 compliance by 2000. The options available for reducing aircraft noise levels at the source include retrofitting, reengining, and replacement. Retrofitting refers to the placement of sound-absorbent material in the engines and nacelles and altering the sound characteristics of intakes and exhausts. Retrofitting a transport with a "hushkit" reduces engine noise and the "footprint" or area affected (Fig. 35.1) but increases weight by about 300 kg per engine. There is also a fuel penalty, since the engines are required to operate at lower, less efficient thrust settings during takeoff and landing (9).

Reengining requires a lowering of the jet exhaust velocity, either with lowered performance of the old engine and reduced efficiency or with replacement with new engines using larger bypass fans around the core gas turbine (10). The option preferred by most people in the aircraft business appears to be replacement over retrofit or reengining.

Expenses Involved With Compliance

The cost of compliance is staggering. The implementation of ICAO Chapter 3 requirements alone are expensive. A 1995 ban throughout Europe cost airlines an estimated $500 million in reengining or new planes. To meet this 1995 deadline worldwide would have cost $9.5 billion; delay until 2005 reduces the cost to $3.5 billion. As one African delegate to the ICAO stated, "The cost to airlines will be an impossible burden, particularly to those of the developing countries" (11). A more competitive environment, along with increased operating costs, will serve as fuel in the fight to delay

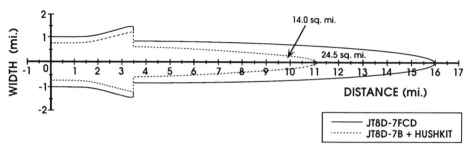

Figure 35.1. Typical 85-dB noise footprints for Boeing 727 on takeoff comparing Pratt and Whitney JT8D engines without and with noise reduction modifications. (From Kandebo SW. Launch of Roll's reengining plan poses challenge to JT8D hushkits. Aviation Week and Space Technology, 131 (20):1124. May 14, 1990.)

implementation of noise restrictions in many countries until old age retires many of the noisier planes.

Coordination and Planning

Controlling aircraft noise at the source has been achieved primarily through the use of turbofan engines. These alone have cut the noise exposure in half since their introduction (12). The long economic life of commercial aircraft (approximately 25 years), means that some limited technology improvements can still be applied, but at increasing cost. Measures to combat aircraft noise at the source are now into diminishing returns with increases in operating costs and fuel expenditures disproportionately large compared to the limited decreases in noise.

Although noise source control is necessary, there must also be planning to ensure that land around airports is not used for purposes incompatible with existing and projected noise levels. State and local governments can control the land use through zoning. They also can take other measures, such as assuring that noise exposure levels are revealed in real estate transactions. Local governments also have the responsibility to take noise levels into account in locating and designing schools, hospitals, and other public buildings and in developing highways, sewers, and other basic services that influence local development. This is greatly preferable to forcing departing aircraft to reduce thrust to minimum

flying requirements, creating unsafe situations in the name of noise abatement.

This twofold approach to the solution of the problem of aircraft noise is the only reasonable way to achieve a reduction in the noise experience of people living in airport environs in the future.

SONIC BOOMS

A unique environmental effect of supersonic flight is the sonic boom. Much like the bow wave of a ship, the wave pattern traveling with the aircraft sweeps over the terrain, similar to the advancing shock wave of a mild explosion. Numerous sonic boom studies have been done during the past three decades due to the increased operation of high-performance military aircraft, the proposed U.S. supersonic transport (SST), and the entry of the Anglo-French Concorde SST into commercial airline service. Documentation of the phenomenon and its effects has been extensively reported (13,14).

Effects of Sonic Boom

Figure 35.2 shows the effect of the atmosphere above and below the aircraft on the development of the primary and secondary carpets. It depicts an aircraft at 20 km altitude flying toward the viewer. The downward rays (solid lines) impact the terrain to form the primary boom carpet, extending to 40 km in this example. A secondary carpet region is depicted at about 120 to 170

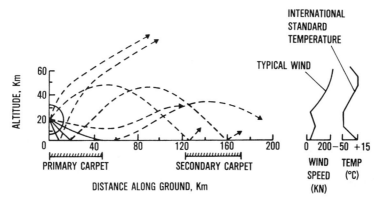

Figure 35.2. Propagation paths of sonic booms.

km from the flight track. The dashed line rays impacting in this carpet may arrive directly as a result of bending in the upper atmosphere, or they may first impact in the primary carpet region, then reflect upward and subsequently bend downward into the secondary region. Between these two carpets there is no boom.

Primary Boom Carpet

The primary boom carpet and its disturbances have been researched intensely and involve only propagation in the lower atmosphere. The disturbances involve high overpressures and steep rise times and have a substantial high-frequency content. Overpressures may reach 700 N/m^2. Levels increase with increasing aircraft size and decrease with increasing altitude. Highest overpressures occur near ground track and are associated with an N- wave-type signature. This is an impact steep rise time followed by straight-line recovery through the negative phase and abrupt cessation. Promulgation distances are typically less than 50 km, and at the lateral cutoff point, the N-wave form is lost and the boom becomes a rumble. Sonic booms in the primary carpet cause adverse community response.

Secondary Boom Carpet

The secondary boom carpet and its disturbances are not as well defined. Only fragmentary obser-

vations and measurements are available. These disturbances involve both the upper and lower levels of the atmosphere during propagation and have low-frequency content. Propagation distances of greater than 150 km are common, and relatively large areas are exposed. Secondary carpet booms are generally not audible (0.1 to 1.0 Hz) but can cause building vibrations that are readily observed. These boomlets were initially observed in coastal New Jersey when Concorde service from Europe to New York was initiated, and were connected with the flights only after much detective work. They remain more of a curiosity and are not likely to cause serious adverse community response.

Community Response

Human response to impulse noise (such as sonic booms) is most complex, involving not only the physical stimulus but also the immediate environment (ambient noise conditions), the experience, attitudes, and opinions of those exposed, and other factors not directly related to the stimulus. Individual and group reactions to sonic booms are summarized by Von Gierke in Figure 35.3 (15). Similar experiences have now been documented in domestic and wild animals (16).

During the mid-1960s, numerous studies of public reactions to sonic booms were conducted in selected metropolitan areas of the United States and France. In these studies, the number

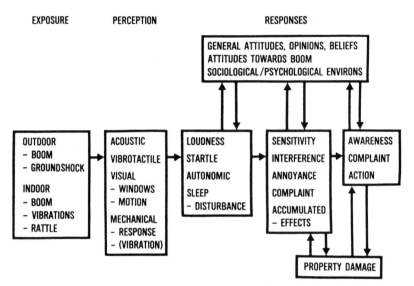

Figure 35.3. Reactions to sonic booms.

of complaints reported was small. Popular notions that sonic booms cause snow avalanches or affect egg hatching and livestock adversely are not supported by scientific data (16,17). Considerably more frequent and just as loud are thunderstorms, which also have little effect. All these notions and resultant studies produced enough concern over annoyance to cause the FAA to prohibit civil aircraft flights at speeds that create a sonic boom over U.S. territory. This action effectively ended intensive sonic boom research in 1972, although observations in military jet training areas continues to supply useful information.

Before this decision was made, many proposals were advanced to decrease the sonic booms of the SSTs. One of the more imaginative approaches suggested an electromagnetic device to elongate the fuselage signature to modify the shock wave. Thousands of megawatts of electrical power, however, were required to achieve a 10% reduction in boom intensity, and the equipment required exceeded the payload capability of the SST. Another proposal would use a second penalty aircraft in formation with the SST so that the shock waves would cancel each other. Neither of these approaches is economically fea-

sible. The latest version is the staged SST, with the noisy SST carried aloft on the back of a larger transport. This old idea has been tried several times over the last 60 years, never with much success (18).

More practical is the oblique wing aircraft, in which one wing sweeps forward and the other sweeps aft during supersonic flight. This arrangement causes the shock waves from each wing to be out of phase and nonreinforcing. A subsonic experimental model, the AD-1, was flight-tested in the late 1980s, defining flight stability and demonstrating the concept. The future probably belongs to hypersonic vehicles flying so high that no appreciable energy reaches ground level, combined with cleaner burning engines that can reduce oxides of nitrogen emissions by 90% (19).

RADIOFREQUENCY RADIATION

Characteristics and Sources

Radiofrequency (RF) radiation occupies the lowest frequency band of the electromagnetic spectrum. RF frequencies range from 10 kilohertz to 300 gigahertz, with wavelengths varying from 30

Table 35.1.
Radiofrequency and Microwave Band Designations

Band Designation			
United States	Wavelengths	Frequencies	Typical Uses
Radiofrequency bands			
Low frequency (LF)	10^4–10^3 m	30–300 kHz	Radionavigation, radio beacon
Medium frequency (MF)	10^3–10^2 m	0.3–3 MHz	Marine radiotelephone, loran, AM broadcast
High frequency (HF)	10^2–10 m	3–30 MHz	Amateur radio, worldwide broadcasting, medical diathermy, radio astronomy
Microwave bands			
Very high frequency (VHF)	10–1 m	30–300 MHz	FM broadcast, television, air traffic control, radionavigation
Ultra high frequency (UHF)	1–0.1 m	0.3–3 GHz	Television, citizens band, microwave point-to-point, microwave ovens, telemetry, tropo scatter, and meteorologic radar
Super high frequency (SHF)	10–1 cm	3–30 GHz	Satellite communication, airborne weather radar, altimeters, shipborne navigational radar, microwave point-to-point
Extra high frequency (EHF)	1–0.1 cm	30–300 GHz	Radio astronomy, cloud detection radar, space research, HCN (hydrogen cyanide) emission

Modified from Wilkening GM. Nonionizing radiation. In: The industrial environment—its evaluation and control. National Institute of Occupational Safety and Health, U.S. Government Printing Office, Washington, D.C., 1973;357–373.

km to about 1 mm. Wavelength determines the amount of RF absorption and greatly defines the use and bioeffects. Table 35.1 displays the features of RF and microwave bands (20).

The growing number of domestic, commercial, and medical applications of RF technology (microwave ovens, materials drying, and diathermy) has resulted in a greater awareness and concern on the part of the public as to potential hazards. The expanded use of RF emitters has also greatly ''polluted'' that part of the spectrum used by radioastronomers and made their work more difficult.

Microwave sources may operate continuously (communication), intermittently (microwave oven), or in a pulsed mode (radar). Natural sources of RF radiation also exist. The movement of a cold front may generate peak field intensities of over 100 V/m at ground level. Solar radiation also includes a relatively small fraction of RF radiation.

Biologic Effects

The photon energy in RF radiation is too low to produce ionizations by knocking electrons off atoms or molecules; the 300 GHz photons have only one ten-thousandth the energy of visible light photons. Instead, the energy is absorbed by the tissues and is manifested as heat, which must then be dissipated. A permissible exposure level (PEL) was originally set at 10 mW/cm^2 across the RF spectrum using the idea that a maximum of 58 W of energy could be absorbed, with a body temperature elevation of 1°C. This rise should be well within the thermoregulatory ability of all individuals. In comparison, the human basal metabolic rate approximates 80 W at rest and increases to 290 W with moderate work.

Absorption at different frequencies is dependent upon the size and orientation of the exposed individual. Due to ground coupling effects, maximum absorption by humans is in the 35- to 80-megahertz range. Accordingly, in 1982 the American National Standards Institute (ANSI) adopted maximum safe PELs for human exposure (averaged over a 6-minute period), which are shown in Table 35.2 (21).

While the ANSI standard is for whole-body exposure, regional irradiation may produce different effects, varying with depth of penetration

Table 35.2.
The American National Standards Institute Human Exposure Limits

Frequency (MHz)	Power Density (mW/cm^2)
0.01–3	100
3–30	900/f
30–300	1.0
300–1500	f/300
1500–100,000	5.0

f, frequency (MHz).
From American National Standards Institute (21).

and absorption of RF energy. Again, tissue penetration varies with wavelength. Wavelengths less than 3 cm are absorbed in the outer skin layer; wavelengths of 3 to 10 cm may penetrate up to 1 cm, and wavelengths of 25 to 100 cm may penetrate more deeply and have the potential of damaging internal organs. The human body is thought to be virtually transparent to wavelengths above 200 cm. At wavelengths less than 1 cm, the depth of penetration declines rapidly with frequency and is only millimeters at micrometer wavelengths (22).

Considerable public interest has been shown in the potential of chronic low-level microwave exposure to cause cataracts and other illnesses. In test animals, lens opacities have been produced under controlled conditions with power densities of 80 to 40 mW/cm^2 (well above the PEL). These levels require anesthesia of the animals and shielding of the head to prevent death due to burns. Case-control epidemiologic studies strongly indicate that there is no greater risk of cataract formation in the exposed groups. Fetal exposure of test animals does not demonstrate increased risk at levels safe for the mother (23).

Athermic effects have been postulated, possibly due to magnetic field induction. This is manifested as ''radiowave sickness'' in eastern European literature but is not recognized as an entity elsewhere. Assessment of this phenomenon continues.

Obsolete, unshielded cardiac pacemakers, particularly the demand type, may be theoretically compromised by nearby microwave radiation at levels far below those causing thermal effects. Shielding of pacemakers and appropriate warning signs have provided the answer. In the medical field, microwave radiation plays a useful and expanding role in therapy. The judicious exposure of humans to diathermy may be as high as 100 mW/cm^2, and is an excellent method for applying localized heat with controlled penetration.

Assessment

Low-level RF radiation appears to pose no real threat to the general environment or to individuals. The PELs at all levels are one tenth the exposure demonstrated to cause biologic effects. Generators and transmitters are ordinarily inaccessible or airborne. Industrial hygiene and safety monitoring are adequate. Many of the systems are low power (less than 25 mW), most are omnidirectional, and some rotate at 12 rpm, keeping area flux down. Standard tower heights are 10 to 20 m, whereas 12 m away from a generator is generally safe. Navigational radar is directed 2° or more above the horizon, posing no threat to the community. The major danger of significant exposure to microwave and RF radiation is to avionics and maintenance personnel if there is a lapse in safety procedures as a generator is energized. The installation of an interlock system, hard-wired to any entryway, will automatically turn off power if a hazardous area is entered. Particular care must be devoted to the development and operation of tracking radar systems due to the lock-on phenomenon.

IONIZING RADIATION

The threat of terrorist bombing or hijacking has mandated the screening of passengers, baggage, and cargo. To minimize delays, most airports and airlines rapidly screen with detailed searches performed only on selected articles. People are screened as they walk through magnetic sensors. Hand baggage is screened using x-ray equipment. A review of baggage x-ray machines revealed that as many as 8% exceeded emissions limits and posed an occupational hazard to the operators. Passengers and other airport employees were not exposed to any significant risk (24).

The future screening of baggage for nonmetallic threats may be done by neutron-scanning devices. The nature, extent, and cost of these techniques is yet to be determined.

ATMOSPHERIC POLLUTION

Aircraft Emission

Aircraft contribute but a small portion of total atmospheric emissions from all sources on a national scale. Aircraft account for about 1% of hydrocarbons, oxides of nitrogen, and carbon monoxide and an even smaller fraction of particulate matter and oxides of sulfur. Commercial aircraft have lower hydrocarbons but higher emissions of oxides of nitrogen than do military aircraft because of their larger and newer engines (Table 35.3). General aviation aircraft contribute the least and have been exempted from emission standards. Tetraethyl lead has been removed from aviation gasoline in the United

States but not in other countries. Because of the long-term, devastating effects of even low lead exposures to children, consideration must be given to completely eliminate any traces of lead from the environment (25).

At the regional and local levels, the contributions of aircraft may be greater. Table 35.3 presents information on the Atlanta, Georgia, region as well as the Atlanta Airport. At the regional level, aircraft contribute about 3% of total emissions. At the airport, aircraft are the predominant source of emissions; surface traffic is second. Dispersion and dilution of aircraft emissions occurs more rapidly than surface traffic emissions in congested terminal areas (26).

In addition to aircraft engine improvements, air pollution at airports can be reduced by changes in ground operations procedures. Among the alternatives available are the following:

1. Controlling the times of departure to minimize the time spent idling in queue on the taxiway
2. Assigning aircraft to runways to minimize

Table 35.3.
Aircraft Contribution to Air Pollution

Source	Hydrocarbons (%)	Oxides of Nitrogen (%)	Carbon Monoxide (%)
National level			
All aircraft	1.2	0.6	0.6
Commercial	0.3	0.4	0.2
Military	0.7	0.2	0.2
General aviation	0.2	—	0.2
All sources	30 MT/y	MT/y	116 MT/y
Regional (Atlanta area)			
Aircraft	3.2	3.1	2.4
Fuel evaporation	0.8	—	—
All sources	89 kt/y	75 kt/y	300 kt/y
Local (Atlanta airport)			
Aircraft	69	75	58
Fuel evaporation	11	—	—
Traffic, other	20	22	42
All sources	3.9 kt/y	2.9 kt/y	9.5 kt/y

Modified from Naugle D, Fox DL. Aircraft and air pollution. Environ Sci Technol 1981;15:342.
MT/y, *metric megatons/year;* kty, *metric kilotons/year.*

taxi distance andtime between gate and runway

3. Shutting down one or more engines during taxi operations
4. Towing aircraft between runways and gates (while considering the emissions of the towing vehicle in assessing the net reduction)

Controversy continues as to whether aircraft emissions directly endanger public health and welfare and whether federal regulation is needed to control aircraft atmospheric pollution. Critics point out that regulations promulgated by the EPA in 1973 under the Clean Air Act are too complex and stringent and have yet to be substantiated by proper air quality studies. Further, significant energy shortages, economic problems, and safety considerations impact on the feasibility of antipollution measures.

Fuel Dumping

Fuel dumping, or fuel jettisoning, is the discharge of unburned fuel directly into the atmosphere by an aircraft while airborne. The basic purpose for jettisoning fuel is to reduce the aircraft's gross weight to permit a safe landing. To perform their missions, many aircraft must take off with a gross weight much higher than their maximum safe landing weight. An emergency or change in operation plans may require the aircraft to land prematurely, and fuel must be jettisoned to reduce the gross weight to a safe level.

When jettisoned, jet fuel quickly breaks up into a small droplets. Within minutes, over 90% dissipates as vapor. When jettisoned 1500 m above ground level at a temperature above freezing, more than 98% of the fuel will evaporate before reaching the ground.

Atmospheric diffusion processes rapidly disperse and dilute the fuel vapors to levels far below those at which they could be harmful in themselves. The principal environmental problem of these hydrocarbon vapors is their contribution to photochemical oxidant pollution

(ozone and smog). This contribution is not important when compared with that of automobiles, aircraft exhausts, and other sources in the region.

The small fraction of fuel persisting in residual droplets may become seed nuclei for the condensation of water, to the extent of causing precipitation. Usually, such droplets settle directly to the ground and are dispersed over a wide area, reducing ground contamination to low levels.

Hydrocarbons released by fuel dumping continue to be dispersed and scrubbed by natural processes until they reach natural background level. Fuel jettisoning does not appear to have any serious environmental implications.

Alternative Fuels

A continuing and increasing interest exists in developing advanced, improved fuels for aircraft propulsion. The environmental pollution potential of each new candidate fuel receives attention along with essential energy and economic considerations.

The aromatic hydrocarbons, in view of their high carbon content, will continue to produce deposit and smoke problems. In contrast, the liquefied hydrocarbon gases are expected to be clean-burning. The alcohols are intermediate as to pollution potential. The nitrogen hydrides, ammonia and hydrazine, are clean-burning in the aviation context.

Beryllium is being substituted for aluminum as the fuel in some solid-propellant rockets destined for use in space. The environmental hazard presented by mishaps during production, testing, or launch should have outweighed the use of beryllium, but the lure of increased energy was too tempting (27).

Liquid hydrogen appears to be the most promising of the alternative fuels evaluated from both the environmental and energy standpoints. The absence of carbon prevents the emission of unburned hydrocarbons, carbon monoxide, carbon dioxide, and most particulates. The only major combustion product is water, which merely returns to the atmosphere. The temperatures involved can give rise to the emission of some oxides of nitrogen but much less than conventional engines. The next generation of supersonic transports, hypersonic and possibly exoatmospheric, may be fueled by liquid hydrogen. The physical properties of hydrogen persist as major obstacles. To remain liquid, hydrogen must be kept below $-253°C$. This intense cold requires special production, handling, and storage techniques. While hydrogen has three times as much energy for the same mass of conventional jet fuel, it has only one fourth the energy density. In other words, a given volume of hydrogen will take an aircraft only one fourth the distance as the same volume of kerosene or Jet A (28).

The major environmental threat in the use of nuclear fuels for aircraft is the potential of a crash landing, with the release of vaporized radioactive materials contaminating a wide area for a long time. A nuclear reactor was tested as a power source in an NB-36 in the 1950s, but the weight of shielding made nuclear-powered aircraft unfeasible. Nuclear reactors and thermal generators may continue to be the key to our future expansion into space, especially for large satellites on extended missions. Adequate safeguards include maintaining the reactor at a subcritical level until orbit is obtained and boosting the reactor into a higher orbit prior to vehicular reentry. The U.S. position is that reactors will only be used for interplanetary exploration missions, but when they are the preferred technical choice, they can be used safely (29). Nuclear fuel wasused extensively by the Soviet Union for Earth-orbiting reconnaissance satellites. To date, three of these have reentered the earth's atmosphere, two over ocean areas. The third, Kosmos 954, crashed in northern Canada on January 24, 1978, contaminating a large area and requiring an extensive cleanup. In each incident, over 50 kg of uranium 235 fuel and radioactive by-products, including cesium, strontium, and cerium, were released (30). As of 1989, 29 Soviet reactors with over 3000 kg of reactor fuel

remain in earth orbit. This constitutes a major environmental concern which must eventually be addressed (31).

Exotic propulsion includes solar-electric power. Improved solar cells, developed for use in space, are finding wider use on Earth. If the relative cost of solar cells drops, they may help to significantly decrease the use of fossil fuels to produce electricity. A solar sail, using the solar wind, is the ultimate low-cost system and is scheduled for testing in the late 1990s.

Contrails

Contrail (condensation trail) formation in the wake of high- flying aircraft is a function of the water-carrying capacity of the ambient atmosphere versus the water content of the exhaust. Whether hydrocarbons, oxides of nitrogen, or other gases in the exhaust make contrails different from regular clouds is not known. It is known that the vapor trails diffuse laterally, suggesting that they may seed the surrounding atmosphere, spawning adjacent new clouds.

Contrails may be causing subtle weather changes in regions with heavy jet traffic, such as the New York-to-Chicago corridor. Local increases in cloud cover have been associated with expanding jet traffic, with a diminishing average difference between daily high and low temperatures. Heavy jet traffic may be causing climatic changes affecting crop production and energy use.

Clouds (regular or contrail) have two main effects: shielding the Earth from the sun by day and reducing radiation heat loss by night. This contributes to a leveling off of diurnal temperature extremes. The apparent trend toward increasing cloud cover in jet- traffic corridors could contribute to cooler summer days and warmer winter nights, thereby reducing costly home heating and cooling requirements and lengthening growing seasons in these regions.

Condensation trail formation introduces the possibility of reducing solar radiation at ground level on the order of 1% in regions with low natural lower cloud cover, adding only a trace to the attenuation of natural cloud cover. The overall effect of contrail formation pales next to industry, power, and ground transportation as the source of midaltitude water.

OZONE DEPLETION

Ozone is both foe and friend to humans. Its presence in the air that surrounds us has adverse effects as a powerful photochemical oxidant on many of the materials we depend on, greatly speeding their deterioration. Animal studies have shown marked pulmonary changes with exposure to ozone, with evidence of decreased resistance to pulmonary infection. Other studies suggest that ozone is a potent mutagenic and carcinogenic agent. As such, ozone in the troposphere is a potentially dangerous pollutant.

On the other hand, without the ozone layer in the stratosphere, life would not be possible on this planet. The recent development of our ability to navigate routinely within the stratosphere has caused concerned debate and scientific investigation as to what effect high-flying, air-breathing machines might have on this protective blanket of ozone.

The total amount of ozone in the atmosphere is small. If it were all accumulated at the earth's surface at standard atmospheric pressure, it would form a layer less than 4 mm thick. Ninety-seven percent of this ozone is distributed in the stratosphere between 19 and 50 km altitude in the lower latitudes and 8 to 50 km near the poles. The amount of ozone normally varies up to 30% from season to season, year to year, and decade to decade, complicating the assessment of environmental factors. However, between 1977 and 1984 there was a 40% decrease in the ozone layer overlying Antarctica, documented first by satellite and later by high-altitude aircraft and balloons (Fig. 35.4) (32).

This stratospheric ozone layer absorbs solar radiation so thoroughly throughout a wide range of wavelengths in the ultraviolet (UV) spectrum that only small amounts reach the earth's sur-face. In the UV-B region (wavelengths from 280 to 320 nm), however, ozone absorbs less than perfectly. A decrease of 10% in ozone would lead to a 20% increase in the UV-B photons reaching ground level.

UV-B radiation causes sunburn and snow blindness, and UV-B is felt to be responsible for most skin cancers and accelerated aging of the skin. Increased UV-B radiation also is associated with decreased agricultural production and with serious damage to certain marine species, particularly surface-dwelling plankton. These plankton form an important source of oxygen and food in the sea. In absorbing the energy of UV radiation, ozone causes a warming of the upper stratosphere and a relative cooling of the troposphere. Thus, it is clear that any major decrease in the stratospheric ozone layer could have serious and far-reaching effects on humans.

To appreciate the effect, if any, that stratospheric flight will have on the ozone layer, it is helpful to review some basic chemical equations that describe the dynamic equilibrium in the natural formation and breakdown of ozone.

Only a generation ago, the ozone equilibrium was thought to be totally described by the following four photochemical equations (the Chapman Reactions) (33, 34):

$$O_2 + UV \text{ (short wave)} = O \qquad (1)$$

$$O + O_2 = O_3 \qquad (2)$$

$$O_3 + UV \text{ (long wave)} = O_2 + O \qquad (3)$$

$$O_3 + O = 2O_2 \qquad (4)$$

Equations 1 and 2 account for the formation of ozone (O_3), which can occur only at high altitudes. In the troposphere, water vapor is present and the reaction becomes:

$$O + H_2O = 2\,OH \qquad (5)$$

and free OH is a highly reactive radical. Therefore, it is imperative that short-wave UV not reach the troposphere. The products of equation

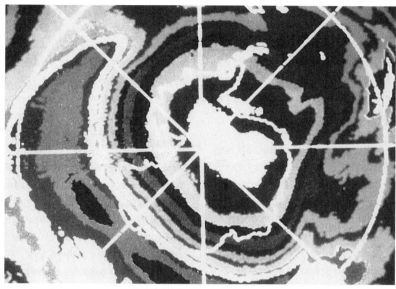

Figure 35.4. The Antarctic ozone hole. Ultraviolet spectrum as viewed by Nimbus 7 (NASA photo).

3 immediately recombine to form ozone, so that only equation 4 accounts for its destruction. When measured, however, the amount of ozone was less than predicted by these equations, so other routes of ozone breakdown were sought.

Around 1970, another method, involving oxides of nitrogen, was proposed to explain a more rapid destruction of ozone:

$$NO_3 + O_3 = NO_2 + O_2 \qquad (6)$$

$$NO_2 + O = NO + O_2 \qquad (7)$$

$$NO + O_2 = NO_3 \qquad (8)$$

Because the catalyst (NO_X) remains unchanged, it is available to "attack" other ozone molecules. Thus, a small amount of NO_X can have a substantial effect in decreasing total ozone. At least 50 other equations are known to involve the ozone layer, but the reactions are judged to be too slow to show any effect.

This information on the link between oxides of nitrogen and ozone depletion coincided with the early SST flights (Concorde and Tupolev 144), which cruise in the low stratosphere (18 to 20 km) and emit large amounts of oxides of nitrogen. This aroused great concern among many environmentalist groups. Consequently, great public pressure was exerted that threatened the existence of the SST program. Based on these equations and a proposed SST fleet of 100 aircraft, it was estimated that the ozone layer would decrease by 10% when equilibrium was reached. This led to alarming predictions, such as an FAA Environmental Impact Statement in 1974 that stated, " . . . the limited flights to be awarded to Concorde would produce an additional 200 cases of skin cancer per year in the United States."

Two years later a reaction was measured by observation which demonstrated that the reaction proceeded 20 times as fast as originally assumed. This reaction is as follows:

$$H_2O + NO_2 = H_2NO_3 \qquad (9)$$

The additional hydration added to the stratosphere reacts with oxides of nitrogen to form nitric acid, which does not react with ozone but is eventually removed by rain. The reaction also removes NO_X so that catalyst reaction terminates.

This last equation (9) reduces the problem of ozone destruction by nitrogen oxides. Results suggest that low-level stratospheric flight (less than 20 km) can actually increase ozone; flight at higher altitudes can decrease ozone but by very small percentages. Thus, stratospheric operation of aircraft is not a significant problem, certainly not as important as other difficulties involved in SST operations. Other major threats to the ozone layer still exist, including the use of nitrogen fertilizers and chlorofluorocarbons(CFCs).

CFCs are synthetic chemicals widely used as refrigerants, aerosol propellants, expanding agents in foams, and electronic parts cleaners. Although highly stable gases, when CFCs are released into the atmosphere, they drift upward until they reach the stratosphere. Once there, UV radiation decomposes the molecules and releases free chlorine. Even in extraordinarily low concentra tions, free chlorine plays havoc with ozone (35). As a catalyst in the reaction:

$$Cl + O_3 = ClO + O_2 \qquad (10)$$

which proceeds as:

$$2ClO = 2Cl + O_2 \qquad (11)$$

Thus the chlorine is not consumed but rather continues to degrade ozone (36). At free chlorine levels of only 1 ppb, ozone is rapidly eliminated. This reaction is only ended when:

$$ClO + NO_2 = ClNO_3 \qquad (12)$$

The effect of ozone layer thinning may already be manifest. In the 1980s, the United States experienced a 7% increase in melanoma cases, but some of this is undoubtedly due to cultural behavior patterns. Recently, arctic ozone depletion has also been detected.

SPACE LAUNCH VEHICLES

Most expendable launch vehicles, such as the Atlas, Ariane, or Proton, are relatively small and have little environmental impact. Larger vehicles, such as the Titan IV, are potentially harmful around the launch site on an order of magnitude less than the space shuttle. Only a low-level destruction of the launch vehicle can cause significant, short-term effects outside the immediate area (37).

The space shuttle is a manned, reusable vehicle: the orbiter, mounted with an expendable external tank containing hydrogen/oxygen propellants and two reusable solid rocket boosters (SRBs), fueled by aluminum/ammonium perchlorate. Integral to the orbiter are three main liquid hydrogen/liquid oxygen rocket engines. An environmental impact occurs during both launch and reentry of the vehicle. At launch, toxic gases are produced in the launch area. As the system penetrates the stratosphere, exhaust products are released that can affect the ozone layer. The orbiter produces sonic booms during both launch and reentry. Table 35.4 shows the exhaust products emitted by the space shuttle into selected atmospheric layers.

Table 35.4.
Exhaust Products Emitted by the Space Shuttle Vehicle Into Selected Atmospheric Layers

Atmospheric Layer	Altitude Range	Hydrogen Chloride (kg)	Chlorine (kg)	Nitric Oxide (kg)	Carbon Monoxide (kg)	Carbon Dioxide (kg)	Water (kg)	Aluminum Oxide (kg)
Surface boundary layer	0 to 500 m	24,666	2741	1697	131	55,075	45,674	39,284
Troposphere	0.5 to 13 km	78,517	9657	4618	839	172,570	152,677	26,385
Stratosphere	13 to 50 km	59,732	11,727	293	2198	147,684	146,393	110,304
Lower mesosphere	50 to 67 km	0	0	0	0	0	15,542	0
Mesosphere thermosphere	Above 67 km	0	0	0	0	0	149,045	0

Modified from Potter AE. Environmental effects of the Space Shuttle, Environ Sci Technol 1978;12:15–21

Table 35.5.
Space Shuttle Exhaust Products

Product	Total per Launch	Launch Site
Aluminum oxide	56 100 kg	10.0 mg/m^3
Hydrogen chloride	35 200 kg	3.9 ppm
Water	65 300 kg	
Carbon dioxide	76 800 kg	
Chlorine	4 000 kg	0.4 ppm
Nitrogen oxides	2 300 kg	0.2 ppm
Carbon monoxide	240 kg	0.02 ppm

TROPOSPHERIC EFFECTS

Exhaust products from the SRB are detailed in Table 35.5. They include significant amounts of hydrogen chloride, chlorine, and nitrogen oxides (38,39–41). This hot exhaust cloud rises rapidly to altitudes of 0.6 to 3 km, then drifts and disperses with the prevailing wind.

A temporary and localized degradation of air quality occurs in regions over which the cloud passes. Surface contaminations are not expected to exceed the allowable limits for humans, wildlife, or plants. Peak concentrations of ground cloud constituents during a standard launch at Kennedy Space Center are also described in Table 35.5 and constitute a significant local acid rainfall.

Acid Rain

The aluminum oxide dust particles form condensation nuclei for the water vapor, resulting in rain. Raindrops falling though the exhaust cloud absorb hydrogen chloride and produce acid rain. The acidity diminishes as hydrogen chloride is washed from the cloud. Near the launch area, the initial rain acidity may reach pH values near 1 and may temporarily damage vegetation. Beyond the immediate launch area, the initial rain is less acidic, and damage is less likely. In any case, the effect is highly localized and temporary in the very wet climate of Florida, where rainfall averages 460 cm per year. If prior to launch, winds threaten to blow exhaust clouds towards inhabited or highly sensitive areas, the launch may be postponed.

Stratospheric Effect

As the space shuttle penetrates the stratosphere, chlorine compounds are introduced into the ozone layer, reducing the ozone level. When the space shuttle program is fully operational at up to 20 launches per year, the mean reduction in ozone level is predicted to be about 0.07%. Further, this 0.07% reduction in ozone is expected to result in about a 0.1% increase in the biologically harmful UV radiation reaching the surface of the earth, a trivial amount compared to the damage wrought by CFCs. The solution is to develop chlorine-free fuel for the SRBs, a project currently under study by the U. S. Air Force.

Sonic Booms

Sonic booms are produced during both launch and reentry of the space shuttle. The intensity of the launch boom approximates 300 N/m^2 over a wide area of the ocean, with a narrow carpet a few hundred meters wide where the focused boom may reach 1500 N/m^2. The launch boom is larger than the orbiter's reentry boom because the total launch vehicle and its exhaust plume are much larger than the orbiter. For launches at Kennedy Space Center, the boom occurs entirely over the Atlantic Ocean and produces no significant environmental impact. The thunderous launch of the shuttle's 6.3 million pounds of thrust exceeds 120 dB at 9 km from the launch pad and 110 dB at 37 k downrange, causing observers to ignore any subsequent boom (42).

The reentry boom of the orbiter is much less, reaching a maximum of 101 N/m^2. The reentry boom, however, occurs over populated areas of California, New Mexico, and Florida. These low-intensity booms have not caused any effect other than a slight startle reaction in some people; for most, it is a signal that the orbiter is passing overhead.

Environmental Factors

Four basic elements are important in the assessment of the environmental impact of any space system:

1. Propulsion-system exhausts associated with the construction and station-keeping activities of the space segment
2. Disposal of waste products while in orbit
3. Physical structure and debris associated with the space segment
4. Launch and landing activities with launches as frequently as every 15 to 30 days

Specific treatment of these environmental concerns is beyond the scope of this chapter. They are presented to provide a perspective on the direction and magnitude of future space exploits and their potential impact on the global and near-Earth environment.

EARTH SYSTEMS SCIENCE

As we have seen, aviation's contribution to pollution and the buildup of greenhouse gases is negligible. Conversely, the understanding of climatic changes is immeasurably due to air- and space-based observations.

Earth systems observations began over a century ago with the use of balloons to measure temperature, pressure, and content of the atmosphere. While aerial photography for military purposes began very early in aviation, organized geographic surveys by aircraft were initiated by a young graduate student, Curtis LeMay, in 1931 (43). Use of color and infrared during World War II has been broadened to include the entire spectrum.

We now have an unparalleled view of our planet. The Earth is a dynamic system driven by the sun. According to space- based observations of the solar cycle by the Solar Maximum Mission (Solar Max, 1977–89), the primacy of insolation is due to variability of the sun's output, now known to have both an 11-year cycle and

a much longer cycle, perhaps varying on the order of centuries. Our sun appears to be near the maximum on the long periodsolar cycle (44).

The Earth Radiation Budget Experiment (ERBE, 1984) helped define the influence of the earth's orbital eccentricity, wobble, and precession upon solar insolation (45). The Upper Atmosphere Research Satellite (UARS, launched in 1991) will help further define the effects greenhouse gas accumulations are having. Laser Geodynamics Satellites (LAGEOS-1, 1976 and LAGEOS-2, 1993), Ocean Topography Satellite (TOPEX, 1992), and Magnetic Survey Satellite (MAGSAT, 1985) have been instrumental in comprehending global norms and fluctuation. Plate tectonics, paleoclimate atmosphere, and ocean dynamics are key drivers in molding the environment. Developing the instruments and techniques to deploy a variety of air and space experiments are part of a comprehensive earth systems observation program (46).

Earth Resources

The ability to monitor the health and condition of large areas of plant life by satellite was vividly demonstrated in the summer of 1988, when forest fires devastated huge areas of Yellowstone National Park in Wyoming. At the same time, a health alert along the beaches of North Carolina gave 3 days' warning of an impending red tide, visible only by satellite. The same ability to use infrared signatures of healthy versus ill plants may be used to monitor crops, estimate harvests, and predict impending failure and famine. Illicit crops, such as marajuana, and insect vector breeding areas have also been identified by space-based observations. Damage by erosion, air pollution, and oil spills are monitored by satellite (Figs. 35.5, 35.6).

New resources such as oil and minerals may be identified by aerial mapping and magnetic surveys. Radar can penetrate jungle and desert to identify hidden water sources or overgrown archaeologic sites. Weather satellites are indispensable for forecast and warning of storms.

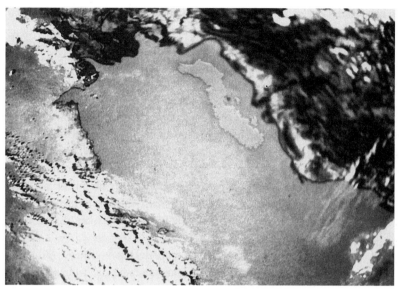

Figure 35.5. Oil spill from war-damaged tanker in the northern Persian Gulf. Infrared viewed by Landsat 4 (NASA photo).

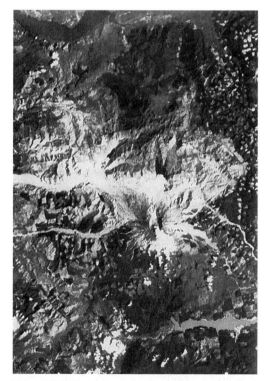

Figure 35.6. Damage to forest and lands surround-ingMount Saint Helens after 1981 eruption (NASA photo).

Even the weather on other worlds, such as Mars, Venus, and Jupiter, is now used to improve models of earth's behavior.

The Greenhouse

Global warming has been observed, with an average rise in world temperature by 0.6°C over the past century. The primary cause of this change is felt to be due to the accumulation of the greenhouse gas, carbon dioxide, along with other less promininant greenhouse gases, such as carbon monoxide and water vapor. Although not as important in the Earth's total energy budget as the variability of the solar flux and orbital deviations, the trapping of heat energy by the Earth's atmosphere raises our planet's temperature by 40°C over what it would be if the Earth had no atmosphere at all. This is more impressive since over 99% of our atmosphere consists of the non-greenhouse gases nitrogen, oxygen, and argon (47).

Further research has led to the knowledge that although carbon dioxide is the most important of the greenhouse gases, methane, carbon monoxide, and nitrogen oxides also have significant ability to trap heat. While a steady state of these gases existed prior to the 18th century, since then there has been a constant increase of greenhouse gases, almost entirely due to human activity. Industry accounts for 75% of the carbon dioxide and 50% of the carbon monoxide increase. Surprisingly, satellite data demonstrate that the remainder comes almost entirely from what would seem to be a minor source—the burning of tropical forests (48,49).

Global warming will cause dramatic changes in the environment. These changes are presaged by significant increases in greenhouse gases. Atmospheric carbon dioxide monitoring started on a pristine mountain in Hawaii only in 1958. Carbon dioxide increased from 315 ppm in the beginning to 353 ppm in 1988, a worldwide atmosheric increase of 5000 million metric tons of newly generated carbon dioxide. Studies of trapped gas in Greenland ice indicate that total atmosheric carbon dioxide has doubled since the beginning of the Industrial Revolution. Estimates based on the effects of the greenhouse gases call for a global warming of 2°C to 5°C average temperature increase over the next century, melting polar icecaps and causing a rise in sea level from 1 to 7 m. A mean sea level rise of only 1 m would create at least 50 million refugees as coastlines flood. Food production would fall as farmland is inundated and rainfall shifts. Some species will face extinction as habitats are eliminated, while others will have population explosions due to expanded ranges. Tropical diseases will expand into temperate zones. Combined with a thinned ozone layer and resulting decline in immune function due to increased UV-B exposure, malnutrition and disease will run rampant (50).

The models that predict these catastrophes have considerable uncertainties, but continued observations are confirming some of these predictions. Ceasing production of CFCs and moving toward their elimination, as directed by the Vienna Convention for the Protection of the Ozone Layer and the Montreal Protocol (1987),

will not produce an actual restoration of the atmosphere for many years after full com pliance.

ENVIRONMENTAL CONCERNS IN PERSPECTIVE

Chicken Little was wrong; the sky is not falling, but it is certainly changing before our eyes. A review of the environmental consequences of our operations within the atmosphere and in space indicates that while we have been prudent and responsible in protecting the ecology as we have ventured higher, faster, and farther, others have not.

Perspective is the key. Although we have contaminated the air with aircraft emissions, our contribution is but a small fraction of the total anthropogenic pollution activity. The emissions of automobiles bringing observers to space launches exceed the atmospheric contamination of the launches themselves. Continued efforts must be made to reduce all of these sources of environmental contamination.

Aviation's impact on the weather (from carbon dioxide and contrails) and on increased UV radiation reaching the earth through catalytic ozone depletion is likewise insignificant. The many contributions of aviation to understanding these phenomena and our environment more than outweighs the harm.

Noise, particularly adjacent to airports, is a significant environmental problem associated with aviation. Its resolution is based on both community and national understanding, cooperation, and action. The economic impact on the commercial aviation industry will depend on how fast regulation is effected. Sonic booms appear to be novelties rather than real problems, with some degree of political overlay.

Statutory provisions and regulatory agencies appear to be adequate to deal with aerospace environmental issues, now and in the future, but we must not become complacent. Research, development, engineering, and operating authorities must remain aware of environmental consequences of their actions and programs. They

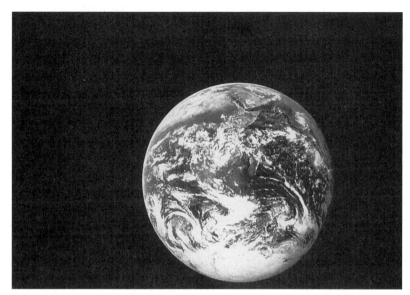

Figure 35.7. The home planet. Viewed by Apollo 8 astronauts en route to the moon, 1968 (NASA photo).

must receive the full and timely professional advice of biomedical personnel who are also dedicated to mission accomplishment within the constraints of a healthy ecology. We must anticipate and respond to state-of- the-art technological developments. The best perspective of the earth was provided by a single photograph, possibly the most important ever taken, by Apollo astronauts on their way to the moon (Fig. 35.7). Our fragile blue planet, our only home, hangs in the sheer blackness of space. Less than a year later, a worldwide ecology movement was born and the first Earth Day celebrated in 1970. Aviation and aerospace developments have been and will continue to be important tools in helping us to understand and save our home.

Ultimately, the quality of life depends upon the quality of the environment.

REFERENCES

1. Public Law 91–190. 42 U.S. Congress 4321–4347, January 1, 1970. Amended by Public Law 94–83, August 9, 1975.
2. U.S. Environmental Protection Agency. Aviation noise: let's get on with the job. Prepared by the Honorable Russell E. Train for delivery before the Inter-Noise 1976 Conference, April 5, 1976. Washington, DC: U.S. Government Printing Office 1976.
3. Noise, vibration and thermal problems. In: Army flight surgeons manual. Fort Rucker, AL: United States Army Aviation School, 1976.
4. Tracor, Inc. Community reaction to airport noise. NASA CR-1761. Washington, DC: U.S. Government Printing Office, 1971.
5. Kryter KD. The effects of noise on man. New York: Academic Press, 1970.
6. Kandebo SW. Restrictions on chapter 2 aircraft could cost airlines billions of dollars. Aviation Week and Space Technolology 1989;131(21):61–66.
7. Intelligence 6. FAA evaluation proposes noise programs. Business and Commercial Aviation 1989;June: 32.
8. Fotos CP. FAA noise rules give carries flexiblity in meeting deadline for stage 2 aircraft. Aviation Week and Space Technology 1991;135(13):65.
9. Kandebo SW. Noise compliance rules boost airline interest in hushkits. Aviation Week and Space Technology 1991;135(5):56–57.
10. Kandebo SW. Launch of Roll's reengining plan poses challenge to JT8D hushkits. Aviation Week and Space Technology 1990;131(20):1124.
11. Kandebo SW. Restrictions on chapter 2 aircraft could cost airlines billions of dollars. Aviation Week and Space Technology, 1989;131(21):61–66.
12. Smith MJT. Aircraft noise—a review. Birmingham, England: Institute of Acoustics, February 1988.
13. Maliger DV. Status of knowledge of sonicb. NASA TM-80113. Washington, DC: U.S. Government Printing Office, June, 1979.
14. Aircraft sonic boom: biological effects. Springfield, VA: National Technical Information Service, 1990.
15. Von Gierke HE. Effects of sonic boom on people: review and outlook. Acoust Soc Am 1966;39:543–550.

16. Manci KM, Gladwin DN, Villella R, et al. Effects of aircraft noise and sonic booms on domestic animals and wildlife. Ft. Collins, CO: National Ecology Research Center, 1988.

17. Kull RC, Fisher AD. Supersonic and subsonic aircraft noise effects on animals, AAMRL TR-87-032. Wright-Patterson Air Force Base, OH: Human Systems Division, 1986.

18. Ruskam J, Rogers D. Is a staged SST the answer? Aerospace Engineering 1990;11(2):17–19.

19. Ott J. Researchers seek technologies for quiet, environmentally safe SST. Aviation Week and Space Technology 1990;132(25):94–98.

20. Wilkening GM. Nonionizing radiation. In: National Institute of Occupational Health and Safety. The industrial environment-its evaluation and control. Washington, DC: U.S. Government Printing Office, 1973.

21. American National Standards Institute. American national standard safety levels with respect to human exposure to radio frequency electromagnetic fields, 300 kHz to 100 GHz. New York: Institute of Electrical and Electronic Engineers, 1982.

22. Graham RB. Medical results of human exposures to radio frequency radiation, OEHL report 85–029CV111ARA. Alexandria, VA: Defense Technical Center, 1985.

23. Erwin D. An overview of the biological effects of radio-frequency radiation. Mil Med 1983;148(2):164–168.

24. Maharaj HP. Stray radiation from baggage x-ray equipment: results and implications. Health Physics 1989; 57(1):141–148.

25. Needleman HL, Schell A, Bellinger D, et L. The long-term effects of exposure to low doses of lead in childhood: an 11-year follow-up report. N Engl J Med 1990; 322(2):83–88.

26. Naugle DF, Fox DL. Aircraft and air pollution. Environ Sci Technol 198115:342.

27. Parmet AJ. Beryllium rocket fuels: a physician's perspective. Joint Army-Navy-NASA-Air Force Symposium, Monterey, California, May 24, 1988.

28. Price RO. Liquid hydrogen—an alternative fuel. Aerospace Engineering 1991;11(2):21–25.

29. Buden D. The Acceptability of reactors in space. Report LA- 8724-MS,Pl. Los Alamos, New Mexico: Los Alamos Scientific Laboratory, April, 1981.

30. Covault C. U.S. assesses hazard of Cosmos fuel. Aviat Week Space Technol 1983;118(5):20–21.

31. Aftergood S, Hafemeister DW, Prilutsky OF, et al. Nuclear power in space. Scientific American 1991;264(6): 42–49.

32. Stolarski RS, Krueger AJ, Schoeberl MR, et al. Nimbus 7 satellite measurements of the springtime antarctic ozone decrease. Nature 1986;322(6082):808–811.

33. Crutzen PJ, Graedel TE. The role of atmospheric chemistry in environment-development interactions. In: Clark WC, Munn RE, eds. Sustainable Development of the Biosphere. Cambridge, U.K.: Cambridge University Press, 1986.

34. Graedel TE, Cruzen PJ. The changing atmosphere. Scientific American 1989;261(3):58–68.

35. Stolarski RS. The antarctic ozone hole. Scientific American 1988;258(1):30–36.

36. Anderson JG, Toohey DW, Brune WH. Free radicals within the antarctic vortex: the role of CFCs in the antarctic ozone hole. Science 1991;251:39–46.

37. Parmet AJ, Morford JM. Medical aspects of a titan missile mishap. Aviat Space Environ Med 1987;58(5):161.

38. Potter AE. Environmental effects of the space shuttle. Environ Sci Tech, 1978;21(March/April):15–21.

39. Potter AE. Ch 19: Environmental effects of shuttle launch and landing. In: Pool SL, Johnson PC Jr, Mason JA, eds. STS-1 medical report. NASA TM-58240, Houston, Texas, 1981.

40. Potter AE. Ch 15: Environmental effects of shuttle launch and landing. In: Pool SL, Johnson PC Jr, Mason JA, eds. STS-2 medical report. NASA TM-58245, Houston, Texas, 1982.

41. Potter AE. Ch 14: Environmental effects of shuttle launch and landing. In: Pool SL, Johnson PC Jr, Mason JA, eds. STS-3 medical report. NASA TM-58247, Houston, Texas, 1982.

42. Environmental impact statement: space shuttle program. National Aeronautics and Space Administration. Washington, DC: U. S. Government Printing Office, 1978.

43. LeMay CE, Kantor M. Mission with LeMay. New York: Doubleday and Co., 1965:84–85.

44. Foukal PV. The variable sun. Scientific American 1990; 262(2):34–41.

45. Broeker WS, Denton GH. What drives glacial cycles. Scientific American 1990;262(1):48–56.

46. Report of the Earth Systems Science Committee. Earth systems science: a closer view. National Aeronautics and Space Administration. Washington, DC: U.S. Government Printing Office, 1988.

47. Schneider SH. Climate modeling, Scientific American 1987;256(5):72–80.

48. Houghton RA, Woodwell GM. Global climate change. Scientific American 1989;260(4):36–44.

49. Newell RE, Reichle HG Jr, Seiler W. Carbon monoxide and the burning earth. Scientific American 1989;261(4): 82–88.

50. Leaf A. Potential health effects of global climatic change and environmental changes. N Engl J Med 1989; 321(23):1577–1583.

Index

Numerals in *italics* indicate a figure; page numbers followed by a "t" indicate a table.

principle of, 4
U.S. Army
  accident rates, 710, 710t
  in other nations, 712
U.S. Navy, squadron and air station
    assignments, 738–740, *739, 740*
Helix, 4
Helmet, protective
  Army, 721, *721*
  development of, 163–164
Hematologic considerations, aerospace
    medicine, 643–646
Hemorrhoids, 649
Henry's Law, 65
Henson, Samuel, 12
Hering-Breuer reflex, 73
Hiatal hernia, 648
High linear energy transfer (LET), 1034
High-sustained G exposures, 201
  recovery from, 244–251
Hirschberg reflex test, tropias, 553, *553*
Hitchock, Fred, 11–12
Human engineering, USAF, 701
Human immunodeficiency virus, spread, air
    travel and, 1008–1009
Human resources
  aerospace medicine, 897–921
  air transport operations, 923–951
Humidity
  composition of atmosphere, 59
  effects on aircrew, 456
Hydrogen, 5–12
Hydrostatic pressure, and bubble growth, in
    decompression sickness, 134
Hyperbaric medicine, 698–699
  Army, 727–728
Hyperbaric oxygen therapy, 83–84, *84–85*
  for decompression sickness, 142–147
    adjuvants to, 153
    tissue oxygen tension after, *145*
Hypercapnia, 105
Hypersonic flight, 40–41, *41*
  aeromedical considerations, 42–45
Hypertension
  arterial, aircrew, 501–503
  intraocular, 558

Hyperthermia, 414
Hyperventilation, 102–105, 616–617
  causes, 102–103
  effects, 103–104, *104*
  hypoxic hypoxia syndrome comparison,
    104t
  prevention, 105
  treatment, 104–105
Hypothermia, 72, 416–417
  localized, 416–417
  rapid decompression and, 115
  systemic, 417
Hypoxia, 12, 89–102
  aircraft accidents and, 885–886
  aircrew, 454–455
  causes of, 90
  characteristics, 96–98
  effects of, 94–95
  histotoxic, 94
  hypoxemic, 92–93
  hypoxic, 90–92
    recovery from, 98–99
  patient in flight environment, 668–669
  prevention, 99–101
  rapid decompression and, 115
  stages, 96–98, 98t
  stagnant, 93–94
  treatment, 98
  vision and, 532

Identification facility, mass disasters, 860
Illumination, 528–531, *529*
Illusions
  coriolis, 355–356, *356*
  in flight, 340
  G-excess effect, *360–361,* 360–362
  inversion, 358–360, *359*
  the leans, 362–364, *363*
  oculogravic, 362
  oculogyral, 354–355
  somatogravic, 356–358, *357*
  somatogyral, 351–354, *351–354*
  vection, 347–348, *348*
  vestibular, 351–364
  visual, 340
Immersion suits, 418